Male Sexual Dysfunction

Male Sexual Dysfunction

Pathophysiology and Treatment

Edited by

FOUAD R. KANDEEL

City of Hope National Medical Center, Duarte, California, USA
David Geffen School of Medicine at the University of California, Los Angeles, USA

Associate Editors

TOM F. LUE

University of California, San Francisco, USA

JON L. PRYOR

University of Minnesota Medical School, Minneapolis, USA

RONALD S. SWERDLOFF

Harbor-UCLA Medical Center, Torrance, California, USA
David Geffen School of Medicine at the University of California, Los Angeles, USA

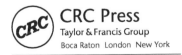

CRC Press
Taylor & Francis Group
Boca Raton London New York

CRC Press is an imprint of the
Taylor & Francis Group, an **informa** business

CRC Press
Taylor & Francis Group
6000 Broken Sound Parkway NW, Suite 300
Boca Raton, FL 33487-2742

First issued in paperback 2019

© 2007 by Taylor & Francis Group, LLC
CRC Press is an imprint of Taylor & Francis Group, an Informa business

No claim to original U.S. Government works

ISBN-13: 978-0-8247-2439-9 (hbk)
ISBN-13: 978-0-367-38909-3 (pbk)

This book contains information obtained from authentic and highly regarded sources. While all reasonable efforts have been made to publish reliable data and information, neither the author[s] nor the publisher can accept any legal responsibility or liability for any errors or omissions that may be made. The publishers wish to make clear that any views or opinions expressed in this book by individual editors, authors or contributors are personal to them and do not necessarily reflect the views/opinions of the publishers. The information or guidance contained in this book is intended for use by medical, scientific or health-care professionals and is provided strictly as a supplement to the medical or other professional's own judgement, their knowledge of the patient's medical history, relevant manufacturer's instructions and the appropriate best practice guidelines. Because of the rapid advances in medical science, any information or advice on dosages, procedures or diagnoses should be independently verified. The reader is strongly urged to consult the relevant national drug formulary and the drug companies' and device or material manufacturers' printed instructions, and their websites, before administering or utilizing any of the drugs, devices or materials mentioned in this book. This book does not indicate whether a particular treatment is appropriate or suitable for a particular individual. Ultimately it is the sole responsibility of the medical professional to make his or her own professional judgements, so as to advise and treat patients appropriately. The authors and publishers have also attempted to trace the copyright holders of all material reproduced in this publication and apologize to copyright holders if permission to publish in this form has not been obtained. If any copyright material has not been acknowledged please write and let us know so we may rectify in any future reprint.

Except as permitted under U.S. Copyright Law, no part of this book may be reprinted, reproduced, transmitted, or utilized in any form by any electronic, mechanical, or other means, now known or hereafter invented, including photocopying, microfilming, and recording, or in any information storage or retrieval system, without written permission from the publishers.

For permission to photocopy or use material electronically from this work, please access www.copyright.com (http://www.copyright.com/) or contact the Copyright Clearance Center, Inc. (CCC), 222 Rosewood Drive, Danvers, MA 01923, 978-750-8400. CCC is a not-for-profit organization that provides licenses and registration for a variety of users. For organizations that have been granted a photocopy license by the CCC, a separate system of payment has been arranged.

Trademark Notice: Product or corporate names may be trademarks or registered trademarks, and are used only for identification and explanation without intent to infringe.

Library of Congress Cataloging-in-Publication Data

Male sexual dysfunction : pathophysiology and treatment / edited by
   Fouad R. Kandeel.
     p. ; cm.
   Includes bibliographical references.
   ISBN-13: 978-0-8247-2439-9 (hardcover : alk. paper)
   ISBN-10: 0-8247-2439-9 (hardcover : alk. paper)
    1. Generative organs, Male--Pathophysiology. 2. Generative organs, Male--Diseases.
3. Importance--Treatment. 4. Sexual disorders. 5. Men--Diseases.
   I. Kandeel, Fouad R. [DNLM: 1. Sexual Dysfunction, Physiological--physiopathology.
2. Sexual Dysfunction, Physiological--diagnosis. 3. Sexual Dysfunction,
Physiological--therapy. WJ 709 M24563 2007]

   RC875.M3559 2007
   616.6'5--dc22
                                 2007006450

Visit the Taylor & Francis Web site at
http://www.taylorandfrancis.com

and the CRC Press Web site at
http://www.crcpress.com

*This volume is dedicated to those aspirations that
have gotten me started, the milestones I have already achieved,
and the life dreams I have yet to fulfill.*

Preface

Sexual interaction is the physical manifestation of our emotional need for acceptance, our need for affirmation, and our need for life. These drives may be as strong in us now as in our earliest ancestors. Such deeply rooted influences have invariably linked a man's self-worth to his ability to perform sexually—making sex a very important concern, indeed.

Many real advances in the understanding of the physiology of male sexual function have been attained in the last three decades. The erectile mechanism has been correctly delineated on molecular, cellular, and functional levels, from the role of the vascular elements involved in the normal sexual response to the progress made in the comprehension of the neuroendocrine, behavioral, and psychological mechanisms that govern sexuality. This greater knowledge has fostered the development of similarly innovative advances in the investigation and treatment of male sexual dysfunction.

Sexual complaints are astonishingly common among men of all ages, ethnicities, and cultural backgrounds. In 1995, it was estimated that more than 152 million men worldwide suffered from some degree of erectile dysfunction, and this number is expected to reach a formidable 322 million by the year 2025. Although erectile dysfunction is the most commonly highlighted type of male sexual dysfunction, there are many other sexual disorders that influence the parameters of desire, ejaculation, orgasm, and penile detumescence. Premature ejaculation, for example, is actually the most frequent male sexual dysfunction, but it is often confused with erectile dysfunction by many patients. Thus, the treating physician must possess a full understanding of all physiological aspects of normal sexual function as well as the manifestations and mechanisms of its disorders. With such a wide range of sexual disorders of varying nature and contributing factors from almost every system of the body, however, the successful practice of sexual medicine can only be delivered by a truly multidisciplinary team that involves the intricate coordination of the andrologist, urologist, sex therapist, psychiatrist, and, often, the radiologist.

This first edition of *Male Sexual Dysfunction: Pathophysiology and Treatment* comprehensively summarizes our most current knowledge of normal and abnormal male sexual function from all clinical aspects, including historical, psychosocial, and behavioral as well as medical and surgical perspectives. The chief goal of this work has been to compile a complete desk reference that will not only educate its reader with the science behind these complex disorders, but will also equip them with practical tools to approach the management of these conditions rationally and effectively. It is hoped that all sexual medicine professionals, both new and seasoned, will benefit from the updated information in this volume. Written by more than sixty world authorities, the book's forty-three chapters are organized into four logically sequential parts addressing the physiology, pathophysiology, investigation and treatments of male sexual disorders. A multitude of original illustrations, step-by-step algorithms, imaging studies, and comprehensive, well-organized tables complement the discussions and further elucidate these complex topics.

While some methods of investigating male sexual dysfunction, such as advanced vascular and neurological assessments, have largely fallen out of general favor since the revolutionary advent and subsequent widespread use of phosphodiesterase inhibitors, these techniques are carefully described in this volume—not simply for historical value, but because they often remain invaluable for patients who do not respond to phosphodiesterase inhibitors and those who cannot tolerate such medications. By taking the time and effort to establish the true etiologic basis and particular nature of an individual's sexual dysfunction, it may be possible to discover psychologically, medically, or even surgically reversible pathologies. For such patients, the selection of appropriate treatment modalities, including other systemic or locally applied drugs, nonsurgical devices, surgical procedures, and psychological or behavioral interventions, is of great importance, and thus is detailed thoroughly.

Some additional highlights of this book are several novel chapters dedicated to the in-depth description of state-of-the-art advances in penile revascularization, phallic reconstruction, and tissue/molecular engineering, as well as often controversial topics, such as male circumcision and the differences and similarities between male and female sexual function and dysfunction. Also critically reviewed is the abundant assortment of complementary and alternative medicine options available to patients without medical sanction.

Above all, it must be remembered that the patient's quality of life is paramount. In order to provide the safest and most effective treatment, the patient must be evaluated as a whole person; thus, judicious consideration of the myriad potentially contributing pathological factors, including family dynamics and interpersonal relationships, should be employed in all cases. Open lines of communication among the patient, his partner, and the treating professional must be achieved and maintained if rendered treatment is to be successful. Yet, many practitioners who do not specialize in sexual medicine may still feel awkward dealing with the intimate nature of sexual dysfunction in the office, as do many patients. It is the professional responsibility of the clinician, however, to bridge this gap of embarrassment by asking appropriate questions and drawing problems into the open with sensitivity and compassion. By providing a solid, scientific foundation of the pathophysiological factors that may cause sexual dysfunction and clearly outlining current practices for the investigation and treatment of these conditions, it is hoped that this book will allow its readers to approach the management of male sexual dysfunction with broader knowledge and greater confidence, so that no further men will have to suffer their sexual inadequacies in silence.

Fouad R. Kandeel

Acknowledgments

The editors are very grateful to the following individuals and would like to acknowledge their assistance in the preparation of this volume: Chakriya Anunta, Jeannette Hacker, Bernard de la Cruz, Karen Ramos, and Angela Hacker.

Contents

Contributors

Sherif R. Aboseif   Division of Neurology and Reconstructive Surgery, Department of Urology, Kaiser Permanente Medical Center, Los Angeles, California, U.S.A.

K. E. Andersson   Wake Forest Institute for Regenerative Medicine, Wake Forest University School of Medicine, Wiston-Salem, North Carolina, U.S.A.

Chakriya D. Anunta   Department of Diabetes, Endocrinology and Metabolism, City of Hope National Medical Center, Duarte, California, U.S.A.

Abdullah Armagan   Department of Urology, Faculty of Medicine, Suleyman Demirel University, Isparta, Turkey

Claudia Avina   Social Science Division, Pepperdine University, Malibu, California, U.S.A.

David Barton   School of Psychology and Psychological Medicine, Monashe University, Melbourne, Victoria, Australia

Armin J. Becker   Department of Urology, Hannover Medical School, Hannover, Germany

Duncan L. Browne   Academic Department of Diabetes, Queen Alexandra Hospital, Portsmouth, U.K.

Culley C. Carson   Division of Urology, Department of Surgery, University of North Carolina School of Medicine, Chapel Hill, North Carolina, U.S.A.

Ratna Chatterjee   Reproductive Medicine Unit, University College London Hospital, London, U.K.

Gary W. Chien   Department of Urology, Kaiser Permanente Medical Center, Bellflower, California, U.S.A.

Raymond A. Costabile   Department of Urology, University of Virginia, Charlottesville, Virginia, U.S.A.

Michael H. Cummings   Academic Department of Diabetes, Queen Alexandra Hospital, Portsmouth, U.K.

Bernard J. de la Cruz   Department of Diabetes, Endocrinology and Metabolism, City of Hope National Medical Center, Duarte, California, U.S.A.

Danielle N. Dienert   Department of Urology, University of Pittsburgh, Pittsburgh, Pennsylvania, U.S.A.

Robert J. Dimitriou   Michigan Institute of Urology, P.C. Oakwood Hospital, Dearborn, Michigan and Providence Hospital, Novi/Southfield, Michigan, U.S.A.

Mark Esensten   Division of Diagnostic Radiology, City of Hope National Medical Center, Duarte, California, U.S.A.

Carlos R. Estrada   Department of Urology, Children's Hospital Boston and Harvard Medical School, Boston, Massachusetts, U.S.A.

Gemma Viola Fantini   Department of Urology, University Vita-Salute San Raffaele, Milan, Italy

William W. Finger   Mountain Home Veterans Affairs Medical Center, James H. Quillen School of Medicine, East Tennessee State University, Johnson City, Tennessee, U.S.A.

Shahram S. Gholami   Department of Urology, University of California, San Francisco, California, U.S.A.

David Goldmeier   Jane Wadsworth Sexual Function Clinic, The Jefferiss Wing, St. Mary's Hospital, Paddington, London, U.K.

Irwin Goldstein   Department of Sexual Medicine, Alvarado Hospital, San Diego, California, U.S.A.

Louis J. Gooren   Department of Endocrinology/Andrology, Vrije University Medical Center, and Genderteam Sex Reassignment Centre, Amsterdam, The Netherlands

Franklynn C. Graves   Department of Psychology and Yerkes National Primate Research Center, Emory University, Atlanta, Georgia, U.S.A.

Alessandra Graziottin   Center of Gynecology and Medical Sexology, Hospital San Raffaele Resnati, Milan; Post-Graduate Course of Sexual Medicine, University of Florence, Florence; Specialty School of Gynecology and Obstetrics, University of Florence and University of Parma, Parma, Italy

Jeannette Hacker   Department of Diabetes, Endocrinology and Metabolism, City of Hope National Medical Center, Duarte, California, U.S.A.

David J. Handelsman   Department of Andrology, Concord Hospital and ANZAC Research Institute, University of Sydney, Sydney, New South Wales, Australia

Wayne J. G. Hellstrom   Department of Urology, Tulane University Health Sciences Center, New Orleans, Louisiana, U.S.A.

Graham Jackson   Cardiothoracic Centre, St. Thomas' Hospital, London, England, U.K.

Emmanuele A. Jannini   Department of Experimental Medicine, University of L'Aquila, L'Aquila, Italy

Lynette Joubert   Department of Social Work, The University of Melbourne, Parkville, Victoria, Australia

Fouad R. Kandeel   Department of Diabetes, Endocrinology and Metabolism, City of Hope National Medical Center, Duarte, California and David Geffen School of Medicine, University of California, Los Angeles, California, U.S.A.

Nabil Koussa   H.C. Healthcare Management and Development, Inc., Long Beach, California, U.S.A.

Vivien Koussa   H.C. Healthcare Management and Development, Inc., Long Beach, California, U.S.A.

Ash Kshirsagar   Division of Urology, Department of Surgery, University of North Carolina School of Medicine, Chapel Hill, North Carolina, U.S.A.

Andrea Lenzi   Department of Medical Pathophysiology, University of Rome "La Sapienza," Rome, Italy

Timothy F. Lesser   Department of Urology, Kaiser Permanente Medical Center, Los Angeles, California, U.S.A.

Laurence A. Levine   Department of Urology, Rush-Presbyterian-St. Luke's Medical Center, Chicago, Illinois, U.S.A.

Peter Y. Liu   Department of Andrology, Concord Hospital and ANZAC Research Institute, University of Sydney, Sydney, New South Wales, Australia

Tom F. Lue   Department of Urology, University of California, San Francisco, California, U.S.A.

Per Olov Lundberg   Neurology, Department of Neuroscience, University Hospital, Uppsala, Sweden

Alvin M. Matsumoto   Department of Medicine, University of Washington School of Medicine, and Clinical Research Unit, Seattle, Washington, U.S.A.

Marita P. McCabe   School of Psychology, Deakin University, Burwood, Victoria, Australia

Manoj Monga   Department of Urologic Surgery, University of Minnesota, Minneapolis, Minnesota, U.S.A.

Harold Mouras   Equipe Développement Social et Affectif, Faculté de Psychologie et des Sciences de l'Education, Université de Genéve, Suisse INSERM U742, Université Pierre et Marie Curie, Paris, France

Mark A. Moyad   Department of Urology, University of Michigan Medical Center, Ann Arbor, Michigan, U.S.A.

John J. Mulcahy   Department of Urology, Indiana University School of Medicine, Indianapolis, Indiana, U.S.A.

Ricardo Munarriz   Department of Urology, Boston University School of Medicine, Boston, Massachusetts, U.S.A.

William T. O'Donohue   Department of Psychology, University of Nevada, Reno, Nevada, U.S.A.

Cynthia S. Osborne   Department of Psychiatry and Behavioral Sciences, Johns Hopkins School of Medicine, Baltimore, Maryland, U.S.A.

Lisa Regev   Kaiser Permanente, Stockton, California, U.S.A.

Daniel Richardson   Royal County Sussex Hospital, Brighton and Sussex University Hospitals NHS Trust, Brighton, U.K.

David L. Rowland   Department of Psychology, Valparaiso University, Valparaiso, Indiana, U.S.A.

Arshad M. Safi   The Franklin County Heart Center, Chambersburg, Pennsylvania, U.S.A.

Edgar J. Schoen   Department of Genetics, Kaiser Permanente Medical Center, Oakland, California, U.S.A.

Judith Shell   Osceola Cancer Center, Kissimmee, Florida, U.S.A.

Mark A. Slagle   Department of Veterans Affairs MidSouth Healthcare Network, Nashville, Tennessee, U.S.A.

David John Smith   Faculty of Medicine, University of New South Wales, Rural Clinical School, Albury, New South Wales, Australia

Richard A. Stein   Cardiology Division, Beth Israel Medical Center, New York, New York, U.S.A.

Christian G. Stief   Department of Urology, Hannover Medical School, Hannover, Germany

Serge Stoléru   INSERM U742 and Université Pierre et Marie Curie, Paris, France

Kirk Tamaddon   Department of Urology, Kaiser Permanente Medical Center, Los Angeles, California, U.S.A.

Michael C. Truss   Department of Urology, Hannover Medical School, Hannover, Germany

Kim Wallen   Department of Psychology and Yerkes National Primate Research Center, Emory University, Atlanta, Georgia, U.S.A.

Joerg Wefer   Department of Urology, Hannover Medical School, Hannover, Germany

Lionel S. Zuckier   New Jersey Medical School, University Hospital, Newark, New Jersey, U.S.A.

Part I

Physiology of Male Sexual Dysfunction

The intricate coordination of physiologic events that enable the repeatable occurrence of male arousal, erection, orgasm, and detumescence is nothing short of biologically extraordinary. Because so many different anatomical, vascular, neurologic, psychologic, endocrine, and systemic factors must function in complete synchrony in order to achieve a total sexual response, defects in any one or more of these individual components may result in sexual dysfunction, as detailed in Part II. Due to breakthroughs in bench research studies and the development of state-of-the-art anatomical and functional imaging techniques, much progress has been made in the understanding of the physiology of male sexual function in the last three decades, resulting in a greater appreciation of the intricate neurovascular and hormonal mechanisms that govern sexual activity. As discussed in Parts III and IV, this knowledge has fueled similarly innovative advances in the investigation and treatment of male sexual dysfunction, including the advent of perhaps the most significant drug class in the history of the field: phosphodiesterase 5 (PDE5) inhibitors. Therefore, it is imperative that sexual health professionals attain (and maintain) a thorough understanding of the current data regarding the physiology of the normal male sexual response before any meaningful determinations can be made about the presence of particular disorders.

A History of the Penis: Images, Worship, and Practices

Bernard J. de la Cruz and Jeannette Hacker
Department of Diabetes, Endocrinology and Metabolism, City of Hope National Medical Center, Duarte, California, U.S.A.

Fouad R. Kandeel
Department of Diabetes, Endocrinology and Metabolism, City of Hope National Medical Center, Duarte, California, and David Geffen School of Medicine, University of California, Los Angeles, California, U.S.A.

□ INTRODUCTION

Man's awe of the miracle of procreation has led him to worship the agents he thought were responsible for life. For ancient peoples, the power to create life was magical and provided a sense of protection. Hence, man fashioned images of the organs of procreation to worship as powerful protectors against death and destruction. Phallic monuments, emblems, festivals, and decorative motifs are found in all parts of the world. Mythologies of all races have elements that are both symbolically and literally phallic in content.

From the post-Renaissance period through the late 1800s, a certain prudery existed, with scholars ignoring or bowdlerizing any sexual content from their studies. In the later Victorian age through the early part of the twentieth century, however, anthropological treatises of primitive "natural" cultures became fixated on sexual imagery and "sex worship" such as those of Westropp [published 1884 (1)] or Brown [published 1916 (2)]. By these interpretations, sex worship represented a natural state unspoiled by contemporaneous Puritanical views.

At the turn of the twentieth century, Freud's work on psychoanalysis returned the subject of sex into the realm of scientific study. Landmark studies by Kinsey et al. (3,4) and by Masters and Johnson (5) have followed, although they each generated significant controversies due to the nature and methods of their investigations. In the late twentieth century and into the beginning of the twenty-first, studies of sex and sexuality have been viewed through the lens of various critical theories [e.g., Foucault (6)]. Contemporary studies of gender, sex, and sexuality from the academic, medical, and lay perspectives have been the subject of volumes and even entire museums (e.g., the Musée de l'Érotisme in Paris).

The full appreciation of contemporary ideas of male sexual function and dysfunction requires reflection on the anthropology, history, and artistry surrounding the penis across the ages. This chapter seeks to provide a broad summary of the penis as a subject of cultural fascination and worship.

□ IMAGES AND SYMBOLOGY
Prehistoric

As described by Dening, paleolithic man (before 12,000 B.C.) was focused on survival: the gathering of food, the finding of shelter, and defending of the tribe (7). The creation of life was viewed as powerful magic, and thus, childbearing women were regarded with awe. Although archeologists and scholars have frequently perceived phallic symbols in artifacts of this period (e.g., cave paintings of hunters following prey), Tannahill warns that "dedicated seekers can recognize phallic intent in designs and objects which were originally (*pace* Freud) unimpeachably innocent" (8).

It was not until humans started to transition from the hunter-gatherer mode into farming and domesticating of animals (circa 10,000 B.C.) did the male role in procreation come into common belief (7). For these people, rocks and other natural objects found to resemble the organs of procreation were revered as manifestations of the gods themselves. Such objects were often placed at the edges of fields to ensure their fertility and as protection against crop diseases and failure. Male symbols included tall upright stones, cones, pyramids, and pointed fingers. In contrast, the female was represented by the crescent moon, earth, darkness, water, and a cup or shallow vessel, amongst many other symbols (7). Figure 1 illustrates such a primitive phallic figurine that is 10,000 years old.

Ancient Egypt

The ancient Egyptians were a polytheistic society, with each god having a role to play, often with sexual or reproductive connotation. For example, one of the creation myths involves the male god Geb (earth) with an upright penis impregnating Nut (heaven) (Fig. 2). Min, god of fertility, harvest, and desert paths, was believed to bestow sexual powers to men (Fig. 3 and on the cover of this volume). Min was particularly popular during the New Kingdom, and orgiastic festivals were held in his honor (9).

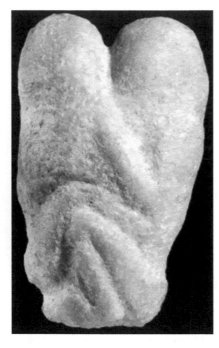

Figure 1 Small sculpture of a human couple engaged in intercourse. About 10,000 years old, this piece may have represented ideas about fertility at the time, reflecting new understanding of the role men played in reproduction. From the cave of Ain Sakhri, Wadi Khareitoun, Judea. *Source*: Courtesy of the British Museum.

Another myth surrounds the gods Isis and Osiris, who were both siblings and lovers, like Nut and Geb. Osiris was the god of the living and ruled with Isis. Another god, Set, became jealous of Osiris, so he tore Osiris's body into many pieces and scattered them throughout the land of Egypt. Isis gathered Osiris's parts, except for the penis, which had been eaten by a river crab, and breathed life back into the body, thus giving birth to their son Horus. Consequently, Horus became god of the living, while Osiris became god of the underworld. Festivals of Isis and Osiris were held in celebration of this story, featuring women carrying puppets portraying the male genitalia on nearly the same size scale as the rest of the body (10).

Interestingly enough, the phallus itself was used as a hieroglyph representing a particular phoneme. This confused historians of the time; for example, Rocco mistakes the hieroglyphs as repetitive phallic images: "Numerous figures of gods and kings on the walls of the temple at Thebes are depicted with the male genital erect. The great temple at Karnac is full of such figures" (11). While the use of the phallus as a glyph was not necessarily sexual, however, it underscores the importance of the male genitalia in ancient Egypt.

Ancient Greece

In her survey of sexual imagery of the ancient Greeks, Keuls contradicts the work of earlier anthropologists—in particular, Bachofen—about sex worship in the prehistoric age and in early civilizations as being focused on adoration of the feminine. Rather, she insists a persistent male dominance was clearly evident within ancient Greece (12).

The Greeks were not ashamed of the sex organs, and in fact revered them piously and with religious reverence. The Greeks were especially phallocentric, idolizing the male genitalia as a source of life and as a representation of the immortality of the Greek race. Worship of the phallus reveled in adoration of inexhaustible fruitfulness (13). Greek cities were studded with statues of gods with phalluses erect. In contrast, female sexuality was feared; women were viewed as caged tigers waiting for a chance to break out of their confinement and take revenge on the male world (e.g., tales of Amazons, women who murder their husbands and sons). This male fear manifested as a social reality and formed part of the justification for a phallocratic society, one derived from and focused on masculine dominance (12).

The men of ancient Greece habitually displayed their genitals. They actually preferred a "dainty" penis that was small and taut. Aristotle outlined a rationale for the preference that the small penis was more fertile than the large one because the seed has a shorter distance to travel; consequently, it does not cool and thus retains

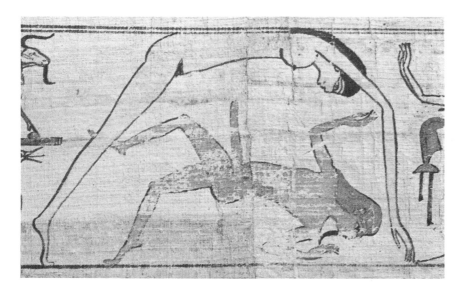

Figure 2 (*See color insert.*) Ancient Egyptian creation myth. Papyrus from the Twenty-first Dynasty. By the order of Ra, the goddess Nut was lifted off her recumbent lover Geb, and her body formed the arch of the sky. Geb, propped on one elbow and with bent knee, formed the earth with its mountains and valleys. He appears green, the usual color given to him as a vegetation god. *Source*: Courtesy of the British Museum.

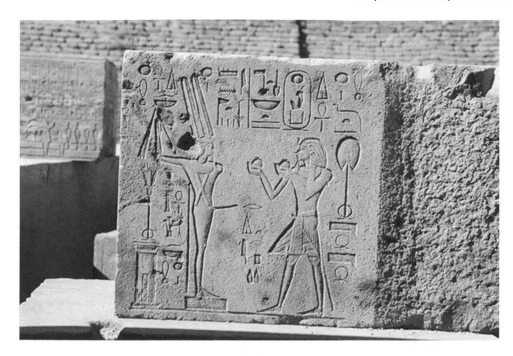

Figure 3 (*See color insert.*) Stone carving from the "Red Chapel" of Hatshepsut and Tuthmosis III depicts the pharoah's worship of Min, ancient god of fertility and sexuality.

vitality. Large sex organs were even considered ugly. Imagery of large phalluses were intended for "the domains of abstraction, of caricature, of satyrs, and of barbarians" (12). Phallic bronzes depicting large, erect penises largely belonged to satyrs and other theatrical creatures (Fig. 4). Although they were long believed to be symbols of fertility, modern reinterpretation indicates they also played a defensive role (i.e., protection from evil) particularly in the case of grotesquely shaped phalluses. In particular, sculpture from the late sixth and fifth centuries B.C. tended to be more fantastical than utilitarian and included figures with double phalluses, phalluses with eyes, and plants and animals shaped as phalluses (12). Also, the Greeks believed the penis should be left intact; circumcision and exposure of the glans was done only by the uncivilized.

Most phallic worship involved Dionysus or Demeter. Dionysus was the god of wine and harvest, and his symbol was the phallus. The retinue of Dionysus consisted of ithyphallic (erect penis) spirits, as well as spirits of fruitfulness and vegetation, and his temples prominently displayed the phallus (Fig. 5). Demeter was the goddess of fertility and home; although her rites focused on women, phalluses were also used (13).

In particular, there was a series of festivals (Dionysia) held over several months in conjunction with the harvesting of grapes and making of wine. These festivals involved solemn processions through the streets carrying one or more giant phalluses (Fig. 6). During the Great Dionysia in Athens, other cities were obligated to send phalluses to be part of the celebration. So important were these Dionysia that in order to secure the phallus procession, wars were temporarily stopped. Also, there were maedas, women in the cult of Dionysus known for their orgiastic dances that were performed while swinging a phallus (13).

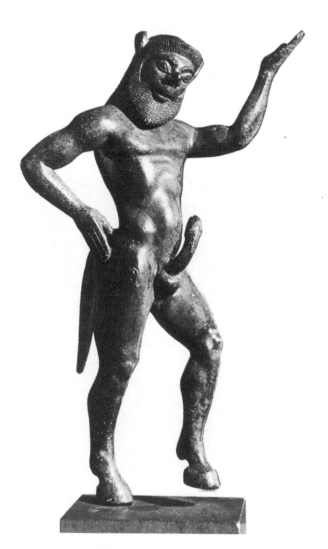

Figure 4 Ancient Greece. Bronze statue of ithyphallic satyr. *Source*: The National Museum, Athens.

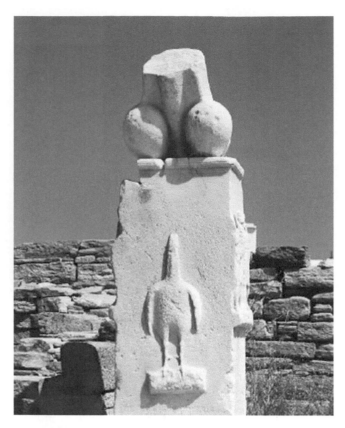

Figure 5 Ancient Greece. Phallic monument with a relief of the phallus-bird, a symbol of the god Dionysus. At the sanctuary of Dionysus, Delos, Greece.

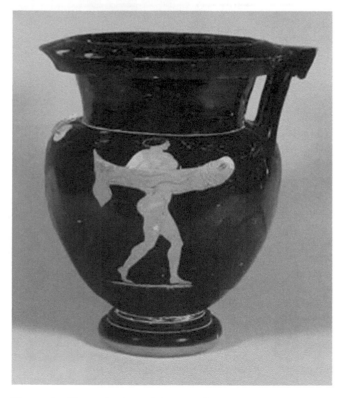

Figure 6 (*See color insert.*) Ancient Greece. Hetera (prostitute) carrying large phallus.

China

Early people in the region of China worshipped fertility and the genitals. The female essence and genitalia were often represented as rings, the double-fish motif, and the frog (due to its having an expansive belly and many offspring). The male was represented by snakes and the heads of birds (the elongated neck and beak being of similar shape to an uncircumcised penis). Often, the male and female images were brought together (e.g., a bird holding a fish in its beak, or a frog entwined by a snake). Stone carvings often had scenes of couples having sex or many naked dancers, the men having exaggerated penises and the women having large hips and breasts (14).

The Chinese pantheon numbers in the thousands, each representing a human aspiration such as prosperity, progeny, or love. There was a focus on cocreation: the male and the female together. One creation myth has the goddess Nu Wa and the god Fu Xi coiling their serpentine tails together and thus producing humanity. Another has Jiang Yuan, the goddess of Earth, giving birth to Ji, the God of Grain (14).

Over time, Chinese polytheism gave way to Confucianism, Buddhism, and Daoism. Broadly speaking, Confucianism was patriarchal and focused on moderation. Buddhism (at least the main form) focused on detachment from the world and asceticism. Daoism reveled in spiritual liberation of the individual, utopian community, and laissez-faire leadership. An underlying shared belief was in various life/energy forces, most notably *qi* (or *chi*, vital energy), *shen* (spirit), and *jing* (sexual energy). Daoists had a combination of group rituals using sexual yoga in order to unite *qi*; these rites are detailed in a surviving text called "Salvation Ritual of the Yellow Book of Highest Purity." In fact, a variety of Daoist texts were focused on "bedroom arts" and presented techniques for husbands to satisfy their wives (while maintaining their *qi*) and produce heirs. With the adoption of Tantric Buddhism, emphasis was placed on the union of the male and the female; again, channeling the feminine energy with male essence. Out of Tantric Buddhism arose much imagery of gods and goddesses in ecstatic embrace. It seemed that through sex that one most approximates the gods (14).

Another belief was that men needed to reserve their sexual power (*ying*) and that by ejaculating, they lost energy. On the other hand, women were thought to have unlimited orgasmic energy (*yang*) (7). Consequently, the practice of *coitus reservatus* or sex without ejaculation was developed; through bodily (tantric) control, men could tap into the abundance held by women thereby building up their own energy (14).

India

Early Indian sculpture had its fertility symbols, which were plainly phallic within a society that regarded sex as a natural and productive function. Much early religious imagery in India was blatantly phallic or

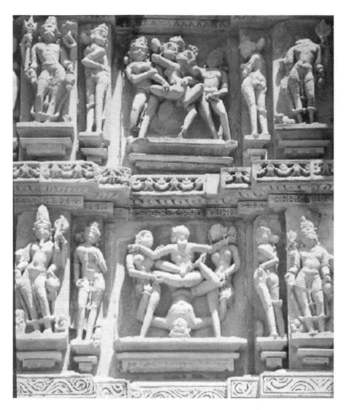

Figure 7 (*See color insert.*) Erotic reliefs from the Indian temple of Khajuraho built by the Tantric Chandela monarchs between 950–1050 A.D. Adherents of Tantrism believe that gratification of earthly desires is a step toward achieving Nirvana.

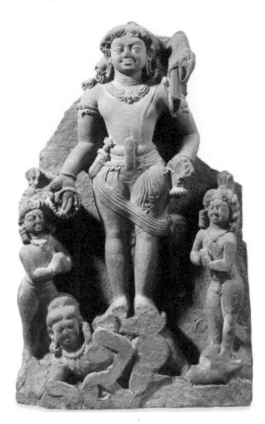

Figure 8 (*See color insert.*) Sandstone aspect of the Hindu god Shiva, circa 700 A.D. The erect phallus represents his omnipotent and creative nature, and he stands upon Apasmara, the vanquished dwarf of ignorance, illusion, and ego.

erotic. The entire walls of temples were filled with figures in the middle of coitus. One of the three great gods of the Hindu triad is the personification of destruction known as Shiva, "the Bright and Shining One" (Figs. 7 and 8). Shiva has also been recognized as a god of fertility and lord of the ghosts and goblins (15).

The Indian tantric form of Buddhism focused on the joining of the *lingam* (penis) and *yoni* (vagina). A common image is that of Shiva in conjunction with a female aspect, Parvati (Divine Mother) or Kali (goddess of death). Through their union arose energies of creation. Furthermore, the sex act not only brought orgasmic bliss but also warded off evil (7).

The famed text of sex rituals, the *Kama Sutra* (16), described several ways of enhancing the penis. For example, it recommends use of "armlets" of gold, silver, or ivory to sheathe the penis. Alternately, the penis may be wrapped with a metal coil to enhance it. One of the more painful treatments involved rubbing the penis with nettles to cause it to swell. Even primitive penile implants that are inserted under the skin were referenced, although they were not clearly described or illustrated (8).

Europe

Like other areas of the world, pre-Christian Europe was polytheistic and included gods representing the male and the female. Again, the phallus was at the center of the sexual value system and was often prominently displayed. For example, there were the Norse tales of the Volsi, often represented as the phallus of a horse. Images of Frey, the Germanic god of sexuality and fertility, depicted him with a large phallus (17).

In the Middle Ages, these pagan gods were displaced by Christianity, with its emphasis on purity and asceticism. The people of medieval Europe were full of fear, seeing the Devil all around them. Sex was associated with the Devil, and was to be repressed within oneself. At this time, original sin came to be sexual in nature (17). The Devil was often possessed of a large phallus for the purpose of defiling women, consorting with witches, and having semen as cold as ice water. An obsession of the age was the idea of the incubus and succubus, the male and female demon seducer. Nocturnal emissions were thought to be a sign of visitation by a succubus in one's dreams (8). Pagan deities came to be regarded as hobgoblins that lurked in the lonely places and in forests and emerged in order to indulge in all sorts of sexual excesses (17).

In the secular realm, men were very focused on the phallus. Rather than overt display of the penis, however, the focus was channeled into clothing. For a while, colorful, long pointy shoes were fashionable; popular belief equated size of the shoe with size of the penis, so men often stuffed the points of their shoes to make them

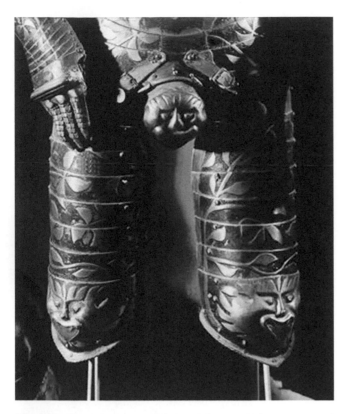

Figure 9 (*See color insert.*) Medieval Europe. Elaborate armored codpiece.

stand upright (17). Also, codpieces were commonly worn. Although initially used to protect the genitals during battle, often they were made extravagantly large, projecting far beyond the suit of armor (Fig. 9) (8).

Practices

There exist a multitude of practices involving the genitals (or their stand-ins). The emotions surrounding reproduction are primitive, powerful, and fundamental. Therefore, it is not difficult to realize that early man should dignify them with rituals and rites. As Brown states, "Sex worship likely was an unconscious expression of longings and desires on the part of the race, representing a phase in man's mental evolution, a process of mental development (2)." Briefly, two practices specific to the male sexual organs are addressed: circumcision and castration.

Circumcision

Circumcision has been said to be the most common surgery performed in the past 100 years (18). The subject of circumcision is fraught with controversy with entire libraries—often shrill—written on the topic. This is not surprising, considering the aura of religion, sexual morality, and medicine surrounding the procedure. To bring some perspective, a brief historical account is provided.

Along with the understanding of man's role in procreation (circa 10,000 B.C.) came rites of passage whereby male adolescents were socially acknowledged as adult men capable of reproduction. Circumcision became a ritual practiced by a variety of primitive and advanced peoples throughout the world. The practice likely arose at different times and in different locations including the Middle East, Africa, North and South America, and Polynesia. It has alternately been speculated that circumcision was done by matriarchal societies as ritualized castration, a mimicking of menstruation, or a form of taking trophies from defeated enemies (8,19,20).

Earliest records of circumcision come from ancient Egypt (21). A bas-relief from the temple of Ankha-ma-Hor in Saqqara circa 2400 B.C. illustrates the procedure (Fig. 10). In the image, a man (priest) holds a child's penis, foreskin extended, in his left hand and an instrument that appears to be made of stone or shaped flint in his right hand. Shokeir and Hussein even speculate the procedure was done using a mild anesthetic [the "Memphis stone," a stone composed of lime, plus an acid (vinegar) would produce carbonic acid on moist skin]. It has been suggested that circumcision in ancient Egypt was done for practical reasons; that is, removal of

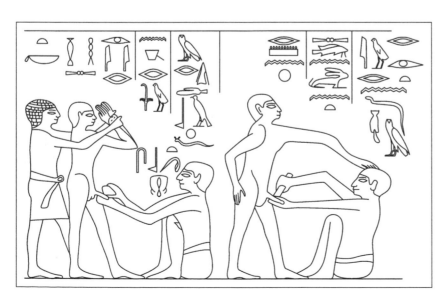

Figure 10 Ancient Egyptian circumcision ritual. Artist's rendition of a bas-relief from Ankha-ma-Hor. *Source*: From Ref. 21.

the foreskin would be more hygienic and comfortable in the sandy environment. It is more likely, however, that removal of the foreskin exposed the glans, making the penis appear less feminine (8). Egyptian statues and mummies of high priests and pharaohs who had undergone circumcision have been found. Yet, incomplete and inconsistent records make it unclear whether circumcision was done to the male populace in general.

The practice of circumcision in modern Western society arises from the Jewish practice as laid out in the Old Testament as part of the Divine Covenant made between God and Abraham (Genesis 17). From this injunction, ritual circumcision is the sacrifice made to God in return for being His Chosen People; from a practical perspective, circumcision marks those within the tribe from those outside. The Arabs have also practiced circumcision since before the birth of Mohammed; however, Islam neither mandates circumcision nor is it mentioned in the Qur'an. It is still traditionally practiced by Muslims for hygienic and purification purposes. In addition, circumcision has been widely adopted by Christians, because St. Paul came to believe that physical evidence of allegiance to the Church was necessary (22).

The transformation of circumcision from religious ritual to routine surgery has circulated around medical (and pseudomedical) issues. Likely, it arose out of hysteria surrounding masturbation (23). In the 1890s, tracts such as that of Remondino outlined the benefits of circumcision, including "better health, greater capacity for labor, longer life, less nervousness, sickness, loss of time, and less doctor bills," and thus urged all parents to circumcise their sons (24). In contemporary times, however, a strong sentiment has arisen that believes neonatal circumcision is tantamount to mutilation and child abuse. Even preliminary evidence indicating a reduction in penile cancers or HIV infection is viewed with skepticism (25) (see Chapter 9).

Castration

Despite Freud's theories on the castration complex and pop culture, the ancient practice of castration typically referred to removal of the testicles. Around 6000 B.C., man began domesticating animals. This included learning to remove the testicles from bulls to make them more docile draft animals. Incidentally, some anthropologists have posited that circumcision may be a ritualized form of castration (8). In Medieval Europe, castration was used as a means of criminal punishment, especially for rape, adultery, and homosexuality. Also, there were the *castrati*, boys in church choirs who had their testicles removed to maintain their angelic voices (26). Examples of self-castration for ascetic or spiritual reasons can be found in both Western and Eastern texts (27); however, such examples were not prevalent, tending to be aberrant rather than the norm. On the other hand, there are two prominent examples of institutionalized castration worth mentioning: the eunuchs in the Middle East and the hijras in India.

Eunuchs

The practice in the Middle East of using eunuchs was carried out primarily in the first millennium. Eunuchs were prisoners/slaves who had their penises and/or testicles cut off (generally, black eunuchs had complete genital removal, whereas white eunuchs only had the testicles removed). They were used primarily as servants and harem guards. Cyrus the Great, in the sixth century A.D., had a preference for eunuchs as personal servants. Eunuchs, being unable to bear children and thus having no family ties, were thought of by Cyrus and other leaders as being highly loyal (8).

Contemporary ideas regarding eunuchs as sexless or effeminate servants likely oversimplify the case. Some eunuchs were valued as powerful men-at-arms to defend the harem; however, there was a role for penis-laden eunuchs to service a harem without fear of impregnating the women. Other perks for being a eunuch included money and power, since their owners were usually socially dominant (27). Thus, some free men seeking to climb the social ladder voluntarily gave up their organs. In fact, in a few cases, eunuchs held the real power of the state. This idea extended into the Byzantine (Eastern) Christian church, which developed a preference for ministers and patriarchs who were eunuchs (8).

Hijras

As mentioned above, Indian culture places the male and the female as complementary opposites. In classic Hinduism, the female principle is considered active, whereas the male is thought inert and latent. The erotic aspect of woman is powerful and dangerous, brought into balance by the male. There is, however, also an underlying acknowledgment of other sexes/genders—most notably, the hijras—who have played an important role in Indian society (28).

There are two types of hijras. There are "real" or "born" hijras who are hermaphroditic at birth. There are also "made" hijras or those who have been castrated. The crucial point is the inability to bear children. Made hijras are often those who are gay or effeminate. Others are impotent men who are called in their dreams by the Mother Goddess to castrate themselves. Through sacrificing of the phallus and testicles, the hijras are connected to Shiva and the Mother Goddess, and thus embody the procreative spirit. Also through ascetic practices and sexual abstinence, they are thought to have access to *tapas*, the power of creation. Thus, they are called upon during births and marriages to perform ritual ceremonies and provide entertainment (usually flamboyant and comic) (28).

Although originally existing outside the Indian caste system, most hijras now tend to come from the lower castes. Some Indian states even granted parcels of land to hijras along with the privilege to collect food and small sums from households. In modern times, the hijras have lost much of their legal status, particularly during the British rule where they were viewed as abominations. In contemporary India, the term is now commonly used to describe not just eunuchs but also gay men and other transgender people. As India has become more westernized, the traditional role for the hijras has diminished, forcing many into prostitution (28).

☐ CONCLUSION

The evolution of phallic symbolization gives us a perspective on the values various cultures place on male sexual and reproductive function. There is a wealth of literature available for the interested reader to pursue a further understanding of the complexities of male sexuality within a given culture. In present-day societies, the maintenance of acceptable levels of male sexual function is of utmost importance; hence, the subsequent chapters in this text are dedicated to the issues surrounding all aspects of this topic.

☐ REFERENCES

1. Westropp HM. Primitive Symbolism, as Illustrated in Phallic Worship or the Reproductive Principle. London: George Redway, 1884.
2. Brown S. The Sex Worship and Symbolism of Primitive Race. Boston: Badger RG, 1916.
3. Kinsey AC, Poneroy WB, Martin CE. Sexual Behavior in the Human Male. Philadelphia: WB Saunders, 1948.
4. Kinsey AC. Sexual Behavior in the Human Female. Philadelphia: WB Saunders, 1953.
5. Masters WH, Johnson VE. Human Sexual Response. Boston: Little Brown, 1966.
6. Foucault M. History of Sexuality (English translation). New York: Random House, 1978.
7. Dening S. The Mythology of Sex. New York: Macmillan, 1996.
8. Tannahill R. Sex in History. New York: Stein and Day, 1980.
9. Manniche L. Sexual Life in Ancient Egypt. New York: Routledge, 1987.
10. Shaw I. The Oxford History of Ancient Egypt. Oxford, UK: Oxford University Press, 2000.
11. Rocco S. The Masculine Cross and Ancient Egypt. London: Kegan Paul, 1889.
12. Keuls EC. The Reign of the Phallus: Sexual Politics in Ancient Athens. New York: Harper and Row, 1985.
13. Licht H, Freese JH, Dawson LH. Sexual Life in Ancient Greece. London: Routledge, 1949.
14. Wile D. Chinese religion. In: Manning C, Zuckerman P, eds. Sex and Religion. Belmont, CA: Thomson Wadsworth, 2005.
15. Martin EO. The Gods of India, Their History, Character and Worship. Delhi, India: Indological Book House, 1972.
16. Vatsyayana. The Kama Sutra of Vatsyayana (English translation by Sir Richard Burton). Benares: Kama Shastra Society, 1885.
17. Murray J. Hiding behind the universal man: male sexuality in the middle ages. In: Bullough VL, Brundage JA, eds. Handbook of Medieval Sexuality. New York: Garland, 1996.
18. Hammond T. A preliminary poll of men circumcised in infancy or childhood. BJU Int 1999; 83(suppl 1):85–92.
19. Wrana P. Historical review: circumcision. Arch Pediat 1939; 56(4):385–392.
20. Bettelheim B. Symbolic Wounds: Puberty Rites and the Envious Male. Glencoe, IL: Free Press, 1954.
21. Shokeir AA, Hussein MI. The urology of Pharonic Egypt. BJU Int 1999; 84(7):755–761.
22. Strage M. The Durable Fig Leaf. New York: William Morrow, 1980.
23. Hall LA. Forbidden by God, despised by men: masturbation, medical warnings, moral panic, and manhood in Great Britian, 1850–1950. In: Fout J, ed. Forbidden History: the State, Society, and the Regulation of Sexuality in Modern Europe. Chicago: University of Chicago Press, 1992.
24. Remondino PC. History of Circumcision: from the Earliest Times to the Present. Philadelphia: Davis FA, 1891.
25. Alanis MC, Lucidi RS. Neonatal circumcision: a review of the world's oldest and most controversial operation. Obstet Gynecol Surv 2004; 59(5):379–395.
26. Kuefler MS. Castration and Eunuchism in the middle ages. In: Bullough VL, Brundage JA, eds. Handbook of Medieval Sexuality. New York: Garland, 1996.
27. Taylor G. Castration: An Abbreviated History of Western Manhood. New York: Routledge, 2000.
28. Nanda S. The Hijras: An Alternative gender in Indian culture. In: Ellingson S, Green MC, eds. Religion and Sexuality in Cross-Cultural Perspective. New York: Routledge, 2002.

Male Sexual Anatomy

Fouad R. Kandeel

Department of Diabetes, Endocrinology and Metabolism, City of Hope National Medical Center, Duarte, California and
David Geffen School of Medicine, University of California, Los Angeles, California, U.S.A.

Nabil Koussa and Vivien Koussa

H.C. Healthcare Management and Development, Inc., Long Beach, California, U.S.A.

☐ INTRODUCTION

Adequate penile erection is of central importance to the physical manifestation of sexual intercourse and therefore to the process of reproduction. Thus, the problem of erectile dysfunction (ED) is a major clinical concern in both sexual and reproductive medicine (1). ED affects many millions of men worldwide (2–5), and although it may not mean a total loss of satisfaction for some, for most, it creates mental stress and anxiety that adversely affects personal relationships and quality of life. The physiology of male penile erection is extremely complex (6–9), and the process is subject to a great number of clinical disorders (see Chapter 10). The achievement of a solid understanding of the anatomy and physiology of the penis is an essential backdrop to the clinical management of male sexual dysfunction. This chapter will provide a brief overview of the anatomy of the main organ responsible for erection and intercourse, the penis.

☐ THE PENIS
Structure

The key structures mediating penile erection are the two functional compartments of the penis: the paired corpora cavernosa and the corpus spongiosum (Fig. 1) (6–10). The corpora cavernosa comprise the bulk of the penis and consist of two cylinders of sponge-like tissue fused distally for approximately three-quarters of their length with a common septum in between, separating at the proximal portion of each corpus cavernosum, which is known as the crus, and this is attached to the inferior surface of the ischial ramus on the respective side. The septum is perforated by vessels that allow free passage of blood from one cylinder to the other, permitting the two cavernosal bodies to function as a single unit.

The erectile tissues of the corpora cavernosa are surrounded by a dense, nondistensible fascial sheath known as the tunica albuginea (Fig. 2) (10). Emissary veins that carry the returned blood from the corporeal bodies traverse the tunica albuginea. Tensing of the tunica albuginea during erection by the expanded corporeal tissue compresses the subtunical plexus and emissary veins, reducing blood outflow.

Inferior to the corpora cavernosa lies the corpus spongiosum (Fig. 3), which contains the urethra and extends distally to form the majority of the glans penis (11). The penile corporeal tissue is surrounded by another dense fascial sheath (Buck's fascia) (Fig. 2), which anchors the penis to the symphysis pubis and compresses the circumflex veins during the erectile responses, thereby further limiting venous drainage (10). Histologically, the tissue of the corpora cavernosa consists of bundles of smooth-muscle fibers intertwined in a collagenous extracellular matrix. Interspersed within this parenchyma is a complex network of endothelial cell-lined sinuses (lacunae), helicine arteries, and nerve terminals (12).

The skin overlying the penis (Fig. 4) is exceptionally mobile; it is capable of expanding to accommodate the considerable increase in girth and length that occurs during erection (10). This lack of adherence makes the penis relatively susceptible to edema. In its distal portion, the penile skin extends forward to form the prepuce before folding backward and attaching to the corona of the glans penis.

The pendulous portion of the penis (Fig. 5) is supported and stabilized by the suspensory ligament (10). Division of this structure makes the penis appear longer in its flaccid state, but it will not enhance the proportions of the organ when erect.

Vasculature

The terminal branches of the paired internal pudendal arteries (Fig. 6) supply the penis with blood (10,14). Each internal pudendal artery arises from the anterior division of the respective internal iliac (hypogastric) artery (10) and arborizes into four branches (Fig. 7) (13,15): the bulbar artery, which supplies the urethral bulb, the posterior portion of the corpus cavernosum, and the bulbourethral gland; the urethral (spongiosal) artery, which supplies the urethral and the corpus spongiosal tissue; the deep penile (corpus cavernosal or profunda) artery, which supplies the corpus

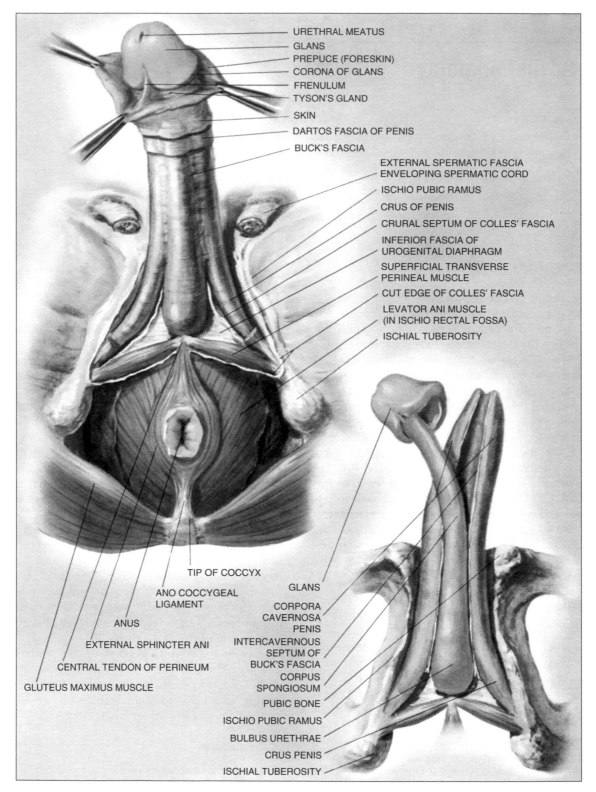

URETHRAL MEATUS
GLANS
PREPUCE (FORESKIN)
CORONA OF GLANS
FRENULUM
TYSON'S GLAND
SKIN
DARTOS FASCIA OF PENIS
BUCK'S FASCIA

EXTERNAL SPERMATIC FASCIA
ENVELOPING SPERMATIC CORD
ISCHIO PUBIC RAMUS
CRUS OF PENIS
CRURAL SEPTUM OF COLLES' FASCIA
INFERIOR FASCIA OF
UROGENITAL DIAPHRAGM
SUPERFICIAL TRANSVERSE
PERINEAL MUSCLE
CUT EDGE OF COLLES' FASCIA
LEVATOR ANI MUSCLE
(IN ISCHIO RECTAL FOSSA)
ISCHIAL TUBEROSITY

TIP OF COCCYX
ANO COCCYGEAL
LIGAMENT
ANUS
EXTERNAL SPHINCTER ANI
CENTRAL TENDON OF PERINEUM
GLUTEUS MAXIMUS MUSCLE

GLANS
CORPORA
CAVERNOSA
PENIS
INTERCAVERNOUS
SEPTUM OF
BUCK'S FASCIA
CORPUS
SPONGIOSUM
PUBIC BONE
ISCHIO PUBIC RAMUS
BULBUS URETHRAE
CRUS PENIS
ISCHIAL TUBEROSITY

Figure 1 (*See color insert.*) Perineum and external male genitalia: deep dissection. *Source*: From Ref. 11. Netter medical illustration used with permission of Elsevier. All rights reserved.

cavernosum; and finally, the deep dorsal artery, which supplies the skin and the glans penis. The deep penile artery lies centrally within the corpus cavernosum and measures 600 to 1000 µm in diameter during the flaccid state. The deep penile artery gives rise to many perpendicular branches called helicine arterioles (150 µm in diameter) that supply the cavernous sinusoidal space (16). During erection, the deep penile artery dilates to twice its diameter in the flaccid state. Several normal anatomic variations in the arterial supply of the penis have been described (17–21), including the presence of an accessorial internal pudendal

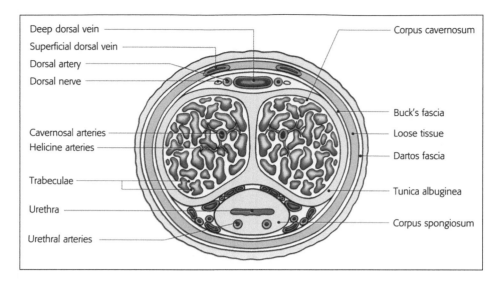

Deep dorsal vein
Superficial dorsal vein
Dorsal artery
Dorsal nerve

Cavernosal arteries
Helicine arteries

Trabeculae

Urethra

Urethral arteries

Corpus cavernosum

Buck's fascia
Loose tissue
Dartos fascia

Tunica albuginea

Corpus spongiosum

Figure 2 (*See color insert.*) Each corpus cavernosum is surrounded by a thick fibrous sheath, the tunica albuginea, which limits the expansion of the erectile tissue, producing a rise in the intracorporal pressure and, ultimately, erections during periods of sexual stimulation. Each corpus has a centrally running cavernosal artery, which supplies blood to the multiple lacunar spaces, which are interconnected and lined by vascular endothelium. *Source*: From Ref. 10.

artery and the presence of bridging, cross-flowing, and collateral routing. The penile arteries are interconnected by anastomoses along their entire course.

The venous drainage of the penis occurs through two major systems, the superficial and the deep (Fig. 8) (6–9,14,22–24). The skin is serviced mainly by the superficial system, which gives rise to a single superficial dorsal penile vein. This eventually empties into the external iliac vein via the external pudendal, saphenous, and femoral veins. The deep venous drainage system drains the corpora cavernosa, the corpus spongiosum, and the urethra. The distal and middle portions of the corpora cavernosa are drained by the subtunical plexus and emissary veins. The emissary veins enter the circumflex veins at the lateral borders of the penis. The circumflex veins empty into a single deep dorsal vein, which drains into the pudendal plexus or periprostatic plexus (Santorini's plexus) (Fig. 9) and finally into the internal iliac vein. The proximal corpora cavernosa are drained via the cavernous and crural veins into the periprostatic plexus and the internal pudendal veins. The superficial dorsal vein has many collaterals to the deep dorsal penile vein. Urethral veins that empty into the internal pudendal vein drain the corpus spongiosum and the urethra. Direct arteriovenous anastomoses also exist. Similarly, the presence of communication between the spongiosal and the cavernosal vascular compartments of the penis has been suggested (10).

Lymphatic Drainage

Lymph is drained from the penis by lymphatics that pass to the superficial and deep inguinal lymph nodes of the femoral triangle (Fig. 10) (10). In turn, these nodes, which may become secondarily involved in patients who have carcinoma of the penis, drain into the external and internal iliac lymphatic chains. Conditions that obstruct these lymphatic channels, such as metastatic prostate cancer, may result in gross penile and scrotal edema.

Innervation

The penis is innervated by somatic and autonomic nerve fibers (Fig. 11) (6,7,9,25–33). Somatic innervation supplies the penis with sensory fibers and the perineal skeletal muscles with motor fibers. The paired dorsal nerve of the penis carries the somatosensory afferent inputs for transmission to the intermediolateral cell column in the lumbosacral spinal cord and subsequently to the brain cortex. The right and left dorsal nerves travel in close (within 1 cm) apposition to one another, directly on the surface of the tunica albuginea of the corpus cavernosum, beneath Buck's fascia. The axons of each nerve are arranged in two populations, one traveling to the glans, and one arborizing over the surface of the penile shaft, with some fibers terminating in the urethra (31). The nerve terminals in the glans penis are numerous and present as free nerve endings (FNEs) in almost all dermal papillae as well as scattered throughout the deep dermis. The ratio of FNEs to corpuscular receptors in the glans is approximately 10:1. Genital end bulbs are also present throughout, but are most abundant in the corona and near the frenulum. The unique corpuscular receptor of the glans consists of axon terminals that resemble a tangled skein of FNEs. The glans is relatively insensitive to tactile and mechanical stimuli but its FNEs can sense deep pressure and pain (25). In contrast, penile skin is rich in fine-touch neuroceptors that carry sensory input from the penile shaft. A band of ridged mucosa, located at the junction of true penile skin with the smooth inner surface of the prepuce, contains more Meissner's corpuscles than does the rest of the smooth preputial mucosa and thus exhibits features of specialized sensory mucosa. This band constitutes an important component of the overall sensory mechanism of the penis (26). Fibers from the urethral innervation appear to carry afferent information necessary for sustaining reflex bulbocavernosus muscle contractions until expulsion of all seminal fluid is complete (29). The dorsal penile nerves have an undulating course to accommodate the significant change in penile length during erection. Proximally, the dorsal nerves pass through the suspensory ligaments,

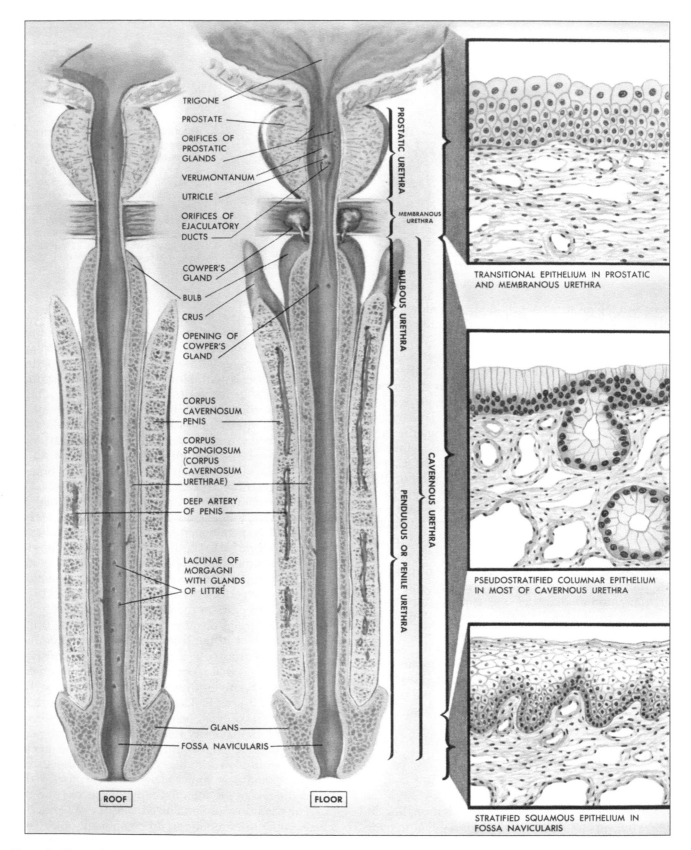

TRIGONE

PROSTATE

ORIFICES OF PROSTATIC GLANDS

VERUMONTANUM

UTRICLE

ORIFICES OF EJACULATORY DUCTS

COWPER'S GLAND

BULB

CRUS

OPENING OF COWPER'S GLAND

CORPUS CAVERNOSUM PENIS

CORPUS SPONGIOSUM (CORPUS CAVERNOSUM URETHRAE)

DEEP ARTERY OF PENIS

LACUNAE OF MORGAGNI WITH GLANDS OF LITTRÉ

GLANS

FOSSA NAVICULARIS

ROOF

FLOOR

PROSTATIC URETHRA

MEMBRANOUS URETHRA

BULBOUS URETHRA

CAVERNOUS URETHRA

PENDULOUS OR PENILE URETHRA

TRANSITIONAL EPITHELIUM IN PROSTATIC AND MEMBRANOUS URETHRA

PSEUDOSTRATIFIED COLUMNAR EPITHELIUM IN MOST OF CAVERNOUS URETHRA

STRATIFIED SQUAMOUS EPITHELIUM IN FOSSA NAVICULARIS

Figure 3 (*See color insert.*) Cross-section of the penis: roof and floor views. *Source*: From Ref. 11. Netter medical illustration used with permission of Elsevier. All rights reserved.

along the inferior pubic ramus on the inferior surface of the urogenital diaphragm, to join other sensory fibers from the perineal and inferior rectal nerves at the pudendal canal, to form the pudendal nerve. Fibers from the somesthetic receptors of the glans penis and frenulum (specialized genital corpuscles and Pacinian corpuscles) as well as those from the penile skin (non-capsulated spray-like FNEs) pass through numerous

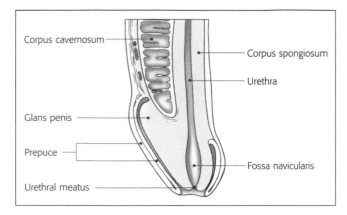

Figure 4 (*See color insert.*) Skin overlying the penis is exceptionally mobile and expandable to accommodate the considerable increase in length and girth that occurs during erection. Distally, the penile skin is reflected forward over the glans penis to form the prepuce before folding back on itself to attach to the corona of the glans penis. *Source*: From Ref. 10.

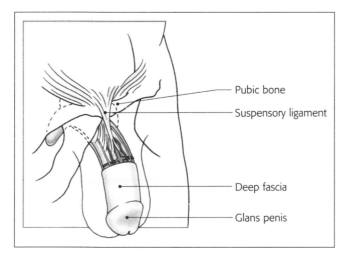

Figure 5 (*See color insert.*) The pendulous portion of the penis is supported by the suspensory ligament, a fibrous condensation that supports and stabilizes the erect penis. Division of this structure makes the penis appear longer in its flaccid state but does not enhance the proportions of the organ when erect. *Source*: From Ref. 10.

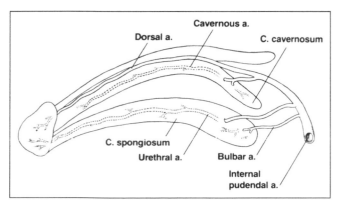

Figure 6 Arterial supply of the penis. *Source*: From Ref. 13.

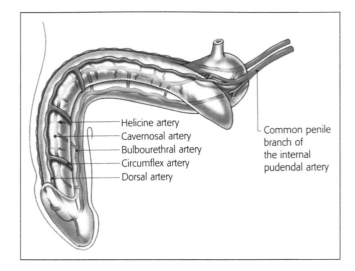

Figure 7 (*See color insert.*) Paired dorsal arteries run along the dorsal aspect of the corpora beneath Buck's fascia, giving off multiple circumflex branches and, eventually, supplying blood to the glans penis. The cavernosal arteries run along the middle of each corpus cavernosum, giving off multiple helicine branches that supply blood to the lacunar spaces. *Source*: From Ref. 10.

networks on the dorsum of the penile shaft to form the right and left dorsal nerves (30). Proximally, the dorsal nerves pass through the suspensory ligaments to follow their respective internal pudendal arteries along the inferior pubic ramus on the inferior surface of the urogenital diaphragm. Additional sensory fibers from other genital nerves, including the perineal and inferior rectal nerves, join in at the pudendal canal to form the pudendal nerve. The pudendal nerve fibers enter the dorsal roots of the sacral spinal cord segment S_2 to S_4. Fibers then ascend into the spinal cord to synapse in the corticomedullary junction and the thalamus, and then terminate in the contralateral primary sensory area deep in the interhemispheric tissue. The somatic motor innervation supplies the perineal skeletal muscles (the bulbocavernosus and ischiocavernosus muscles that surround the corporeal bodies), the external sphincter, and the levator ani muscles. The motor fibers originate from the sacral segments S_2 to S_4 and exit the spinal cord together with the pudendal nerve in the posterior portion of the pudendal canal to form the deep perineal nerve, which passes alongside the perineal artery (31). Contraction of the perineal skeletal muscles during erection leads to a temporary increase in corporeal body pressure to a level above the mean systolic pressure and thus helps to increase penile firmness.

The autonomic innervation of the penis is both parasympathetic and sympathetic. The major efferent parasympathetic pathway originates in the intermediolateral aspect of the sacral cord (S_2–S_4), traveling in the pelvic nerve (Nervi Erigentes) to supply a vasodilating innervation to the corporeal bodies. The higher centers for the parasympathetic pathway include the cingulate gyrus, the gyrus rectus, the medial forebrain bundle, the anterior medial portion of the thalamus, the hippocampus, the septum pellucidum, the paraventricular nucleus, and the mamillothalamic tracts.

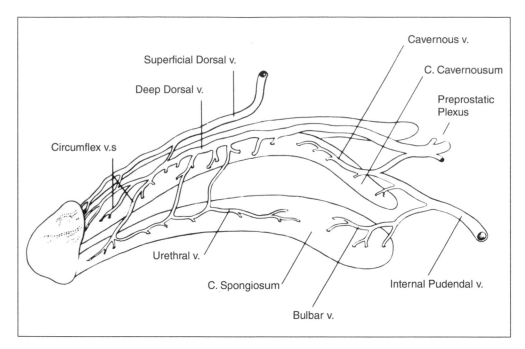

Figure 8 Venous return of the penis. *Source*: From Ref. 13.

Outflow neural messages travel through the substantia nigra to the ventrolateral portion of the pons and descend to the sacral parasympathetic nuclei. After the parasympathetic nerve fibers exit the spinal cord, they run in the retroperitoneal space in the lateral aspect of the rectum and bladder, then pass inferiorly and laterally toward the prostate and urogenital diaphragm. The cavernous nerve enters the corporeal body alongside the cavernous artery at the crura of the corpora as preganglionic nerve fibers. The most likely neurotransmitter at the synaptic end of these fibers is acetylcholine. The postganglionic nerve fiber segments terminate either on the vascular smooth muscle of the corporeal arterioles or on the nonvascular smooth muscle of trabecular tissue surrounding the corporeal lacunae (31). The sacral parasympathetic neurons are chiefly responsible for the erectile function and are influenced by a cortical–sacral efferent pathway. Penile erection can be initiated with a single episode of pelvic nerve electrical stimulation. Maintenance of erection for an extended period of time without significant changes in corporeal body blood gases can be achieved with repetitive stimulation for 40 to 50 seconds, with each stimulus having a minimum latency period between stimuli of 50 seconds (31). The sympathetic outflow originates in the thoracolumbar region of the spinal cord (T11-L2) and passes through the inferior mesenteric, hypogastric, and pelvic plexuses. The

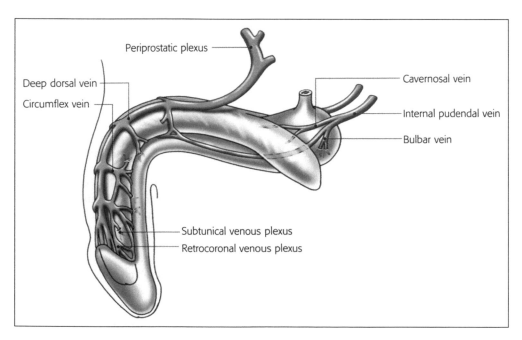

Figure 9 (*See color insert.*) Venous drainage from the corpora cavernosa takes place mainly through the deep dorsal vein, which lies dorsally in the groove between the corpora and passes beneath the pubic arch to join the dorsal venous complex at the urethroprostatic junction. The less surgically accessible bulbar and cavernosal veins join to form the internal pudendal vein. *Source*: From Ref. 10.

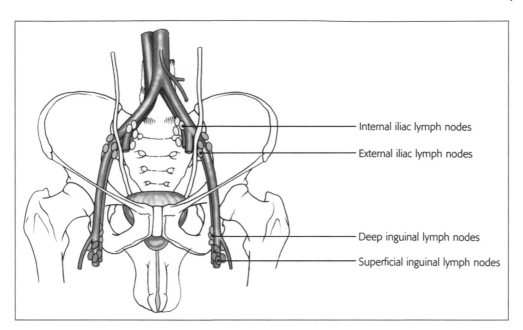

Internal iliac lymph nodes

External iliac lymph nodes

Deep inguinal lymph nodes

Superficial inguinal lymph nodes

Figure 10 (*See color insert.*) Lymphatic drainage of the penis is accomplished by the superficial and deep inguinal nodes, which, in turn, drain into the iliac and para-aortic nodes. *Source*: From Ref. 10.

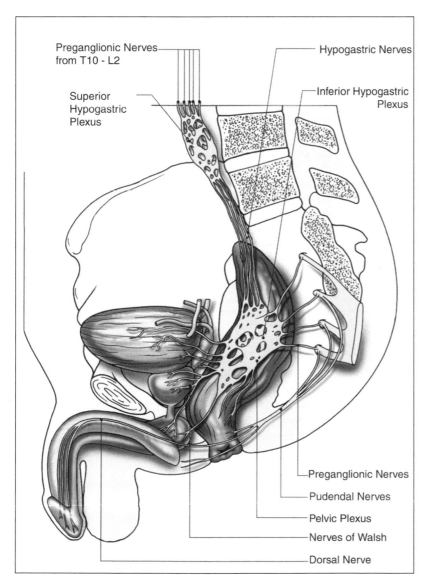

Preganglionic Nerves from T10 - L2

Superior Hypogastric Plexus

Hypogastric Nerves

Inferior Hypogastric Plexus

Preganglionic Nerves

Pudendal Nerves

Pelvic Plexus

Nerves of Walsh

Dorsal Nerve

Figure 11 (*See color insert.*) The hypogastric nerves are vulnerable during retroperitoneal lymph-node dissection. Both sympathetic and parasympathetic nerves merge in the pelvic plexus and pass posterolaterally to the prostate gland in the so-called bundles of Walsh, where they may be damaged during radical prostatectomy and cystoprostatectomy. *Source*: From Ref. 10.

sympathetic innervation of the penis mediates the detumescence following the orgasmic relief, and in the absence of sexual arousal, it maintains the penis in the flaccid state. Evidence suggests that activation of the postsynaptic α-1 and α-2 adrenergic receptors by norepinephrine and epinephrine is involved in the local control of corpus cavernosum smooth-muscle tone (24,25). The sympathetic innervation to the prostate, the seminal vesicles, and the related structures is the chief neural system involved in regulation of ejaculation. Stimulation of the postganglionic fibers leads to contraction of the ejaculatory duct with a concomitant contraction of the bladder neck musculature, resulting in expulsion of the seminal fluid and prevention of the seminal fluid from retrograde deposition into the bladder.

□ NORMAL PENILE SIZE IN ADULT MALES

Wessells et al. (34) have reviewed the normative data on penile size of the adult human male. The studies ranged in sample size from 50 to 2770 subjects with an age range between 17 and 91 years. The average unstretched flaccid length ranges from 8.85 to 10.7 cm, stretched flaccid length ranges from 12.45 to 16.74 cm, and erection length ranges from 12.89 to 15.5 cm.

Reports on penile volume are limited and have relied either upon the measurement of penile circumference manually (35–37) or upon penile cross-section by ultrasound techniques (34,38,39). In these latter studies, the average penile volume ranged from 17.15 to 43.62 mL in the flaccid state and from 69.41 to 80.16 mL in the erect state (induced by intracorporeal injection of vasoactive agents). The average volume increase between these two phases of the erectile cycle ranged from 27.87 to 56.35 mL. The average mid-shaft circumference for the flaccid and erect penises was 9.71 and 12.30 cm, respectively. Average pubic fat-pad

depth was 2.85 cm, which when added to the average erect penis length, rendered the average functional penile length 15.74 cm. Stretched, flaccid penile length correlated strongly with the erect length in this series. Further, pubic fat-pad was greater in depth in men older than 40 years of age. The increase in central obesity may contribute to the occasionally reported decrease in penile length with age. Differences in methods of data gathering (subject self-reporting, single vs. multiple examiners, single vs. repeated stretching of the penis prior to measurement) and/or differences in populations studied (men with normal sexual function vs. men with sexual dysfunction, different ethnic or age groups) could have contributed to some of the differences seen in the average values reported in the above studies. There is a loss of tensile strength of the tunica as men grow older but no loss of the tunica albuginea itself.

Based on the available data, Wessells et al. (34) considered adult men with penile length of greater than 4 cm in the unstretched flaccid state or greater than 7.5 cm in the stretched flaccid state or the erect state to have a normal penile length. No parallel suggestions were made for penile girth or volume.

□ CONCLUSION

The widespread prevalence of ED has made this particular complaint a primary clinical concern for adult males of any age. Although it was once commonly believed that psychogenic problems were the predominant cause of ED, it has become evident that organic causes are more common, especially in middle-aged to older men. The brief overview of the anatomy of the penis presented in this chapter is intended to clarify the basic knowledge necessary for the diagnosis and management of male sexual dysfunction.

□ REFERENCES

1. The American Society of Andrology. Handbook of Andrology. San Francisco: American Society of Andrology, 1995.
2. Ayta IA, McKinlay JB, Krane RJ. The likely worldwide increase in erectile dysfunction between 1995 and 2025 and some possible policy consequences. Br J Urol Int 1999; 84(1):50–56.
3. Frank E, Anderson C, Rubinstein D. Frequency of sexual dysfunction in "normal" couples. N Engl J Med 1978; 299(3):111–115.
4. Furlow WL. Prevalence of impotence in the United States. Med Aspects Hum Sex 1985; 19:13–16.
5. Feldman HA, Goldstein I, Hatzichristou DG, et al. Impotence and its medical and psychosocial correlates: results of the Massachusetts Male Aging Study. J Urol 1994; 151(1):54–61.
6. Myer JK. Disorders of sexual function. In: Wilson JD, Foster DW, eds. Williams Textbook of Endocrinology. 7th ed. Philadelphia: WB Saunders Company, 1985:476–491.
7. Newman HF. Physiology of erection: Autonomic consideration. In: Krane RF, Siroky MB, Goldstein I, eds. Male Sexual Dysfunction. Boston: Little, Brown and Company, 1983:1–7.
8. Krane RJ. Sexual function and dysfunction. In: Walsh PC, ed. Campbell's Urology. 5th ed. Philadelphia: WB Saunders Company, 1986:700–735.
9. Rivard DJ. Anatomy, physiology, and neurophysiology of male sexual function. In: Bennett AH, ed. Management of Male Impotence. Int Perspect Urol. Vol. 5. Baltimore: Williams & Wilkins, 1982:1–25.

10. Kirby RS. An Atlas of Erectile Dysfunction: An Illustrated Textbook and Reference for Clinicians. New York: The Parthenon Publishing Group, 1999.

11. Netter FH. Oppenheimer E, eds. The CIBA Collection of Medical Illustrations: A Compilation of Paintings on the Normal and Pathologic Anatomy of the Reproductive System. Vol. 2. Summit, NJ: CIBA Pharmaceutical Products, Inc., 1954.

12. Lerner SE, Melman A, Christ GJ. A review of erectile dysfunction: new insights and more questions. J Urol 1993; 149(5 Pt 2):1246–1255.

13. Lue TF, Tanagho EA. Hemodynamics of erection. In: Tanagho EA, Lue TF, McClure RD, eds. Contemporary Management of Impotence and Infertility. Baltimore: Williams & Wilkins, 1988:28–38.

14. Wagner G. Erection: physiology and endocrinology. In: Wagner G, Green R, eds. Impotence: Physiological, Psychological, Surgical Diagnosis and Treatment. New York: Plenum Press, 1981:25–36.

15. Krysiewicz S, Mellinger BC. The role of imaging in the diagnostic evaluation of impotence. AJR 1989; 153(6): 1133–1139.

16. Krane RJ, Goldstein I, Saenz de Tejada I. Impotence. N Engl J Med 1989; 321(24):1648–1659.

17. Aboseif SL, Lue TF. Hemodynamics of penile erection. Urol Clin North Am 1988; 15(1):1–7.

18. Rosen MP, Schwartz AN, Levine FJ, Greenfield AJ. Radiologic assessment of impotence: angiography, sonography, cavernosography, and scintigraphy. Am J Roentgenol 1991; 157(5):923–931.

19. Bookstein JJ, Lang EV. Penile magnification pharmacoarteriography: details of intrapenile anatomy. AJR 1987; 148(5):883–888.

20. Gray RR, Keresteci AG, Louis ELS, et al. Investigation of impotence by internal pudendal angiography: experience with 73 cases. Radiology 1982; 144(4): 773–780.

21. Rosen MP, Greenfield AJ, Walker TG, et al. Arteriogenic impotence: findings in 195 impotent men examined with selective internal pudendal angiography. Radiology 1990; 174(3):1043–1048.

22. Bodner D. Impotence: evaluation and treatment. Prim Care 1985; 12(4):719–733.

23. Althof S, Seftel A. The evaluation and management of erectile dysfunction. Psychiatr Clin North Am 1995; 18(1):171–192.

24. Klein E. The anatomy and physiology of the normal male sexual function. In: Montague D, ed. Disorders of Male Sexual Function. Chicago: Year Book Medical Publishers Inc., 1988:2–19.

25. Federman DD. Impotence: etiology and management. Hosp Prac 1982; 17(3):155–159.

26. Siroky MB, Krane RJ. Neurophysiology of erection. In: Krane RJ, Siroky MB, Goldstein I, eds. Male Sexual Dysfunction. Boston: Little, Brown and Company, 1983:9–20.

27. Siroky MB, Krane RJ. Physiology of male sexual function. In: Krane RJ, Siroky MB, eds. Clinical Neuro-Urology. Boston: Little, Brown and Company, 1979:45–62.

28. Steers WD. Current perspectives in the neural control of penile erection. In: Lue TF, ed. World Book of Impotence. London/Niigata-Shi: Smith-Gordon/Nishimura, 1992: 23–32.

29. Gupta S, Moreland RB, Yang S, et al. The expression of functional postsynaptic alpha2-adrenoceptors in the corpus cavernosum smooth muscle. Br J Pharmacol 1998; 123(6):1237–1245.

30. Traish AM, Moreland RB, Huang YH, Goldstein I. Expression of functional alpha2-adrenergic receptor subtypes in human corpus cavernousm and in cultured travecular smooth muscle cells. Recept Signal Transduct 1997; 7(1):55–67.

31. Goldstein I. Evaluation of penile nerves. In: Tanagho EA, Lue TF, McClure RD, eds. Contemporary Management of Impotence and Infertility. Baltimore: Williams & Wilkins, 1988:70–83.

32. Giuliano FA, Benoit G, Rampin O, Jardin A. Neural control of penile erection. Urol Clin North Am 1995; 22(4):747–766.

33. Saenz de Tejada I, Goldstein I, Krane RJ. Local control of penile erection. Nerves, smooth muscle, and endothelium. Urol Clin North Am 1988; 15(1):9–15.

34. Wessells H, Lue TF, McAninch JW. Penile length in the flaccid and erect states: guidelines for penile augmentation. J Urol 1996; 156(3):995–997.

35. Virag R, Bouilly P, Virag H. Dimensions, volume and rigidity of the penis. Fundamental elements in the study of the erection and its dysfunctions. [Article in French]. Ann Urol (Paris) 1986; 20(4):244–248.

36. Gobec CJ, Cass AS. Quantification of erection. J Urol 1981; 126:345–357.

37. Bancroft J, Bell C. Simultaneous recording of penile diameter and penile arterial pulse during laboratory-based erotic stimulation in normal subjects. J Psychosom Res 1985; 29(3):303–313.

38. Chen KK, Chou YH, Chang LS, Chen MT. Sonographic measurement of penile erectile volume. J Clin Ultrasound 1992; 20(4):247–253.

39. Nelson RP, Lue TF. Determination of erectile penile volume by ultrasonography. J Urol 1989; 141(5):1123–1126.

3

Normal Male Sexual Response Cycle

Fouad R. Kandeel

Department of Diabetes, Endocrinology and Metabolism, City of Hope National Medical Center, Duarte, California and David Geffen School of Medicine, University of California, Los Angeles, California, U.S.A.

Vivien Koussa

H.C. Healthcare Management and Development, Inc., Long Beach, California, U.S.A.

□ INTRODUCTION

Many significant advances in the understanding of the physiology of male sexual function have been attained in the last three decades. The individual nature and function of the elements involved in the normal sexual response have been delineated. Additional progress has been made in the comprehension of the intricate neural mechanisms that govern sexual activity. This greater knowledge has enabled similarly innovative advances in the investigation and treatment of male sexual dysfunction. It is hoped that the information provided in this chapter will serve to familiarize clinicians and other health professionals with this topic and to provide them with a means of better understanding the physiological basis of their patients' sexual concerns.

□ LOCAL CONTROL OF PENILE FUNCTION
Parasympathetic Control of Penile Erection

Acetylcholine appears to be the neurotransmitter of the preganglionic parasympathetic neurons. The neurotransmitters for the short postganglionic neurons have not been fully defined. Acetylcholine does not appear to influence the contractility of the corporeal smooth-muscle fibers directly but does so through activation of cholinergic receptors on the endothelial cells (Fig. 1) (2). Nitric oxide (NO) has been identified in the corporeal tissue (3) and is believed to be the endothelial-derived relaxation factor(s). NO is also produced by pre- and postsynaptic neuronal structures including the brain and the preganglionic sympathetic and the postganglionic parasympathetic neuronal fibers. In many of these structures, it colocalizes with other classical (acetylcholine) and nonclassical [vasoactive intestinal polypeptide (VIP)] neurotransmitters (4). Unlike the classical neurotransmitters that accumulate in secretory vesicles of producing cells prior to release and exert their action through the binding to a specific cell-surface receptor, NO is a membrane-permeable gas, that diffuses out rapidly to act on neighboring cellular elements, including

the presynaptic nerve endings and astrocytes (5). Within these target cells, it activates a soluble guanylate cyclase to stimulate the formation of cyclic guanosine monophosphate (cGMP).

NO participates in a number of key processes within the central nervous system (CNS), including certain forms of synaptic plasticity and memory formation (6), thalamic and cerebral cortical processing of afferent sensory information (7), striatal dopaminergic transmission (8), hypothalamic gonadotropin releasing hormone (GnRH) gene expression (9) and cerebral blood flow regulation (10). It also participates in modulation of synaptic vesicle docking/fusion reactions (11) and in mediating the effects of certain autonomic muscarinic (12,13) and nicotinic (14) neurotransmissions. NO is synthesized from its precursor, L-arginine, by the enzyme nitric oxide synthase (NOS). Both constitutive and inducible NOS isoforms are produced in the cavernosal tissues (15,16). Constitutive NOS is produced by the endothelial cells and the nerve terminals, whereas the inducible NOS appears to be produced by the corporeal smooth-muscle cells only (Fig. 2).

The catalytic activity of the constitutive NOS isoform is stimulated by the presence of calcium and calmodulin (a calcium-binding protein), reduction in nicotinamide adenine dinucleotide phosphate, activation of cholinergic receptors, increase in oxygen tension subsequent to an increase in blood inflow, and mechanical stretching (shear stress) due to dilatation of the helicine arterioles and engorgement of the sinusoidal spaces with incoming blood (17–20). Conversely, the catalytic effect of NOS is inhibited by the presence of arginine derivatives (15). When intracellular calcium increases, calcium binds to calmodulin, and the calcium–calmodulin complex binds to and activates the constitutive NOS (21,22). NOS then converts L-arginine and oxygen into L-citrulline and NO. Once stimulated, small quantities of NO continue to be produced in pulses until the calcium level drops and the catalytic effect of NOS diminishes. NO produced by the sinusoidal endothelial cells and by the noncholinergic parasympathetic neurons diffuses into the adjacent smooth-muscle cells and activates soluble guanylate

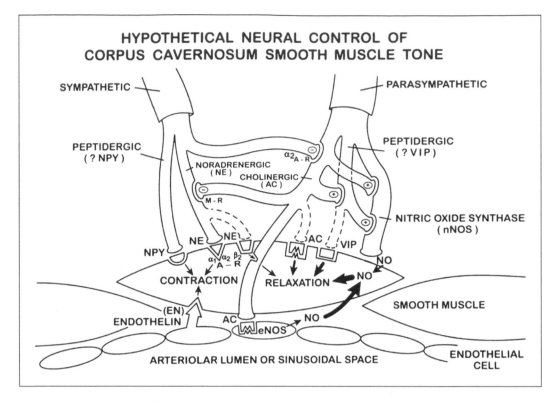

Figure 1 Proposed neural control of the corporeal smooth-muscle function. Parasympathetic fibers directly innervate the corporeal smooth muscle and sinusoidal endothelial cells. AC is the parasympathetic neuromediator at the endothelial cells and it activates the production of constitutive endothelial NOS and consequently stimulates NO production. Parasympathetic innervation of the smooth-muscle cells, on the other hand, is mediated largely by NOS-containing fibers, and, to a lesser extent, by VIP-containing fibers. NO, produced locally in the smooth-muscle cell or reaching it by diffusion from adjacent endothelial cell(s), is the major mediator of smooth-muscle relaxation via stimulation of cGMP production. VIP plays a lesser role in the direct stimulation of corporeal smooth-muscle relaxation. The sympathetic innervation of smooth-muscle cells includes NE and nonadrenergic (most likely NPY) fibers. α-1 and α-2 A-R activation, together with NPY and EN-1 actions, are responsible for smooth-muscle cell contraction. Cross talk between the two divisions of the autonomic innervation appears to exist, via an α-2 A-R and an M-R on the parasympathetic and the sympathetic divisions, respectively. This aids in the inhibition of each division when the other is activated. Arrow size reflects the relative importance of innervation or neurotransmission. *Abbreviations*: AC, acetylcholine; NOS, nitric oxide synthase; NO, nitric oxide; VIP, vasoactive intestinal polypeptide; NE, norepinephrine; A-R, adrenoreceptor; NPY, neuropeptide Y; EN-1, endothelin-1; M-R, muscarinic receptor; +, stimulatory or positive effect; −, inhibitory or negative effect. *Source*: From Ref. 1.

cyclase to increase the intracellular cGMP concentration (15). The cGMP appears to be the major intracellular effector of the smooth-muscle cell relaxation (23–25) via a biochemical cascade of protein kinases.

A putative mechanism for cGMP-induced corporeal smooth-muscle relaxation involves protein kinase phosphorylation of myosin light chains directly or as a consequence of lowering intracellular calcium stores (15). Although several types of phosphodiesterase (PDE) isoenzymes have been identified in the human corpora cavernosa, type 5 was found to be the predominant isoenzyme responsible for the inactivation of cGMP (26). Sildenafil (Viagra) inhibits this PDE, which is also found in vascular smooth muscles and platelets (27). Sildenafil also inhibits PDE type 6 to a lesser extent in the retinal rod photoreceptors (responsible for metabolism of the light-stimulated cGMP) and has little or no effect on the calcium/calmodulin-dependent PDE-1 and the calcium/calmodulin-independent PDE-3 isoenzymes in the cardiac muscles (responsible for metabolism of cGMP that is involved in regulation of cardiac contractility) (27). Sildenafil has come to be viewed as an attractive physiological means for the

induction and/or prolongation of erection in man (28). For further information on sildenafil and other PDE5 inhibitors, see Chapter 29.

In addition to stimulation of cGMP production, NO itself may also directly influence the contractility of the corporeal smooth-muscle fibers by altering the transcellular ion flux through activation of the sodium/potassium-adenosinetriphosphatase (Na/K-ATPase) (29,30) and the potassium-conductive membrane hyperpolarization pathway (31).

It has been shown that inducible NOS isoform is expressed by rat corporeal smooth-muscle cells (32). Typically, this form of NOS is expressed by macrophages after stimulation with specific cytokines and results in synthesis of NO in large quantities, which in tissues other than the penis could have pathogenic effects. The exact role of this inducible NOS and its catalyzed product NO in the control of erectile function in the human remains to be elucidated.

NO half-life in biological fluids is short, ranging between 2 and 30 seconds. Further, formation and/or action of NO can be inhibited by a number of factors including the presence of oxyhemoglobin or

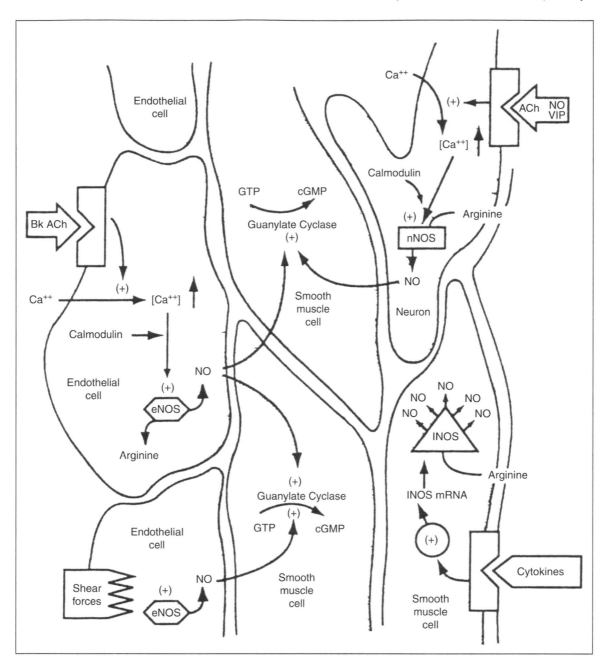

Figure 2 Proposed mechanisms for NO synthesis, regulation, and action in the penis. NO is constitutionally formed from its precursor, L-arginine, in endothelial cells and neurons by catalytic action of eNOS and nNOS, respectively. Whereas messenger molecules commonly activate these enzymes by signaling influx of calcium and its binding with calmodulin, other biochemical or mechanical factors may interact with this process, influencing production of NO. Once synthesized, NO diffuses to local smooth-muscle cells, where it primarily activates guanylate cyclase to convert 5'-GTP to 3',5'-cGMP. Smooth-muscle cells represent another source of NO, but these appear to require cytokine stimulation of iNOS expression. *Abbreviations*: Bk, bradykinin; Ach, acetylcholine; VIP, vasoactive intestinal peptide; NO, nitric oxide; eNOS, endothelial NOS; nNOS, neuronal NOS; GTP, guanosine triphosphate; cGMP, cyclic guanosine monophosphate; iNOS, inducible NOS. *Source*: From Ref. 15.

superoxide anions, hypoxia, low intracellular calcium stores, extreme acid-base conditions, advanced glycosylation end products, and androgen deficiency (33–37). High levels of the tissue superoxide dismutase enzyme appear to protect NO from destruction by superoxide anions (38). In addition, the hypothesis of testosterone dependence of penile NO synthesis is gaining support from observations in which both testosterone and NO levels were lower in penile venous blood than in the brachial blood of

men with psychogenic impotence, and androgen replacement restored NOS production and action of the penis in castrated rats (36,39).

Other noncholinergic parasympathetic neurotransmitters capable of promoting smooth-muscle relaxation, and hence the erectile response, include VIP, bradykinin, peptide histidine methionine, pituitary adenylate cyclase–activating polypeptide, helospectin, galanin, calcitonin gene-related peptide, and prostaglandin E$_1$ (PGE$_1$) (40–44). Prior to the identification of

NO in the penile tissue, VIP was thought to be the chief neuromediator of the erectile function because of its presence in relatively large quantities in neurons supplying the corporeal tissue. More recently, VIP was found to colocalize with NOS in penile neurons of rats and humans (45,46). Further, its relaxation effect on the corporeal smooth-muscle fibers appears to be mediated by the NO–cGMP pathway as inhibitors of NOS or guanylate cyclase can attenuate this action (47,48). Similarly, the relaxation effect of bradykinin on corporeal smooth muscles is via stimulation of the endothelial NOS pathway to generate NO (49). The exact mechanisms by which other neuropeptides participate in regulation of the erectile function, however, remain to be determined.

Sympathetic Control of Penile Detumescence and Flaccidity

The major functions of the sympathetic innervation of the penis are to maintain the flaccid state and to produce detumescence following orgasmic relief. Norepinephrine is responsible for the regulation of corpus cavernosum smooth-muscle tone via the interaction with α-1 and α-2 adrenergic receptors (50,51). Observations supporting a role for α-adrenergic receptors in mediating this effect are summarized in the following: first, α-1a (predominant), α-1b, and α-1d adrenergic receptor subtypes were shown by mRNA measurement to be expressed in human corpus cavernosum tissue (52); second, α-adrenergic receptors were shown by radiological binding assays to be present in human corpus cavernosum tissue in higher quantity than β-adrenergic receptors (53,54); third, norepinephrine induced a concentration-dependent contraction of isolated strips of corporeal tissue, and this contraction was attenuated or blocked by α-adrenergic receptor blockers (55–57); and fourth, the level of norepinephrine in penile blood of patients with psychogenic erectile dysfunction was significantly higher than in normal controls or in patients with vasculogenic erectile dysfunction. Further, patients with psychogenic erectile dysfunction who failed the erectile response to intracavernous injection of papaverine hydrochloride (smooth-muscle relaxant) had even higher penile blood norepinephrine than those who elicited an erectile response (58). Other neurotransmitters capable of promoting smooth-muscle contraction, and hence detumescence, include endothelin-1, substance-P, prostaglandin $F_{2\alpha}$, thromboxane A_2, angiotensin II, and calcium (2,17–20,25,40,42,43,47,54,59–63). Some of these agents exert their effect through modulation of the presynaptic α-2 adrenergic receptors. Evidence obtained from equine penile resistance arteries suggests that presynaptic α-2 adrenergic receptor stimulation can inhibit electric field stimulation-induced relaxation. Since the latter effect can also be blocked by N^G-Nitro-L-arginine "methyl ester (L-NAME)," a NOS inhibitor, it is thought that α-2 adrenergic receptor stimulation leads to inhibition of NO release (64). A role for sympathetic innervation of the penis in mediation of psychologically provoked erection has been suggested, but the validity of such a belief has been disputed based upon the observation of full retention of erectile capacity in men who undergo bilateral complete sympathectomy (65,66). Yet, recent in vitro studies demonstrating the relaxation effect of the β-2 adrenergic receptor agonist, isoproterenol, on noradrenaline-precontracted human penile smooth-muscle cells (67) suggest that, at least in some situations, β-adrenergic innervation could participate in the mediation of human erection. The relaxation effect of β-agonists on penile smooth muscles has been corroborated by at least one other study (68).

Differences in the relative preponderance of α-adrenergic receptor subtypes appear to exist among human corporeal trabecular tissue, cavernosal arteries, and cavernosal veins. α-1 adrenergic receptor is the preponderant subtype in corporeal smooth muscles (57,69) and the deep dorsal penile vein (70), whereas α-2 receptors dominate in the cavernosal arteries (57,69). No quantitative differences in the prevalence of the two subtypes, however, were found in the circumflex veins of either potent or impotent men (71). The functional significance of these differences in the distribution of α-adrenergic receptor subtypes remains to be conclusively elucidated. Crowe et al. (72) used immunohistochemical techniques to determine the presence of peptide-containing nerves in the human deep dorsal penile vein. They found the greatest density of nerves supplying the deep dorsal vein and the vasa vasorum were neuropeptide-Y (NPY) followed (in a decreasing order) by VIP- and dopamine-β-hydroxylase-containing nerves. These investigators proposed that NPY may aid in penile erection via its prolonged vasoconstricting effect, and that VIP may also be involved in facilitating the drainage of penile blood during detumescence via its vasodilating effect. A series of in vitro experiments by Segarra et al. (73), using ring segments of human penile dorsal vein, has provided additional evidence for an active role of the deep dorsal vein in the total penile vascular resistance through the release of NO from both neural and endothelial elements.

Role of Trabecular Smooth Muscle in Penile Erection and Detumescence

It has been increasingly recognized that trabecular smooth-muscle cells play an important role in mediating the erection and detumescence of the penis through their intrinsic compliance and adequate relaxation and contraction response to the neuronal control in both human and animal penises (25,40,74). During erection, the complete relaxation of corporeal smooth-muscle fibers allows the entrapment of a large amount of circulating blood and subsequent increase in intrasinusoidal pressure to a supradiastolic level, which leads to the tensing of the fibroelastic tunica albuginea and closure of the emissary veins. This, in turn, leads to the development of an erectile state adequate for coitus. Conversely, sufficient contraction of the trabecular smooth muscles limits the capacity of the intracorporeal

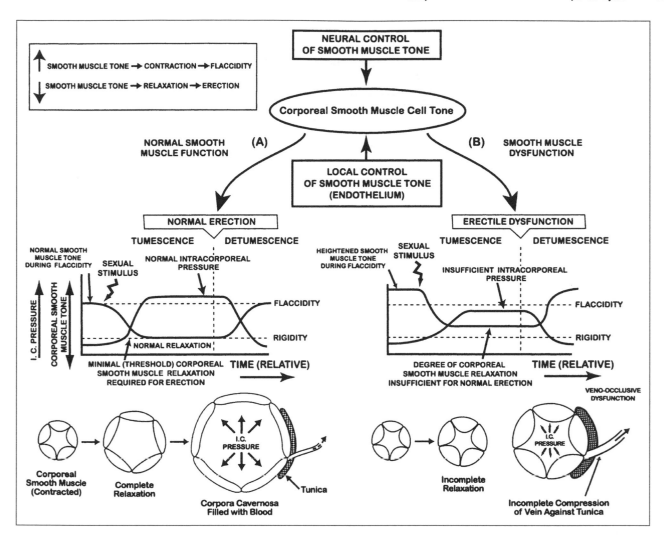

Figure 3 The illustration depicts the effects of normal (**A**) and abnormal (**B**) balance between smooth-muscle contraction and relaxation on the entire erectile process. Normal smooth-muscle tone during flaccidity and sufficient relaxation during tumescence permits the rise in intracorporeal pressure to the level needed for full erection to occur. Any physiological perturbation that results in heightened contractility during flaccidity and impaired relaxation of the corporeal smooth muscle during tumescence will shift the delicate balance in favor of flaccidity over erection. *Abbreviation*: I.C. pressure, intracorporeal pressure. *Source*: From Ref. 1.

vascular bed and increases venous return and hence induces penile detumescence. The presence of a critical balance of smooth muscle to connective tissue has been suggested for the successful veno-occlusion and the manifestation of erectile response to occur. A potential role for transforming growth factor β-1 and PGE_1 in maintaining this critical balance of smooth muscle/connective tissue and a role for intracorporeal oxygen tension in regulation of synthesis of these regulatory factors have also been suggested (75). Thus, neuronal dysregulation or poor intrinsic compliance of the corporeal smooth-muscle cells could be a significant factor in the pathogenesis of erectile dysfunction (Fig. 3) (74).

Another aspect of the control of corporeal smooth-muscle cell function that has recently been described is the role played by the gap junction (Fig. 4) (40,55, 74–78). Gap junction channels interconnect the corpus cavernosum smooth-muscle cells and allow them to function as a coordinated network with synchronous myographic activity. This occurs as a result of rapid intercellular propagation of local neural or hormonal signals. Certain second messengers such as calcium ion and inositol triphosphate (IP_3) are transported between corporeal smooth-muscle cells through these junctions. Therefore, cell-to-cell communication is a likely means for synchronization and integration of the corporeal smooth-muscle activity that occurs despite the paucity of nerve supply to individual smooth-muscle cells. The exact role played by the gap junction in coordinating the corporeal smooth-muscle function into a single syncytial tissue response, however, has yet to be fully elucidated. Similarly, a recent patch clamp study indicated the presence of a stretch-sensitive chloride channel in 5% of smooth-muscle cells of human corpus cavernosum (79). The specific details of how this channel regulates penile smooth-muscle contraction/relaxation remains to be determined.

□ NORMAL MALE SEXUAL CYCLE

Sexual stimulation of the human male results in a series of psychological, neuronal, vascular, and local genital

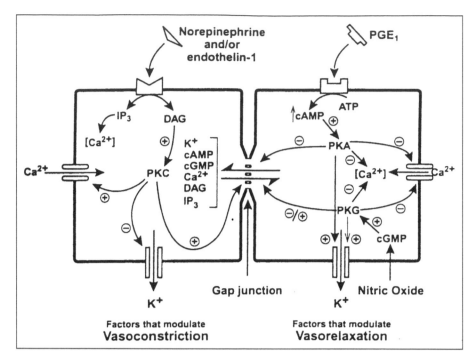

Figure 4 Role of gap junction in regulating smooth-muscle tone: the interaction of important second messenger systems in the regulation of gap junction, K+, and Ca^{2+} channels and thus in modulation of corporeal smooth-muscle tone in vitro and in vivo. Two corporeal smooth-muscle cells, interconnected by a gap junction plaque at their lateral borders are shown. The left cell depicts the series of intracellular events linked to corporeal smooth-muscle contraction (an elevation in intracellular calcium levels). In the corpora, this might be accomplished following activation of the α-1 adrenergic receptor by norepinephrine or by ET-1 activation of the ET$_A$ receptor. In both cases, receptor activation leads to Ca^{2+} mobilization. Specifically, activation of these receptors by norepinephrine or ET-1 leads to activation of phospholipase C, which cleaves membrane-bound PIP$_2$ into IP$_3$ and DAG. Conversely, the right cell depicts the series of intracellular events linked to corporeal smooth-muscle relaxation (a diminution of transmembrane Ca^{2+} flux, sequestration of intracellular Ca^{2+}, membrane hyperpolarization, and smooth-muscle relaxation). In this example, PGE-1 activates the PGE-1 receptor to stimulate the adenylate cyclase enzyme, which then catalyzes the conversion of ATP to cAMP. Increased cAMP then stimulates PKA. Alternatively, smooth-muscle relaxation can be achieved by nitric oxide, released from the endothelial or neuronal sources. Nitric oxide diffuses into smooth-muscle cells to activate soluble guanylate cyclase, which catalyzes the conversion of GTP to cGMP. Elevated cGMP levels activate PKG. The effects of PKA, PKG, and PKC on gap junction, K channels, and Ca channels are thought to be mediated via phosphorylation of specific amino acid residues on target proteins. The result of their actions is illustrated. *Abbreviations*: +, stimulatory, positive, or increasing effect; –, inhibitory or negative effect; ET-1, endothelin-1; PIP$_2$, phosphatidyl inositol; IP$_3$, inositol triphosphate; DAG, diacylglycerol; PGE-1, prostaglandin E-1; cAMP, cyclic adenosine monophosphate; PKA, protein kinase A; cGMP, cyclic guanosine monophosphate; PKG, protein kinase G. *Source*: From Ref. 74.

changes. At least three different classification schemes for these changes have been offered, and each has its particular utility depending on the application, be it psychosexual, penodynamic, or functional.

In the middle part of the twentieth century, gynecologist William Howell Masters and psychologist Virginia Eshelman Johnson were pioneers in the field of sexual medicine, recording some of the first human physiological data from the sex organs during sexual excitation (80,81). Their four-stage model of sexual response remains one of the most enduring and important aspects of their work, defined by excitement, plateau, orgasm, and resolution. Sexual excitement occurs as the result of external sensual (visual, auditory, tactile, or olfactory) and internal psychic stimuli to the limbic system, leading to activation of the sacral parasympathetic pathway and inhibition of the thoracolumbar sympathetic pathway. This produces relaxation of the penile corporeal smooth muscles and helicine arterioles, allowing increased arterial blood inflow and, thus, increased penile volume due to its filling with blood. The fall of resistance within the corporeal vascular bed and the subsequent increase in arterial

inflow are the major vascular events leading to erection of the penis. Central to these events is the corporeal contractile system, which is composed of bundles of smooth muscles, vascular endothelium, and elastic fibers. Relaxation of the smooth muscles with a concomitant stretching of the endothelium leads to enlargement of the sinusoidal or lacunar spaces and an increase in their capacity for blood storage. Distention of the sinusoidal spaces within the corpora cavernosa with arterial blood tenses the surrounding tunica albuginea and compresses the subtunical and emissary veins, thereby reducing venous drainage. The progressive increase in intracorporeal pressure leads to penile expansion, tumescence, and rigidity. The pressure in the lacunar spaces during erection is the result of an equilibrium between the perfusion pressure in the cavernosal artery and the helicine arterioles and the resistance to blood outflow through the compressed subtunical venules.

Activation of the sacrospinal reflex subsequent to direct genital stimulation during the plateau phase leads to contraction of the ischiocavernosus muscles and stimulation of the corpus spongiosum and the accessory Cowper's and Littre's glands. Contraction of the pelvic floor muscles augments the intracavernous pressure, resulting in decreased venous blood outflow. The coordination of these activities produces a state of full erection and rigidity. Further, stimulation of the corpus spongiosum and accessory glands leads to the dilatation of the urethral bulb and the secretion of a lubricating fluid, respectively. As sexual pleasure approaches its climax, activation of the thoracolumbar spinal reflex occurs, leading to the contraction of vas deferens, ampulla, seminal vesicle, and prostate. This results in the deposition of the seminal fluid in the posterior urethra. Rhythmic contractions of the bulbocavernosus and the pelvic floor muscles, usually at 0.8-second intervals, lead to expulsion of the seminal fluid (ejaculation), which is accompanied by concomitant closure of the bladder neck to prevent the retrograde fall of semen into the bladder cavity. After the release of sexual tension and at the onset of the resolution phase, a thoracolumbar sympathetic pathway acts to contract the corporeal smooth muscles and the arterial tree, thereby limiting blood inflow and augmenting venous outflow, producing penile flaccidity. A refractory period, during which a subsequent full erection or repeated orgasm is nearly impossible, ensues.

With the advent of modern imaging and examination techniques, a second classification scheme has emerged that characterizes the penodynamic changes during the sexual cycle (82,83) such that each of the psychosexual phases is divided into two interrelated events: excitement into latency and tumescence; plateau into erection and rigidity; orgasm into emission and ejaculation; and, resolution into detumescence and refractoriness.

A dramatic increase in penile arterial blood flow to about 25 to 60 times that of the flaccid state occurs during the rapid period of tumescence (84). Pulse Doppler analysis studies with intracavernous vasoactive drug injections have established that a peak cavernosal artery systolic flow greater than 25 mL/sec is required for erection to occur (85–94). At full rigidity, an increase in penile length of 7.5 cm usually requires the entrapment of 80 to 115 mL of blood. As the penile volume increases to near maximum (from less than 10 mL in the flaccid state to about 60 mL in the erect state), the arterial influx declines and plateaus at a level that is sufficient to keep the penis in the rigid (full erection) state. Dynamic infusion cavernosometry and cavernosography (DICC) studies showed that a fluid flow rate between 5 and 40 mL/min is required to maintain a normal penis in the erect state (95–101). Further, at these minimum flow rates of full erection, the cavernosal artery occlusion pressure equilibrates with the intracavernous pressure. With maximum rigidity induced with pelvic muscle contraction, suprasystolic pressures are generated, and cavernosal artery flow ceases transiently. The initial increase in blood inflow during sexual excitement is associated with a transient increase in venous return. As penile tumescence ensues and compression of the subtunical venous

plexus and emissary veins against the nonstretchable tunica albuginea occurs, venous return falls and the end diastolic cavernosal artery flow reverses (up to 7 mL/sec). At the conclusion of ejaculation, a rapid increase in venous outflow occurs as a result of the contraction of the corporeal smooth muscles and diminution in the compression pressure to the subtunical and emissary veins. The rate of venous flow returns to that of the flaccid state at the conclusion of the detumescence phase.

The intracorporeal pressure during the flaccid state is between 10 and 15 mm Hg. Intrapenile pressure changes are modest during the initial phase of the sexual cycle and remain so until near-maximum changes in circumference and volume are attained. As the penis becomes erect, the penile body pressure increases rapidly to about 90 mm Hg. Perineal muscle contraction results in further increase in penile body pressure to greater than 120 mm Hg (suprasystolic pressure), which results in full rigidity and elevation of the penis to greater than 90° from the plane of the lower extremities (80,81,101). Following orgasm, penile body pressure declines rapidly and penile volume returns to the flaccid size. The DICC studies suggested that the intrapenile pressure normally drops at a rate of less than 1 mmHg/sec during the detumescence, as reflected by the rate of drop in intrapenile pressure when fluid infusion is discontinued. Figure 5 depicts these psychosexual and penodynamic classifications of the male sexual cycle and the accompanying local hemodynamic and physical changes. Table 1 summarizes the relationships among the phases of the sexual response cycle, neural pathways, end-organ and hemodynamic changes, and genital functional responses.

Magnetic resonance imaging (MRI) has recently been used as a diagnostic tool to study erectile dysfunction. MRI has been particularly attractive in this application since it produces images with exquisite anatomical detail that are much more clear than those obtained via ultrasonography or radiography. Additionally, MRI appears to be relatively safe. In a remarkable study, Schultz et al. (102) tested the limits of MRI technology by taking images of both male and female genitals during coitus in order to determine whether former and current ideas regarding anatomy during sexual intercourse are based on fact or assumption (Fig. 6A and B). The results of the study revealed several unusual findings regarding the anatomy of intercourse, such as the striking engorgement that occurs in the anterior vaginal wall of the female, including lengthening of the anterior wall and a rising of the uterus without a change in size; the observation was also made that when in the so-called "missionary" sexual position, the penis is not straight, as had been assumed in the past by historic anatomists such as Leonardo da Vinci, but in fact has the shape of a "boomerang." For further information on the modalities used to elucidate penile hemodynamics, see Chapter 25.

Yet a third classification focuses on the functional activities of the sexual cycle (103), adding an initial phase of desire or libido that encompasses sex-seeking behavior while pooling together excitement and

Table 1 Male Sexual Function: Relationships Among the Phase of Sexual Response Cycle, Neural Pathways, End-Organ and Hemodynamic Changes, and Genital Functional Responses

Phase of sexual response cycle	Neural pathways	End-organ changes	Penile hemodynamic changes	Genital functional responses
Excitement	Inputs from external sensual (visual, auditory, tactile, olfactory) and internal psychic stimuli to the limbic system resulting in activation of sacral parasympathetic and inhibition of thoracolumbar sympathetic pathways	Relaxation of smooth muscles and helicine arterioles of corpora cavernosa	Increase in arterial blood flow without change in intracavernous pressure	Penile filling (latency) Tumescence
Plateau	As above plus: Activation of the sacrospinal reflex	As above plus: Contraction of ischiocavernousus muscle. Stimulation of corpus spongiosum. Stimulation of accessory glands (Cowper's and Litter's)	Rise in intracavernous pressure to 85% of systolic and decrease in arterial inflow. Rise in intracavernous pressure to above systolic and further decrease in arterial inflow	Full erection and dilatation of urethral bulb Rigidity and secretion of fluid from accessory glands
Orgasm	As above plus: Activation of the thoraco-lumbar spinal reflex Neuronal discharge to somatic efferent pudenal nerve. Activation of CNS orgasmic sensations	As above plus: Contraction of vas deferens, ampulla, seminal vesicle and prostate. Contraction of bulbocavernosus and pelvic-floor muscles —	Maintenance of intracavernous pressure above systolic — —	Emission Ejaculation —
Resolution	Activation of thoracolumbar sympathetic pathway —	Contraction of smooth muscles and arterioles of corpora cavernosa —	Increase in venous return Arterial and venous blood flow returns to minimum	Detumescence Refractoriness and flaccidity

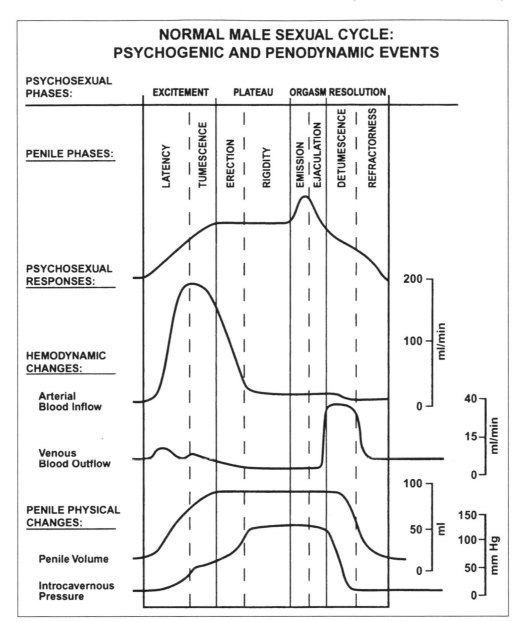

NORMAL MALE SEXUAL CYCLE: PSYCHOGENIC AND PENODYNAMIC EVENTS

Figure 5 Normal male sexual cycle: psychogenic and penodynamic events. The psychosexual response cycle has four major phases: excitement, plateau, orgasm, and resolution. They are represented by the solid vertical lines and by the top diagram. Each of the psychosexual phases comprises two interrelated physical events, which are represented by the vertical dashed lines. The penile hemodynamic changes associated with the sexual cycle (arterial and venous flow rates) are depicted in the middle portion, and the penile physical changes (volume and intracorporeal pressure) are depicted in the lower portion of the graph. Arterial blood inflow rate increases dramatically during latency, tumescence, and early stages of erection. This increase in arterial inflow is accompanied by an earlier increase in venous return, and results in gradual expansion of the cavernous tissue, increase in intracorporeal pressure, obliteration of emissary veins, and ultimately the restriction of venous return. The rise in intracavernous pressure, in turn, leads to a progressive decline in the arterial inflow to a temporary cessation during full penile rigidity. Venous drainage also completely ceases with full penile rigidity. As the corporeal smooth-muscle cells begin to contract in late ejaculation, venous return increases sharply and remains high during the detumescence phase until the entrapped blood is fully drained and the intracorporeal pressure declines to its baseline level, which is maintained during the flaccid state. Penile volume expands maximally during late erection, and intracavernous pressure rises maximally during full rigidity. Data are compiled from several sources referenced in this chapter. *Source*: From Ref. 1.

plateau into a single phase of erection. Further, the orgasmic phase is split into the physical function of ejaculation and the psychological sensation of orgasmic pleasure. In this manner, the normal male sexual response cycle can be divided functionally into five interrelated events that occur in a defined sequence: libido, erection, ejaculation, orgasm, and detumescence. Since the functional classification of the male sexual

cycle is the most clinically relevant one, it will constitute the basis for the following discussion.

Libido or Sexual Desire

Libido is defined as the biological need for sexual activity (the sex drive) and is expressed frequently as "sex-seeking" behavior. The intensity of libido is highly variable

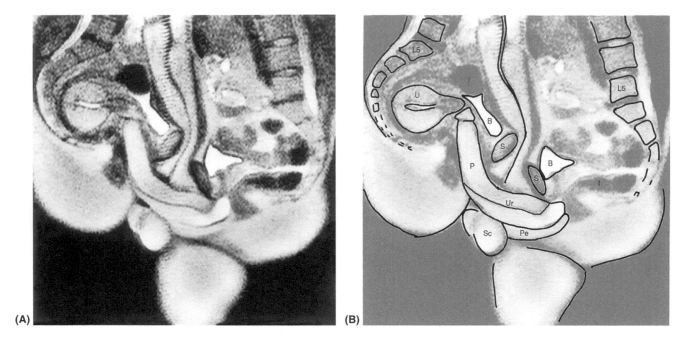

Figure 6 (**A**) Mid-sagittal MRI of the anatomy of sexual intercourse. (**B**) Schematic diagram of Figure 6A. *Abbreviations*: MRI, magnetic resonance imaging; P, penis; Ur, urethra; Pe, perineum; U, uterus; S, symphysis; B, bladder; I, intestine; L5, fifth lumbar vertebra; Sc, scrotum. *Source*: From Ref. 102.

between individuals as well as within an individual over a given period of time. Little is known about the physiological basis of libido; however, past and current sexual activity, psychosocial background, brain and spinal cord dopaminergic receptor activation, and gonadal hormones are among the factors that are believed to participate in the regulation of male sexual desire.

Role of Dopaminergic Neurotransmissions

The medial preoptic area has been identified as the site of integration of sexual functioning and response (see Chapter 4). This area contains dopaminergic neurons and receives innervation from serotonergic and norepinephrine neurons. It has interconnections with the cerebral cortex and other areas of the diencephalon and limbic system, which is believed to be a major regulator of libido and sexual drive (104). In animal studies, stimulation of this area increases sexual behavior, and lesioning produces the opposite effect.

Several lines of evidence in animal and human males support a role for central dopaminergic neurotransmission in mediating sexual behavior and erection (105). Dopamine is released before or during copulation in three integrated neuronal systems with distinct sexual roles: in the nigrostriatal system, dopamine enhances readiness for the sexual response; in the mesolimbic system, it promotes sexual appetitive behaviors; finally, in the medial preoptic area, it increases sexual motivation, genital reflexes, and copulation. Further, testosterone promotion of copulation appears to be mediated by an increase in dopamine release in the medial preoptic area, possibly via upregulation of NO synthesis (106). Evidence in rodents implicates the D2-dopamine rec-

eptor as the subtype mediating these central dopaminergic effects (107). The following observations further support the role of dopaminergic activation in the stimulation of human sexual behavior: the administration of the dopamine agonists apomorphine, bromocriptine, and pergolide mesylate frequently elicits spontaneous penile erection; the use of the dopamine precursor levodopa is associated with increased libido (108–110), the return of spontaneous erection (111,112), or the onset of nocturnal emissions (113) in 20% to 30% of patients with Parkinson's disease who were treated with this agent; also, the use of pharmacological agents with antidopaminergic effects such as reserpine, methyldopa, and many neuroleptics, including chlorpromazine, pimozide, thiothixene, thioridazine, sulpiride, haloperidol and fluphenazine, is associated with decreased libido and erectile dysfunction in up to 50% of the cases. Caution must be exerted in interpreting some of these data for the following reasons, however: (*i*) a lack of consistency in the results of many investigations; (*ii*) pharmacological agents used may stimulate or inhibit other central neuromediator systems, including adrenergic, cholinergic, serotonergic, histaminic, and peptidergic systems; (*iii*) the use of many neuroleptics increases prolactin secretion, which can decrease libido through inhibition of the hypothalamic-pituitary-gonadal axis, inhibition of 5-α-reductase activity, or by a direct effect of prolactin on the CNS (114).

Role of Androgens

Mooradian et al. (115) have reviewed evidence for the role of androgens in the regulation of human male sexual behavior. Higher serum testosterone appears to be associated with greater sexual activity in healthy older (116), but not younger (117,118), men. Further, higher testosterone levels may also shorten the latency of erection stimulated by the exposure to erotic material (119), and testosterone replacement of hypogonadal males restores sexual interest (120–123), shortens latency, and increases frequency and magnitude of nocturnal penile tumescence (121,124). Conversely, withdrawal of androgen therapy in hypogonadal males leads to a decline of libido within three to four weeks (125,126), and unreplaced hypogonadal men have impairment in spontaneity of erection (127). Despite these androgen-deficiency–related abnormalities, hypogonadism does not appear to compromise the ability for erection in response to viewing erotic films (124,128). Both ethinyl estradiol and the antiandrogen cyproterone acetate can impair the erectile response to fantasy (129). The mechanism(s) of such effects is not entirely clear. Since ethinyl estradiol can lower testosterone production and antiandrogens may block testosterone action, it is not currently known whether such impairment is caused by a reduction in testosterone action or is the result of intrinsic effects of estrogen and antiandrogen preparations.

Erection

Erection is the ultimate response to multiple psychogenic and sensory stimuli from imaginative, visual, auditory, olfactory, gustatory, tactile, and genital reflexogenic sources. As previously mentioned, such psychogenic and sensory stimuli initiate several neurological and vascular cascades that lead to penile tumescence and rigidity sufficient for vaginal penetration. Further, erection is associated with significant psychological and physical changes, including: heightened sexual arousal, full testicular assent and swelling, dilatation of the urethral bulb, an increase in glans and coronal size, cutaneous flush over the epigastrium, chest, and buttocks, nipple erection, tachycardia, elevation in blood pressure, hyperventilation, and generalized myotonia (80,81,130). The local penile changes are effected by a vasodilating parasympathetic discharge subsequent to CNS inputs and/or as the result of reflex actions in response to local afferent stimulation of the sacral parasympathetic nuclei.

Role of Dopaminergic and Cholinergic Neurotransmissions

Evidence discussed above supports a role for dopaminergic neurotransmission in mediating the erectile response, although the precise receptors involved in humans remain unclear. The fact that many drugs with anticholinergic effects, such as tricyclic antidepressants and neuroleptics, cause impotence suggests a role for cholinergic transmission in facilitating the erectile response. Several case reports in which the cholinergic drug bethanechol chloride was able to restore potency in patients with erectile difficulty (131,132) support

this theory. Currently, however, it is not clear if any of these effects are exerted at the CNS level.

Role of Androgens and NO Secretion

New data implicate gonadal androgens in the modulation of penile erection through local regulation of NO secretion and/or action. Experiments have shown reduced penile tissue NOS content in castrated rats, with a restoration of NOS production and action with subsequent androgen replacement (34), casting doubt on the older dogma that androgens act only centrally to modulate sexual libido. Data in which androgens were shown to influence the frequency of nonerotic or "reflex" erections support a role for peripheral androgen actions in the human (133). Moreover, a study in rats by Lugg et al. (39) implicates dihydrotestosterone, and not testosterone, as the local modulating androgen of the NO–cGMP pathway. The fact that androgens can enhance nocturnal penile tumescence but not erection in response to erotic stimuli (133), however, may suggest the presence of both androgen-sensitive and androgen-insensitive central pathways for erectile control.

Ejaculation

The ejaculation phase is controlled by sympathetic innervation of the genital organs and occurs as a result of a spinal cord reflex arc. There is a considerable voluntary inhibitory control over this phase of the sexual response, which consists of two sequential processes. The first of these processes, "emission," is associated with deposition of seminal fluid into the posterior urethra. Emission is mediated by simultaneous contractions of the ampulla of the vas deferens, the seminal vesicles, and the smooth muscles of the prostate (83,103). The second process is "true" ejaculation, and it results in the expulsion of seminal fluid from the posterior urethra through the penile meatus, involving a rhythmic contraction of the pelvic floor musculature, particularly the bulbocavernosus and ischiocavernosus muscles, usually at 0.8-second intervals. The force of seminal expulsion is related to the intermittent closure and relaxation of the external urethral sphincter and the buildup of pressure in the posterior urethra. Concomitant closure of the bladder neck prevents the retrograde passage of semen into the bladder. Androgens are required for the production of normal seminal fluid volume ($\geq$ 2 mL) (134).

Role of Serotonergic Neurotransmissions

Evidence reviewed by Segraves (105) suggests that serotonergic neurotransmission has an inhibitory effect on male sexual function and ejaculation. Lowering of brain serotonin levels in laboratory animals enhances the mounting behavior (135). In humans, it is therefore possible that increased serotonergic receptor activation, such as with the use of selective serotonin reuptake inhibitors, could lead to orgasmic inhibition.

The inhibitory action of serotonin neurotransmission on ejaculation is likely to be mediated by the serotonergic tracts in the medial forebrain bundle. Absence of pure serotonergic agonists and antagonists (135), heterogeneity of serotonergic receptors (5HT-1 vs. 5HT-2 receptors) (136), and varying sites of action (spinal cord vs. brain) (137) may account for the seemingly inconsistent results frequently encountered in human studies (105).

Orgasm

Both physiologic and psychogenic elements contribute to genesis of the orgasmic phase (80,103). Afferent stimuli that transmit via the pudendal nerve induce the following physiologic events: smooth-muscle contraction of the accessory sex organs; buildup and release of pressure in the posterior urethra; sensation of the ejaculatory inevitability; contraction of the urethral bulb and perineum; rhythmic contractions of the pelvic floor muscles; semen emission and ejaculation; and finally, the reversal of the generalized physiologic changes and sexual tension. Sensory cortical neurons perceive these events as pleasurable. Factors that influence the subjective sensation of orgasmic pleasure include the degree of sexual excitement, recency of sexual activity, and the psychosexual makeup of the individual. Depending on the site and degree of defect in the elements of the male sexual cycle, orgasm can occur without being preceded by the previous two phases—that is, erection and ejaculation. Conversely, contractions of the pelvic musculature and ejaculation can occur in the absence of orgasmic sensations.

Detumescence

During this phase, the penis returns to the flaccid state. Vasoconstriction of the arterioles and the reversal of events within the contractile corporeal units divert the blood away from the cavernous sinuses and allow an increase in the venous drainage of their contents. Initially, the rate of blood outflow increases by about tenfold, following which the rate decreases progressively until it reaches the pretumescence level (Fig. 5) (83). A period of inhibition follows before the resumption of normal erectile and ejaculatory functions. The length of this refractory phase is dependent upon many variables including the age of the individual, his physical state, and the psychological environment (80,83,103). Interestingly, the traditional assumption that the male orgasm is instantly followed by detumescence and refractoriness has been challenged by observations in which some men were found to be multiorgasmic and by the ability of men to learn to have repeated orgasms without intervening detumescence and refractoriness (138). Local penile α-adrenergic receptor activation is the most important neuromediator mediating detumescence, and interference with this function, such as with α-1-receptor blockade, can lead to the development of priapism (44).

□ MALE SEXUAL FUNCTION AND AGING

Males typically reach peak sexual capacity in their late teens. With advancement of age, however, a gradual decrease in sexual responsiveness occurs (139) that is characterized by a prolongation of the time required to achieve full erection as well as a decrease in the effectiveness of psychic and tactile stimuli in initiating an erection. The plateau phase is also prolonged, and the maintenance of erection requires continuing direct genital stimulation. Orgasm and the feeling of ejaculatory inevitability frequently become less intense. Penile detumescence occurs more rapidly and the refractory period is prolonged, as well. Further, the ejaculatory volume decreases with age.

Studies in rats have shown that advanced age is associated with a decrease in the number of NOS-containing penile nerve fibers, the erectile response to apomorphine stimulation, and the maximum intracavernous pressure attained. It is not yet clear whether some of these changes are related to the age-associated decline in serum testosterone concentrations.

The effects of age on male reproductive physiology have been reviewed (140,141). Aging is associated with decreased total serum and bioavailable testosterone concentrations, decreased testosterone-to-estradiol ratio, increased sex hormone–binding globulin (SHBG) leading to increased plasma protein binding of circulating testosterone and decreased testosterone clearance, decreased luteinizing hormone (LH) pulse frequency, and diminished accumulation of 5-α-reduced steroids in reproductive tissues. Some of these changes are related to the increased incidence of idiopathic hypogonadotropic hypogonadism and/or a decline in serum levels of growth hormone, insulin-like growth factor-1 (IGF-1) and dehydroepiandrosterone sulfate (DHEA-S) (140,141). Normally, IGF-1 enhances the Leydig-cell response to LH and DHEA-S provides a precursor for testosterone production.

The Massachusetts Male Aging Study showed that between the ages of 40 and 70 years, both serum levels of free and albumin-bound testosterone decrease annually by about 1% (142). Korenman (141) has suggested that 90% of older men with reduced testosterone concentration show evidence of hypothalamic–pituitary dysfunction as reflected by a low-normal serum LH and reduced LH response to GnRH stimulation. Several other studies have established a role for obesity in the decline of androgen levels of aging men (143). Both aging-related and obesity-related reductions in gonadal hormones are caused by a parallel decline in the functional capacity of the hypothalamic–pituitary axis (143,144). A decrease in testicular Leydig cell number (145) and in their secretory capacity for testosterone in response to hCG injections (146) in aging men has also been shown. Recent studies have implicated leptin (the obese *ob* gene product) in the development of some of these abnormalities. Decreased testosterone production with age could be due to a decrease in dehydroepi-androsterone (DHEA) and DHEA-S formation (147) as a result of a differential decrease in the side chain cleavage (17,20 lyase activity) rather than in the 17-α-hydroxylation of the cytochrome P450$_{C17}$ enzyme system. This decrease in 17,20 lyase activity restricts the metabolic conversion of 17-α-hydroxy progesterone to DHEA and its steroid derivatives, including testosterone.

Although some studies have shown the absence of correlation between erectile dysfunction and testosterone concentration (148–150), it is widely believed that severe testosterone deficiency is likely to be the primary cause of sexual dysfunction in many cases of combined hypogonadism and erectile dysfunction. Such beliefs are supported by observations in which long-standing hypogonadal men usually complain of loss of sexual interest and activity, decrease in seminal emission volumes, loss of nocturnal and morning erections, and loss of energy and sense of well-being, whereas testosterone replacement is associated with improved self-reported libido, sexual potency, and both subjective (126,127,151) and objective measures of nocturnal erections (152).

□ CONCLUSION

Great advances have been made in improving the understanding of cognitive, neural, and hemodynamic aspects of the physiology of normal adult male sexual function. The information gained has led to the development of several classifications of the male sexual cycle and thus the definition and quantification of its various components. Future research and the development of effective investigative and therapeutic interventions will likely encompass both molecular and cellular structural levels in order to further our understanding of the myriad factors involved in the regulation of the normal male sexual cycle. This will also include the delineation of the complex interactions within the CNS neural networks, the elucidation of a number of vasoactive and neuroactive peptides and amines found in the penis, and the clarification of the relevance of activated gene products throughout the body, particularly those influencing neural, vascular, and endocrine functions. The true complexity of this field will continue to necessitate the interdigitation of multiple disciplines, including endocrinology, radiology, neurology, urology, and psychology.

□ REFERENCES

1. Kandeel FR, Koussa VK, Swerdloff RS. Male sexual function and its disorders: physiology, pathophysiology, clinical investigation, and treatment. Endocr Rev 2001; 22(3):342–388.
2. Saenz de Tejada I, Goldstein I, Krane RJ. Local control of penile erection. Nerves, smooth muscle, endothelium. Urol Clin North Am 1988; 15(1):9–15.
3. Bloch W, Klotz T, Sedlaczek P, et al. Evidence for the involvement of endothelial nitric oxide synthase from smooth muscle cells in the erectile function of the human corpus cavernosum. Urol Res 1998; 26(2):129–135.
4. Lundberg JM. Pharmacology of cotransmission in the autonomic nervous system: integrative aspects on amines, neuropeptides, adenosine triphosphate, amino acids and nitric oxide. Pharmacol Rev 1996; 48(1):113–178.
5. Garthwaite J. Glutamate, nitric oxide and cell-cell signaling in the nervous system. Trends Neurosci 1991; 14(2):60–67.
6. Bohme G, Bon C, Lemaireet M, et al. Altered synaptic plasticity and memory formation in nitric oxide synthase inhibitor-treated rats. Proc Natl Acad Sci USA 1993; 90(19):9191–9194.
7. Salter M, Strijobs PJ, Neale S, et al. The nitric oxide-cyclic GMP pathway is required for nociceptive signalling at specific loci within the somatosensory pathway. Neuroscience 1996; 73(3):649–655.
8. Lin AMY, Kao LS, Chai CY. Involvement of nitric oxide in dopaminergic transmission in rat striatum—an in vivo electrochemical study. J Neurochem 1995; 65(5): 2043–2049.
9. Belsham DD, Wetsel WC, Mellon PL. NMDA and nitric oxide act through the cGMP signal transduction pathway to repress hypothalamic gonadotropin-releasing hormone gene expression. EMBO 1996; 15(3):538–547.
10. Li J, Ladecola C. Nitric oxide and adenosine mediate vasodilation during functional activation in cerebellar cortex. Neuropharmacology 1994; 33(11):1453–1461.
11. Meffert MK, Calakos NC, Scheller RH, et al. Nitric oxide modulates synaptic vesicle docking/fusion reactions. Neuron 1996; 16(6):1229–1236.
12. Zhu BS, Gibbins IL, Blessing WW. Preganglionic parasympathetic neurons projecting to the sphenopalatine ganglion contain nitric oxide synthase in the rabbit. Brain Res 1997; 769(1):168–172.
13. Ando M, Tatmatsu T, Kunii S, et al. The intercellular communication via nitric oxide and its regulation in coupling of cyclic GMP synthesis upon stimulation of muscarinic cholinergic receptors in rat superior cervical sympathetic ganglia. Brain Research 1994; 650(2):283–288.
14. Quinson N, Catalin D, Miolan JP, et al. Nerve-induced release of nitric oxide exerts dual effects on nicotinic transmission within the coeliac ganglion in the rabbit. Neuroscience 1998; 84:229–240.
15. Burnett AL. Nitric oxide in the penis: physiology and pathology. J Urol 1997; 157(1):320–324.
16. Lowenstein CJ, Dinerman JL, Snyder SH. Nitric oxide: a physiologic messenger. Ann Intern Med 1994; 120(3):227–237.

17. Rubanyi GM, Romero JC, Vanhoutte PM. Flow-induced release of endothelium-derived relaxing factor. Am J Physiol 1986; 250(6 Pt 2):H1145–H1149.

18. Rodger RS, Fletcher K, Dewar JH, et al. Prevalence and pathogenesis of impotence in one hundred uremic men. Uremia Invest 1984; 8(2):89–96.

19. Nonnast-Daniel B, Creutzig A, Kuhn K, et al. Effect of treatment with recombinant human erythropoietin on peripheral hemodynamics and oxygenation. Contrib Nephrol 1988; 66:185–194.

20. Wein AJ, Arsdalen KNV, Hanno PM, et al. Penis: a physiology of male sexual function. In: Rajfer J, ed. Urologic Endocrinology. Philadelphia: WB Saunders Company, 1986:249–274.

21. Bredt DS, Snyder SH. Isolation of nitric oxide synthetase, a calmodulin-requiring enzyme. Proc Natl Acad Sci USA 1990; 87(2):682–685.

22. Long CJ, Stone TW. The release of endothelium-derived relaxant factor is calcium-dependent. Blood Vessels 1985; 22(4):205–208.

23. Ignarro LJ, Bush PA, Buga GM, et al. Nitric oxide and cyclic GMP formation upon electrical field stimulation cause relaxation of corpus cavernosum smooth muscle. Biochem Biophys Res Commun 1990; 170(2):843–850.

24. Rajfer J, Aronson WJ, Bush PA, et al. Nitric oxide as a mediator of relaxation of the corpus cavernosum in response to nonadrenergic, noncholinergic neurotransmission. N Engl J Med 1992; 326(2):90–94.

25. Saenz de Tejada I. Mechanism for regulation of penile smooth muscle contractility. In: Lue TF, ed. World Book of Impotence. London/Niigata-Shi: Smith-Gordon/Nishimura, 1992:39–48.

26. Boolell M, Allen MJ, Ballard SA, et al. Sildenafil: an orally active type 5 cyclic GMP-specific phosphodiesterase inhibitor for the treatment of penile erectile dysfunction. Int J Impot Res 1996; 8(2):47–52.

27. Wallis RM, Corbin JC, Francis SH, et al. Tissue distribution of phosphodiesterase families and the effects of sildenafil on tissue cyclic nucleotides, platelet function, and the contractile responses of trabeculae carneae and aortic rings in vitro. Am J Cardiol 1999; 83(5A):3c–12c.

28. Boolell M, Gepi-Attee S, Gingell JC, et al. Sildenafil, a novel effective oral therapy for male erectile dysfunction. Br J Urol 1996; 78(2):257–261.

29. Schmidt PS, Gupta S, Daley J, et al. Mechanisms of nitric oxide-induced relaxation of rabbit corpus cavernosum smooth muscle. J Urol 1995; 153:442A [Abstract].

30. Gupta S, Moreland RB, Schmidt PS, et al. Nitric oxides, Na(+)-K(+)-ATPase and human corpus cavernosum smooth muscle contractility. Br J Pharmacol 1995; 116(4):2201–2206.

31. Seftel AD, Viola KA, Kasner SE, et al. Nitric oxide relaxes rabbit corpus cavernosum smooth muscle via a potassium-conductive pathway. Biochem Biophys Res Commun 1996; 219(2):382–387.

32. Hung A, Vernet D, Xie Y, et al. Expression of the inducible nitric oxide synthase in smooth muscle cells from rat penile corpora cavernosa. J Androl 1995; 16(6):469–481.

33. Hoffman D, Seftel AD, Hampel N, et al. Advanced glycation end-products quench cavernosal nitric oxide. J Urol 1995; 153:441A [Abstract].

34. Kim N, Vardi Y, Padma-Nathan H, et al. Oxygen tension regulates the nitric oxide pathway. Physiological role in penile erection. J Clin Invest 1993; 91(2):437–442.

35. Mills TM, Wiedmeier VT, Stopper VS. Androgen maintenance of erectile function in the rat penis. Biol Reprod 1992; 46(3):342–348.

36. Lugg JA, Rajfer J, Gonzalez-Cadavid NF. Dihydrotestosterone is the active androgen in the maintenance of nitric oxide-mediated penile erection in the rat. Endocrinology 1995; 136(4):1495–1501.

37. Chamness SL, Ricker DD, Crone JK, et al. The effect of androgen on nitric oxide synthase in the male reproductive tract of the rat. Fertil Steril 1995; 63(5):1101–1107.

38. Martin W, McAllister KH, Paisley K. NANC neurotransmission in the bovine retractor penis muscle is blocked by superoxide anion following inhibition of superoxide dismutase with diethyldithiocarbamate. Neuropharmacology 1994; 33(11):1293–1301.

39. Lugg JA, Schlunt K, Rajfer J, et al. Modulation of nitric oxide synthase activity in the penis by electrical stimulation of the cavernosal nerve. J Urol 1995; 153:509A [Abstract].

40. Lerner SE, Melman A, Christ GJ. A review of erectile dysfunction: new insights and more questions. J Urol 1993; 149(5 Pt 2):1246–1255.

41. Hedlund P, Alm P, Ekstrom P, et al. Pituitary adenylate cyclase-activating polypeptide, helospectin, and vasoactive intestinal polypeptide in human corpus cavernosum. Br J Pharmacol 1995; 116(4):2258–2266.

42. Sjostrand NO, Klinge E, Himberg JJ. Effects of VIP and other putative neurotransmitters on smooth muscle effectors of penile erection. Acta Physiol Scand 1981; 113(3):403–405.

43. Stief CG, Wetterauer U, Schaebsdau FH, et al. Calcitonin-gene-related peptide: a possible role in human penile erection and its therapeutic application in impotent patients. J Urol 1991; 146(4):1010–1014.

44. Ruffolo RR, Nichols AJ, Stadel JM, et al. Pharmacologic and therapeutic applications of alpha 2-adrenoceptor subtypes. Annu Rev Pharmacol Toxicol 1993; 33:243–279.

45. Ehmke H, Junemann KP, Mayer B, et al. Nitric oxide synthase and vasoactive intestinal polypeptide colocalization in neurons innervating the human penile circulation. Int J Impot Res 1995; 7(3):147–156.

46. Tamura M, Kagawa S, Kimura K, et al. Coexistence of nitric oxide synthase, tyrosine hydroxylase and vasoactive intestinal polypeptide in human penile tissue—a triple histochemical and immunohistochemical study. J Urol 1995; 153(2):530–534.

47. Azadzoi KM, Kim N, Brown ML, et al. Endothelium-derived nitric oxide and cyclooxygenase products modulate corpus cavernosum smooth muscle tone. J Urol 1992; 147(1):220–225.

48. Kim YC, Choi HK, Ahn YS, et al. The effect of vasoactive intestinal polypeptide (VIP) on rabbit cavernosal smooth muscle contractility. J Androl 1994; 15(5):392–397.

49. Kimoto Y, Kessler R, Constantinou CE. Endothelium-dependent relaxation of human corpus cavernosum by bradykinin. J Urol 1990; 144(4):1015–1017.

50. Gupta S, Moreland RB, Yang S, et al. The expression of functional postsynaptic alpha2-adrenoceptors in the corpus cavernosum smooth muscle. Br J Pharmacol 1998; 123(6):1237–1245.

51. Traish AM, Moreland RB, Huang YH, et al. Expression of functional alpha2-adrenergic receptor subtypes in human corpus cavernosum and in cultured trabecular smooth muscle cells. Recept Signal Transduct 1997; 7(1):55–67.

52. Dausse JP, Leriche A, Yablonsky F. Patterns of messenger RNA expression for alpha1-adrenoceptor subtypes in human corpus cavernosum. J Urol 1998; 160(2):597–600.

53. Christ GJ, Maayani S, Valcic M, et al. Pharmacological studies of human erectile tissue. Characteristics of spontaneous contractions and alterations in alpha-adrenoreceptor responsiveness with age and disease in isolated tissues. Br J Pharmacol 1990; 101(2):375–381.

54. Levin RM, Wein AJ. Adrenergic alpha receptors outnumber beta receptors in human penile corpus cavernosum. Investig Urol 1980; 18(3):225–226.

55. Christ GJ, Moreno AP, Parker ME, et al. Intercellular communication through gap junctions: a potential role in pharmacomechanical coupling and syncytial tissue contraction in vascular smooth muscle isolated from the human corpus cavernosum. Life Sci 1991; 49(24): PL195–PL200.

56. Hedlund H, Andersson KE. Comparison of the responses to drugs acting on adrenoreceptors and muscarinic receptors in human isolated corpus cavernosum and cavernous artery. J Auton Pharmacol 1985; 5(1):81–88.

57. Imagawa A, Kimura K, Kawanishi Y, et al. Effect of moxisylyte hydrochloride on isolated human penile corpus cavernosum tissue. Life Sci 1989; 44(9):619–623.

58. Kim SC, Oh MM. Norepinephrine involvement in response to intracorporeal injection of papaverine in psychogenic impotence. J Urol 1992; 147(6): 1530–1532.

59. Saenz de Tejada I, Carson MP, Morenas ADL, et al. Endothelin: localization, synthesis, activity, and receptor types in human penile corpus cavernosum. Am J Physiol 1991; 261(4 Pt 2):H1078–H1085.

60. Holmquist F, Andersson KE, Hedlund H. Actions of endothelin on isolated corpus cavernosum from rabbit and man. Acta Physiol Scand 1990; 139(1):113–122.

61. Roy AC, Tan SM, Kottegoda SR, et al. Ability of human corpora cavernosa muscle to generate prostaglandins and thromboxane in vitro. IRCS J Med Sci 1984; 12:608–609.

62. Kifor I, Williams GH, Vickers MA, et al. Tissue angiotensin II as a modulator of erectile function: I. Angiotensin peptide content, secretion and effects in the corpus cavernosum. J Urol 1997; 157(5): 1920–1925.

63. Sparwasser C, Schmelz HU, Drescher P, et al. Role of intracellular Ca2+ stores in smooth muscle of human penile erectile tissue. Urol Res 1998; 26(3):189–193.

64. Simonsen U, Prieto D, Hernandez M, et al. Prejunctional alpha 2-adrenoceptors inhibit nitrergic neurotransmission in horse penile resistance arteries. J Urol 1997; 157(6):2356–2360.

65. Siroky MB, Krane RJ. Physiology of male sexual function. In: Krane RJ, Siroky MB, eds. Clinical Neuro-Urology. Boston: Little, Brown and Company, 1979:45–62.

66. Siroky MB, Krane RJ. Neurophysiology of erection. In: Krane RJ, Siroky MB, Goldstein I, eds. Male Sexual Dysfunction. Boston: Little, Brown and Company, 1983:9–20.

67. Costa P, Soulie-Vassal ML, Sarrazin B, et al. Adrenergic receptors on smooth muscle cells isolated from human penile corpus cavernosum. J Urol 1993; 150(3): 859–863.

68. Adaikan PG, Kottegoda SR, Ratnam SS. Is vasoactive intestinal polypeptide the principal transmitter involved in human penile erection? J Urol 1986; 135(3):638–640.

69. Hedlund H, Andersson KE, Mattiasson A. Pre- and postjunctional adreno- and muscarinic receptor functions in the isolated corpus spongiosum urethrae. J Auton Pharmacol 1984; 4(4):241–249.

70. Fontaine J, Schulman CC, Wespes E. Postjunctional alpha-1- and alpha-2-like adrenoceptors in human isolated deep dorsal vein of the penis. Br J Pharmacol 1986; 89:493P[Abstract].

71. Kirkeby HJ, Forman A, Sorensen S, et al. Alpha–adrenoceptor function in isolated penile circumflex veins from potent and impotent men. J Urol 1989; 142(5):1369–1371.

72. Crowe R, Burnstock G, Dickinson IK, et al. The human penis: an unusual penetration of NPY-immunoreactive nerves within the medial muscle coat of the deep dorsal vein. J Urol 1991; 145(6):1292–1296.

73. Segarra G, Medina P, Domenech C, et al. Neurogenic contraction and relaxation of human penile deep dorsal vein. Br J Pharmacol 1998; 124(4):788–794.

74. Christ GJ. The penis as a vascular organ. The importance of corporal smooth muscle tone in the control of erection. Urol Clin North Am 1995; 22(4):727–745.

75. Moreland RB. Is there a role of hypoxemia in penile fibrosis: a viewpoint presented to the Society for the Study of Impotence. Int J Impot Res 1998; 10(2): 113–120.

76. Moreno AP, Campos de Carvalho AC, Christ GJ, et al. Gap junctions between human corpus cavernosum smooth muscle cells in primary culture: electrophysiological and biochemical characteristics. Int J Impot Res 1990; 2:55–56.

77. Christ GJ, Moreno AP, Melman A, et al. Gap junction-mediated intercellular diffusion of Ca2+ in cultured human corporal smooth muscle cells. Am J Physiol 1992; 263(2 Pt 1):C373–C383.

78. Christ GJ, Spray DC, Melman A, Brink P. Electrophysiological studies of ion channels in cultured human corporal smooth muscle cells in culture. Int J Impot Res 1992; 4(supp 2):A40 [Abstract].

79. Fan SF, Christ GJ, Melman A. A stretch-sensitive Cl$^-$ channel in human corpus cavernosal myocytes. Int J Impot Res 1999; 11(1):1–7.

80. Masters WH, Johnson VE. Male Sexual Response. Boston: Little, Brown and Company, 1966.

81. Kolodny RC, Masters WH, Johnson VE. Sexual Anatomy and Physiology. Boston: Little, Brown and Company, 1979.

82. Govier FE, Asase D, Hefty TR, et al. Timing of penile color flow duplex ultrasonography using a triple drug mixture. J Urol 1995; 153(5):1472–1475.

83. Lue TF, Tanagho EA. Hemodynamics of erection. In: Tanagho EA, Lue TF, McClure RD, eds. Contemporary Management of Impotence and Infertility. Baltimore: Williams & Wilkins, 1988:28–38.

84. Wagner G. Erection: physiology and endocrinology. In: Wagner G, Green R, eds. Impotence: Physiological, Psychological, Surgical Diagnosis and Treatment. New York: Plenum Press, 1981:25–36.

85. Lue TF. Functional evaluation of penile arteries with papaverine. In: Tanagho EA, Lue TF, McClure RD, eds. Contemporary Management of Impotence and Infertility. Baltimore: Williams & Wilkins, 1988:57–64.

86. Fitzgerald SW, Erickson SJ, Foley WD, et al. Color Doppler sonography in the evaluation of erectile dysfunction. Radiographics 1992; 12(1):3–17.

87. Benson CB, Aruny JE, Vickers MA. Correlation of duplex sonography with arteriography in patients with erectile dysfunction. Am J Roentgenol 1993; 160(1):71–73.

88. Brock G, Breza J, Lue TF. Intracavernous sodium nitroprusside: inappropriate impotence treatment. J Urol 1993; 150(3):864–867.

89. Kim SH, Paick JS, Lee SE, et al. Doppler sonography of deep cavernosal artery of the penis: variation of peak systolic velocity according to sampling location. J Ultrasound Med 1994; 13(8):591–594.

90. Wegner HE, Andresen R, Knispel HH, et al. Evaluation of penile arteries with color-coded duplex sonography: prevalence and possible therapeutic implications of connections between dorsal and cavernous arteries in impotent men. J Urol 1995; 153(5):1469–1471.

91. Montorsi F, Bergamaschi F, Guazzoniet G, et al. Morphodynamic assessment of penile circulation in impotent patients: the role of duplex and color Doppler sonography. Scand J Urol Nephrol 1993; 27(3):399–408.

92. Mancini M, Bartolini M, Maggi M, et al. The presence of arterial anatomical variations can affect the results of duplex sonographic evaluation of penile vessels in impotent patients. J Urol 1996; 155(6):1919–1923.

93. Mills RD, Sethia KK. Reproducibility of penile arterial colour duplex ultrasonography. Br J Urol 1996; 78(1):109–112.

94. Nisen HO, Edgren J, Ruutu ML, et al. Duplex Doppler scanning with high-dose prostaglandin E1 stimulation in the diagnosis of arteriogenic impotence. Eur Urol 1993; 24(1):36–42.

95. Lue TF. Functional study of penile veins. In: Tanagho EA, Lue TF, McClure RD, eds. Contemporary Management of Impotence and Infertility. Baltimore: Williams & Wilkins, 1988:65–69.

96. Goldstein I. Vasculogenic impotence: its diagnosis and treatment. Probl Urol 1987; 1:547–563.

97. Padma-Nathan H. Dynamic infusion cavernosometry and cavernosography (DICC) and the cavernosal artery systolic occlusion pressure gradient: a complete evaluation of the hemodynamic events of a penile erection. In: Lue TF, ed. World Book of Impotence. London/Niigata-Shi: Smith-Gordon/Nishimura, 1992:101–103.

98. Sasso F, Gulino G, Basar M, et al. Could standardized cavernosometry be helpful in therapeutic management of veno-occlusive dysfunction? J Urol 1996; 155(1):150–154.

99. Kaufman JM, Borges FD, Fitch WP, et al. Evaluation of erectile dysfunction by dynamic infusion cavernosometry and cavernosography (DICC). Multi-institutional study. Urology 1993; 41(5):445–451.

100. Glina S, Silva MF, Puech-Leao P, et al. Veno-occlusive dysfunction of corpora cavernosa: comparison of diagnostic methods. Int J Impot Res 1995; 7(1):1–10.

101. DePalma RG. New developments in the diagnosis and treatment of impotence. West J Med 1996; 164(1):54–61.

102. Schultz WW, van Andel P, Sabelis I, et al. Magnetic resonance imaging of the male and female genitals during coitus and female sexual arousal. BMJ 1999; 319(7225):1596–1600.

103. Walsh PC, Wilson JD. Impotence and infertility in men. In: Braunwald E, Isselbacher KJ, Petersdorf RS, et al., eds. Harrison's Principals of Internal Medicine. 11 ed. New York: Mc Graw-Hill Book Company, 1987:217–220.

104. Harvey KV, Balon R. Clinical implications of antidepressant drug effects on sexual function. Ann Clin Psychiatry 1995; 7(4):189–201.

105. Segraves RT. Effects of psychotropic drugs on human erection and ejaculation. Arch Gen Psychiatry 1989; 46(3):275–284.

106. Hull EM, Du J, Lorrain DS, et al. Testosterone, preoptic dopamine, and copulation in male rats. Brain Res Bull 1997; 44(4):327–333.

107. Gessa GL, Tagliamonte A. Role of brain monoamines in male sexual behavior. Life Sci 1974; 14(3):425–436.

108. Barbeau A. L-dopa therapy in Parkinson's disease: a critical review of nine years' experience. Can Med Assoc J 1969; 101(13):59–68.

109. Hyyppa M, Rinne UK, Sonninen V. The activating effect of L-dopa treatment on sexual functions and its experimental background. Acta Neurol Scand 1970; 46(suppl 43):223.

110. Jenkins RB, Groh RH. Mental symptoms in Parkinsonian patients treated with L-dopa. Lancet 1970; 2(7665):177–179.

111. O'Brien CP, DiGiacomo JN, Fahn S, et al. Mental effects of high-dosage levodopa. Arch Gen Psychiatry 1971; 24(1):61–64.

112. Sathananthan G, Angrist BM, Gershon S. Response threshold to L-dopa in psychiatric patients. Biol Psychiatry 1973; 7:139–146.

113. Bowers MB, van Woert M, Davis L. Sexual behavior during L-dopa treatment for Parkinsonism. Am J Psychiatry 1971; 127(12):1691–1693.

114. Carter JN, Tyson JE, Tolis G, et al. Prolactin-screening tumors and hypogonadism in 22 men. N Engl J Med 1978; 299(16):847–852.

115. Mooradian AD, Morley JE, Korenman SG. Biological actions of androgens. Endocr Rev 1987; 8(1):1–28.

116. Toone BK, Wheeler M, Nanjee M, et al. Sex hormones, sexual activity and plasma anticonvulsant levels in male epileptics. J Neurol Neurosurg Psychiatry 1983; 46(9):824–826.

117. Kraemer HC, Becker HB, Brodie HK, et al. Orgasmic frequency and plasma testosterone levels in normal human males. Arch Sex Behav 1976; 5(2):125–132.

118. Brown WA, Monti PM, Corriveau DP. Serum testosterone and sexual activity and interest in men. Arch Sex Behav 1978; 7(2):97–103.

119. Lange JD, Brown WA, Wincze JP, et al. Serum testosterone concentration and penile tumescence changes in men. Horm Behav 1980; 14(3):267–270.

120. O'Carroll R, Shapiro C, Bancroft J. Androgens, behavior and nocturnal erection in hypogonadal men: the effects of varying the replacement dose. Clin Endocrinol 1985; 23(5):527–538.

121. Morley JE. Impotence. Am J Med 1986; 80(5):897–905.

122. Armstrong EG, Villee CA. Characterization and comparison of estrogen and androgen receptors of calf anterior pituitary. J Steroid Biochem 1977; 8(4):285–292.

123. Lloyd RV, Karavolas HJ. Uptake and conversion of progesterone and testosterone to 5alpha-reduced products by enriched gonadotropic and chromophobic rat anterior pituitary cell fractions. Endocrinology 1975; 97(3):517–526.

124. Kwan M, Greenleaf WJ, Mann J, et al. The nature of androgen action on male sexuality: a combined laboratory-self-report study on hypogonadal men. J Clin Endocrinol Metab 1983; 57(3):557–562.

125. Luisi M, Franchi F. Double-blind group comparative study of testosterone undecanoate and mesterolone in hypogonadal male patients. J Endocrinol Invest 1980; 3(3):305–308.

126. Skakkebaek NE, Bancroft J, Davidson DW, et al. Androgen replacement with oral testosterone undecanoate in hypogonadal men: a double-blind controlled study. Clin Endocrinol 1981; 14(1):49–61.

127. Salmimies P, Kockott G, Pirke KM, et al. Effects of testosterone replacement on sexual behaviour in hypogonadal men. Arch Sex Behav 1982; 11(4):345–353.

128. Bancroft J, Wu FC. Changes in erectile responsiveness during androgen replacement therapy. Arch Sex Behav 1983; 12(1):59–66.

129. Bancroft J, Tennent G, Loucas K, et al. The control of deviant sexual behavior by drugs. I. Behavioral changes following oestrogens and antiandrogens. Br J Psychiatry 1974; 125:310–315.

130. Kinsey AC, Pomeroy WB, Martin CE. Early sexual growth and activity. Sexual Behavior in the Human Male. Philadelphia: WB Saunders Company, 1948:157–192.

131. Gross MD. Reversal by bethanechol of sexual dysfunction caused by anticholinergic antidepressants. Am J Psychiatry 1982; 139(9):1193–1194.

132. Yager J. Bethanechol chloride can reverse erectile and ejaculatory dysfunction induced by tricyclic antidepressants and mazindol: case report. J Clin Psychiatry 1986; 47(4):210–211.

133. Davidson JM, Chen JJ, Crapo L, et al. Hormonal changes and sexual function in aging men. J Clin Endocrinol Metab 1983; 57(1):71–77.

134. WHO normal ranges for semen analysis. Mortimer D. Practical Laboratory Andrology. New York: Oxford University Press, 1994.

135. Tucker TC, Ale SE. Serotonin and sexual behavior. In: Wheatley D, ed. Psychopharmacology and Sexual Disorders. Oxford, New York: Oxford University Press, 1983:22–49.

136. Fuller RW. Pharmacologic modification of serotonergic function: drugs for the study and treatment of psychiatric and other disorders. J Clin Psychiatry 1986; 47(suppl):4–8.

137. Paul SM, Janowsky A, Skolnick P. Monoaminergic neurotransmitters and antidepressant drugs. In: Hales RE, Frances AJ, eds. Psychiatry Update: American Psychiatric Association Annual Review, Vol. 4. Washington, D.C.: American Psychiatric Press, 1985:37–48.

138. Dunn ME, Trost JE. Male multiple orgasms: a descriptive study. Arch Sex Behav 1989; 18(5):377–387.

139. Schiavi RC, Rehman J. Sexuality and aging. Urol Clin North Am 1995; 22(4):711–726.

140. Kaiser FE, Viosca SP, Morley JE, et al. Impotence and aging: clinical and hormonal factors. J Am Geriatr Soc 1988; 36(6):511–519.

141. Korenman SG. Androgen function after age 50 years and treatment of hypogonadism. In: Bardin CW, ed. Current Therapy in Endocrinology and Metabolism. 5th ed. St. Louis: Mosby Year Book, 1994:585–587.

142. Gray A, Feldman HA, McKinlay JB, et al. Age, disease, and changing sex hormone levels in middle-aged men: results of the Massachusetts Male Aging Study. J Clin Endocrinol Metab 1991; 73(5):1016–1025.

143. Erfurth EM, Hagmar LE. Decreased serum testosterone and free triiodothyronine levels in healthy middle-aged men indicate an age-effect at the pituitary level. Eur J Endocrinol 1995; 132(6):663–667.

144. Vermeulen A. Decreased androgen levels and obesity in men. Ann Med 1996; 28(1):13–15.

145. Neaves WB, Johnson L, Porter JC, et al. Leydig cell numbers, daily sperm production, and serum gonadotropin levels in aging men. J Clin Endocrinol Metab 1984; 59(4):756–763.

146. Harman SM, Tsitouras PD. Reproductive hormones in aging men. I. Measurement of sex steroids, basal luteinizing hormone, and Leydig cell response to human chorionic gonadotropin. J Clin Endocrinol Metab 1980; 51(1):35–40.

147. Morley JE, Kaiser F, Raum WJ, et al. Potentially predictive and manipulable blood serum correlates of aging in the healthy human male: progressive deceases in bioavailable testosterone, dehydroepiandrosterone sulfate, and the ratio of insulin-like growth factor 1 to growth hormone. Proc Natl Acad Sci 1997; 94(14):7537–7542.

148. Feldman HA, Goldstein I, Hatzichristou DG, et al. Impotence and its medical and psychosocial correlates: results of the Massachusetts Male Aging Study. J Urol 1994; 151(1):54–61.

149. Schiavi RC, White D, Mandeli J, et al. Hormones and nocturnal penile tumescence in healthy aging men. Arch Sex Behav 1993; 22(3):207–215.

150. Rowland DL, Greenleaf WJ, Dorfman LJ, et al. Aging and sexual function in men. Arch Sex Behav 1993; 22(6):545–557.

151. Davidson JM, Camargo CA, Smith ER. Effects of androgen on sexual behavior in hypogonadal men. J Clin Endocrinol Metab 1979; 48(6):955–958.

152. Cunningham GR, Hirshkowitz M, Korenman SG, et al. Testosterone replacement therapy and sleep-related erections in hypogonadal men. J Clin Endocrinol Metab 1990; 70(3):792–797.

4

Functional Neuroanatomy of Sexual Arousal

Harold Mouras
Equipe Développement Social et Affectif, Faculté de Psychologie et des Sciences de l'Education, Université de Genève, Suisse INSERM U742, Université Pierre et Marie Curie, Paris, France

Serge Stoléru
INSERM U742, and Université Pierre et Marie Curie, Paris, France

☐ INTRODUCTION

Sexual behavior is considered to be one of the most important forms of goal-directed behaviors necessary for the long-term survival of any species. In all animals, there are three distinct phases of sexual behavior in which the brain plays an essential role: (*i*) an appetitive phase, which serves to bring animals and humans into contact with sexual incentives, (*ii*) a precopulatory phase, consisting of solicitation and courtship behavior, and (*iii*) a consummatory phase, comprised of copulatory responses (1,2). In humans, sexual desire and arousal (SDA) may be further categorized into a series of distinct cognitive, motivational, emotional, and autonomic components (3). Although animal studies have facilitated the identification of key cerebral areas involved in animal sexual behavior, these experiments still cannot explain the features of sexual behavior uniquely developed in humans, such as the cognitive aspects of SDA (2). Although neuropsychological and neurological studies have been of great importance in elucidating the cerebral basis of human sexual motivation, their essential focus on pathological conditions has resulted in only a partial understanding of the normal physiologic brain processes underlying SDA (4,5). For further information on these processes, see Chapter 3.

In the last 10 years, tremendous progress in the development of neuroimaging techniques has made possible the more accurate investigation of the cerebral processes involved in many different forms of normal human behavior, making it possible to investigate the neural networks that process emotionally or motivationally relevant information. For example, Phan et al. have reviewed 55 positron emission tomography (PET) and functional magnetic resonance imaging (fMRI) studies of the neural correlates of emotion in healthy human subjects (6). The study of the neural correlates of SDA using neuroimaging techniques is one specific aspect of this broad field of research.

This chapter first outlines the basic biophysical principles of the two main neuroimaging techniques currently in use, PET and fMRI, and then reviews the studies of SDA that have been performed using neuroimaging techniques. Included in this review is a consideration of the methodological approaches used across studies and a comparison of their results. Finally, a tentative neurobehavioral model of SDA is presented.

☐ BASIC PRINCIPLES OF NEUROIMAGING TECHNIQUES
Overview

PET and fMRI share two main technical characteristics. First, the variable used to reflect cerebral activation and deactivation in each type of imaging modality is regional cerebral blood flow (rCBF). Second, both PET and fMRI have relatively poor temporal resolutions, although the temporal resolution of fMRI (approximately one second) is 60 times greater than that of PET (one minute). Thus, in comparison with PET, the greater temporal resolution of fMRI enables a better and more precise understanding of the successive steps of SDA and of the temporal dynamics of neural circuits involved in processing sexual information. Another advantage of fMRI over PET is that it allows the analyses of single individuals, while analyses of PET data must be performed at a group level.

Because of their overall poor quality of temporal resolution, however, both PET and fMRI are more suited to localize cerebral activation and deactivation than to define cerebral activation and deactivation dynamics over time. This issue may be remedied in the near future by the improvement of other imaging techniques such as magnetoencephalography (MEG), which has a significantly higher temporal resolution (of the order of 1 msec). Although MEG has only been used in one study of the neural correlates of SDA to date, this technique could prove to be of great future value in elucidating the finer complexities of the neural mechanisms involved in SDA (7).

One of the disadvantages of fMRI is its susceptibility to the presence of artifacts at the air–fluid interfaces between the skull sinuses and the water-laden brain tissues. Such interfaces often result in signal loss, making it difficult to image cerebral activation in some parts of the temporal and the frontal lobes—particularly the medial portion of the orbito-frontal cortex (OFC). This limitation is significant since the temporal lobes and the OFC play important roles in processing sexual information (8). Technical advances in acquisition sequences, however, should help alleviate this problem in the coming years (9).

Although brain responses are being recorded with PET and fMRI, it is possible to measure other physiologic responses characteristic of SDA concurrently—in particular, penile tumescence (8,10,11). Although the higher temporal resolution of fMRI allows the performance of finer-grain temporal correlation studies between brain activity and peripheral responses (12), it must be noted that experimental options are very constrained in the magnetic resonance imaging (MRI) environment because of the fact that no metal can be introduced. Thus, the apparatuses used in obtaining experimental measurements with concurrent fMRI data acquisition must be adapted accordingly.

The Physics of PET

Water represents 55% to 65% of total body mass in the average human male (13). Each water molecule contains two atoms of hydrogen and one atom of oxygen; the oxygen nucleus consists of eight protons and eight neutrons. In so-called "activation studies" performed with PET, subjects typically receive an intravenous injection of water in which a small proportion of molecules contains a radioactive isotope of oxygen called oxygen 15, or [^{15}O], whose nucleus consists of eight protons and only seven neutrons. This radioactive water mixes with the bloodstream and diffuses into body tissues, including the brain.

When a cerebral area gets activated, blood flow increases with a corresponding increase of [^{15}O] H_2O

disintegrations in the activated area. The disintegration of [^{15}O] atoms leads to the emission of positrons. After traveling for a few millimeters in the surrounding tissues, positrons encounter electrons, which leads to the annihilation of both particles and the liberation of two photons. These two photons are emitted in exactly opposite directions (Fig. 1A).

Detectors capable of recognizing such photons are placed around the subject's head. Due to the special electronic coupling circuits between detectors, only those photons detected simultaneously by a pair of detectors are taken into account (Fig. 1B). This pair of detectors allows the determination of the location from which the photons have been emitted. In an activated cerebral region, several disintegrations occur at the same point, resulting in as many pairs of photons detected by several pairs of detectors. The integration of the simultaneous activation of pairs of detectors thus allows the three-dimensional reconstruction of the point of emission.

The Physics of fMRI

Because water constitutes 77% to 78% of the cerebral mass (15), hydrogen is the most abundant atom in the brain. Each hydrogen atom follows a rotational movement called the "spin," and it is this property that is utilized by MRI technology (Fig. 2A). When placed in the magnetic field of the scanner, B_0, the spins of all the atoms of the body, including those of the brain, become oriented in one of two directions: the same direction as B_0 ("spin-up"), or the opposite direction ("spin-down"). Because the "spin-up" population is slightly larger, the scanner thus confers a non-null magnetic moment, M_0, to the tissues. Essentially, the subject becomes a magnet. This process is called "magnetization."

Because the M_0 and B_0 magnetic fields are oriented in the same direction, the value of M_0 is not readily measurable. A perpendicular magnetic field, B_1, is then applied based on the resonance principle described

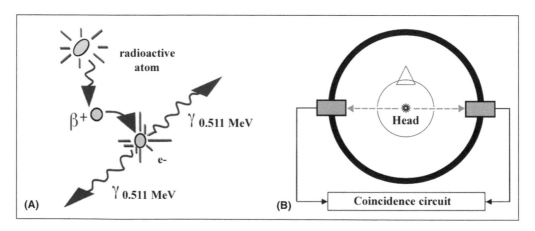

Figure 1 Basic principles of the PET technique. (**A**) The meeting of a positron from the radioactive molecule used in the study, e.g., [^{15}O] in H_2O, and a neighboring electron leads to the emission of two photons in opposite directions. (**B**) A crown of receivers placed around the subject's head allow the detection of pairs of photons coming from oxygen 15 disintegration. Because of a complex electronic coupling system between receivers, only photons detected simultaneously by pairs of receivers will be counted. Any detection leads to a straight line on which the emission point is located. Several lines coming from several disintegrations from the same spatial point allow the detection of the exact localization of an activated cerebral area. *Abbreviation*: PET, positron emission tomography. *Source*: Adapted from Ref. 14.

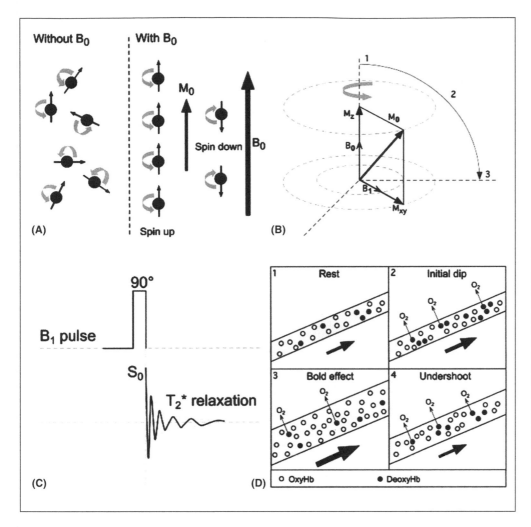

Figure 2 Basic principles of the fMRI technique: recording cerebral activations. (**A**) Influence of the magnetic field of the scanner on the spin movement of hydrogen atoms. (**B**) The application of a second magnetic field, perpendicular to the first, changes the direction of the magnetic moment of tissues in the scanner. (**C**) Relaxation. (**D**) Basis of BOLD signal. *Abbreviations*: BOLD, blood-oxygen level-dependent; B_0, magnetic field of the scanner; B_1, magnetic field perpendicular to B_0; M_0, magnetic moment of tissues in the scanner; M_{xy}, transversal component of M_0; T2*, temporal constant of relaxation process. *Source*: Adapted from Ref. 14.

by Purcell and Bloch in 1952 (Fig. 2B) (65,66). When the rotation frequency of the B_1 field is the same as the frequency of the spins (the Larmor frequency), it can modify the M_0 direction up to a certain angle. Generally, B_1 is applied until M_0 is flipped by 90° (flip angle of 90°), resulting in the appearance of an M_0 transversal component, M_{xy}.

By measuring M_{xy}, it is then possible to calculate M_0. To do so, the B_1 magnetic field has to be removed so that B_0 can once again influence M_0. From its flipped perpendicular direction, M_0 will regain its initial position—that is, the M_{xy} component will approach zero. This process is called "relaxation."

Due to complex biophysical processes, relaxation is exponential with respect to a temporal constant, T2* (Fig. 2C). Because respective differences in tissue water concentration cause the value of T2* to vary from one tissue to another, in order to construct an accurate anatomic image (structural MRI), T2* must be measured in all points of the brain.

In order to understand the nature of the signal recorded in fMRI, it is necessary to present the main principles of the blood-oxygen level-dependent (BOLD) contrast. The increased activity of a neuronal assembly is coupled with an increase in rCBF, providing the oxygen supply necessary for neuronal activity.

Hemoglobin, which carries oxygen in the blood, exists in two forms: deoxyhemoglobin and oxyhemoglobin. When placed into a magnetic field, these two molecules exhibit different magnetic properties in that only deoxyhemoglobin produces local field inhomogeneities due to the fact that it contains an iron atom in the Fe^{2+} form. For this reason, deoxyhemoglobin is tantamount to an endogenous tracer for the fMRI technique, making fMRI a noninvasive study in comparison with PET. When a brain area becomes activated, the rCBF increase is so high that the increased concentration of oxyhemoglobin leads to a relative decrease in the local blood deoxyhemoglobin concentration. This constitutes the basis of the BOLD response (Fig. 2D). On a macroscopic scale, inhomogeneities due to these variations concentrations produce a reduction in the T2* value detectable with fMRI.

☐ METHODOLOGY OF SDA NEUROIMAGING STUDIES

In order to identify studies of the neural correlates of sexual arousal that were based on functional brain imaging techniques, several bibliographical requests were addressed to large databases listing English-language manuscripts, including: PsychInfo, MEDLINE, Pascal Biomed, Biological Abstracts, FRANCIS, Current Contents, and BiomedCentral. In April 2004, 18 studies had been published (Tables 1 and 2). This review focuses on the methodological aspects of these studies regarding (i) neuroimaging techniques, (ii) samples of volunteers, (iii) the experimental paradigms used to induce SDA, and (iv) functional data analysis.

Subject Samples

Since the use of neuroimaging techniques in the investigation of SDA is quite recent, most studies have been performed on healthy male volunteers (8,10,11,16–19, 21–23,25). Regarding the samples of subjects used in the different studies listed in Tables 1 and 2, it must be noted that (i) in some studies, sexual orientation was not specified; (ii) the mean age was relatively young, often less than 35 years; (iii) the subjects' physical health was sometimes not verified with biological assays. Subclinical biological anomalies, however, such as an elevated prolactin plasma level, should have resulted in the exclusion of subjects from these studies (3).

Experimental Paradigms Used for SDA Induction

Across SDA neuroimaging studies, most experimental paradigms have been of the "block-type," meaning that stimuli—most commonly of a visual type, such as photographs or film clips—are presented during a "block" of time extending from 20 to 1200 seconds. For "block-type" paradigms involving experimental stimulation, subtractive analyses are often used to compare the response of the brain to blocks of different stimuli. In order to obtain a precise study of the brain response to sexual stimuli, the reference stimuli should be "emotionally neutral" and have the same properties as the sexual stimuli, differing only in the sexual nature of their content. For example, the number and age of the people shown in photographs should be matched across all categories of photographs.

In some studies, several types of sexual stimuli are used in the same experiment. For example, still photographs are used in addition to film clips in one PET study, with the rationale being to: (i) control for the cerebral process of moving targets (thus avoiding any confusion between cerebral activation related to moving stimuli and cerebral activation related to SDA—e.g., in the occipitotemporal cortex); (ii) perform correlational analyses between cerebral activation and graded intensity of SDA—a gradation that is easy to implement with photographs (8).

Another study modification involves control conditions that are not restricted to "emotionally neutral" stimuli. Bearing in mind the emotional component of SDA, the use of reference stimuli that include content such as exciting sports highlights (10,25), humorous material (8), or scenarios of nonsexual, amicable social interactions between males and females (24) is meant to control for cerebral activation as the result of the emotionally salient but nonsexual properties of stimuli.

The length of exposure to sexually explicit stimuli, especially visual sexual stimuli (VSS), is also a very important factor regarding the intensity of the SDA and the corresponding cerebral activation that subjects experience. In most SDA neuroimaging studies, the presentation of sexual stimuli lasts from about 30 seconds (22) to several minutes (18).

Analysis of Functional Data

In most SDA neuroimaging studies, and more generally in neuroimaging experiments, analyses conducted on functional data are subtractive analyses. In PET experiments, for example, each successive scan corresponds to a distinct experimental condition. In fMRI experiments, however, "runs" of continuous data acquisition typically traverse several different experimental conditions. Thus, in the case of SDA neuroimaging studies, stimuli pertaining to different experimental conditions, such as neutral and sexually explicit stimuli are presented as sequential "blocks" within the same run.

A typical subtractive analysis involves the subtraction of cerebral activity recorded in one experimental condition from cerebral activity recorded in another experimental condition, with the difference termed "activation" or "deactivation." Thus, in order to study the brain areas that are more activated in a sexual condition than in a neutral condition, for each "voxel," or volume element of the brain, the activity recorded during the presentation of neutral stimuli is subtracted from the activity recorded during the presentation of sexual stimuli.

Another possible statistical approach is to study the correlation between cerebral hemodynamic signals and other measures recorded in the same experiment. Such analyses are performed with two different types of measures: (i) with subjective ratings—e.g., of perceived sexual arousal, or (ii) with objective measures of SDA, such as penile tumescence or heart rate. This approach may reveal cerebral activation that is not demonstrated by subtractive analyses.

Studies in Males with Disturbances of SDA

At present, few studies have used neuroimaging techniques to investigate the neural correlates of SDA in sexual disorders. Included for review in this chapter are (i) a study on patients with hypoactive sexual desire disorder (HSDD) in which PET was used to compare the cerebral responses of patients and healthy control subjects to VSS of graded intensity (3); (ii) three studies in which apomorphine, a dopamine agonist with proerectile properties, was sublingually administered to patients presenting with psychogenic erectile dysfunction (26,27,29); and (iii) a study on patients with hypogonadism (28).

Table 1 Methodological Features of the Neuroimaging Studies of Sexual Desire and Arousal in Samples of Healthy Volunteers

Study (Ref.)	Participants				Sexual condition		Control condition		Measures	
	M/F	Age range (mean)	Sexual orientation	NT	Stimulation type	Length (s)	Control condition(s)	Length (s)	Objective measures	Subjective measures
Rauch 1999 (16)	8/0	21–32 (25)	NI	PET	Script-driven imagery	30–40	Neutral, competitive arousal	30–40	HR, ER, lat. front. EMG	Valence, general arousal, sexual arousal, competitive arousal, happiness
Stoléru 1999 (11)	8/0	21–25 (23)	Hetero	PET	Sexually explicit clip	600	Documentary, humorous clips	600	Phallometry, plasma testosterone, HR, RR	PSA, humor
Redouté 2000 (8)	9/0	21–39 (30.7)	Hetero	PET	Sexually arousing clips/three types of photographic stimuli of graded intensity	120	Documentary, humorous clips/nonsexually arousing photographs	120	Phallometry, plasma testosterone, HR, BP	PSA, humor
Beauregard 2001 (17)	10/0	20–42 (23.5)	NI	fMRI	Sexually arousing clip	39 s-blocks	Emotionally neutral clips	39 s-blocks	No	Intensity of sexual arousal or primary emotions
Bocher 2001 (18)	10/0	24–32 (27)	Hetero	PET	Sexually arousing clip	600, 1200, 1800	Baseline, nature, talk-show clips	NI	No	Sexual thoughts, PSA, perceived erection
Park 2001 (19)	12/0	21–25 (23)	NI	fMRI	Sexually arousing clip	120 s-blocks	Documentary clip	60	No	PSA, perceived erection
Park 2001 (20)	0/6	25–41 (33)	NI	fMRI	Erotic clip	240	Documentary clip	60	No	PSA
Arnow 2002 (10)	14/0	18–30	Hetero	fMRI	Sexually arousing clip	108–543	Relaxing scenes, sports highlights	30–129	Circ. phallometry; HR; RR	Sexual interest, onset of erection, loss of interest
Karama 2002 (21)	20/20	M: 21–29/F: 21–27	Hetero	fMRI	Sexually arousing clip	179	Emotionally neutral clips	179	No	PSA, surprise, amusement, sadness, fear, disgust, anger
Mouras 2003 (22)	8/0	24–29 (26)	Hetero	fMRI	Sexually arousing photographs	21	Emotionally neutral photographs	21	No	See table notes
Holstege 2003 (23)	11/0	19–45 (33)	Hetero	PET	Ejaculation by manual stimulation by partner	120	Penile stimulation without ejaculation	120	Visual control of ejaculation by experimenter	None
Hamann 2004 (24)	14/14	M: 25.9/F:25	Hetero	fMRI	Sexually arousing clip	20	Pleasant social interaction stimuli; fixation cross	20	No	Sexual attractiveness, physical arousal
Ferretti 2005 (25)	10/0	21–25	NI	fMRI	Sexually arousing clip/photographic stimuli	180/3	Neutral and sport clips	Neutral: 30/sport: 120	Circ. phallometry	Beginning and end of sexual interest

For Mouras et al. (22), the subjective ratings were as follows: perceived beauty; desire to engage in sexual behavior; desire to engage in sexual behavior; degree of pleasure/displeasure; degree of erection; degree of pleasure/displeasure; degree of interest; and degree of tenderness.

Abbreviations: NT, neuroimaging technique; NI, not indicated; Circ. phallometry, circumferential phallometry; EMG, electromyogram; PSA, perceived sexual arousal; HR, heart rate; RR, respiratory rate; BP, blood pressure; ER, electrodermal response; M/F, males/females; PET, positron emission tomography; lat., lateral; fMRI, functional magnetic resonance imaging.

Table 2 Methodological Features of the Neuroimaging Studies of SDA in Pathological Conditions

Study (Ref.)	Participants				NT	Sexual condition		Control condition		Measures	
	M/F	P/H	Age range (mean)	Sexual orientation		Stimulation type	Dur. (sec)	Control condition(s)	Dur. (sec)	Objective measures	Subjective measures
Hagemann 2003 (29)[a]	12/0	12/0	24–41 (35)	NI	PET	Sexually arousing clip	30	Emotionally neutral clips	30	Penile rigidity	No
Montorsi 2003a (26)[a]	12/0	8/4	Patients: 25–58 (43)/ healthy: 22–28 (25)	NI	FMRI	Erotic clip	40	Emotionally neutral clips	40	No	No
Montorsi 2003b (27)[a]	16/0	10/6	Patients: NI (49)/ controls: NI	NI	FMRI	Erotic clip	40	Emotionally neutral clips	40	No	No
Stoléru 2003 (3)[b]	15/0	7/8	Patients: 26–47 (37.2)/ controls 21–39 (30.2)	Hetero	PET	Sexually arousing clips/three types of photographic stimuli of graded intensity	120	Documentary, humorous clips/nonsexually arousing photographs	120	Circ. phallom-etry, HR, BP	Perceived sexual arousal, humor
Redouté 2005 (28)[c]	17/0	9/8	Patients: 24–49 (35.4)/ controls 21–39 (30.2)	Hetero	PET	Sexually arousing clips/three types of photographic stimuli of graded intensity	120	Documentary, humorous clips/nonsexually arousing photographs	120	Circ. phallom-etry, HR, BP	Perceived sexual arousal, humor

[a]Studies on the modulation of neural correlates of SDA in participants with psychogenic erectile dysfunction treated by apomorphine administration.
[b]Study on the neural correlates of SDA in patients with hypoactive sexual desire disorder.
[c]Study on the neural correlates of SDA in patients with hypogonadism.

Abbreviations: SDA, sexual desire and arousal; NT, neuroimaging technique; NI, not indicated; Circ. phallometry, circumferential phallometry; EMG, electromyogram; PSA, perceived sexual arousal; HR, heart rate; RR, respiratory rate; BP, blood pressure; ER, electrodermal response; M/F, males/females; P/H, patients/healthy; Dur, duration; PET, positron emission tomography; fMRI, functional magnetic resonance imaging.

Table 3 Brain Areas Reported as Activated in Response to Sexual Stimuli in Healthy Men and Women

Study (Ref.)	SPL	IPL	Insula	ACC	LOFC	LOccTC	InfTC	Claustrum	CN	Put.	Amyg.	Hyp.	Thal.	Cereb.
Studies in healthy male volunteers														
Rauch 1999 (16)	–	–	–	R (32, r)	–	–	–	L	–	–	–	–	–	–
Stoléru 1999 (11)	–	–	R	L (24, 32, c)	R(47)	R	–	R	R	–	–	–	–	–
Redouté 2000 (8)	R (7)	R (7)	–	L–R(24,32,r/c)	R(11,47)	–	–	L–R	R	L–R	L	midline	L–R	L–R
Beauregard 2001 (17)	L(7)–R(7)	–	–	–	–	L(19)–R(19)	R(37)	–	–	–	R	R	–	L
Bocher 2001 (18)	L–R	L	–	–	–	L/R	L	–	–	–	–	–	–	–
Park 2001a (19)	–	–	L–R	L–R(r/c)	–	L–R	L–R	L–R	L–R	L–R	–	–	L–R	–
Arnow 2002 (10)	–	–	L–R	L(24,32)–R(32) (r/c)	–	R(37,19)	–	R	L	–	–	R	–	–
Karama 2002 (21)	L(7)–R(7)	–	L–R	L(24)–R(24)[c]	L(47)–R(47)	L(21)–R(37)	–	–	–	L–R	L–R	L–R	L–R	–
Mouras 2003 (22)	–	L(40)	R	–	R(47)	R(19)	R-L	L–R	–	–	–	–	R	L–R
Holstege 2003 (23)	–	R(40)	–	–	–	–	R(20/21)	–	–	–	–	L–R	–	R
Hamann 2004 (24)	L–R	L–R	L–R	L–R	R	L–R	L–R	–	–	L–R	L–R	L–R	L–R	–
Ferretti 2005 (25)	–	L–R	–	L–R	R	–	–	–	–	–	L–R	R	L–R	R
Total/11	5	6	6	8	6	7	6	5	4	3	5	6	6	4
Studies in healthy female volunteers														
Park 2001b (20)	–	–	L–R	L–R[r]	U	–	L–R	–	L–R	–	–	–	–	–
Karama 2002 (21)	–	–	L–R	L(24)–R(24)[c]	L(47)–R(47)	L(39)–R(21)	–	–	–	–	L–R	–	L–R	–
Hamann 2004 (24)	L–R	L–R	–	L–R	R	L–R	–	–	–	–	L–R	–	–	R

Numbers in parentheses noted after site of activation refer to Brodmann area. For the study by Hamann et al. (24), areas more strongly activated in men than in women are in italics.
Abbreviations: SPL, superior parietal lobule; IPL, inferior parietal lobule; ACC, anterior cingulate cortex; LOFC, lateral orbitofrontal cortex; LOccTC, lateral occipitotemporal cortex; InfTC, inferotemporal cortex; CN, caudate nucleus; Put, putamen; Amyg, amygdala; Hyp, hypothalamus; Thal, thalamus; Cereb, cerebellum; L, left hemisphere; R, right hemisphere; r, rostral part; c, caudal part; U, undetermined.

Other Studies

Table 1 illustrates some studies that investigate the neural correlates of female sexual response (20,21). Others compare the brain responses of males and females to VSS and odorous sex hormone–like compounds (24,30). In nonhuman primates, neural responses of males to the odor of ovulating females have been reported (31,32).

Caveats

It is important to keep in mind that the successful implementation of neuroimaging techniques for the identification of activated brain areas in SDA depends on the threshold of statistical certainty adopted by the investigator. Lowering the threshold will create more regions that are statistically significant, whereas raising the threshold will reduce the number of significant regions. The choice of threshold is not an absolute standard and is largely determined by convention among researchers. Thus, reports of brain activation patterns are primarily statistical interpretations of very complex data sets, and they may be interpreted differently by different researchers (33).

☐ COMPARING THE RESULTS OF SDA STUDIES

This section focuses on studies involving the main brain areas where responses to VSS have been demonstrated. Table 3 illustrates details of the activated areas. Both similarities and inconsistencies between results across studies are examined.

Subtractive Analyses
Occipitotemporal and Inferotemporal Cortices

One of the most consistent findings in SDA studies is the activation of the occipitotemporal and inferotemporal areas. These are cortical regions corresponding to the "ventral stream" of visual processing that contains the "what" aspect of visual stimuli—that is, the content of the visual stimuli, as opposed to the aspects of shape and location that are processed along the so-called "dorsal stream." In fact, such activation has been reported in a majority of visually induced emotional or motivational states, regardless of the specific nature of the emotion or motivation induced by the stimuli (6). Thus, occipitotemporal and inferotemporal activations may not be related specifically to the sexual content of stimuli but rather to the fact that they are emotionally arousing visual stimuli. One possible interpretation is that the occipitotemporal and inferotemporal regions are under the control of other areas, particularly those related to focused, attentional processes elicited by VSS (34).

Orbitofrontal Cortex

OFC activation was reported in the very first SDA neuroimaging study (11). Since that time, this finding

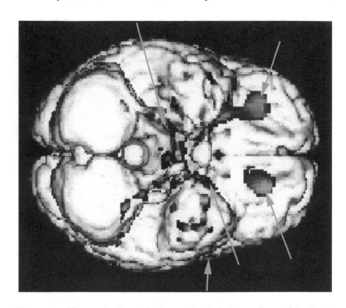

Figure 3 (*See color insert.*) View of the inferior surface of the brain showing orbitofrontal activations in both hemispheres. Clusters of voxels with higher regional cerebral blood flow in the sexual condition than in the humor condition.

has been replicated in five studies, with activation appearing to be more common in the right hemisphere than the left (Fig. 3) (8,21,23–25). Redouté et al. demonstrated that activation of the OFC was actually greater in response to sexual stimuli of moderate intensity than to highly arousing sexual stimuli (8). In fact, OFC response was found to be greater overall when stimuli showed women than other targets, regardless of the pictures being sexually stimulating or otherwise. On debriefing, subjects commented on the beauty of women only in the moderately sexually arousing pictures. These results are consistent with both reports of OFC activation in response to facial attractiveness (35,36) and the well-documented role of this region in the appraisal of motivationally relevant stimuli (37). Thus, OFC activation may be more related to the process of evaluation than to SDA per se. In the proposed model (see below), the OFC mediates the cognitive component of SDA, whereby stimuli are qualitatively labeled as sexual and then quantitatively evaluated as such. This interpretation is consistent with two case reports: (*i*) a patient presenting with acquired pedophilia, who was subsequently found to have a right orbitofrontal tumor (38), and (*ii*) a patient presenting with pedophilia in whom fMRI demonstrated right OFC activation in response to pictures of children wearing underwear (39).

Anterior Cingulate Cortex

Activation in the anterior cingulate cortex (ACC) has often been reported across SDA neuroimaging studies (Fig. 4). Many of these studies have confirmed the distinction between a rostral "affective" division and a caudal "cognitive" division of the ACC (40). The rostral

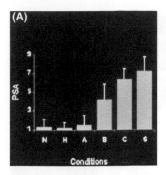 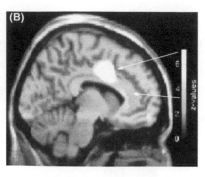

Figure 4 (*See color insert.*) PSA and rCBF in left anterior cingulate gyrus means and standard deviations of PSA in each condition. Parasagittal section (4 mm left of midline) showing the positive correlation between rCBF in the left anterior cingulate gyrus (Brodmann area 24) and PSA. Height threshold: $z = 3.71$, $p < 0.0001$, uncorrected. Anterior is to the right. *Abbreviations*: PSA, perceived sexual arousal; rCBF, regional cerebral blood flow; N, neutral clips; H, humor clips; S, sexual clips; A, neutral photographs; B, moderately arousing photographs; C, highly arousing photographs. *Source*: From Ref. 8.

division has strong connections to subcortical structures such as the amygdala and the hypothalamus and is linked to both the autonomic and the endocrine systems. The caudal division may be involved in the motivational component of SDA—i.e., the production of the impulse to act upon the presentation of sexual stimuli. The functional similarities between the caudal part of the ACC and the premotor and supplementary motor cortices has led to the hypothesis that activation of the caudal ACC in response to VSS could reflect motor preparation processes associated with SDA (8). In addition to its role in the mediation of SDA, the ACC may also be involved in processes that inhibit SDA. The caudal part of the ACC has been clearly shown to monitor conflicts between contradictory signals or intentions (41). It is speculated that the pronounced activation of the caudal part of the left ACC may be the result of multiple conflicting inputs to this area: on the one hand, inputs of the "go" type, correlated with the perceived urge to enact SDA, and, on the other hand, inputs of the "no-go" type, correlated with the perceived need to withhold any overt sexual behavior in the context of the experiment (8). Further, the observed activation of the rostral part of the right ACC in an inhibition condition compared to a sexual arousal condition demonstrates the complex involvement of this region in the control of SDA (17).

In summary, both the rostral affective part and the caudal cognitive part of the ACC are activated in response to VSS. Within these regions, certain areas seem to have an activating role in SDA, while others may have an inhibiting one.

Parietal Lobules
Superior Parietal Lobule
Activation of the superior parietal lobule (SPL) has been related to attentional processes elicited by VSS. In a recent fMRI study, still pictures and relatively short periods of VSS presentation were used to investigate the early cerebral processes involved in the emergence of SDA (22). When comparing the periods of sexual visual stimulation with periods of neutral visual stimulation, it was found that an early bilateral activation of SPLs occurred at the beginning of the VSS presentation, followed by a bilateral sustained activation of SPLs. These results could reflect an early increase in attentional processes in response to VSS.

They are also consistent with other results showing very early onset of appraisal processes: first, Spiering et al. (42) reported very fast reaction times (between 526 and 738 msec) in a picture categorization task involving sexual and neutral pictures, and second, Pizzagalli et al. (43) reported very early parietal activation in response to attractive faces as compared to unattractive ones. These results demonstrate how quickly the brain may become involved in the processing of sexual information. Although fMRI seems to be able to identify such cerebral responses, techniques with better temporal resolution such as MEG could assist in the elucidation of these early responses in greater detail.

Inferior Parietal Lobule
In neuroimaging studies focusing on tasks with no sexual content, inferior parietal lobule (IPL) activation has been associated with tasks involving mental imagery, in which subjects must imagine themselves grasping visually presented objects (44) or manipulating imaginary joysticks with their hands (45). In a study comparing HSDD patients with healthy controls, IPL activation in response to sexual visual stimulation was found only in controls (3). When coupled with the fact that a much higher percentage of control subjects (62.5%) than patients (14.3%) reported sexual motor imagery in response to VSS, this finding suggests the involvement of IPL in motor imagery processes.

Amygdala
Five studies have reported activation of the amygdala in response to VSS (8,17,21,24,25). In a recent review on the induction of emotion, it was reported that amygdalar activation has been widely associated with detecting, generating, and maintaining fear-related emotions (6). Although many neuroimaging studies have also reported amygdalar activation in response to positive emotional stimuli, this activation is far less consistent than activation induced by negative emotional stimuli.

Arousal and motivation are important for the recruitment of the amygdala, as the level of arousal seems to influence amygdalar response to emotional stimuli, with a higher response associated with greater arousal (46). This relationship seems to be more complex for positive emotional stimuli than for negative ones, as only the former can be experienced as being either arousing or relaxing (46).

Amygdalar responses were also reported in studies involving motivationally relevant stimuli other than sexually explicit ones (46). Thus, the sexual nature of motivationally relevant stimuli may not be necessary to provoke amygdalar response.

Hamann et al. reported that given identical sexual stimuli, both the right and the left amygdalae were more strongly activated in men than in women, indicating the possibility of gender-specific amygdalar function (24).

Finally, because the claustrum and some parts of the amygdala may arise from the same embryological origin (47), the role of the amygdala in reward-related processes could be shared in part by the claustrum, where activation in response to VSS has been reported as consistently as in the amygdala.

Deactivated Areas in SDA Neuroimaging Studies

In a recent review of neuroimaging studies of emotion, neural deactivation was not taken into account due to the lack of consistency across studies (6). It should be noted, however, that in some of the studies—particularly those using PET—decreased blood flow was reported in some cerebral regions in response to VSS (Fig. 5). These results have been integrated into the proposed model of SDA (see below).

First, temporal lobe deactivation in response to VSS has been reported. In one study (8), almost all of the cerebral areas in which activity was negatively correlated with markers of sexual arousal—i.e., perceived sexual arousal and penile tumescence—were localized to the temporal lobes. Additionally, surgical removal of the temporal lobes produces the hypersexuality manifestations of Klüver-Bucy syndrome (48). Such findings suggest that physiologically, the temporal regions exert an inhibition on SDA development. If this were the case, deactivation within the temporal lobes would cause a reduction in inhibitory function, resulting in the more ready development of SDA in response to sexual stimulation.

The medial OFC and posterior cingulate gyrus have also been reported to show deactivation in response to VSS; these regions may exert similar inhibitory influences on SDA (8). A review of nine PET studies with no relation to sexual behavior reported that the posterior cingulate cortex was consistently deactivated in active visual tasks in comparison to passive visual tasks, even while there was increased activation in the visual areas of the brain (49). Thus, such deactivation of the posterior cingulate cortex could be related to an increased attentional focus on VSS.

Correlational Analyses

Some experimental studies have focused on the cerebral areas involved in mediating the penile response occurring during SDA. The studies considered here are (*i*) those in which penile tumescence was assessed concurrently with functional data acquisition (8,10,25) and (*ii*) studies on the influence of apomorphine administration on the cerebral activation during SDA in patients with erectile dysfunctions (Fig. 6) (26,27,29).

Numerous studies have shown the major role played by the brain in erectile response (50). Although the use of neuroimaging techniques in the investigation of the neural correlates of SDA is relatively recent, many improvements have been made in the recording and integration of penile tumescence data in neuroimaging analyses.

The first approach is based on recording the subjective ratings of the perceived degree of erection reported by the subjects during or after acquisition of functional cerebral data (18,19,22). As expected, subjective ratings of the perceived degree of erection were significantly higher during sexual conditions than control conditions. In one recent study, subjects were requested to press a button to signal their perception of penile tumescence while both cerebral data acquisition and objective measurements of penile response were being performed; button presses were closely coupled with objective recordings (10).

Bocher et al. (18) studied the relationship between rCBF and the subjects' ratings of their perceived degree of erection, noting a correlation between subjective ratings of erection and rCBF on the right side of the brain in the inferior temporal, occipitotemporal, and inferior occipital gyri and the midbrain, as well as on the left side of the brain in the medial frontal, postcentral,

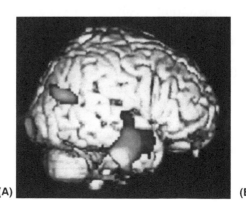
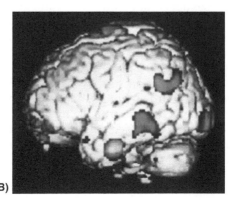

(A) (B)

Figure 5 (*See color insert.*) Deactivations in temporal regions and in medial orbitofrontal cortex. (**A**) Right view; anterior is to the right. (**B**) Left view; anterior is to the left. The most anterior cluster corresponds to the deactivated medial orbitofrontal cortex.

TURGIDITY-CORRELATED ACTIVATIONS

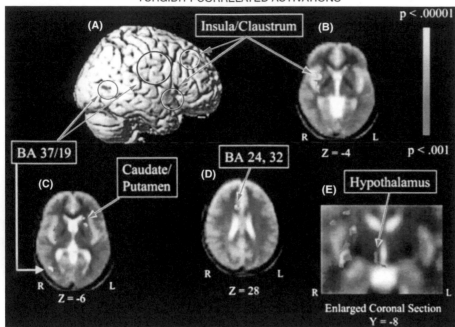

Figure 6 (*See color insert.*) Brain regions where activation was correlated with penile tumescence in a group of 11 healthy male volunteers. (**A**) SPM99 surface reconstruction depicting projections of activation on the right side of the brain. (**B**) Axial section showing right insula and claustrum activation. (**C**) Axial section showing left caudate/putamen activation. (**D**) Right cingulate cortex activation. (**E**) Right hypothalamus activation. *Source*: From Ref. 10.

medial occipital, and inferior temporal gyri and precuneus. It is possible that the strong correlation between midbrain activation and the subjects' rating of their perceived degree of erection is related to the activity of the dopaminergic neuronal structures in this region, which transmit motivationally relevant information to the forebrain. Moreover, the midbrain is connected to the hypothalamus, whose role in the erectile response has clearly been demonstrated in animals. Finally, the midbrain is a relay point for genital sensory information being transmitted to other cerebral areas such as the insula.

Curiously, midbrain activation has rarely been observed in SDA neuroimaging studies. The length of the sexual stimulation used by Bocher et al. was the longest among all reviewed studies; thus, it is conceivable that midbrain activation might occur only after a long period of continuous sexual stimulation (18). In another recent study, PET was used to study cerebral activation recorded during ejaculation induced by penile stimulation (23). The strongest activation was observed in the midbrain, specifically in the mesodiencephalic transition zone; this confirms that strong sexual stimulation may induce activation of the midbrain.

The second correlational approach is based on using penile plethysmography with concurrent cerebral data acquisition (8,10,11,25). Circumferential phallometry performed during PET data acquisition has been used since the first published SDA neuroimaging study (11). Notably, this device was also used in a more recent study performed in a larger sample of subjects with an improved PET scanner, using films and photographs of sexually explicit stimuli of graded intensity (8). Arnow et al. also used circumferential phallometry during fMRI data acquisition to investigate the temporal

aspects of the correlation between the BOLD response and penile tumescence; interestingly, both subtractive analyses and correlational analyses were performed for the same subjects (10). Although no cerebral activation was observed in the case of contrasting sexual conditions and control conditions (sports clips), the activation of several brain areas was correlated with the recorded penile response (Table 3).

Circumferential phallometry with concurrent PET cerebral data acquisition has also been used to study patients presenting with psychogenic erectile dysfunctions (29) and patients with HSDD (3).

Anterior Cingulate Cortex

In one PET study, a high correlation was found between the magnitude of penile tumescence and rCBF in the rostral part of the left ACC (8). Similarly, the magnitude of the BOLD signal in the left ACC was found to correlate with tumescence in a separate fMRI study (10). In another PET study investigating the neural correlates of SDA in a group of patients with erectile dysfunction, a significant positive correlation was reported between penile rigidity and activity in the right rostral ACC (29). Additionally, it was determined that the coefficient of correlation between tumescence and rCBF in the caudal part of the ACC was significantly higher in control subjects than in HSDD patients (3). The involvement of the ACC in erectile processes is further supported by other experimental results: (*i*) lesion and electrical stimulation studies have demonstrated the role of the rostral portion of the ACC in autonomic responses and in the expression of affect (51) and (*ii*) electrical stimulation of the rostral portion of the ACC elicits erection in monkeys (52,53).

Hypothalamus

Although subtractive analyses between experimental conditions have often failed to show activation of the hypothalamus, correlational analyses between cerebral activation and penile tumescence have demonstrated hypothalamic involvement. Both a PET study and an fMRI study have demonstrated a positive correlation between rCBF and tumescence, which was recorded in the posterior hypothalamus (8,10). Interestingly, the correlation between tumescence and rCBF in the posterior hypothalamus demonstrated in control subjects was not found in HSDD patients (3). Nonetheless, a study by Hagemann et al. did not find any correlation between penile rigidity and hypothalamic rCBF (29). It was suggested in a recent review that the lack of consistency of reported hypothalamic activation could be a result of the relatively low level of arousal attained in many SDA neuroimaging studies (54). It must be noted, however, that the studies utilizing the longest sexual stimulation periods reported no hypothalamic activation (11,18). Further, a case study noted that activation of the hypothalamus actually started 30 seconds prior to the initiation of the penile response (55).

Brain imaging studies that report correlations between hypothalamic activation and penile tumescence are consistent with neurophysiological data illustrating the fundamental role of the hypothalamus in the erectile mechanism. Animal studies have revealed that while electrical stimulation of the hypothalamus in rats (56) and monkeys (57) will induce erection or copulative behavior in various species, lesions in the medial preoptic area will impair male copulative behavior (2). Hypothalamic activation in response to the odors of periovulatory females was also reported in two studies of the neural correlates of SDA performed in monkeys (31,32).

The Insula and Bordering Claustrum

In a recent review of neuroimaging studies of SDA, bilateral activation of the insula and the bordering claustrum was reported as "one of the most robust findings" (54). One PET study (8) has shown bilateral activation of the claustrum to correlate strongly with penile tumescence, while bilateral activation of both the claustrum and the insula correlate positively with penile tumescence in fMRI (10). Preliminary results based on volumetric plethysmography performed in one subject with concurrent fMRI demonstrated a correlation between penile erection and left insular activation in response to VSS (55). These results are consistent with recent data on the involvement of the insula in somatosensory and neuroendocrine processes. First, MEG has shown that stimulation of the dorsal penile nerve, which supplies sensory axons to a major portion of the penis, elicits a bilateral but predominantly left-hemispheric activation of the secondary somatosensory cortex (58) in an area that lies very close to the insula and contains many reciprocal connections with it (59). Second, in a recent fMRI study of neural correlates of penile sensory stimulation, Kell et al. (60) established a mediolateral sequence of somatosensory foot, penis, and lower abdominal wall representation on the contralateral postcentral gyrus in primary sensory cortex and a bilateral secondary somatosensory representation in the parietal operculum. Third, neuromorphological studies using a transsynaptic viral tracing technique showed pituitary-independent neural pathways between the insular cortex and the testis. Such pathways could allow for pituitary-independent brain control—particularly insular control—over testicular secretion, with gonadal feedback on cerebral structures via the effects of plasma testosterone (61,62).

The Putamen

Although the putamen resides within the territory of the basal ganglia, two studies testing the correlation between cerebral responses and penile tumescence have demonstrated activation within the putamen (8,10). Such results are consistent with another study showing that electrical stimulation of the putamen in monkeys most frequently evoked erection, genital manipulation behavior, or both (53).

Areas Where BOLD Response Is Negatively Correlated with Penile Tumescence

Some studies have distinguished negative correlations between penile response and rCBF in some brain regions—i.e., these areas show more deactivation as the strength of the erectile response increases. One PET study has reported such deactivation in temporal lobe areas (8). Studies using fMRI, however, have not revealed any areas where the BOLD response was negatively correlated with penile tumescence. Yet, in patients presenting with erectile dysfunction, a negative correlation was reported between penile tumescence and rCBF response in the medial inferior temporal cortex, 50 minutes after apomorphine administration (29). In another study of patients with erectile dysfunction, apomorphine administration also induced the deactivation of limbic areas of the temporal cortex (26). These responses may be related to the inhibitory processes that are part of the proposed multicomponent neurobehavioral model of SDA (8) described below in "Proposed Model of Cerebral Processing of VSS."

Inconsistencies Between Studies

With regard to the activation of parietal lobules, Rauch et al. have reported a significantly lower signal of activation in a sexual imagery condition than in a neutral imagery condition; as the focus of this study was the valence of arousal, however, script-driven imagery was used in the same way to induce both the sexual and the neutral conditions (16). Thus, the apparent lack of activation of the inferior parietal lobules in the sexual condition should not be regarded as definitive evidence against their role in mediating motor imagery.

Although activation of the ACC is one of the most frequently reported results across SDA neuroimaging studies, such activation has not been reported during the initial cerebral responses to VSS (22). Bocher et al. reported deactivation bilaterally of the ACC when contrasting sexual and baseline conditions, but not when the sexual condition was contrasted with other control conditions such as nature and talk-show clips. Considering that Mouras et al. (22) used the shortest VSS presentation and Bocher et al. (18) the longest, it is possible that the ACC activations are present until a certain degree of SDA is reached, at which point the ACC activity decreases as SDA intensity increases. For example, Beauregard et al. reported right ACC activation when subjects had to inhibit induced sexual arousal (17). This study suggests the existence of contrasting roles played by the left ACC, which is often activated in response to VSS, and the right ACC, which gets activated in the inhibition condition.

Preliminary Results on the Neural Correlates of SDA in Healthy Females

Among the published neuroimaging studies listed in Table 1, three have investigated the neural correlates of female sexual response (20,21,24). Sexual arousal was induced in these women in the fMRI environment, albeit at a significantly lower level than in comparable male sample populations. On a five-point scale, Park et al. (20) reported a mean score of perceived sexual arousal of 2.7 (compared to 3.0 on the same scale for the male sample), while on a scale ranging from 0 to 8, Karama et al. (21) reported a mean perceived sexual arousal of 2.6 in the female sample (compared to 3.8 on the same scale for the male sample). Interestingly, one study found the level of sexual arousal to be similar both in females and in males when photographic stimuli representing couples were selected so that they would be maximally attractive to females (24). Preliminary data obtained on the neural correlates of female sexual arousal in these studies demonstrate a high degree of similarity in the brain responses to VSS between male and female samples—i.e., bilateral activation in the medial prefrontal, orbitofrontal, insular, and occipitotemporal cortices, the anterior cingulate gyrus, the ventral striatum, and the amygdala (21). Park et al. reported additional activations in the thalamus, caudate, globus pallidus, inferior temporal, and frontal lobes (20). In contrast, Karama et al. reported that the significant activation in the thalamus and the hypothalamus associated with the processing of erotic film segments was observed only in males, despite identical stimulation paradigms between male and female samples (21). Recently, Hamann et al. compared neural correlates of human male and female sexual arousal, reporting that the amygdala and hypothalamus are less strongly activated in women than in men, even when viewing exactly identical sexual stimuli (24). Yet, in conditions involving reward stimuli, men and women showed similar activation patterns across multiple brain regions, including those of the ventral striatum involved in the reward. For further details on the similarities and differences between male and female sexual function, see Chapter 11.

The studies of Park et al., Karama et al., and Hamann et al. have underlined the relevance of using neuroimaging to investigate the cerebral processes involved in the female sexual response. As in male samples, objective measures of female genital responses may prove to be an additional correlational method in the investigation of female SDA.

Preliminary Results on SDA Neural Correlates in Monkeys

Two studies by Ferris et al. have demonstrated that fMRI can be used to study the neural responses of fully conscious monkeys to female odors (31,32). Using a baseline condition as a reference, an assessment was made of the number of voxels in various brain regions that showed an increased or a decreased BOLD signal in response to odors from periovulatory and ovariectomized females. It was reported that an increased BOLD signal in response to periovulatory females' odors was represented by a higher number of voxels mainly in the preoptic and anterior hypothalamic areas, as well as in the striatum, hippocampus, septum, periaqueductal gray matter, and cerebellum. The highest number of voxels showing a decreased BOLD signal in response to ovariectomized females' odors were localized to the temporal cortex, cingulate cortex, putamen, hippocampus, substantia nigra, medial preoptic area, and cerebellum. It is important to note that in several areas, such as the medial preoptic area, there were both a higher number of voxels showing an increased BOLD signal in response to periovulatory females' odors and a higher number of voxels showing a decreased BOLD signal in response to ovariectomized females' odors. Based on these results, the authors of this study have suggested that the odor-driven enhancement and suppression of sexual arousal may affect neuronal activity in many of the same general brain areas.

☐ A PROPOSED MODEL OF CEREBRAL PROCESSING OF VSS Components

In order to provide an integrated view of the cerebral areas known to demonstrate activation or deactivation across SDA neuroimaging studies, a four-component neurobehavioral model of the brain processes involved in SDA has been proposed (3,8).

Cognitive Component

Activation of the cognitive component may be considered the earliest step in the unfolding process of SDA, and according to this model, comprises (*i*) the initial processes of appraisal that lead to the categorization of stimuli as sexually relevant for the ultimate purpose of evaluating their intensity, related to the activation of the right lateral OFC; (*ii*) the attentional processes that focus on stimuli categorized as sexual, related to the activation of the SPLs; (*iii*) motor imagery processes, related to the activation of areas within the domain of motor imagery networks—e.g., the inferior parietal lobules, the left anterior cingulate gyrus, the supplementary motor areas, the ventral premotor areas, and the caudate nuclei.

Motivational Component

The motivational component of SDA comprises the processes directing behavior to a sexual goal. According to the proposed model, this component is related to the activation of the caudal part of the left ACC and to the activation of the claustrum bilaterally. The motivational component is also closely related to motor imagery processes and their supporting neural network.

Autonomic and Neuroendocrine Component

The autonomic and neuroendocrine component includes peripheral aspects of SDA such as cardiovascular, respiratory, and genital responses. As summarized above, this component has been associated with the activation of the rostral portion of the left ACC and the hypothalamus, with possible relation to the insular control of testicular secretion.

Emotional Component

The emotional component of SDA comprises the pleasure associated with increasing arousal and penile tumescence. This activity has been related to the activation of the right insula and secondary somatosensory cortex.

Inhibitory Influences

The four components of SDA are conceived as being closely interrelated, and it is more than likely that a brain area that is preferentially involved in one component could also be involved in the activity of other components. This model also proposes mechanisms for the inhibitory processes that control the various components, comprising (*i*) inhibitory processes operating in the resting state that are exerted by the temporal lobes to inhibit the initiation of SDA; (*ii*) processes that limit the development of SDA once it has been initiated, particularly in the realm of active expression, as mediated by the caudate nucleus and the putamen; (*iii*) a lack of deactivation in the medial OFC that may result in cognitive processes of devaluation of potential sexual partners, providing a

possible explanation for the pathology related to HSDD (3).

□ PERSPECTIVES ON THE USE OF PENILE PLETHYSMOGRAPHY IN NEUROIMAGING EXPERIMENTS

Analyses investigating the correlation between penile responses and brain activation have major importance. For example, while no activation was found in one fMRI study with the use of subtractive analyses, the activity of numerous regions correlated positively with penile tumescence (10).

It is important to mention that, with the exception of Stoléru et al. (55), in all the studies reviewed above, penile plethysmography relied on a circumferential method of measurement and not a volumetric one, the latter being the only method that takes into account changes in both penile length and circumference. This is an important distinction, as many psychophysiological studies have reported considerable differences between penile circumference variations and penile volume variations in response to VSS, most notably in the early phase of genital response. Kuban et al. compared circumferential and volumetric measures in a sample of 42 healthy males, reporting an inverse relation between penile volume variations (increase) and penile circumference variations (decrease) during the early phase of sexual arousal, defined as "the mirror effect" (63). Thus, for low levels of response, volumetric methods result in more sensitive and accurate measures of penile tumescence, allowing a better assessment of SDA, especially in its early phase. A case study based on volumetric plethysmography has indicated that measures obtained through this technique were significantly and meaningfully correlated with the BOLD signal level in the rostral part of the ACC (55).

Some experimental results have shown that penile responses can occur very quickly in response to VSS. McConaghy has underlined that variations in penile volume generally occur rapidly, with exposure to a short 10-second stimulus being sufficient to induce a response (64). In fact, a study (58) revealed that a primary somatosensory cerebral response can occur within the first 100 msec after genital nerve stimulation, with accompanying responses in the secondary somatosensory cortex occurring at 107 and 126 msec after stimulation. These results illustrate the importance of monitoring penile volumetric response in SDA neuroimaging studies, not only for the purpose of assessing SDA objectively, but also to enable the accurate monitoring of the temporal profile of SDA with fine-grain resolution.

In view of the preceding studies, it is possible to consider the potential of specific approaches in correlational analyses between cerebral activation and the genital response. Based on the hypothesis that neural activation related to erectile response precedes the actual genital response, a series of correlational analyses between the BOLD signal and penile volumetric plethysmography measures was performed using various time lags between the two variables. In this preliminary case study, the highest number of cerebral areas correlating with a volumetric penile response was found when the BOLD signal preceded the penile response by 30 seconds (55).

In spite of a generally good correlation between objective penile plethysmography data and the subjectively perceived degree of erection, differences are likely to exist in the cerebral areas involved in the development of the genital response and in its conscious perception. By using both correlational analyses and functional cerebral data, it may be possible to distinguish the areas involved in the two phenomena.

☐ CONCLUSION

This review indicates that the process of SDA is not mediated by a single brain center, or even several brain centers, but by a large, intricate network of brain areas that are likely involved in the mediation of all the cognitive, motivational, emotional, and autonomic aspects of this complex biobehavioral state. Consistent as well as discrepant findings have been reported regarding the involvement of each specific brain region implicated in SDA. It is likely that methodological advances in terms of experimental design, statistical analysis, and technology will allow for an improved understanding of the brain areas involved in SDA and their complex interactions. A greater knowledge of the basic neurophysiologic building blocks will pave the way for the eventual development of new therapeutic approaches to the disorders of sexual arousal and desire.

☐ REFERENCES

1. Pfaus JG. Homologies of animal and human sexual behaviors. Horm Behav 1996; 30(3):187–200.

2. Meisel RL, Sachs BD. The physiology of male sexual behavior. In: E Knobil, JD Neill, eds. The Physiology of Reproduction. Vol. 2. New York: Raven Press, 1994: 3–105.

3. Stoléru S, Redoute J, Costes N, et al. Brain processing of visual sexual stimuli in men with hypoactive sexual desire disorder. Psychiatry Res 2003; 124(2):67–86.

4. Sandel ME, Williams KS, Dellapietra L, et al. Sexual functioning following traumatic brain injury. Brain Inj 1996; 10(10):719–728.

5. Krueger RB, Kaplan MS. Disorders of sexual impulse control in neuropsychiatric conditions. Semin Clin Neuropsychiatry 2000; 5(4):266–274.

6. Phan KL, Wager T, Taylor SF, et al. Functional neuroanatomy of emotion: a meta-analysis of emotion activation studies in PET and fMRI. Neuroimage 2002; 16(2):331–348.

7. Costa M, Braun C, Birbaumer N. Gender differences in response to pictures of nudes: a magnetoencephalographic study. Biol Psychol 2003; 63(2):129–147.

8. Redoute J, Stoléru S, Gregoire MC, et al. Brain processing of visual sexual stimuli in human males. Hum Brain Mapp 2000; 11(3):162–177.

9. Wilson JL, Jenkinson M, de Araujo I, et al. Fast, fully automated global and local magnetic field optimization for fMRI of the human brain. Neuroimage 2002; 17(2): 967–976.

10. Arnow BA, Desmond JE, Banner LL, et al. Brain activation and sexual arousal in healthy, heterosexual males. Brain 2002; 125(Pt 5):1014–1023.

11. Stoléru S, Gregoire MC, Gerard D, et al. Neuroanatomical correlates of visually evoked sexual arousal in human males. Arch Sex Behav 1999; 28(1):1–21.

12. Moseley ME, Glover GH. Functional MR imaging. Capabilities and limitations. Neuroimaging Clin N Am 1995; 5(2):161–191.

13. Murray RK, Granner DK, Mayes PA, et al. Harper's Biochemistry. 23rd ed. Norwalk: Appleton & Lange, 1993.

14. Houdé O, Mazoyer B, Tzourio-Mazoyer N. Cerveau et Psychologie. Paris: Presses Universitaires de France, 2002:609.

15. McIlwain H, Bachelard HS. Biochemistry and the Central Nervous System. Edinburgh: Churchill Livingstone, 1985.

16. Rauch SL, Shin LM, Dougherty DD, et al. Neural activation during sexual and competitive arousal in healthy men. Psychiatry Res 1999; 91(1):1–10.

17. Beauregard M, Levesque J, Bourgouin P. Neural correlates of conscious self-regulation of emotion. J Neurosci 2001; 21(18):RC165.

18. Bocher M, Chisin R, Parag Y, et al. Cerebral activation associated with sexual arousal in response to a pornographic clip: a ^{15}O–H$_2$O PET study in heterosexual men. Neuroimage 2001; 14(1):105–117.

19. Park K, Seo JJ, Kang HK, et al. A new potential of blood oxygenation level dependent (BOLD) functional MRI for evaluating cerebral centers of penile erection. Int J Impot Res 2001; 13(2):73–81.

20. Park K, Kang HK, Seo JJ, et al. Blood-oxygenation-level-dependent functional magnetic resonance imaging for evaluating cerebral regions of female sexual arousal response. Urology 2001; 57(6):1189–1194.

21. Karama S, Lecours AR, Leroux JM, et al. Areas of brain activation in males and females during viewing of erotic film excerpts. Hum Brain Mapp 2002; 16(1):1–13.

22. Mouras H, Stoléru S, Bittoun J, et al. Brain processing of visual sexual stimuli in healthy men: a functional magnetic resonance imaging study. Neuroimage 2003; 20(2):855–869.

23. Holstege G, Georgiadis JR, Paans AM, et al. Brain activation during human male ejaculation. J Neurosci 2003; 23(27):9185–9193.

24. Hamann S, Herman RA, Nolan CL, et al. Men and women differ in amygdala response to visual sexual stimuli. Nat Neurosci 2004; 7(4):411–416.

25. Ferretti A, Caulo M, Del Gratta C, et al. Dynamics of male sexual arousal: distinct components of brain activation revealed by fMRI. Neuroimage 2005; 26(4):1086–1096.

26. Montorsi F, Perani D, Anchisi D, et al. Apomorphine-induced brain modulation during sexual stimulation: a new look at central phenomena related to erectile dysfunction. Int J Impot Res 2003; 15(3):203–209.

27. Montorsi F, Perani D, Anchisi D, et al. Brain activation patterns during video sexual stimulation following the administration of apomorphine: results of a placebo-controlled study. Eur Urol 2003; 43(4):405–411.

28. Redouté J, Stoléru S, Pugeat M, et al. Brain processing of visual sexual stimuli in treated and untreated hypogonadal patients. Psychoneuroendocrinology 2005; 30(5):461–482.

29. Hagemann JH, Berding G, Bergh S, et al. Effects of visual sexual stimuli and apomorphine SL on cerebral activity in men with erectile dysfunction. Eur Urol 2003; 43(4):412–420.

30. Savic I, Berglund H, Gulyas B, et al. Smelling of odorous sex hormone-like compounds causes sex-differentiated hypothalamic activations in humans. Neuron 2001; 31(4):661–668.

31. Ferris CF, Snowdon CT, King JA, et al. Functional imaging of brain activity in conscious monkeys responding to sexually arousing cues. Neuroreport 2001; 12(10):2231–2236.

32. Ferris CF, Snowdon CT, King JA, et al. Activation of neural pathways associated with sexual arousal in non-human primates. J Magn Reson Imaging 2004; 19(2):168–175.

33. Canli T, Amin Z. Neuroimaging of emotion and personality: scientific evidence and ethical considerations. Brain Cogn 2002; 50(3):414–431.

34. Corbetta M, Miezin FM, Shulman GL, et al. A PET study of visuospatial attention. J Neurosci 1993; 13(3):1202–1026.

35. O'Doherty J, Winston J, Critchley H, et al. Beauty in a smile: the role of medial orbitofrontal cortex in facial attractiveness. Neuropsychologia 2003; 41(2):147–155.

36. Aharon I, Etcoff N, Ariely D, et al. Beautiful faces have variable reward value: fMRI and behavioral evidence. Neuron 2001; 32(3):537–551.

37. Rolls ET. The Brain and Emotion. New York: Oxford University Press, 1999:367.

38. Burns JM, Swerdlow RH. Right orbitofrontal tumor with pedophilia symptom and constructional apraxia sign. Arch Neurol 2003; 60(3):437–440.

39. Dressing H, Obergriesser T, Tost H, et al. Homosexual pedophilia and functional networks—An fMRI case report and literature review. [Article in German]. Fortschr Neurol Psychiatr 2001; 69(11):539–544.

40. Bush G, Luu P, Posner MI. Cognitive and emotional influences in anterior cingulate cortex. Trends Cogn Sci 2000; 4(6):215–222.

41. Kerns JG, Cohen JD, MacDonald AW III, et al. Anterior cingulate conflict monitoring and adjustments in control. Science 2004; 303(5660):1023–1026.

42. Spiering M, Everaerd W, Elzinga B. Conscious processing of sexual information: interference caused by sexual primes. Arch Sex Behav 2002; 31(2):159–164.

43. Pizzagalli DA, Lehmann D, Hendrick AM, et al. Affective judgments of faces modulate early activity (approximately 160 ms) within the fusiform gyri. Neuroimage 2002; 16(3 Pt 1):663–677.

44. Decety J, Perani D, Jeannerod M, et al. Mapping motor representations with positron emission tomography. Nature 1994; 371(6498):600–602.

45. Grafton ST, Arbib MA, Fadiga L, et al. Localization of grasp representations in humans by positron emission tomography. 2. Observation compared with imagination. Exp Brain Res 1996; 112(1):103–111.

46. Zald DH. The human amygdala and the emotional evaluation of sensory stimuli. Brain Res Rev 2003; 41(1):88–123.

47. Swanson LW, Petrovich GD. What is the amygdala? Trends Neurosci 1998; 21(8):323–331.

48. Kluver H, Bucy PC. Preliminary analysis of functions of the temporal lobes in monkeys. 1939. J Neuropsychiatry Clin Neurosci 1997; 9(4):606–620.

49. Shulman GL, Fiez JA, Corbetta M, et al. Common blood flow changes across visual tasks: II. Decreases in cerebral cortex. J Cogn Neurosci 1997; 9:648–663.

50. McKenna KE. Neural circuitry involved in sexual function. J Spinal Cord Med 2001; 24(3):148–154.

51. Devinsky O, Morrell MJ, Vogt BA. Contributions of anterior cingulate cortex to behaviour. Brain 1995; 118(Pt 1):279–306.

52. Dua S, Maclean PD. Localization for penile erection in medial frontal lobe. Am J Physiol 1964; 207:1425–1434.

53. Robinson BW, Mishkin M. Penile erection evoked from forebrain structures in Macaca mulatta. Arch Neurol 1968; 19(2):184–198.

54. Sumich AL, Kumari V, Sharma T. Neuroimaging of sexual arousal: research and clinical utility. Hosp Med 2003; 64(1):28–33.

55. Stoléru S, Mouras H, Rouxel R, et al. Neuroanatomical correlates of penile tumescence recorded through volumetric phallometry in an fMRI environment [abstract]. 9th International Conference on Functional Mapping of the Human Brain, Poster 78, New York, 2003.

56. Caggiula AR. Analysis of the copulation-reward properties of posterior hypothalamic stimulation in male rats. J Comp Physiol Psychol 1970; 70(3): 399–412.

57. Perachio AA, Marr LD, Alexander M. Sexual behavior in male rhesus monkeys elicited by electrical stimulation of preoptic and hypothalamic areas. Brain Res 1979; 177(1):127–144.

58. Makela JP, Illman M, Jousmaki V, et al. Dorsal penile nerve stimulation elicits left-hemisphere dominant activation in the second somatosensory cortex. Hum Brain Mapp 2003; 18(2):90–99.

59. Augustine JR. Circuitry and functional aspects of the insular lobe in primates including humans. Brain Res Rev 1996; 22(3):229–244.

60. Kell CA, von Kriegstein K, Rosler A, et al. The sensory cortical representation of the human penis: revisiting somatotopy in the male homunculus. J Neurosci 2005; 25(25):5984–5987.

61. Gerendai I, Toth IE, Boldogkoi Z, et al. Central nervous system structures labelled from the testis using the transsynaptic viral tracing technique. J Neuroendocrinol 2000; 12(11):1087–1095.

62. Lee S, Miselis R, Rivier C. Anatomical and functional evidence for a neural hypothalamic-testicular pathway that is independent of the pituitary. Endocrinology 2002; 143(11):4447–4454.

63. Kuban M, Barbaree HE, Blanchard R. A comparison of volume and circumference phallometry: response magnitude and method agreement. Arch Sex Behav 1999; 28(4):345–359.

64. McConaghy N. Validity and ethics of penile circumference measures of sexual arousal: a critical review. Arch Sex Behav 1989; 18(4):357–369.

5

Neuroendocrine Control of Male Erectile Function

K. E. Andersson

Wake Forest Institute for Regenerative Medicine, Wake Forest University School of Medicine, Winston-Salem, North Carolina, U.S.A.

□ INTRODUCTION

Penile erection is mediated by coordinated spinal activity in the autonomic pathways to the penis and in the somatic pathways to the perineal striated muscles. The process is initiated by the recruitment of afferent impulses, and after central processing and integration of tactile, visual, olfactory, and imaginative stimuli, the signals to the peripheral tissues involved are generated. This central regulation of penile erection (Fig. 1) involves many transmitters and transmitter systems, the details of which are still not completely known. Some of the anatomical areas of the brain that relate to sexual function have been defined, including the medial amygdala, medial preoptic area (MPOA), paraventricular nucleus (PVN), periaqueductal gray, and ventral tegmentum (1–3). Studies in rats have revealed that electrical stimulation of the MPOA (4), the PVN (5), or the hippocampal formation (6) can elicit an erectile response.

In the spine, there seems to be a network consisting of primary afferents from the genitals, spinal interneurons, and sympathetic, parasympathetic, and somatic nuclei. This network appears capable of integrating information from the periphery and eliciting reflexive erections and also of being the recipient of supraspinal information (7).

The balance between factors that control the degree of contraction of the smooth muscle of the corpora cavernosa determines the functional state of the penis. Despite intensive research during the last decade, many details of neurotransmission, impulse propagation, and intracellular transduction of signals in penile smooth muscles are yet to be elucidated.

As evidenced by several recent reviews, the information on both central and peripheral control mechanisms involved in erection is rapidly expanding, and new details are continuously added (1,8–15).

□ CENTRAL NEUROMEDIATION

The central mechanisms controlling erection include supraspinal as well as spinal pathways. The current knowledge about these mechanisms is largely based on experimental data from animals—mainly rats, in which oxytocin, dopamine, adrenocorticotropic hormone (ACTH)/α-melanocyte-stimulating hormones (α-MSH), and nitric oxide (NO) have a facilitatory role on erection, whereas serotonin may be either facilitatory or inhibitory, and enkephalins are inhibitory. Erections evoked by stimulation via dopamine agonists, oxytocin, ACTH/α-MSH, excitatory amino acids, and 5-hydroxytryptamine (5-HT) agonists are all dependent on the effects of androgens (Fig. 2) and disappear after castration. They are also dependent on NO (see below).

Oxytocin

Oxytocinergic spinal projections from the supraoptic and paraventricular nuclei of the hypothalamus are likely to influence the sacral autonomic outflow more than the somatic outflow (16,17). The finding that immunoreactive oxytocin-containing spinal neurons associate with sacral preganglionic neurons supports the idea that oxytocin has an important role in the autonomic spinal circuitry that mediates penile erection (18,19).

Oxytocin is a potent inducer of penile erection when injected into the lateral cerebral ventricle, the PVN, or the hippocampus of laboratory animals; intrathecal (i.t.) oxytocin can also initiate an erection. These erections can be blocked by the administration of oxytocin antagonists given intracerebroventricularly (i.c.v.) or intrathecally, or by electrolytic lesion of the PVN. Additionally, noncontact erections can be reduced by a selective oxytocin receptor antagonist administered into the lateral ventricles, which supports the view that oxytocin mediates this response (20).

Oxytocin increases NO production in the PVN (14,21), and NO synthase (NOS) inhibitors prevent penile erection and yawning in rats induced by oxytocin and also by dopamine, excitatory amino acids, the 5-HT$_{2C}$ receptor agonist, m-chlorophenylpiperazine (5-HT$_{2C}$ agonist, trazodone metabolite), and ACTH/α-MSH (Fig. 2). Yawning is a phylogenetically old, stereotyped event that occurs alone or associated with stretching and/or penile erection in humans and animals under different conditions (22). It has been suggested that NO acts as an intracellular, rather than an intercellular, modulator inside the paraventricular oxytocinergic neurons in which NO is formed to facilitate the expression of this phylogenetically old event

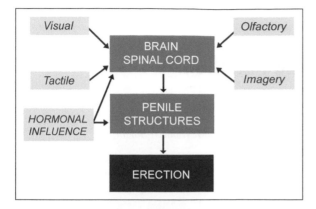

Figure 1 Penile erection is basically a spinal reflex controlled supraspinally, where erectile stimuli can be generated in response to visual, olfactory, and imaginative stimuli. Both centrally and peripherally, sexual hormones can influence erectile responses.

by guanylate cyclase-independent mechanisms (22,23). It is likely that this involves the parvocellular neuron population within the nucleus (24).

Plasma oxytocin concentrations are known to be elevated following sexual stimulation in humans (1); however, the relevance of the oxytocinergic pathway has never been established. This makes it of interest to explore the therapeutic potential of this system.

Dopamine

Central dopaminergic neurons project to the MPOA and the PVN (25). Furthermore, dopaminergic neurons that travel from the caudal hypothalamus to innervate the autonomic and somatic nuclei in the lumbosacral spinal cord have been identified (26,27). Thus, dopamine can be expected to participate in the regulation of both the autonomic and the somatic components of penile reflexes.

Both the major families of dopamine receptors, D1- (D1, D5) and D2-like receptors (D2, D3, and D4) (28), have been associated with central erectile functions;

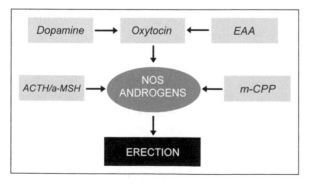

Figure 2 Androgens and nitric oxide play an essential role for erections evoked by central transmitters/mediators, including dopamine, oxytocin, EAA, ACTH/α-MSH, and 5-HT$_{2C}$ agonists (m-CCP). *Abbreviations*: EAA, excitatory amino acids; ACTH, adrenocorticotropic hormone; α-MSH, α-melanocyte–stimulating hormones; 5-HT, 5-hydroxytryptamine; m-CPP, m-chlorophenylpiperazine.

however, the D2-like receptor subtype seems to have the predominating effect. The nonselective dopamine receptor agonist, apomorphine, when administered systemically to male rats, was found to induce penile erection (29), simultaneously producing yawning and seminal emission. Similarly, low-dose systemic administration of other dopamine agonists initiates erection (1). The effects of these agonists can be attenuated by centrally, but not peripherally, acting dopamine receptor antagonists.

Injection of apomorphine into the MPOA demonstrated that low levels of dopaminergic stimulation, via D1 receptors in particular, facilitated erections (30). In contrast, dopaminergic antagonists injected into the MPOA decreased the number of penile reflexes (31,32). In the PVN, similar experiments have established that D2-like receptors rather than D1-like receptors primarily facilitate erections (1).

The erection following paraventricular D2-like-receptor stimulation apparently involves oxytocinergic neurotransmission. Dopaminergic neurons impinge on oxytocinergic cell bodies in the PVN (33,34), and apomorphine-induced penile erection is prevented dose dependently by oxytocin receptor antagonists (35) or by electrolytic lesions of the PVN that deplete the oxytocin content (36–38). Conversely, injection of oxytocin into the PVN induced erections that were not attenuated by dopamine receptor blockade, suggesting that dopaminergic neurons activate oxytocinergic neurons in the PVN and that released oxytocin then accounts for the erectile response. Martino et al. (39) investigated central oxytocinergic and dopaminergic mechanisms regulating penile erection in conscious rats and concluded that proerectile activity mediated via D2-like (D4?) receptors may be dependent on supraspinal and spinal oxytocin receptors, and that oxytocin-mediated erection (supraspinal and spinal) requires basal D2-like (D4) receptor activation. Brioni et al. (40) reported that the dopamine D4 receptor plays a role in the regulation of penile function using a selective dopamine D4 receptor agonist, ABT-724, with no effect on dopamine D1, D2, D3, or D5 receptors. ABT-724 dose-dependently facilitated penile erection when given subcutaneously (s.c.) to conscious rats, an effect that was blocked by haloperidol and clozapine (acting centrally and peripherally) but not by domperidone (acting only peripherally). A proerectile effect was observed after intracerebroventricular but not i.t. administration, suggesting a supraspinal site of action. The drug seemed to be without emetic effects in a ferret model of emesis (41), and it was suggested that ABT-724 could be useful for the treatment of erectile dysfunction (ED).

Injection of apomorphine into the lumbosacral subarachnoid space was reported to impair ex copula (i.e., outside the context of copulation) penile reflexes, slow the rate of copulation, and decrease the number of intromissions preceding ejaculation (42,43), suggesting an inhibitory effect on spinal erectile mechanisms. This is in contrast to recent findings showing that i.t.

injection of apomorphine in rats evokes erection in both normal animals and animals in which the spinal cord has been transected (44,45). Most likely, stimulation of the dopaminergic system can produce erection both at the supraspinal and at the spinal sites.

As mentioned above, systemically administered apomorphine enhances seminal emission. Pehek et al. (43) found that apomorphine injected into the PVN, but not in the MPOA, enhanced seminal emission. Recording of intracavernosal pressure in the nonanesthetized rat after systemic administration of apomorphine showed that the pressure response consisted of both smooth and striated muscle components (46). This implies that systemically given apomorphine has effects not only on the sacral parasympathetic output but also on somatic pathways.

ACTH and Related Peptides

Administered i.c.v., the ACTH and α-MSH are able to induce penile erection—along with grooming, stretching, and yawning (1,2,47). These effects are most probably mediated via stimulation of melanocortin (MC) receptors, of which five different subtypes have been cloned and characterized (48,49). α-MSH/ACTH seem to act in the hypothalamic periventricular region, and grooming, stretching, and yawning, but not penile erection, was reported to be mediated by MC_4 receptors (47,50). It is unclear, however, what MC receptor subtype(s) can be linked to the erectile responses. For example, the MC_3 receptor is found in high density in the hypothalamus and limbic systems (38), regions known to be important for erectile functions. The site and mechanism of action of α-MSH/ACTH seem to be different from those involving dopamine or oxytocin (8).

Martin and MacIntyre (51) concluded that current evidence indicates that the MC_4 receptor subtype contributes to the proerectile effects observed with MC pan-receptor agonists; however, the putative receptor subtypes, pathways, and mechanisms implicated in mediating the proerectile effects of MCs are yet to be fully elucidated.

Melanotan II, a synthetic analogue of α-MSH, when given s.c., was shown to have proerectile effects in men with psychogenic impotence (52). Still, the therapeutic potential of α-MSH analogues remains to be established (53–55).

Excitatory Amino Acids

Microinjections of L-glutamate into the MPOA elicit an increase in intracavernous pressure (4), and behavioral studies have shown that N-methyl-D-aspartate (NMDA) increases the number of penile erections when injected into the PVN (56–58). Furthermore, NMDA, amino-3-hydroxy-5-methyl-isoxazole-4-propionicacid, or trans-1-amino-1,3-cyclo-pentadicarboxylic acid increases intracavernosal pressures when injected into the PVN (59). The effect of NMDA was prevented by intracerebroventricular administration of an oxytocin antagonist (56). The NOS signal transduction pathway is considered to mediate the effect of NMDA. Injection of the amino acid leads to an increased concentration of NO metabolites in the PVN (60), and the administration of NOS inhibitors into the PVN and i.c.v. blocked the NMDA effect (56,61).

Nitric Oxide

Several investigators have shown that within the central nervous system (CNS), NO can modulate sexual behavior and penile erection (23,62–65). NO may act in several discrete brain regions, e.g., in the MPOA (64,65) and the PVN (5,50). NO production increases in the PVN of male rats during noncontact penile erections and copulation, confirming that NO is a physiological mediator of penile erection at the level of the PVN (63).

As mentioned previously, injection of NOS inhibitors i.c.v. or in the PVN prevents penile erectile responses induced by dopamine agonists, oxytocin, and NMDA in rats. NO may also mediate the actions of ACTH/α-MSH and $5-HT_{2C}$ agonists, which elicit erections when injected into the intracerebroventricular system, according to mechanisms unrelated to oxytocinergic neurotransmission (23). The inhibitory effect of NOS inhibitors was not observed when these compounds were injected concomitantly with L-arginine, the substrate for NO (23).

Serotonin

Neurons containing serotonin (5-HT) can be found in the medullary raphe nuclei and ventral medulla reticular formation, including the rostral nucleus paragigantocellularis, and bulbospinal neurons containing 5-HT project to the lumbar spinal cord in the rat and cat (1). Some serotonergic fibers occur in close apposition with sacral preganglionic neurons and motoneurons, and synapses were demonstrated at the ultrastructural level (19). These morphological findings support the involvement of 5-HT in both the supraspinal and the spinal pharmacology of erection, with participation in both the sympathetic and parasympathetic outflow mechanisms.

In animals, 5-HT seems to exert a general inhibitory effect on male sexual behavior (66), although the amine may be inhibitory or facilitatory depending upon its action at different sites and at different 5-HT receptors within the CNS (67,68). This may explain conflicting reports of 5-HT agonists either enhancing or depressing sexual function. Yonezawa et al. (69) found that p-chloroamphetamine, an indirect 5-HT agonist, elicited penile erection and ejaculation simultaneously in anesthetized rats. It was suggested that these effects were mainly produced by the release of 5-HT as limited to the lower spinal cord and/or peripheral sites. The use of selective 5-HT receptor agonists and antagonists can reveal different components of male copulatory behavior (11).

$5-HT_{2C}$ receptors seem to mediate erectile responses (70), and stimulation of $5-HT_{2C}$ receptors increased circulating oxytocin (71). NOS inhibitors given i.c.v. prevents 5-HT$_{2C}$ receptor–mediated erectile responses (23). These findings suggest that both oxytocin and NO are involved in 5-HT$_{2C}$ receptor–mediated erections.

Noradrenaline

The information on noradrenergic mechanisms involved in the central neuromediation of penile erection is sparse; however, the current data suggest that increased noradrenergic activity stimulates sexual function, whereas decreased noradrenergic activity inhibits it (66,72,73).

γ-Amino Butyric Acid

Cumulative data resulting from investigations on the role of γ-aminobutyric acid (GABA) in penile erection indicate that this neurotransmitter may function as an inhibitory modulator in the autonomic and somatic reflex pathways involved in penile erection (74). Activation of GABA (A) receptors in the PVN reduced apomorphine-, NMDA-, and oxytocin-induced penile erection and yawning in male rats (74).

Opioid Peptides

Available information supports the hypothesis that opioid μ receptor stimulation centrally prevents penile erection by inhibiting mechanisms that converge upon central oxytocinergic neurotransmission (1). In rats, morphine injected into the PVN prevents noncontact penile erections (i.e., when penile erection is induced in the male by the presence of an inaccessible receptive female) and impaired copulation. These morphine effects are apparently mediated by prevention of the increased NO production that occurs in the PVN during sexual activity (75). Morphine also prevents apomorphine- oxytocin-, NMDA- and noncontact-induced penile erection and yawning by inhibiting NOS activity in the PVN (76–78).

Prolactin

Long-term hyperprolactinemia can depress sexual behavior, reduce sexual potency in men, and depress genital reflexes in rats (67,79). Acute and chronic central prolactin treatment in rats, however, may have stimulatory and inhibitory effects on male sexual behavior, respectively (80). Correspondingly, striatal dopaminergic activity was shown to be increased and decreased by acute and five-day central prolactin treatment (80), supporting the view that the effects of prolactin are associated with changes in striatal dopaminergic activity. Prolactin has been shown to inhibit the dopaminergic incertohypothalamic pathway to the MPOA (81).

In humans, it is still unclear whether the negative effects of hyperprolactinemia on erectile function are mediated centrally by way of reduction in sexual interest and sex drive (82) or through a direct effect of prolactin on corpus cavernosum smooth muscle

contractility. In dogs, a direct effect on the corpus cavernosum was suggested (83). In any case, the effect seems independent of circulating testosterone levels and gonadal axis function (84).

Sexual Hormones

Androgens, particularly testosterone, are necessary (though not sufficient) for sexual desire in men. They are essential in the maintenance of libido and have an important role in regulating erectile capacity (85–89). In men with normal gonadal function, however, there is no correlation between circulating testosterone levels and measures of sexual interest, activity, or erectile function (90). Following castration in the male, which may reduce plasma testosterone levels by 90% (91), or other causes leading to a reduction in androgen levels, there is generally a decline in libido and sometimes in erectile and ejaculatory functions. Testosterone administration restores sexual interest and associated sexual activity in hypogonadal or castrated adult men (92–94). The testosterone dose–response relationships for sexual function and visuospatial cognition differ in older and young men, higher testosterone doses needed in the elderly for normal sexual functioning (89). When castration has been performed in humans, the resultant sexual function may range from a complete loss of libido to continued normal sexual activity. Thus, the role of androgens in erectile function is complex, and androgen deprivation may not always cause erectile impotence, either in man (95) or in rats (96).

In hypogonadal individuals, it is known that exogenous testosterone administration stimulates both sleep-related erections and erectile responses to visual erotic stimulation (97–99). Serum testosterone levels, however, have to fall to well below the lower end of the normal laboratory range before nocturnal penile tumescence is impaired (100). In healthy men, testosterone enhances sexual desire and the rigidity of nocturnal penile tumescence and leads to more rigid spontaneous erections with longer duration (99,101). It is therefore possible that testosterone acts on the motor neurons that supply the striated muscles of the penis. Spontaneous nocturnal erections are androgen dependent (85,102); they are impaired in states of androgen deficiency and restored with androgen replacement. Erections in response to visual erotic stimuli, on the other hand, are partly independent of androgens (102,103). They persist in hypogonadal men and are not altered by androgen replacement (104,97). Thus, there may be one androgen-dependent system in the brain subserving sexual arousability and sexual desire, and one androgen-independent system involving response to moving visual stimuli (85). Further, in normal individuals, it has been shown that there is a relationship between bioavailable testosterone and the frequency, duration, and degree of nocturnal penile tumescence (101,105). Other studies performed in eugonadal men have shown that high testosterone may promote sexual arousal with no significant changes in sexual activity (106). Several studies, however, suggest that testosterone replacement therapy in relatively modest deficiency states may improve erections in a minority of the patients (103,104,107,108).

Sexual hormones can induce structural changes in the nervous system, including alterations in cell size and number, neural connectivity, and neural sprouting (109–112). These changes, which may result in sex differences (sexual dimorphism), are obvious in most mammalian species during the prenatal or early postnatal periods. There is evidence, however, that brain regions containing sexual hormone–accumulating neurons in adult animals possess a considerable plasticity in response to sexual steroids, and that androgens have the potential to stimulate the growth of neuronal processes and remodel neural circuits also in the adult brain (113–115). Naturally occurring and socially induced changes in androgen levels were not shown to induce morphological changes of the motoneurons of the spinal nucleus of the bulbocavernosus muscle (116).

The MPOA of rats and the spinal nucleus of the bulbocavernosus (1) are sexually dimorphic model systems that have been well investigated. In humans, the localization and morphology of neurons innervating the small, striated pelvic muscles correspond to that of Onuf's nucleus X (117,118). This nucleus, similar to its rat homologue (the spinal nucleus of the bulbocavernosus), contains fewer motoneurons in the female than the male (119).

□ PERIPHERAL NEUROMEDIATION

The different structures of the penis receive sympathetic, parasympathetic, somatic, and sensory innervation (1,120). The nerves contain different transmitters, and the nerve populations have been categorized as adrenergic, cholinergic, and nonadrenergic, noncholinergic (NANC). It should be stressed that these nerves often contain more than one transmitter or transmitter/modulator generating enzymes, such as NOS and heme oxygenases. One important population of nerves in the corpora cavernosa contains not only acetylcholine (ACh), but also NOS, vasoactive intestinal polypeptide (VIP), and neuropeptide Y (121,122). If co-released, the different transmitters/modulators may interact, implying that the end result may be more complex than would be suggested from an experimental situation, where often the effect of a single agent is investigated.

It is not only the nerves but also the endothelium of the vasculature of the penis that produces and releases transmitters and modulators that can influence the contractile state of the corpus cavernosum smooth muscle. In addition, they may also have other important functions.

Noradrenaline and α-Adrenoceptors

It is generally accepted that the penis is kept in the flaccid state mainly via a tonic activity in adrenergic nerves

releasing noradrenaline (NA) (123). NA stimulates α-adrenoceptors (ARs) in the penile vasculature and in the corpus cavernosum, producing contraction. Both α_1- and α_2-ARs have been demonstrated in human corpus cavernosum tissue, but available information supports the view of a functional predominance of α_1-ARs. This may be the case also in the penile vasculature, although a contribution of α_2-ARs to the contraction induced by NA and electrical stimulation of nerves cannot be excluded (1).

The mRNAs of all the subtypes of α_1-AR with a high affinity for prazosin, α_{1A}, α_{1B} and α_{1D}, have been demonstrated in human corporal tissue. Goepel et al. (124), however, have shown that α_{1A}, α_{1B}, and α_{2A} receptor protein were predominantly expressed, and that the α_{1D} AR is present only at the mRNA level. The functional α_1-AR proteins in human corpus cavernosum tissue were characterized by Traish et al. (125) using receptor binding and isometric tension experiments. Their results demonstrated the presence of α_{1A}-, α_{1B}-, and α_{1D}-ARs, and they suggested that the NA-induced contraction in this tissue is mediated by two, or possibly three, receptor subtypes.

An additional α_1-AR subtype with low affinity for prazosin (α_{1L}), and which probably represents a conformational state of the α_{1A}-AR, has been suggested to be of importance in human penile erectile tissues (126). In rats, α_{1B}- and α_{1L}-AR subtypes seem functionally relevant for erectile function, and α_{1B}-, and/or α_{1L}-AR subtype selective antagonists were suggested to represent advantages in the treatment of ED (127). The distribution of α_1-AR subtypes in the penis and systemic vasculature, however, may not be the same in rats and humans, and the method of study may influence the results. For example, Hussain and Marshall (128) found that the α_{1D}-AR predominated in several systemic rat vessels in vitro, which may not be the case in humans (129). Similarly, Tong and Cheng (130) found α_{1A}-ARs to be responsible for the contractile response of rat corpus cavernosum, which does not seem to be in agreement with the in vivo data.

Expression of mRNA for α_{2A}-, α_{2B}-, and α_{2C}-ARs in whole human corpus cavernosum tissue has been demonstrated. Radioligand binding revealed specific α_2-AR binding sites, and functional experiments showed that the selective α_2-AR agonist, UK 14,304, induced concentration-dependent contractions of isolated strips of human corpus cavernosum smooth muscle (131). Whether or not these α_2-ARs are of importance for the contractile regulation of tone in corpus cavernosum smooth muscle is still unclear. Prejunctional α_2-ARs have been shown to inhibit stimulus-evoked release of NA from nerves in the human corpus cavernosum. Stimulation of prejunctional α_2-ARs in horse penile resistance arteries was also shown to inhibit NANC-transmitter release (132). This might be one of the mechanisms by which NA maintains detumescence.

Endothelins and Endothelin Receptors

Endothelins (ETs) have been demonstrated in penile erectile tissues and may contribute to the maintenance of corporal smooth muscle tone (1). Cultured endothelial cells from the human corpus cavernosum, but not non-endothelial cells, express ET-1 mRNA. In the endothelium of human cavernous tissue, intense ET-like immunoreactivity has been observed; immunoreactivity has also been observed in the cavernous smooth muscle. Binding sites for ET-1 have been demonstrated by autoradiography in the vasculature and cavernous tissue. As both ET_A and ET_B receptors have been found in human corporal smooth muscle membranes, it cannot be excluded that both receptor subtypes are functional.

ET-1 potently induces slowly developing, long-lasting contractions in different smooth muscles of the penis: corpus cavernosum, cavernous artery, deep dorsal vein, and penile circumflex veins (1). Contractions can also be evoked in human corpus cavernosus tissue by ET-2 and ET-3, although these peptides have a lower potency than ET-1 (133). The contractions induced by ET-1 are dependent on both transmembrane calcium flux (through voltage-dependent and/or receptor-operated calcium channels) and on the mobilization of inositol trisphosphate-sensitive intracellular calcium stores (1).

Even if much available in vitro information suggests that ETs may be of importance in erectile physiology and pathophysiology, the role of the peptides in vivo is unclear. Blockade of the ET_A or the ET_B receptor have no effect on the erectile response induced by maximal ganglionic stimulation in rats (134). This may seem to reflect a minimal role of ET-1 in the erectile response in the rat; however, the results do not rule out that ETs may play a role in keeping the penis in a flaccid state or that ETs may be associated with ED.

ETs may function not only as a long-term regulator of corporal smooth muscle tone but also as a modulator of the contractile effect of other agents, e.g., NA (135–137), or as a modulator of cellular proliferation and phenotypic expression (138).

ACh and Cholinergic Receptors

The importance of parasympathetic nerves for producing penile erection has been well established (1). Penile tissues from humans and several animal species are rich in cholinergic nerves (97–106), from which ACh can be released by transmural electrical field stimulation. In isolated corpus cavernosum cells, carbachol consistently produces contraction. This means that relaxation induced by ACh can be obtained either by inhibition of the release of a contractant factor, e.g., NA, and/or is produced by the release of a relaxation-producing factor, e.g., NO.

It is important to stress that parasympathetic nerve activity is not equivalent with the actions of ACh; other transmitters may be released from cholinergic nerves (121,122). Parasympathetic activity may produce penile tumescence and erection by inhibiting the release of NA through stimulation of muscarinic receptors on adrenergic nerve terminals, and/or by releasing NO and vasodilating peptides from nerves and endothelium.

NO and the Guanylate Cyclase/cGMP Pathway

It is widely accepted that NO plays an important role in the relaxation of the corpus cavernosum smooth muscle and vasculature (1,139). In vitro, several investigators have shown that both ACh- and neuronally mediated relaxation in animal and human corpus cavernosum involves the release of NO or an NO-like substance (1). Both the nerves (neuronal nNOS) and the endothelium (endothelial eNOS) of the corpus cavernosum may be the source of the NO, the former initiating erection, and the latter providing sustained maximal erection (140–142). The relative contribution of the different forms of NOS to erection has not been definitely established; however, more than one isoform of nNOS may be involved (141).

Mice lacking both eNOS and nNOS have erections, show normal mating behavior, and respond with erection to electrical stimulation of the cavernous nerves (141,143,144). Surprisingly, isolated corporal tissue from both wild-type and NOS-deleted animals have demonstrated similar responses to electrical stimulation; however, Hurt et al. (141) showed that alternatively spliced forms of nNOS are major mediators of penile erection.

Cyclic guanosine monophosphate (cGMP) signals via different receptors in eukaryotic cells, including ion channels, phosphodiesterases, and protein kinases. At present, the molecular targets that are activated by cGMP in order to execute the relaxation of penile smooth muscle are not known. Two different cGMP-dependent protein kinases (cGK I and II) have been identified in mammals. Inactivation of cyclic GMP-dependent protein kinase I (cGKI) in mice abolishes both NO/cGMP-dependent relaxation of vascular and intestinal smooth muscle and the inhibition of platelet aggregation, causing hypertension, intestinal dysmotility, and abnormal hemostasis (145).

Male mice deficient in cGKI seem to have very low reproductive capability, likely due to the markedly reduced ability of their corpus cavernosum tissues to relax in response to NO, whether it is neuronally or endothelially released or exogenously administered (146). Analysis of the NO/cGMP-induced relaxation clearly shows that cGKI is the major mediator of the cGMP-signaling cascade in murine corpus cavernosum tissue. Its absence cannot be compensated for by the cyclic adenosine monophosphate (cAMP) signaling cascade (146). Taken together, these findings suggest that activation of cGKI is a key step in the signal cascade leading to penile erection.

VIP and VIP Receptors

Mammalian penises are richly supplied with nerves containing VIP (120). The majority of these nerves also contain immunoreactivity to NOS, and colocalization of NOS and VIP within nerves innervating the penis of both animals and humans has been demonstrated by many investigators. It seems that most of these NO- and VIP-containing neurons are cholinergic, since they also contain vesicular acetylcholine transporter (121,122), which is a specific marker for cholinergic neurons. VIP receptors (types 1 and 2), linked via a stimulatory G protein to adenylyl cyclase, are considered to mediate the actions of the peptide (147). The importance of the different subtypes of VIP in penile tissues has not been clarified. VIP-related peptides (such as pituitary adenylyl cyclase-activating peptide, which has been found to be colocalized with VIP in penile nerves) seem to act through one of the VIP receptors. The stimulatory effect of VIP on adenylyl cyclase leads to an increase in cAMP, which in turn activates cAMP-dependent protein kinase.

Undeniably, VIP has both an inhibitory and a relaxing effect on strips of human corpus cavernosum tissue and cavernosal vessels in vitro, but it has been difficult to show convincingly that VIP released from nerves is responsible for relaxation of penile smooth muscle in vitro or in vivo (1,148). Thus, the role of VIP as a neurotransmitter or modulator of neurotransmission in the penis has not been established. Even if its physiological role in penile erection and in ED remains to be settled, VIP receptors in the penis are an interesting therapeutic target.

Prostanoids and Prostanoid Receptors

Human corpus cavernosum tissue has the ability to synthetize various prostanoids and the additional ability to metabolize them locally (1,149,150). The production of prostanoids can be modulated by oxygen tension and suppressed by hypoxia. Corresponding to the five primary active prostanoid metabolites [Prostaglandin D_2 (PGD_2), prostaglandin E_2 (PGE_2), prostaglandin $F_{2\alpha}$ ($PGF_{2\alpha}$), prostaglandin E_2 (PGI_2), and thromboxane A_2 (TXA_2)], there are five major groups of receptors that mediate their effects—the receptor for PGD_2 (DP), receptor for PGE_2 (EP), receptor for $PGF_{2\alpha}$ (FP), receptor for PGI_2 (IP), and receptor for TXA_2 (TP). cDNAs encoding representatives of each of these groups of receptors have been cloned, including several subtypes of EP receptors.

Penile tissues may contain most of these groups of receptors; however, their role in penile physiology is still far from established (149,150). Prostanoids may be involved in contraction of erectile tissues via $PGF_{2\alpha}$ and TXA_2, stimulating FP and TP receptors and initiating phosphoinositide turnover, as well as in relaxation via PGE_1 and PGE_2, stimulating EP receptors (EP2/EP4), and initiating an increase in the intracellular concentration of cAMP. Prostanoids may also be involved in the inhibition of platelet aggregation and white-cell adhesion, and recent data suggest that prostanoids and transforming growth factor-β_1 may have a role in the modulation of collagen synthesis and in the regulation of fibrosis of the corpus cavernosum (151).

The RhoA/Rho-Kinase Pathway

A major mechanism of the Ca^{2+} sensitization of smooth muscle contraction is through the inhibition of the smooth muscle myosin phosphatase (MLCP). The resulting myosin phosphorylation and subsequent smooth-muscle contraction therefore occurs without a change in sarcoplasmic Ca^{2+} concentration. Several studies have revealed important roles for the small GTPase RhoA and its effector, Rho-associated kinase (Rho kinase), in Ca^{2+}-independent regulation of smooth muscle contraction. The RhoA/Rho-kinase pathway modulates the level of phosphorylation of the myosin light chain of myosin II, mainly through inhibition of myosin phosphatase (152,153). This calcium-sensitizing RhoA/Rho-kinase pathway may also play a synergistic role in cavernosal vasoconstriction to maintain penile flaccidity (154). Rho-kinase is known to inhibit myosin light chain phosphatase, and to phosphorylate myosin light chains directly, altogether resulting in a net increase in activated myosin and the promotion of cellular contraction. Although Rho-kinase protein and mRNA have been detected in cavernosal tissue, the role of Rho-kinase in the regulation of cavernosal tone is not established. Using the Rho-kinase antagonist Y-27632, Chitaley et al. (155) examined the role of Rho-kinase in cavernosal tone, based on the hypothesis that antagonism of Rho-kinase results in increased corpus cavernosum pressure, initiating the erectile response independently of NO. They found that Rho-kinase antagonism stimulated rat penile erection independently of NO, and suggested that this principle could be a potential alternate avenue for the treatment of ED.

Since RhoA/Rho-kinase-mediated Ca^{2+} sensitization is important for regulation of smooth muscle contraction, increased RhoA/Rho-kinase activity may lead to abnormal contractility of the corpora cavernosa. Evidence has been presented that elevated RhoA/Rho-kinase activity contributes to the pathogenesis of diseases such as diabetes and hypertension and possibly to other conditions associated with ED, such as hypogonadism and aging (154). Several studies have suggested that NO inhibits RhoA/Rho-kinase activity (156–158), but the detailed mechanisms by which this regulation occurs are yet to be determined.

Theoretically, suppression of increased RhoA/Rho-kinase activity is an attractive therapeutic principle in ED; however, the ubiquitous occurrence of the Rho/Rho-kinase pathway limits the use of Rho-kinase inhibitors. If regulators of RhoA/Rho-kinase uniquely expressed in penile tissue can be demonstrated, they may be targets for drugs. This will potentially lead to the development of new therapeutic agents for the treatment of ED.

Sexual Hormones

The peripheral effects of sexual hormones on penile smooth muscle have not been established (86,87). Penile erectile tissue from patients undergoing gender reassignment operations after estrogen treatment have been used in several studies, including those focusing on receptor-mediated responses in human corpus cavernosum tissue. It has been claimed that hormonal treatment does not qualitatively change responses to drugs and electrical field stimulation (159,160); however, this is still open to discussion, since systematic comparisons between tissues from these patient groups and normal subjects have not been performed.

In vivo studies of castrated dogs suggest that androgen deficiency has direct effects on the function of the erectile tissues, resulting in a higher tonus of the detumescence factors that could be explained by an incomplete relaxation of the trabecular smooth muscle (161). In isolated human corpus cavernosum pretreated with testosterone for 30 minutes, testosterone appeared to have no effect on contraction or relaxation (162). On the other hand, castration enhanced NANC nerve-mediated relaxation in corpus cavernosum tissue from rabbits (163,164). Since the response to the NO donor morpholinosydnonimine (SIN-1) was the same in corpus cavernosum tissue from controls and castrated animals, it may be assumed that the responsiveness of the penile erectile tissue to NO was not changed. In castrated animals, however, there was a reduction in the release of NA from adrenergic nerves caused by electrical stimulation (164). The hormonal changes caused by castration, which include a change in the balance between androgens and estrogens, may additionally stimulate the synthesis and/or release of NO. The influence of androgens on erectile function may be mediated by the NO/cGMP pathway to a significant extent, even if non–NO-dependent pathways have been demonstrated (86,87).

The effects of castration and testosterone replacement on peripheral autonomic control of penile erection have been studied in dogs (165) and rats (166). The findings in the dog study suggest that castration and/or the resulting low plasma testosterone levels did not directly affect penile erectile ability through actions on peripheral nerves or corpora cavernosa. In the rat study, it was shown that castration reduced the erectile response and that testosterone could restore it. It was concluded from these experiments, which included preganglionic axotomy of the pelvic nerves, that testosterone enhances the erectile response to cavernous nerve stimulation acting peripherally to the spinal cord, with proerectile postganglionic parasympathetic neurons as the hormonal target (166).

Androgens may regulate the α-AR responsiveness of cavernous smooth muscle. Compared to normal rats, castrated animals showed an enhanced reactivity to α_1-AR stimulation (167). Androgens may also have important functions in the intrapenile mechanisms of erection. In the penis, androgen deprivation leads to smooth muscle cell apoptosis, a relative increase in connective tissue content, and a consequently reduced relaxation of the erectile tissue (86,168–171).

☐ CONCLUSION

The central regulation of the erectile process is still only partly known. Central transmitter systems, which seem to be dependent on androgens as well as NO, may be the targets of future drugs aimed at the treatment of ED. In penile erectile tissues, the different steps involved in neurotransmission, impulse propagation, and intracellular transduction of neural signals require further investigation. Increased knowledge of the central and peripheral changes associated with ED may lead to an increased understanding of these pathogenetic mechanisms and, therefore, new treatments and possibly even prevention of the disorder.

☐ REFERENCES

1. Andersson K-E, Wagner G. Physiology of penile erection. Physiol Rev 1995; 75(1):191–236.
2. Argiolas A. Neuropeptides and sexual behaviour. Neurosci Biobehav Rev 1999; 23(8):1127–1142.
3. Heaton JP. Central neuropharmacological agents and mechanisms in erectile dysfunction: the role of dopamine. Neurosci Biobehav Rev 2000; 24(5):561–569.
4. Giuliano F, Rampin O, Brown K, et al. Stimulation of the medial preoptic area of the hypothalamus in the rat elicits increases in intracavernous pressure. Neurosci Lett 1996; 209(1):1–4.
5. Chen KK, Chan SH, Chang LS, et al. Participation of paraventricular nucleus of hypothalamus in central regulation of penile erection in the rat. J Urol 1997; 158(1):238–244.
6. Chen KK, Chan JY, Chang LS, et al. Elicitation of penile erection following activation of the hippocampal formation in the rat. Neurosci Lett 1992; 141(2):218–222.
7. Giuliano F, Rampin O. Central neural regulation of penile erection. Neurosci Biobehav Rev 2000; 24(5):517–533.
8. Argiolas A, Melis MR. Neuromodulation of penile erection: an overview of the role of neurotransmitters and neuropeptides. Prog Neurobiol 1995; 47(4–5):235–255.
9. Rampin O, Bernabe J, Giuliano F. Spinal control of penile erection. World J Urol 1997; 15(1):2–13.
10. McKenna KE. Central nervous system pathways involved in the control of penile erection. Annu Rev Sex Res 1999; 10:157–183.
11. Andersson K-E, Burnett AL, Chen KK, et al. Current research and future therapies. In: Jardin A, Wagner G,

eds. 1st International Consultation on Erectile Dysfunction. UK: Plymbridge Distributors Ltd, 2000: 139–203.

12. Steers WD. Neural pathways and central sites involved in penile erection: neuroanatomy and clinical implications. Neurosci Biobehav Rev 2000; 24(5):507–516.

13. Andersson K-E, Argiolas A, Burnett A, et al. Future treatment targets. In: Lue TF, Basson R, Rosen R, et al., eds. Sexual Medicine. Sexual Dysfunctions in Men and Women. France: Health Publications, 2004:569–603.

14. Argiolas A, Melis MR. Central control of penile erection: role of the paraventricular nucleus of the hypothalamus. Prog Neurobiol 2005; 76(1):1–21.

15. Toda N, Ayajiki K, Okamura T. Nitric oxide and penile erectile function. Pharmacol Ther 2005; 106(2):233–266.

16. Tang Y, Rampin O, Giuliano F, et al. Spinal and brain circuits to motoneurons of the bulbospongiosus muscle: retrograde transneuronal tracing with rabies virus. J Comp Neurol 1999; 414(2):167–192.

17. Argiolas A, Melis MR. The role of oxytocin and the paraventricular nucleus in the sexual behaviour of male mammals. Physiol Behav 2004; 83(2):309–317.

18. Tang Y, Rampin O, Calas A, et al. Oxytocinergic and serotonergic innervation of identified lumbosacral nuclei controlling penile erection in the male rat. Neuroscience 1998; 82(1):241–224.

19. Veronneau-Longueville F, Rampin O, Freund-Mercier MJ, et al. Oxytocinergic innervation of autonomic nuclei controlling penile erection in the rat. Neuroscience 1999; 93(4):1437–1447.

20. Melis MR, Spano MS, Succu S, et al. The oxytocin antagonist d(CH2)5Tyr(Me)2-Orn8-vasotocin reduces noncontact penile erections in male rats. Neurosci Lett 1999; 265(3):171–174.

21. Melis MR, Succu S, Iannucci U, et al. Oxytocin increases nitric oxide production in the paraventricular nucleus of the hypothalamus of male rats: correlation with penile erection and yawning. Regul Pept 1997; 69(2):105–111.

22. Argiolas A, Melis MR. The neuropharmacology of yawning. Eur J Pharmacol 1998; 343(1):1–16.

23. Melis MR, Argiolas A. Role of central nitric oxide in the control of penile erection and yawning. Prog Neuropsychopharmacol Biol Psychiatry 1997; 21(6):899–922.

24. Kita I, Yoshida Y, Nishino S. An activation of parvocellular oxytocinergic neurons in the paraventricular nucleus in oxytocin-induced yawning and penile erection. Neurosci Res 2006; 54(4):269–275.

25. Björklund A, Lindvall O, Nobin A. Evidence of an incerto-hypothalamic dopamine neuron system in the rat. Brain Res 1975; 8(1)9:29–42.

26. Skagerberg G, Bjorklund A, Lindvall O, et al. Origin and termination of the diencephalo-spinal dopamine system in the rat. Brain Res Bull 1982; 9(1–6):237–244.

27. Skagerberg G, Lindvall O. Organization of diencephalic dopamine neurones projecting to the spinal cord of the rat. Brain Res 1985; 342(2):340–341.

28. Sibley DR. New insights into dopaminergic receptor function using antisense and genetically altered animals. Annu Rev Pharmacol Toxicol 1999; 39:313–341.

29. Benassi-Benelli A, Ferrari F, Quarrantotti BP. Penile erection induced by apomorphine and N-n-propylnorapomorphine in rats. Arch Int Pharmacodyn 1979; 242(2):241–247.

30. Hull EM, Eaton RC, Markowski VP, et al. Opposite influence of medial preoptic D1 and D2 receptors on genital reflexes: implications for copulation. Life Sci 1992; 51(22):1705–1713.

31. Pehek EA, Thompson JT, Eaton RC, et al. Apomorphine and haloperidol, but not domperidone, affect penile reflexes in rats. Pharmacol Biochem Behav 1988; 31(1):201–208.

32. Warner RK, Thompson JT, Markowski VP, et al. Microinjection of the dopamine antagonist cis-flupenthixol into the MPOA impairs copulation, penile reflexes and sexual motivation in male rats. Brain Res 1991; 540(1–2):177–182.

33. Buijs RM. Intra- and extrahypothalamic vasopressin and oxytocin pathways in the rat. Pathways to the limbic system, medulla oblongata and spinal cord. Cell Tissue Res 1978; 192(3):423–435.

34. Lindvall O, Björklund A, Skagerberg G. Selective histochemical demonstration of dopamine terminal systems in rat di- and telencephalon: new evidence for dopaminergic innervation of hypothalamic neurosecretory nuclei. Brain Res 1984; 306(1–2):19–30.

35. Argiolas A, Collu M, D'Aquila P, et al. Apomorphine stimulation of male copulatory behavior is prevented by the oxytocin antagonist d(CH2)5 Tyr(Me)-Orn8-vasotocin in rats. Pharmacol Biochem Behav 1989; 33(1):81–83.

36. Lang RE, Heil J, Ganten D, Herman K, et al. Effects of lesions in the paraventricular nucleus of the hypothalamus on vasopressin and oxytocin content in the brainstem and spinal cord of rat. Brain Res 1983; 260(2):326–329.

37. Hawthorn J, Ang VT, Jenkins JS. Effects of lesions in the hypothalamic paraventricular, supraoptic and suprachiasmatic nuclei on vasopressin and oxytocin in rat brain and spinal cord. Brain Res 1985; 346(1):51–57.

38. Argiolas A, Melis MR, Mauri A, et al. Paraventricular nucleus lesion prevents yawning and penile erection induced by apomorphine and oxytocin, but not ACTH 1–24. Brain Res 1987; 421:349–352.

39. Martino B, Hsieh GC, Hollingsworth PR, et al. Central oxytocinergic and dopaminergic mechanisms regulating penile erection in conscious rats. Pharmacol Biochem Behav 2005; 81(4):797–804.

40. Brioni JD, Moreland RB, Cowart M, et al. Activation of dopamine D4 receptors by ABT-724 induces penile erection in rats. Proc Natl Acad Sci USA 2004; 101(17):6758–6763.

41. Osinski MA, Uchic ME, Seifert T, et al. Dopamine D2, but not D4, receptor agonists are emetogenic in ferrets. Pharmacol Biochem Behav 2005; 81(1):211–219.

42. Pehek EA, Thompson JT, Hull EM. The effects of intracranial administration of the dopamine agonist apomorphine on penile reflexes and seminal emission in the rat. Brain Res 1989; 500(1–2):325–332.

43. Pehek EA, Thompson JT, Hull EM. The effects of intrathecal administration of the dopamine agonist apomorphine on penile reflexes and copulation in the male rat. Psychopharmacology (Berl) 1989; 99(3):304–308.

44. Giuliano FA, Allard J, Rampin O, Bernabé J. Proerectile effects of apomorphine delivered at the spinal level in anesthetized rat. Int J Imp Res 2000; 12(suppl 3):S66 [abstract A22].

45. Giuliano FA, Allard J, Rampin O, et al. Proerectile effects of systemic apomorphine: existence of a spinal site of action. 9th World Meeting on Impotence Research, Perth, Western Australia, Nov. 26–30, 2000; Int J Impotence Res 2000; 34:69.

46. Andersson K-E, Gemalmaz H, Waldeck K, et al. The effect of sildenafil on apomorphine-evoked increases in intracavernous pressure in the awake rat. J Urol 1999; 161(5):1707–1712.

47. Argiolas A, Melis MR, Murgia S, et al. ACTH- and alpha-MSH-induced grooming, stretching, yawning and penile erection in male rats: site of action in the brain and role of melanocortin receptors. Brain Res Bull 2000; 51(5):425–431.

48. Wikberg JE. Melanocortin receptors: perspectives for novel drugs. Eur J Pharmacol 1999; 375(1–3):295–310.

49. Wikberg JE, Muceniece R, Mandrika I, et al. New aspects on the melanocortins and their receptors. Pharmacol Res 2000; 42(5):393–420.

50. Vergoni AV, Bertolini A, Mutulis F, et al. Differential influence of a selective melanocortin MC4 receptor antagonist (HS014) on melanocortin-induced behavioral effects in rats. Eur J Pharmacol 1998; 362(2–3):95–101.

51. Martin WJ, MacIntyre DE. Melanocortin receptors and erectile function. Eur Urol 2004; 45(6):706–713.

52. Wessels H, Levine N, Hadley ME, et al. Melanocortin receptor agonists, penile erection, and sexual motivation: human studies with Melanotan II. Int J Imp Res 2000; 12(suppl 4):S74–S79.

53. Giuliano F. Control of penile erection by the melanocortinergic system: experimental evidences and therapeutic perspectives. J Androl 2004; 25(5):683–691.

54. Wessells H, Blevins JE, Vanderah TW. Melanocortinergic control of penile erection. Peptides 2005; 26(10): 1972–1977.

55. Giuliano F, Clement P, Droupy S, et al. Melanotan-II: Investigation of the inducer and facilitator effects on penile erection in anaesthetized rat. Neuroscience 2006; 138(1):293–301.

56. Melis MR, Stancampiano R, Argiolas A. Penile erection and yawning induced by paraventricular NMDA injection in male rats are mediated by oxytocin. Pharmacol Biochem Behav 1994; 48(1):203–207.

57. Melis MR, Stancampiano R, Argiolas A. Nitric oxide synthase inhibitors prevent N- methyl-D-aspartic acid-induced penile erection and yawning in male rats. Neurosci Lett 1994; 179(1–2):9–12.

58. Melis MR, Succu S, Spano MS, et al. Effect of excitatory amino acid, dopamine, and oxytocin receptor antagonists on noncontact penile erections and paraventricular nitric oxide production in male rats. Behav Neurosci 2000; 114(4):849–857.

59. Zahran AR, Vachon P, Courtois F, et al. Increases in intracavernous penile pressure following injections of excitatory amino acid receptor agonists in the hypothalamic paraventricular nucleus of anesthetized rats. J Urol 2000; 164(5):1793–1797.

60. Melis MR, Succu S, Iannucci U, et al. N-methyl-D-aspartic acid-induced penile erection and yawning: role of hypothalamic paraventricular nitric oxide. Eur J Pharmacol 1997; 328(2–3):115–123.

61. Argiolas A. Nitric oxide is a central mediator of penile erection. Neuropharmacology 1994; 33(11): 1339–1344.

62. Lorrain DS, Matuszewich L, Howard RV, et al. Nitric oxide promotes medial preoptic dopamine release during male rat copulation. Neuroreport 1996; 8(1): 31–34.

63. Melis MR, Succu S, Mauri A, et al. Nitric oxide production is increased in the paraventricular nucleus of the hypothalamus of male rats during non-contact penile erections and copulation. Eur J Neurosci 1998; 10(6): 1968–1974.

64. Sato Y, Horita H, Kurohata T, et al. Effect of the nitric oxide level in the medial preoptic area on male copulatory behavior in rats. Am J Physiol 1998; 274(1 Pt 2): R243– R247.

65. Sato Y, Christ GJ, Horita H, et al. The effects of alterations in nitric oxide levels in the paraventricular nucleus on copulatory behavior and reflexive erections in male rats. J Urol 1999; 162(6): 2182–2185.

66. Bitran D, Hull EM. Pharmacological analysis of male rat sexual behavior. Neurosci Biobehav Rev 1987; 11(4):365–389.

67. de Groat WC, Booth AM. Neural control of penile erection. In: Maggi CA, ed. The Autonomic Nervous System. Nervous Control of the Urogenital System. Vol. 6., London, UK: Harwood Academic Publishers, 1993:465–524.

68. Rehman J, Christ GJ, Melman A, et al. Intracavernous pressure responses to physical and electrical stimulation of the cavernous nerve in rats. Urology 1998; 51(4):640–644.

69. Yonezawa A, Watanabe C, Ando R, et al. Characterization of p-chloroamphetamine-induced penile erection and ejaculation in anesthetized rats. Life Sci 2000; 67(25):3031–3039.

70. Bancila M, Verge D, Rampin O, et al. 5-Hydroxytryptamine2C receptors on spinal neurons controlling penile erection in the rat. Neuroscience 1999; 92(4): 1523–1537.

71. Bagdy G, Kalogeras KT, Szemeredi K. Effect of 5-HT1C and 5-HT2 receptor stimulation on excessive grooming, penile erection and plasma oxytocin concentrations. Eur J Pharmacol 1992; 229(1):9–14.

72. Giuliano F, Rampin O. Central noradrenergic control of penile erection. Int J Impot Res 2000; 12(suppl 1): S13–S19.

73. Rampin O. Pharmacology of alpha-adrenoceptors in male sexual function. Eur Urol 1999; 36(suppl 1): 103–106.

74. Melis MR, Spano MS, Succu S, et al. Activation of gamma-aminobutyric acid(A) receptors in the paraventricular nucleus of the hypothalamus reduces apomorphine-, N-methyl-D-aspartic acid- and oxytocin-induced penile erection and yawning in male rats. Neurosci Lett 2000; 281(2–3):127–130.

75. Melis MR, Succu S, Spano MS, et al. Morphine injected into the paraventricular nucleus of the hypothalamus prevents noncontact penile erections and impairs copulation: involvement of nitric oxide. Eur J Neurosci 1999; 11(6):1857–1864.

76. Melis MR, Stancampiano R, Gessa GL, et al. Prevention by morphine of apomorphine- and oxytocin-induced penile erection: Site of action in the brain. Neuropsychopharmacology 1992; 6(1):17–21.

77. Melis MR, Succu S, Argiolas A. Prevention by morphine of N-methyl-D-aspartic acid-induced penile erection and yawning: involvement of nitric oxide. Brain Res Bull 1997; 44(6):689–694.

78. Melis MR, Succu S, Iannucci U, et al. Prevention by morphine of apomorphine- and oxytocin-induced penile erection and yawning: involvement of nitric oxide. Naunyn Schmiedebergs Arch Pharmacol 1997; 355(5):595–600.

79. Rehman J, Christ G, Alyskewycz M, et al. Experimental hyperprolactinemia in a rat model: alteration in centrally mediated neuroerectile mechanisms. Int J Impot Res 2000; 12(1):23–32.

80. Cruz-Casallas PE, Nasello AG, Hucke EE, et al. Dual modulation of male sexual behavior in rats by central prolactin: relationship with in vivo striatal dopaminergic activity. Psychoneuroendocrinology 1999; 24(7): 681–693.

81. Lookingland KJ, Moore KE. Effects of estradiol and prolactin on incertohypothalamic dopaminergic neurons in the male rat. Brain Res 1984; 323(1):83–91.

82. Carani C, Granata AR, Fustini MF, et al. Prolactin and testosterone: their role in male sexual function. Int J Androl 1996; 19(1):48–54.

83. Ra S, Aoki H, Fujioka T, et al. In vitro contraction of the canine corpus cavernosum penis by direct perfusion with prolactin or growth hormone. J Urol 1996; 156 (2 Pt 1):522–525.

84. Sato F, Aoki H, Nakamura K, et al. Suppressive effects of chronic hyperprolactinemia on penile erection and yawning following administration of apomorphine to pituitary-transplanted rats. J Androl 1997; 18(1):21–25.

85. Everitt BJ, Bancroft J. Of rats and men: the comparative approach to male sexuality. Annu Rev Sex Res 1991; 2:77–117.

86. Mills TM, Reilly CM, Lewis RW. Androgens and penile erection: a review. J Androl 1996; 17(6):633–638.

87. Mills TM, Lewis RW. The role of androgens in the erectile response: A 1999 perspective. Mol Urol 1999; 3:75–86.

88. Gooren LJ, Saad F. Recent insights into androgen action on the anatomical and physiological substrate of penile erection. Asian J Androl 2006; 8(1):3–9.

89. Gray PB, Singh AB, Woodhouse LJ, et al. Dose-dependent effects of testosterone on sexual function, mood, and visuospatial cognition in older men. J Clin Endocrinol Metab 2005; 90(7):3838–3846.

90. Krause W, Muller HH. Relation of sexual dysfunction to hormone levels, diseases and drugs used in andrological patients. Urol Int 2000; 64(3):143–148.

91. Walsh PC. Physiologic basis for hormonal therapy in carcinoma of the prostate. Urol Clin N Am 1975; 2(1): 125–140.

92. Davidson JM, Camargo CA, Smith ER. Effects of androgen on sexual behavior in hypogonadal men. J Clin Endocrinol Metab 1979; 48(6):955–958.

93. Skakkebaek NE, Bancroft J, Davidson DW, et al. Androgen replacement with oral testosterone undecanoate in hypogonadal men: a double blind controlled study. Clin Endocrinol (Oxf) 1981; 14(1):49–61.

94. O'Carroll R, Shapiro C, Bancroft J. Androgens, behaviour and nocturnal erection in hypogonadal men: the effects of varying the replacement dose. Clin Endocrinol (Oxf) 1985; 23(5):527–538.

95. Ellis WJ, Grayhack JT. Sexual function in aging males after orchiectomy and estrogen therapy. J Urol 1963; 89:895–899.

96. Hart BL. Testosterone regulation of sexual reflexes in spinal male rats. Science 1967; 155(767):1283–1284.

97. Kwan M, Greenleaf WJ, Mann J, et al. The nature of androgen action on male sexuality: a combined laboratory-self-report study on hypogonadal men. J Clin Endocrinol Metab 1983; 57(3):557–562.

98. Cunningham GR, Hirshkowitz M, Korenman SG, et al. Testosterone replacement therapy and sleep-related erections in hypogonadal men. J Clin Endocrinol Metab 1990; 70(3):792–797.

99. Rakic Z, Starcevic V, Starcevic VP, et al. Testosterone treatment in men with erectile disorder and low levels of total testosterone in serum. Arch Sex Behav 1997; 26(5):495–504.

100. Granata AR, Rochira V, Lerchl A, et al. Relationship between sleep-related erections and testosterone levels in men. J Androl 1997; 18(5):522–527.

101. Carani C, Zini D, Baldini A, et al. Effects of androgen treatment in impotent men with normal and low levels of free testosterone. Arch Sex Behav 1990; 19(3):223–234.

102. Carani C, Bancroft J, Granata A, et al. Testosterone and erectile function, nocturnal penile tumescence and rigidity, and erectile response to visual erotic

stimuli in hypogonadal and eugonadal men. Psychoneuroendocrinology 1992; 17(6):647–654.

103. Carani C, Granata AR, Bancroft J, et al. The effects of testosterone replacement on nocturnal penile tumescence and rigidity and erectile response to visual erotic stimuli in hypogonadal men. Psychoneuroendocrinology 1995; 20(7):743–753.

104. Bancroft J, Wu FC. Changes in erectile responsiveness during androgen therapy. Arch Sex Behav 1983; 12(1):59–66.

105. Schiavi RC, Schreiner-Engel P, White D, et al. The relationship between pituitary-gonadal function and sexual behavior in healthy aging men. Psychosom Med 1991; 53(4):363–374.

106. Anderson RA, Bancroft J, Wu FC. The effects of exogenous testosterone on sexuality and mood of normal men. J Clin Endocrinol Metab 1992; 75(6):1503–1507.

107. Morales A, Johnston B, Heaton JP, et al. Testosterone supplementation for hypogonadal impotence: assessment of biochemical measures and therapeutic outcomes. J Urol 1997; 157(3):849–854.

108. Morales A. Testosterone replacement: when is there a role? Int J Impot Res 2000; 12(suppl 4):S112–S118.

109. MacLusky NJ, Naftolin F. Sexual differentiation of the central nervous system. Science 1981; 211(4488): 1294–1302.

110. Arnold AP, Gorski RA. Gonadal steroid induction of structural sex differences in the central nervous system. Annu Rev Neurosci 1984; 7:413–442.

111. Kurz EM, Sengelaub DR, Arnold AP. Androgens regulate the dendritic length of mammalian motoneurons in adulthood. Science 1986; 232(4748):395–398.

112. Danzer SC, McMullen NT, Rance NE. Testosterone modulates the dendritic architecture of arcuate neuroendocrine neurons in adult male rats. Brain Res 2001; 890(1):78–85.

113. Arnold AP, Breedlove SM. Organizational and activational effects of sex steroids on brain and behavior: a reanalysis. Horm Behav 1985; 19(4):469–498.

114. Leedy MG, Beattie MS, Bresnahan JC. Testosterone-induced plasticity of synaptic inputs to adult mammalian motoneurons. Brain Res 1987; 424(2):386–390.

115. Matsumoto A, Micevych PE, Arnold AP. Androgen regulates synaptic input to motoneurons of the adult rat spinal cord. J Neurosci 1988; 8(11):4168–4176.

116. Beversdorf DQ, Kurz EM, Sengelaub DR. Sexual activity and the morphology of steroid-sensitive rat spinal motoneurons. Physiol Behav 1990; 47(1):11–17.

117. Onuf (Onufrowicz) B. On the arrangement and function of the cell groups of the sacral region of the spinal cord in man. Arch Neurol Psychpathol 1901; 3:387–412.

118. Schröder HD. Onuf's nucleus X: a morphological study of a human spinal nucleus. Anat Embryol (Berl) 1981; 162(4):443–453.

119. Forger NG, Breedlove SM. Sexual dimorphism in human and canine spinal cord: role of early androgen. Proc Natl Acad Sci USA 1986; 83(19):7527–7531.

120. Dail WG. Autonomic innervation of male reproductive genitalia. In Maggi CA, ed. The Autonomic Nervous System. Nervous Control of the Urogenital System. Vol. 6. London, UK: Harwood Academic Publishers, 1993:69–101.

121. Hedlund P, Alm P, Andersson K-E. NO synthase in cholinergic nerves and NO-induced relaxation in the rat isolated corpus cavernosum. Br J Pharmacol 1999; 127(2):349–360.

122. Hedlund P, Ny L, Alm P, Andersson K-E. Cholinergic nerves in human corpus cavernosum and spongiosum contain nitric oxide synthase and heme oxygenase. J Urol 2000; 164(3 Pt 1):868–875.

123. Andersson KE, Hedlund P, Alm P. Sympathetic pathways and adrenergic innervation of the penis. Int J Impot Res 2000; 12(S1):S5–S12.

124. Goepel M, Krege S, Price DT, et al. Characterization of alpha-adrenoceptor subtypes in the corpus cavernosum of patients undergoing sex change surgery. J Urol 1999; 162(5):1793–1799.

125. Traish AM, Netsuwan N, Daley J, et al. A heterogeneous population of alpha 1 adrenergic receptors mediates contraction of human corpus cavernosum smooth muscle to norepinephrine. J Urol 1995; 153(1): 222–227.

126. Davis B, Chapple C, Chess-Williams R. The a1L-adrenoceptor mediates contraction in human erectile tissue. Eur J Urol 1999; 35(suppl 2):102 [abstract 406].

127. Sironi G, Colombo D, Poggesi E, et al. Effects of intracavernous administration of selective antagonists of alpha(1)-adrenoceptor subtypes on erection in anesthetized rats and dogs. J Pharmacol Exp Ther 2000; 292(3):974–981.

128. Hussain MB, Marshall I. Characterization of alpha1-adrenoceptor subtypes mediating contractions to phenylephrine in rat thoracic aorta, mesenteric artery and pulmonary artery. Br J Pharmacol 1997; 122(5): 849–858.

129. Rudner XL, Berkowitz DE, Booth JV, et al. Subtype specific regulation of human vascular alpha(1)-adrenergic receptors by vessel bed and age. Circulation 1999; 100(23):2336–2343.

130. Tong YC, Cheng JT. Subtyping of alpha1-adrenoceptors responsible for the contractile response in the rat corpus cavernosum. Neurosci Lett 1997; 228(3): 159–162.

131. Gupta S, Moreland RB, Yang S, et al. The expression of functional postsynaptic alpha2-adrenoceptors in the corpus cavernosum smooth muscle. Br J Pharmacol 1998; 123(6):1237–1245.

132. Simonsen U, Prieto D, Hernandez M, et al. Prejunctional alpha 2-adrenoceptors inhibit nitrergic neurotransmission in horse penile resistance arteries. J Urol 1997; 157(6):2356–2360.

133. Saenz de Tejada I, Carson MP, De las Morenas A, et al. Endothelin: localization, synthesis, activity, and receptor types in human penile corpus cavernosum. Am J Physiol 1991; 261(4 Pt 2):H1078–H1085.

134. Dai Y, Pollock DM, Lewis RL, et al. Receptor-specific influence of endothelin-1 in the erectile response of the rat. Am J Physiol Regul Integr Comp Physiol 2000; 279(1):R25–R30.

135. Holmquist F, Andersson K-E, Hedlund H. Actions of endothelin on isolated corpus cavernosum from rabbit and man. Acta Physiol Scand 1990; 139(1):113–122.

136. Christ GJ, Lerner SE, Kim DC, et al. Endothelin-1 as a putative modulator of erectile dysfunction: I. Characteristics of contraction of isolated corporal tissue strips. J Urol 1995; 153(6):1998–2003.

137. Kim DC, Gondre CM, Christ GJ. Endothelin-1-induced modulation of contractile responses elicited by an alpha 1-adrenergic agonist on human corpus cavernosum smooth cells. Int J Impot Res 1996; 8(1):17–24.

138. Zhao W, Christ GJ. Endothelin-1 as a putative modulator of erectile dysfunction. II. Calcium mobilization in cultured human corporal smooth muscle cells. J Urol 1995; 154(4):1571–1579.

139. Burnett AL. Nitric oxide in the penis: physiology and pathology. J Urol 1997; 157(1):320–324.

140. Hurt KJ, Musicki B, Palese MA, et al. Akt-dependent phosphorylation of endothelial nitric-oxide synthase mediates penile erection. Proc Natl Acad Sci USA 2002; 99(6):4061–4066.

141. Hurt KJ, Sezen SF, Champion HC, et al. Alternatively spliced neuronal nitric oxide synthase mediates penile erection. Proc Natl Acad Sci USA 2006; 103(9): 3440–3443.

142. Musicki B, Burnett AL. eNOS function and dysfunction in the penis. Exp Biol Med (Maywood). 2006; 231(2):154–65.

143. Burnett AL, Nelson RJ, Calvin DC, et al. Nitric oxide-dependent penile erection in mice lacking neuronal nitric oxide synthase. Mol Med 1996; 2(3):288–296.

144. Burnett AL, Chang AG, Crone JK, et al. Noncholinergic penile erection in mice lacking the gene for endothelial nitric oxide synthase. J Androl 2002; 23(1):92–97.

145. Pfeifer A, Klatt P, Massberg S, et al. Defective smooth muscle regulation in cGMP kinase I-deficient mice. EMBO J 1998; 17(11):3045–3051.

146. Hedlund P, Aszodi A, Pfeifer A, et al. Erectile dysfunction in cyclic GMP-dependent kinase I-deficient mice. Proc Natl Acad Sci USA 2000; 97(5):2349–2354.

147. Fahrenkrug J. Transmitter role of vasoactive intestinal peptide. Pharmacol Toxicol 1993; 72(6):354–363.

148. Okamura T, Ayajiki K, Toda N. Monkey corpus cavernosum relaxation mediated by NO and other relaxing factor derived from nerves. Am J Physiol 1998; 274 (4 Pt 2):H1075–H1081.

149. Minhas S, Cartledge J, Eardley I. The role of prostaglandins in penile erection. Prostaglandins Leukot Essent Fatty Acids 2000; 62(3):137–146.

150. Khan MA, Thompson CS, Sullivan ME, et al. The role of prostaglandins in the aetiology and treatment of erectile dysfunction. Prostaglandins Leukot Essent Fatty Acids 1999; 60(3):169–174.

151. Moreland RB, Traish A, McMillin MA, et al. PGE1 suppresses the induction of collagen synthesis by transforming growth factor beta 1 in human corpus cavernosum smooth muscle. J Urol 1995; 153(3 Pt 1): 826–834.

152. Somlyo AP; Somlyo AV. Signal transduction by G-proteins, rho-kinase and protein phosphatase to smooth muscle and non-muscle myosin II. J Physiol 2000; 522(Pt 2):177–185.

153. Fukata Y, Amano M, Kaibuchi K, et al. Rho-Rho-kinase pathway in smooth muscle contraction and cytoskeletal reorganization of non-muscle cells. Trends Pharmacol Sci 2001; 22(1):32–39.

154. Jin L, Burnett AL. RhoA/Rho-kinase in erectile tissue: mechanisms of disease and therapeutic insights. Clin Sci (Lond) 2006; 110(2):153–165.

155. Chitaley K, Wingard CJ, Clinton Webb R, et al. Antagonism of Rho-kinase stimulates rat penile erection via a nitric oxide-independent pathway. Nat Med 2001; 7(1):119–122.

156. Sauzeau V, Le Jeune H, Cario-Toumaniantz C, et al. Cyclic GMP-dependent protein kinase signaling pathway inhibits RhoA-induced Ca^{2+} sensitization of contraction in vascular smooth muscle. J Biol Chem 2000; 275(28):21722–21729.

157. Sauzeau V, Rolli-Derkinderen M, Marionneau C, et al. Rho A expression is controlled by nitric oxide through cGMP-dependent protein kinase activation. J Biol Chem 2003; 278(11):9472–9480.

158. Sawada N, Itoh H, Yamashita J, et al. cGMP dependent protein kinase phosphorylates and inactivates RhoA. Biochem Biophys Res Commun 2001; 280(3):798–805.

159. Adaikan PG, Karim SM. Adrenoreceptors in the human penis. J Auton Pharmacol 1981; 1(3):199–203.

160. Hedlund H, Andersson KE. Comparison of the responses to drugs acting on adrenoreceptors and muscarinic receptors in human isolated corpus cavernosum and cavernous artery. J Auton Pharmacol 1985; 5(1):81–88.

161. Muller SC, Hsieh JT, Lue TF, et al. Castration and erection. An animal study. Eur Urol 1988; 15(1–2): 118–124.

162. Kimura K, Hashine K, Tamura M, et al. Effect of testosterone on contraction and relaxation of isolated human corpus cavernosum tissue. Int J Impotence Res 1990; 2(suppl 1):53.

163. Andersson KE, Holmquist F, Bodker A. Castration enhances NANC nerve-mediated relaxation in rabbit isolated corpus cavernosum. Acta Physiol Scand 1992; 146(3):405–406.

164. Holmquist F, Persson K, Bodker A, et al. Some pre- and postjunctional effects of castration in rabbit isolated corpus cavernosum and urethra. J Urol 1994; 152(3):1011–1016.

165. Lin SN, Yu PC, Huang JK, et al. Castration may not affect the penile erection ability in terms of peripheral neurocavernous mechanism in dogs. J Urol 1990; 143(1):172–174.

166. Giuliano F, Rampin O, Schirar A, et al. Autonomic control of penile erection: modulation by testosterone in the rat. J Neuroendocrinol 1993; 5(6):677–683.

167. Reilly CM, Stopper VS, Mills TM. Androgens modulate the alpha-adrenergic responsiveness of vascular smooth muscle in the corpus cavernosum. J Androl 1997; 18(1):26–31.

168. Baskin LS, Sutherland RS, DiSandro MJ, et al. The effect of testosterone on androgen receptors and human penile growth. J Urol 1997; 158(3 Pt 2):1113–1118.

169. Shabsigh R. The effects of testosterone on the cavernous tissue and erectile function. World J Urol 1997; 15(1):21–26.

170. Shabsigh R, Raymond JF, Olsson CA, et al. Androgen induction of DNA synthesis in the rat penis. Urology 1998; 52(4):723–728.

171. Traish AM, Park K, Dhir V, et al. Effects of castration and androgen replacement on erectile function in a rabbit model. Endocrinology 1999; 140(4): 1861–1868.

6

Sex Hormones and Male Sexual Behavior

Kim Wallen and Franklynn C. Graves

Department of Psychology and Yerkes National Primate Research Center, Emory University, Atlanta, Georgia, U.S.A.

☐ INTRODUCTION

The study of sexual behavior is subjected to the same scientific analysis as any other behavioral system. This objectivity about sexual behavior has allowed investigators to divest the subject of some of its social trappings, enabling the clearer understanding and analysis of the role of hormones in modulating sexual behavior. It is becoming increasingly apparent that, aside from regulating fertility, the most profound effects of gonadal hormones on both males and females are psychological. Hormones influence both sexual interest in others and the willingness to engage in sexual activity. The former, heavily mechanistic view of the endocrinology of sexual behavior, in which hormones statically regulated the expression of stereotyped sexual patterns, has been enlarged and adapted to a more modern view in which hormones set the basic responsiveness of individuals to their sexual environment, with the final pattern of response then to be determined by the current context and the individual's history and motivational state. According to this view, hormones are not seen as the sole regulators of sexual behavior but instead are integral parts of the complex of social and physiological systems that coordinate sexual behavior within the contexts of society and the biology of reproduction.

Traditionally, the study of male sexual behavior has been predominantly focused on the conspicuous physical changes that occur in males during sexual arousal. Thus, the occurrence of penile erection has been the focus of many studies of male sexual activity. Because sexual intercourse for males requires erections, the effects of specific drugs or hormonal preparations tend to be assessed for their impact on erectile function. It has only been in the last 20 years, however, that male sexual motivation has been investigated independently of erectile function. The increased focus on male sexual desire has resulted primarily from the finding that hypogonadal males have significantly lower frequencies of spontaneous nocturnal erections [nocturnal penile tumescence (NPT)] but are able to produce erections in response to erotic stimuli as readily as do males with normal gonadal function (1–4). Conversely, androgen therapy of hypogonadal males increases NPT frequency but has no effects on erectile response to erotic stimuli

(1,2,5); notably, androgen therapy also increases both maximum penile rigidity and circumference attained (4). The suppression of male androgens to those levels seen in castrated males significantly reduces their sexual desire (6,7). Thus, androgens do not appear to be responsible for making it physically possible for a male to engage in sexual activity but instead influence the male's interest in engaging in sexual activity. In this regard, the role of steroid hormones in modulating sexual activity is remarkably similar in men and women, even though the physical differences in genital changes during sexual activity are markedly different.

Male sexual behavior has been extensively studied in a number of mammalian species. In all these species, testicular function has been found to be necessary for the full male copulatory pattern of mounting, intromission, and ejaculation. Species do differ, however, in the extent to which the removal of testicular androgens will eliminate the facets of male sexual function. The case in human males is less well understood, but strong similarities to many aspects of the nonhuman data are suggested.

☐ TESTICULAR FUNCTION, SEXUAL MOTIVATION, AND PENILE STRUCTURE
Rodents

It has long been known that in nonprimate species, male sexual behavior is completely dependent upon the functioning of the male testes. Castration produces a complete disappearance of sexual behavior, but unlike the effect of ovariectomy in nonprimate females, male sexual behavior gradually declines following gonadectomy rather than ceasing immediately (8). Early quantification of postcastration behavioral change in male rats (9) noted that sexual behavior declined in an orderly progression, with ejaculation disappearing first, followed by intromission, mounting, and finally interest in a sexually receptive female. Another early study noted that the decline in behavior was associated with a change in the surface of the glans penis, which is normally rough due to the presence of keratinaceous penile papillae (10). Castration causes these spines to slough off, and their failure to regenerate results in the eventual appearance of a smooth glans penis (10). When testosterone therapy is given to castrated males, sexual behavior is reinstated, with the components returning in the reverse of the order in which they disappeared, restoring penile papillae to the male's glans penis. The orderly disappearance of the components of sexual behavior and associated changes to the glans penis combined with the restoration of both behavior and penile morphology by testosterone has led to the suggestion that the postcastration decline in behavior results from reduced sensory feedback from a penis deprived of testosterone stimulation (9). This view suggests an important role for penile sensitivity and function for male sexual behavior and the consequently lesser role of hormones in influencing male sexual motivation. Although other work in male rats has described the importance of arousal mechanisms in male sexual behavior (11), the connection between male testicular function and male sexual interest in females was not made until relatively recently (12).

When it was discovered that androgens other than testosterone are responsible for the maintenance of penile structure without maintaining male sexual behavior, it became apparent that male testicular hormones only partially influence penile sensory feedback. Whalen and Luttge (13) found that although 5α-dihydrotestosterone (DHT)—an androgen that cannot be metabolized to estrogen—restored penile morphology following castration, it did not reinstate male sexual behavior. In contrast, 19-hydroxytestosterone—an androgen that can be converted to estrogen, but not DHT—restored male sexual behavior without completely reinstating penile structure. These findings suggest that conversion of testosterone to estrogen is important for the maintenance of male sexual functioning. This idea, termed the "aromatization hypothesis," has gained support in a number of species in which it has been shown that aromatization blockers administered to intact males eliminate sexual behavior [Japanese quail (14); zebra finches (15); hamsters (16); ferrets (17); rats (18,19)].

Although the effects of androgens on penile structure may not be of primary importance in maintaining male rat sexual behavior, penile feedback is of critical importance to male rats. If penile sensitivity is reduced by anesthetic (20,21) or dorsal nerve transection (22), male rats will continue to mount but will fail to achieve erections, resulting in decreased intromissions and ejaculations. Thus, penile feedback is important for the full copulatory sequence, but cannot account for changes in mounting and interest in the female following castration.

There is evidence that testosterone directly affects the sexual motivation of male rats. Sachs and colleagues (23) determined that male rats will display erections in response to estrous females, even if the females are inaccessible. Males with intact gonads display noncontact erections (NCE) in approximately 50% of the exposures to inaccessible estrous females; however, following castration, the males no longer show any response (24). Males that were given any type of androgen replacement (testosterone, DHT, or DHT + estradiol) showed a restoration of NCE, while males treated with estradiol or a control treatment did not differ from castrated males (24). These data suggest that androgens, and not estrogens, are the important steroid for male sexual motivation in rats.

In male guinea pigs, the role of penile sensitivity in the maintenance of male sexual behavior is less apparent. Reducing penile sensitivity via topical anesthetic only affects the temporal patterning of male copulatory behavior but does not eliminate either ejaculation or intromissions (Slimp JC. Personal communication. Sept. 1976). As in the rat, castration in this species produces a gradual disappearance of male sexual behavior that is reinstated with testosterone therapy (25). In contrast to the male rat, treatment of castrated male guinea pigs with either testosterone or DHT reinstates male sexual behavior (26). Similarly, treatment of castrated male guinea pigs with testosterone and an aromatase blocker still reinstated sexual behavior (27,28). Thus, aromatization is apparently not involved in the maintenance or restoration of male guinea pig sexual behavior.

Nonhuman Primates

Nonhuman primates show both similarities and marked differences to the previously described rodent species in the regulation of male sexual behavior. As with rodents, aspects of male primate sexual function are dependent upon testicular function. The exact relationship, however, continues to elude investigators, because no one has convincingly demonstrated that the level of male sexual activity can be predicted from circulating steroid levels. The most striking difference between nonprimates and primates has been reported for macaque males in relation to the effect of castration. Castration reduces overall frequencies of mating in three species of macaques—rhesus monkeys (29,30), stumptail macaques (31), and cynomolgous monkeys (32); however, rhesus males continue to intromit and show ejaculatory reflexes even after castration for at least six years (33). Castration does not remove the ability of the male to produce erections, and, unlike the rat, transection of the dorsal nerves of the penis does not interfere with erections and intromissions, although it virtually eliminates ejaculation (34). Whether more subtle changes in penile sensory feedback, such as those produced by local anesthesia, would affect male sexual behavior has not been investigated. One new world monkey, the common marmoset, possesses penile spines similar to those found in male rats that may possibly provide genital sensory feedback. In this species, neonatal castration completely eliminates adult sexual activity, which is reversed by testosterone administration (35). The removal of the penile spines in intact males, however, does not eliminate either intromission or ejaculation but does significantly increase the amount of time needed to intromit after mounting as well as the number of mountings in which the males fail to achieve intromission (36). Unlike male rats, transection of the penile nerves or spine removal in male marmosets does not alter the occurrence of mountings or erections (36,37). Thus, it appears that genital sensory feedback may be less critical in primates for erections than in some rodent species.

In contrast to many rodents but similar to guinea pigs, either DHT or testosterone restores male sexual behavior after castration in nonhuman primates (29,33). In addition, the androgen 19-hydroxytestosterone, which can be aromatized to estrogen but cannot be 5α-reduced to DHT, does not restore sexual behavior in castrated male rhesus macaques, suggesting that aromatization is not important for rhesus male sexual behavior (38). Similarly, estradiol does not maintain the sexual behavior of castrated rhesus males and actually interferes with their ability to intromit (39). Therefore, estrogenic metabolites of testosterone do not appear to have a role in male rhesus sexual behavior. Responsiveness to DHT for the restoration of male sexual behavior, however, is not necessarily a primate characteristic, because physiological levels of DHT do not restore the sexual behavior of castrated crab-eating macaques (*Macaca cynomolgous*) (40). The poorer restoration of male sexual behavior with DHT in cynomolgous monkeys possibly stems from a role in this species of estrogenic metabolites of testosterone in male sexual behavior. Although the evidence is not particularly convincing, blocking the production of estrogenic metabolites of testosterone with a nonsteriodal aromatase inhibitor, fadrozole, significantly reduces ejaculatory frequency (32). In only three of six males, however, did supplementary estradiol reverse the decrement in ejaculations. The degree to which estrogenic metabolites of testosterone are necessary for the maintenance of male sexual behavior in this species is still unclear. It seems apparent that testosterone acting on an androgen receptor is probably the primary gonadal steroid influencing male sexual behavior in nonhuman primates.

Work using gonadotropin-releasing hormone (GnRH) agonists and antagonists to suppress testicular function in rhesus monkeys has demonstrated that, at least for this species, the extent to which the suppression of testicular function will reduce or eliminate sexual behavior depends upon the social context. When male testicular function is suppressed in a multimale group, it produces a significant reduction in male sexual behavior within one week (41). This is in contrast to the seven-week minimum required to produce a significant decline following castration in male–female pairs (29). Interestingly, testicular suppression in a single-male/multiple-female group setting requires a period of time intermediate to that required in pair tests and multimale groups to produce a significant decline in behavior (42). This social context effect is observed most clearly in two males who were used in the following testicular suppression studies (41,42). In the multifemale social group, these males continued to routinely mate even after four weeks of testicular suppression. These same males, however, stopped mating one week after testicular suppression when tested in a multimale group (41). Thus, the opportunity for intrasexual competition seems to influence how tightly coupled sexual behavior is to gonadal function.

Humans

The regulation of sexual behavior in human males shares much in common with the findings from rhesus monkeys: there is no clear relationship between circulating levels of androgen and frequency of sexual activity. The administration of exogenous testosterone to eugonadal men does not increase levels of sexual activity or sexual interest (43,44). It is only when androgen titers fall into the castrated range that a relationship between androgens and sexual activity becomes apparent (45), despite the fact that castrated males often continue to engage in sexual activity—albeit at a reduced level (46). Empirical evidence does strongly support the idea that testicular hormones primarily influence male sexual interest and not the ability to perform sexually. Castrated male sex offenders were asked to estimate their level of sexual intercourse and masturbation before and after castration (46). Although castration reduced both types of sexual activity significantly, the effect on masturbation was significantly greater than that on intercourse. Since masturbation is more dependent upon the male's own sexual desire while intercourse can be in response to the interest of his partner, this finding suggests that castration primarily affects sexual interest and not the ability to engage in sex.

Recently, there has been an increasing focus on the effects of declining levels of androgens in older men. From puberty through old age, men experience a marked decline in circulating androgen levels (47). An increase in symptoms spanning physical, psychological, and sexual domains in aging men has been dubbed "andropause," and testosterone replacement therapy has been suggested as a means of treatment (48). It is unclear, however, if the decline in androgens is truly the causative agent in the increase of these symptoms, or if the symptoms are related to the aging process either directly or through other factors associated with aging, such as complications of illnesses. In aging men, there is no apparent correlation between circulating levels of total testosterone and NPT, but there is a significant correlation between bioavailable testosterone and NPT (49,50); the total amount of testosterone in circulation does not predict erectile function, but rather it is the amount of testosterone that is unbound, or readily accessible for cellular use, that is critical. These data suggest that although the total level of androgens decline with age, as long as the bioavailable testosterone remains sufficient, the relationship between androgens and sexual function seen in young men can be seen in aging men, as well. Nevertheless, some aspect of the aging process itself appears to influence sexual functioning. Although aging males report greater difficulties with erectile function, these symptoms are not related to androgen levels (51–53). Thus, androgen replacement therapy in aging men is not likely to improve erectile function. Sexual desire, however, is correlated with levels of bioavailable testosterone (48). Thus, the hormonal relationship between androgens and sexual interest appears to be the same in aging men as is seen in young men.

The view that testicular steroids regulate male sexual motivation has received support in studies demonstrating that hypogonadal males with castrate levels of testosterone developed erections to sexually explicit films as rapidly as and maintained the erections longer than normal control males (1,2,4,5). These hypogonadal males, who readily responded to erotic stimulation, showed lower frequencies of NPT. Interestingly, androgen therapy increased NPT to control levels but did not influence the occurrence of erections to erotic stimuli. In addition, androgen therapy did not affect penile circumference to stimulation, but it did increase the rigidity of the erection (4). These results demonstrate that the basic capacity to produce an erection in response to erotic stimulation is not under gonadal control, although androgens influence some of the specific characteristics of the erection. In contrast, the frequency of NPT appears to be regulated by an androgen-dependent mechanism (1,2,4,5). The relationship between androgen-regulated spontaneous erection and male sexual function is unclear. The spontaneous occurrence of NPT suggests that it is psychogenically generated and thus may be an external indicator of the male's underlying level of sexual motivation—which itself is strongly influenced by gonadal steroids.

Studies of male sexual function have only recently begun to focus specifically on male sexual motivation instead of measures such as erection or sexual intercourse frequency. When investigators have measured male sexual interest, they have consistently found it to be influenced by androgen levels. Two studies have examined the effect of androgen replacement in hypogonadal males on measures of sexual motivation. The use of testosterone gel or injections of gonadotropin or testosterone enanthate (TE) have all resulted in a reported increase in libido, sexual motivation, and desire (3,54). Although intriguing, these data provide no information on the role of endogenous testosterone in healthy men. The most striking evidence of the effect of testicular androgens on male sexual motivation comes from studies investigating GnRH antagonists as possible male contraceptives. In human males, as in monkeys, these compounds rapidly suppress testicular function by blocking the release of luteinizing hormone and follicle-stimulating hormone from the anterior pituitary. Circulating androgen levels fall to castrated levels within the first week after GnRH antagonist administration (6). Castrated levels of testosterone can also be attained with GnRH agonists (55). Male sexual interest and desire, frequency of sexual fantasy, and sexual intercourse decline rapidly

following the decline in testosterone (7,55,56). Exogenously maintaining testosterone at intact levels during GnRH antagonist therapy prevents any significant decline in male libido (6,7,55).

A study by Bagatell (7) presented evidence that estrogenic metabolites of testosterone are not involved in human male sexual motivation. Suppression of testicular function with a GnRH antagonist produced a significant drop in male sexual desire within four weeks that could be prevented by concurrent administration of 50 to 100 mg of TE. Administration of the aromatization inhibitor Teslac to males receiving the GnRH antagonist and TE reduced circulating estradiol levels by 60% to levels comparable to the GnRH antagonist group without TE treatment. Yet, even with significantly reduced estradiol levels, these males reported no significant decreases in sexual desire or any other measure of male sexual motivation or behavior. Further, a review of case studies indicated that men with congenital estrogen deficiency have no sexual dysfunction (57), suggesting that estrogen does not influence male sexual functioning. Thus, it appears that, like the rhesus monkey and the guinea pig, sexual motivation in human males does not rely upon the aromatization of testosterone to its estrogenic metabolites. Unfortunately, no one has yet undertaken clinical studies of the capacity of DHT to prevent a decline in male sexual motivation during GnRH antagonist treatment. Thus, it is still unclear whether DHT acting as testosterone can stimulate male sexual motivation in man, similar to what has been observed in the male guinea pig.

Considered together, these studies demonstrate that the primary effect of androgen is to modulate male sexual motivation, with minimal effect on the male's capacity to engage in sex. This finding is of particular importance when considering possible endocrine therapies to deal with both erectile difficulties and male sex offenders. Erectile failure in response to erotic stimulation is highly unlikely to result from androgen insufficiency or be responsive to androgen therapy. In contrast, if erectile difficulties in a sexual context are also associated with low frequencies of NPT, this may be amenable to androgen therapy, unless the organic difficulty physically prevents blood-flow changes necessary to produce an erection. Similarly, treatments for sex offenders designed to reduce sexual motivation may effectively employ manipulations of gonadal function and androgen action. Such treatments, however, are unlikely to remove the male's capacity to become aroused in a sexual context or prevent the capacity to engage in penetrative sexual offenses.

☐ PHARMACOLOGICAL INTERFERENCE WITH TESTICULAR FUNCTION

The discovery of androgen receptor blockers such as cyproterone acetate (CA) and flutamide have ushered in an era of pharmacological methods to control male sexual functioning in the hopes of creating humane treatments for male sex offenders. Although these compounds dramatically eliminate male sexual behavior when administered to rats and guinea pigs, their effects in primates, both nonhuman and human, are less clear. The single study in rhesus monkeys reports that daily administration of CA reduces but does not eliminate male ejaculatory behavior after several weeks of treatment (58). In contrast, long-term administration of CA to male stumptail macaques had no detectable effect upon their sexual behavior (59). Administration of medroxyprogesterone acetate (MPA) to castrated testosterone-treated male cynomolgous monkeys significantly reduced but did not eliminate male sexual behavior (60). Some of this lack of effect may result from the social conditions of testing or may reflect the incomplete action of these compounds. The results in humans suggest these compounds influence male sexual interest but may have little effect on the ability to engage in sex.

Bancroft et al. (61) studied the effect of administering CA to males who had voluntarily admitted themselves for various sexual concerns, ranging from pedophilia to excessive sexual demands upon their wives. CA treatment markedly decreased sexual desire and interest, but it had no effect on erections in response to sexually explicit materials. Similarly, Cooper (62) found that CA reduced sexual interest besides reducing spontaneous sexual activity. Thus, the treatment of sex offenders with androgen receptor blockers may decrease the male's interest in seeking out sexual situations but may have no effect on his responsiveness if he is in the presence of his preferred sexual stimulus. The hope for a simple treatment that will make males uninterested in sex as well as incapable of producing erections seems unlikely.

Hypersexuality, as described in the clinical literature, typically refers to deviant or compulsive sexual behavior. The exact meaning of the term, however, is unclear because it has been used to refer to the selection of socially inappropriate sexual stimuli, a discordance between levels of sexual desire in a couple and even extremely frequent masturbation (62,63). This lack of precision in the use of this term makes it difficult to reach general conclusions about its cause or treatment. However, if hypersexuality refers to compulsive sexual behavior of high frequency or disturbing intensity, it seems that therapies that reduce endogenous testosterone production or action may reduce the compulsive aspects of this sexuality. The androgen receptor blocker CA, as previously described, reduces male sexual desire and has been reported to effectively reduce compulsive sexual behavior (62,63). Similarly, Gagne's study (64) of MPA treatment in sexual offenders reported a reduction in the compulsive aspects of these male's behavior and fantasies. Treatment with a GnRH agonist suppressed testicular function, reduced reported sexual desire and fantasy, and reduced the occurrence of male paraphilias within the first month of treatment (65–67). Thus, to the extent to which hypersexuality results from

excessive or compulsive sexual desire, antiandrogen therapies reduce the occurrence or intensity of this hypersexuality.

It is interesting that hypersexuality is almost exclusively a male domain, with exceedingly few reports of female compulsive sexuality. This may partly reflect the fact that male hypersexuality can easily take the form of illegal, assaultive–insertive sexual activity, whereas female hypersexuality, if it exists, is not viewed as potentially dangerous, and thus it is of less social concern. Alternatively, male deviant hypersexuality may be an extreme manifestation of an underlying gender difference in sexual desire. For example, in a study of Danish women, almost one-third reported having never experienced spontaneous sexual desire (68). Similarly, the National Health and Social Life Survey (69) reported that 33.4% of women reported a "… period of several months or more …" in which they lacked sexual interest, in contrast to 15.7% of men. Additionally, women are significantly more likely than men to report hypoactive sexual desire disorder (HSDD) (70). A difference between males and females in the routine level of sexual desire could also influence the frequency of sexual activity. Supporting evidence comes from a comparison of the frequency of sexual activity between heterosexual and lesbian couples in whom the sexual activity of the latter is uninfluenced by male sexual motivation. Two-thirds of long-term heterosexual couples had sex weekly; in contrast, only one-third of long-term lesbian couples had sexual encounters that frequently (71). Furthermore, 85% of heterosexual couples but only 53% of lesbian couples engaged in sex once per month or more (71). While these results may reflect differences in sexual motivation between lesbian and heterosexual women, it is more likely that these differences actually reflect the influence of male sexual interest on the occurrence of sex. This possible sex difference in sexual motivation is probably not one of degree but of constancy (72,73). Males, exposed to relatively constant levels of gonadal steroids, experience relatively constant levels of sexual desire. In contrast, women experience marked cyclical changes in gonadal steroids that produce dramatic changes in the level of sexual desire (72,73). Thus, peak sexual desire probably does not differ between men and women, but longer periods of relative sexual disinterest experienced by women may psychologically buffer them from developing the sort of hypersexuality sometimes seen in males. For further information on sexual differences between males and females, see Chapter 11.

□ MALE SEXUAL DYSFUNCTION

Historically, male sexual dysfunction has been synonymous with erectile failure. In fact, male erectile capacity is so intimately identified with male sexual identity that erectile failure is often referred to as impotence, even though it should not realistically have such a profound impact on a male's life. Although female sexual dysfunction is no longer referred to as "frigidity," the use of "impotence" is still common, illustrating how penile functioning is still intrinsically connected to other psychological aspects of male experience (74). In addition, though much attention has been devoted to many aspects of female sexual dysfunction, including orgasmic dysfunction, arousal difficulties, and low sexual desire, male sexual dysfunction has primarily focused on erectile difficulties, and to a lesser extent, low sexual desire.

Erectile failure now appears to be completely unrelated to steroid levels but may, in fact, be either psychogenic in origin or related to organic causes such as the circulatory consequences of diabetes or other disorders affecting the control of blood flow through the penis. Studies demonstrating undiminished erectile capacity in hypogonadal males have clearly demonstrated that in normal males, androgen levels are not required to produce erections capable of intromitting (1,2,4,5). Erectile failure in a sexual context similarly appears to be completely unrelated to steroid levels. Bancroft and Wu (5) suggest that the erectile failure seen by clinicians in hypogonadal males may be psychogenically induced as a result of performance anxiety in males with low sexual interest. This finding is further supported by studies in aging men. Although erectile dysfunction becomes more likely with increasing age, there is no apparent relationship between erectile function and circulating hormone levels (49,51). Thus, although erection and male hormones are intimately linked in common parlance, there actually appears to be little relationship between these two male characteristics.

A more recently characterized male sexual dysfunction is HSDD. The classification of this problem as a dysfunction of desire has been valuable in that it focuses attention on sexual interest and avoids the catchall term "impotence," which confounds sexual desire and sexual performance, making it difficult to determine the primary dysfunction. HSDD occurs significantly less frequently in males than in females, and males tend to experience HSDD when older than females (70). Unlike female cases, HSDD in males appears to be related to lower levels of androgen. This may be the result of hypogonadism or age-related declines in testicular function (49). Schiavi et al. (75) reported significantly lower nocturnal erections and nocturnal levels of testosterone in 17 HSDD males than in 17 matched controls. Furthermore, nocturnal testosterone level in HSDD males, but not in control males, was positively correlated to sexual behavior frequency, suggesting a role for androgen deficiency in this disorder for males. In cases in which HSDD appears related to declines in androgen, hormonal therapy often successfully reverses HSDD (76). There are, however, cases of HSDD in which hypoandrogenicity can be ruled out as well as other endocrinopathies such as hyperprolactinemia (77), and no clear cause can be determined. Clearly, as in the female, male sexual desire is determined by multiple causes, but there does appear to be a more direct relationship between androgen levels and sexual desire for men, even if the two are not always strictly correlated.

□ CONCLUSIONS

Separating male sexual desire from erectile functioning has transformed the understanding of the role of hormones in male sexuality. Although the published information is only slowly becoming generally known, the evidence now overwhelmingly supports the notion that androgens primarily affect male sexual desire and not erectile capacity. Thus, gonadal hormones in humans act primarily on motivational systems and not on the physical mechanisms that allow sexual intercourse to occur. In this regard, human males differ from males of many mammalian species but may yet bear striking similarities to nonhuman primates in the way that hormones regulate sexual behavior. Unlike nonhuman primates, human male sexuality also is strongly influenced by social expectations that may be adversely affected by an individual male's expectations and his need to function normally. Hormonal therapy still appears to be effective only in those cases with clear evidence of endocrine deficiency, and many aspects of male sexuality are unresponsive to hormonal treatment. An understanding of the pivotal role that hormones play in male sexual motivation, but not erectile capability, should result in the reevaluation of expectations for the effectiveness of antiandrogen treatments for male sex offenders. It is unwarranted to think that these treatments will ever prevent a sexually aggressive male from committing further offenses when presented with provocative circumstances. More realistically, it is possible that these treatments, by reducing the male's level of sexual interest, will reduce the likelihood that the male sex offender will seek out the contexts in which such offenses previously occurred, thus reducing recidivism.

☐ REFERENCES

1. Kwan M, Greenleaf WJ, Mann J, et al. The nature of androgen action on male sexuality: a combined laboratory-self-report study on hypogonadal men. J Clin Endocrinol Metab 1983; 57(3):557–562.
2. Carani C, Bancroft J, Granata A, et al. Testosterone and erectile function, nocturnal penile tumescence and rigidity, and erectile response to visual erotic stimuli in hypogonadal and eugonadal men. Psychoneuroendocrinology 1992; 17(6):647–654.
3. Clopper RR, Voorhess ML, MacGillivray MH, et al. Psychosexual behavior in hypopituitary men: a controlled comparison of gonadotropin and testosterone replacement. Psychoneuroendocrinology 1993; 18(2): 149–161.
4. Carani C, Granata AR, Bancroft J, et al. The effects of testosterone replacement on nocturnal penile tumescence and rigidity and erectile response to visual erotic stimuli in hypogonadal men. Psychoneuroendocrinology 1995; 20(7):743–753.
5. Bancroft J, Wu FC. Changes in erectile responsiveness during androgen replacement therapy. Arch Sex Behav 1983; 12(1):59–66.
6. Pavlou SN, Brewer K, Farley MG, et al. Combined administration of a gonadotropin-releasing hormone antagonist and testosterone in men induces reversible azoospermia without loss of libido. J Clin Endocrinol Metab 1991; 73(6):1360–1369.
7. Bagatell CJ, Dahl KD, Bremner WJ. The direct pituitary effect of testosterone to inhibit gonadotropin secretion in men is partially mediated by aromatization to estradiol. J Androl 1994; 15(1):15–21.
8. Young WC. The hormones and mating behavior. In: Young WC, ed. Sex and Internal Secretions. Baltimore: Williams & Wilkins, 1961:1173–1239.
9. Beach F, Levinson G. Effects of androgen on the glans penis and mating behavior of castrated rats. J Exp Zool Lond 1950; 114:159–171.
10. Phoenix CH, Copenhaver KH, Brenner RM. Scanning electron microscopy of penile papillae in intact and castrated rats. Horm Behav 1976; 7(2):217–227.
11. Beach FA. Analysis of the stimuli adequate to elicit mating behavior in the sexually inexperienced male rat. J Comp Psychol 1942; 33:163–207.
12. Everitt BJ. Sexual motivation: a neural and behavioural analysis of the mechanisms underlying appetitive and copulatory responses of male rats. Neurosci Biobehav Rev 1990; 14(2):217–232.
13. Whalen RE, Luttge WG. Testosterone, androstenedione and dihydrotestosterone: effects on mating behavior of male rats. Horm Behav 1971; 2:117–125.
14. Watson JT, Adkins-Regan E. Testosterone implanted in the preoptic area of male Japanese quail must be aromatized to activate copulation. Horm Behav 1989; 23(3):432–447.
15. Walters MJ, McEwen BS, Harding CF. Estrogen receptor levels in hypothalamic and vocal control nuclei in the male zebra finch. Brain Res 1988; 459(1): 37–43.
16. Steel E, Hutchison JB. Behavioral action of estrogen in male hamsters: effect of the aromatase inhibitor, 1,4,6-androstatriene-3,17-dione (ATD). Horm Behav 1988; 22(2):252–265.
17. Carroll RS, Weaver CE, Baum MJ. Evidence implicating aromatization of testosterone in the regulation of male ferret sexual behavior. Physiol Behav 1988; 42:457–460.
18. Sodersten P, Eneroth P, Hansson T, et al. Activation of sexual behaviour in castrated rats: the role of oestradiol. J Endocrinol 1986; 111(3):455–462.
19. Kaplan ME, McGinnis MY. Effects of ATD on male sexual behavior and androgen receptor binding: a reexamination of the aromatization hypothesis. Horm Behav 1989; 23(1):10–26.
20. Adler N, Bermant G. Sexual behavior of male rats: effects of reduced sensory feedback. J Comp Physiol Psychol 1966; 61(2):240–243.
21. Carlsson SG, Larsson K. Mating in male rats after local anesthetization of the glans penis. Z Tierpsychol 1964; 21:854–856.
22. Larsson K, Sodersten P. Mating in male rats after section of the dorsal penile nerve. Physiol Behav 1973; 10(3):567–571.
23. Sachs BD, Akasofu K, Citron JH, et al. Noncontact stimulation from estrous females evokes penile erection in rats. Physiol Behav 1944; 55(6):1073–1079.
24. Manzo J, Cruz MR, Hernandez ME, et al. Regulation of noncontact erection in rats by gonadal steroids. Horm Behav 1999; 35(3):264–270.
25. Grunt J, Young WC. Consistency of sexual behavior patterns in individual male guinea pigs following castration and androgen therapy. J Comp Physiol Psychol 1953; 46(2):138–144.
26. Alsum P, Goy RW. Actions of esters of testosterone, dihydrotestosterone, or estradiol on sexual behavior in castrated male guinea pigs. Horm Behav 1974; 5(3):207–217.
27. Roy MM, Goy RW. Sex differences in the inhibition by ATD of testosterone-activated mounting behavior in guinea pigs. Horm Behav 1988; 22(3):315–323.
28. Roy MM. Effects of prenatal testosterone and ATD on reproductive behavior in guinea pigs. Physiol Behav 1992; 51(1):105–109.
29. Phoenix CH, Slob AK, Goy RW. Effects of castration and replacement therapy on sexual behavior of adult male rhesuses. J Comp Physiol Psychol 1973; 84(3):472–481.
30. Michael RP, Wilson M. Effects of castration and hormone replacement in fully adult male rhesus monkeys (Macaca mulatta). Endocrinology 1974; 95(1): 150–159.

31. Schenck PE, Slob AK. Castration, sex steroids, and heterosexual behavior in adult male laboratory-housed stumptailed macaques (*Macaca arctoides*). Horm Behav 1986; 20(3):336–353.

32. Zumpe D, Bonsall RW, Michael RP. Effects of the nonsteroidal aromatase inhibitor, fadrozole, on the sexual behavior of male cynomolgus monkeys (*Macaca fascicularis*). Horm Behav 1993; 27(2):200–215.

33. Phoenix CH. Effects of dihydrotestosterone on sexual behavior of castrated male rhesus monkeys. Physiol Behav 1974; 12(6):1045–1055.

34. Herbert J. The role of the dorsal nerves of the penis in the sexual behaviour of the male rhesus monkey. Physiol Behav 1973; 10:293–300.

35. Dixson AF. Effects of testosterone propionate upon the sexual and aggressive behavior of adult male marmosets (Callithrix jacchus) castrated as neonates. Horm Behav 1993; 27(2):216–230.

36. Dixson AF. Penile spines affect copulatory behaviour in a primate (Callithrix jacchus). Physiol Behav 1991; 49(3):557–562.

37. Dixson AF. Effects of dorsal penile nerve transection upon the sexual behaviour of the male marmoset (Callithrix jacchus). Physiol Behav 1988; 43(2):235–238.

38. Phoenix CH. Sexual behavior of castrated male rhesus monkeys treated with 19-hydroxytestosterone. Physiol Behav 1976; 16(3):305–310.

39. Michael RP, Zumpe D, Bonsall RW. Estradiol administration and the sexual activity of castrated male rhesus monkeys (*Macaca mulatta*). Horm Behav 1990; 24(1):71–88.

40. Michael RP, Bonsall RW, Zumpe D. Testosterone and its metabolites in male cynomolgus monkeys (Macaca fascicularis): behavior and biochemistry. Physiol Behav 1987; 40(4):527–537.

41. Wallen K, Eisler JA, Tannenbaum PL, et al. Antide (nallys GnRH antagonist) suppression of pituitary-testicular function and sexual behavior in group-living rhesus monkeys. Physiol Behav 1991; 50(2):429–435.

42. Davis-daSilva M, Wallen K. Suppression of male rhesus testicular function and sexual behavior by a gonadotropin-releasing-hormone agonist. Physiol Behav 1989; 45(5):963–968.

43. Anderson RA, Bancroft J, Wu FC. The effects of exogenous testosterone on sexuality and mood of normal men. J Clin Endocrinol Metab 1992; 75(6):1503–1507.

44. Schiavi RC, White D, Mandeli J, et al. Effect of testosterone administration on sexual behavior and mood in men with erectile dysfunction. Arch Sex Behav 1997; 26(3):231–241.

45. Davidson JM, Camargo CA, Smith ER. Effects of androgens on sexual behavior in hypogonadal men. J Clin Endocrin Metab 1979; 48:955–958.

46. Heim N. Sexual behavior of castrated sex offenders. Arch Sex Behav 1981; 10(1):11–19.

47. Dabbs JM Jr. Age and seasonal variation in serum testosterone concentration among men. Chronobiol Int 1990; 7(3):245–249.

48. Lund BC, Bever-Stille KA, Perry PJ. Testosterone and andropause: the feasibility of testosterone replacement therapy in elderly men. Pharmacotherapy 1999; 19(8):951–956.

49. Schiavi RC, Schreiner-Engel P, White D, et al. The relationship between pituitary-gonadal function and sexual behavior in healthy aging men. Psychosom Med 1991; 53(4):363–374.

50. Schiavi RC, White D, Mandeli J, et al. Hormones and nocturnal penile tumescence in healthy aging men. Arch Sex Behav 1993; 22(3):207–215.

51. Rhoden EL, Teloken C, Mafessoni R, et al. Is there any relation between serum levels of total testosterone and the severity of erectile dysfunction? Int J Impot Res 2002; 14(3):167–171.

52. T'Sjoen G, Goemaere S, De Meyere M, et al. Perception of males' aging symptoms, health and well-being in elderly community-dwelling men is not related to circulating androgen levels. Psychoneuroendocrinology 2004; 29(2):201–214.

53. Christ-Crain M, Mueller B, Gasser TC, et al. Is there a clinical relevance of partial androgen deficiency of the aging male? J Urol 2004; 172(2):624–627.

54. Steidle C, Schwartz S, Jacoby K, et al. AA2500 testosterone gel normalizes androgen levels in aging males with improvements in body composition and sexual function. J Clin Endocrinol Metab 2003; 88(6):2673–2681.

55. Schmidt PJ, Berlin KL, Danaceau MA, et al. The effects of pharmacologically induced hypogonadism on mood in healthy men. Arch Gen Psychiatry 2004; 61: 997–1004.

56. Loosen PT, Purdon SE, Pavlou SN. Effects on behavior of modulation of gonadal function in men with gonadotropin-releasing hormone antagonists. Am J Psychiatry 1994; 151(2):271–273.

57. Rochira V, Balestrieri A, Madeo B, et al. Congenital estrogen deficiency: in search of the estrogen role in human male reproduction. Mol Cell Endocrinol 2001; 178(1–2):107–115.

58. Michael RP, Plant TM, Wilson MI. Preliminary studies on the effects of cyproterone acetate on sexual activity and testicular function in adult male rhesus monkeys (*Macaca mulatta*). Adv Biosci 1972; 10:197–208.

59. Slob AK, Schenck PE. Chemical castration with cyproterone acetate (Androcur) and sexual behavior in the laboratory-housed male stumptailed macaque (*Macaca arctoides*). Physiol Behav 1981; 27(4):629–636.

60. Michael RP, Zumpe D. Medroxyprogesterone acetate decreases the sexual activity of male cynomolgus monkeys (*Macaca fascicularis*): an action on the brain? Physiol Behav 1993; 53(4):783–788.

61. Bancroft J, Tennent TG, Loucas K, et al. Control of deviant sexual behaviour by drugs. I. Behavioural changes following oestrogens and anti-androgens. Brit J Psychiat 1974; 125(0):310–315.

62. Cooper AJ. A placebo-controlled trial of the antiandrogen cyproterone acetate in deviant hypersexuality. Compr Psychiatry 1981; 22(5):458–465.

63. Cooper AJ, Ismail AA, Phanjoo AL, et al. Antiandrogen (cyproterone acetate) therapy in deviant hypersexuality. Br J Psychiatry 1972; 120(554):59–63.

64. Gagne P. Treatment of sex offenders with medroxyprogesterone acetate. Am J Psychiatry 1981; 138(5):644–646.

65. Thibaut F, Cordier B, Kuhn JM. Effect of a long-lasting gonadotrophin hormone-releasing hormone agonist in six cases of severe male paraphilia. Acta Psychiatr Scand 1993; 87(6):445–450.

66. Rosler A, Witztum E. Treatment of men with paraphilia with a long-acting analogue of gonadotropin-releasing hormone. N Engl J Med 1998; 338(7):416–422.

67. Briken P, Nika E, Berner W. Treatment of paraphilia with luteinizing hormone-releasing hormone agonists. J Sex Marital Ther 2001; 27(1):45–55.

68. Garde K, Lunde I. Female sexual behaviour. A study in a random sample of 40-year-old women. Maturitas 1980; 2(3):225–240.

69. Laumann EO, Gagnon JH, Michael RT, et al. The Organization of Sexuality. Chicago: University of Chicago Press, 1994.

70. Segraves KB, Segraves RT. Hypoactive sexual desire disorder: prevalence and comorbidity in 906 subjects. J Sex Marital Ther 1991; 17(1):55–58.

71. Blumenstein P, Schwartz P. American Couples: Money, Work, Sex. New York: Morrow, 1983.

72. Wallen K. The evolution of female sexual desire. In: Abramson PR, Pinkerton SD, eds. Sexual Nature, Sexual Culture. Chicago: The University of Chicago Press, 1995:57–79.

73. Wallen K. Sex and context: hormones and primate sexual motivation. Horm Behav 2001; 40(2):339–357.

74. Tieffer L. In pursuit of the perfect penis: the medicalization of male sexuality. Am Behav Sci 1986; 29:579–599.

75. Schiavi RC, Schreiner-Engel P, White D, et al. Pituitary-gonadal function during sleep in men with hypoactive sexual desire and in normal controls. Psychosom Med 1988; 50(3):304–318.

76. Segraves RT. Hormones and libido. In: Leiblum R, Rosen RC, eds. Sexual Desire Disorders. New York: The Guilford Press, 1988:271–311.

77. Franks S, Jacobs HS, Martin N, et al. Hyperprolactinaemia and impotence. Clin Endocrinol (Oxf) 1978; 8(4):277–287.

7

Cardiovascular Response to Sexual Activity in the Male

Richard A. Stein

Cardiology Division, Beth Israel Medical Center, New York, New York, U.S.A.

Arshad M. Safi

The Franklin County Heart Center, Chambersburg, Pennsylvania, U.S.A.

☐ INTRODUCTION

Response of the cardiovascular system to coitus and other sexual activity has been the subject of a number of studies in the recent past. These studies have been conducted against the backdrop of a popular "mythology" in both the lay and health-care provider communities concerning the intensity of the physiologic response to coitus and orgasm, and the belief that sexual activity represents a significant risk in patients with known or occult coronary artery disease. In part, this perception was fostered by the work of Bartlett in 1956 (1) and Masters and Johnson in 1966 (2). These groups were among the first to study heart rate and blood pressures (BPs) in unmarried student couples engaging in coitus in a "private" laboratory room.

☐ UNDERSTANDING CARDIAC WORKLOAD AND STRESS

The cardiac workload and "stress" of sexual activity can be best understood in the context of the cardiovascular response to a more usual exercise task such as running on a treadmill at increasing speeds or elevations or pedaling a bicycle against increasing resistance. The increased work of the leg muscles must be met by an increase in adenosine triphosphate production. Although this need can be met in part by shunting blood from nonworking muscles and by increasing the extraction of oxygen by working muscles, the major response is an increase in cardiac output; that is, the amount of blood pumped by the heart each minute. This is achieved by a modest increase in the amount of blood ejected with each beat (stroke volume) and a major increase in the heart rate (upward of 300%).

Increasing the heart rate, stroke volume, and generating a higher peak BP necessitates an increase in the oxygen requirement of the heart muscle. Thus, the workload of an activity (sexual or other) can be evaluated by measuring the amount of oxygen the body consumes during the activity. This is expressed as the minute oxygen (O_2) consumption in mL/kg/min, or METS (metabolic equivalent). (One MET equals 3.5/mL O_2/kg/min. An example of the use of the term METS is as follows: a person who, during exercise, is consuming 14 mL O_2/kg/min is exercising at a 4 METS level.) Workload of the heart can be estimated by the increase in its oxygen requirement as calculated by the double product (achieved peak heart rate × achieved peak systolic BP).

☐ CARDIOVASCULAR RESPONSE TO SEXUAL ACTIVITY

Below, a number of important studies regarding sex and cardiovascular response are reviewed: first are the key investigations in healthy subjects used to establish our understanding of a "normal" response; second are the studies done in men who have had heart attacks [post-myocardial infarction (post-MI)]; third are studies investigating "myths" surrounding the heart and sex. Key findings are summarized in Table 1. Afterward, limitations of the studies are outlined, and finally, other (noncardiovascular) physiological responses to sexual activity are explored (1–9).

Normal Cardiovascular Response

Over the years, various studies have sought to measure cardiovascular response during sex. In 1956, Bartlett published a study of three couples engaged in coitus within an experimental room equipped with wires going through the wall (1). The couples signaled the stages of coitus (intromission, orgasm, and withdrawal) via handheld buttons. A mean peak heart rate of 170 beats/min (bpm) occurred at orgasm. A follow-up study was performed with couples wearing mouthpieces permitting the collection and analysis of expired air during coitus. Respiratory rates and tidal volumes were noted to increase in all subjects. The highest respiratory rate noted during orgasm was over 60/min in some subjects. The minute volumes were in the range expected during moderate-to-severe exertion.

Table 1 Summary of Cardiovascular Responses to Sexual Activity

Author[a]	Mean peak heart rate (bpm)	Heart rate range (bpm)	Blood pressure (mmHg)	Mean age (yr)	Oxygen consumption
Bartlett (1)	170 (orgasm)	–	–	–	–
Masters, Johnson (2)	–	140–180	+ 80 (systolic) + 50 (diastolic)	–	–
Hellerstein, Friedman (6)	117.4 (coitus)	90–144	162/89	47.5	16 mL/kg/min
Stein (5)	127 (week 1) 120 (week 16)	120–130	– –		2.7 L/min (week 1) 3.0 L/min (week 16)
Nemec et al. (7)	114 (man on top) 117 (woman on top)	–	163/81 (man on top) 161/77 (woman on top)	29.3	– –
Masini et al. (9)	127 (men) 137 (women)	–	– –	– –	– –
Bohlen et al. (3)	102 (self-stimulation)	–	–	33.2	1.7 MET (self-stimulation)
	102 (partner stimulation)	–	–		1.8 MET (partner stimulation)
	127 (man on top)	–	–		3.3 MET (man on top)
	120 (woman on top)	–	–		2.5 MET (woman on top)
Sanderson et al. (4)	117 (men) 120 (women)	–	– –	28.2 (men) 28.2 (women)	–
Mann et al. (8)	124 (men)	–	155/87 (rest) 237/138 (coitus)	–	–

[a]Reference is given in parentheses.
Abbreviation: MET, metabolic equivalent (1 MET equals 3.5 mL O_2/kg/min).

In 1966, Masters and Johnson published their seminal work on sexuality (2). They measured heart rates and BP of men during sex and found heart rates in men ranged from 140 to 180 bpm. This represented, for example, 93% of age-predicted maximum heart rate for a 27-year-old man (calculated as 220 – age). BP was measured via a "through the wall" sphygmomanometer tube, and mean values for systolic BP increased by 80 mm Hg and diastolic by 50 mm Hg. Impact of potential confounding factors such as performance anxiety, coitus among non-long-term sex partners, and having their data "observed" in the next room during the coitus were not fully addressed. Nonetheless, these heart rates and BPs became the "working numbers" for the next several years.

One of the few studies to include women was conducted by Masini et al. (9). Ten normal couples were studied during coitus at home using ambulatory electrocardiograph (EKG). The women's age range was 20 to 37 years. The men's age range was 25 to 49 years. Data was separated into an "initial phase" of sexual activity and a "realization phase" including coitus and orgasm. Heart rate elevated to 137 bpm in the women and was significantly elevated for a mean of 2.8 minutes, whereas in men heart rate rose to a mean of 127 bpm with the elevation lasting for a mean of 2.1 minutes. These heart rates represented 60% to 70% age-predicted maximum heart rates and were often exceeded during daily activities. The higher heart rates achieved by the women in their study may be related to the young age of their women subjects as compared to the men.

In 1984, Bohlen et al. (3) did the most comprehensive study to date using a highly instrumented protocol in order to study the physiological response to coitus in the laboratory setting. Ten married couples participated in four sexual activities on different days in a laboratory room with data recording tubes and cables passing through a wall. The men were young (mean age 33.2 years) and very fit (mean VO_2max 54/mL/kg). Data collected included heart rates, BP, and VO_2max. The four sexual activities included coitus with husband-on-top, coitus with wife-on-top, noncoital stimulation of the husband by the wife, and self-stimulation of the husband when alone. Stages of sexual activity that were recorded included: baseline resting, foreplay, stimulation, and orgasm. Heart rates were noted to increase at each stage of sexual activity with peak values occurring at orgasm. Mean peak heart rates at orgasm with self- and partner stimulation were 102 bpm; with wife-on-top coitus, 120 bpm; and with husband on top coitus, 127 bpm. Double products, reflecting myocardial oxygen demand, were increased about two fold during self- and partner stimulation and were not significantly different from this value in either of the coital positions. Minute oxygen consumption obtained during the protocol included resting baseline, foreplay, and stimulation orgasm. The latter two stages were included as one since peak heart rate elevations at orgasm lasted only 10 to 16 seconds and expired air collection utilized a 60-second sample. The authors expressed VO_2 in terms of METs (1 MET = 3.5 mL O_2/kg/min). VO_2 was only modestly increased during self- and partner stimulation (1.7 and 1.8 METs); it was 2.5 METs for woman on top and 3.3 METs for man on top during coitus. The later value represents a VO_2 of 11.7 mL/kg/min, which interestingly is near the value obtained by Hellerstein and Friedman in their study using bicycle exercise to peak coital heart rates (described below). Of note is a study by Sanderson et al. (4) that recorded somewhat higher heart rates than Bohlen et al. during self-stimulation to orgasm among 11 men (mean age 28.2 years) and 11 women (mean age 28.2 years). In this study, the mean peak heart rate among the men was 117 bpm and among the women, it was 120 bpm.

Although the Bohlen study is highly comprehensive, its clinical application may be limited. First, the subjects were exceptionally fit young men (vs. average, middle-aged men). Second, data is from a "laboratory setting" using highly sophisticated equipment (e.g., facemasks to collect expired air). The lower heart rates they noted most probably reflect the high level of fitness of their subjects, consistent with Stein's data (5), demonstrating a reduced peak coital heart rate after exercise training and consequent enhancement in VO_2max.

Cardiovascular Response in Post-MI Men

In 1970, Hellerstein and Friedman of the Cleveland Clinic published their findings on men who were enrolled in a Cardiac Rehabilitation Program and were sexually active with their spouses (6). Ninety-one patients responded to a questionnaire regarding sexual activity and wore ambulatory EKG. Fourteen subjects with atherosclerotic heart disease were monitored by ambulatory EKG for 24 to 48 hours around days when the couples engaged in coitus at home (usual place, time, partner, position, and foreplay). Hellerstein and Friedman noted significantly lower peak heart rates (mean of 117.4 bpm, with a range of 90–144 at orgasm in 14 subjects) than were reported by Bartlett and by Masters and Johnson. The Hellerstein–Friedman patients were older (mean age 47.5 years) and their cardiorespiratory fitness, as assessed by the measurement of maximum oxygen consumption during a maximal exercise EKG testing, was similar to that reported for ambulatory, middle-aged normal subjects. Of interest is that the 24-hour ambulatory EKG recording often noted that heart rates during occupational or home recreational activities exceeded those achieved during coitus.

Hellerstein and Friedman did not measure BP directly at home because no practical device existed at the time; however, BPs and minute oxygen consumption were obtained by having these 14 patients perform a graded bicycle ergometer exercise EKG examination. In a limited fashion, measuring the BPs during cycle ergometry at heart rates equivalent to those achieved during coitus and orgasm approximated BPs during coitus and orgasm. Relatively modest values (mean 162/89 mm Hg) were found, but it was noted that this value might significantly underestimate the peak BP achieved during coitus because it does not take into consideration the neuroendocrine responses associated with arousal and coitus. The minute oxygen consumption during bicycle exercise to peak coital heart rates was 16 mL O_2/kg/min. This value corresponded to 60% of their subject's maximum oxygen consumption.

Hellerstein and Friedman's data is important to our understanding of the physiologic response to coitus in the "usual" patient of interest, i.e., a middle-aged, normally active male who engages in coitus with a long-term, stable sex partner. Their finding of a peak heart rate and, by extrapolation, peak myocardial oxygen requirement [estimated from changes in the "double product" (heart rate × systolic BP)], was well below maximum values and frequently exceeded during daily activities. Their measurement of minute oxygen consumption at coital heart rates denotes that coitus, in the usual manner in middle-aged men, imposes only a modest physiologic cost.

In 1977, Stein published a study on coital heart rates and maximum oxygen consumption in post-MI men before and after a 16-week bicycle ergometer exercise program (5). Six post-MI patients comprised a control group not given exercise training. To permit acclimation, the couples were introduced to the ambulatory EKG, watched a playback of an ambulatory EKG recording, and wore the device during coitus once prior to the data collection phase of the protocol. Data was collected on two occasions before and two occasions after completion of the 16-week exercise program. Prior to the exercise program, mean peak coital heart rate was 127 bpm (range 120–130). After the 16-week exercise program, a training effect was confirmed by an 11.5% increase in mean minute oxygen consumption from 2.7 pretraining to 3.0 L/min posttraining. There was also an average decrease of 5.5% in peak coital heart rate to a mean of 120 bpm. In the control group, VO_2max and peak coital heart rates were not significantly changed. A training effect is expected to reduce peak heart rates at given exercise levels due to an enhanced oxygen extraction capacity of the trained muscles with consequent reduction in the cardiac output requirement. The reduction in coital heart rates suggests that the heart rate achieved during coitus is responsive, at least in part, to the same demands as endurance training "aerobic" activities.

In another study, Nemec et al. examined the impact of coital position (man on top vs. woman on top) on peak coital heart rates achieved (7). This was of interest since clinicians were counseling post-MI patients to use the women-on-top position on the assumption that it would be associated with a lower work level and a lower cardiac oxygen requirement. In addition to the ambulatory EKG recording device, the male subjects wore sphygmomanometer cuffs attached to an automatic BP machine utilizing an ultrasonic detection device. They triggered the BP machine prior to coitus and at orgasm. Their subjects were eight adult males (mean age 29.3 years, range 24–40 years), who engaged in a total of 35 episodes of coitus with their spouses in their own homes. Of them, 16 were in the man-on-top position and 19 were in the women-on-top position. Peak coital heart rates were not significantly changed with position (mean of 114 bpm with man on top and 117 with woman on top). BP and double product (heart rate×systolic BP) also did not change significantly (163/81 mmHg for man on top and 161/77 for woman on top). The mean peak coital heart rates were 61% of the age-predicted maximum heart rates for their subject. Thus, they concluded that there is no physiologic rationale for counseling men to alter the man-on-top coital position.

In 1979, Johnston and Fletcher published their findings from ambulatory EKG recording during the at-home, usual-partner sexual activity in 24 patients either post-MI or post-coronary artery bypass graft (CABG) surgery (10). The peak heart rates in the post-CABG surgery patients were higher during coitus (90–118 bpm) than in the post-MI patients (74–108 bpm). Of interest is their finding that 12 of the 24 patients had arrhythmias associated with coitus. In 5 of these 12 patients, this abnormality was noted only during coitus and not during the rest of the ambulatory EKG recording.

Drory et al. addressed this issue in 88 male outpatients (ages 36–66 years) with stable coronary artery disease (11). Ambulatory EKG recordings included sexual activity and near maximum ergometric test in all subjects. Arrhythmia was found during intercourse in 56% of the patients and during exercise in 38% of the patients. The most frequently observed arrhythmia during exercise was the occurrence of or an increase in the frequency of ectopic beats; during coitus this occurred in only 11% of the patients. In 12% of the patients, a complex ventricular arrhythmia was noted during coitus. The authors concluded that, in most patients, existing rhythm disturbances were not exacerbated during coitus and most arrhythmias noted during coitus were simple.

Myths

Various health "myths" surround the sex act. Of clinical (and social) interest is the possibility that the physiological response to coitus with extramarital partners may be significantly elevated compared to coitus with marital partners and this may be associated with enhanced risk of acute cardiac events. The data in this regard is very limited and, more importantly, confounded. In 1993, Dr. Ueno, a pathologist from Japan, reviewed 5559 cases of sudden death (12). Thirty-four cases were recorded as having occurred during or immediately after coitus. At autopsy and case evaluation, 18 of these deaths were determined to be cardiac in origin. The relatively low incidence of coitus reported as proximate to sudden death was noted (0.06%), but of particular interest was that 27 of the 34 cases occurred with coitus involving extramarital sex partners. This data implies that extramarital sex may be associated with a greater physiologic demand and greater risk of a cardiac event than is sex with a spouse. It seemed that we had finally arrived at a physiologic and medical basis for marital fidelity. This concept was consistent with the cultural mythology, supported by the reported deaths of prominent figures, and television dramas in which characters had cardiac events during extramarital coitus.

One case notation regarding this is contained in a report by Cantwell (13). Heart rates were recorded during coitus by ambulatory EKG in cardiac rehabilitation patients from the Georgia Baptist Medical Center. The authors noted that one subject had intercourse with his girlfriend at noon and his heart rate rose from 96 to 150 bpm. He then had intercourse with his wife in the evening with a more modest increase in heart rate from 72 to 92 bpm.

Another myth is the connection between sex and physical or mental performance. Boone and Gilmore address this question specifically (14). They tested 11 male subjects under maximal treadmill exercise before sex and 12 hours after sex. Aerobic power, oxygen pulse, and double product were measured. Boone and Gilmore found no significant reduction in maximum athletic output. Another study by Sztajzel et al. (15) has explored the relationship of coitus on mental and athletic endeavors. Fifteen high-level male athletes underwent two maximal ergometer exercise EKG examinations and an arithmetic mental concentration test on a day when the subject had engaged in coitus prior to the exercise study and on a day without coitus prior to the exercise study. One exam was timed to follow coitus by two hours and the second by 10 hours. At two hours, significantly higher recovery heart rates at 5 and 10 minutes were found after the maximal ergometer exercise EKG testing on the coital day as compared to the noncoital day. This difference was not seen in the 10-hour postcoital studies. Sexual activity had no impact on maximum achieved workload or mental concentration. The higher post-effort heart rates after maximal stress testing on the morning of sexual intercourse is intriguing, suggesting recovery following athletic endeavors may be impacted if such an event is carried out shortly after sexual intercourse.

Study Limitations

Several limitations of the studies above should be noted. In particular with earlier studies, where tubes through a wall were used to do stethoscope or other measurements, peak orgasm might be missed. Also, use of automatic BP devices at home may be inaccurate due to certain postures or the forceful use of the extremity wearing the BP cuff.

In addition, the time needed for cuff inflation and deflation may miss transient post-orgasmic BP changes as suggested from data collected by Mann et al. (8). Indwelling radial artery catheters were used to record continuous BP for a 24-hour period in a significant number of untreated hypertensive patients. Eighteen of their subjects engaged in coitus during the recording period (14 men and 4 women). The men had elevated resting BPs (mean values of 155/87 mm Hg), and achieved peak coital heart rates of a mean value of 124 bpm and achieved peak coital BPs of a mean of 237/138 mm Hg, representing a 55% increase in systolic BP that lasted only seconds. This suggests that normal subjects or treated hypertensive patients may also have very brief significant elevations of BP. Although the physiological significance of such very brief elevation in BP is minor, there is concern that this may create shear forces across an atherosclerotic plaque, which could "trigger" plaque fracture or erosion and subsequent thrombus formation and acute MI.

Perhaps of greatest concern is that although the most accurate measurements are obtained in a laboratory setting, it is not a natural setting for sex. The sense of being monitored during coitus could significantly impact on the usual coital practice and intensity. The correlation of peak heart rates in recent laboratory and ambulatory settings decrease this concern to some degree. Later studies measured physiological response to coitus under more natural conditions (i.e., at home). The strength of "at home" studies is the relevance of their findings to real-life coitus. The weakness of "at home" measurements is loss of accuracy. As previously mentioned, BP measurement may be compromised by cuff inflation/deflation times. Also, timing is left to the subjects, who may miss orgasm by important seconds. Furthermore, oxygen consumption, the most definitive method of establishing coitus workload and percentage of peak exercise capacity, cannot be measured in this setting.

Other Physiological Responses

A series of recent studies (16) has addressed the role of changes in hormonal levels during sexual activity and orgasm.

The hormone oxytocin is well known in promoting lactation in women (17); however, Carmichael et al. (18) obtained continuous blood levels for oxytocin analysis during self-stimulation to orgasm in 13 men and 10 women. BP, anal electromyography, and anal photoplethysmography (to assess anal contractions) were also continuously measured. In both men and women, there is a direct correlation between the increase in oxytocin observed and the peak achieved systolic BP and a subjective measurement of orgasm intensity. Other molecular studies have identified oxytocin receptors in the penis and changes in expression levels, suggesting a role in detumescence after orgasm (19,20).

Another hormone associated with lactation, prolactin, also has an effect in male sexual response. Kruger et al. administered drugs to increase (protirelin) or decrease (cabergoline) prolactin levels in healthy male subjects (21). They found that greater than physiological levels of prolactin had a minimal effect, but lower than physiological levels corresponded with enhanced sexual drive, function, and shortened refractory period.

Another area of study is the role of sex steroids and coronary artery disease. Wranicz et al. looked at 88 post-MI men measuring heart rate variability using Holter monitoring along with various hormone parameters including testosterone level, estradiol level, free testosterone index, and estradiol/testosterone ratio (22). They conclude testosterone may have positive influence on autonomic regulation of the heart.

☐ CONCLUSION

By and large, the many studies addressing heart rates and BP, as well as those measuring workload and minute oxygen consumption, have reported consistent results. Usual cardiovascular responses to sexual activity include increases in heart rate, BP, double product, and myocardial oxygen consumption. These responses gradually increase, with peak rates occurring during the orgasm phase of sexual activity. Peak coital heart rates are noted to be in the range of 114 to 130 beats/min, with the higher values noted in the younger subjects. The percentage of age-predicted maximum heart rate was near 60% in several studies. When heart rates during the day were compared to those at peak sexual activity, there were usually several instances of higher values during daily activity as compared to peak coital values. BPs raised approximately 40 mm Hg in both the home ambulatory setting and the laboratory setting. The data presented by Mann et al. (8) is a source of concern because it suggests that a transient yet significant elevation (above 220 mm Hg) in systolic BP may accompany orgasm; however, workloads measured in a laboratory setting with on-line minute oxygen consumption as well as estimated measurements during ergometer exercise to coital heart rates are remarkably similar, indicating a moderate MET workload of 3 to 4.

In addition, epidemiological data suggest only a small incremental risk of cardiovascular events (MI, unstable angina, or cardiac-related sudden death) coincident to sexual activity. This risk is similar to that of a moderately intense exercise event and can be reduced by engaging in regular physical activity.

Finally, studies addressing hormonal and chemical changes during coitus and their relationship to sexual performance, satisfaction, and physiology may significantly enhance our understanding of the physiologic response of the male to sexual activity.

☐ REFERENCES

1. Bartlett RG Jr. Physiologic responses during coitus. J Appl Physiol 1956; 9(3):469–472.
2. Masters WH, Johnson VE. Human Sexual Response. Boston: Little Brown, 1966.
3. Bohlen JG, Held JP, Sanderson MO, et al. Heart rate, rate-pressure product, and oxygen uptake during four sexual activities. Arch Intern Med 1984; 144(9):1745–1748.
4. Sanderson MO, Held JP, Bohlen JG. Heart rate during masturbation. J Cardiac Rehab 1982; 2:542–546.
5. Stein RA. The effect of exercise training on heart rate during coitus in the post myocardial infarction patient. Circulation 1977; 55(5):738–740.
6. Hellerstein HK, Friedman EH. Sexual activity and the postcoronary patient. Arch Intern Med 1970; 125(6):987–999.
7. Nemec ED, Mansfield L, Kennedy JW. Heart rate and blood pressure responses during sexual activity in normal males. Am Heart J 1976; 92(3):274–277.
8. Mann S, Craig MWM, Gould B, et al. Coital blood pressure in hypertensives [Abstract]. Circulation 1980; 62(suppl 3):111–137.
9. Masini V, Romei E, Fiorella AT. Dynamic electrocardiogram in normal subjects during sexual activity. G Ital Cardiol 1980; 10(11):1442–1448.
10. Johnston BL, Fletcher GF. Dynamic electrocardiographic recording during sexual activity in recent post-myocardial infarction and revascularization patients. Am Heart J 1979; 98(6):736–741.
11. Drory Y, Fisman EZ, Shapira Y, et al. Ventricular arrhythmias during sexual activity in patients with coronary artery disease. Chest 1996; 109(4):922–924.
12. Ueno M. The So-Called Coition Death [Japanese]. Nihon Hoigaku Zasshi 1963; 17:330–340.
13. Cantwell JD. Sex and the heart. Med Aspects Hum Sex 1981; 15:14–23.
14. Boone T, Gilmore S. Effects of sexual intercourse on maximal aerobic power, oxygen pulse, and double product in male sedentary subjects. J Sports Med Phys Fitness 1995; 35(3):214–217.
15. Sztajzel J, Periat M, Marti V, et al. Effect of sexual activity on cycle ergometer stress test parameters, on plasmatic testosterone levels and on concentration capacity. A study in high-level male athletes performed in the laboratory. J Sports Med Phys Fitness 2000; 40(3):233–239.
16. Bancroft J. The endocrinology of sexual arousal. J Endocrinol 2005; 186(3):411–427.
17. Buhimschi CS. Endocrinology of lactation. Obstet Gynecol Clin North Am 2004; 31(4):963–979, xii.
18. Carmichael MS, Warburton VL, Dixen J, et al. Relationships among cardiovascular, muscular, and oxytocin responses during human sexual activity. Arch Sex Behav 1994; 23(1):59–79.
19. Vignozzi L, Filippi S, Luconi M, et al. Oxytocin receptor is expressed in the penis and mediates an estrogen-dependent smooth muscle contractility. Endocrinology 2004; 145(4):1823–1834.
20. Vignozzi L, Vannelli GB, Morelli A, et al. Identification, characterization and biological activity of oxytocin receptor in the developing human penis. Mol Hum Reprod 2005; 11(2):99–106.
21. Kruger TH, Haake P, Haverkamp J, et al. Effects of acute prolactin manipulation on sexual drive and function in males. J Endocrinol 2003; 179(3):357–365.
22. Wranicz JK, Rosiak M, Cygankiewicz I, et al. Sex steroids and heart rate variability in patients after myocardial infarction. Ann Noninvasive Electrocardiol 2004; 9(2):156–161.

8

Psychological and Social Influences on Male Sexual Function

David John Smith
Faculty of Medicine, University of New South Wales, Rural Clinical School, Albury, New South Wales, Australia

David Barton
School of Psychology and Psychological Medicine, Monashe University, Melbourne, Victoria, Australia

Lynette Joubert
Department of Social Work, The University of Melbourne, Parkville, Victoria, Australia

☐ INTRODUCTION

This chapter reviews the various psychological and social factors that influence a man's sexual functioning throughout the course of his life.

Sexuality is a complex phenomenon, determined by anatomy, physiology, and psychology together with culture, relationships with others, and developmental experiences throughout the life cycle. Sex and procreation are associated with some of the great joys of existence. Perceptions, thoughts, feelings and behaviors connected with sexual gratification and reproduction, and the attraction of one person for another are influential determinants of a man's sexual function. A new relationship, a successful lifelong relationship, a newborn child, and sex itself, are all deeply appreciated experiences; however, sexuality can also be associated with feelings of sadness, shame, or guilt, perhaps due to disappointing early sexual encounters, sexual misbehavior, a lost relationship, betrayal, or death of a partner. In fact, few individuals have a sexual life that is completely free of negative feelings.

The clinician assessing a man's sexual function is entering an area where different aspects of human behavior converge. It is a subject that reaches into the heart of the individual. The clinician's own sexuality will color the thinking of even the most objective observer. Everyone from the celibate to the promiscuous has preconceived ideas and notions about sex. Nowhere is this more so than with sexual morality.

It is usually the context of sexual behavior that defines its morality. What would be considered wholesome in one context is defiling in another, with many shades of gray in between. Even the libertine has boundaries beyond which sexual behavior should not transgress. For most men, morality—both their own and their partners'—is a central aspect of their sexual functioning.

Male sexual life can be fascinating, puzzling, contradictory, and perplexing. Its complexity belies the simplicity of its expression. It is the meeting place of the mental and physical. Penile tumescence and subsequent erection occurs through the combined activity of the parasympathetic nervous system functioning at a spinal reflex level and the sympathetic nervous system. The neural control of erection is influenced by the cerebral cortex, including the limbic system and hypothalamus. It is therefore subject to psychologically induced stimulation as well as external factors such as stress and drugs. The sympathetic nerves are solely responsible for ejaculation, making this function particularly vulnerable to psychological events and external factors (1).

☐ DEVELOPMENT AND NATURAL HISTORY OF SEXUAL FUNCTION
Developmental Factors
Psychological Developmental Factors

Becoming a sexually mature man involves the thoughts, feelings, and behaviors, both conscious and unconscious, that result from the interplay between unfolding biology and experiences of life. There are many psychological factors that are thought to be associated with sexual development. These include the parent–child bond, competition with father for mother's attention, competition with siblings, and the early association of the genitals with privacy and shame. Early erotic experiences during puberty and adolescence may have an imprinting effect (2). Gender identity issues, early masturbatory activity and associated fantasies, initial sexual activity, fear of pregnancy or disease, and adult role expectations all play their parts (3).

Testosterone is essential for the prenatal development required to produce a male. In the absence of sex hormones, the individual develops as a female (4).

Testosterone is also needed at other critical times in masculine psychological and behavioral development (5). It is believed that men may have a greater risk for physical and behavioral developmental disorders than women because of this dependence on testosterone.

In addition, there are stages in the life cycle that require satisfactory resolution, such as the psychosocial stages described by Erickson, including the identity versus role confusion stage between the ages of 13 and 21 years. This is of particular importance in sexual development (6). Failure to satisfactorily negotiate life-cycle stages may lead to sexual dysfunction.

Family Developmental Factors

A normal family life is essential for the proper learning of sexuality, including relationships with siblings and the success of the parent(s) in establishing a satisfactory home environment (7). Learning begins with parent–child interactions meeting the infant boy's needs. Personal closeness and warmth bring trust and positive feelings towards his body, contributing to a healthy body image that is to be a part of a strong sexual self-esteem. Bolstering or avoidance of appropriate gender-associated activities reinforces the genotype gender identity. From birth, girls and boys are treated differently. Boys are treated more ruggedly and spoken to in a different way. They are encouraged to accept adversity more readily than girls. Boys are dressed in a masculine manner and encouraged to be competitive. During male development, sexuality is vulnerable to negative influences such as verbal, physical, and sexual abuse.

Learned male behavior depends on interactions with the father and other significant adult males as well as with other boys (8). There is increasing concern in Western society over the developmental effects on boys growing up in single-parent families, where the adult is usually the mother, and where there is no regularly available male on whom the boy may model his masculine behavior (9).

Social and Cultural Development Factors

The culture in which a boy is brought up has effects on his sexual development through familial and social norms, cultural rights of passage, and the accepted manner in which the genders relate to each other. In Western culture, sexual activity among young people and single people of any age is now more common. Factors that have influenced this change include earlier puberty, delayed marriage, a decline in the influence of the family leading to more autonomy, exposure to sexual stimuli through the mass media, and travel across cultural boundaries (10). There also have been changes in Western culture concerning attitudes toward gender identity difficulties and acceptance of homosexuality.

There is considerable variation in cultural and ethnic behavioral norms relating to sex and reproduction (11). In one study of students (median age 14) in a society with two principal cultures (Maori and European), boys in one cultural group were nearly three times more likely to be sexually active as boys in the other (12). In multicultural societies, differences of this nature can be expected to lead to both internal and external tensions for the developing male. A young man from an immigrant family may need to resolve conflicting feelings originating from his own desires, the expectations of the society in which he lives, and loyalty to family and culture. For example, his family may require him to enter an arranged marriage, while the society in which he has grown up expects him to choose a partner.

Influence of the Life Cycle

The stages of sexual expression are among some of the more significant events on the journey through life: puberty, first sexual activity, marriage or its equivalent, the birth of children, and sexual involution are all momentous events, although the significance of these may not be fully understood by each individual at the time. Sexual difficulties often present in the context of one of these life stages.

Sexuality is a core human behavior; yet, it varies considerably between individuals and even within the same man because he learns throughout life. Sexual learning and experimentation continue throughout the life cycle, the repertoire of sexual behavior expands, and, in general, is compatible with cultural norms.

Attitudes toward the events of the life cycle vary between individuals and in the family and society at large. This can be seen in a family's response to the first youthful expression of lust or the aging man's extant sexuality. Performance anxieties may be associated with a wide variety of developmental stages, with different responsibilities and in contexts as varied as early sexual activity and long-term relationships. These anxieties may occur of themselves or in connection with the physical changes associated with aging and disease, particularly when illnesses such as disorders of the genital tract have a direct influence on sexual function.

Testosterone is considered to be the hormone associated with libido in men as well as women. Testosterone levels fall throughout adult life and certain behaviors, stress, sleep, mood and lifestyle influence its levels (13). These influences vary according to age and circumstances. In turn, testosterone level has a feedback effect on the factors that influence its production (14).

Marriage

In Western culture, societal attitudes toward premarital sex have become considerably more permissive. Even so, marriage remains a central feature of everyday life—although it is not as popular as it once was. From a high point in the 1960s, there has been a decline in marriage rates throughout the Western world. In Europe (especially northern Europe), the proportion of the population marrying has declined and the age of marriage has increased. These trends have been most pronounced in Sweden (15), where a significant proportion of men and women will not marry; however, many will live in "de facto" relationships, meaning that they are not married in law but in "fact."

When men form lasting relationships, they continue to follow more traditional patterns of behavior. In one study in a developed Western society, most adults between 25 and 60 years of age reported monogamous behavior. Of all heterosexually active men, 80% and of all heterosexually active women, 90% reported having had only one sex partner in the preceding year (16).

As a result of the increased prevalence of divorce, a man may now have more than one wife during his lifetime. Obviously, women have the same options. A man is likely to regard each relationship as permanent at the time; yet, there may be variations in sexual life with different spousal expectations and possible disappointments. He may have had experiences in one marriage that carry over with him to the next. He may have experienced sexual betrayal or may have himself committed sexual indiscretions. A man may compulsively repeat mistakes and not address his underlying problems, leading to successive failed marriages and relationships.

Influences of Modern Social Structure
Economic Influences

What both society and family may expect from a man by way of economic functioning and financial responsibilities varies according to cultural context and over time. Modern social structure continues to normalize the principal economic role of men in family life despite the increased contribution made by women. In addition, the male is expected to play a greater role in the family. This arrangement will vary significantly between family units to the extent that men in some families function in the day-to-day care of their children. Economic success can boost a man's libido, while stress associated with economic hardship can interfere with his sexual functioning.

Media Influences

Media plays a large part in the influences on modern society. Through the media, a man is exposed to the lives of many others, both real and fictional, many more than if he was restricted to those in his immediate environment. Concerns have been raised about the effect of media on the sexual development of adolescents (17). Since there is little consensus on sexual education, erotica may be the primary agent of sexual socialization (18).

A significant part of modern media is directly or indirectly concerned with sex. The guiltless expression of sexuality is a central theme of the entertainment media. It is also true that in recent times there has been a great deal of accurate information about sex in the media, thus bringing knowledge and greater sexual sophistication; however, books, magazines, television, and movies often have sexual content promoting fantasy over reality. The portrayal of idealized sexual relationships raises the expectations of men and women. This is not by any means confined to Western culture as exemplified in the Indian film industry.

The Internet is the latest medium to have effects on the sex lives of men, with sexually themed and pornographic material available at the "click of a mouse." Although this brings more knowledge, it may further heighten expectations and lead to feelings of frustration and inadequacy. The "safe sex" of Internet chat rooms introduces new pleasures and temptations.

Advertising Influences

In advertising, the commercialization of sex may direct new, and as yet little understood, influences on sexual development. The association of sexual gratification with consumer behavior influences the developing libido as well as the mature observer. It is possible that images of unrealistic perfection in sexual objects may diminish arousal toward the more everyday person.

Divorce Practices

Separation and divorce enable the formation of more than one long-term relationship in an individual's life through socially sanctioned ways of expressing dissatisfaction with these relationships. Divorce and the threat of divorce bring many new stressors to family life and may lead to an increasing sense of uncertainty that can impact a man's sexual functioning. Failure to resolve the feelings associated with divorce can impinge on sexual functioning in a new relationship. Furthermore, new relationships formed in middle age may carry expectations of the kinds on libidinal practices that normally would be expressed earlier in life. A man presenting at this time may be faced with anticipations of youthfulness from his new partner that results in increased anxiety and decreased sexual performance.

Aging

Greater longevity resulting from modern advances in medical practices has brought sexual function into a new era. There are many myths surrounding the sexual inadequacies of aging men and women. These myths are confounded by the elderly person's sexual performance. Good health and an available sexual partner are as much related to potency as age.

Nevertheless, there is a steady reduction in the frequency of intercourse in both sexes with advancing age, though individual variations are quite large. The prevalence of erectile dysfunction (ED) increases with age. One study showed an increase from about 5% in the fourth decade to around 65% in the seventh decade (19). Despite the presence of performance problems, many men look to continue a sexual life into their later years. The ready acceptance of the use of medications to assist men in this area is an indication of these expectations (20). Age is not a barrier to treatment, nor should it be presumed that age is the cause of a problem without other causes having been investigated.

☐ SEXUALITY IN MEN

Internal and external influences synthesize male sexual function in a mixture of psychological and relationship fundamentals. Tensions and problems result from conflict between inner psychic needs and the needs of others. Sexual attraction, the need for intimacy and trust, and the struggle for dominance interact in a cauldron of passion cooled by personal, family, and societal values. Normal sexuality also results from innate biologically determined drives, satisfactory self-esteem, memories of previously good sexual experiences, and the availability of an appropriate person as a sexual object for a man's desire. This desire is further enhanced when the man shares a good relationship with that other person in areas in addition to sex.

Development of Sexuality

A boy learns much of his sexual behavior by example, assisted by the presence of balanced family attitudes to sexual learning with appropriate boundaries and expressions of intimacy. This includes a sound family approach to philosophical issues and religious life. A strict upbringing may lead to problems resulting from the internalization of guilt and shame at levels that inhibit normal sexual function. Societal values expressed in ultraconservative or religious orthodoxy with severe control of sexual and social development or the formulation of ideas that link sexuality with "sin" or uncleanness can detrimentally affect sexual functioning (21).

An appropriate level of sexual control is important, however. Exposure of children to certain sexual influences can also be to their detriment; hence, the censorship on media and the seriousness with which society considers the problem of pedophilia, even to the extent of the notification of the residency of offenders in some neighborhoods.

Psychological Theory

Freudian psychoanalytic theories are as much about psychopathology as they are about sexuality. When Freud involved sex in his ideas on psychotherapy, he was referring to the complex organization of the human mind. Freud placed sexuality and libido at the center of human development when he conceptualized the oral, anal, urethral, and phallic stages, and introduced ideas such as the Oedipal conflict. His references to sex verge on the allegorical, however, and by no means constitute a global theory of sexuality (22).

Classic psychodynamic theory considers adequate sexual functioning to have its origins in early family life with feelings of being loved or unloved. Necessary communication skills are learned in the family and society, and the development of sexuality is seen as part of general emotional and cognitive development. It would be equally reasonable to maintain, however, that adults are able to adjust sexually and develop the capacity to be intimate over and above the events of childhood. Interpersonal events of adult life also lead to feelings of adequacy or inadequacy or engender trust or distrust.

Social Influences

There are many new influences on sexuality in contemporary Western society, including the women's movement, acceptance of gay and lesbian lifestyles, converging gender roles, and the separation of the pleasures of sex from those of procreation. Other influential factors are economic, scientific, and social (e.g., drug use).

Masters and Johnston reported fear of sexual inadequacy in almost all men over 40 (23). Many factors, organic, psychological, and social contribute to this finding. The impact of social context on sexual activity is demonstrated when some men are able to have coitus in certain circumstances in a relationship but not in others. In ongoing relationships, ejaculatory inhibition frequently reflects interpersonal difficulties.

In considering sexuality, it is not possible to avoid the concept of normality. Conceptions of human behavior as being either inside or outside certain boundaries are subjective and bound by culture. Civilized individuals would judge some of these boundaries inviolable, such as the prohibitions on incest and bestiality; yet, within these borders, there are uncertainties. For instance, it is not always clear who constitutes an incestuous partner. Some would take a first cousin to be an acceptable partner but others would not. Similarly, in areas of same-gender sexual practices, individuals vary in the degree to which they consider these to be normalized. Not only is there variability in attitudes and values concerning normality between cultures and individuals but also in the same culture or individual over time.

Many factors are responsible for maintaining social behavior within boundaries. The private feelings of shame and guilt bound up with internalized cultural norms are central to sexual expression. Sexual functioning is made possible by good health, both physical and mental. Thus, physical and mental impairments may predispose an individual to develop socially unacceptable sexual behaviors.

The law is an important instrument of social control and the legal system has become increasingly involved with sexual function. Laws governing sexuality are generally a reflection of underlying social and cultural sexual norms. Criminal law controls forced sexual penetration, indecent dealings, public display of sexuality, and victimizing paraphilias. Family and divorce laws control established relationships and other laws oversee contraception and abortion. More laws control the sex industry and censorship, and still additional laws are concerned with sexual behavior in the workplace.

This depth of involvement indicates the level to which society engages itself in the sexual behavior of individuals. The law is constantly evolving. Controversies continue as old laws lose their relevance and new laws emerge. This varies from jurisdiction to jurisdiction, but one underlying theme is constant: sex is the business of the wider society, and its rules play a central role in the development of a man's sexual attitudes, values, and behavior.

Homosexuality

Although well established and accepted in some cultures, homosexuality continues to attract controversy. The "gay" lifestyle is a social phenomenon that has accompanied the growth of tolerance in Western culture. However, not all men who are practicing homosexuals participate in this stereotypic behavior. In general, sexuality is relatively safe for heterosexual men, but less safe for homosexual men, who have an increased risk of illness—in particular HIV/AIDS, a disorder that in Western societies appears largely confined to the homosexual population and intravenous drug users. Homosexual men also have a greater incidence of psychiatric disorders and increased suicide rates (24,25).

Different forms of sexual expression may be understood by considering all people as sexual with different objects for their carnal desires. The erotic feelings that a heterosexual man would have for a woman are similar to the feelings a homosexual man would have for another man. How this variation originates is a source of long-standing debate, but it is generally thought to occur either as part of development or through genetic predisposition. Opinions vary as to the relative importance of these two factors.

Existing diagnostic categories of sexual dysfunction and disorders have a heterosexual bias, and a broader understanding of the disorder at hand may be required when managing problems associated with sexual function in gay men (26). Dealing with the specific sexual concerns of gay men may be difficult because of unfamiliarity and possible disapproval of same sex behavior. An open mind and commitment to the process will allow for a satisfactory completion (27).

Paraphilias

In most people, the complexity of sexual intention is rarely consciously considered. The acting out of sexual desire involves cooperation with another individual in the mutual pursuit of pleasure including orgasm. In these circumstances, coercion, when it is present, is subtle and received by either party as part of consensual sexual behavior. In persons with a paraphilia, sexual intentions frequently intrude into consciousness often to the extent of preoccupation. Sexual activity is usually selfish and one-sided and may involve aggression and victimization. Mutuality is not considered.

Persons with a paraphilia have compulsive sexual urges or sexual behaviors requiring an unusual stimulus that is either personally or socially unacceptable. They are necessarily fixated and dependent on this stimulus for the optimal initiation or maintenance of sexual arousal and the facilitation or attainment of orgasm. The stimulus is either perceived directly or imagined as intensely arousing sexual fantasies. Sexual behaviors that are part of a paraphilia may involve children, nonconsenting adults, nonhuman objects, or the suffering of another person or the self (28).

Paraphilias are in general not common, although they are often profoundly disturbing manifestations of sexuality. Pedophilia, sexual activity with children or adolescents, is universally condemned and illegal. Some paraphilias are well known, such as exhibitionism (exposing the genitals), voyeurism (viewing sexual activities), and tranvestophilia (cross-dressing). There are many others that are less well known. Formicophilia is the use of crawling things such as ants and cockroaches for sexual pleasure. Autonepiophilia is when the paraphilic individual behaves like a child, usually in wearing diapers as a necessary part of sexual activity. Asphyxiophilia is a sometimes lethal activity in which self-strangulation is used to enhance erotic arousal either with or without a partner.

Gender Identity Disorders

Almost all men, regardless of sexual orientation, have a gender role congruent with their biological gender. A man with a gender identity disorder is distressed or is impaired in his everyday functions because he believes he should not be a man but rather a woman. The small number of men who have a gender identity disorder may go to the extent of gender reorientation surgery to cross over to the opposite gender. Men with this disorder may present with sexual dysfunction when they attempt sexual relations functioning in the role of a man against their inner desires to be a woman (29).

□ PSYCHOPATHOLOGY AND SEXUALITY
Psychiatric Disorders

From a psychiatric perspective, sexual dysfunction exists either as a primary psychiatric disorder or secondary to a general medical condition, another psychiatric disorder, or as an effect of medication or drug abuse. Primary sexual dysfunction is classified as a specific sexual disorder. Sexual dysfunction secondary to a psychiatric condition may be caused by anxiety disorders, mood disorders (depression and bipolar disorder), schizophrenia, or a number of other conditions.

Psychiatric disorders, particularly anxiety and mood disorders, are among some of the most common causes of sexual dysfunction in men. Psychiatric disorders may coexist with sexual dysfunction due to organic causes. An undiagnosed psychiatric disorder may be a cause of treatment resistance. Due to the high prevalence of psychiatric disorders, it is recommended that a brief psychiatric assessment be done for every patient presenting with a sexual dysfunction. For further information on this topic, see Chapter 24. It is also important to note that a man's partner may also have a psychiatric problem that could be negatively impacting his sex life.

Specific Sexual Disorders

Concerns about sexuality are ubiquitous. Concern over penis size is practically universal among men (30). An estimated 30% to 40% of the normal population has sexual dissatisfaction or dysfunction (31). Men may complain of a loss of sexual pleasure or suffer from a form of sexual addiction. Sexual addiction can be the final expression of a number of sexual disorders and paraphilias.

In psychiatry, the classification of sexual dysfunction is based on the human sexual physiological response described by Masters and Johnson (Chapter 3). They described four stages: drive, arousal, release, and resolution. One or more of these four phases of sexual response may be disturbed. Sexual desire disorders, sexual arousal disorders, and orgasm disorders represent the first three phases. To be considered a psychiatric disorder, the disturbance must cause marked distress or interpersonal difficulties and the sexual dysfunction must not be secondary to another psychiatric condition, medical condition, or substance abuse (32). The psychological and social variables that commonly impact sexual function at each of these stages are outlined briefly below and are discussed in further detail (Chapter 12).

Sexual Desire Disorders
There are two sexual desire disorders, hypoactive sexual desire disorder and sexual aversion disorder. In the first, there is a deficiency or absence of sexual fantasies or desire for sexual activity. In the second, there is persistent or recurrent aversion to and avoidance of all, or almost all, genital sexual contact with a sexual partner. Sexual desire disorders are often associated with psychological or social circumstances and may disguise another sexual problem.

Sexual Arousal Disorders
Arousal disorders in a man present as difficulties with erectile function. ED is defined as the inability to attain or to maintain an adequate erection until the completion of sexual activity, provided the impotence is not the result of a medical condition, another psychiatric condition, or substance abuse.

The underlying causes of ED are often multifactorial and there is a significant overlap of psychological and medical factors. The presence of impotence causes considerable anxiety and other psychological symptoms that further contribute to the problem. Estimates vary, but impotence is considered to have some organic medical basis in 50% to 80% of men (33).

Orgasmic disorders
Orgasmic disorders include premature ejaculation, delayed/absent ejaculation, and anorgasmia. Since the sympathetic nervous system is responsible for ejaculation, this phase of the sexual cycle is particularly vulnerable to psychological and social influence. The most common orgasmic disorder in men is premature ejaculation. Premature ejaculation is present when ejaculation occurs with minimal sexual stimulation before, on, or shortly after penetration and before the man wishes it to occur. Some men may have a biological predisposition to this condition, but premature ejaculation has been considered as usually having a psychological or social cause and can also be a learned behavior.

Anxiety about sex may cause difficulty with ejaculatory control. Other psychological factors that have been implicated are sexual guilt, a background of parent–child conflict, interpersonal hypersensitivity, and perfectionism or unrealistic expectations about sexual performance (34).

Anxiety Disorders

Anxiety disorders are common and are often associated with sexual dysfunction. They have a prevalence rate estimated to be between 2% and 5% and include generalized anxiety disorder, agoraphobia, other phobias, panic disorder, obsessive compulsive disorder, post-traumatic stress disorder, and acute stress disorder (35). Anxiety disorders may lead to sexual dysfunction involving all four stages of the human sexual physiological response. A further complicating factor for those men with agoraphobia and social phobia is that their disorder may inhibit social contact and therefore the opportunity to express their sexuality. About one-third of patients with obsessive compulsive disorder report obsessions experienced as recurrent intrusive thoughts that are sexual in nature (36). Associated compulsive behavior, such as repeated questioning concerning a partner's past sexual experiences, may severely affect relationships.

Stress is a potent and common cause of decreased sexual functioning. The rapid pace of change, unemployment, work stress, parenting, and financial burdens in the modern world contribute to sexual difficulties.

Post-traumatic stress disorder may occur after either experiencing or witnessing a life-threatening event that endangers either the person or someone close to them. Men who have been in combat are at risk of developing this condition and symptoms of sexual dysfunction may be part of their presentation.

Mood Disorders
Depression
Depression is a common, frequently recurrent, and sometimes chronic disorder of mood where the patient experiences either persistent sadness or a loss of interest in their normal activities for a period of weeks. Clinical features include fatigue, weight loss, and sleep disturbance. People who are depressed may feel worthless

and have inappropriate shame and guilt. They may have constant thoughts about death with suicidal ideas or actions (37). Some patients do not report feeling sad, but present with somatic complaints including sexual dysfunction. In fact, sexual dysfunction is common in depression, with decreased libido being the most likely symptom. Approximately 30% to 70% of patients with major depression experience decreased libido, and depression is a significant treatable cause of sexual disorder (38). Ejaculatory and erectile dysfunctions may also occur, either separately or together (39).

Mania

Bipolar disorder is characterized by episodes of mania (or hypomania) and depression. These mood disturbances are usually separated by periods of normal functioning. A manic episode is characterized by elevated, expansive, irritable or agitated mood, inflated self-esteem or grandiosity, sleep disturbance, talkativeness, racing thoughts, distractibility, disinhibition, and increased goal-directed activity either socially, at work, or sexually, together with excessive involvement in pleasurable activities that may have a high potential for painful consequences. Psychotic phenomena of a grandiose nature may be part of the symptoms of mania. Hypomania is a less severe form of mania.

During periods of elevated mood, the patient may have a heightened sexual drive, which, in the presence of disinhibition, may lead to reckless and sometimes self-destructive behavior. Once treated, the bipolar man may have profound guilt concerning his behavior when he was manic. This may affect future sexual and social functioning. Also he may have contracted a sexually transmitted disease.

Manic episodes may have intense effects on intimate relationships, possibly adversely affecting one's attractiveness to a partner. These effects may be both positive and negative. Certain aspects of manic behavior (e.g., hypersexuality or overgenerosity) can be attractive; indeed, a man in a manic phase may be charming. On the other hand, his partner may blame him for his unacceptable behavior or sexual indiscretions when in a manic or hypomanic state.

Other Psychiatric Disorders

Schizophrenia is a psychotic disorder characterized by delusions, hallucinations, and disorganized speech or behavior together with social or occupational decline (40). Delusions may exist separate from or as part of schizophrenia. The patient maintains a fixed false belief that is held despite evidence and reassurance to the contrary. A patient may present with what superficially might be a reasonable concern but it then proves to be without basis in reality. This delusion may be of a sexual nature and may be hypochondriacal, somatic, dysmorphic, or nihilistic. The delusion may also concern a psychotic false belief about a partner as part of the particularly dangerous psychiatric disorder of morbid jealousy.

A high frequency of sexual dysfunction has been found in patients with schizophrenia, whether treated or not (41). Desire, in particular, is decreased in untreated schizophrenia. Inappropriate or impaired social functioning may also preclude sexual activity even if there is no sexual dysfunction.

Substance Abuse

The effects of alcohol on sexual function are well known, and drugs of abuse have similar effects. In low doses, their use decreases inhibition and anxiety and sometimes leads to elation of mood, all of which increases sexual performance; however, erectile and/or orgasmic dysfunctions often result from continued use (42). Substance-induced sexual dysfunction is recognized as a specific disorder with sexual pain and impaired desire, arousal, or orgasm. In most people, abuse of all drugs, particularly opioids, suppresses desire in due course.

Cocaine and amphetamines give a subjective feeling of increased energy and may initially prolong an erection while impairing ejaculation; however, this is followed by ED. The hallucinogens can cause an artificial heightening of the sexual experience as part of their general affect but may also cause anxiety, delirium, and psychosis. Sadly, long-term substance abuse in adolescence may lead to diminished sexual functioning as well as difficulties in forming intimate personal relationships as a result of problems during crucial years of personality development.

Long-term alcohol abuse also impairs the ability of the liver to metabolize estrogens, leading to feminization, with testicular atrophy and breast development.

Psychiatric Aspects of Neurological Disorders
Dementia

Dementia or global cerebral impairment has many causes including Alzheimer's disease, cerebrovascular disease, trauma, infection, and substance abuse. It is most commonly seen in association with aging. Indifference to sexual activity is reported by about 70% of the spouses of Alzheimer's sufferers and sexual behavioral modifications in approximately 50% (43). The early changes of dementia can be subtle and difficult to demonstrate and may include a loss of the ability to judge the consequence of actions. Occasionally, this may be associated with the development of perverse disinhibited behavior.

Cerebrovascular Disease

Cerebrovascular disease produces localized and generalized cerebral lesions. Sexual dysfunction may result from a localized neurological deficit or a generalized manifestation of the disease process (i.e., dementia or depression). It is not unusual for a marked change in sexual activities to follow a cerebrovascular accident and its sequelae, and this change may be overlooked during rehabilitation (44).

Head Injury

Sexual dysfunction after head injury is prevalent. The consequences of head injury may have profound effects on an established relationship, and changes involving sexual functioning may be overlooked during rehabilitation. Such changes after head injury include impulsiveness, inappropriateness, changes in libido and sexual frequency, global sexual difficulties, and specific sexual dysfunctions (45).

Epilepsy

Disturbance of sexual functioning is common in men with partial seizures and is sometimes present, although less frequent, in those with generalized epilepsy. Between one- and two-thirds of men with partial seizures have hyposexuality (reduced sexual functioning), compared with less than one in ten who have generalized epilepsy. The most common complaint is general lack of sexual drive and disinterest. The specific problems of erectile and orgasmic dysfunction also occur. Occasionally, patients with partial seizures present with hypersexuality (increased sexual functioning) (46,47).

Psychopharmacological Factors

One of the major causes of sexual dysfunction is medication. Almost every pharmacological agent, particularly those used in psychiatry, has been associated with an effect on sexuality. Most currently prescribed antidepressants cause sexual dysfunction in up to half of the patients who take them (48). Sexual problems associated with antidepressant use include decreased libido and anorgasmia (49,50). Lithium, a mood stabilizer, can decrease sexual desire and erectile capabilities, although most patients on Lithium report normal pleasure and satisfaction with their sexual performance (51). Antipsychotics may directly cause erectile problems, including prolonged erection, also known as the "bicycle kickstand" phenomenon (52), retrograde ejaculation, and other orgasmic problems. In addition, certain antipsychotic agents cause weight gain, which can negatively affect a person's confidence, self-esteem, and sense of attractiveness and may decrease libido and cause orgasmic difficulties. Sexual side effects to psychiatric medications can lead to noncompliance, resulting in a recurrence of the patient's disorder. For more information on the sexual effects of psychiatric medications and other drugs, see Chapter 19.

□ **DYSFUNCTIONAL SOCIAL INFLUENCES**
Relationship Difficulties

Human relationships are at the interchange of economic, moral, and cultural life. Societal, familial, interpersonal, and individual elements contribute to the development of human relationships. In a time of increased individuality, interpersonal relationships have been affected but nevertheless remain an important domain for the expression of that individuality.

Relationship difficulties may be the cause of sexual problems or alternatively may be caused by them. Sexual functioning may be the barometer of a relationship and it usually expresses the depth of love two people have for each other. An intimate relationship that has good sex as one of its foundations has a greater chance of success. Deterioration in sexual functioning in a successful relationship may be experienced as a significant loss. When relationship problems occur, usually there is an effect on the couple's sex life that may be expressed as dysfunction in one of the partners.

Family Dysfunction
Family Events as Stressors

Many stressors originate directly or indirectly from family life. One example would be the serious illness, injury, or death of a child. This is a particularly disturbing event that may have long-term effects on a man's well-being. A man expects of himself and is expected by others to cope with his feelings and be supportive of other family members. Living up to these important expectations can come at a price. In general, men take their family responsibilities seriously and when things go wrong may internalize blame and guilt. Stressors such as these are known to cause psychological problems and may disturb a man's sexual function.

Domestic Violence

Domestic violence is a demonstration of pathology in an individual (usually a man) in the relationship. It is a poorly understood phenomenon that has serious consequences. Domestic violence may coexist with a healthy sex life or it may be the product of a disturbed sex life. It may be part of a psychiatric disturbance or the result of a sociopathic personality. The same psychological determinates that lead to violence may also bring about disturbances of sexual functioning. Episodes of domestic violence occur in all social and ethnic sections of society.

Sexual Abuse

When sexually compulsive persons seek relief for their urges, they may victimize others. Unfortunately, this may occur in family life. Campaigns to educate children on the dangers of sexual abuse usually have a "stranger danger" theme, when often the threat comes not from a stranger, but another family member. It may even be an adolescent or a female rather than an adult male. Unraveling the complex psychological and social determinants and effects of sexual abuse is a daunting clinical task.

Traumatic events associated with sexual abuse or rape have significant sexual as well as other consequences. Men are often the forgotten victims of these crimes. Although the occurrence of these events in men has been reported less frequently than in women, when they do occur, they have a profound effect on the psychological well-being of the male victim. The perpetrator already has a sexual dysfunction that leads to the victim developing problems of his own. Victims may have low sex drive and aversion to certain sexual activities that were part of the abuse-(53). They may also have specific symptoms of post-traumatic stress disorder, including flashbacks, nightmares, emotional numbing, and phobic avoidance. Most of the published data refers to women victims of sexual abuse, but the clinical experience of the authors supports its generalization to men.

Social Deprivation

Many people have limited economic resources. Sexual problems may not receive attention due to lack of availability of these resources and impoverishment may be one of the stressors contributing to the problems. Changes in economic circumstances brought about by business failures or unemployment, when combined with a man's sense of duty and responsibility, may result in psychiatric disorder and psychological disturbances including those of sexual functioning.

Sexual Crime

Abhorrent sexual acts such as rape are well established as crimes attracting severe punishments. In addition, there has been an increased recognition of the need to protect girls and boys from sexual victimization, along with a growth in the importance of the enforcement of criminal laws prohibiting sexual behavior with children and adolescents. Coupled with this is an increased tendency to see perpetrators not only as criminal but also as ill, with a shift in emphasis on treatment as part of rehabilitation. Nonviolent perpetrators of offences such as voyeurism or exhibitionism are more likely to be referred for treatment.

Other sexual acts that were previously considered criminal such as anal intercourse have been removed from the laws of many criminal jurisdictions, although this varies between countries and states.

☐ MANAGEMENT

Sexual functioning is psychosomatic, and for each man, the relative importance of social, psychological, and organic factors is to some extent unknown. Men with a disturbance of sexual functioning invariably develop an increased fear of failure and a self-consciousness about performance irrespective of the cause. In the clinical management of these disorders, a broad perspective assists in achieving satisfactory outcomes.

☐ REFERENCES

1. Sadock V. Normal human sexuality. In: Sadock BJ, Sadock VA, eds. Kaplan and Sadock's Comprehensive Textbook of Psychiatry. 7th ed. Philadelphia: Lippincott Williams & Wilkins, 2000:1577–1608.
2. Katchadourian H. Adolescent sexuality. Pediatr Clin North Am 1980; 27(1):17–28.
3. Leitenberg H, Detzer MJ, Srebnik D. Gender differences in masturbation and the relation of masturbation experience in preadolescence and/or early adolescence to sexual behavior and sexual adjustment in young adulthood. Arch Sex Behav 1993; 22(2):87–98.
4. Wiener JS, Marcelli M, Lamb DJ. Molecular determinants of sexual differentiation. World J Urol 1996; 14(5):278–294.
5. Hiort O, Holterhus PM, Nitsche EM. Physiology and pathophysiology of androgen action. Baillieres Clin Endocrinol Metab 1998; 12(1):115–132.
6. Erikson E. Identity and the Life Cycle. New York: International Universities Press, 1959:50–100.
7. Scharff DE. Sex is a family affair: sources of discord and harmony. J Sex Marital Ther 1976; 2(1):17–31.
8. Blos P. Son and father. J Am Psychoanal Assoc 1984; 32(2):301–324.
9. Golombok S, Tasker F, Murray C. Children raised in fatherless families from infancy: family relationships and the socioemotional development of children of lesbian and single heterosexual mothers. J Child Psychol Psychiatry 1997; 38(7):783–791.
10. Friedman HL. Changing patterns of adolescent sexual behavior: consequences for health and development. J Adolesc Health 1992; 13(5):345–350.
11. Broude G. The cultural management of sexuality. In: Munroe R, Munroe R, Whiting B, eds. Handbook of Cross-Cultural Human Development. New York: Garland STPM, 1981:633–673.
12. Fenwicke R, Purdie G. The sexual activity of 654 fourth form Hawkes Bay students. NZ Med J 2000; 113(1121): 460–464.
13. Tenover JL. Testosterone and the aging male. J Androl 1997; 18(2):103–106.
14. Zitzmann M, Nieschlag E. Testosterone levels in healthy men and the relation to behavioural and physical characteristics: facts and constructs. Eur J Endocrinol 2001; 144(3):183–197.
15. Hall R. Households, families and fertility. In: Hall R, White P, eds. Europe's Population: Toward the Next Century. London: UCL Press, 1995:38–42.
16. Seidman SN, Rieder RO. A review of sexual behavior in the United States. Am J Psychiatry 1994; 151(3): 330–341.
17. Brown JD. Adolescents' sexual media diets. J Adolesc Health 2000; 27(suppl 2):35–40.

18. Zillmann D. Influence of unrestrained access to erotica on adolescents' and young adults' dispositions toward sexuality. J Adolesc Health 2000; 27(suppl 2):41–44.

19. Pinnock CB, Stapleton AM, Marshall VR. Erectile dysfunction in the community: a prevalence study. Med J Aust 1999; 171(7):353–357.

20. Boyce EG, Umland EM. Sildenafil citrate: a therapeutic update. Clin Ther 2001; 23(1):2–23.

21. White SD, DeBlassie RR. Adolescent sexual behavior. Adolescence 1992; 27(105):183–191.

22. Gabbard G. Psychodynamic Psychiatry in Clinical Practice. Washington, D.C.: American Psychiatric Press, 1990:19–48.

23. Masters W, Johnson V. Human Sexual Response. Boston: Little Brown, 1966:260–270.

24. Sandfort TG, de Graaf R, Bijl RV, et al. Same-sex sexual behavior and psychiatric disorders: findings from the Netherlands Mental Health Survey and Incidence Study (NEMESIS). Arch Gen Psychiatry 2001; 58(1):85–91.

25. Cochran SD, Mays VM. Lifetime prevalence of suicide symptoms and affective disorders among men reporting same-sex sexual partners: results from NHANES III. Am J Public Health 2000; 90(4):573–578.

26. Rosser BR, Short BJ, Thurmes PJ, et al. Anodyspareunia, the unacknowledged sexual dysfunction: a validation study of painful receptive anal intercourse and its psychosexual concomitants in homosexual men. J Sex Marital Ther 1998; 24(4):281–292.

27. Stein T. Homosexuality and homosexual behavior. In: Sadock B, Sadock V, eds. Kaplan and Sadock's Comprehensive Textbook of Psychiatry. 7th ed. Philadelphia: Lippincott Williams & Wilkins, 2000:1608–1631.

28. Money J. Gay, Straight, and In-between: The Sexology of Erotic Orientation. New York: Oxford University Press, 1988:126–183.

29. Green R, Blanchard R. Gender identity disorders. In: Sadock B, Sadock V, eds. Kaplan & Sadock's Comprehensive Textbook of Psychiatry. 7th ed. Philadelphia: Lippincott Williams & Wilkins, 2000:1646–1662.

30. Murtagh J. The 'small' penis syndrome. Aust Fam Physician 1989; 18(3):218, 220.

31. Kessler RC, McGonagle KA, Zhao S, et al. Lifetime and 12-month prevalence of DSM-III-R psychiatric disorders in the United States. Results from the National Comorbidity Survey. Arch Gen Psychiatry 1994; 51(1):8–19.

32. American Psychiatric Association. Sexual and gender identity disorders. In: Diagnostic and Statistical Manual of Mental Disorders: DSM-IV, 4th ed. Washington, D.C.: American Psychiatric Publishing Inc., 1994:493–538.

33. McKinlay J. The worldwide prevelance and epidemiology of erectile dysfunction. Int J Impt Res 2000; 12(suppl 4): S6–S11.

34. Hartmann U. Psychological stress factors in erectile dysfunctions. Causal models and empirical results. Urologe A 1998; 37(5):487–494.

35. American Psychiatric Association. Anxiety Disorders. In: Diagnostic and Statistical Manual of Mental Disorders: DSM-IV, 4th ed. Washington, D.C.: American Psychiatric Publishing Inc., 1994:393–442.

36. Freund B, Steketee G. Sexual history, attitudes and functioning of obsessive-compulsive patients. J Sex Marital Ther 1989; 15(1):31–41.

37. American Psychiatric Association. Mood Disorders. Diagnostic and Statistical Manual of Mental Disorders: DSM-IV. 4th ed. Washington, D.C.: American Psychiatric Publishing Inc., 1994:317–391.

38. Clayton AH. Recognition and assessment of sexual dysfunction associated with depression. J Clin Psychiatry 2001; 62(suppl 3):5–9.

39. Phillips RL Jr, Slaughter JR. Depression and sexual desire. Am Fam Physician 2000; 62(4):782–786.

40. American Psychiatric Association. Schizophrenia and other psychotic disorders. In: Diagnostic and Statistical Manual of Mental Disorders: DSM-IV, 4th. Washington, D.C.: American Psychiatric Publishing Inc., 1994: 273–315.

41. Aizenberg D, Zemishlany Z, Dorfman-Etrog P, et al. Sexual dysfunction in male schizophrenic patients. J Clin Psychiatry 1995; 56(4):137–141.

42. Barton D, Joubert L. Psychosocial aspects of sexual disorders. Aust Fam Physician 2000; 29(6):527–531.

43. Derouesne C, Guigot J, Chermat V, et al. Sexual behavioral changes in Alzheimer disease. Alzheimer Dis Assoc Disord 1996; 10(2):86–92.

44. Sjogren K, Fugl-Meyer AR. Adjustment to life after stroke with special reference to sexual intercourse and leisure. J Psychosom Res 1982; 26(4):409–417.

45. Elliott ML, Biever LS. Head injury and sexual dysfunction. Brain Inj 1996; 10(10):703–717.

46. Lishman W. Organic Psychiatry: The Psychological Consequences of Cerebral Disorder. 2nd ed. Malden, MA: Blackwell Science, 1987.

47. Herzog AG. Psychoneuroendocrine aspects of temporolimbic epilepsy. Part I. Brain, Reproductive Steroids, and Emotions. Psychosomatics 1999; 40(2):95–101.

48. Balon R, Yeragani VK, Pohl R, et al. Sexual dysfunction during antidepressant treatment. J Clin Psychiatry 1993; 54(6):209–212.

49. Gelenberg AJ, Delgado P, Nurnberg HG. Sexual side effects of antidepressant drugs. Curr Psychiatry Rep 2000; 2(3):223–227.

50. Monteiro WO, Noshirvani HF, Marks IM, et al. Anorgasmia from clomipramine in obsessive-compulsive disorder. A controlled trial. Br J Psychiatry 1987; 151(1):107–112.

51. Aizenberg D, Sigler M, Zemishlany Z, et al. Lithium and male sexual function in affective patients. Clin Neuropharmacol 1996; 19(6):515–519.

52. Gold DD Jr, Justino JD. "Bicycle kickstand" phenomenon: prolonged erections associated with antipsychotic agents. South Med J 1988; 81(6):792–794.

53. Cahill C, Llewelyn SP, Pearson C. Long-term effects of sexual abuse which occurred in childhood: a review. Br J Clin Psychol 1991; 30(Pt 2):117–130.

9

Male Circumcision

Edgar J. Schoen

Department of Genetics, Kaiser Permanente Medical Center, Oakland, California, U.S.A.

□ DEFINITION

Circumcision (from the Latin *circumciseo*, to cut around) is defined as removal of part or all of the prepuce (foreskin). In the United States, about 80% of the male population—120 million boys and men—have been circumcised (1–4). Circumcision in the United States is usually done during the immediate neonatal period and consists of removing the foreskin from the preputial opening at the tip of the penis to the coronal sulcus at the base of the glans (Figs. 1 and 2) (5).

□ EMBRYOLOGY OF THE PENIS AND FORESKIN

Development of the penis and formation of the foreskin occur at 8 to 16 weeks' gestation (6–11). The male external genitalia are initially undifferentiated, arise from the genital tubercle, and masculinize by the 10th week of gestation under the influence of testosterone produced by the fetal testes. The genital tubercle develops into the phallus, which elongates and enlarges to become the penis. Beginning at 11 weeks' gestation, the spongy, endoderm-derived urethra of the body of the penis extends distally to meet the distal urethral opening (derived from ectoderm) and extends inward from the distal urethral orifice. The primitive foreskin arises in the region of the corona. The skin on the penile shaft grows faster than the shaft itself and folds itself dorsally to form a hood (the foreskin) over the glans. The foreskin then grows ventrally to completely encircle the glans. The frenulum is formed by the preputial and urethral folds as they fuse on the ventrum of the glans. Formation of the anterior aspect of the urethra is dependent on preputial development. Incomplete preputial development accounts for the hooded prepuce and lack of frenulum seen in hypospadias.

Keratinization between the preputial and the glanular epithelia occurs by six months of gestation and leads to pearl formation. The pearl cavities coalesce, thus allowing the foreskin in full-term infants to be mechanically retracted from the glans at birth without tearing the epithelia, although complete separation and easy retraction of the foreskin can take months or even years.

□ FUNCTION OF THE FORESKIN

The postnatal role of the foreskin is ill defined because definitive data are lacking. The foreskin protects the glans from trauma, and therefore might have been important in earlier times, when men lived naked in a hostile environment; however, the current value of the foreskin is questionable. Preputial secretions combine with epithelial debris to form smegma, a substance of unknown function that collects in the preputial space. Smegma has been thought to serve as a lubricant with an antibacterial role but has also been described as an effective bacterial culture medium that increases the chance of balanoposthitis (inflammation/infection of the glans and foreskin; a condition distinct from balanitis, inflammation/infection of the glans only) (Fig. 3) (5). Balanoposthitis occurs in about 3.5% of uncircumcised males at some time, is recurrent in many cases, and can lead to chronic irritation of the glans (12–14). Balanoposthitis can also lead to penile dermatoses and penile cancer later in life.

Smegma was shown to be carcinogenic when applied to the skin of animals (15). In horses, a species of animal in which the male produces large amounts of smegma, penile cancer accounts for 23% of carcinomas in males. Moreover, because geldings lack erections (which aid in the removal of smegma), geldings are 10 times more likely to develop penile cancer than are stallions (16). Evidence in both humans and monkeys (17–20) suggests that the foreskin is rich in phagocytic cells (Langerhans cells) to which the human immunodeficiency virus (HIV) can attach. These cells are target cells for HIV transmission and infection.

The appearance and odor of smegma have led to findings that many women esthetically prefer a circumcised penis and that the improved cleanliness made possible by circumcision encourages more varied sexual activity such as oral sex (21). But those favoring the uncircumcised state have claimed that the foreskin leads to improved sexual pleasure. (Sexual aspects of the foreskin are addressed in a separate section.)

Thus, the fetal foreskin plays an important embryologic role in genital differentiation and in complete development of the penis, particularly the glans and the anterior aspect of the urethra. By

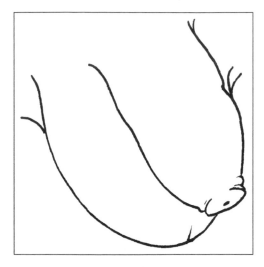

Figure 1 Normal uncircumcised penis in a newborn. The preputial opening appears small. The foreskin usually adheres to the glans and separates later.

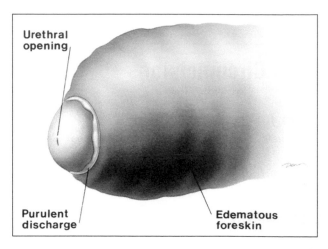

Figure 3 Balanoposthitis. Balanoposthitis is an infection of foreskin and glans resulting in edema, redness, pain, and purulent preputial discharge. *Source*: From Ref. 4.

contrast, presence of the foreskin has no proven benefit after birth and becomes a risk factor in development of urinary tract infection (UTI) (22–29), penile cancer (30–39), human papilloma virus (HPV) infection (40), cervical cancer in female partners (40,41), HIV (42–49), certain other sexually transmitted diseases (STDs) including chlamydia (46–62), local infections of the foreskin (11,57–60), and penile dermatoses (60), and makes genital hygiene more difficult (57–60). Newborn circumcision is therefore a preventive health measure that protects against these conditions later in life.

□ PREVALENCE, TIMING, AND METHOD OF CIRCUMCISION
Neonatal Circumcision

As shown by the diagnostic code assigned at the birth hospital, about 65% of boys born in the United States

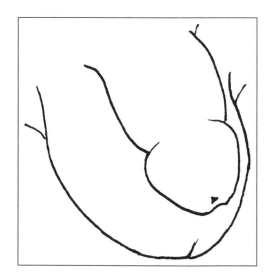

Figure 2 Circumcised penis in a newborn. The foreskin has been removed from the preputial opening to the coronal sulcus.

are circumcised as newborns (1,63), before they are discharged. This prevalence varies markedly across different geographic sections of the country and depends largely on cultural factors (63,64). The lowest circumcision rates are found on both coasts and are highest in middle America (64). Hispanic and Asian immigrants are uncircumcised, which accounts for the fact that the circumcision rate in California is under 40%. Hispanics currently account for more than half of the almost 600,000 infants each year who are born in California (65). Among nonimmigrants in California, the circumcision rate continues to be above 70% (66). The overall newborn circumcision rate was found to be about 65% among male subscribers to Kaiser Permanente of Northern California (28), a large health maintenance organization with more than 3 million members. Midwestern states have newborn circumcision rates of about 80% (2,3,8). In one Wisconsin community, 92% of newborn boys were circumcised (67).

The discrepancy between the 65% rate recorded from the hospital of birth and the 80% to 85% prevalence observed in older males (2,3,64,66,68–70) is explained by the fact that in about 15% of newborn males, the circumcision was performed in the birth hospital but not coded on the discharge sheet used for national statistics (68,70). Another 7% to 9% of males are circumcised postnatally for medical reasons (usually balanoposthitis or phimosis) (71,72).

Newborn circumcision is done by any of three acceptable methods: the Plastibell (Fig. 4), Gomco clamp (Fig. 5) (73), or Mogen clamp techniques (Fig. 6). Local anesthesia should be used with all three methods and may include dorsal penile nerve block (DPNB) (Fig. 7) (74), ring block, and/or anesthetic cream (most often a eutectic mixture of local anesthetic) (75–77). DPNB is probably the most effective and most widely used method. One weakness of anesthetic cream is that it must be applied approximately an hour before

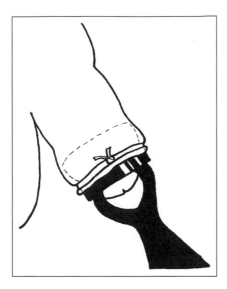

Figure 4 Plastibell method of circumcision. After separation and retraction of the foreskin, a plastic bell is fitted over the glans, and a suture is tied around the foreskin over a groove in the bell. The distal foreskin is excised, and the Plastibell handle is removed. The Plastibell is left in place and drops off after five to seven days. This figure shows the Plastibell in place after the foreskin has been excised.

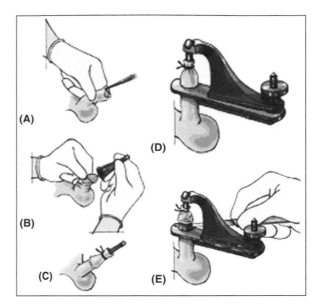

Figure 5 Gomco method of circumcision. (**A**) Foreskin is separated from the glans and a dorsal slit is often made to allow placement of the metal dome. (**B**) Metal dome is placed over the glans. (**C**) A suture is made around the foreskin (or a clamp is applied) to keep the foreskin in place. (**D**) Gomco clamp is slipped over the foreskin and then tightened and left in place for one to two minutes. (**E**) Distal foreskin over dome is excised; Gomco clamp is removed. *Source*: From Ref. 73.

circumcision. Having the newborn infant suck on a 20% sucrose solution has also been shown to decrease the pain response (78).

Of these three methods of newborn circumcision, the Mogen clamp method is the quickest and least traumatic (79); however, the author's experience has shown the Plastibell method to be the safest. The key to quick, safe, painless circumcision depends more on the experience of the practitioner than on the method used. Complication rates for properly performed circumcision are low (0.2–0.6%), and complications are usually minor (e.g., local infection and minor bleeding) (80–82). Severe complications (e.g., penile amputation) are extremely rare and are usually caused by improperly performed surgery. Reported deaths have almost all been secondary to general anesthesia. Hence, the author's opinion is that general anesthesia should never be used for elective circumcision.

Postneonatal Circumcision

In Finland, circumcision is not routinely performed in newborns and is instead done only when medically indicated (usually for local infection, phimosis, or both). Approximately 7.1% of males are circumcised after the newborn period in Finland, and 50% of these are boys younger than 15 years of age [Gissler M, National Research and Development Centre for Welfare and Health (STAKES), Helsinki, Finland, personal communication, February 7, 2000]. The author's experience is similar: from 1996 through 1998, 9.6% of uncircumcised male Kaiser Permanente subscribers required postneonatal circumcision for medical indications, and more than 50% of these patients received the procedure before the age of 15 years (71). Rates of postneonatal

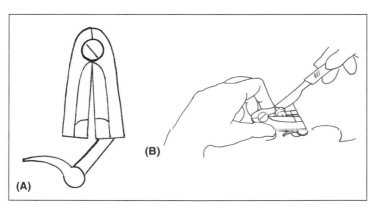

Figure 6 Mogen clamp method of circumcision. (**A**) Mogen clamp. (**B**) The procedure: after separation, the foreskin is pinched between the surgeon's fingers. The open Mogen clamp is slid across, and the clamp is closed, locked, and left in place for about 60 seconds. The distal foreskin is then excised with a scalpel (as shown) before reopening the clamp.

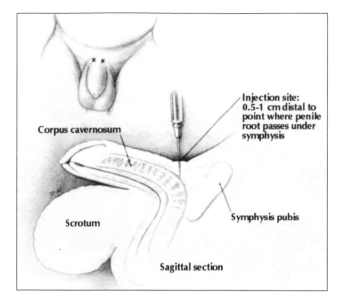

Figure 7 DPNB. Procedure: a 26-gauge needle is used to inject 0.5 to 1 mL of 1% lidocaine solution (without epinephrine) into two locations (10:30-hour position and 1:30-hour position) at the base of penis near pubic symphysis. Allow about two minutes before beginning the circumcision. *Abbreviation*: DPNB, dorsal penile nerve block. *Source*: From Ref. 74.

circumcision in England appear to be in the same range. Rickwood et al. (83) found that 3.8% of British boys under the age of 15 years required postneonatal circumcision. If the age distribution of patients receiving postneonatal circumcision in England is similar to the age distribution in Finland and in Kaiser Permanente (approximately 50% in boys less than 15 years of age), then the total rate of postneonatal circumcision for male patients of all ages would be about 7.5%, a figure remarkably similar to the Finnish finding.

Compared with newborn circumcision, post-neonatal circumcision is surgically more difficult and is about 10 times more expensive (71). The procedure is generally done by a urologist using a "freehand" technique, which takes more time than newborn circumcision and requires sutures. General anesthesia (which adds to the risk) may be used, and convalescence is more prolonged.

The difficulties presented by postneonatal circumcision emphasize that the newborn period is a window of opportunity for circumcision. Newborns who have so recently undergone the great trauma of birth have high levels of stress hormones (epinephrine, corticosteroids, thyroid hormones, and sex hormones), which increase the newborn's ability to cope with the surgical effects (stress) of circumcision. Newborns also heal quickly and are resilient. Use of local anesthesia prevents pain. Many medical providers are adept at the procedure, and an array of mechanical surgical equipment has been designed for newborn circumcision (e.g., the Gomco, Mogen, and Plastibell devices noted previously). The inner and outer layers of the thin foreskin adhere to each other after the clamp is applied, and sutures are rarely required. Circumcision

is more traumatic, disruptive, and expensive for older boys and men than for infants. Although no data are available on rates of complications after postneonatal circumcision, when performed in older boys and men, the procedure requires placement of sutures, requires more time, and leads to slower healing as well as greater potential for complications.

□ LIFETIME MEDICAL BENEFITS OF CIRCUMCISION

As is true of childhood immunization, newborn circumcision is a preventive health measure whose medical benefits accrue throughout life. In the case of newborn circumcision, these medical benefits continue from infancy through old age. Medical benefits of newborn circumcision in infancy and childhood include: prevention of severe UTI (22–29), avoidance of local infection (balanoposthitis), phimosis (unretractable foreskin due to preputial constriction) (Fig. 8), and paraphimosis (tight preputial ring, which allows foreskin retraction but prevents its return) (Fig. 9), three conditions that are often seen in childhood (12,57–60). In early adulthood, circumcised men benefit from reduction in susceptibility to HIV infection (42–49) and other STDs (49,50,53–60), including HPV and chlamydia infection (Fig. 10) (41,61). Evidence has shown that neonatal circumcision also helps prevent penile cancer (Fig. 11) in later life (30–39) and cervical cancer in female partners of circumcised men (40,41). Throughout life, newborn circumcision promotes ease of genital hygiene (57–60) and prevents penile dermatoses (62). Data on the multiple lifetime benefits extending from infancy through old age have appeared in the literature of different disciplines (pediatrics, geriatrics, urology, and infectious disease), and interpretation of these data has thus been compartmentalized. Nonetheless, separately considering the data on each preventive

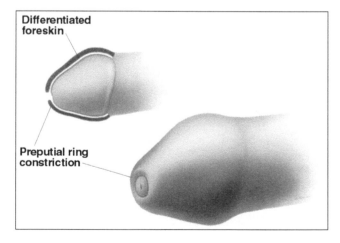

Figure 8 Phimosis. Phimosis is a constriction of the preputial opening (sometimes to pinpoint size) that prevents foreskin retraction despite separation of the foreskin from the glans.

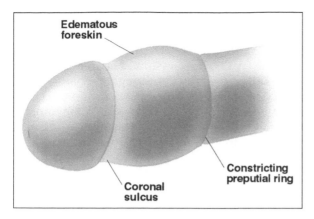

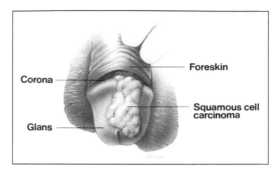

Figure 9 Paraphimosis. In paraphimosis, the preputial opening is tight but the foreskin can still be retracted over the glans, albeit with difficulty. Particularly in the case of erection, however, the foreskin cannot be brought back over the glans. The tight preputial ring interferes with circulation, causing edema. This further prevents return of the foreskin to a normal position.

Figure 11 Carcinoma of the penis. In most cases of penile carcinoma, invasive disease arises on the glans and is almost exclusively found in uncircumcised men.

health effect may help clinicians appreciate the overall medical evidence favoring newborn circumcision.

Reduced Risk of UTI

In the first year of life, serious UTI is about 10 times more likely to occur in uncircumcised boys than in circumcised infants (22,23,28,29). Multiple studies (22–29) comparing the odds ratio of UTI in uncircumcised versus circumcised infants have shown that the mean prevalence of UTI in uncircumcised infants is tenfold greater than in circumcised infants. UTI is most dangerous in the first three months of life, when UTI often leads to hospitalization (18 times more likely in uncircumcised than in circumcised infants) (28) and can result in sepsis and its consequences (23). In addition, UTI in infants can have long-term as well as acute effects, such as renal scarring, which has been found in about 40% of boys who had UTI as infants (84,85). Evidence (mainly from Europe, where infant circumcision is not routinely done) has shown that UTI in infants may be accompanied by disturbed renal and

hormonal function, including natriuresis, decreased glomerular filtration rate, hyperreninemia, and hyperaldosteronemia (86–88). The author has found similar cases in the United States (89). These findings raise concern that hypertension and renal failure might develop as late complications in patients who had UTI early in life.

Experimental evidence has elucidated the mechanism by which the foreskin predisposes males to UTI. Uropathic bacteria (mainly fimbriated *Escherichia coli*) bind preferentially to the moist mucosal undersurface of the foreskin and then ascend the urinary tract to cause UTI, including pyelonephritis (27,90–93).

Reduced Risk of Invasive Penile Cancer

For more than a century, invasive penile cancer has been recognized as extremely rare among circumcised men (94). Multiple reported series from major academic and cancer institutes have shown that essentially all invasive penile cancer occurs in uncircumcised men (30–42). In a study that reported an odds ratio of 3 for penile cancer in uncircumcised men (95), circumcision had a less complete protective effect; however, that study was flawed in that it invalidly combined carcinoma in situ (CIS), a benign condition, with invasive penile cancer, a devastating disease. More recently, an odds ratio of 22 was shown for invasive penile cancer in uncircumcised versus circumcised men, and only a threefold increased risk of CIS was found in uncircumcised men (28). These findings confirm earlier evidence of almost complete protection against invasive penile cancer in circumcised men.

Of about 1200 cases of penile cancer reported in the United States annually, more than 200 result in death, predominantly among uncircumcised men aged a mean of 60 years at diagnosis (96). In many underdeveloped countries, where poor hygiene is combined with lack of circumcision, penile cancer is one of the most common malignant conditions in men (97). In the United States, invasive penile cancer confers a lifetime risk of 1 in 600 in uncircumcised men (98) and is thus much less common than breast cancer, for which the lifetime risk is 1 in 11. However, invasive penile cancer is at least as devastating in several ways. Penile cancer

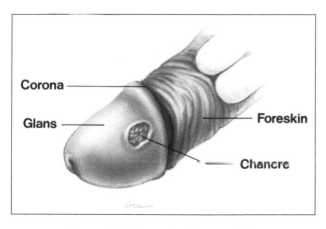

Figure 10 Chancre in primary syphilis.

has a lower five-year survival rate (72%) than breast cancer (89%), and treatment is at least as traumatic physically and emotionally (39,96). Partial or total penectomy is often required, and, as in breast cancer, chemotherapy and radiation may be part of the therapeutic regime. Invasive penile cancer is one of the most preventable (if not the most preventable) of all cancers: The odds ratio (at least 22) of uncircumcised men versus circumcised men (39) indicates that the protective effect of circumcision against invasive penile cancer is equivalent to the protective effect conferred by nonsmoking behavior on lung cancer and heart disease.

Reduced Risk of HPV Infection in Males and for Cervical Cancer in Female Partners of Circumcised Men

Although a link between male circumcision, penile cancer, cervical cancer, and HPV infection has long been known (99–101), the role of confounders has prevented definitive conclusions. The issue was clarified in 2002 by analyzing data from seven case-control studies in five countries and by correcting for confounders (40,41). Circumcised men were found to be less likely to have HPV infection, and their female partners were found to have a reduced risk of cervical cancer.

Reduced Susceptibility to HIV Infection and Other STDs

Circumcision has long been known to have a protective effect against certain STDs, particularly those (such as syphilis and chancroid) in which infection is promoted by disruption of the delicate foreskin mucosal surface (46,47,53–60,94). In the past 15 years, however, most excitement has been engendered by evidence (mainly from Africa) that circumcision has a protective effect against heterosexual transmission of HIV. More than 40 separate studies (including eight prospective series and one randomized controlled trial) have shown that uncircumcised men are two to eight times more likely to contact HIV infection after heterosexual exposure than are circumcised men (42–49,102,103). One prospective study involved couples in whom the woman was HIV positive and the man was HIV negative. Of the 137 couples in whom the man was uncircumcised, 40 men became HIV positive after 30 months, whereas none of the 50 circumcised men tested HIV positive. This difference in HIV incidence is highly significant ($p < 0.001$) (102). Potts estimated that universal circumcision in Africa and Asia would have prevented 8 million cases of HIV infection (104). Most convincing is a randomized controlled trial (RCT) from South Africa which showed that uncircumcised men were twice as likely to contract HIV on exposure as were circumcised men (49); the results were so convincing that the study was terminated early on ethical grounds. Publication is pending for two similar RCTs,

which also had to be terminated early when it was found that the uncircumcised men were at greater risk.

HIV infection and acquired immunodeficiency syndrome (AIDS) have assumed epidemic proportion in sub-Saharan Africa. Although the areas of sub-Saharan Africa where HIV infection is most prevalent contain only 2% of the world's population, more than 25 million HIV cases have been identified there (105), and more than 25% of adults between the ages of 15 and 45 years are HIV positive in some regions (106). Adult circumcision is being increasingly performed in some African countries in an attempt to control this HIV epidemic.

The situation differs in the United States, where most reported HIV/AIDS cases occur in homosexual (gay) men. Intravenous drug use accounts for a smaller number of cases, and heterosexually transmitted HIV disease is least common. An obvious observation is that if a man contracts HIV infection as the receptor of anal intercourse or through intravenous drug usage, his circumcision status is irrelevant. These factors make it difficult to evaluate the role of circumcision in HIV transmission among homosexual men, because men who are receptors of anal intercourse are at higher risk than are initiators. Despite this experimental problem, a Seattle (Washington) study of 502 homosexual men (107) showed that uncircumcised men had twice the risk of becoming HIV positive as did circumcised homosexual men.

The preponderance of other types of STDs in uncircumcised men is most evident in cases of syphilis and chancroid and is supported by data extending back before the turn of the twentieth century (47,94,108,109). A recent analysis of multiple studies of non-HIV STDs in Africa (46) showed that uncircumcised men are at increased risk of gonorrhea, syphilis, and chancroid. In cases of genital herpes and HPV infection, evidence was not conclusive (46) but more recent studies showed significant increases in risk of HPV (41) as well as for chlamydia (49) in uncircumcised men.

Reduced Risk of Foreskin Infection, Phimosis, and Penile Dermatoses

The preputial space offers a warm, moist environment for bacterial growth, a situation that leads to increased bacterial colonization in uncircumcised males (23,90,91). Bacterial colonization is promoted by adherence of fimbriated E. coli and other uropathic bacteria to the inner, moist surface of the foreskin and can lead not only to ascending UTI but also to balanoposthitis, local infection of the foreskin and glans (balanoposthitis) (Fig. 3) (5) with swelling, pain, and purulent discharge (12). In children, balanoposthitis is most common between the ages of two to five years (12). At this "in-between age," when the foreskin may not yet have completely separated from the glans, a greater likelihood of poor hygiene exists because the child is still learning to wash himself and because parents may no longer maintain proper cleansing habits. Balanoposthitis is also more likely to develop in those living under poor hygienic conditions (57–60). This situation was evident in World War II, particularly during the North African desert campaign, where a profusion of sand and lack of water resulted in severe local foreskin infections. More than 146,000 U.S. servicemen required hospitalization for local infection, phimosis, and other problems related to the foreskin (60). Servicemen "were unable to maintain adequate local hygiene under combat conditions. The man hours lost as a result of circumcisions and adjuvant therapy were costly to the war effort and exasperated the commanding officers. Time and money could have been saved had prophylactic circumcision been performed before the men were shipped overseas" (60). This loss of soldiers from active duty led the armed services to perform prophylactic circumcision in many young recruits as well as therapeutic circumcision in men who were on active duty. A similar problem occurred in Iraq during the military operation known as "Desert Storm."

Phimosis ("to tie with a string") (94) is defined as constriction of the preputial opening at the tip of the foreskin so that the foreskin cannot be retracted, even when it has separated from the glans (Fig. 8). A common misconception among many professionals and laymen is that phimosis is simply inability to retract the foreskin due to adherence of the foreskin to the glans (67). Inability to retract the foreskin may be due either to physiologic adhesion of the prepuce to the gland or to fibrous adhesion (Fig. 12). Phimosis consists of a permanent preputial constriction, often a pinpoint opening. Because of trapped secretions and buildup of smegma, phimosis predisposes affected men to early local infection as well as to penile cancer later in life. Phimosis also results in painful erections because the foreskin is unable to retract over the glans. The most famous case of phimosis was that of King Louis XVI of France, husband of Marie Antoinette (110). When this couple married as teenagers, the young king had painful erections due to phimosis, preventing sexual activity with a consequent lack of heirs. The condition was remedied when, at age 22, the king was circumcised and sexual pleasure and offspring resulted. (The story ended sadly for the king, however: The circumcision was followed by decapitation a few years later.) True phimosis necessitates circumcision for medical reasons.

Circumcision also reduces the incidence of local skin disorders. Types of penile dermatoses ranging from eczema to psoriasis to lichen planus are more common among uncircumcised males at all ages than among circumcised males (62).

Improved Genital Hygiene

As noted previously, balanoposthitis, phimosis, and local problems often occur in uncircumcised men and boys (12–14,57–60,111). By retracting and properly cleaning under the foreskin, risk of balanoposthitis can be minimized. The likelihood of penile cancer also can be decreased by good genital hygiene. However, even in developed countries with high standards of hygiene and a low rate of penile cancer, this rate remains about 10 times higher in uncircumcised men (39,96,112). In cases of true phimosis, adequate genital hygiene is impossible because the constricted preputial opening prevents retraction.

The importance of good genital hygiene in uncircumcised males is widely recognized but is often not achieved. A study of British middle-class schoolboys attending private schools showed that poor genital hygiene was the rule despite easy availability of facilities for washing and cleansing (13). When adequate sanitary facilities are unavailable, such as in underdeveloped countries or in unusual situations (e.g., war), acute and chronic penile problems occur frequently (57–60). In areas of poverty, penile cancer is much more prevalent in uncircumcised men than in circumcised men despite the equally low living standards maintained by both groups (31,39,112). Similar findings were reported for increased cervical cancer rates in the wives of uncircumcised men and in the wives of men with penile cancer (100,113), although confounding factors make these findings less compelling than those for penile cancer alone. A more recent, comprehensive study supports the preventive effect of circumcision against cervical cancer (40,41).

Adequate genital hygiene is also difficult to achieve in elderly men, particularly those in nursing homes where they cannot care for themselves. The problem of having others retract the foreskin and properly clean the genitals is not only an embarrassment but can also have a sexual connotation to a confused older man. This problem has been observed in facilities that house U.S. veterans (114).

Clearly, circumcision promotes genital hygiene throughout life, particularly in childhood and in old age (i.e., when washing is done mostly by others) and when adequate sanitary care is unavailable. But even in

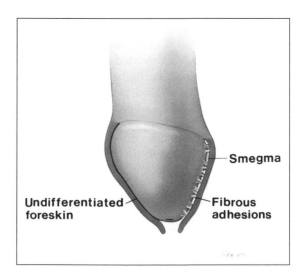

Figure 12 Adherent foreskin. Undifferentiated foreskin with physiologically delayed separation of the foreskin from the glans and adhesion of the foreskin to the glans by fibrous bonds. As in true phimosis, these conditions can result in an inability to retract the foreskin.

developed countries, genital hygiene is often inadequate among uncircumcised males (13,57–60,114).

□ CIRCUMCISION AND SEXUAL FUNCTION

Although anticircumcision groups claim that presence of the foreskin enhances sexual pleasure, the proof offered consists of anecdotes and testimonials. No objective evidence indicates that uncircumcised men have more sexual pleasure than circumcised men do. Indeed, there is no reason to believe that U.S. men (most of whom are circumcised) do not enjoy sex at least as much as do Europeans, who traditionally are not circumcised. Immediately after World War II, when U.S. forces occupied European and Asian countries, the attractiveness of "Yanks" to European and Asian women was shown by the high number of foreign brides of servicemen and by the success of these soldiers in competing for the favors of women in countries where circumcision is not routinely done. Similarly, there is no evidence showing better sexual function in Hindu men (uncircumcised) than in Moslem or Jewish men (circumcised) or better sexual function among men born in Europe (uncircumcised) than in those born in the United States (mostly circumcised).

The lack of a sexually important role of the foreskin is not surprising in view of the complexity of erectile function (115,116). Sexual behavior and penile erection are controlled by the nervous system (i.e., the hypothalamus, cerebral cortex, and spinal cord). Erection is a neurovascular event that involves sensory, motor, and autonomic nerves and neurotransmitters, the cavernosal structures of the penis, the penile circulation, and hormonal factors. The foreskin does have sensory nerve endings that have a role in initiating erectile function, but these nerve endings are also present in large numbers in the rest of the penile skin, glans, and urethra. The glans itself is the site of numerous afferent terminations with free nerve endings and corpuscular receptors present in a ratio of 10:1. There is no objective clinical or experimental data indicating that the foreskin is needed for initiation of sexual play, and certainly the foreskin is not one of the multiple important factors required in erectile function.

Recent reports (117–121) show no clinically significant differences in sexual function or penile sensitivity in circumcised versus uncircumcised men. Some studies have shown an advantage of circumcision in sexual activity. Laumann et al. (1) found that circumcised men have more varied sexual experiences, and uncircumcised men are more likely to have sexual dysfunction later in life. A survey of midwestern U.S. women (21) showed that the circumcised penis was preferred by 75% of these women, mainly because of improved genital hygiene. Circumcised men were preferred for sexual intercourse and for fellatio. When the women who preferred the circumcised penis were asked their reasons for this preference, they answered that it was cleaner (92%), looked sexier (90%), felt nicer (85%) and, most interestingly, seemed more natural (77%).

□ RELIGIOUS, HISTORICAL, AND CULTURAL ASPECTS

Circumcision is the first known surgical procedure, having been performed for millennia. In the Jewish religion, as recorded in *Genesis*, circumcision is performed on the eighth day of life as a covenant between Abraham and God. Muslim boys are usually circumcised later in childhood, depending on the culture of the particular region. Ancient Egyptian paintings depict circumcision. In Africa, certain tribes practice circumcision as a rite of passage into manhood, and boys in the Philippines are circumcised in the preadolescent period, usually at about 10 years of age.

Circumcision in the United States

In the United States, widespread circumcision began at the end of the nineteenth and beginning of the twentieth century. This trend was greatly influenced by a monograph (originally published in 1891 with two subsequent editions) in which a prominent California physician, Peter Remondino, thoroughly reviewed the medical aspects of circumcision (94). Remondino recognized the health benefits of circumcision (prevention of penile cancer, syphilis, phimosis, and other local problems) as well as improved genital hygiene. Although he was mistaken in overemphasizing the clinical significance of the foreskin in masturbation (a practice feared at the time), most of Remondino's observations have been confirmed and were probably responsible for the increasing popularity of circumcision in the United States. An epidemiologic study of penile cancer by Wolbarst in 1932 (30) and observations in the same year by Dean et al. (31) at Memorial Hospital in New York City (currently Memorial Sloan-Kettering Cancer Center) proved that invasive penile cancer was found almost exclusively in uncircumcised men; this finding was reported also in subsequent studies (37–39). The popularity of circumcision continued to increase in the United States as a result of the writings of Remondino, of the clinical findings of Wolbarst, Dean, and others on penile cancer, and of the then current emphasis on genital hygiene and avoidance of local infection. By the mid-1930s, about half of all U.S. male newborns were circumcised. This number increased to about 90% in the 1950s and 1960s (i.e., after World War II), when the Armed Forces demonstrated the health advantages of the procedure (57–60). However, in the late 1960s and early 1970s, with the increased popularity of techniques for promoting infant bonding, advocacy of ways to avoid causing discomfort to newborns was sought. Emphasis was placed on eliminating intervention during the newborn period, and newborn circumcision became unpopular in some middle-class families, mainly on the East and West Coasts. The wisdom of this course was challenged in the mid-1980s by Wiswell et al. (22), who indicated that uncircumcised infant boys under the age of one year were about 10 times more likely to get severe UTI as were those who had been circumcised. With subsequent publication of multiple studies confirming these observations on infant UTI (22–29) as well as evidence (mainly from Africa) of increased risk of heterosexual HIV infection among uncircumcised men (46–56), the popularity of newborn circumcision stabilized, and there is evidence that it increased between 1988 and 2000 (2,122).

☐ THE ANTICIRCUMCISION MOVEMENT

The activist anticircumcision movement began in the early 1970s coincidentally with both the popularity of the infant bonding movement and the publication of anticircumcision statements issued by the American Academy of Pediatrics (123,124). A number of lay anticircumcision groups with descriptive acronyms have formed over the past 30 years, including NOCIRC (National Organization of Circumcision Resource Centers), NOHARMM (National Organization to Halt Abuse and Routine Mutilation of Males), and various "foreskin restoration" groups such as NORM (National Organization of Restoring Males), RECAP (Recover a Penis) and BUFF (Brothers United for Future Foreskins).

The anticircumcision groups have successfully promoted their message in newspapers and on radio and television. Anticircumcision websites dominate the topic of circumcision on the Internet. The most remarkable achievement of the lay anticircumcision groups has been their success in encouraging and contributing to a 1999 supplemental issue of a major medical journal, *BJU International* (125), to advance their cause. Although the editors of the *BJU International* supplement stated that their aim was "the dissemination of varying convictions" (126), many of the contributors were lay leaders and members of the anticircumcision organizations mentioned above. Moreover, although many investigators have conducted major studies relating circumcision to prevention of diseases (including UTI, penile cancer, and HIV), none were represented in the supplement. Over the years, the leaders of the anticircumcision movement have managed to increase their influence through mass media–based activism despite the mounting clinical evidence confirming the health benefits of circumcision. They have been successful in convincing 16 states not to cover the cost of newborn circumcision in welfare patients, thus depriving poor boys of the protective effect of circumcision.

☐ CONCLUSION

During fetal life, the foreskin plays an important embryologic role in the development of the distal aspect of the penis, including the glans and the anterior aspect of the urethra. After birth, however, the foreskin is a risk factor for a variety of local and systemic disorders from infancy to old age, including: phimosis, balanoposthitis, UTI, HIV, HPV and chlamydia infection, and penile cancer, and cervical cancer in female partners of uncircumcised men. Although the foreskin has been claimed to increase sexual pleasure, no clinical evidence exists to support this contention. Indeed, data show that women prefer the circumcised penis esthetically, mainly because of improved cleanliness.

When properly performed by an experienced practitioner using local anesthesia, newborn circumcision is quick, safe, and virtually painless. A large body of compelling published medical evidence, particularly from the last two decades, shows that newborn circumcision is a valuable preventive health measure that protects against a wide variety of disorders throughout life.

☐ ACKNOWLEDGMENTS

The author would like to acknowledge the assistance of Trinh T. To, B.S. with graphics preparation and bibliographic research, as well as the editorial assistance of the Medical Editing Service of The Permanente Medical Group Physician Education and Development Department.

☐ REFERENCES

1. Laumann EO, Masi CM, Zuckerman EW. Circumcision in the United States: prevalence, prophylactic effects, and sexual practice. JAMA 1997; 277(13): 1052–1057.
2. Schoen E. Ed Schoen, MD on Circumcision: Timely Information for Parents and Professionals from America's #1 Expert on Circumcision. Berkeley, CA: RDR Books, 2005.
3. Schoen EJ. Re: the increasing incidence of newborn circumcision: data from the nationwide inpatient sample [letter]. J Urol 2006; 175(1):394–395; author reply 395.
4. Xu F, Markouitz L, Sternberg M, Aral S. Prevalence of circumcision in the United States: data from the National Health and Nutritional Examination Survey. (NHANES), 1999–2002. XVI International AIDS conference, 2006 (Abstract TUPEO 395).
5. Newborn Circumcision [videotape]. Oakland, CA: Northern California Innovation Program, Regional Health Education, Multimedia Communications (California Division), Kaiser Permanente, 1998.
6. Moore KL, Persaud TV. The Developing Human: Clinically Oriented Embryology. 6th ed. Philadelphia: WB Saunders, 1998.
7. Brooks JD. Anatomy of the lower urinary tract and male genitalia. In: Walsh PC, Retik AB, Vaughan ED, et al., eds. Campbell's Urology. 7th ed. Philadelphia: WB Saunders, 1998:89–128.
8. Maizels M. Normal and anomalous development of the urinary tract. In: Walsh PC, Retik AB, Vaughan ED, et al., eds. Campbell's Urology. 7th ed. Philadelphia: WB Saunders, 1998:1545–1600.
9. Tanagho EA. Anatomy of the genitourinary tract. In: Tanagho EA, McAninch JW, eds. Smith's General Urology. 15th ed. New York: Lange Medical Books/ McGraw-Hill, 2000:1–16.
10. Tanagho EA. Embrology of the genitourinary system. In: Tanagho EA, McAninch JW, eds. Smith's General Urology. 15th ed. New York: Lange Medical Books/ McGraw-Hill, 2000:17–30.
11. Altemus AR, Hutchins GM. Development of the human anterior urethra. J Urol 1991; 146(4):1085–1093.
12. Escala JM, Rickwood AM. Balanitis. Br J Urol 1989; 63(2):196–197.
13. Kalcev B. Circumcision and personal hygiene in school boys. Med Officer 1964; 112:171–173.
14. Oster J. Further fate of the foreskin: incidence of preputial adhesions, phimosis, and smegma among Danish school-boys. Arch Dis Child 1968; 43(228):200–203.
15. Plaut A, Kohn-Speyer AC. The carcinogenic action of smegma. Science 1947; 105(2728):391–392.
16. Schoberlein W. Significance and frequency of phimosis and smegma. Muchener Medizinische Wochenschrift 1966; 7:373–377. (Translated by Kasper JP, 1997; edited by Bailis SA, 1997.)
17. Szabo R, Short RV. How does male circumcision protect against HIV infection? BMJ 2000; 320:1592–1594.
18. Miller CJ. Localization of Simian immunodeficiency virus-infected cells in the genital tract of male and female Rhesus macaques. J Reprod Immunol 1998; 41(1–2):331–339.
19. Hussain LA, Lehner T. Comparative investigation of Langerhans' cells and potential receptors for HIV in oral, genitourinary and rectal epithelia. Immunology 1995; 85(3):475–484.
20. Patterson BK, Landay A, Siegel JN, et al. Susceptibility to human immunodeficiency virus-1 infection of human foreskin and cervical tissue grown in explant culture. Am J Pathol 2002; 161(3):867–873.
21. Williamson ML, Williamson PS. Women's preferences for penile circumcision in sexual partners. J Sex Educ Ther 1988; 14(2):8–12.
22. Wiswell TE, Enzenauer RW, Holton ME, et al. Declining frequency of circumcision: implications for changes in the absolute incidence and male to female sex ratio of urinary tract infections in early infancy. Pediatrics 1987; 79:338–342.
23. Wiswell TE. John K. Lattimer lecture. Prepuce presence portends prevalence of potentially perilous periurethral pathogens. J Urol 1992; 148(2 Pt. 2): 739–742.
24. Roberts JA. Does circumcision prevent urinary tract infection? J Urol 1986; 135(5):991–992.
25. Spach DH, Stapleton AE, Stamm WE. Lack of circumcision increases the risk of urinary tract infection in young men. JAMA 1992; 267(5):679–681.
26. Shaw KN, Gorelick M, McGowan KL, et al. Prevalence of urinary tract infection in febrile young children in the emergency department. Pediatrics 1998; 102(2):e16.
27. Lohr JA. The foreskin and urinary tract infections. J Pediatr 1989; 114(3):502–504.
28. Schoen EJ, Colby CJ, Ray GT. Newborn circumcision decreases incidence and costs of urinary tract infections during the first year of life. Pediatrics 2000; 105(4 Pt 1):789–793.
29. Jakobsson B, Esbjorner E, Hansson S. Minimum incidence and diagnostic rate of first urinary tract infection. Pediatrics 1999; 104(2 Pt 1):222–226.
30. Wolbarst AL. Circumcision and penile cancer. Lancet 1932; 1:150–153.
31. Dean AL Jr. Epithelioma of the penis. J Urol 1935; 33:252–283.
32. Lenowitz H, Graham AP. Carcinoma of the penis. J Urol 1946; 56:458–484.
33. Hardner GJ, Bhanalaph T, Murphy GP, et al. Carcinoma of the penis: analysis of therapy in 100 consecutive cases. J Urol 1972; 108(3):428–430.

34. Dagher R, Selzer ML, Lapides J. Carcinoma of the penis and the anti-circumcision crusade. J Urol 1973; 110(1):79–80.

35. Persky L, deKernion J. Carcinoma of the penis. CA Cancer J Clin 1986; 36(5):258–273.

36. Leiter E, Lefkovitis AM. Circumcision and penile carcinoma. NY State J Med 1975; 75:1520–1522.

37. Heyns CF, van Vollenhoven P, Steenkamp JW, et al. Cancer of the penis—a review of 50 patients. S Afr J Surg 1997; 35(3):120–124.

38. Schoen EJ. The relationship between circumcision and cancer of the penis. CA Cancer J Clin 1991; 41(5):306–309.

39. Schoen EJ, Oehrli M, Colby CJ, et al. The highly protective effect of newborn circumcision against invasive penile cancer. Pediatrics 2000; 105(3):E36.

40. Adami HO, Trichopoulos D. Cervical cancer and the elusive male factor. N Engl J Med 2002; 346(15): 1160–1161.

41. Castellsagué X, Bosch FX, Muños N, et al. Male circumcision, penile human papillomavirus infection, and cervical cancer in female partners. N Engl J Med 2002; 346(15):1105–1112.

42. Cameron DW, Simonsen JN, D'Costa LJ, et al. Female to male transmission of human immunodeficiency virus type 1: risk factors for seroconversion in men. Lancet 1989; 2(8660):403–407.

43. Simonsen JN, Cameron DW, Gakinya MN, et al. Human immunodeficiency virus infection among men with sexually transmitted diseases. Experience from a center in Africa. N Engl J Med 1988; 319(5):274–278.

44. Moses S, Plummer FA, Bradley JE, et al. The association between lack of male circumcision and risk for HIV infection: a review of the epidemiological data. Sex Transm Dis 1994; 21:201–210.

45. Kelly R, Kiwanuka N, Wawer MJ, et al. Age of male circumcision and risk of prevalent HIV infection in rural Uganda. AIDS 1999; 13(3):399–405.

46. Moses S, Bailey RC, Ronald AR. Male circumcision: assessment of health risks and benefits. Sex Transm Infect 1998; 74(5):368–373.

47. Caldwell JC, Caldwell P. The African AIDS epidemic. Sci Am 1996; 274:62–63:66–68.

48. Halperin DT, Bailey RC. Male circumcision and HIV infection: 10 years and counting. Lancet 1999; 354(9192):1813–1815.

49. Auvert B, Taljaard D, Lagarde E, et al. Randomized, controlled intervention trial of male circumcision for reduction of HIV infection risk: the ANRS 1265 Trial. PLoS Med 2005; 2(11):e298. Epub 2005 Oct 25.

50. Wilson RA. Circumcision and venereal disease. Can Med Assoc 1947; J 56:54–56.

51. Bailey RC, Moses S, Parker CB, et al. Male circumcision for HIV prevention in young men in Kisumu, Kenya: a randomized controlled trial. Lancet 2007; 369:643–656.

52. Gray RH, Kigozi G, Serwadda D, et al. Male circumcision for HIV prevention in men in Rakai, Uganda: randomized trial. Lancet 2007; 369:657–666.

53. Sawires SR, Dworken SL, Flamma A, et al. Viewpoint. Male circumcision and HIV/AIDS: challenges and opportunities. Lancet 2007; 869:707–713.

54. Parker SW, Stewart AJ, Wren MN, et al. Circumcision and sexually transmissible disease. Med J Aust 1983; 2(6):288–290.

55. Taylor PK, Rodin P. Herpes genitalis and circumcision. Br J Vener Dis 1975; 51(4):274–277.

56. Thirumoorthy T, Sng EH, Doraisingham S, et al. Purulent penile ulcers of patients in Singapore. Genitourin Med 1986; 62(4):253–255.

57. Patton JF. Venereal disease. United States Army. Medical Dept. Surgery in World War II: Urology. Washington, D.C.: Office of the Surgeon General and Center of Military History, United States Army, 1987: 45–88.

58. Stewart CM. Infections and related conditions. United States Army. Medical Dept. Surgery in World War II: Urology. Washington, D.C.: Office of the Surgeon General and Center of Military History, United States Army, 1987:99–146.

59. Vermooten V. Genitourinary neoplasms. United States Army. Medical Dept. Surgery in World War II: Urology. Washington, D.C.: Office of the Surgeon General and Center of Military History, United States Army, 1987:167–192.

60. Culp OS, Patton JF. Reflections. United States Army. Medical Dept. Surgery in World War II: Urology. Washington, D.C.: Office of the Surgeon General and Center of Military History, United States Army, 1987:485–490.

61. Castellsagué X, Peeling RW, Franceschi S, et al. *Chlamydia trachomatis* infection in female partners of circumcised and uncircumcised adult men. Am J Epidemiol 2005; 162(9):907–916. Epub 2005 Sep 21.

62. Mallon E, Hawkins D, Dinneen M, et al. Circumcision and genital dermatoses. Arch Dermatol 2000; 136(3): 350–354.

63. National Center for Health Statistics (United States). Trends in circumcisions among newborns. http:// www.cdc.gov/nchs/products/pubs/pubd/hestats/ circumcisions/circumcisions.htm (accessed November 11, 2001).

64. Adler R, Ottaway S, Gould S. Circumcision: we have heard from the experts; now let's hear from the parents [abstract]. Pediatrics 2001; 107(2):395.

65. California. Department of Health Services. Vital Statistics Data Tables, 1999. Sacramento, CA: Department of Health Services, 2001. http://www.dhs. ca.gov/; select "Statistical Resources"; "Vital Statistics" (accessed May 4, 2001).

66. Ciesielski-Carlucci C, Milliken N, Cohen NH. Determinants of decision making for circumcision. Camb Q Healthc Ethics 1996; 5(2):228–236.

67. Van Howe RS. Variability in penile appearance and penile findings: a prospective study. Br J Urol 1997; 80(5):776–782.

68. O'Brien TR, Calle EE, Poole WK. Incidence of neonatal circumcision in Atlanta, 1985–1986. South Med J 1995; 88 (4):411–415.

69. Binner SL, Mastrobattista JM, Day NC, et al. Effect of parental education ib decision-making about neonatal circumcision. South Med J 2002; 95(4): 457–461.

70. Lyon J. Neonatal circumcision in Anchorage 1985–1990. Alaska Med 1992; 34(2):94–95.

71. Schoen EJ, Colby CJ, To TT. Cost analysis of neonatal circumcision in a large health maintenance organization. J Urol 2006; 175(3 Pt 1):1111–1115.

72. Colby CJ, Schoen EJ, Ray GT, et al. Cost analysis of newborn circumcision (NC) in a large health maintenance organization (HMO). Pediatr Res 2001; 49(Part 2):395.

73. Bennett PC. Circumcision. Dr. Paul.co.nz [website]. http://www.drpaul.co.nz; select "Procedures"; then "Circumcision" (accessed March 3, 2004).

74. Fontaine P, Toffler WL. Dorsal penile nerve block for newborn circumcision. Am Fam Physician 1991; 43(4):1327–1333.

75. Stang HJ, Snellman LW, Condon LM, et al. Beyond dorsal penile nerve block: a more humane circumcision. Pediatrics 1997; 100(2):E3.

76. Butler-O'Hara M, LeMoine C, Guillet R. Analgesia for neonatal circumcision: a randomized controlled trial of EMLA cream versus dorsal penile nerve block. Pediatrics 1998; 101(4):E5.

77. Taddio A, Pollock N, Gilbert–Macleod C, et al. Combined analgesia and local anesthesia to minimize pain during circumcision. Arch Pediatr Adolesc Med 2000; 154(6):620–623.

78. Blass EM, Hoffmeyer LB. Sucrose as an analgesic for newborn infants. Pediatrics 1991; 87(2):215–218.

79. Kurtis PS, DeSilva HN, Bernstein BA, et al. A comparison of Mogen and Gomco clamps in combination with dorsal penile nerve block in minimizing the pain of neonatal circumcision. Pediatrics 103(2):E23.

80. American Academy of Pediatrics Report of the Task Force on Circumcision. Pediatrics 1989; 84(2):388–391. Published erratum appears in Pediatrics 1989; 84(5):761.

81. Circumcision policy statement. American Academy of Pediatrics. Task Force on Circumcision. Pediatrics 1999; 103(3):686–693.

82. Gee WF, Ansell JS. Neonatal circumcision: a ten-year overview: with comparison of the Gomco clamp and the Plastibell device. Pediatrics 1976; 58(6):824–827.

83. Rickwood AM, Kenny SE, Donnell SC. Towards evidence based circumcision of English boys: survey of trends in practice. BMJ 2000; 321:792–793.

84. Rushton HG, Majd M, Jantausch B, et al. Renal scarring following reflux and nonreflux pyelonephritis in children: evaluation with 99mtechnetium-dimercaptosuccinic acid scintigraphy. J Urol 1992; 147(5):1327–1332. (Published erratum appears in J Urol 1992; 148(3):898.)

85. Stokland E, Hellstrom M, Jacobsson B, et al. Renal damage one year after first urinary tract infection: role of dimercaptosuccinic acid scintigraphy. J Pediatr 1996; 129(6):815–820.

86. Melzi ML, Guez S, Sersale G, et al. Acute pyelonephritis as a cause of hyponatremia/hyperkalemia in young infants with urinary tract malformations. Pediatr Infect Dis J 1995; 14(1):56–59.

87. Rodriguez-Soriano J, Vallo A, Quintela MJ, et al. Normokalaemic pseudohypoaldosteronism is present in children with acute pyelonephritis. Acta Paediatr 1992; 81(5):402–406.

88. Rodriguez-Soriano J, Vallo A, Oliveros R, et al. Transient pseudohypoaldosteronism secondary to obstructive uropathy in infancy. J Pediatr 1983; 103(3): 375–380.

89. Schoen EJ, Bhatia S, Ray GT, et al. Transient pseudohypoaldosteronism with hyponatremia-hyperkalemia in infant urinary tract infection. J Urol 2002; 167(2 Pt 1): 680–682.

90. Fussell EN, Kaack MB, Cherry R, et al. Adherence of bacteria to human foreskins. J Urol 1988; 140(5): 997–1001.

91. Schoolrik GK. How *Escherichia coli* infects the urinary tract. N Engl J Med 1989; 320(12):804–805.

92. Schlager TA, Hendley JO, Dudley SM, et al. Explanation for false-positive urine cultures obtained by bag technique. Arch Pediatr Adolesc Med 1995; 149(2): 170–173.

93. Wiswell TE, Miller GM, Gelston HM Jr, et al. Effect of circumcision status on periurethral bacterial flora during the first year of life. J Pediatrc 1988; 113(3): 442–446.

94. Remondino PC. History of Circumcision from the Earliest Times to the Present: Moral and Physical Reasons for its Performance, with a History of Eunuchism, Hermaphrodism, etc., and of the Different Operations Practiced upon the Prepuce. (Physicians' and students' ready reference series, no. 11). Philadelphia: FA Davis, 1900.

95. Maden C, Sherman KJ, Beckmann AM, et al. History of circumcision, medical conditions, and sexual activity and risk of penile cancer. J Natl Cancer Inst 1993; 85(1):19–24.

96. Ries LAG, Kosary CL, Hankey BF, et al., eds. SEER Cancer Statistics Review, 1973–1995. Bethesda, MD: National Cancer Institute, 1998.

97. Owor R. Carcinoma of the penis in Uganda. IARC Sci Publ 1984; 63:493–497.

98. Kochen M, McCurdy S. Circumcision and the risk of cancer of the penis: a life-table analysis. Am J Dis Child 1980; 134:484–486.

99. zur Hausen H. Genital papillomavirus infections. Prog Med Virol 1985; 32:15–21.

100. Gajalakshmi CK, Shanta V. Association between cervical and penile cancers in Madras, India. Acta Oncologica 1993; 32(6):617–620.

101. Cannistra SA, Niloff JM. Cancer of the uterine cervix. N Engl J Med 1996; 334(16):1030–1037.

102. Quinn TC, Wawer MJ, Sewankambo N, et al. Viral load and heterosexual transmission of human immunodeficiency virus type 1. Rakai Project Study Group. N Engl J Med 2000; 342(13):921–929.

103. Cohen MS. Preventing sexual transmission of HIV—new ideas from sub-Saharan Africa. N Engl J Med 2000; 342(13):970–972.

104. Potts M. Male circumcision and HIV infection [letter]. Lancet 2000; 355(9207):926–927, author reply 927.

105. Short RV. New ways of preventing HIV infection: thinking simply, simply thinking. Philos Trans R Soc Lond B Biol Sci [electronic serial] 2006; FirstCite e-publishing, [cited 2006 Apr 5]. Available from: http://www.journals.royalsoc.ac.uk/media/l2t6d-dyxyhcrrmtvxceg/contributions/t/8/0/5/t8051p68662p820h.pdf.

106. Ngom P, Clark S. Adult Mortality in the Era of HIV/AIDS: Sub-Saharan Africa [monograph on the Internet]. New York: United Nations Secretariat, Department of Economic and Social Affairs, Population Division, 2003 [cited 2006 Apr 5]. Available from: http://www.un.org/esa/population/publications/adultmort/CLARK_Paper3.pdf.

107. Kreiss JK, Hopkins SG. The association between circumcision status and human immunodeficiency virus infection among homosexual men. J Infect Dis 1993; 168(6):1404–1408.

108. Cook LS, Koutsky LA, Homes KK. Circumcision and sexually transmitted diseases. Am J Public Health 1994; 84(2):197–201.

109. Lavreys L, Rakwar JP, Thompson ML, et al. Effect of circumcision on incidence of human immunodeficiency virus type-1 and other sexually transmitted diseases: a prospective cohort study of trucking company employees in Kenya. J Infect Dis 1999; 180(2):330–336.

110. Shearn MA, Shearn L. Profile: Louis XVI. Medical Aspects of Human Sexuality 1983; 17:139–140.

111. Wiswell TE. The prepuce, urinary tract infections, and the consequences. Pediatrics 2000; 105(4 Pt 1):860–862.

112. Cancer Incidence in Five Continents. Age-standardized incidence rates, four-digit rubrics, and age-standardized and cumulative incidence rates, three-digit rubrics. IARC Sci Publ 1992; 120: 871–1011.

113. Dhar GM, Shah GN, Naheed B, et al. Epidemiological trend in the distribution of cancer in Kashmir Valley. J Epidemiol Community Health 1993; 47(4): 290–292.

114. Frank R. Circumcision and hygiene in geriatric patients [letter]. J Am Geriatr Soc 1999; 47(9):1155.

115. Brendler CB. Evaluation of the urologic patient: history, physical examination, and urinalysis. In: Walsh PC, Retik AB, Vaughan ED, et al., eds. Campbell's Urology. 7th ed. Philadelphia: WB Saunders, 1998:131–157.

116. Lue TF. Physiology of penile erection and pathophysiology of erectile dysfunction and priapism. In: Walsh PC, Retik AB, Vaughan ED, et al., eds. Campbell's Urology. 7th ed. Philadelphia: WB Saunders, 1998:1157–1180.

117. Collins S, Upshaw J, Rutchik S, et al. Effects of circumcision on male sexual function: debunking a myth? J Urol 2002; 167(5):2111–2112.

118. Fink KS, Carson CC, DeVellis RF. Adult circumcision outcomes study: effect on erectile function, penile sensitivity, sexual activity and satisfaction. J Urol 2002; 167(5):2113–2116.

119. Bluestein CB, Eckholdt H, Arezzo JC, et al. Effects of circumcision on male penile sensitivity [abstract]. J Urol 2003; 169(suppl 4):324.

120. Senkul T, Iseri C, Sen B, et al. Circumcision in adults: effect on sexual function. Urology 2004; 63(1):155–158.

121. Waldinger MD, Quinn P, Dilleen M, et al. A multinational population survey of intravaginal ejaculation latency time. J Sex Med 2005; 2:492–497.

122. Nelson CP, Dunn R, Wan J, et al. The increasing incidence of newborn circumcision: data from the nationwide inpatient sample. J Urol 2005; 173(3):978–981.

123. American Academy of Pediatrics. Committee on Fetus and Newborn. Standards and Recommendations for Hospital Care of Newborn Infants. 5th ed. Evanston, IL: American Academy of Pediatrics, 1971.

124. Thompson HC, King LR, Knox E, et al. Report of the ad hoc task force on circumcision. Pediatrics 1975; 56(4):610–611.

125. Circumcision Supplement Released by the British Journal of Urology. BJU Int 1999; 83(suppl 1):1–113.

126. Whitfield HN, Frank JD, Williams G, et al. Editorial. BJU Int 1999; 83(suppl 1):v.

Part II

Pathophysiology of Male Sexual Dysfunction

Male sexual dysfunction may be largely classified as being either of psychogenic or organic etiology; in many cases, it may be a combination of both. While there are no universally acknowledged defining criteria, persistence over a period of three months has been suggested as a reasonable guideline for clinical concern. Isolated dysfunction of the erectile mechanism is the most common clinical problem, but disturbances may occur in one or more of the phases of the male sexual response cycle (described in Part I), including some or all of the subjective components of desire (hypo- or hyperactive), physical arousal (erectile dysfunction, including arterial insufficiency, venous leakage, structural lesions, or neuropathy), and the experience of pleasure (anxiety and/or other mood disorders). There may also be defects in the objective components of sexual performance (premature, absent, or delayed ejaculation), orgasm (delayed or absent), and detumescence (priapism), although any of these may be affected independently. The sexual health professional must not discount the significant roles that a past medical history, concomitant systemic disease such as diabetes or diffuse cardiovascular disease, and any pharmacological or surgical treatments thereof, may play in the etiology of any sexual dysfunction present. Identification of such factors is relevant to guiding future investigations and the development of personalized therapeutic strategies, as detailed in Parts III and IV.

Disorders of the Male Sexual Response Cycle

Fouad R. Kandeel

Department of Diabetes, Endocrinology and Metabolism, City of Hope National Medical Center, Duarte, California and David Geffen School of Medicine, University of California, Los Angeles, California, U.S.A.

Vivien Koussa

H.C. Healthcare Management and Development, Inc., Long Beach, California, U.S.A.

□ INTRODUCTION

Normal male sexual function depends on the sexual response cycle, which consists of an anticipatory libidinous state (sexual motive or desire), effective vasocongestive arousal (erection), orgasm, and resolution (detumescence). Libido is defined as the biological need for sexual activity and frequently is expressed as sexseeking behavior. Its intensity is variable between individuals as well as within an individual over a given period of time. Little is known about the physiological basis of libido. Erection, however, is associated with significant psychological and physical changes. This is the ultimate response to multiple psychogenic and sensory stimuli from imaginative, visual, auditory, olfactory, gustatory, tactile, and genital reflexogenic sources, which trigger several neurological and vascular cascades that produce penile tumescence and rigidity sufficient for vaginal penetration. The sensation of orgasm is accompanied by two sequential functions: emission and ejaculation. Emission, mediated by contractions of the prostate, seminal vesicles, and urethra, produces a sensation of ejaculatory inevitability and deposition of semen in the posterior urethra. Generalized muscular tension, perineal contractions, and involuntary pelvic thrusting (every 0.8 seconds) usually follow and lead to the expulsion of semen from the urethral meatus. The resolution phase returns the penis to the flaccid state and provides a sense of general pleasure, well-being, and muscular relaxation. During this period, men are physiologically refractory to subsequent erection and orgasm for a variable amount of time. (For further information on normal male sex physiology, see Chapter 3.)

Disorders of the sexual response may involve one or more of the cycle's phases; these may be generalized or limited to certain situations or partners or may be lifelong (i.e., there has been no evidence of any effective sexual performance, generally due to persistent intrapsychic conflicts) or acquired (dysfunction arises after a period of normal function). Although there are no universally acknowledged defining criteria, a period of persistence over three months has been suggested as a reasonable guideline for clinical concern. Isolated dysfunction of the erectile mechanism is the most common problem, but generally, disturbances may occur in some or all of the subjective components of desire, arousal, and pleasure and the objective components of performance, vasocongestion, and orgasm, although any of these may be affected independently.

Historically, the inability to develop or sustain an erection sufficient for penetrative sexual intercourse was labeled "impotence." However, as this term connotes a loss of prowess in mental and physical domains that may be unrelated to sexual functioning, "erectile dysfunction" (ED) is now the preferred expression.

ED is a significant male health matter, affecting more than 160 million men worldwide. The Massachusetts Male Aging Study determined that ED was present in about 52% of men aged 40 to 70 years. Although there is evidence of an increased prevalence with age, the presence of ED is often incorrectly assumed to be an inevitable part of getting older. In fact, ED is frequently the result of some systemic illness such as diabetes mellitus or hypertension, or it is the consequence of the treatment of such diseases with pharmacologic agents. Appropriate treatment of the underlying physical disorder often results in the resolution or amelioration of the sexual dysfunction.

Any specific sexual dysfunction may have a psychologic, physiologic, or combined etiology. It should be noted that the distinction between what is purely "physiologic" or "psychologic" is frequently blurred in many situations. Although the presence of ED may not always result in a complete loss of sexual satisfaction or reproductive capability, in most men, it creates psychological stress (loss of self-esteem and fear of humiliation and rejection) that negatively impacts their willingness to initiate or continue sexual relationships, which, in fact, often compounds the physical problem. Thus, ED has a major impact not only on the quality of life of the male patient but also on that of his partner. The correct diagnosis of ED depends on an accurate history elicited in a sympathetic manner that takes into account the likelihood that physical dysfunction may comprise only a part

Table 1 Causes of Male Sexual Dysfunction Classified by Etiologic Category

Psychologic/psychiatric conditions	Pharmacologic agents	Organic dysfunctions

Situational conditions
  Partner discord or ambivalence
  Delayed grief
  Unexpressed anger, anxiety, or guilt
  Discord with attachment figures
  Gender identity conflict
Psychiatric disorders
  Character pathology
  Bipolar disorders
  Schizophrenia
	Antihypertensives
	  Central sympatholytics (e.g., methyl-dopa)
	  Ganglion blockers
	  Postganglionic blockers (e.g., guanethidine, guanadrel, reserpine)
	  β-receptor blockers (e.g., propranolol, atenolol, metoprolol)
	  Central α agonists (e.g., clonidine and guanabenz)
	  Diuretics (e.g., chlorthalidone, hydrochlorothiazide, spironolactone)
	  Calcium channel antagonists (e.g., nifedipine verapamil)
	  Angiotensin converting enzyme (ACE) inhibitors (e.g., enalapril, lisinopril)
	Anticholinergics
	  Atropine
	  Scopolamine
	  Benztropine
	  Trihexyphenidyl
	Antidepressants
	  Tricyclic antidepressants (e.g., clomipramine, amitriptyline, doxepin, dothiepin, imipramine)
	  Monoamine oxidase inhibitors (e.g., isocarboxazid, phenelzine)
	  Selective serotonin receptor inhibitors (e.g., fluoxetine, sertraline)
	Antipsychotics
	  Phenothiazines (e.g., chlorpromazine, flupheazine, thioridazine)
	  Thioxanthenes
	  Butyrophenone
	  Lithium
	  Heterocyclic antipsychotics (e.g., pimozide)
	  Dopamine antagonists (e.g., sulpiride)
	Sedatives and drug abuse
	  Barbiturates
	  Diazepam
	  Chlordiazepoxide
	  Tobacco
	  Alcohol
	  Cannabis (marijuana)
	  Methadone
	  Heroin
	  Cocaine
	  Lysergic acid (LSD)
	Others
	  Cardiac glycosides (e.g., digoxin)
	  Chemotherapeutic agents
	  Antihyperlipidemics (e.g., clofibrate, niacin)
	  H2 blockers (e.g., cimetidine)
	  Antihistamines (e.g., diphenhydramine, hydroxyzine)
	  Carbonic anhydrase inhibitors (e.g., acetazolamide, dichlorphenamide, methazolamide)
	  Imidazoles (e.g., ketoconazole)
	  Progestins (e.g., norethindrone, danazol)
	  Estrogens (e.g., ethinyl estradiol)
	  Aminocaproic acid
	  Baclofen
	  Ethionamide
	  Perhexiline
		Systemic
		  Hepatic failure
		  Renal failure
		  Congestive heart failure
		  Angina pectoris
		Endocrine
		  Primary or secondary hypogonadism
		  Androgen resistance
		  Diabetes mellitus
		  Hypothyroidism
		Vascular
		  Large-, medium-, and small-vessel atherosclerosis
		  Cavernosal artery anomalies
		  Corporal venous leak
		  Corporeal trabecular smooth-muscle dysfunction due to sympathetic overtone or intrinsic defect
		Neurologic
		  Temporal lobe lesions
		  Diseases of spinal cord
		  Loss of sensory input
		  Postoperative disturbances of nervi erigentes
		  Nutritional neuropathies
		  Parkinsonism
		  Poststroke
		  Alzheimer's disease
		  Shy-Drager syndrome
		Penile Diseases
		  Congenital malformation
		  Peyronie's disease
		  Previous priapism
		  Phimosis
		  Cold abscess
		  Penile trauma
		  Penile schwannoma
		  Pelvic irradiation

Abbreviations: ACE, angiotensin converting enzyme; LSD, lysergic acid.
Source: From Ref. 1.

Table 2 Mechanisms of Action for Drugs Commonly Associated with Male Sexual Dysfunction

Sexual dysfunction	Drugs	Mechanism of action
Hypoactive sexual desire	Antihypertensives, alcohol, narcotics, major and minor tranquilizers, barbiturates, baclofen	Sedation and/or central neurogenic blockade
	Antiandrogens, GnRH analogs, 5-α-reductase inhibitors, alcohol, marijuana, spironolactone, cimetidine, estrogen, digoxin, clofibrate	Testosterone deficiency and antagonism
Erectile dysfunction	Narcotics, phenothiazine, methyldopa	Elevation of prolactin
	Atropine, benztropine, propantheline, disopyramide, metoclopramide, anti-Parkinsonian drugs, antihistamines	Parasympatholysis
Absence of emission and/ or retrograde ejaculation	Antihypertensives, monamine oxidase inhibitors, antipsychotics	Sympatholysis
Delayed ejaculation and/or orgasmic dysfunction	Selective serotonin reuptake inhibitors	Serotonergic agonists

of the problem. Careful physical examination and the judicious use of targeted investigations help to complete the assessment. For further information on the investigation of male sexual dysfunction, please refer to Chapter 22.

A range of safe and effective treatment options is now available for patients that suffer from ED. Too often, however, these treatments are not utilized adequately because both clinicians and patients alike remain too embarrassed to address the highly prevalent and distressing problem of ED in a serious and sympathetic manner. There are few comparable areas of medicine in which there is so much potential to improve the quality of life for the millions of affected patients and their partners. (For further information on this topic, please refer to Part IV of this volume.) This chapter will focus on providing an overview of the different clinical categories of sexual dysfunction that can arise. Tables 1 to 3 summarize the content of this chapter.

□ DISORDERS OF DESIRE
Hypoactive Sexual Desire

The Diagnostic and Statistical Manual-IV (DSM-IV) (2) defines hypoactive sexual desire (HSD) as the persistently or recurrently deficient (or absent) sexual fantasy and desire for sexual activity, leading to marked distress or interpersonal difficulty (3–5). Disorders of desire are highly prevalent in both men and women. Although prevalence rates have varied widely from one study to another, it is generally estimated that more than 15% of adult men and 30% of adult women have HSD. The diagnosis of primary desire loss in men can only be made after eliminating the presence of factors known to affect the sexual function. These include major psychological disorders, chronic medical conditions, intake of contributing pharmacological agents, or existing substance abuse. The most common causes of secondary disorders of sexual desire are psychogenic etiologies and androgen deficiency (6–9).

Psychogenic Factors

Psychogenic conditions leading to a desire deficiency state in men (previously termed desire inhibition) include psychiatric illnesses such as depression or psychosis, preoccupation with life crisis or grief, maternal transference to sexual partners, gender identity conflicts, and aging-related psychological issues (10–12). Another form of secondary desire disorder caused by psychological factors is termed excitement inhibition and is seen in patients who have sexual drive but cannot maintain excitement. It is commonly seen in patients with performance anxiety due to the fear of sexual failure and the vigilant preoccupation with erection during lovemaking (10,12). (For further details on this topic, see Chapter 12).

Endocrine Factors

Evidence reviewed above suggests that a certain critical level of blood androgens is required for the maintenance of normal sexual desire, nocturnal penile tumescence (NPT), and nonerotic penile erections in most men. A certain concentration of androgens is also required for initiation and maintenance of spermatogenesis and for maximum stimulation of growth and function of the prostate and seminal vesicles (13,14). The amount of androgens required for these latter effects is greater than that needed for maintenance of libido. Thus, states of androgen deficiency manifested by desire disorders are always associated with some decrease in seminal volume (13,14).

Not all the studies that examined the relationship between serum testosterone (T) and sexual desire in aging men have reported a robust relationship. For example, a recent retrospective study of 108 men (mean age 59.5 years) attending a hospital-based ED clinic found low, but not statistically different, serum total and free T concentrations in men with low, moderate, and high sexual desire (means of 2.8, 3.2, and 3.4 mg/mL for total T, and means of 9.1, 9.5, and 11.4 pg/mL for free T, respectively) (15). Such results suggest that total or free T levels may not be an adequate measure of sexual drive, at least in some populations.

Table 3 Causes of Sexual Dysfunction in the Male Classified by Clinical Manifestation

Clinical manifestation	Most common causes	Examples
Disorders of desire HSD	Psychogenic	Depression Marital discord leading to desire deficiency Performance anxiety leading to excitement inhibition
	CNS disease	Partial epilepsy Parkinson's disease Post-stroke Adrenoleukodystrophy

	Endocrinopathies	Androgen deficiency (primary or secondary hypogonadism
		    and androgen resistance)
		Other endocrinopathies (adrenal insufficiency, hypo- or
		    hyperthyroidism)

	Drugs	Antihypertensives Psychotropics Alcohol Narcotics Dopamine blockers Antiandrogens
Compulsive sexual behaviors	Psychogenic	Obsessive-compulsive sexuality Excessive sex seeking associated with affective disorders Addictive sexuality Sex impulsivity
Erectile dysfunction	Psychogenic	Depression Marital discord leading to desire deficiency Performance anxiety leading to excitement inhibition
	Drugs	Antihypertensives Anticholinergics Psychotropics Cigarette smoking Substance abuse
	Systemic diseases	Cardiac Hepatic Renal Pulmonary Cancer Metabolic Post organ transplant Pelvic irradiation

	Endocrinopathies	Androgen deficiency (primary or secondary hypogonadism
		    and androgen resistance)
		Other endocrinopathies (adrenal insufficiency and
		    hypo- or hyperthyroidism)

	Vascular insufficiency	Atherosclerosis Pelvic steal syndrome Penile Raynaud's syndrome Venous leakage
	Neurological disorders	Parkinson's disease Alzheimer's disease Shy-Drager syndrome Encephalopathy Spinal-cord or nerve injury
	Penile disease	Peyronie's disease Priapism Phimosis Smooth-muscle dysfunction Trauma
Disorders of ejaculation Premature ejaculation (primary or secondary)	Psychogenic	Neurotic personality Anxiety/depression Partner discord Other situational factors

(Continued)

Table 3 Causes of Sexual Dysfunction in the Male Classified by Clinical Manifestation (*Continued*)

Clinical manifestation	Most common causes	Examples
	Organic	Increased central dopaminergic activity Increased penile sensitivity
Absent or retarded emission	Sympathetic denervation	Diabetes Surgical injury Irradiation
	Drugs	Sympatholytics CNS depressants
	Androgen deficiency	Primary or secondary hypogonadism Androgen resistance
Postejaculation pain	Psychogenic	Depression Marital discord leading to desire deficiency Performance anxiety leading to excitement inhibition
Orgasmic dysfunction Loss of orgasmic sensation	Drugs	Selective serotonin reuptake inhibitors Tricyclic antidepressants Monoamine oxidase inhibitors Substance abuse
	CNS disease	Multiple sclerosis Parkinson's disease Huntington's chorea Lumbar sympathectomy
Orgasmic inhibition	Psychogenic	Performance anxiety Conditioning factors Fear of impregnation HSD
Failure of detumescence Structural penile disease	Penile structural abnormalities	Peyronie's disease Phimosis
Priapism (primary or secondary)	Primary priapism	Idiopathic
	Secondary priapism	Hematologic (Sickle-cell anemia) Infiltrative (Faber's disease and amyloidosis) Inflammatory (Tularemia and mumps) Other (Neurologic diseases, solid tumors and trauma)
	Priapism secondary to drugs	Phenothiazines Trazodone Cocaine Intrapenile vasoactive injections

Abbreviations: CNS, central nervous system; HSD, hypoactive sexual desire.
Source: From Ref. 1.

Hypogonadism

A more clear androgen deficiency state can be due to primary gonadal failure as the result of conditions such as Klinefelter's syndrome (47,XXY) or other sex chromosome disorders (XYO mixed gonadal dysgenesis and XX males or XYY males), uncorrected cryptorchidism, orchitis, autoimmune polyglandular failure, and exposure to ionizing radiation or cytotoxic agents (16,17). Leydig cells are more resistant to the effect of irradiation than the germinal epithelium and generally can withstand doses up to 800 rads before their capacity for steroid biosynthesis is compromised. In contrast, germinal epithelium is irreversibly damaged when doses of irradiation reach 400 rads (17). Similarly, seminiferous tubule failure occurs more readily than Leydig-cell dysfunction with the exposure to chemotherapy. Failure of androgen production could also be secondary to deficiency in pituitary secretion of gonadotropins (hypogonadotropic hypogonadism)

(16,17). The latter condition could arise from disorders of the hypothalamus or the pituitary. Hypothalamic abnormalities lead to partial or complete deficiency in secretion of the gonadotropin-releasing hormone (GnRH) and occur as a result of congenital defects (Kallmann's syndrome, adiposogenital dystrophy, Prader-Willi syndrome, Lawrence-Moon-Bardet-Biedl syndrome) or subsequent to trauma, infiltrative disease (sarcoid, tuberculosis), fungal infection, severe malnutrition, systemic disease (uremia or liver failure) or drug therapy (see below). Common pituitary lesions include tumors, more frequently prolactin-secreting adenomas, and diseases such as hemochromatosis and autoimmune hypophysitis (16,17). Decreased sexual libido and activity have been reported in many patients with these conditions of androgen deficiency due to primary or secondary hypogonadism (18–25). Some patients with Klinefelter's syndrome, particularly those with 46XY and/or 47XXY, however, were reported to have normal sexual libido and sexual activity (26,27).

Androgen Resistance

The effects of androgen resistance, due to 5-α-reductase deficiency or due to androgen receptor defects (Reinfenstein syndrome), on sexual desire and sexual activity have not been well studied. Conceivably, these states of androgen resistance could be associated with sexual dysfunction despite the presence of normal-to-elevated androgen blood concentrations (28). Congenital androgen resistance is associated with a range of clinical manifestations from complete feminization of the external genitalia to various grades of perineoscrotal hypospadias. Acquired androgen resistance may manifest merely as a disturbance in spermatogenesis or sperm function with little or no other sexual phenotypic abnormalities (17). Structural or functional defects of the cytosolic androgen receptor in androgen-sensitive tissues can be elicited in most cases of androgen resistance. The structural defects in androgen receptors are usually caused by point mutations in the hormone-binding domain (18). The functional defects in androgen receptors cause a concomitant rise in luteinizing hormone and T, characteristic of the androgen resistance syndromes (16). Improvement in sexual performance with high-dose androgen therapy has been reported in some males with pseudohermaphroditism due to incomplete 5-α-reductase deficiency or androgen receptor defects (28).

Pharmacological Factors

A number of pharmacologic agents or drugs of addiction could potentially induce libido dysfunction, including antihypertensives (chlorthalidone, guanadrel, guanethidine, methyldopa, reserpine, and spironolactone), psychiatric medications (fluoxetine, barbiturates, clomipramine, and fluphenazine), and others (including danazol, digoxin, ethinyl-estradiol, ketoconazole, methadone, niacin, alcohol, diazepam, and marijuana) (6–9,29–33). Multiple mechanisms are involved in the development of desire dysfunction (Table 1). Antihypertensives, alcohol, narcotics, and phenothiazine decrease libido through their sedative effects. Antidopaminergic agents including dopamine-receptor blockers such as haloperidol, dopamine storage inhibitors such as reserpine, and dopamine synthesis–competitive inhibitors such as methyldopa decrease libido through the central blockade of dopamine neurotransmission. In addition, narcotics, phenothiazines, and methyldopa reduce T production via elevation of prolactin, whereas 5-α-reductase inhibitors block the conversion of T to dihydrotestosterone, the most biologically active androgen. Ketoconazole, on the other hand, suppresses both the adrenal and the gonadal steroidogenesis by blocking the 17-α hydroxylase and 17,20-desmolase activities. In contrast, digoxin, cimetidine, spironolactone, estrogens, alcohol, and marijuana act as T antagonists. Digoxin is

among the 10 most frequently dispensed medications associated with male sexual dysfunction (34). Further, analysis of data on multiple antihypertensive, vasodilator, and cardiac medications in 1709 men from the Massachusetts Male Aging Study found that digoxin use had the highest association with complete ED (3,35,36). In addition to the diminution in sexual desire, chronic use of digoxin was also reported to cause a decrease in sexual excitement and a reduction in the frequency of sexual relations (37). Digoxin-associated ED was reported to be caused, in part, by an inhibition of the corporeal smooth-muscle sodium pump activity, which promotes smooth-muscle contraction and impedes nitric oxide (NO)-induced relaxation (34). It should be noted that not all men taking digoxin are suffering from sexual dysfunction, and patients with well-compensated cardiac states may not necessarily experience impotence. Cimetidine has also been reported to cause diminished libido (38) and ED (39–41). In one prospective study in 22 male patients with gastric hypersecretory states, cimetidine administration was associated with development of impotence, breast tenderness, or gynecomastia in 50% of cases (impotence in nine, gynecomastia in nine, and both impotence and gynecomastia in seven patients). Further, the side effects disappeared when cimetidine was replaced with ranitidine, another H2-receptor blocker that does not block androgen secretion or action (40). Besides androgen antagonism, cimetidine was also reported to inhibit pituitary responsiveness to GnRH and to prevent the normal gonadotropin response to stimulation with clomiphene citrate (42) and to cause a reversible defect in 17-β-hydroxysteroid dehydrogenase (43). The latter effect leads to a decrease in T production. (For further details on this topic, see Chapter 19.)

Neurologic Factors

Patients with a primary central nervous system (CNS) disease such as partial epilepsy (44–47), Parkinsonism (48), post stroke (49,50), and adrenoleukodystrophy (51) may have diminished sexual arousal. The pathogenesis of desire insufficiency in these disorders appears to be multifactorial in origin. For example, patients with epilepsy frequently have low serum concentrations of gonadotropins and sex hormones. However, treatment of the primary disease was shown to improve sexual desire and, in some cases, normalize reproductive hormone serum levels (52), suggesting that the primary CNS neuronal changes, at least in some cases, may also be responsible for the changes in reproductive hormones. In addition, the improvement in the sense of well-being of the patient may contribute to a further improvement in his sexual function. In keeping with this is the observation that proper counseling and rehabilitation of patients with stroke frequently lead to an improvement in libido and other sexual disorders (49). (For further information on this topic, see Chapter 15.)

Hyperactive Sexual Desire

Another group of desire disorders with psychological bases is known as compulsive sexual behaviors (53–56). These constitute a wide range of complex sexual behaviors that have strikingly repetitive, compelling, or driven qualities, and usually manifest as one or more of several aberrant sexual behaviors, including: obsessive-compulsive sexuality (e.g., excessive masturbation and promiscuity), excessive sex seeking in association with affective disorders (e.g., major depression or mood disorders), addictive sexuality (e.g., attached to another person, object, or sensation for sexual gratification to the exclusion of everything else), and sexual impulsivity (failure to resist an impulse or temptation for sexual behavior that is harmful to self or others such as exhibitionism, rape, or child molestation). Detailed discussion of these disorders is beyond the scope of this review and can be found elsewhere (53–56), including Chapters 12 and 24.

□ DISORDERS OF ERECTION

ED is usually defined as the persistent failure to generate sufficient penile body pressure to achieve vaginal penetration and/or the inability to maintain this degree of penile rigidity until ejaculation (57,58). Although the exact prevalence of impotence in the U.S. male population is not known, it is estimated to range from 12% of males above age 18 in the report of Furlow (59) to 25% to 30% of men between ages 60 and 70 in the surveys of Kinsey et al. (60), Schiavi et al. (61), and Diokno et al. (62), to 52% in the Massachusetts Male Aging Study (3). In the last study, the disorder was strongly related to age. The prevalence increased from 40% at age 40 to 67% at age 70. The prevalence of impotence in France was reported as 12% in the age group of 18 to 24 years and 29% in the age group of 55 to 69 years, and the overall prevalence of impotence among men 18 to 69 years of age was 20% (63). A much smaller study in England reported a similar overall prevalence rate of impotence (17%) among men attending primary care facilities (64). Further, in the Massachusetts Male Aging Study in the United States, 19.6% of a cohort of 255 men without ED at baseline was reported to have developed moderate-to-severe ED during a follow-up interval of eight years. Significant baseline predictors of this new-onset ED included cigarette smoking, serum high-density lipoprotein (HDL)-cholesterol, and obesity (65,66).

Psychogenic Factors

The current literature on the relationship between sexual dysfunction and psychiatric disorders in men is not extensive, and much of the older literature is limited by methodological flaws. Several studies, however, have established some association between sexual dysfunction and psychological disorders. In the Massachusetts Male Aging Study, male ED was found to be associated with depressive symptoms as measured by a score of 16 or greater on the Center for Epidemiology Studies-Depression Scale, after controlling for potential cofounders (odds ratio 1.82) such as demographic, anthropometric and life style factors, health status, medication use, and hormones (67). Similar results were reported by at least two other studies. In the first, ED was found to be associated with a high incidence of depressive symptoms, regardless of age, marital status, or comorbidities. In addition, patients with ED had lower libido and were more likely to discontinue treatment for their erectile problem than other patients without depressive symptoms (68). In the second study, depressed men reported significantly lower sexual interest and satisfaction, but no less sexual activity, on both retrospective questionnaires and prospective daily logs, than healthy control men. Depressed men also showed significantly more negative body image and less "manly" sexual role function as measured by the Derogatis Sexual Functioning Inventory (see below). Significant partial correlations (controlling for the effect of anxiety) were also found between severity of depression and sexual interest, satisfaction, and role (69). Further, in the cross-sectional Massachusetts Male Aging Study, the incidence of moderate-to-complete ED was estimated to be nearly 90%, 60%, and 25% in men with severe, moderate, and minimal depression, respectively (67). In addition, older studies have estimated that approximately one-third of all patients with untreated depression have reported sexual dysfunction (70,71). Another study, which focused on the relationship between psychogenic disorder and sexual function in older men reported diagnosable psychological difficulties that were assumed to be related to the sexual difficulties in 52.8% of patients and, a second large group (39.9%) had psychological factors (although not diagnosable disorders) that were assumed to contribute to the current manifestation of sexual dysfunction (72). A high frequency of sexual dysfunction was also reported in males with schizophrenia. Reduced sexual desire parameters were found in both untreated and neuroleptic-treated patient groups. Further, reductions in the frequency of sexual thoughts were confined to the untreated patients, and impairments in arousal (erection) and orgasm were reported by the treated patients. Moreover, the schizophrenic patients were more involved in masturbatory activity as compared with control subjects (73). The association between male ED and panic disorder (74) and perfectionism (75) has also been reported. Surprisingly, however, long-lasting adverse familial relationship to attachment figures were found to be more influential to later sexual dysfunction than are childhood sexual abuse experiences in the nonclinical male student sample. Premature ejaculation and sexual desire disorders were the frequent reported problems in this young adult male population (76). Premature ejaculation was also found to be associated with anxiety in a recent survey of 789 men in England (77). (For further information on this topic, see Chapter 12.)

Organic Factors

The organic causes of erectile failure can be grouped into endocrine, neurologic, vascular, systemic, or local penile disorders (Table 2) (14).

Endocrine Factors

In addition to a deficiency of androgen secretion and/or action that has already been addressed in the preceding section, diabetes mellitus has increasingly been recognized as a major cause for erectile failure (78–82). Surveys by various investigators suggest that ED is encountered by about 50% of diabetic males (11,83), which is twice the incidence in nondiabetic normal males (59). Moreover, the frequency of impotence in diabetics increases with age, from about 25% at age 35 to greater than 70% after age 60, and among patients with autonomic neuropathy. This frequency, however, does not correlate with the duration of diabetes, the mode of treatment, or the manifestation of retinopathy, nephropathy, or hypertension. Although diabetics can suffer from psychogenic erectile failure, current evidence suggests that neurologic and vascular abnormalities are the predominant etiologies. Recent data in rats also implicate a decrease in penile tissue neuronal nitric oxide synthase (NOS) content and a marked decrease in penile NOS activity in both insulin-dependent and non–insulin-dependent diabetes in the development of ED (84,85). Similar data were reported for insulin-dependent diabetic men (86). Androgen deficiency (84–89) and accumulation of advanced glycosylation end products (90) and raised reactive oxygen species (85) were thought to be responsible for the decrease in cavernosal NO formation and/or action in diabetics. (For further information on this topic, see Chapter 14.)

Neurologic Factors

ED can also accompany a variety of CNS and peripheral nervous system diseases (13,91–102). Table 1 lists some of these conditions. Parkinson's disease, Alzheimer's disease, Shy-Drager syndrome, encephalopathy, stroke, and spinal-cord injury or disease are among the many neurological disorders that cause male sexual dysfunction.

Spinal-cord injuries deserve special comment. Loss of erectile or ejaculatory functions in these conditions depends upon the level and extent of the damage. Upper motor neuron lesions diminish the erectile response to psychogenic stimuli but leave the reflexogenic erections intact. The degree of diminution in psychogenic erections is directly related to the extent of the lesion. In contrast, lower motor neuron lesions abolish the reflexogenic response without altering the psychogenic erections except when the lesion is complete. When the latter occurs, psychogenic erections diminish in about 75% of the patients (94,96,97). (For further information on this topic, see Chapters 15, 26, and 38.)

Vascular Factors

Vascular Insufficiency

Vascular insufficiency is probably the most common cause of organic male sexual dysfunction (13,79,103–120). Atherosclerosis of the large pelvic arteries (common iliac, hypogastric, or pudendal) could lead to inadequate perfusion of the penis. In some instances of unilateral disease, erection is achievable while the patient is in the supine position but is lost upon initiation of active pelvic movements. Shunting of blood from the penis to the hip muscles constitutes the pathogenic mechanism for this "steal" phenomenon (107,108). Other examples of large vessel disease are Leriche syndrome (104) and penile Raynaud's phenomenon (120). In the former condition, impedance of penile blood supply occurs as a result of obstruction of the distal aorta and presents with claudication of lower back, buttocks, and thighs, whereas the latter condition is due to a vasospastic disorder superimposed on borderline penile arterial flow. Obliteration of the small vessels of the cavernous tissue, on the other hand, is frequently implicated in the diminution of erectile rigidity in aged men and in men with diabetes (13,78,105,114).

Diabetes, hyperlipidemia, and hypertension are other major risk factors for arterial diseases. After adjusting the Massachusetts Male Aging Study data for age, men treated for diabetes (28%), heart disease (39%), and hypertension (15%) had significantly higher probabilities for erectile insufficiency than the whole sample (9.6%). Also, the probability of dysfunction correlated inversely to HDL but not total cholesterol (36). In another study in 3250 men, followed for a period of 6 to 48 months, high levels of total cholesterol and low levels of HDL cholesterol were found to be risk factors for ED, even after adjustment for other potential confounders (121). Hypercholesterolemia may impair endothelial NOS-dependent mechanisms of erectile function (122). (For further information, see Chapters 13 and 14.)

Venous Leakage

Impotence secondary to excessive venous leakage is being reported with significant frequency in clinical studies (35,111–113,115,123–128); however, studies in animal models and the low success rate of venous ligation surgery in humans (28–73% of patients recover their erectile function after surgery) suggest that the primary defect is likely to be related to an abnormal function (incomplete relaxation) of trabecular smooth-muscle cells of the corpora cavernosa rather than due to a pathological process inflecting the penile veins themselves (129). (For further information on this topic, see Chapters 25 and 33.)

Systemic Factors

A variety of advanced states of systemic diseases are associated with sexual dysfunctions (11,130), including chronic liver disease (131), renal failure (132,133), chronic obstructive pulmonary disease (134), sleep apnea (135,136), cancer (137,138), and postorgan transplantation (139). Hepatic cirrhosis and renal failure adversely affect androgen production and/or metabolism. Other chronic debilitating diseases may interfere with sexual functioning even though the erectile mechanism per se remains intact. (For further information on this topic, see Chapter 13.)

Surgery/Radiation Treatment

Loss of erectile function is also common following a variety of abdominal, pelvic, and urologic surgeries and following therapeutic radiation of the pelvic organs (13,130,140–143). Nerve injury is the major cause of sexual dysfunction in most of these cases. In addition, studies in rats showed that radiation (2000 cGy over the prostate bed) causes a reduction in NOS-containing nerve fibers in the cavernous tissue and a defect in the vascular supply of the penis (144). (For further information, see Chapters 16 and 20.)

Pharmacologic Agents

Many commonly prescribed pharmacologic agents can adversely influence sexual function of the male (31,33,145,146). Antihypertensives, anticholinergics, psychotropics, and many of the other agents listed in Table 1 are common causes for erectile failure. Table 2 provides the common mechanisms of action for drugs commonly associated with sexual dysfunction. The percentage of men with complete erectile failure in the Massachusetts Male Aging Study, who were taking hypoglycemic agents (26%), antihypertensive drugs (14%), vasodilators (36%), and cardiac drugs (28%) was significantly higher than the 9.6% observed for the sample as a whole (3). The cause of impotence in many of these patients may not be related to the intake of the pharmacological agent but to the underlying disease. Another possibility in the case of antihypertensives is the reduction of blood pressure in the face of penile arterial atherosclerosis (147).

Two recent prospective studies evaluated the effects of different classes of antihypertensive agents on sexual function in men. Rosen et al. (148) studied the effects of β-blockers (propranolol and atenolol), central α-agonists (methyldopa), diuretics (hydrochlorothiazide-triamterene), and placebo in 21 males with sexual dysfunction presumed related to prior use of antihypertensives. Each study drug was administered for a one-month treatment period, followed by a two-week, single-blind washout phase, according to a randomized, Latin-square crossover design. Results indicated a lack of consistency in drug effects on measures of sexual response, although more frequent sexual and nonsexual side effects were observed with methyldopa and propranolol. The study, however, relied on a small number of observations and did not include a direct comparison of sexually functional and dysfunctional males. In the second study, Grimm et al. (149) determined the long-term effects of five antihypertensive drugs on sexual function in 557

men with mild hypertension. Patients were evaluated at baseline prior to treatment, and thereafter annually, for up to four years of therapy with one of five antihypertensive agents (acebutolol, amlodipine, chlorthalidone, doxazosin, and enalapril) or placebo. At baseline, 12.2% reported problems with obtaining and/or maintaining erections and the erectile failure was positively related to age, systolic pressure, and previous antihypertensive drug use. The incidence of erection dysfunction during followup was 9.5% and 14.7% at two and four years of therapy, respectively. Patients taking chlorthalidone reported a significantly higher incidence of erection problems at two years than patients randomized to placebo (17.1% vs. 8.1%). Incidence rates of ED at four years were more similar among treatment groups and not significantly different from placebo-treated groups. Interestingly, disappearance of erection problems during treatment was common in all groups but greatest in the doxazosin group. Limitations of this study include the small sample size (approximately 70 men per treatment group free of erection problems at baseline), the limited nature of sexual evaluation including the prior knowledge of sexual activity of participants, and the use of drugs that have not been previously associated with ED (cardioselective β-blocker, calcium-channel blocker, angiotensin-converting enzyme blocker, and α-blocker).

Mechanisms by which medications can induce ED may include central and/or peripheral neurologic blockade or stimulation of prolactin secretion. Hyperprolactinemia may reduce T concentration and action through a variety of mechanisms including disruption of the anatomic integrity of the hypothalamic–pituitary axis, interference with GnRH action on the pituitary (150), inhibition of gonadotropin secretion (151), and reduction of T conversion to the more active metabolite dihydrotestosterone (152). Hypogonadism has been shown to be associated with decreased NO formation and action in the penis and thus reduced erectile capacity (88,89). Priapism as a mechanism for erectile failure may be invoked by the intake of phenothiazines (e.g., thioridazine and chlorpromazine) (145, 153) or the newer antidepressant trazodone (33,145). At present, it is not clear whether drugs of addiction such as alcohol, methadone, and heroin reduce sexual potency by influencing the secretion and metabolism of androgens or through the associated deterioration in the general physical and psychological status of the addict (14,31,145). ED may accompany any psychiatric disorder or situational condition listed in Table 1 (12,11). A substantial number of patients with affective disorder, chronic depression, and obsessive personality may also develop a desire disorder. (For further information on this topic, see Chapter 19.)

Local Penile Diseases

Penile diseases such as congenital malformation (154), Peyronie's disease (155–157), priapism (158–163), phimosis (164), and, rarely, cold abscess (165) may interfere with the erectile function.

Phimosis

Phimosis, balanitis, and balanoposthitis inhibit sexual function by causing painful sensation and restricting the movement of the glans. Older uncircumcised men have a higher incidence of sexual dysfunction and are less apt to be involved in masturbatory or heterosexual oral activities (166). Further, uncircumcised men have a significantly greater risk of acquiring HIV infection (up to eightfold increase) (167), genital herpes, and cancer of the penis (168) than do circumcised men. Also, women whose sexual partners are uncircumcised have increased risk of cervical cancer secondary to human papilloma virus infection (169). Surgical removal of the prepuce, on the other hand, may result in loss of the majority of fine-touch neuroceptors found in the penis (170). (For further information on this topic, see Chapters 9 and 21.)

Peyronie's Disease

Peyronie's disease is a chronic inflammatory disorder of unknown etiology. Pain and obstruction of blood flow to normal tissue distal to the lesion are major factors in causing the erectile failure. Priapism is manifested by persistent painful erection and is usually due to blood clotting within the penile vasculature. Peyronie's disease is a condition characterized by the development of fibrous plaques on the penile shaft and results in its dorsal or lateral curvature, particularly during the erectile phase. When the curvature is severe, erection becomes painful and coitus becomes difficult or impossible. The disease has an age-adjusted annual incidence rate of 25.7 and prevalence rate of 388.6 per 100,000 population (171,172) and occurs in all races but predominates among Caucasians. More than 90% of cases occur between the ages of 40 and 70 years (173). The hallmark of Peyronie's disease is the formation of fibrous plaques in the tunica albuginea and the subtunical tissue with subsequent ossification and/or invasion of the cavernous bodies (174–176). Although the etiology of the disease is still unclear, acute or chronic mild sexual trauma, vascular inflammation (vasculitis), diffuse collagen disease (most notably Dupuytren's contracture), autoimmune process, and hereditary disorders have been implicated in its genesis (172,173,177). The disease also occurs in association with carcinoid syndrome, use of vacuum constriction devices, penile irradiation, and therapy with β-blocking agents such as propranolol. Devine et al. (177) favor the hypothesis that Peyronie's disease is caused by repetitive microvascular injury, with fibrin deposition and trapping in tissue space that is not adequately cleared during the normal remodeling and repair of the tear in the tunica. According to their postulate, fibroblast activation and proliferation, and enhanced vessel permeability and generation of chemotactic factors for leukocytes, which are stimulated by fibrin deposition in the normal process of wound healing, do not appear to be effective in Peyronie's disease; instead, the lesion fails to resolve either due to an inability to clear the original stimulus or due to further deposition of fibrin subsequent to repeated trauma. Collagen is also trapped and pathological fibrosis ensues (177). Somers and Dawson (178) examined Peyronie's disease plaque tissue for collagen and elastic fiber and fibrin content and distribution. Fibrin deposition was detected histochemically in plaque tissue from 18 of 19 patients (95%), but it was not detected in normal or scarred tunica from control subjects. The presence of authentic fibrin accumulation in plaque tissue was confirmed by immunoblot analysis. A recent study in 100 patients with Peyronie's disease found 43 patients with one or more circulating autoantibodies (24% of the patients were positive for antinuclear antibody and 11% for rheumatoid factor). Patients with active disease were found to have immunoglobulin M antibody deposition, marked T lymphocytic and macrocytic infiltration in the subtunical space, increased expression of adhesion molecules by the endothelial cells, and increased lymphocyte antigen class 2 expression by the cellular infiltrate (157). Other studies demonstrated the association of Peyronie's disease with the presence of the human leukocyte antigen (HLA)-B7 (179), HLA-DQ5 (180), and HLA-B27 (181) antigens. Such findings are supportive of a role for autoimmunity in genesis of the disease, particularly by the cell-mediated process. The progression of the disease is quite unpredictable and can either advance very rapidly or evolve slowly over several years (182). The natural history of the disease suggests a spontaneous improvement in 13% to 50% of the patients one to two years after onset of symptoms (183), but 10% to 30% require surgical treatment (182). (For further information on this topic, see Chapters 17 and 34.)

Etiology of Local Penile Diseases

Local penile disease such as Peyronie's disease, phimosis, or genitourinary trauma that results in rupture of the corpora cavernosa or the encapsulating connective tissue sheaths, formation of traumatic occlusion of multiple arteries, post-traumatic aneurysmal dilatation with arteriovenous fistulae, resection of the cavernosal nerves during pelvic surgery, pelvic irradiation, or penile schwannoma can all be causes for ED (155–164,184–191). Radiation exposure has been shown to decrease the number of NOS-containing nerves in the rat penis (144), and regeneration of penile NOS-containing nerves was shown to coincide with the recovery of erectile function in animals with unilateral cavernous nerve injury (192). Such observations suggest that NO pathway abnormalities are involved in the pathogenesis of erectile failure following unilateral cavernosal nerve injury or pelvic radiation in man (122). Painful erections and/or venous incompetence are thought to be the bases for erectile insufficiency in Peyronie's disease, and mechanical interference and/ or pain are the mechanisms for impotence associated with phimosis. Sporadic reports of congenital anomalies such as absent communication between the corpora cavernosa (isolated cavernous bodies), the corporeal veno-occlusive dysfunction, and/or the hypoplastic cavernous arteries leading to primary ED have also been reported (154,193–195). Moreover, increased expression of a 68-kDa nonionic detergent extraction-resistant protein was demonstrated in tissues of more than half of 38 patients with vasculogenic ED, compared to one out of nine patients without erectile insufficiency (196). Increased expression of this protein was not related to a specific type of vascular insufficiency, aging, or presence of diabetes. Histochemical and immunochemical evaluations suggested that the expressed protein is not structurally related to nervous, smooth-muscle, or collagen tissues.

Smoking and Erectile Dysfunction

There is convincing evidence that smoking is a major risk factor for the development of impotence (82). The results of the Massachusetts Male Aging Study showed the association of impotence with certain risk factors to be greatly amplified in cigarette smokers (3). Similarly, in the secondary analysis of a cross-sectional survey of 4462 U.S. Army Vietnam-era veterans aged 31 to 49 years, who took part in the Vietnam Experience study in 1985–1986, cigarette smoking was found to be an independent risk factor for impotence (197). In a study of incidence of cigarette smoking in a sample of 178 patients with impotence, 58.4% were current smokers and 81% were current/ex-smoker combined, an incidence that was significantly higher than would be expected among males in the general population. Also, penile blood pressure was lower among smokers compared with nonsmoking patients (198). Further, recent statistical studies have shown that the relative risk of developing arterial atherosclerosis in the penis, and subsequent impotence, is 1.31 for each 10 pack-years of smoking (199), and that 86% of smokers have an abnormal penile vascular evaluation (200). Moreover, penile rigidity during NPT inversely related to the number of cigarettes inhaled, and the duration of NPT in 314 men with ED was reduced in smokers of more than 40 cigarettes/day (201). Long-term smoking also caused ultrastructural damage to the corporeal tissue in impotent men (202). Acute vasospasm of penile arteries in response to cigarette smoking, possibly subsequent to excessive release of catecholamines, was also reported (203). Nicotine and cotinine were shown to inhibit steroidogenesis in mouse Leydig cells (204). Moreover, long-term passive smoking in the rat was shown to cause an age-independent moderate hypertension as well as considerable decrease in penile NOS activity and neuronal NOS content (205). Thus, smoking impairs erection through a variety of mechanisms, including enhancing atherogenesis, reduction in T production, inappropriate adrenergic stimulation, and inhibition of local vasodilator(s) release.

☐ DISORDERS OF EJACULATION

There exists a spectrum of disorders of ejaculation ranging from mild premature to severely retarded or absent ejaculation. Normally, by the age of 17 or 18 years, 75% of men are able to control their ejaculation (206).

Premature Ejaculation

Premature ejaculation is the most common male sexual dysfunction (207). Several surveys among different populations estimate its prevalence at 29%, with a range between 1% and 75%, depending on the population and criteria used to define the condition (65,207–209). The DSM-IV (2) defines the diagnostic criteria for premature ejaculation as follows: (*i*) persistent or recurrent ejaculation with minimum sexual stimulation that occurs before, upon, or shortly after penetration and before the person wishes it; (*ii*) marked distress or interpersonal difficulty; and, (*iii*) the condition does not arise as a direct effect of substance abuse such as opiate withdrawal. Premature ejaculation and sexual desire disorders were frequently reported problems in young adult males with adverse familial relationships to attachment figures (76). Premature ejaculation was also found to be associated with anxiety in a recent survey of 789 men in England (77). Table 3 delineates other common causes of disorders of ejaculation.

Several classifications of premature ejaculation have been reported. In one, premature ejaculation was classified into primary and secondary disorders (208). Primary premature ejaculation describes the inability to control the ejaculatory function since the beginning of sexual experience, whereas secondary premature ejaculation describes individuals who develop the condition after years of satisfactory sexual activity. Further, primary premature ejaculation appears to be associated with high anxiety states but relatively normal sex drive, whereas secondary premature ejaculation is more associated with ED and decreased arousal (208). In another classification, premature ejaculation was thought to arise from either biological or psychological etiologies (207). The psychological theory stemmed from the association of premature ejaculation with neurotic personality traits, presence of anxiety and/or depression, lack of shared awareness between partners, or a high prevalence of other situational factors such as low self-esteem, frustration, guilt, sexual fear, hostility, or unrealistic expectations (14,65,207–213). The conflicting results of many existing studies, the absence of supporting evidence from controlled ones, and the poor treatment outcome of behavioral trials cast doubt on the validity of a pure psychological basis for this common sexual disorder. The biological theory, on the other hand, stemmed from observations in which ejaculation was delayed or inhibited by the intake of pharmacological agents that act centrally to block the action of dopamine (e.g., neuroleptics or antipsychotics), to increase the accumulation of serotonin (e.g., serotonin reuptake inhibitors), or to increase the brain levels of serotonin and norepinephrine by blocking their uptake (e.g., tricyclic agents that have anticholinergic and α-adrenergic antagonistic properties), or by the intake of pharmacological agents that act peripherally to block the α-adrenergic activation of the ejaculatory reflex (e.g., phenoxybenzamine) (207); however, several investigations of the possibility that increased penile sensitivity (low sensitivity threshold) is etiologically important in the development of premature ejaculation, using a variety of physical or electrical stimuli, have reported conflicting results (210,211).

Absent/Delayed Ejaculation

Absence or delay of emission or ejaculation is frequently caused by an identifiable organic pathology such as sympathetic denervation, androgen deficiency, or drug treatment side effects (14,29,30,33,145,213–216). Disruption of sympathetic supply to the ejaculatory apparatus is a frequent sequela of chronic metabolic disturbances (diabetes), surgical procedures (bladder neck, perineal, or retroperitoneal), or abdominal and pelvic irradiation. The loss of sympathetic innervation abolishes the ejaculatory apparatus contractions and results in a decrease of seminal secretion as well as retrograde seminal fluid flow into the bladder. Sympatholytic drugs (guanadrel, guanethidine, labetalol, methyldopa, phenoxybenzamine, and reserpine), antidepressants (fluoxetine, phenelzine, and venlafaxine) and other centrally acting agents and drugs of addiction (barbiturates, clomipramine, perphenazine, thioridazine, methadone, amphetamine, cocaine, diazepam and the designer drug 3,4-methylenedioxymethamphetamine (MDMA); a phenethylamine derivative with CNS excitant and hallucinogenic properties) have been implicated in causing ejaculatory failure either by sympatholysis or by central accumulation of serotonin (29,30,33,145,214). Androgen deficiency, on the other hand, is associated with a decrease in semen volume (13,14). In the absence of an identifiable organic or pharmacologic etiology, the failure of ejaculation is probably due to a psychogenic factor (217,218).

Painful Ejaculation

Painful ejaculation has been reported as a side effect of tricyclic antidepressants in at least two patients (219). Psychogenic postejaculatory pain syndrome is a rare sexual disorder of male dyspareunia that was first described in 1979 (220). The chief clinical feature is a persistent and recurrent pain in the genital organs during ejaculation or immediately afterward. The location of the pain is usually deep in the shaft of the penis but can be near the tip, and it may radiate to the testicles or the perineum. The pain is variable in intensity, occurs under certain circumstances, and may have a negative impact on sexual functioning by causing anticipatory distraction and sexual avoidance. The source of the pain appears to involve the involuntary spasm of certain muscles of the male genitalia and can be triggered by a variety of psychosexual conflicts. Detailed descriptions of clinical features, pathogenesis, and treatment of this syndrome have been reviewed by Kaplan (221).

Ejaculatory pain in the testicular region may result from epididymal congestion after vasectomy (222) or from duct obstruction and/or infection (223,224), testicular torsion, mass lesion or prostatitis (225). In some cases, specific etiologic factors other than psychological stress cannot be identified (226).

☐ DISORDERS OF ORGASM

Male orgasmic disorder is defined as a persistent or recurrent delay in, or absence of, orgasm following a normal sexual-excitement phase during sexual activity (2,227). The disorder is relatively rare, occurring in 3% to 10% of patients presenting with sexual dysfunction (227–230). Commonly, orgasmic inhibitions occur as a result of the intake of psychotropic agents, most often the serotonin reuptake inhibitors (fluoxetine, phenelzine, sertraline, and venlafaxine). Some tricyclic antidepressants, monoamine oxidase inhibitors, and drugs of addiction (alprazolam, clomipramine, methadone, MDMA, and alcohol) are also common offenders (29,30,33,92,145,229–238). In fact, most of the antidepressants approved for use in the United States, with the possible exception of bupropion and nefazodone, have been associated with drug-induced anorgasmia, with the rate of sexual problems including orgasmic disturbances ranging from 24% to 75% in men taking fluoxetine (233). Both the antagonism of central adrenergic mechanisms that underlie normal orgasm by 5-hydroxytryptamine-2 receptor activation and the downregulation of postsynaptic serotonin receptors have been implicated in the pathogenesis of antidepressant-induced orgasmic dysfunctions (233,239). Absence of the orgasmic sensations with normal ejaculation has been reported in several neurological disorders including multiple sclerosis, Parkinson's disease, and Huntington's chorea (240). Loss of orgasmic sensations can also occur after lumbar sympathectomy during retroperitoneal lymph-node dissection, bilateral anterolateral cordotomy for the relief of pain, and prostatectomy (241–243). The ejaculatory process is compromised, however, in a significant number of patients with these conditions. In the absence of offending drugs, neurological condition, or history of prior surgery, loss of orgasmic sensations in patients with normal libido and erectile and ejaculatory functions is almost always due to a psychogenic condition. These include performance anxiety, conditioning factors, fear of impregnation, and lack of desire or arousal (16–18,227). Table 3 delineates the most common causes of orgasmic dysfunction.

☐ FAILURE OF DETUMESCENCE

Persistent painful erections could be caused by structural penile conditions such as Peyronie's disease or phimosis or by the presence of other systemic or local conditions that could lead to the development of priapism. Priapism is a prolonged (greater than four hours' duration) and extremely painful erection unaccompanied by sexual desire and is often preceded by usual sexual stimuli. The condition is self-perpetuating and is characterized by diminished perfusion of the corporeal bodies. When chronically present, corporeal fibrosis and ED occur. At least two classifications of priapism have been described (158). The first is etiologically based and classifies the condition into primary (idiopathic) and secondary priapism. The latter condition could be precipitated by causes listed in Table 3. Of particular note, drug-induced priapism lasting for more than 48 hours frequently leads to the development of corporeal fibrosis (244) and cocaine-induced priapism can be refractory to treatment (245). The second classification is pathophysiologically based and depends on measurement of penile blood gases and pressures. It classifies priapism into low-blood-flow (ischemic) and high-blood-flow (nonischemic) conditions. In the majority of ischemic priapism cases, erection probably starts with a normal- or high-blood-flow state (particularly in cases induced with intrapenile drug injection) and ischemia ensues when a large number of emissary veins become occluded. Recent studies in rabbits (246) showed that acidosis impairs trabecular smooth-muscle contractility, probably secondary to the interference of $[H^+]$ with the intra- and extracellular mechanisms that regulate homeostasis of $[Ca^{2+}]$. Since acidosis is an early complication of ischemic priapism, it was thought that the reduced contractility of trabecular smooth muscle is a significant factor in the perpetuation of the ischemic state (246). A variant of high-flow priapism that is caused by perineal or penile trauma occurs as a result of arterial-lacunar fistula. In this condition, blood bypasses the helicine artery and passes directly into the lacunar spaces. Characteristically, there is no pain or tenderness in this form of priapism, and the penis is incompletely but constantly rigid with a focal area of high-flow turbulence on color-flow Doppler ultrasound examination and high-oxygen tension (160). Sexual stimulation may cause a further increase in penile rigidity. (For further information on this topic, see Chapter 18.)

☐ CONCLUSION

Sexual dysfunction is a highly prevalent set of disorders that is frequently associated with a loss of self-esteem and a reduced quality of life in both male patients and their partners. Many recent advances in the understanding of erectile mechanisms and the pathophysiology of various types of sexual dysfunction have resulted in the development of a wide array of safe and effective treatment options; to date, the field's crowning achievement has been the widespread implementation of phosphodiesterase inhibitors, which has realized the possibility of providing practical solutions for the problem of sexual dysfunction for its many millions of sufferers. Unfortunately, the advent of such a successful drug for the majority of men has resulted in far less diagnostic effort in discovering the cause of each individual case of sexual dysfunction. It should be remembered that phosphodiesterase inhibitors do not work for all men, particularly those who have concomitant systemic disorders with vascular complications such as diabetes. In these patients, practitioners should perform a detailed clinical history and physical exam and be willing to utilize the many state-of-the-art diagnostic procedures now available in order to elucidate the specific nature of the sexual dysfunction. As patients may often be too embarrassed to raise sexual concerns in the clinical setting, it is doubly important for healthcare providers to initiate these discussions routinely in order to establish the means for restoring sexual activity and improving the quality of life, including couple relationships.

☐ REFERENCES

1. Swerdloff RS, Kandeel FR. Approach to sexual dysfunction in the male. In: Kelly WN, ed. Textbook of Internal Medicine. 2nd ed. Vol. 2. Philadelphia: Lippincott Company, 1992:2098–2100.

2. American Psychiatric Association. Diagnostic and Statistical Manual of Mental Disorders, 4th ed. Washington, D.C., 1994.

3. Feldman HA, Goldstein I, Hatzichristou DG, et al. Impotence and its medical and psychosocial correlates: results of the Massachusetts Male Aging Study. J Urol 1994; 151(1):54–61.

4. Rosen RC, Leiblum SR. Hypoactive sexual desire. Psychiatr Clin North Am 1995; 18(1):107–121.

5. Beck JG. Hypoactive sexual desire disorder: an overview. J Consult Clin Psychol 1995; 63(6):919–927.

6. Benet AE, Melman A. The epidemiology of erectile dysfunction. Urol Clin North Am 1995; 22(4):699–709.

7. Morley JE, Kaiser FE. Impotence: the internist's approach to diagnosis and treatment. Adv Intern Med 1993; 38:151–168.

8. O'Keefe M, Hunt DK. Assessment and treatment of impotence. Med Clin North Am 1995; 79(2):415–434.

9. Schiavi RC, Segraves RT. The biology of sexual function. Psychiatr Clin North Am 1995; 18(1):7–23.

10. Salmimies P, Kockott G, Pirke KM, et al. Effects of testosterone replacement on sexual behaviour in hypogonadal men. Arch Sex Behav 1982; 11(4):345–353.

11. Segraves RT, Schoenberg HW. Diagnosis and treatment of erectile problems: current status. In: Segraves RW, Schoenberg HW, eds. Diagnosis and Treatment of Erectile Disturbances: A Guide for Clinicians. New York: Plenum Medical Book Company, 1985:1–21.

12. Levine SB. The psychological evaluation and therapy of psychogenic impotence. In: Seagraves RT, Schoenberg HW, eds. Diagnosis and Treatment of Erectile Disturbances: A Guide for Clinicians. New York: Plenum Medical Book Company, 1985: 87–104.

13. Myer JK. Disorders of sexual function. In: Wilson JD, Foster DW, eds. Williams Textbook of Endocrinology. 7 ed. Philadelphia: WB Saunders Company, 1985: 476–491.

14. Walsh PC, Wilson JD. Impotence and infertility in men. In: Braunwald E, Isselbacher KJ, Petersdorf RS, et al., eds. Harrison's Principals of Internal Medicine. 11th ed. New York: McGraw-Hill Book Company, 1987:217–220.

15. Ansong KS, Punwaney RB. An assessment of the clinical relevance of serum testosterone level determination in the evaluation of men with low sexual drive. J Urol 1999; 162(3 Pt 1):719–721.

16. Handelsman DJ, Swerdloff RS. Male gonadal dysfunction. Clin Endocrinol Metab 1985; 14(1):89–124.

17. Clifton DK, Bremner WJ. The effect of testicular x-irradiation on spermatogenesis in man. A comparison with the mouse. J Androl 1983; 4(6):387–392.

18. Arver S, Dobs AS, Meikle AW, et al. Improvement of sexual function in testosterone deficient men treated for 1 year with a permeation enhanced testosterone transdermal system. J Urol 1996; 155(5):1604–1608.

19. Nicholls DP, Anderson DC. Clinical aspects of androgen deficiency in men. Andrologia 1982; 14(5): 379–388.

20. Sorensen K, Nielsen J, Froland A, et al. Psychiatric examination of all eight adult males with the karyotype 46,XX diagnosed in Denmark till 1976. Acta Psychiatr Scand 1979; 59(2):153–163.

21. McClure RD, Oses R, Ernest ML. Hypogonadal impotence treated by transdermal testosterone. Urology 1991; 37(3):224–228.

22. Nachtigall LB, Boepple PA, Pralong FP, et al. Adult-onset idiopathic hypogonadotropic hypogonadism-treatable form of male infertility. N Engl J Med 1997; 336(6): 410–415.

23. Raboch J, Mellan J, Starka L. Klinefelter's syndrome: sexual development and activity. Arch Sex Behav 1979; 8(4):333–339.

24. Raboch J, Mellan J. Sexual development and activity of men with disturbances of somatic development. Andrologia 1979; 11(4):263–271.

25. Zini D, Carani C, Baldini A, et al. Sexual behavior of men with isolated hypogonadotropic hypogonadism or prepubertal anterior panhypopituitarism. Horm Behav 1990; 24(2):174–185.

26. Wu FC, Bancroft J, Davidson DW, et al. The behavioural effects of testosterone undecanoate in adult men with Klinefelter's syndrome: a controlled study. Clin Endocrinol 1982; 16(5):489–497.

27. Yoshida A, Miura K, Nagao K, et al. Sexual function and clinical features of patients with Klinefelter's syndrome with the chief complaint of male infertility. Int J Androl 1997; 20(2):80–85.

28. Price P, Wass JA, Griffin JE, et al. High dose androgen therapy in male pseudohermaphroditism due to 5 alpha-reductase deficiency and disorders of the androgen receptor. J Clin Invest 1984; 74(4):1496–1508.

29. Harvey KV, Balon R. Clinical implications of antidepressant drug effects on sexual functio. Ann Clin Psychiatry 1995; 7(4):189–201.

30. Segraves RT. Effects of psychotropic drugs on human erection and ejaculation. Arch Gen Psychiatry 1989; 46(3):275–284.

31. Segraves RT, Madison R, Carter CS, et al. Erectile dysfunction associated with pharmacological agents. In: Segraves RT, ed. Diagnosis and Treatment of Erectile Disturbances: A Guide for Clinicians. New York: Plenum Medical Book Company, 1985:23–63.

32. Crenshaw TL, Goldberg JP. Drugs That Affect Sexual Functioning. New York: WW Norton & Company, 1996.

33. Finger WW, Lund M, Slagle MA. Medications that may contribute to sexual disorders. A guide to assessment and treatment in family practice. J Fam Pract 1997; 44(1):33–43.

34. Gupta S, Salimpour P, Saenz de Tejada I, et al. A possible mechanism for alteration of human erectile function by digoxin: inhibition of corpus cavernosum sodium/potassium adenosine triphosphatase activity. J Urology 1998; 159(5):1529–1536.

35. Goldstein I. Vasculogenic impotence: its diagnosis and treatment. Probl Urol 1987; 1:547–563.

36. Feldman HA, Goldstein I, Hatzichristou DG, et al. Construction of a surrogate variable for impotence in the Massachusetts male aging study. J Clin Epidemiol 1994; 47(5):457–467.

37. Neri A, Aygen M, Zuckerman Z, et al. Subjective assessment of sexual dysfunction of patients on long-term administration of digoxin. Arch Sex Behav 1980; 9(4):343–347.

38. Biron P. Diminished libido with cimetidine therapy. Can Med Assoc J 1979; 121(4):404–405.

39. Wolfe MM. Impotence on cimetidine treatment. N Engl J Med 1979; 300(2):94 (Letter).

40. Jensen RT, Collen MJ, Pandol SJ, et al. Cimetidine-induced impotence and breast changes in patients with gastric hypersecretory states. N Engl J Med 1983; 308(15):883–887.

41. Peden NR, Cargill JM, Browning MCK, et al. Male sexual dysfunction during treatment with cimetidine. Br Med J 1979; 1(6164):659.

42. Van Thiel DH, Gavaler JS, Smith WI Jr, et al. Hypothalamic-pituitary-gonadal dysfunction in men using cimetidine. N Engl J Med 1979; 300(18): 1012–1015.

43. Lardinois CK, Mazzaferri EL. Cimetidine blocks testosterone synthesis. Arch Intern Med 1985; 145(5): 920–922.

44. Mancini M, Bartolini M, Maggi M, et al. The presence of arterial anatomical variations can affect the results of duplex sonographic evaluation of penile vessels in impotent patients. J Urol 1996; 155(6):1919–1923.

45. Morrell MJ, Sperling MR, Stecker M, et al. Sexual dysfunction in partial epilepsy: a deficit in physiologic sexual arousal. Neurology 1994; 44(2): 243–247.

46. Shukla GD, Srivastava ON, Katiyar BC. Sexual disturbances in temporal lobe epilepsy: a controlled study. Br J Psychiatry 1979; 134:288–292.

47. Toone BK, Edeh J, Nanjee MN, et al. Hyposexuality and epilepsy: a community survey of hormonal and behavioral changes in male epileptics. Psychol Med 1989; 19:937–943.

48. Koller WC, Vetere-Overfield B, Williamson A, et al. Sexual dysfunction in Parkinson's disease. Clin Neuropharmacol 1990; 13(5):461–463.

49. Hawton K. Sexual adjustment of men who have had strokes. J Psychosom Res 1984; 28(3):243–249.

50. Agarwal A, Jain DC. Male sexual dysfunction after stroke. J Assoc Physicians India 1989; 37(8):505–507.

51. Powers JM, Schaumburg HH. A fatal cause of sexual inadequacy in men: adreno-leukodystrophy. J Urol 1980; 124(5):583–585.

52. Spark RF, Wills CA, Royal H. Hypogonadism, hyperprolactinaemia and temporal lobe epilepsy in hyposexual men. Lancet 1984; 1(8374):413–417.

53. Travin S. Compulsive sexual behaviors. Psychiatr Clin North Am 1995; 18(1):155–169.

54. Kaplan HS. Erotic obsession: relationship to hypoactive sexual desire disorder and paraphilia. Am J Psychiatry 1996; 153(suppl 7):30–41.

55. Kafka MP. Sertraline pharmacotherapy for paraphilias and paraphilia–related disorders: an open trial. Ann Clin Psychiatry 1994; 6(3):189–195.

56. Greenberg DM, Bradford JM, Curry S, et al. A comparison of treatment of paraphilias with three serotonin reuptake inhibitors: a retrospective study. Bull Am Acad Psychiatry Law 1996; 24(4):525–532.

57. Wagner G. Erection: physiology and endocrinology. In: Wagner G, Green R, eds. Impotence: Physiological, Psychological, Surgical Diagnosis and Treatment. New York: Plenum Press, 1981:25–36.

58. Metz P, Wagner G. Penile circumference and erection. Urology 1981, 18(3):260–270.

59. Furlow WL. Prevalence of impotence in the United States. Med Aspects Hum Sex 1985; 19:13–16.

60. Kinsey AC, Pomeroy WB, Martin CE. Early sexual growth and activity. Sexual Behavior in the Human Male. Philadelphia: WB Saunders Company, 1948:157–192.

61. Schiavi RC, Schreiner-Engel P, Mandeli J, et al. Healthy aging and male sexual function. Am J Psychiatry 1990; 147(6):766–771.

62. Diokno AC, Brown MB, Herzog AR. Sexual function in the elderly. Arch Intern Med 1990; 150(1):197–200.

63. Bejin A, Colomby PD, Spira A, et al. Epidemiology of male sexual disorders in France. [Abstr 529]. J Urol 1998; 159(suppl):140.

64. Read S, King M, Watson J. Sexual dysfunction in primary medical care: prevalence, characteristics and detection by the general practitioner. J Public Health Med 1997; 19(4):387–391.

65. Laumann EO, Gagnon JH, Michael RT, et al. Sex, health and happiness. Chicago: University of Chicago Press, 1994.

66. Feldman HA, McKinlay JB, Goldstein I, et al. Erectile dysfunction, cardiovascular disease, and cardiovascular risk factors: prospective results in a large random sample of Massachusetts men. [Abstr 347]. J Urol 1998; (suppl) 159:91.

67. Araujo AB, Durante R, Feldman HA, et al. The relationship between depressive symptoms and male erectile dysfunction: cross-sectional results from the Massachusetts Male Aging Study. Psychosom Med 1998; 60(4):458–465.

68. Shabsigh R, Klein KT, Seidman S, et al. Increased incidence of depressive symptoms in men with erectile dysfunction. Urology 1998; 52(5):848–852.

69. Howell JR, Reynolds CF III, Thase ME, et al. Assessment of sexual function, interest and activity in depressed men. J Affect Disord 1987; 13(1):61–66.

70. Casper RC, Redmond DE Jr, Katz MM, et al. Somatic symptoms in primary affective disorder. Presence and relationship to the classification of depression. Arch Gen Psychiatry 1985; 42(11):1098–1104.

71. Matthews RJ, Weinman M, Claghorn JL. Tricyclic side effects without tricyclics in depression. Psychopharmacol Bull 1980; 16(3):58–60.

72. Zeiss RA, Delmonico RL, Zeiss AM, et al. Psychologic disorder and sexual dysfunction in elders. Clin Geriatr Med 1991; 7(1):133–151.

73. Aizenberg D, Zemishlany Z, Dorfman-Etrog P, et al. Sexual dysfunction in male schizophrenic patients. J Clin Psychiatry 1995; 56(4):137–141.

74. Sbrocco T, Weisberg RB, Barlow DH, et al. The conceptual relationship between panic disorder and male erectile dysfunction. J Sex Marital Ther 1997; 23(3): 212–220.

75. DiBartolo PM, Barlow DH. Perfectionism, marital satisfaction, and contributing factors to sexual dysfunction in men with erectile disorder and their spouses. Arch Sex Behav 1996; 25(6):581–588.

76. Kinzl JF, Mangweth B, Traweger C, et al. Sexual dysfunction in males significance of adverse childhood experiences. Child Abuse Negl 1996; 20(8):759–766.

77. Dunn KM, Croft PR, Hackett G. Association of sexual problems with social, psychological, and physical problems in men and women: a cross sectional

population survey. J Epidemiol Community Health 1999; 53(3):144–148.

78. Goldstein I, Siroky MB, Krane RJ. Impotence in diabetes mellitus. In: Krane RJ, Goldstein I, eds. Male Sexual Dysfunction. Boston: Little, Brown and Company, 1983:77–86.

79. Podolsky S. Diagnosis and treatment of sexual dysfunction in the male diabetic. Med Clin North Am 1982; 66(6):1389–1396.

80. Bancroft J, Bell C, Ewing DJ, et al. Assessment of erectile function in diabetic and non–diabetic impotence by simultaneous recording of penile diameter and penile arterial pulse. J Psychosom Res 1985; 29(3):315–324.

81. Lin JT, Bradley WE. Penile neuropathy in insulin-dependent diabetes mellitus. J Urol 1985; 133(2): 213–215.

82. Virag R, Bouilly P, Frydman D. Is impotence an arterial disorder? A study of arterial risk factors in 440 impotent men. Lancet 1985; 1(8422):181–184.

83. Kaiser FE, Korenman SG. Impotence in diabetic men. Am J Med 1988; 85(suppl 5A):147–152.

84. Vernet D, Cai L, Garban H, et al. Reduction of penile nitric oxide synthase in diabetic BB/WORdp:(type I) and BBZ/WORdp (type II) rats with erectile dysfunction. Endocrinology 1995; 136(12):5709–5717.

85. Keegan A, Cotter MA, Cameron NE. Effects of diabetes and treatment with the antioxidant alpha-lipoic acid on endothelial and neurogenic responses of corpus cavernosum in rats. Diabetologia 1999; 42(3):343–350.

86. Ehmke H, Junemann KP, Mayer B, et al. Nitric oxide synthase and vasoactive intestinal polypeptide colocalization in neurons innervating the human penile circulation. Int J Impot Res 1995; 7(3):147–156.

87. Mills TM, Wiedmeier VT, Stopper VS. Androgen maintenance of erectile function in the rat penis. Biol Reprod 1992; 46(3):342–348.

88. Chamness SL, Ricker DD, Crone JK, et al. The effect of androgen on nitric oxide synthase in the male reproductive tract of the rat. Fertil Steril 1995; 63(5): 1101–1107.

89. Lugg JA, Rajfer J, Gonzalez-Cadavid NF. Dihydrotestosterone is the active androgen in the maintenance of nitric oxide-mediated penile erection in the rat. Endocrinology 1995; 136(4):1495–1501.

90. Hoffman D, Seftel AD, Hampel N, et al. Advanced glycation end–products quench cavernosal nitric oxide. [Abstr 849]. J Urol 1995; 153(Pt 2):441A.

91. Karacan I, Salis PJ, Williams RL. The role of the sleep laboratory in diagnosis and treatment of impotence. In: Williams RL, Karacan I, ed. Sleep Disorders: Diagnosis and Treatment. New York: John Wiley & Sons, 1978:353–382.

92. Yalla SV. Sexual dysfunction in the paraplegic and quadriplegic. In: Bennett AH, ed. Management of Male Impotence. Int Perspect Urol, Vol. 5. Baltimore: Williams & Wilkins, 1982:181–191.

93. Goldstein I. Neurologic impotence. In: Krane RJ, Siroky MB, Goldstein I, eds. Male Sexual Dysfunction. Boston: Little, Brown and Company, 1983:193–201.

94. Bennett CJ, Seager SW, Vasher EA, et al. Sexual dysfunction and electroejaculation in men with spinal cord injury: review. J Urol 1988; 139(3):453–457.

95. Beckerman H, Becher J, Lankhorst GJ. The effectiveness of vibratory stimulation in anejaculatory men with spinal cord injury. Review article. Paraplegia 1993; 31(11):689–699.

96. Courtois FJ, Charvier KF, Leriche A, et al. Sexual function in spinal cord injury men. I. Assessing sexual capability. Paraplegia 1993; 31(12):771–784.

97. Smith EM, Bodner DR. Sexual dysfunction after spinal cord injury. Urol Clin North Am 1993; 20(3): 535–542.

98. Betts CD, Jones SJ, Fowler CG, et al. Erectile dysfunction in multiple sclerosis. Associated neurological and neurophysiological deficits, and treatment of the condition. Brain 1994; 117(Pt 6):1303–1310.

99. Ghezzi A, Malvestiti GM, Baldini S, et al. Erectile impotence in multiple sclerosis: a neurophysiological study. J Neurol 1995; 242(3):123–126.

100. Barak Y, Achiron A, Elizur A, et al. Sexual dysfunction in relapsing-remitting multiple sclerosis. Magnetic resonance imaging, clinical, and psychological correlates. J Psychiatry Neurosci 1996; 21(4):255–258.

101. Mathias CJ. Autonomic nervous system disorders and erectile dysfunction. Int J STD AIDS 1996; 7(suppl 3):5–8.

102. Korpelainen JT, Nieminen P, Myllyla VV. Sexual functioning among stroke patients and their spouses. Stroke 1999; 30(4):715–719.

103. Hattery RR, King BF, Lewis RW, et al. Vasculogenic impotence. Duplex and color Doppler imaging. Radiol Clin North Am 1991; 29(3).

104. Leriche R, Morel A. The syndrome of thrombotic obliteration of the aortic bifurcation. Ann Surg 1948; 127:193–206.

105. Ruzbarsky V, Michal V. Morphologic changes in the arterial bed of the penis with aging. Relationship to the pathogenesis of impotence. Invest Urol 1977; 15(3).

106. Herman A, Adar R, Rubinstein Z. Vascular lesions associated with impotence in diabetic and nondiabetic arterial occlusive disease. Diabetes 1978; 27(10):975–981.

107. Michal V, Kramar R, Pospichal J. External iliac "steal syndrome." J Cardiovasc Surg 1978; 19(4):355–357.

108. Goldstein I, Siroky MB, Nath RL, et al. Vasculogenic impotence: role of the pelvic steal test. J Urol 1982; 128(2):300–306.

109. Virag R. Arterial and venous hemodynamics in male impotence. In: Bennett AH, ed. Management of Male Impotence. Int Prospect Urol, Vol. 5. Baltimore: Williams & Wilkins, 1982:108–126.

110. Jevtich M. Vascular non-invasive diagnostic techniques. In: Krane J, Goldstein I, ed. Male Sexual Dysfunction. Boston: Little, Brown and Company, 1983:139–163.

111. Buvat J, Lemaire A, Dehaene JL, et al. Venous incompetence: critical study of the organic basis of high maintenance flow rates during artificial erection test. J Urol 1986; 135(5):926–928.

112. Freidenberg DH, Berger RE, Chew DE, et al. Quantitation of corporeal venous outflow resistance in man by corporeal pressure flow evaluation. J Urol 1987; 138(3):533–538.

113. Wespes E, Schulman CC. Cavernovenous leakage: its diagnosis, treatment and importance as a cause of impotence. Probl Urol 1987; 1:487–495.

114. Benvenuti F, Boncinelli L, Vignoli GC. Male sexual impotence in diabetes mellitus. Vasculogenic versus neurogenic factors. Neurourol Urodyn 1993; 12(2):145–151.

115. Wespes E, Schulman C. Venous impotence: pathophysiology, diagnosis and treatment. J Urol 1993; 149:1238–1245.

116. Derouet H, Eckert R, Trautwein W, et al. Muscular cavernous single cell analysis in patients with venoocclusive dysfunction. Eur Urol 1994; 25(2):145–150.

117. Forstner R, Hricak H, Kalbhen CL, et al. Magnetic resonance imaging of vascular lesions of the scrotum and penis. Urology 1995; 46(4):581–583.

118. Meuleman EJ, Diemont WL. Investigation of erectile dysfunction. Diagnostic testing for vascular factors in erectile dysfunction. Urol Clin North Am 1995; 22(4):803–819.

119. Sharaby JS, Benet AE, Melman A. Penile revascularization. Urol Clin North Am 1995; 22(4):821–832.

120. Mooradian AD, Viosca SP, Kaiser FE, et al. Penile Raynaud's phenomenon: a possible cause of erectile failure. Am J Med 1988; 85(5):748–750.

121. Wei M, Macera CA, Davis DR, et al. Total cholesterol and high density lipoprotein cholesterol as important predictors of erectile dysfunction. Am J Epidemiol 1994; 140(10):930–937.

122. Burnett AL. Nitric oxide in the penis: physiology and pathology. J Urol 1997; 157:320–324.

123. Lue TF. Functional evaluation of penile arteries with papaverine. In: Tanagho EA, Lue TF, McClure RD, eds. Contemporary Management of Impotence and Infertility. Baltimore: Williams & Wilkins, 1988: 57–64.

124. Padma–Nathan H. Dynamic infusion cavernosometry and cavernosography (DICC) and the cavernosal artery systolic occlusion pressure gradient: a complete evaluation of the hemodynamic events of a penile erection. In: Lue TF, ed. World Book of Impotence. Nishimura, London, Niigata-Shi: Smith-Gordon, 1992: 103–101.

125. Sasso F, Gulino G, Basar M, et al. Could standardized cavernosometry be helpful in therapeutic management of veno-occlusive dysfunction? J Urol 1996; 155(1):150–154.

126. Kaufman JM, Borges FD, Fitch WP, et al. Evaluation of erectile dysfunction by dynamic infusion cavernosometry and cavernosography (DICC). Multi-institutional study. Urology 1993; 41:445–451.

127. Glina S, Silva MF, Puech-Leao P, et al. Veno-occlusive dysfunction of corpora cavernosa: comparison of diagnostic methods. Int J Impot Res 1995; 7(1):1–10.

128. DePalma RG. New developments in the diagnosis and treatment of impotence. West J Med 1996; 164(1):54–61.

129. Bensen GS. Vascular evaluation: is it useful in 1992? In: Lue TF, ed. World Book of Impotence. Nishimura, London, Niigata-Shi: Smith-Gordon, 1992:85–90.

130. Kuhr CS, Heiman J, Cardenas D, et al. Premature emission after spinal cord injury. J Urol 1995; 153(2):429–431.

131. Jensen SB, Gluud C. Sexual dysfunction in men with alcoholic liver cirrhosis. A comparative study. Liver 1985; 5(2):94–100.

132. Kaufman JM, Hatzichtristou DG, Mulhall JP, et al. Impotence and chronic renal failure: a study of the hemodynamic pathophysiology. J Urol 1994; 151(3):612–618.

133. Palmer BF. Sexual dysfunction in uremia. J Am Soc Nephrol 1999; 10(6):1381–1388.

134. Aasebo U, Glytnes A, Bremnes RM, et al. Reversal of sexual impotence in male patients with chronic obstructive pulmonary disease and hypoxemia with long-term oxygen therapy. J Steroid Biochem Mol Biol 1993; 46(6):799–803.

135. Hirshkowitz M, Karacan I, Gurakar A, et al. Hypertension, erectile dysfunction, and occult sleep apnea. Sleep 1989; 12(3):223–232.

136. Schiavi RC, Stimmel B, Mandeli J, et al. Diabetes, sleep disorders, and male sexual function. Biol Psychiatry 1993; 34:171–177.

137. Andersen BL. Sexual functioning morbidity among cancer survivors. Current status and future research directions. Cancer 1985; 55(8):1835–1842.

138. Cull AM. The assessment of sexual function in cancer patients. Eur J Cancer 1992; 28A(10):1680–1686.

139. Barry JM. The evaluation and treatment of erectile dysfunction following organ transplantation. Semin Urol 1994; 12(2):147–153.

140. Walsh PC, Donker PJ. Impotence following radical prostatectomy: insight into etiology and prevention. J Urol 1982; 128(3):492–497.

141. Samdal F, Vada K, Lundmo P. Sexual function after transurethral prostatectomy. Scand J Urol Nephrol 1993; 27(1):27–29.

142. Kim ED, Blackburn D, McVary KT. Post-radical prostatectomy penile blood flow. Assessment with color flow Doppler ultrasound. J Urol 1994; 152(6 Pt 2).

143. Hall SJ, Basile G, Bertero EB, et al. Extensive corporeal fibrosis after penile irradiation. J Urol 1995; 153(2):372–377.

144. Havenga K, Enker WE, McDermott K, et al. Male and female sexual and urinary function after total mesorectal excision with autonomic nerve preservation for carcinoma of the rectum. J Am Coll Surg 1996; 182(6):495–502.

145. Crenshaw TL, Goldberg JP. Sexual Pharmacology: Drugs That Affect Sexual Function. New York: WW Norton & Company, 1996.

146. Barnes TR, Bamber RW, Watson JP. Psychotropic drugs and sexual behaviour. Br J Hosp Med 1979; 21(6):594–600.

147. Jensen J, Lendorf A, Stimpel H, et al. The prevalence and etiology of impotence in 101 male hypertensive outpatients. Am J Hypertens 1999; 12(3):271–275.

148. Rosen RC, Kostis J, Jekelis A, et al. Sexual sequelae of antihypertensive drugs: treatment effects on self-report and physiological measures in middle-aged hypertensives. Arch Sex Behav 1994; 23(2):135–152.

149. Grimm RHJ, Grandits GA, Prineas RJ, et al. Long-term effects on sexual function of five antihypertensive drugs and nutritional hygienic treatment in hypertensive men and women. Treatment of Mild Hypertension Study (TOMHS). Hypertension 1997; 29(1 Pt 1):8–14.

150. Garcia A, Herbon L, Barkan A, et al. Hyperprolactinemia inhibits gonadotropin-releasing hormone (GnRH) stimulation of the number of pituitary GnRH receptors. Endocrinology 1985; 117(3):954–959.

151. Kandeel FR, Butt WR, Rudd BT, et al. Oestrogen modulation of gonadotropin and prolactin release in women with anovulation and their responses to clomiphene. Clin Endocrinol 1979; 10:619–635.

152. Margrini G, Pallaton M, Felber JP. Prolactin-induced modification of testosterone metabolism in man. [Abstr 234]. Acta Endocrinol 1977; 85(suppl 212):143.

153. Gottlieb JI, Lustberg T. Phenothiazine-induced priapism: a case report. Am J Psychiatry 1977; 134(12): 1445–1446.

154. Matter LE, Hailemariam S, Huch RA, et al. Primary erectile dysfunction in combination with congenital malformation of the cavernous bodies. Urol Int 1998; 60(3):175–177.

155. Carrier S, Hricak H, Lee SS, et al. Radiation-induced decrease in nitric oxide synthase-containing nerves in the rat penis. Radiology 1995; 195(1):95–99.

156. Vahlensieck WKJ, Schaefer HE, Westenfelder M. Penile ossification and acquired penile deviation. Eur Urol 1995; 27(3):252–256.

157. Ralph DJ, Mirakian R, Pryor JP, et al. The immunological features of Peyronie's disease. J Urol 1996; 155(1):159–162.

158. Weidner W, Schroeder-Printzen I, Weiske WH, et al. Sexual dysfunction in Peyronie's disease: an analysis of 222 patients without previous local plaque therapy. J Urol 1997; 157:325–328.

159. Hellstrom WJG, McAninch JW, Lue TF. Priapism: physiology and treatment. Probl Urol 1987; 3:518–529.

160. Torok A, Jilling A, Gotz F. Induced priapism and its management. Int Urol Nephrol 1991; 23(2):191–194.

161. Bastuba MD, Saenz de Tejada I, Dinlenc CZ, et al. Arterial priapism: diagnosis, treatment and long-term follow up. J Urol 1994; 151(5):1231–1237.

162. Soni BM, Vaidyanathan S, Krishnan KR. Management of pharmacologically induced prolonged penile erection with oral terbutaline in traumatic paraplegics. Paraplegia 1994; 32(10):670–674.

163. Hakim LS, Kulaksizoglu H, Mulligan R, et al. Evolving concepts in the diagnosis and treatment of arterial high flow priapism. J Urol 1996; 155(2):541–548.

164. Alexander WD. Phimosis and treatment for erectile failure. Diabet Med 1993; 10(8):782 (Letter).

165. Murali TR, Raja NS. Cavernosal cold abscess: a rare cause of impotence. Br J Urol 1998; 82(6):929–930.

166. Laumann EO, Masi CM, Zuckerman EW. Circumcision in the United States. Prevalence, prophylactic effects, and sexual practice. J Am Med Assoc 1997; 277(13):1052–1057.

167. Royce RA, Sena A, Catas W, et al. Sexual transmission of HIV. N Engl J of Med 1997; 336(15):1072–1078.

168. Warner E, Strashin E. Benefits and risks of circumcision. Can Med Assoc J 1981; 125(9):967–976, 992.

169. Agarwal S, Sehgal A, Sardana S, et al. Role of male behavior in cervical carcinogenesis among women with one lifetime sexual partner. Cancer 1993; 72(5):1666–1669.

170. Halata Z, Munger BL. The neuroanatomical basis for the protopathic sensibility of the human glans penis. Brain Res 1986; 371(2):205–230.

171. Lindsay MB, Schain DM, Grambsch P, et al. The incidence of Peyronie's disease in Rochester, Minnesota, 1950 through 1984. J Urol 1991; 146(4):1007–1009.

172. Ganabathi K, Dmochowski R, Zimmern PE, et al. Peyronie's disease: surgical treatment based on penile rigidity. J Urol 1995; 153(3 Pt 1):662–666.

173. Vorstman B, Lockhart J. Peyronie's disease. Probl Urol 1987; 1:507–517.

174. Davis CJ. The microscopic pathology of Peyronie's disease. J Urol 1997; 157(1):282–284.

175. Brock G, Hsu GL, Nunes L, et al. The anatomy of the tunica albuginea in the normal penis and Peyronie's disease. J Urol 1997; 157(1):276–281.

176. Ehrlich HP. Scar contracture: cellular and connective tissue aspects in Peyronie's disease. J Urol 1997; 157(1):316–319.

177. Devine CJJ, Somers KD, Jordan SG, et al. Proposal: trauma as the cause of the Peyronie's lesion. J Urol 1997; 157(1):285–290.

178. Somers KD, Dawson DM. Fibrin deposition in Peyronie's disease plaque. J Urol 1997; 157(1):311–315.

179. Willscher MK, Cwazka WF, Novicki DE. The association of histocompatibility antigens for the B7 cross-reacting group with Peyronie's disease. J Urol 1979; 122(1):34–35.

180. Nachtsheim DA, Rearden A. Peyronie's disease is associated with an HLA class II antigen, HLA-DQ5, implying an autoimmune etiology. J Urol 1996; 156(4):1330–1334.

181. Ralph DJ, Schwartz G, Moore W, et al. The genetic and bacteriological aspects of Peyronie's disease. J Urol 1997; 157(1):291–294.

182. Bailey MJ, Yande S, Walmsley B, et al. Surgery for Peyronie's disease. A review of 200 patients. Br J Urol 1985; 57(6):746–74.

183. Gelbard MK, Dorey F, James K. The natural history of Peyronie's disease. J Urol 1990; 144(6):1376–1379.

184. Armenakas NA, McAninch JW, Lue TF, et al. Posttraumatic impotence: magnetic resonance imaging

and duplex ultrasound in diagnosis and management. J Urol 1993; 149:1272–1275.

185. Mertens C, Merck L, Derluyn M, et al. Iatrogenic femoral arteriovenous fistula as a cause of erectile dysfunction. Eur Urol 1994; 26(4):340–341.

186. Lehmann K, Schopke W, Hauri D. Subclinical trauma to perineum: a possible etiology of erectile dysfunction in young men. Eur Urol 1995; 27(4):306–310.

187. Licht MR, Lewis RW, Sershon PD. Immediate impotence after penetrating perineal trauma: restoration of erections with penile artery revascularization, corpus cavernosum aneurysm repair, and deep penile venous ligation. Urology 1995; 46(4):577–580.

188. Mayersak JS, Viviano CJ, Babiarz JW. Schwannoma of the penis. J Urol 1995; 153(6):1931–1932.

189. Asgari MA, Hosseini SY, Safarinejad MR, et al. Penile fractures: evaluation, therapeutic approaches and long-term results. J Urol 1996; 155(1):148–149.

190. Crook J, Esche B, Futter N. Effect of pelvic radiotherapy for prostate cancer on bowel, bladder, and sexual function: the patient's perspective. Urology 1996; 47(3):387–394.

191. Goldman HB, Dmochowski RR, Cox CE. Penetrating trauma to the penis: functional results. J Urol 1996; 155(2):551–553.

192. Carrier S, Zvara P, Nunes L, et al. Regeneration of nitric oxide synthase-containing nerves after cavernous nerve neurotomy in the rat. J Urol 1995; 153(5): 1722–1727.

193. Teloken C, Busato WFS Jr, Neto JF, et al. Congenital abnormality of corpora cavernosa and erectile dysfunction: a case report. J Urol 1993; 149(5):1135–1136.

194. Bar-Moshe O, Oboy G, Timmermans CH, et al. Megalourethra and abnormalities of the cavernous bodies: cause of erectile dysfunction. Eur Urol 1995; 27(3):249–251.

195. Montague DK, Lakin MM, Angermeier KW, et al. Primary erectile dysfunction in a man with congenital isolation of the corpora cavernosa. Urology 1995; 46(1):114–116.

196. Van der Ven PF, Wei AY, Jap PH, et al. Increased expression of a 68-kDa protein in the corpus cavernosum of some men with erectile dysfunction. J Androl 1995; 16(3):242–247.

197. Mannino DM, Klevens RM, Flanders WD. Cigarette smoking: an independent risk factor for impotence? Am J Epidemiol 1994; 140(11):1003–1008.

198. Condra M, Morales A, Owen JA, et al. Prevalence and significance of tobacco smoking in impotence. Urology 1986; 27(6):495–498.

199. Rosen MP, Greenfield AJ, Walteret TG, et al. Cigarette smoking: an independent risk factor for atherosclerosis in the hypogastric-cavernous arterial bed of men with arteriogenic impotence. J Urol 1991; 145(4):759–763.

200. Shabsigh R, Fishman IJ, Schum C, et al. Cigarette smoking and other vascular risk factors in vasculogenic impotence. Urology 1991; 38(3):227–231.

201. Hirshkowitz M, Karakan I, Howell JW, et al. Nocturnal penile tumescence in cigarette smokers with erectile dysfunction. Urology 1992; 39(2):101–107.

202. Mersdorf A, Goldsmith PC, Diederichs W, et al. Ultrastructural changes in impotent penile tissue: a comparison of 65 patients. J Urol 1991; 145(4):749–758.

203. Levine LA, Gerber GS. Acute vasospasm of penile arteries in response to cigarette smoking. Urology 1990; 36(1):99–100 (Letter).

204. Patterson TR, Stringham JD, Meikle AW. Nicotine and cotinine inhibit steroidogenesis in mouse Leydig cells. Life Sci 1990; 46(4):265–272.

205. Xie Y, Garban H, Ng C, et al. Effect of long-term passive smoking on erectile function and penile nitric oxide synthase in the rat. J Urol 1997; 157(3):1121–1126.

206. Richardson JD. Male sexual dysfunction. Ejaculatory problems. Aust Fam Physician 1993; 22:1367–1370.

207. Metz ME, Pryor JL, Nesvacil LJ, et al. Premature ejaculation: a psychophysiological review. J Sex Marital Ther 1997; 23(1):3–23.

208. Cooper AJ, Cernovsky ZZ, Colussi K. Some clinical and psychometric characteristics of primary and secondary premature ejaculators. J Sex Marital Ther 1993; 19(4):276–288.

209. Frank E, Anderson C, Rubinstein D. Frequency of sexual dysfunction in "normal" couples. N Engl J Med 1978; 299(3):111–115.

210. Rowland DL, Haensel SM, Blom JH, et al. Penile sensitivity in men with premature ejaculation and erectile dysfunction. J Sex Marital Ther 1993; 19(3): 189–197.

211. Grenier G, Byers ES. Rapid ejaculation: a review of conceptual, etiological, and treatment issues. Arch Sex behav 1995; 24(4):447–472.

212. Semmens JP, Semmens FJ. Premature ejaculation and impotence: male problems with gynecologic implications. Clin Obstet Gynecol 1978; 21(1):223–233.

213. Goldstein I. Impotence. In: Tayor RB, ed. Difficult Diagnosis. Philadelphia: WB Saunders Company, 1985:300–309.

214. O'Meara J, White WB. Ejaculatory failure and urinary dysfunction secondary to labetalol. J Urol 1988; 139(2): 371–372.

215. Murphy JB, Lipshultz LI. Abnormalities of ejaculation. Urol Clin North Am 1987; 14(3):583–596.

216. Gilja I, Parazajder J, Radej M, et al. Retrograde ejaculation and loss of emission: possibilities of conservative treatment. Eur Urol 1994; 25(3):226–228.

217. Levine SB. Marital sexual dysfunction: ejaculation disturbances. Ann Intern Med 1976; 84(5):575–579.

218. Hendry WF. Disorders of ejaculation: congenital, acquired and functional. Br J Urol 1998; 82(3): 331–341.

219. Aizenberg D, Zemishlany Z, Hermesh H, et al. Painful ejaculation associated with antidepressants in four patients. J Clin Psychiatry 1991; 52(11):461–463.

220. Kaplan HS. Disorders of sexual desire and other new concepts and techniques in sex therapy. New York: Brunner/Mazel, 1979.

221. Kaplan HS. Post-ejaculatory pain syndrome. J Sex Marital Ther 1993; 19(2):91–103.

222. Schwingl PJ, Guess HA. Safety and effectiveness of vasectomy. Fertil Steril 2000; 73(5):923–936.

223. True LD, Berger RE, Rothman I, et al. Prostate histopathology and the chronic prostatitis/chronic pelvic pain syndrome: a prospective biopsy study. J Urol 1999; 162(6):2014–2018.

224. Alexander RB, Ponniah S, Hasday J, et al. Elevated levels of proinflammatory cytokines in the semen of patients with chronic prostatitis/chronic pelvic pain syndrome. Urology 1998; 52(5):744–749.

225. Litwin MS, McNaughton-Collins M, Fowler FJ, et al. The National Institutes of Health chronic prostatitis symptom index: development and validation of a new outcome measure. Chronic Prostatitis Collaborative Research Network. J Urol 1999; 162(2): 369–375.

226. Miller HC. Stress prostatitis. Urology 1988; 32(6): 507–510.

227. Rosen RC, Leiblum SR. Treatment of sexual disorders in the 1990s: an integrated approach. J Consult Clin Psychol 1995; 63(6):877–890.

228. Spector IP, Carey MP. Incidence and prevalence of the sexual dysfunctions: a critical review of the empirical literature. Arch Sex Behav 1990; 19(4):389–408.

229. Sovner R. Anorgasmia associated with imipramine but not desipramine: case report. J Clin Psychiatry 1983; 44(9):345–346.

230. McCormick S, Olin J, Brotman AW. Reversal of fluoxetine-induced anorgasmia by cyproheptadine in two patients. J Clin Psychiatry 1990; 51(9):383–384.

231. Zajecka J, Fawcett J, Schaff M, et al. The role of serotonin in sexual dysfunction: fluoxetine-associated orgasm dysfunction. J Clin Psychiatry 1991; 52(2): 66–68.

232. Walker PW, Cole JO, Gardner EA, et al. Improvement in fluoxetine-associated sexual dysfunction in patients switched to bupropion. J Clin Psychiatry 1993; 54:459–465.

233. Segraves RT. Antidepressant-induced orgasm disorder. J Sex Marital Ther 1995; 21(3):192–201.

234. Margolese HC, Assalian P. Sexual side effects of antidepressants: a review. J Sex Marital Ther 1996; 22:209–217.

235. Monteiro WO, Noshirvani HF, Marks IM, et al. Anorgasmia from clomipramine in obsessive-compulsive disorder. A controlled trial. Br J Psychiatry 1987; 151:107–112.

236. Keller A, Hamer R, Rosen RC. Serotonin reuptake inhibitor-induced sexual dysfunction and its treatment: a large-scale retrospective study of 596 psychiatric outpatients. J Sex Martial Ther 1997; 23(3):165–175.

237. Lane RM. A critical review of selective serotonin reuptake inhibitor-related sexual dysfunction; incidence, possible aetiology and implications for management. J Psychopharmacol 1997; 11:72–82.

238. Rosen RC, Lane RM, Menza M. Effects of SSRIs on sexual function: a critical review. J Clin Psychopharmacol 1999; 19(1):67–85.

239. Murphy M. Down-regulation of post-synaptic serotonin receptors as a mechanism for clomipramine-induced anorgasmia. Br J Psychiatry 1987; 151:704 (Letter).

240. Federoff JP, Peyser C, Franz ML, et al. Sexual disorders in Huntington's disease. J Neuropsychiatry Clin Neurosci 1994; 6:147–153.

241. Tomic R, Sjodin JG. Sexual function in men after radical cystectomy with or without urethrectomy. Scand J Urol Nephrol 1992; 26(2):127–129.

242. Brindley GS. Pathophysiology of erection and ejaculation. In: Whitfield HN, Hendry WF, eds. A Textbook of Genitourinary Surgery. London: Churchill Livingstone, 1988:1083–1094.

243. Koeman M, Driel MF, Schultz WC, et al. Orgasm after radical prostatectomy. Br J Urol 1996; 77(6):861–864.

244. Kulmala RV, Tamella TL. Effects of priapism lasting 24 hours or longer caused by intracavernosal injection of vasoactive drugs. Int J Impot Res 1995; 7(2):131–136.

245. Altman AL, Seftel AD, Brown SL, et al. Cocaine associated priapism. J Urol 1999; 161(6):1817–1818.

246. Saenz de Tejada I, Kim NM, Daley JT, et al. Acidosis impairs rabbit trabecular smooth muscle contractility. J Urol 1997; 157(2):722–726.

11

Comparing Male and Female Sexual Function and Dysfunction

Alessandra Graziottin

Center of Gynecology and Medical Sexology, Hospital San Raffaele Resnati, Milan; Post-Graduate Course of Sexual Medicine, University of Florence, Florence; Specialty School of Gynecology and Obstetrics, University of Florence and University of Parma, Parma, Italy

☐ INTRODUCTION

The anatomic, somatic, and psychological differences that exist between men and women have largely been responsible for the striking sociocultural gender disparities—and discriminations—that have endured over centuries and into the present day throughout the majority of the world's civilizations. Even in the field of modern sexual research, this deep-seated dichotomy has generated some major consequences. First, in the medical sciences, a traditionally male-dominated perspective has influenced the development of interpretative models of sexual function based on a basic male frame. This resulted in the essential "overgenitalization" of dysfunctional states and the consequent design of disappointing classification systems, with their associated diagnostic and therapeutic approaches (1–3). Second, because women tend to enjoy greater representation in the humanistic sciences such as psychology and psychosexology, the sum product of these particular occupational gender biases has resulted in the misconception that while the mechanisms of sexual function are biologically determined in men, they are chiefly driven by psychology in women (4). The deleterious perspectives of "medicine without soul" and "psychology without body" only serve to deprive each gender of a more comprehensive understanding of the continuous interactions between biology, psychology, and context-dependent factors (5–7).

It should be noted that beyond the inescapable differences in reproductive anatomy, secondary sexual characteristics, and reproductive behaviors, human extragenital anatomy and systemic functions are indeed very similar in both sexes, differing more in quantitative than qualitative respects; these similarities include the vital components of the nervous, vascular, metabolic, immune, muscular, and endocrine systems, with the exception of sexual hormones. For example, other than the smaller average dimensions of nonsexual female organs, male and female internal anatomy is exactly the same: there are no dimorphic livers, lungs, or hearts (8,9). It is often overlooked that the fundamental mechanisms of the sexual response depend upon little else but the integrity of major organ function, including vascular, metabolic, and hormonal considerations. Even the gender prevalence of certain disorders such as postpubertal depression or postmenopausal osteoarthritis is more frequently due to differences in sex-specific endocrine modulation rather than substantial anatomic or functional differences. Consider the fact that of the 46 chromosomes physiologically present in humans, men and women differ in only one sex chromosome. The simple substitution of a Y for an X is the sole factor responsible for the production of the male instead of the female of the species, with all of the associated striking sexual differences in anatomy, function, reproductive capability, psychology—and, not in the least, sociocultural standing.

These scientific truths suggest that, biologically speaking, men and women have far more in common than not. The fundamental similarities that exist initially, however, become diametrically polarized over time as the result of lifelong exposure to a steeply conflicted societal construct, with obvious macroscopic and cultural differences overshadowing the less apparent similarities in sexual function. All of this may be evidence to support why (*i*) until recently, sexual research on males and females followed widely disparate paths and methodologies; (*ii*) many effective treatments for sexual dysfunction have been developed and marketed for men (4–6) whereas very few have become available to women (7); (*iii*) organic sexual pain disorders such as dyspareunia have been labeled as "psychogenic" for decades, depriving women of correct diagnoses and effective treatments (10,11–14); and (*iv*) the exaggerated current focus on differences between male and female sexual responses may be obfuscating key biological parallels in pathophysiology—similarities that could be researched more effectively using analogous methods and data.

This chapter organizes comparative male and female sexual function into four main sections: (*i*) the basic physiological factors that lead to similarities in sexual function between genders; (*ii*) the key dimorphic differences in the central nervous system function that determine most of the gender variations in the endocrine milieu and the psychosexual, behavioral, and endocrine-dependent somatic aspects of sexual function and dysfunction; (*iii*) the new, neuropsychological insights on the biological basis of sexual desire and behavior in both sexes, focusing on the similarities and differences in the four "basic emotional command systems" that coordinate the complex interactions of instinctual drive and the motivational-affective and cognitive aspects of the sexual response; and (*iv*) the clinical similarities and differences between male sexual dysfunction (MSD) and female sexual dysfunction (FSD) (1–24).

☐ GENERAL SIMILARITIES IN SEXUAL PHYSIOLOGY OF MEN AND WOMEN

In both genders, sexuality encompasses three major dimensions: sexual identity, sexual function, and sexual relationships, although the lines between each category may become blurred through their partially overlapping interactions in both functional and dysfunctional conditions (Fig. 1).

A brief review of physiology is included to underscore many of the frequently overlooked similarities between male and female sexuality. Special attention is given to the role of the brain, which coordinates both biological and psychosexual dimensions of sexual function and dysfunction, particularly in the domain of desire and central arousal. (For further information on normal male anatomy and sexual response, see Chapters 2 and 3.)

Sexual Desire and the Limbic System

Sexual function is rooted in biological, psychosexual, and context-dependent factors. Focusing first on the biological aspects, a normal sexual response requires the anatomic and functional integrity of the brain's entire limbic system rather than a particular anatomic structure within it (8). Indeed, the limbic system is a comprehensive network involving the hypothalamus and the thalamus (both within the diencephalon), the anterior cingulate gyrus, and many structures

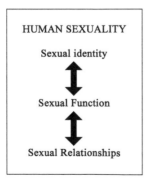

HUMAN SEXUALITY

Sexual identity

↕

Sexual Function

↕

Sexual Relationships

Figure 1 Human sexuality. Three major dimensions interact and partially overlap in both physiologic and pathologic conditions. *Source*: From Ref. 25.

of the temporal lobes, including the amygdala, the mammillary bodies, the fornix, and the hippocampus, a phylogenetically ancient type of cortex (8,22,26). Together with the prefrontal lobe, which has a predominantly inhibitory role over the basic instinctual drives, the limbic system is essential in both sexes for initiation of sexual desire and related sexual phenomena such as sexual fantasies, sexual daydreams, erotic dreams, mental sexual arousal, and the initiation of the cascade of neurovascular events triggering all of the somatic and genital responses of sexual function as well as the associated socially appropriate behaviors. It is thought that the amygdala maintains a key role as the control center for the four "basic emotional command systems" described by Panksepp; the disruption of any level of the limbic system, however, may cause sexual dysfunction in both sexes, particularly in the domains of desire, central arousal, and socially appropriate sexual behavior (8,9,26–30). For further information on the four basic emotional command systems, see below.

Neurotransmitters

In men and women, the sexual response is coordinated by the same neurotransmitters, with the most studied being monoamines (dopamine, norepinephrine, and serotonin) and neuropeptides (opioid peptides, oxytocin, and vasopressin) (9,20,22–24,29). Regional and quantitative differences in neurotransmitter activities reflect brain sexual dimorphisms that are modulated by prenatal and postnatal endocrine milieus and their interactions with environmental factors.

Neural Pathways

At the level of the spine, the neural pathways of sympathetic and parasympathetic sexual responses in both genders follow the same anatomic distributions until their termination in different male and female target sexual organs. These pathways involve the superior hypogastric plexus, the middle hypogastric plexus (which gives rise to the hypogastric nerves joining the testicular or ovarian plexus), the ureteric plexus, the internal iliac arterial plexus, and the inferior hypogastric plexus (which receives mostly sympathetic afferent and efferent fibers from the hypogastric nerves, the postganglionic sympathetic fibers derived from the sacral splanchnic nerves, and the parasympathetic fibers derived from pelvic splanchnic nerves—the nervi erigentes in both sexes—that have their cell bodies in the S2, S3, and S4 segments of the spinal cord) (31,32). These similarities in neural pathways have important implications for oncologic surgeries in which the sparing of the vesical nerve plexus fibers that accompany the vesical artery to the bladder may significantly reduce both sexual and urinary morbidity in both men and women (33).

The prostatic plexus and the uterovaginal plexus are simply the terminal ramifications of the lower part of the inferior hypogastric plexus. In men, the prostatic plexus innervates the prostate, seminal vesicles, prostatic urethra, corpora cavernosa, corpus spongiosum, both the membranous and the penile portions of the urethra, and the bulbourethral glands. In women, the uterovaginal plexus supplies the uterus, salpinges, ovaries, vagina, erectile tissue of the clitoris and vestibular bulbs (via the cavernous nerves of the clitoris), urethra, and greater vestibular glands (31,32).

In both genders, the perineum receives its primary somatic innervation from the pudendal nerve (derived from S2, S3, and S4) and its sympathetic innervation from the sacral portion of the sympathetic chain (31,32). The anatomic pathway of the pudendal nerve is very similar in both men and women, forming a single trunk that runs approximately 1 cm posterior to the ischial spine through the greater sciatic foramen inferior to the piriformis muscle. It then reenters the pelvic cavity through the lesser sciatic foramen and proceeds anteriorly through Alcock's canal, passing posterior to the junction between the ischial spine and the sacrospinous ligament and anterior to the sacrotuberous ligament and medial to the internal pudendal vessels. At this point, the pudendal nerve branches into its three main pathways: the inferior hemorrhoidal nerve, the perineal nerve, and the dorsal nerve of the clitoris (in women) or penis (in men). The similarities in these pathways help explain the equal risks of numbness, reduced sensibility, and arousal difficulties of the external genitalia secondary to compression of the pudendal nerve experienced by both men and women who ride bicycles for long periods of time without adequate protection or frequent position changes (34).

Urogenital Triangle

The pelvic floor muscles in both men and women have the same composition: the pubococcygeous and the coccygeous muscles form the muscular diaphragm that supports the pelvic viscera and opposes the downward thrust produced by increases in intra-abdominal pressure.

In both genders, the urogenital region consists of superficial and deep spaces created by the bulbospongiosus, ischiocavernosus, sphincter urethrae, and the transversus perinei superficialis and profundus (31,32).

In men, the middle fibers of the medially located bulbospongiosus assist erection of the penile corpus spongiosum by compressing the erectile tissue of the bulb. The anterior fibers insert into and are continuous with the deep fascia covering the deep dorsal vein of the penis, and thus they contribute to erection via compression of the deep dorsal vein.

In women, the bulbospongiosus surrounds the orifice of the vagina, covering lateral parts of the vestibular bulb. Anteriorly, it becomes attached to the body of the clitoris and similarly compresses the female deep dorsal vein, enabling erection of the clitoral tissue.

The ischiocavernosus muscle, also called the erector penis muscle, is bilaterally present and, in men,

covers the crura of the penis, compressing them and helping to maintain erection.

The ischiocavernosus is typically smaller in women and covers the unattached surface of the crura clitoridis, compressing these and retarding the outflow of venous blood during sexual arousal to assist in maintaining clitoral erection. Similarly, the transversus perinei profundus and the sphincter urethrae perform identical functions in both genders.

Vasculature

The main vessels that supply the genital organs arise from branches of the left and right internal iliac arteries, each of which has an anterior and posterior division. The anterior branch nourishes most of the pelvic viscera and gives rise to the following arteries: obturator, inferior gluteal, umbilical, superior vesical, middle vesical, inferior vesical, and internal pudendal. The posterior division produces three parietal branches: the iliolumbar, the lateral-sacral, and the superior gluteal arteries. Although similar up until this point in both genders, further divisions of these arteries occupy anatomic distributions representative of their pelvic visceral dimorphisms. The chemoregulatory similarities in vasoconstriction and vasodilation of the primary vascular supply of the genital organs, however, suggests a comparable vulnerability in both men and women to common circulatory impairments such as smoking, cholesterol, and hypertension, although the effects of these factors have been investigated much more thoroughly in men than in women.

Sexual Hormones

The production rates, pattern of secretion, and circulatory levels of sex hormones such as androgens, estrogens, and progesterones across the phases of life are very different between males and females. At menopause, a dramatic reduction in estrogen and progesterone secretion occurs in women, with or without concomitant changes in androgen concentration, depending on the particular type of menopause (spontaneous or iatrogenic); surgically induced menopause acutely deprives a woman of greater than 50% of presurgical total testosterone and androstenedione levels. In contrast, men usually experience a very gradual decline in androgen concentration with age. Sex hormones alone are responsible for most of the striking anatomic and functional differences between men and women.

□ PATHOPHYSIOLOGY
Similarities

Similarities in MSDs and FSDs stem from basic physiologic similarities. All of the sexual dysfunctions seen in both men and women may have biological, motivational-affective, and cognitive etiologies (5–7, 10–24,26–30). They may be lifelong or acquired, generalized or situational, and may, in fact, be of mixed or unknown etiology (1–3,5–7). It should be emphasized, however, that in either gender, a psychogenic diagnosis may, in fact, have a biological basis.

Comorbidities with other physical or psychosocial disorders may negatively impact various aspects of sexual function in both genders but with higher frequency in women (3,5,7,11,12,15,16). For example, hyperprolactinemia, as well as drugs that induce a hyperprolactinemic state, have been associated with the loss of sexual desire in both men and women (9,22). Similarly, central and peripheral nervous system disturbances such as depression, anxiety, obsessive compulsive disorders, schizophrenia, multiple sclerosis, Parkinson's disease, and paraplegia often adversely affect the sexual response in both men and women, causing a variety of disorders—including those of desire, arousal, and orgasm (6,7,22). Considering that orgasm is a neuromuscular reflex modulated by corticomedullary serotoninergic fibers in both men and women (19), the use of selective serotonin reuptake inhibitors (SSRIs) and other antidepressants such as clomipramine, can delay or block orgasm with a dose-dependent effect (14,35,36). In fact, iatrogenic sexual disorders secondary to radiotherapy, chemotherapy, prescription drugs, or postsurgical side effects such as vascular, nervous, or anatomic disruptions are very common in both sexes, often employing identical mechanisms of action (6,10,20,11,37,38). Dopaminergic drugs, on the other hand, reportedly increase sexual desire in both men and women (9,22).

Age is the worst natural enemy of sexual function in both men and women, particularly with sexual desire disorders (15,17), arousal disorders with a multisystemic basis (vascular, neurogenic, hormonal, etc.) that lead to erectile dysfunction (ED) in men (20), dyspareunia secondary to vaginal dryness in women (10,11), and orgasmic disorders (19). Additionally, age-dependent involution of the corpora cavernosa has been demonstrated in both sexes (20,39).

In both men and women, testosterone is the single most important trigger of sexual desire and central arousal, acting as a central "initiator" (5,9,15,20,22). The higher native concentration of testosterone in males (up to 10 times the average level in women) may explain not only the higher levels of desire seen in men but also the functional mental dimorphisms in many sexual behaviors that may occur as a result. Further proof of this correlation comes from the fact that low serum testosterone levels are associated with reduced sexual drive in both genders, although the initiation of testosterone therapy often restores the deficit (40–43).

Androgen receptors have been demonstrated in the corpora cavernosa and in the female vagina, where their activation appears to facilitate nitric oxide production and/or action (20,22). This may explain why the absence or significant reduction of testosterone could be associated with the reduction of genital arousal in both sexes. It should be noted, however, that the vagina also contains estrogen receptors that exert similar effects on neurons responsive to vasoactive intestinal polypeptide (VIPergic neurons). Phosphodiesterase type 5, a key enzyme in the male erectile process, has also been demonstrated in the anterior vaginal wall (44).

Because the genital blood vessels arise from the same vascular branches and respond to identical somatic and autonomic nerve stimuli, vascular etiology may perhaps be regarded as the most important etiological factor in ED. While circulatory compromise is widely recognized as a leading cause of sexual dysfunction in men, vascular factors are frequently overlooked in the clinical evaluation of female sexual disorders.

The integrity of the pelvic floor muscles is important in both sexes, although its vulnerability to anatomic and functional damages is higher in women as the result of reproductive events. Comorbidity of urologic, proctologic, and pelvic floor-related conditions adversely influences sexual function in men and women (45).

In both sexes, satisfaction with prior sexual experiences can significantly enhance the sexual response in subsequent encounters whereas prior dissatisfaction can just as significantly inhibit future sexual responses (Figs. 2 and 3) (46,47).

Sexual Dimorphisms

One exciting challenge in modern sexual medicine is the recognition of the functional similarities and differences between men and women that share a solid biological basis in the context of the many sociocultural constructs that have historically polarized sexual

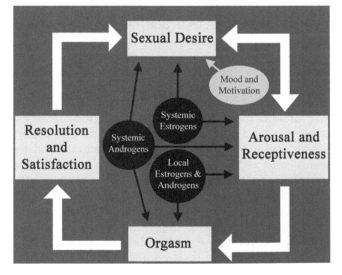

FEMALE SEXUAL FUNCTION

Figure 2 Circular model of female sexual function. The model indicates the interdependence of different dimensions of the female sexual response: the possibility of positive or negative feedbacks in the sexual circuit according to the quality of sexual experience and the reciprocity between sexual desire and arousal, inclusive of the possibility that genital arousal due to direct genital stimulation may trigger and/or increase both mental arousal and sexual desire. The model suggests that mood and motivation are major modulators of sexual desire, further stressing the importance of sexual hormones as central initiators (androgens) and peripheral modulators (androgens and estrogens) in women. *Source*: From Ref. 15.

MALE SEXUAL FUNCTION

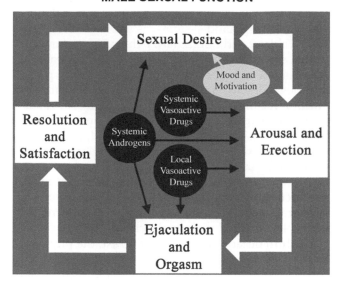

Figure 3 Circular model of male sexual function. The model indicates the interdependence of different dimensions of the male sexual response: the possibility of positive or negative feedbacks in the sexual circuit according to the quality of sexual experience and the reciprocity between sexual desire and arousal, inclusive of the possibility that genital arousal due to direct genital stimulation may trigger and/or increase both mental arousal and sexual desire. The model suggests that mood and motivation are major modulators of sexual desire in men as well, further stressing the importance of androgens as central initiators and of vasoactive drugs as peripheral modulators. *Source*: From Ref. 25.

responses and rights by gender. This section will focus on the discussion of biological sexual functions and their psychosexual correlates, with minor notes on the cultural framework of these events.

Many aspects of adult sexual life, both functional and dysfunctional, can claim their origins in the very earliest steps of "sexual dimorphism." For example, the gene sequences of chromosomes have two functions: the ability to replicate, termed the "template" function, and the expression of genes, called "transcription." The process of activating and expressing genes results in the genotype becoming the phenotype, that is, the transformation of the potential, virtual DNA code into actual, functional tissue (8,9,22,48). Interestingly, the "default" phenotypic expression for the human organism, including its brain, is female (8). Unless a specific substance called testis-determining factor (TDF) is expressed by a short sequence of genes on the Y-chromosome during the maturation process of the fetus, every baby born would have a female body structure.

TDF acts on the gonads to influence cell gene transcription. During the second trimester of pregnancy, the testicles begin to produce testosterone, which appears to be responsible for the developmental differences that distinguish males from females, by acting on a wide range of organ systems including the brain (8,48). Although the interaction of testosterone with an appropriate receptor is a prerequisite for the activation of the cascade of genomic and nongenomic

events, in order to produce certain responses, testosterone must first be converted into its more active metabolite, dihydrotestosterone, by the enzyme 5α-reductase (48). The subsequent activation of testosterone receptors results in the varying gene expression of cells in different organ systems, which in turn causes a myriad of anatomical changes including the formation of external and internal male genitalia, the development of male secondary sexual characteristics at puberty, and the development of other phenotypic differences in the overall size and shape of the body.

It should be noted that the neurons of men and women share all the basic anatomic and functional characteristics. Similarly, neurotransmitters and neurohormones have exactly the same structure and roles in both men and women, with some quantitative differences as well as some variability in regional distribution (8,9,22,48). Even the potential for neuroplasticity—that is, the ability to increase and modulate connections among neurons through neuronal sprouting and the creation of dendritic spines, and the morphological correlate of psychoplasticity—is shared equally in both genders. It appears, then, that the major neurologic differences between men and women lie mainly in their respective degrees of brain dimorphism—differences caused by the action of testosterone on the brain. Quite interestingly, many of the central nervous system effects of testosterone are mediated by estrogen, as a result of the aromatization of testosterone by the enzyme aromatase (8,48).

First, it must be mentioned that sexually dimorphic variations in overall brain weight (which is higher, on an average, in men) do not appear to be of importance in human sexuality. The past claim that a larger brain represented greater intellectual abilities has since been discounted because recent research has shown that intelligence in both sexes depends not on the total number of neurons but on the complex pattern of connections between cells, their continuous plasticity, and the intensity by which they are stimulated through affective events, educational level, and environmental challenges (8,49).

For example, since the region of the corpus callosum is proportionately larger in the average female brain than in the male brain, it seems that masculinization of the brain produces at least a partial suppression of these fibers. This implies that the left and right cerebral hemispheres of an average female are more closely connected than in their male counterparts. A larger corpus callosum is thought to result in less lateral specialization, providing a possible anatomic explanation for the functional correlate that women commonly have superior language abilities—that is, they speak at an earlier age and have greater ultimate adult fluency and vocabulary—while men generally have better visuospatial abilities, as represented by the topographical skills required to remember and describe a particular route or to understand and translate a two-dimensional map into three-dimensional space (8,48). It is not yet clear why an increased interhemispheric interaction produces these particular effects;

nevertheless, the differences are well established and are, in fact, the most widely studied cognitive features in terms of major gender-based mental traits. Of course, it must be recognized that individual men or women may deviate from these largely general trends (49).

Hemispheric asymmetry has manifest implications in male and female sexual function, as well. For example, the most important sexual cues in women for increasing mental arousal—as well as the mental awareness of that arousal—typically involve verbal intimacy such as having her partner's receptive and attentive ear or having affectionate or erotic words spoken to her. Men, on the other hand, rely much more strongly on visual stimulation, either in reality or in fantasy, for mental and genital arousal. Much disappointment and frustration results when these two primary sexual cues are polarized in a couple; the consequent mental dissatisfaction may then potentially contribute to sexual dysfunction and even to sexual avoidance.

Another main neuroanatomical difference between men and women lies in the medial preoptic area of the hypothalamus, the key center of the autonomic nervous system in both sexes. Located within this region is a set of nuclei known as the interstitial nuclei of the anterior hypothalamus that express their products in a "tonic" or relatively continuous secretory state in men, whereas they exhibit a "cyclic" pattern of secretion in fertile, ovulating women. This variability has many important consequences on brain function and sexual behavior as well as many other somatic effects. Notably, while the hypothalamic hormone oxytocin is the primary peptide in female sexual circuitry, the male sexual cycle is most represented by vasopressin (8,9,22,26).

"Need detectors" located within the hypothalamus are responsible for the activation of the four "basic emotional command systems" of the brain: seeking, rage, fear, and panic (Table 1) (26). These hypothalamic detectors are typically switched on and off by different hypothalamic regions. Prefrontal connections also influence the hypothalamic detectors, typically to inhibit the basic drives. Many additional cognitive and perceptual inputs and cues serve to regulate the basic emotional command systems, as well.

Tables 2 and 3 summarize the primary functional sexual similarities and differences between males and females based on hypothalamic dimorphisms. Although likely amplified by environmental and cultural factors, the mere fact that these reproducible variations exist remains hallmark evidence of a true biological basis for commonly observed, gender-wide trends. For example, male sexual behavior is typically stable over the entire adult male lifespan; this may potentially be explained by a typical male's lifelong production of testosterone at a relatively tonic, constant rate (notwithstanding the gradual decrease in serum levels that has been described from the second to the fifth decades of life). In contrast, the physiology of female sexuality is highly discontinuous, both during the regular menstrual cycle and during major reproductive life events such as pregnancy, puerperium, abortion, and menopause (5). Interestingly, it has also been shown that receptivity to pheromones remains relatively stable over life in men, whereas there is a peak in pheromone receptivity during ovulation in women as well as an overall greater level of odor discrimination ability during the years of fertility. After menopause, odor discrimination ability in women decreases significantly and much resembles physiologic male levels (50). Pheromones may be responsible for mediating interactions in the midcycle variations observed in women, which may in turn be triggered by the ovulatory androgen peak, promoting the atresia of nondominant follicles in the ovary as well as a mental and physical peak in sexual desire and receptivity. The biologic ramification of these relationships is to increase female sexual receptivity when the likelihood of conception is at its highest.

Table 1 Gender-Based Differences Among the Four Basic Emotional Command Systems

Basic emotion command system	Men	Women
Seeking (appetite and lust)	Higher	Lower
Rage (anger)	Higher	Lower
Fear-anxiety	Lower	Higher
Panic (separation-distress)	Lower	Higher

Note: The basic emotional command systems may influence the perception and expression of sexual desire and sexual arousal as well as their associated behaviors. These systems may also modulate gender-based vulnerabilities to hypersexual disorders and sexually aggressive or abusive behaviors in men, and loss of sexual desire, sexual avoidance behavior, and panic-related sexual disorders such as vaginismus in women. Individual divergences from group traits should be acknowledged, such as men who are less biologically driven to sex, men who are more vulnerable to sexual performance anxiety, or women who express high levels of anger-driven sexually abusive behaviors.

Table 2 Gender Similarities in the Seeking Component of the Four Basic Emotional Command Systems that Contribute to the Biological Basis of Sexual Desire

Hormone	Testosterone—primes the seeking appetitive pathway
Neurotrasmitter	Dopamine—seeking/appetitive Endorphin—consummatory/satisfaction
Heavily activated	By mental sexual arousal and appetitive states
Perceptive side	"I need/want/can get something good in the environment"
Motor side	"I'll do something to get it" In males: proceptive behavior In females: receptive behavior
Inhibited	By antidopaminergic drugs
Activated	By dopaminergic drugs; e.g., L-dopa, in patients suffering from Parkinson's disease
Drug sensitivity	Cocaine and amphetamines—generate pseudoappetitive behaviors Opiates—generate pseudoconsummatory feelings
Depression	Inhibits sexual desire and correlated behaviors

Table 3 Sexual Desire and Its Clinical Correlates in Men and Women

Parameter	Male	Female
Basic SD	Generally higher	Generally lower
SD and hormonal modulation	High	Higher than suspected (the role of androgens are under active investigation even during the fertile age)
SD in early dating	High	High/normal/low
SD in stable relationships	Usually remains constant for many years	Vulnerable to early decrease
SD in abusive relationship	May be high (aggressiveness may act as an aphrodisiac up to the point of frank sadism)	Verbal, physical, and sexual abuse have a major negative impact on SD (with the exception of masochism)
The presence of comorbid sexual disorders	Variable	Very high
Prevalence of hypersexuality states	High	Very low
Prevalence of paraphilias and paraphilia-related disorders	High	Very low

Abbreviation: SD, sexual desire.

Central nervous system dimorphisms may well represent the biological basis for the differences in sexual desire, perception, and expression experienced by men and women, including the disparities in the frequency, content, and intensity of erotic fantasies, nocturnal erotic dreams, and sexual daydreams; the perception of central arousal; the quality and quantity of expression of the sexual response, and the likelihood and emotional resonance of orgasm (5–7,15–19). Although the most important central sexual effects are correlated to the degree of brain dimorphism, it is likely that different environmental factors in development as well as the relative influence of the four "basic emotional command systems" in each gender play roles, as well (8,49).

Because of the delicate nature of the biochemical processes that are responsible for these sexual dimorphisms, exposure to various environmental conditions before and after birth may serve to manipulate or modulate them, with important consequences on human sexuality. Yet, it must also be acknowledged that hard, biological science exerts a significant influence on the manner in which humans respond to environmental stimuli despite the current trend that defines sexual behavior as the result of solely psychosocial, cultural, and environmental events (8,26,48). A more dynamic understanding of the continuous interactions between the somatic body and the psychic mind and how these processes differ between men and women will help to clarify the similarities that are popularly denied by the polarized focus on contextual factors in women and on biological factors in men.

☐ THE FOUR BASIC EMOTIONAL COMMAND SYSTEMS IN MEN AND WOMEN

As described by Panksepp, the four "basic emotional command systems" represent the biological correlates of the instinctual sexual drive and appetitive urges present in both genders (26). Disorders of the amygdala—a key control center for these systems—may have unexpected consequences on sexual functions, although both genders may present with identical clinical pictures (9,26). The observed similarities and differences in the basic emotional command systems between males and females may have consequent sexual implications in both functional and dysfunctional states. The study of these systems may prove to be very useful in attaining a greater understanding of the complex, dynamic interactions between basic biological mechanisms and human behaviors associated with them, particularly in the realm of sexual desire.

Seeking

The first of the four systems, "seeking," describes a positive, appetitive feeling that is mediated by the neurotransmitter dopamine in both sexes (8,9,22,26). This system is responsible for curiosity, interest, and expectancy, and it has been long regarded as the mechanism for reward-oriented behavior. There are two main aspects of the seeking system: the emotional, or perceptive side, which generates the expectation that something "good"—be it food, water, sex, protection, or shelter—will happen or will be obtained, and the motor side, which promotes exploratory behavior in lieu of achieving the benefits proposed by the emotional/perceptive side, since all emotions must have a motor correlate through which they may be enacted (8,9,22,26).

The seeking system is heavily activated during sexual arousal and other appetitive states. Dopaminergic drugs, such as those used in Parkinsonian patients, further activate the system, whereas antidopaminergic drugs, or other drugs that effectively increase prolactin levels, exert an inhibitory effect (22).

Testosterone also plays an important role in priming and maintaining the intensity of arousal in the hypothalamic/limbic seeking system. Since plasma testosterone levels are, on an average, 10 times higher in adult men than in premenopausal, cycling females, this biological difference may contribute to the discrepancy in strength between the instinctual basic seeking behaviors exhibited by men and women.

Another important part of the seeking pathway is what Panskepp describes as the "lust" subsystem

(26). Lust is associated with the feeling of gratification that occurs when the consummation of the appetites is realized. The command neuropeptide of this gratification system is endorphin, which can be considered the chemical correlate of the human sensations of satisfaction and emotional well-being in both sexes.

The clinical implications of biological gender variations in the construction of seeking systems are that men tend to express their sexual desires more in the lust domain, articulating stronger sexual drives that are more biologically driven and genitally focused whereas women more commonly express their sexual desires as passion, emphasizing the aspects of relationship intimacy (17). Consequently, men are much more likely to present with disturbances of the seeking system that manifest as hypersexuality states, including paraphilia and paraphilia-related disorders (2,28). In contrast, as many as 32% of women present with the opposite malady—a lack of desire—with a prevalence that is twice as common as the 16% figure reported by men (51). The differential modulation of male and female seeking pathways may be an important contributing factor to the specific desire vulnerabilities experienced by both sexes during the earlier phases of relationship with a partner as well as in long-term marriages (52). Women, for example, seem to be particularly susceptible to issues that fall into the categories of interest and frequency. It is interesting to note, however, that the level of female sexual pleasure appears to remain relatively stable over time, indicating the responsive nature of women's sexual response within the context of a stable relationship (53).

From a clinical point of view, it is important to note that illicit drugs such as cocaine and amphetamine also stimulate the seeking system in both sexes, albeit by the artificial generation of positive expectancies and the enhancement of the perception of sexual drive that result in what is termed "pseudoappetitive" behaviors (8,22). Opiates, however, directly stimulate the pleasure centers of the lust subsystem, mimicking a "pseudoconsummatory" gratification state that has already been obtained and effectively blunting sexual drive in both men and women.

The sustained hypoarousal of the seeking system that is typical of depressed patients is well correlated with a diminution or complete loss of sexual drive (2,5–7,15–17). On average, women are more vulnerable to depression from puberty onward; when this statistic is combined with a lower native sexual drive, women become far more prone to the further inhibition of sexual drive by depression than men. The frequent comorbidity of these conditions in women can be explained by the fact that depression and the loss of sexual desire are often triggered concomitantly as the result of frustration stemming from a lack of basic emotional needs such as intimacy and attachment. In men, an observed loss of the appetitive or motivational aspects of sexual desire may, in fact, be the very first symptom of a borderline clinical depression.

Rage

As opposed to the positive emotions represented by the seeking system, the "rage" or "anger-rage" system is characterized by negative emotions that are activated by the perception of frustration when goal-directed actions are thwarted. "Fight" is the motor correlate of this system (8,26,48). Although aggression is an important component of the rage system (54), an important distinction must be made in that the rage system is activated during what is termed "hot" aggression; the "cold" aggression that is typical of predatory behavior actually implies activation of the seeking system (8,26). A third type of aggression associated with the social emotions of male dominance behavior, however, seems to be related to both the seeking and the rage pathways.

Typically, the anger-rage system is discontinuously activated. When it is tonically activated at a low level, however, a state of irritability is generated. Like anger-rage, irritability is caused by chronic frustration of goal-directed activities.

The interactions between the seeking and the rage systems, especially as related to their influence on male dominance behavior—typically heightened by more frequent access to females—suggest that these pathways may be important factors in human male sexual drive, as well as in that of lower mammals (26,55).

Similarly, the author's clinical observations suggest that these interactions may also explain why male sexual aggressiveness can be perceived as highly arousing in both normal and pathologic conditions. The anger-rage activation associated with male dominance behavior may, in fact, represent the biological basis of the sexual drive and arousal associated with the violent sexual abuse of women, especially during circumstances of war. In everyday life, irritability may induce men to seek sex in order to relieve physical and emotional tensions. Conversely, irritability in women has an overall inhibitory effect on sexual desire and response, particularly if the involved partner is believed to be responsible for the irritation.

Fear-Anxiety

The fear-anxiety system is another negative basic emotional command system for which the primary mediating hormone is adrenaline (8,26,48). The primary emotion governing the perceptual side of this system is fear-anxiety, while its motor correlate is the "flight" response. In animals, the flight response can only be displayed as a physical attempt to run away from the object of fear, but in humans, the escape route may be either of the concrete or of the psychological variety because physical actions in response to fears are often socially inhibited.

Quite interestingly, anxiety disorders are much more common in women, with up to three times greater prevalence during transitional periods such as adolescence and perimenopause when higher fluctuations of plasma estrogen levels destabilize the hypothalamic adrenergic set point (56,57).

The fear-anxiety system also activates when sexual performance anxiety occurs; however, flight is biologically incompatible with the evolutionary need to maintain physical contact during the act of intercourse. Because the basic pathways do not distinguish between real and symbolic frightening objects or situations—that is, the apprehension of imminent inadequate sexual performance—shame and embarrassment resulting from real or perceived sexual shortcomings may trigger the instinct to flee. Activation of the fear-anxiety system results in a powerful vasoconstriction of the genital blood vessels as mediated by the effects of adrenaline. This process results in a diminished ability to develop or maintain erection in men and is a leading causative mechanism of ED (5–7,20).

In women, sexual performance anxiety is less frequently diagnosed, but its presence may similarly inhibit the sexual response (51). Although experimental studies have revealed that feelings of anxiety may actually be arousing in women (58), it is possible that observations made within a laboratory environment are not representative of a true activation of the fear-anxiety system.

A clinical pattern known as Klüver-Bucy syndrome has been described in male and female patients with lesions of the amygdala, a brain region that is a vital center of the basic emotional command systems (8,26). These patients, who appear otherwise normal from a cognitive point of view, experience neither fear nor anger. As demonstrated by evidence from amygdalectomized laboratory animals, Klüver-Bucy patients also exhibit hypersexuality. There is a dramatic increase in the amount and variety of sexual behaviors, including masturbatory activity, such that individuals or things that were not previously sexually attractive to them are subsequently found to be so (e.g., members of the same sex, other animal species, and even inanimate objects). In women, this syndrome is also associated with the display of indiscriminately gregarious behavior that may unduly expose them to possible sexual abuse. Both men and women also exhibit hyperorality (59), meaning that objects are explored by mouth indiscriminately; this behavior has also been observed in some bulimic patients. The author proposes that the relationship between hypersexuality and hyperorality deserves further research, particularly as some degree of psychoplasticity between the two behaviors may be modulated by biological dysfunctions in these basic emotional systems.

Panic or Separation-Distress System

The panic or separation-distress system is associated not only with feelings of panic but also with emotions of loss and sorrow. This may explain why panic disorders typically respond well to antidepressant medications. The operation of the panic system seems to be connected intimately with social bonding and the process of parenting (8,26,48). The neurochemistry of this system is dominated by opioids, with further evidence indicating that oxytocin and prolactin are also involved (9,22). This suggests a close link between the panic system and maternal behavior, which is well documented in animal research.

The panic system, like the fear-anxiety system, seems to be more active in women than in men—most likely due to the typically stronger social bonding and parenting patterns exhibited in and socially expected of females. The biological correlates of both the need for intimacy and the dynamics of attachment in women may be important in determining their ability to access arousal states. According to Basson, in stable relationships many women are induced to respond to sexual cues when they are motivated by reasons other than those of frank sexual desire, such as the needs for intimacy and reinforcing partner bonds (16). These nonsexual needs may actually open the mental door for arousal in women, thus triggering actual sexual desire.

Discussion

Although usually attributed to purely psychosocial causes, the dimorphic constructs of sexual desire and arousal in men and women could, in fact, be rooted in the biology of the basic emotional command systems. First, each individual is differentially "primed" by native sexual hormones, and then the subsequent development of male and female sexual systems is further potentiated by psychosocial as well as cultural factors. Although these connections have not yet been described in the literature, it seems that the likely relationship between the basic emotional commands systems and the effect of subsequent social and environmental factors warrants further investigation.

☐ MSDs AND FSDs: CLASSIFICATIONS, SIMILARITIES, AND DIFFERENCES

Leading sexual symptoms in men and women according to the fourth edition of the *Diagnostic and Statistical Manual of Mental Disorders* (DSM-IV) are summarized in Table 4 (2). The brevity and relative simplicity of this list indicates the current inadequacy of this classification in its failure to address the many other sexual dysfunctions reported by patients in the clinical setting (Table 5). A more extended clinical description of these dysfunctions, focusing on the similarities and differences between male and female presentations, is elaborated in this section. (For further information on MSD, see Chapter 10.)

Sexual Desire Disorders
Hypoactive Sexual Desire Disorders

Hypoactive sexual desire disorders are reported twice as frequently in women than in men (50). In both men

TABLE 4 Classification of Sexual Dysfunction According to the DSM-IV

Type 1
Sexual desire disorders
Hypoactive sexual desire
Sexual aversion disorder
Sexual arousal disorder
Female sexual arousal disorder
Erectile disorder
Orgasmic disorder
Female/male orgasmic disorder
Premature (or rapid) ejaculation
Type 2
Pain disorders
Dyspareunia
Vaginismus

Source: From Ref. 2.

and women, they may be lifelong or acquired, generalized or situational, and of organic, psychogenic, mixed, or unknown etiology (1–3,5–7,15–17,35,36). Historically, women with sexual dysfunction have been diagnosed with comorbid physical, psychosocial, or other sexual disorders with higher frequency than men have been, but the presence of comorbid disorders in men could be higher than is currently reported (5,7,10,15,16,18). The inordinate focus on the mechanics of erection has overshadowed many other key features of the sexual experience, such as the intensity of sexual drive and the feeling of orgasmic pleasure. Subsequent dissatisfaction with this approach may provide a possible

Table 5 Clinical Classification of Male and Female Sexual Dysfunctions with the Likelihood of Each Disorder by Gender

Sexual dysfunction	Men	Women
Desire disorders		
Hypoactive sexual desire	+	++
Hyperactive sexual desire	++	–/+
Sexual aversion	–/+	++
Arousal disorders		
Inadequate mental arousal	+	++
Inadequate genital arousal	++	++
Mixed arousal disorder	+	++
Persistent genital arousal	?	–/+
Painful arousal	+	–/+
Orgasmic disorders		
Early (premature) orgasm	++	?
Delayed/impossible orgasm	+	++
Hypoanhedonic orgasm (orgasm of impaired intensity)	++	++
Painful orgasm	+	–/+
Anejaculation with preserved orgasm	+	0
Ejaculation with anorgasmia	+	0
Retrograde ejaculation with hypoanedonia	+	0
Sexual pain disorders		
Dyspareunia	–/+	++
Vaginismus	0	+
Satisfaction disorders	++	++

Note: +, infrequent; ++, frequent; –/+, case report or anecdotal evidence; 0, absent anatomic difference; ?, not reported but worth investigation.

explanation for the fact that at least 40% and up to 70% of men who receive adequate pharmacologic treatment for ED discontinue therapy within two years' time (20,60).

Hyperactive Sexual Desire Disorders

Hyperactive sexual desire disorder leading to hypersexuality states, either paraphilic in nature or within the normative range of sexual behavior (61), has been well described in men whereas it is either miscategorized as "nymphomania" or even entirely ignored in women (62). Hyperactive sexual desire disorders and hypersexual behavior with solid biological etiology do present with the same characteristics in both sexes, however, as has been discussed with Klüver-Bucy syndrome (8,28). For further information on Klüver-Bucy syndrome, see above in "Fear-Anxiety."

Sexual Aversion Disorders

Sexual aversion disorders are more frequent in women than in men (3). This is perhaps due to the higher vulnerability of women to the panic or separation-distress basic emotional command system (8,26). Vaginismus often overlaps with sexual aversion in the most severe cases, which are typically characterized by intense, systemic arousal of the panic state (5,10,11,63,64). (For further information on vaginismus, please see "Female Sexual Pain Disorders" below.)

Sexual Arousal Disorders

Sexual desire may either precede mental arousal or occur concomitantly with mental arousal, making it difficult to distinguish the two states. It is also possible for sexual desire to occur after an individual's positive evaluation of genital arousal as the result of sexual stimuli, departing from previous models in which it was thought that sexual desire always preceded physical arousal (2,6).

Inadequate Arousal Disorders—Mental, Genital, or Mixed

In sexually healthy men, the assessment of obvious genital engorgement provides both visual and proprioceptive pleasure, confirming and compounding further sexual excitation. Thus, the most often reported arousal disorder in men is that of genital arousal, whose epiphenomenon is termed ED. Subtypes of this disorder are classified purely on an etiologic basis as being organic, psychogenic, or mixed (5–7,20). Only recently has low central (mental) arousal been examined as a causative mechanism for ED, possibly occurring before, with, or after the event of a sexual desire disorder. For example, performance anxiety, likely due to the activation of the fear-anxiety basic emotional command system, is one of the most common causes of inadequate mental arousal in men. Activation of the fear-anxiety system likely deactivates the seeking system, and the resulting hyperadrenergic tone acts centrally and peripherally to inhibit arousal as well as the development of a full, sustained, and satisfactory erection.

Men with chronic situational ED typically underrate penile engorgement due to the lack of reinforcing stimuli, even if penile firmness is substantial because the perceived lack of engorgement is distracting in itself. Because it is likely that a diagnosis of chronic male performance anxiety indicates the presence of other sexual disorders, the potential spectrum of comorbid sexual dysfunction results in a broad negative impact on all the dimensions of the sexual response. This leads to a state of lower sexual drive and poor central and peripheral arousal that ultimately results in the induction and maintenance of ED and an impoverished quality of orgasm. The presence of comorbid disorders thus becomes an important diagnostic aspect that should be addressed comprehensively in the clinical setting if a positive outcome is to be pursued effectively.

In women, an accurate awareness of genital engorgement is usually lacking; so, this direct confirmatory stimulus is absent (16). This may explain why many women complain of inadequate genital arousal in spite of objective congestion and lubrication, manifesting in disorders categorized as inadequate mental arousal, inadequate genital arousal, or female mixed arousal disorders, in which both mental and genital arousal responses are deemed inadequate (3,5,16,30,65). It should be noted, however, that the indirect confirmation of genital arousal is possible through the increase in sexual pleasure derived from repeated, direct genital stimulation.

In both sexes, aging is associated with the need for longer, stronger, and more mentally and genitally focused stimulation in order to achieve adequate genital arousal and orgasm, even in the absence of major neurovascular disturbances.

Persistent Sexual Arousal Disorder

On the opposite end of the spectrum, persistent genital arousal syndrome presents as an equally distressing problem, and this typically occurs in the absence of sexual desire (30,65). A diagnosis of increasing clinical frequency in women is the complaint of intrusive, spontaneous, and unwanted genital arousal (e.g., tingling, throbbing, pulsating) in the absence of sexual interest and desire that is unrelieved by orgasm (66). Previously misclassified as "nymphomania" or "hypersexuality," one precise criterion that may be used to distinguish persistent sexual arousal disorder (PSAD) is a lack of sexual desire and interest. This low or absent sexual interest is completely in opposition to the high levels of desire that typically lead to "excess" sexual behavior, with respect to standard behavioral norms for gender, age and sociocultural context. PSAD may have an organic etiology, a psychosexual etiology, or both. First described by Leiblum and Nathan in 2002 (30), this disorder has not yet been reported in men.

Painful Arousal Disorders

Painful arousal is reported in women suffering from clitoralgia of either idiopathic or neurogenic etiology. Although typically the result of pudendal nerve entrapment syndrome, other neurogenic disorders have been described in association with painful arousal. In men, this disorder also occurs at the height of full erection in patients who suffer from Peyronie's disease, priapism, or phimosis, and it may be further associated with painful orgasm (67,68). (For further information on Peyronie's disease, priapism, and phimosis, please see below in "Male Sexual Pain Disorders.")

Orgasmic Disorders

Since the urologist and andrologist tend to be more focused on the quality and competence of erection than on the quality of pleasure, patients most frequently present with orgasmic disorders to the sexologist. Attention to the different characteristics of orgasm, such as timing and intensity of pleasure, is of increasing importance in both genders (5,6,7,19). These aspects may, in fact, overlap. For the sake of clarity, however, it may be useful to classify orgasmic disorders into distinct subtypes.

Early (Premature) Orgasmic Disorder

This type of orgasmic disorder is most frequently seen in men and is associated with early or premature ejaculation. Most professionals who treat premature ejaculation define this condition as the occurrence of ejaculation prior to the wishes of both sexual partners (69). This broad definition thus avoids specifying a precise duration for sexual relations and the achievement of climax, which is quite variable and depends on many factors specific to the individuals engaging in intimate relations. Although an occasional instance of premature ejaculation might not be cause for concern, if the problem occurs in more than 50% of attempted sexual relations, then a dysfunctional pattern usually exists for which treatment may be appropriate (69).

Delayed or Impossible Orgasmic Disorder

Delayed or impossible orgasmic disorder is frequent in women and rare in men. If present, this condition is usually associated in both genders with reduced mental arousal or mental arousal disorder. Specifically in women, it is often also associated with inadequate genital arousal or mixed arousal disorder. Attention to the quality of mental or genital arousal is therefore mandatory when patients complain of this condition. Comorbidity between inadequate arousal and orgasmic disorders is frequent and unfortunately too often overlooked. Iatrogenic causes of orgasmic disorders—e.g., secondary to antiserotoninergic drugs—should be likewise acknowledged and investigated (35,36). In both genders, the use of SSRIs may be associated not only with delayed or impossible orgasm but also with reduced sexual desire, arousal difficulties, and reduced intensity of the orgasm itself, if it occurs (5,7,35,36). (For further information on the effect of SSRIs on sexual function, see Chapter 19).

In diabetic subjects, there is often a gap reported between the time of orgasm and the time of ejaculation. There are several different clinical presentations: an ejaculation with preserved orgasm (usually hypoanhedonic), ejaculation with anorgasmia, and retrograde ejaculation with diminished orgasm. For further information on hypoanhedonic orgasmic disorder, please see below in "Hypoanhedonic Orgasmic Disorder" (For further information on sexual dysfunction in diabetic patients, see Chapter 14).

Hypoanhedonic Orgasmic Disorder

Hypoanhedonic orgasmic disorder occurs when the pleasure associated with erotic orgasm is markedly reduced or is entirely absent, including a reported dissatisfaction with the quality, intensity, or duration of the orgasmic pleasure. In both sexes, this condition may accompany the process of aging, with an associated involution of the corpora cavernosa (34). In women, reduced intensity of orgasm is increasingly reported after menopause, with the loss of sexual hormones having a further detrimental effect on the aging process (70). Typically, a younger age at menopause results in a more severe negative impact on the quality of sexual response and the intensity of orgasm, for both biological and psychosexual reasons (71). In both genders, hypoanhedonic orgasmic disorder may also be associated with psychosexual factors such as low desire levels, low mental arousal, limited or absent erotic foreplay, sexual boredom, repetitive sexual scripts, and a lack of emotional interest, love, or passion. In men, an impoverished quality of orgasm is often associated with premature ejaculation and an erectile deficit.

Painful Orgasm Disorder

In men, painful orgasm is more frequently associated with Peyronie's disease, priapism, or phimosis and less often with neurologic disease and neuropathic genital pain (67). In women, painful orgasm is increasingly reported in postmenopausal women who are not taking hormone replacement therapy, typically presenting as a type of painful uterine cramping (70). For further information on male and female sexual pain disorders, please see below.

Sexual Pain Disorders
Male Sexual Pain Disorders

In men, painful arousal and/or orgasm may be associated with Peyronie's disease, as mentioned previously in the sections "Painful Arousal Disorders" and "Painful Orgasmic Disorder." (For further information on Peyronie's disease, see Chapters 17 and 34.)

Priapism of either spontaneous or iatrogenic etiology is usually associated with neither sexual desire nor mental arousal at the time of diagnosis. In fact, it may or may not be related to sexual function at all because it has been reported in patients with sickle-cell anemia or leukemia that have little to do with genital arousal. Further, there have been other cases of nocturnal priapism that occur during the rapid-eye-movement (REM) phases of sleep. The use of oral (rare) or intracavernosal (more frequent) vasoactive drugs, however, has resulted in priapism after the initiation of active genital arousal (72). (For further information on priapism, see Chapter 18.)

Although all males are born with congenital phimosis, this benign condition often resolves spontaneously in late infancy—usually by the age of five years (73). Phimosis may be considered pathologic when it persists into older childhood or adulthood, usually secondary to poor hygiene or an underlying condition such as diabetes mellitus. Besides causing physical discomfort during sexual relations, phimosis also potentially predisposes patients to paraphimosis, urinary tract infections, sexually transmitted diseases, and penile carcinoma. Elective circumcision may reduce the risk of these complications (73). (For further information on circumcision, see Chapter 9.)

Female Sexual Pain Disorders

In women, sexual pain disorders are classified according to the revised standards of the International Consensus Conference on FSD (12,74). These conditions include (i) dyspareunia, defined as the recurrent or persistent genital pain associated with intercourse, and (ii) vaginismus, the recurrent or persistent involuntary spasm of the musculature of the outer third of the vagina, interfering with vaginal penetration and causing personal emotional distress. Although noncoital sexual pain disorders were formerly included in this classification scheme (3), it has since been deleted by the most recent consensus (74).

A consistent difference in pain perception between men and women has become increasingly evident (68). Epidemiological and psychophysical studies, together with disease prevalence estimates, consistently reveal that the burden of pain is greater, more varied, and more variable for women than for men. Sexual differences in pain are brought about by a confluence of genetic, physiological, anatomical, neural, hormonal, lifestyle and cultural factors. The very existence of these factors, however, has provided women with a wide array of sex-specific biological and sociocultural mechanisms that act to reduce pain. Thus, although women are generally more vulnerable to pain than men are, they also have more ways in which to combat it.

In particular, community epidemiological studies reveal that women report more levels of pain, more frequent pain, pain in more areas of the body, and pain of longer duration than men do (75,76). Differences in pelvic organ structures and arrangement provide further cause for variable gender-specific pain perception. Sexual abuse, which is four times more common in women than in men, may also increase vulnerabilities to pain and its associated emotional consequences (51).

Dysmenorrhea, abortion, and delivery may further target the female genital area with negative physical and emotional pain signals that may further increase female vulnerability to sexual pain (77–82).

Satisfaction Disorders

Although not yet included in any male or female classification systems, satisfaction disorders represent a key, qualitative aspect of sexual dysfunction in both men and women. Although they may or may not be associated with any overt sexual dysfunction, satisfaction disorders remain one of the most important causes of decreased sexual affection in many couples, in spite of adequate basic sexual functioning in both partners. Satisfaction disorders are more likely to occur when one partner, termed the "symptom inducer," is dysfunctional, while the other partner, termed the "symptom carrier," becomes increasingly dissatisfied. The interplay between the inducer and the carrier is potentially present in all forms of MSD and FSD, either as a leading or as a partial cofactor. Even in stable relationships, the potential existence of carrier/inducer interactions stresses the need to regard a couple as a "sexual dyad," whose particular

dynamics may act to produce specific vulnerabilities, precipitating factors, or maintenance factors in sexual dysfunction (11).

Treatment strategies should address the feeling of satisfaction in both partners because overall dissatisfaction is one of the leading causes of treatment discontinuation (5,7,20).

☐ CONCLUSION

One of the most exciting challenges in current sexual medicine involves the elucidation of a solid biological background for gender-based similarities and differences. Hard science is but a prerequisite for the deeper and less biased understanding of the relative influence of organic etiologies on sexual function in the face of the multitudinous sociocultural and religious constructs and dynamics that have so greatly polarized male and female sexual responses and sexual rights over time. A closer dialogue between clinicians who work in the field of MSD and those who work in the field of FSD will certainly prove to be of rich reciprocal inspiration. It is hoped that shared knowledge and increased attention to the interactions amongst the organic and psychogenic components of sexual function will improve clinicians' diagnostic and therapeutic skills, leading to more satisfactory therapeutic outcomes for individual women, men, and couples.

☐ REFERENCES

1. International Statistical Classification of Diseases and Related Health Problems (The) ICD-10. Geneva: World Health Organization, 1992.
2. Diagnostic and Statistic Manual of Mental Disorders (DSM-IV). 4th ed. Washington, DC: American Psychiatric Association, 1994.
3. Basson R, Berman J, Burnett A, et al. Report of the international consensus development conference on female sexual dysfunction: definitions and classifications. J Urol 2000; 163(3):889–893.
4. Graziottin A. The challenge of sexual medicine for women: overcoming cultural and educational limits and gender biases (review). J Endocrinol Invest 2003; 26(suppl 3):139–142.
5. Plaut M, Graziottin A, Heaton J. Sexual Dysfunctions: Fast Fact Series. Oxford: Health Press, 2004.
6. Masters WH, Johnson VE, Kolodny RC. Heterosexuality. New York: Harper Collins, 1994.
7. Leiblum SR, Rosen RC, eds. Principles and Practice of Sex Therapy. 3rd ed. New York: The Guilford Press, 2000.
8. Solms M, Turnbull O. The Brain and the Inner World. London: Karnac Books, 2002.

9. Pfaus JG, Everitt BJ. The psychopharmacology of sexual behaviour. In: Bloom FE, Kupfer D, eds. Psychopharmacology: The Fourth Generation of Progress. New York: Raven Press, 1995:743–758.
10. Graziottin A. Clinical approach to dyspareunia. J Sex Marital Ther 2001; 27(5):489–501.
11. Graziottin A. Etiology and diagnosis of coital pain. J Endocrinol Invest 2003; 26(suppl 3):115–121.
12. Graziottin A, Brotto LA. Vulvar vestibulitis syndrome: a clinical approach. J Sex Marital Ther 2004; 30(3): 125–139.
13. Bergeron S, Binik YM, Khalife S, et al. Vulvar vestibulitis syndrome: a critical review. Clin J Pain 1997; 13(1):27–42.
14. Pukall CF, Binik YM, Khalife S, et al. Vestibular tactile and pain thresholds in women with vulvar vestibulitis syndrome. Pain 2002; 96(1–2):163–175.
15. Graziottin A. Libido: the biologic scenario. Maturitas 2000; 34(suppl 1):S9–S16.
16. Basson R. Women's desire deficiencies and avoidance. In: Levine SB, Risen CB, Althof SE, eds. Handbook of Clinical Sexuality for Mental Health Professionals. New York: Brunner Routledge, 2003:111–130.
17. Levine SB. The nature of sexual desire: a clinician's perspective. Arch Sex Behav 2003; 32(3):279–285.

18. Meston CM, Frohlich PF. The neurobiology of sexual function. Arch Gen Psychiatry 2000; 57(11):1012–1030.

19. Mah K, Binik YM. The nature of human orgasm: a critical review of major trends. Clin Psychol Rev 2001; 21(6):823–856.

20. Jardin A, Wagner G, Khoury S, eds. Erectile Dysfunction. Plymouth, UK: Health Publications, Ltd., 2000.

21. Wilson SK, Delk JR 2nd, Billups KL. Treating symptoms of female sexual arousal disorder with the Eros–Clitoral Therapy Device. J Gend Specif Med 2001; 4(2):54–58.

22. Bloom FE, Kupfer D, eds. Psychopharmacology: The Fourth Generation of Progress. New York: Raven Press, 1995.

23. Levin RJ. Human male sexuality: appetite and arousal, desire and drive. In: Legg C, Booth D, eds. Appetite: Neural and Behavioural Bases. London: Oxford University Press, 1994:127–164.

24. Levin RJ. The mechanism of human female sexual arousal. Ann Rev Sex Res 1992; 3:1–48.

25. Graziottin A, Maraschiello T. Farmaci e Sessualità. Milano: Airon Editore, 2002.

26. Panksepp J. Affective Neuroscience: The Foundations of Human and Animal Emotions (Series in Affective Science). New York: Oxford University Press, 1998.

27. Anderson SW, Bechara A, Damasio H, et al. Impairment of social and moral behavior related to early damage in human prefrontal cortex. Nat Neurosci 1999; 2(11): 1032–1037.

28. Kafka MP. Hypersexual desire in males: an operational definition and clinical implications for males with paraphilias and paraphilia-related disorders. Arch Sex Behav 1997; 26(5):505–526.

29. Kandel ER, Schwartz JH, Jessell TM, eds. Principles of Neural Science. Norwalk: Appleton & Lange, 2000.

30. Leiblum SR, Nathan S. Persistent sexual arousal syndrome in women: a not uncommon but little recognized complaint. Sex Relationship Ther 2002; 17(2):191–198.

31. Gray H. Clemente CD, ed. Gray's Anatomy of the Human Body. 30th ed. Philadelphia: Lea & Febiger, 1985.

32. Netter FH. The Ciba Collection of Medical Illustrations: Reproductive System. Vol. 2. Summit, New Jersey: Ciba Pharmaceuticals, 1979:89–123.

33. Killeen KP, Libertino JA, Sughayer MA, et al. Pathologic review of consecutive radical prostatectomy specimens. Never sparing versus nonnerve sparing. Urology 1991; 38(3):212–215.

34. Tarcan T, Park K, Goldstein I, et al. Histomorphometric analysis of age-related structural changes in human clitoral cavernosal tissue. J Urol 1999; 161(3):940–944.

35. Frohlich PF, Meston CM. Evidence that serotonin affects female sexual functioning via peripheral mechanisms. Physiol Behav 2000; 71(3–4):383–393.

36. Rosen RC, Lane RM, Menza M. Effects of SSRIs on sexual function: a critical review. J Clin Psychopharmacol 1999; 19(1):67–85.

37. Graziottin A. Sexual function in women with gynecologic cancer: a review. It J Gynecol Obstet 2001; 2:61–68.

38. Graziottin A, Castoldi E. Sexuality and breast cancer: a review. In: Studd J, ed. The Management of the Menopause: The Millennium Review 2000. Pearl River, NY: Parthenon Publishing, 2000:211–220.

39. Andersen KV, Bovim G. Impotence and nerve entrapment in long distance amateur cyclists. Acta Neurol Scand 1997; 95(4):233–240.

40. Sherwin BB, Gelfand MM, Brender W. Androgens enhances sexual motivation in females: a prospective, crossover study of sex steroid administration in surgical menopause. Psychosom Med 1985; 47(4):339–351.

41. Davis SR, McCloud P, Strauss BJ, et al. Testosterone enhances estradiol's effects on postmenopausal bone density and sexuality. Maturitas 1995; 21(3):227–236.

42. Miller KK. Androgen deficiency in women. J Clin Endocrinol Metab 2001; 86(6):2395–2401.

43. Bachmann G, Bancroft J, Braunstein G, et al. Female androgen insufficiency: the Princeton consensus statement on definition, classification, and assessment. Fertil Steril 2002; 77(4): 660–665.

44. D'Amati G, di Gioia CR, Bologna M, et al. Type 5 phosphodiesterase expression in the human vagina. Urology 2002; 60(1):191–195.

45. Wesselmann U, Burnett AL, Heinberg LJ. The urogenital and rectal pain syndromes. Pain 1997; 73(3):269–294.

46. Renshaw DC. Coping with an impotent husband. IMJ Ill Med J 1981; 159(1):29–33.

47. Barnes T. The female partner in the treatment of erectile dysfunction: what is her position? J Sex Marital Ther 1998; 13(3):233–238.

48. LeVay S. The Sexual Brain. Cambridge, Massachusetts: MIT press, 1994.

49. Springer SP, Deutsch G. Left Brain, Right Brain: Perspectives from Cognitive Neuroscience. New York: WH Freeman, 1988.

50. Arimondi C, Vannelli GB, Balboni GC. Importance of olfaction in sexual life: morpho-functional and psychological studies in man. Biomed Res (India) 1993; 4:43–52.

51. Laumann EO, Paik A, Rosen RC. Sexual dysfunction in the United States: prevalence and predictors. JAMA 1999; 281(6):537–544.

52. Liu C. Does quality of marital sex decline with duration? Arch Sex Behav 2003; 32(1):55–60.

53. Graziottin A, Koochaki P. Self-reported distress associated with hypoactive sexual desire in women from four European countries. Poster presented at the North American Menopause Society (NAMS) meeting, Miami, FL, 2003. Abstract book, poster no. 126:105.

54. Winkler O, Pjrek E, Kasper S. Anger attacks in depression—evidence for a male depressive syndrome. Psychother Psychosom 2005; 74(5):303–307.

55. LeDoux J. The Emotional Brain. London: Weidenfeld & Nicolson, 1996.

56. Hamann S. Sex differences in the responses of the human amygdala. Review. Neuroscientist 2005; 11(4): 288–293.

57. Graziottin A, Leiblum SR. Biological and psychosocial etiology of female sexual dysfunction during the menopausal transition. J Sex Med 2005; 2(suppl 3):133–145.

58. Bradford A, Meston CM. The impact of anxiety on sexual arousal in women. Behav Res Ther 2006; 44(8):1067–1077.

59. Janszky J, Fogarasi A, Magalova V, et al. Hyperorality in epileptic seizures: periictal incomplete Kluver-Bucy syndrome. Epilepsia 2005; 46(8):1235–1240.

60. Althof SE. Erectile dysfunction: psychotherapy with men and couples. In: Leiblum SR, Rosen R, eds. Principles and Practice of Sex Therapy. 3rd ed. New York: Guilford Press, 2000:242–275.

61. Kafka MP, Hennen J. The paraphilia-related disorders: an empirical investigation of nonparaphilic hypersexuality disorders in outpatient males. J Sex Marital Ther 1999; 25(4):305–319.

62. Brotto LA, Graziottin A. Hyperactive sexual desire in women: myth or reality? Urodinamica 2004; 14(2): 84–88.

63. Reissing ED, Binik YM, Khalife S. Does vaginismus exist? A critical review of the literature. J Nerv Ment Dis 1999; 187(5):261–264.

64. Leiblum SR. Vaginismus: a most perplexing problem. In: Leiblum SR, Rosen R, eds. Principles and Practice of Sex Therapy. 3rd ed. New York: Guilford Press, 2000:181–204.

65. Basson R, Leiblum SR, Brotto L, et al. Definitions of women's sexual dysfunction reconsidered: advocating expansion and revision. J Psychosom Obstet Gynaecol 2003; 24(4):221–229.

66. Leiblum SR. Arousal disorders in women: complaints and complexities. Review. Med J Aust 2003; 178(12): 638–640.

67. Pryor JP, Ralph DJ. Clinical presentations of Peyronie's disease. Int J Impot Res 2002; 14(5):414–417.

68. Berkley KJ, Holdcroft A. Sex and gender differences in pain. In: Wall PD, Melzack R, eds. Textbook of Pain. Edinburgh: Churchill Livingstone, 1999:951–965.

69. Noble MJ, Lakin M. Premature ejaculation. eMedicine Clinical Knowledge Base, 2004: www.emedicine.com/med/topic643.htm (accessed October, 2005).

70. Graziottin A. Sexuality in postmenopause and senium. In: Lauritzen C, Studd J, eds. Current Management of the Menopause. London: Martin Dunitz, 2004:185–203.

71. Graziottin A, Basson R. Sexual dysfunction in women with premature menopause. Menopause 2004; 11(6 Pt 2):766–777.

72. Perimenis P, Athanasopoulos A, Geramoutsos I, et al. The incidence of pharmacologically induced priapism in the diagnostic and therapeutic management of 685 men with erectile dysfunction. Urol Int 2001; 66(1):27–29.

73. Choe JM, Kim H. Phimosis, adult circumcision, and buried penis. eMedicine Clinical Knowledge Base, 2005: www.emedicine.com/med/topic2873.htm (accessed October, 2005).

74. Basson R, Leiblum S, Brotto L, et al. Revised definitions of women's sexual dysfunction. J Sex Med 2004; 1(1):40–48.

75. Unruh AM. Gender variations in clinical pain experience. Pain 1996; 65(2–3):123–167.

76. Berkley KJ. Sex differences in pain. Behav Brain Sci 1997; 20(3):371–380.

77. Goldstein I, Berman JR. Vasculogenic female sexual dysfunction: vaginal engorgement and clitoral erectile insufficiency syndromes. Int J Impot Res 1998; 10(suppl 2):S84–S90.

78. Travell JG, Simons DG. Myofascial Pain and Dysfunction: The Trigger Points Manual. Vol. 2. The Lower Extremities. Media, PA: Williams & Wilkins, 1991.

79. Kegel AH. Sexual functions of the pubococcygeus muscle. West J Surg Obstet Gynecol 1952; 60(10): 521–524.

80. DeLancey JO, Sampselle CM, Punch MR. Kegel dyspareunia: levator ani myalgia caused by overexertion. Obstet Gynecol 1993; 82(4 Pt 2 suppl):658–659.

81. Laan E, Everaerd W. Determinants of female sexual arousal: psychophysiological theory and data. Ann Rev Sex Res 1995; 6:32–76.

82. Jensen MK. Surgery for phimosis with Plastibell. A follow-up study. [Article in Danish]. Ugeskr Laeger 1998; 160(26):3920–3923.

12

Psychological Factors in Male Sexual Dysfunction

David L. Rowland
Department of Psychology, Valparaiso University, Valparaiso, Indiana, U.S.A.

Cynthia S. Osborne
Department of Psychiatry and Behavioral Sciences, Johns Hopkins School of Medicine, Baltimore, Maryland, U.S.A.

□ OVERVIEW

In this chapter, the multiple ways in which psychological functioning can interact with sexual response are presented and discussed. As with physiological systems, psychological factors affecting sexual response can range from the broad and nonspecific (those that impact overall psychological functioning) to the highly detailed and selective (those that are very specific to sexual functioning). For example, a major psychopathology may impact multiple facets of psychological functioning, one of which happens to include sexual response. In contrast, other psychological factors, such as those arising from cognitive and affective responses within the dyadic relationship, may be linked specifically to sexual situations via the man's past and current experiences with his partner. Unlike major psychopathology, however, these latter processes may have little or no observable effect on psychological functioning outside the sexual or relational context.

□ IDENTIFYING THE RELEVANT DOMAINS OF SEXUAL DYSFUNCTION: MODELS OF SEXUAL INTERACTION

Sexual response is complex, requiring specific preconditions, incorporating multiple behavioral responses, and including an array of psychosocial factors that relate to affective, cognitive, and relationship dimensions. Masters and Johnson (1) succeeded in providing a rudimentary characterization of sexual response, breaking it down into arousal, plateau, orgasmic, and resolution phases. Subsequent models introduced a role for sexual interest and desire as a component of the sexual response (2). More recent refinement distinguishes between such constructs as spontaneous desire and arousability, the latter referring to sexual interest derived from a specific individual, object, or context. Further conceptualization has included separate pain-pleasure dimensions (3), as well as attention to a variety of other subjective factors such as the feelings, motivations, and attitudes that surround the sexual act (4). Most recently, emphasis has turned to the role of

the dyadic relationship, an approach that seeks to understand and treat sexual response in its relational context (5,6).

Such complex interactions do not easily lend themselves to the simple one-dimensional sequential model (e.g., desire → arousal → orgasm) often employed in the conceptualization and diagnosis of sexual dysfunction. Rather, they suggest the need to view sexual response according to the recent and frequently cited "biopsychosocial" or systemic model. That is, sexual response can be viewed as the culmination of three interacting domains: the biological (the physiological mechanisms that prepare and enable genital response); the psychological (the affective and cognitive predispositions and interpretations that lead to and sustain the response); and the relational (the dyadic interactions that promote intimacy, meaning, and mutually satisfying outcomes in sex) (Table 1). Consideration of functioning within each domain is important to understanding overall sexual response. Not only can functioning within one domain affect another (e.g., negative feelings toward a sexual partner or situation may inhibit erectile response) but factors within domains may interact with each other as well. For example, knowledge of past sexual failures may result in a negative predisposition toward future sexual situations (7,8).

□ INTEGRATION OF THE BIOPSYCHOSOCIAL DOMAINS

Although the new pharmacotherapies have led to record numbers of men seeking treatment for their sexual problems, they have underscored a position long held by sex therapists. Namely, although improved genital response and overall sexual satisfaction are often related, they are not synonymous. Indeed, restoration of genital response in the absence of improved sexual satisfaction (and perhaps even relationship satisfaction) would seem pointless (9). Yet men often simplify their sexual experiences when they try to give language to them, identifying their problems mainly with the physiological endpoints of sexual

Table 1 Major Domains Relevant to Sexual Response in Men: The Biopsychosocial Model

Domain	Components	Subdomain examples
Biological	General somatic health	Fatigue
		Aging
		Drug use
		Various diseases
	Endocrine	Testosterone
	Erectile response	Vascular and neural integrity
	Ejaculation (orgasm)	Neural reflex
Psychological	General mental health	Major psychiatric disorders
	Effects associated with sex	Positive (enjoyment, intimacy)
		Negative (anxiety/fear, guilt, anger)
	Cognitions	Interpretation of sexual experiences
		Attribution of cause
		Attentional cues, self-monitoring
Relational	Nonsexual	Overall quality
		Emotional Intimacy
	Sexual	Partner expectations
		Partner stimulation
		Mutual satisfaction
		Partner dysfunctions

response. They attribute their problem to a "dysfunctional" body and/or penis—one that fails to achieve erection (erectile dysfunction or impotence) or that ejaculates before desired (premature ejaculation) (10). Accordingly, they often seek solutions aimed primarily, sometimes exclusively, at this level of functioning. Less frequently, men seek help because they suspect psychological or interpersonal factors may be contributing to, sustaining, or even exacerbating the sexual dysfunction.

Even when the problem derives from an undeniable medical condition (e.g., radical prostatectomy), the patient's level of psychological functioning may be critical to understanding his overall sexual response and health. While some psychological factors impacting sexual response may be severe and nonspecific, as with a major psychopathology such as clinical depression, more often they involve subtle and complex cognitive and affective processes commonly manifested as significant emotional or relational distress over the problem (11). Such problems, for example, may involve the cognitive capacity for attending simultaneously to one's own and one's partner's shifting kinesthetic responses to physical and emotional stimulation. Or they may relate to the subjective experiences of pleasure and deep meaning commonly attributed to human intimate interactions (6), factors frequently disrupted by dysfunctional sexual response.

Equally common, psychological distress may arise from specific dynamics occurring within the dyadic relationship. Both erectile dysfunction and premature ejaculation involve complex relational processes, including increasingly intense sequences of partner-to-partner reactivity that often follow and serve to maintain or exacerbate the problem (7,8). In other words, psychological and relational processes not only impact the formation and course of the problem, the sexual problem itself has the potential to impact the physiological, psychological, and relational functioning of the individual and his partner.

As an example, it is not uncommon for a female partner to develop hypoactive desire in response to the man's ejaculatory difficulties. The partner may "personalize" the man's premature ejaculation, convincing herself that his problem is a direct reflection of some inadequacy of her own or his selfish failure to consider her needs. The relational tension that emerges in such scenarios is further exacerbated when the male becomes even more severely symptomatic, perhaps developing comorbid erectile difficulties in response to his partner's disappointment. In such a scenario, a clear understanding of the man's sexual dysfunction requires attention to the complex interplay among these physiological, psychological, and relationship processes.

☐ RELATIONSHIP BETWEEN PSYCHOLOGICAL PROBLEMS AND SEXUAL RESPONSE

Because psychological factors are many and varied, they have the potential to interact with sexual response through a variety of processes. For example, major psychiatric disorder such as clinical depression or schizophrenia (DSM-IV, Axis I) is likely to affect sexual response in a different manner than personality or developmental disorders (DSM IV, Axis II) (12). These may differ substantially from the way in which a lack of self-confidence stemming from anxiety about performance impacts sexual response. In the next sections, we briefly review the literature regarding possible relationships between psychological factors and sexual dysfunction.

Sexual Dysfunction Secondary to Major Psychological Disorders

Chronic psychopathology has long been a suspected cause of sexual dysfunction. Both depression and schizophrenia are associated with diminished sexual desire, impairment of arousal, and loss or delay of ejaculation. Reports that sexual dysfunction occurs in a high percentage of depressed and schizophrenic patients, estimated from 35% to 75% (13–17), provide a strong link between the two. Furthermore, recent research indicating that sexual dysfunction is related to the severity of the depression and is lower in medication-treated (vs. placebo-treated) patients (16) argues that sexual problems are specific to the psychopathological states rather than other concomitants of mental illness (e.g., hospitalization). In one of the few controlled studies investigating the issue, Philipp et al.

(16) reported improvement in libido, erectile response, and orgasmic function following monoamine oxidase inhibitor treatment, noting that sexual dysfunction tended to persist only in men not responding to treatment. The complexity of the relationship between depression and sexual dysfunction, however, is underscored by other studies reporting a higher level of sexual problems in treated depressed and schizophrenic patients (14,18). Whether the specific pharmacotherapy was responsible for the increased dysfunction or whether improved psychological functioning unmasked a previously ongoing sexual dysfunction in these men is not clear.

Somewhat elusive is the extent to which the psychopathology actually causes the dysfunction. Few studies have documented sexual functioning prior to the onset of the mental illness or adequately separated the effects of antidepressant treatment through medication, which itself may have antisexual effects, from those of the depression itself. Furthermore, the extent to which the effect on sexual response represents general malaise, social withdrawal, or inability to experience pleasure rather than a specific effect on a psychosexual process is undetermined. Although the definitive studies have yet to be done, the bulk of the research suggests that the primary effect on sexual dysfunction is mediated through diminished interest in sex, which in turn affects arousal/erectile and orgasmic response. Thus, for individuals manifesting major mental disorders, treatment should first focus on alleviating the psychological condition consistent with DSM-IV (12). For example, an individual should generally not be diagnosed with a psychosexual problem when there is a concomitant Axis "I" disorder such as depression or schizophrenia. However, in some cases a sexual disorder may predate the onset of the major mental disorder. Therefore, a reasonable approach is to give careful consideration to the time of onset and other contextual variables before diagnosing an individual with a psychosexual disorder when there is a concomitant Axis I condition.

Psychosocial Stressors and Concomitant Sexual Problems

Significant life events that result in long term or acute depression may also lead to sexual dysfunction. Populations of aging and diabetic men, for example, often show a higher incidence of depression and anxiety than younger or healthier counterparts; they are also more likely to exhibit low sexual desire and erectile difficulties (19–23). In these men, the relationship between the severity of the depression and the likelihood of sexual dysfunction is less clear, and men exhibiting symptoms of both anxiety and depression do not necessarily have higher levels of sexual dysfunction than men exhibiting only depression (24). Furthermore, because nonpsychotic depression and anxiety are not easily separated from the pathophysiological effects of aging, illness, and stress, it is not clear which factors might be responsible for the sexual dysfunction: the pathophysiological condition itself or the associated psychological states of depression and anxiety. Perhaps it is safest to conclude that sexual dysfunction is most likely compounded by the depression and anxiety in these men, but not solely due to it. Indeed, depression and anxiety associated with various life events may just as likely result from the sexual problems as cause them.

Personality Profiles of Men with Sexual Dysfunctions

The above studies have generally evaluated clinical populations with psychological disorders and determined the prevalence of sexual dysfunction within them. Another approach toward investigating the relationship between sexual dysfunction and psychological disorders has been to select groups of sexually dysfunctional men and determine whether the incidence of psychiatric disorders in these groups is higher than that of randomly selected samples. Apropos to this latter strategy, a number of efforts have attempted to profile the type of male personality prone to sexual dysfunction. Although results are mixed, the most consistent pattern to emerge is that men seeking help for sexual problems exhibit higher levels of depression and anxiety than sexually functional counterparts (24–30). In contrasting the different kinds of sexual dysfunction, Tondo et al. (26) suggest that men with erectile problems manifest their anxiety primarily through negative self-image and low self-esteem, whereas men with premature ejaculation do so through symptoms more characteristic of hypomanic states such as anxiety, agitation, and mild obsession. The relationship between depression, anxiety, and sexual dysfunction appears to extend beyond erectile and ejaculatory disorders. For example, couples (one or both partners) indicating low sexual interest (inhibited sexual desire) have a higher propensity for past or current chronic depression than might typically be expected (21), a finding that may mirror the low sex interest in depressed populations.

When depression and anxiety are excluded from the picture, however, no single personality profile consistently characterizes men with sexual dysfunction. In fact, there is some debate as to whether the incidence of personality disorders is higher in men reporting sexual dysfunction than in the normal population. Several studies report no difference in psychometrically assessed personality disorders between sexually dysfunctional and functional men (31,24). In contrast, Maurice and Guze (32), and more recently Fagan et al. (33), investigated the association between neuroticism and sexual dysfunction for men without concurrent depression. Both groups report concomitant personality disorders in the neighborhood of 30% to 35%, a rate substantially higher than expected within the normal population; however, personality profiles were varied and not particularly consistent, supporting the hypothesis that male sexual dysfunction is not associated with any particular personality trait or cluster of traits. A tendency toward greater self-consciousness and vulnerability and lower openness seemed most consistently to describe dysfunctional men (27), characteristics that may lead to diminished appreciation of varied experiences and act to sustain performance anxiety associated with male sexual dysfunction. Furthermore, men who score low in warmth may have difficulty with intimacy or commitment, suggesting treatment focusing on establishing greater interpersonal intimacy.

Perhaps the most important conclusion from these studies, however, is that no matter which findings are accepted, the large majority of men seeking treatment from sex clinics do not exhibit concomitant personality disorders. For those that do, the personality profiles tend to represent rather subtle deviations from the norm. Fagan et al. (33) suggest that despite the apparent normal personalities of the majority of men with sexual dysfunction, attending to their individual profiles may reveal subtle departures from the norm that could guide the diagnostician in devising more effective treatment plans.

In summarizing the relationship between psychological disorders and sexual impairment, a modest association has been established, with depression and anxiety most consistently implicated. Nevertheless, it is difficult to arrive at a clear interpretation of this association. The fact that such studies have generally relied on clinical groups of one form or another introduces obvious sampling biases. Furthermore, different types of clinics specializing in sexual problems (e.g., private vs. hospital based; psychiatric vs. urological) appear to select from different populations of sexually-dysfunctional men (25,32,34). As a result, the incidence of concomitant psychological disorders may vary according to the specific clinic subpopulation under investigation. More problematic is the fact that little is known regarding cause-effect relationships from these broad psychometric investigations, particularly for men with nonpsychotic disturbances. Nonetheless, the finding that psychological problems are more common among men reporting sexual dysfunctions emphasizes the need to understand and treat the sexual problem within the larger context of the man's psychological health. Indeed, a clinician who lacks an understanding of the potential role of depression and anxiety on sexual functioning, or conversely, simplistically attributes the sexual dysfunction to a psychological disorder such as depression, foregoes the opportunity to provide the best treatment options to the man experiencing a sexual dysfunction.

☐ PSYCHOLOGICAL PROCESSES AND SEXUAL DYSFUNCTION

While various psychological disorders may interact with sexual dysfunction, it is also well known that normal psychological processes associated with sexual response may contribute to or exacerbate an ongoing problem. Despite attempts to de-emphasize the performance aspects of sex, the reality is that sexual response is an "evaluated" behavior for many men, not only by the man himself, but (at least in his view), his partner as well (10). As with the performance of any behavior subject to both self and other's evaluation (e.g., sports performance, public speaking, etc.), sexual response in men is influenced by a variety of affective and cognitive processes that may interfere with or enhance the response. Although these cognitive and affective predispositions vary across individuals, they are specific to the sexual situation and typically sensitive to the presence of the partner. Such factors are discussed in more detail in Chapter 24.

Cognitive Factors

The cognitive component of sexual arousal refers to the way in which information about the sexual situation is processed and interpreted. Three cognitive factors accounting for variation in sexual response have frequently been identified in the clinical and experimental literature over the past 20 years: perceptual (how the man perceives his physiological response), attentional (what stimuli the man attends to), and attributional (to what the man attributes his response or lack of response).

Self-perceptions of physiological response are an important part of information processing during sexual arousal. In comparison with sexually functional counterparts, men with erectile problems tend to underestimate their level of genital response (35). There is no widely accepted explanation for this phenomenon, specifically whether it represents an actual perceptual distortion, a strategy of catastrophizing (i.e., seeing things in their worst possible light), self-defined low expectations (perhaps to minimize embarrassment), or inaccuracy resulting from lack of cues (36). Regarding this last point, men with erectile or ejaculatory problems may have fewer bodily cues to which they can attend, as they show diminished (as with erectile problems) or abbreviated (as with premature ejaculation) physical response. With fewer bodily cues or less time to evaluate them, such men may be less able to accurately assess their physical levels of arousal.

Attentional processes also have been related to sexual response and dysfunction (37,38). Since no one can attend to all the information in the environment, selectivity is required. Within most sexual situations, attention is focused on those cues that elicit or enhance arousal; however, as with any performance-based response, sexual response may take on task-like characteristics, that is, the man may view the goal of arousal as that of producing a usable and/or sustainable erection (10). In such situations, the man's attention may be diverted away from erotic cues provided by the partner or situation and redirected toward his own genital response. Such self-monitoring of genital response (i.e., spectating) becomes the means through which the man is able to determine progress on the "task" of achieving or sustaining his erection. It also, however, can interfere with the arousal process and lead to a cycle of sexual failure. Specifically, men may set unrealistic expectations and become discouraged and anxious when they fail to meet them with the intended erectile or ejaculatory response. As might be expected, men with erectile problems may benefit from mild distractors that draw their attention away from their own bodily responses. At the same time, while it may lessen performance anxiety, overuse of distraction may result in emotional disconnection to one's partner, diminishing intimacy and meaning.

The factors to which the man attributes his sexual arousal are also known to affect his sexual response. A recent experimental literature dealing with performance anxiety in a variety of situations (e.g., sports, public speaking) indicates that attributing failure at a task to internal causes is likely to be associated with poor performance during future attempts. Studies by Weisberg et al. (39) have generalized this finding to sexual response. Specifically, sexually dysfunctional men are more likely to attribute their ability to get an erection to internal factors than sexually functional men, and further, the more internal the attribution even in sexually functional men, the greater the negative impact on future performance. Such attributions have the potential to lead to self-blame and diminished self-esteem, responses that often correlate with sexual dysfunction in men.

Although much of the research on attribution of sexual failure is pertinent mainly to men with psychogenic sexual problems, our own data (Rowland and Burnett, unpublished data) provide further clarification of the relationship between the man's perceived attribution of cause and his response to sexual situations. Men who are able to attribute the cause of their erectile problem to a specific somatic origin are less bothered emotionally by it than men who are uncertain of the cause or who perceive the cause as one of psychological origin. Specifically, whereas those who see their dysfunction as somatic are no different from sexually functional men in their affective response to sexual situations, those who are uncertain of the cause or consider it psychological approach sex with diminished positive feelings. Thus, internal attribution seems to disrupt sexual response primarily under conditions where the man assumes those internal factors are under his control and, thus, his responsibility for the sexual failure.

Affective Factors

As mentioned previously, personality profiles verify that anxiety and other negative affects are commonly associated with male dysfunctional sexual response. Masters and Johnson (1), Kaplan (2), Barlow (40), and others (37,38,41,42) have provided both theoretical and empirical evidence indicating a role for high negative and low positive affect in men with either erectile or ejaculatory problems. Indeed, because tension/anxiety and penile tumescence appear to represent incompatible response domains, cognitive-behavioral approaches to the treatment of sexual dysfunction typically emphasize tension reduction and relaxation. Negative emotional states such as tension and anxiety may well have a physiological underpinning that can account for dysfunctional sexual response, since strong emotional arousal mediated via sympathetic activation appears to be incompatible with erectile response. At the same time, sympathetically-mediated emotional arousal may trigger ejaculation prematurely, a reflex response that is also sympathetically mediated (9,43). Given this possible scenario, it is not surprising that erectile problems and premature ejaculation frequently coexist.

Role of Dyadic Interaction

The above psychological processes are most relevant (and perhaps greatly magnified) within the context of the sexual dyad, where such factors as performance evaluation, expectation, and satisfaction naturally come into play. The man's response *to* his partner and the response *of* his partner introduce potential factors that can explain much of the variance in sexual response. As such, they suggest that a comprehensive understanding of the man's sexual response is not possible without some attention to the systemic (relationship) functioning of the couple. Such an approach also counters the bias in the sexual dysfunction field toward an exclusive individual etiology.

A sexually dysfunctional partner represents a potential source of a sexual problem for men. For example, a partner indicating a sexual aversion, low interest in or desire for sex, or inorgasmia may lead to difficulty with erection or even premature ejaculation so as to terminate intercourse quickly. More subtle dynamics within the relationship may also play an important role: a common consequence of sexual difficulty is frustration, which may lead to suppressed sexual interest on the man's part and subsequent diminished intimacy with the partner. In turn, these may affect a variety of other relationship dynamics. Withdrawal of sexual and emotional intimacy and lack of communication by one partner may lead to bewilderment, reduced trust, and feelings of diminished attractivity by the other partner. Further withdrawal by the partner along with discontentment and anger may alter the relationship in such a way that treatment focused exclusively on genital response is no longer highly effective. In other words, the psychological and relational consequences of the sexual problem may effectively neutralize most of the benefits received from improvement in genital response since such relationship dynamics are not readily reversed by attending solely to the genital problem (8,9).

In view of the importance of conceptualizing sexual response from a systemic approach, Schnarch (6) has proposed a reformulation of the human sexual response cycle that emphasizes the interactive or relational nature, as opposed to the common compartmentalization and polarization, of the physiological and psychological components of sexual functioning. The model proposes assessing *total stimulation level*—defined as the sum total of both physiological or tactile stimulation and psychological or emotional/relational processes—in relation to the patient's threshold levels for genital vasocongestive responses associated with arousal and orgasm. Schnarch examines both the quality and quantity of the patient's and his partner's behaviors that provide *physical stimulation*, and the physiological factors that influence the body's capacity to "transmit" the stimulation, such as aging or the presence of an interfering medical condition (Fig. 1). He also examines the *psychological processes* that either support or interfere with stimulus transmission, such as the individual's ability to attend to sensation, the impact of anxiety, and the relational or interactive patterns that influence response. Both in assessment and in planning treatment, this model challenges the clinician to consider both physiological and psychological processes and to recognize that intervention in either or both domains may be necessary in order to maximize the total level of stimulation and the patient's capacity to reach arousal or ejaculatory thresholds (5,6). Only when clinicians assess both processes can they accurately determine the extent to which interventions in either or both domains may be restorative.

Relational/behavioral interventions that alter sexual style and expand the sexual repertoire have the potential of compensating for the reduced physiological potential that naturally occurs with age or with a medical condition. The total level of stimulation reflects the combination of both physiological and psychological stimulation, and interventions can take place at either or both levels in order to maximize the patient's potential for reaching the threshold level of arousal needed for adequate genital response.

Figure 1A represents Schnarch's (6) systemic formulation of a common etiology of erectile dysfunction in aging men. The need for increasing levels of stimulation to reach arousal and orgasmic threshold occurs naturally with age. At the same time, the total level of transmitted stimulation often decreases due to illness, poor technique, limited repertoire, sexual boredom, decreasing levels of intimacy, performance anxiety, or other psychological or relational processes.

A different scenario occurs for many men with premature ejaculation. As their problems develop over time, these men learn to condition themselves, as well as their spouses or partners, to avoid physical stimulation for fear of triggering the unwanted symptom. For the same reason, they may also avoid psychological stimulation by reducing emotional connection and intimacy during sexual interactions. This anxiety-driven sexual interaction style is organized around the mutual, although most often unspoken, agreement to avoid or minimize both tactile stimulation and intimacy (psychological stimulation). The risk of continuing or worsening dysfunction along with diminishing satisfaction is high in such scenarios. Rather than decreasing stimulation through avoidance and distraction, Schnarch (6) argues for the need to raise ejaculatory threshold by increasing intimacy and stimulation tolerance in these men, inducing, perhaps, a form of arousal "habituation."

As depicted in Figure 1B, the male with premature ejaculation has a low ejaculatory threshold requiring minimal total stimulation to achieve orgasm. The man may report that the psychological stimulation

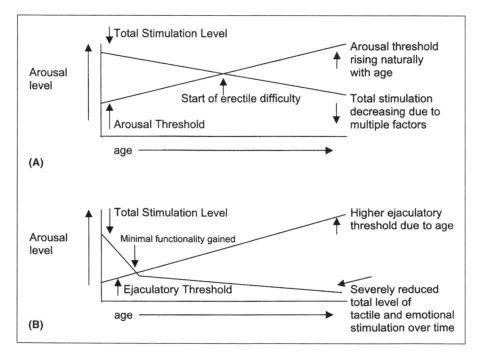

Figure 1 (A) Common etiology of erectile dysfunction in aging men as proposed by Schnarch. (B) Common course of premature ejaculation. *Source*: From Ref. 5.

generated by kissing an attractive woman for the first time takes him to threshold and he spontaneously ejaculates during the kiss. The "conditioning" effect of the problem leads him, and his partner, to reduce tactile stimulation and intimacy over time in order to avoid the problem. These men and their partners "resolve" the problem when they, through stimulation avoidance, gain minimally adequate functioning—an erection long enough to allow penetration for a very brief time, but at the cost of a level stimulation—both physical and psychological—that is minimally satisfying at best, and that increases the odds of developing other dysfunctions over time.

Although studies indicate an unchanging prevalence of premature ejaculation across age cohorts, the prevailing wisdom is that over the lifespan a naturally rising ejaculatory threshold will mitigate the problem and men with premature ejaculation are likely to become less symptomatic. However, psychological and tactile stimulation may both have been so reduced by a couple's long history of avoidance and diminishing satisfaction that there is too little emotional–erotic connection or shared motivation to enjoy the natural benefits of aging on ejaculation latency. The couple manages the premature ejaculation problem by engaging in minimal stimulation, which inevitably leads to an emotional-erotic disconnection, mutually low levels of desire and often erectile difficulties as well. Indeed, secondary conditions of erectile dysfunction in the male and low desire in one or both partners are often predictable long-term outcomes in such couples.

☐ CONCLUSION

It is important to recognize that psychological factors interact with sexual response at multiple levels. Specifically, broad psychological dysfunction is associated with a number of sexual problems, with general psychopathology, severe anxiety, and depression typically related to lack of sexual interest and erectile problems. Moreover, the fact that personality disorders appear with greater frequency in sexually dysfunctional men suggests that specific identifiable characteristics may render some men more vulnerable to sexual problems than others. Nevertheless, the majority of men presenting with a sexual dysfunction manifest no severe pathology or specific personality traits. In such men, various cognitive, affective, and relationship factors may be most important to understanding the etiology of the sexual problem.

The relationship between psychological states and sexual response is compounded by its bi-directional nature, such that each domain has the potential to influence the other. As a consequence, evaluation of psychological functioning in men with sexual dysfunction, as discussed in Chapter 24, must not only address the multiple ways in which psychological factors might impact sexual response, but also must do so in a manner that helps clarify their causal, contributing, or consequential roles. In elucidating such relationships, the clinician is better positioned to devise an optimal program of treatment for the patient.

☐ REFERENCES

1. Masters WH, Johnson VE. Human Sexual Response. Boston: Little Brown, 1966.
2. Kaplan HS. Disorders of Sexual Desire and Other New Concepts and Techniques in Sex Therapy. New York: Brunner/Mazel, 1979.
3. Schover LR, Friedman JM, Weiler SJ, et al. Multiaxial problem-oriented system for sexual dysfunctions: an alternative to DSM-III. Arch Gen Psychiatry 1982; 39(5): 614–619.
4. Byrne D, Schulte L. Personality dispositions as mediators of sexual response. In: Bancroft J, Davis CM, Weinstein D, eds. Annual Review of Sex Research. Vol. 1. Allentown, PA: Society for the Scientific Study of Sexuality, 1990:93–118.
5. Schnarch D. Talking to patients about sex—Part II. Med Aspects Hum Sex 1988; 22:97–106.
6. Schnarch DM. Constructing the Sexual Crucible: An Integration of Sexual and Marital Therapy. New York: Norton, 1991.
7. Bancroft J. Human Sexuality and its Problems. 2nd ed. New York: Churchill Livingstone, 1989.
8. Rowland DL. The psychosocial context of sexual dysfunction. Am J Managed Care 1999; 5(suppl 1):S40–S47.
9. Rowland DL, Burnett AL. Pharmacotherapy in the treatment of male sexual dysfunction. J Sex Res 2000; 37(3):226–243.
10. Zilbergeld B. The man behind the broken penis: social and psychological determinants of erectile failure. In: Rosen R, Leiblum SR, eds. Erectile Disorders: Assessment and Treatment, New York: Guilford Press, 1992:27–55.
11. Wincze J, Carey M. Sexual Dysfunction: A Guide for Assessment and Treatment. New York: Guilford Publications, 1991.
12. American Psychiatric Association. Sexual and gender identity disorders. In: Diagnostic and Statistical Manual of Mental Disorders: DSM-IV, 4th ed. Washington, D.C.: American Psychiatric Publishing Inc., 1994:493–538.
13. Casper RC, Redmond DE Jr, Katz MM, et al. Somatic symptoms in primary affective disorder. Presence and relationship to the classification of depression. Arch Gen Psychiatry 1985; 42(11):1098–1104.
14. Baldwin DS. Depression and sexual function. J Psychopharm 1996; 10(suppl 1):30–34.

15. Clayton AH, McGarvey EL, Clavet GJ, et al. Comparison of sexual functioning in clinical and nonclinical populations using the changes in sexual functioning questionnaire (CSFQ). Psychopharmacol Bull 1997; 33(4): 747–753.

16. Philipp M, Delini-Stula A, Baier D, et al. Assessment of sexual dysfunction in depressed patients and reporting attitudes in routine daily practice: results of the postmarketing observational studies with moclobemide, a reversible MAO-A inhibitor. Intl J Psy Clin Prac 1999; 3(4):257–264.

17. Michael A, O'Keane V. Sexual dysfunction in depression. Hum Psychopharmacol 2000; 15(5):337–345.

18. Lilleleht E, Leiblum SR. Schizophrenia and sexuality: a critical review of the literature. In: Bancroft J, Davis CM, Ruppel HJ Jr, eds. Annual Review of Sex Research. Vol. 4, Allentown, PA: Society for the Scientific Study of Sexuality, 1993:93–118.

19. Tsitouras PD, Alvarez RR. Etiology and management of sexual dysfunction in elderly men. Psychiatr Med 1984; 2(1):43–55.

20. Wise TN, Rabins PV, Gahnsley J. The older patient with a sexual dysfunction. J Sex Marital Ther 1984; 10(2): 117–121.

21. Schreiner-Engel P, Schiavi RC. Lifetime psychopathology in individuals with low sexual desire. J Nerv Ment Dis 1986; 174(11):646–651.

22. Fagan PJ, Wise TN, Schmidt CW Jr, et al. Inhibited sexual excitement in the aging male. J Geriatr Psychiatry 1987; 20(2):153–164.

23. Harland R, Huws R. Sexual problems in diabetes and the role of psychological intervention. Sex Marital Ther 1997; 12(2):147–157.

24. Kennedy SH, Dickens SE, Eisfeld BS, et al. Sexual dysfunction before antidepressant therapy in major depression. J Affect Disord 1999; 56(2–3):201–208.

25. Munjack DJ, Oziel LJ, Kanno PH, et al. Psychological characteristics of males with secondary erectile failure. Arch Sex Behav 1981; 10(2):123–131.

26. Tondo L, Cantone M, Carta M, et al. An MMPI evaluation of male sexual dysfunction. J Clin Psychol 1991; 47(3):391–396.

27. Costa PT Jr, Fagan PJ, Piedmont RL, et al. The five-factor model of personality and sexual functioning in outpatient men and women. Psychiatr Med 1992; 10(2):199–215.

28. Hawton K, Catalan J, Fagg J. Sex therapy for erectile dysfunction: characteristics of couples, treatment outcome, and prognostic factors. Arch Sex Behav 1992; 21(2):161–175.

29. O'Donoghue F. Psychological management of erectile dysfunction and related disorders. Intl J STD AIDS 1996; 7(suppl 3):9–12.

30. Angst J. Sexual problems in healthy and depressed persons. Int Clin Psychopharmacol 1998; 13(suppl 6): S1–S4.

31. Cooper AJ. A clinical study of "coital anxiety" in male potency disorders. J Psychosom Res 1969; 13(2): 143–147.

32. Maurice WL, Guze SB. Sexual dysfunction and associated psychitric disorders. Compr Psychiatry 1970; 11(6): 539–543.

33. Fagan PJ, Schmidt CW Jr, Wise TN, et al. Sexual dysfunction and dual psychiatric diagnoses. Compr Psychiatry 1988; 29(3):278–284.

34. Fagan PJ, Wise TN, Schmidt CW, et al. A comparison of five–factor personality dimensions in males with sexual dysfunction and males with paraphilia. J Pers Assess 1991; 57(3):434–448.

35. Rowland DL, Heiman JR. Self-reported and genital arousal changes in sexually dysfunctional men following a sex therapy program. J Psychosom Res 1991; 35(4–5):609–619.

36. Rowland DL. Issues in the laboratory study of human sexual response: a synthesis for the nontechnical sexologist. J Sex Res 1999; 36(1):3–15.

37. Beck JG, Barlow DH. The effects of anxiety and attentional focus on sexual responding—I: Physiological patterns in erectile dysfunction. Behav Res Ther 1986; 24(1):9–17.

38. Beck JG, Barlow DH. The effects of anxiety and attentional focus on sexual responding—II: Cognitive and affective patterns in erectile dysfunction. Behav Res Ther 1986; 24(1):19–26.

39. Weisberg RB, Brown TA, Wincze JP, et al. Causal attributions and male sexual arousal: the impact of attributions for a bogus erectile difficulty on sexual arousal, cognitions, and affect. J Abnorm Psychol 2001; 110(2): 324–334.

40. Barlow DH. Causes of sexual dysfunction: the role of anxiety and cognitive interference. J Consult Clin Psychol 1986; 54(2):140–148.

41. Rowland DL, Cooper SE, Heiman JR. A preliminary investigation of affective and cognitive response to erotic stimulation in men before and after sex therapy. J Sex Marital Ther 1995; 21(1):3–20.

42. Rowland DL, Cooper SE, Slob AK. Genital and psychoaffective response to erotic stimulation in sexually functional and dysfunctional men. J Abnorm Psychol 1996; 105(2):194–203.

43. Ertekin C, Colakoglu Z, Altay B. Hand and genital sympathetic skin potentials in flaccid and erectile penile states in normal potent men and patients with premature ejaculation. J Urol 1995; 153(1):76–79.

13

Impact of Systemic Disease on Male Sexual Function

Peter Y. Liu

Department of Andrology, Concord Hospital and ANZAC Research Institute, University of Sydney, Sydney, New South Wales, Australia

Louis J. Gooren

Department of Endocrinology/Andrology, Vrije University Medical Center, and Genderteam Sex Reassignment Centre, Amsterdam, The Netherlands

David J. Handelsman

Department of Andrology, Concord Hospital and ANZAC Research Institute, University of Sydney, Sydney, New South Wales, Australia

□ INTRODUCTION

Sexual activity is a key component of the human experience representing both a deep personal need and a highly valued aspect of adult daily living. As such, men have an often unstated but nevertheless strong expectation of preserving their sexual function, and its loss due to medical illness may be greatly regretted. Accordingly, the biology and pathology of sexual function should be considered as an integral part of the comprehensive medical care of the ill.

Male sexual function is generally divided into motivational (libido) and physical (erectile and ejaculatory function) components as well as into central (mental) and peripheral (neurovascular) events. (For more information, see Chapter 3.) Although the final common pathway produces the erectile and ejaculatory functions, social and other learned constraints modulate the transition from desire and sexual arousal to penile erection, ejaculation, and detumescence. Sexual dissatisfaction may occur when any component is dysfunctional (1) and is associated with decreased quality of life and life satisfaction (2). The development of valid assessment tools (3), theoretical frameworks (2), and effective oral therapies (4) means that early detection and empathic treatment of male sexual dysfunction are feasible and should be considered part of adequate medical treatment of systemic diseases.

Systemic disease may cause sexual dysfunction by altering motivational, physical, or both components. Although erectile and ejaculatory function can be independently affected, particularly by drugs or abdominal surgery, synchronous dysfunction is more usual, possibly due to overlapping risk factors (5). Systemic disease alters sexual function by mechanisms that include nonspecific effects of chronic illness (e.g., fatigue, anemia, lethargy, pain, depression, disability), neurovascular dysfunction (e.g., accelerated atherosclerosis, autonomic neuropathy), and androgen deficiency.

In addition, drug or surgical treatment (and even some investigations) of underlying disease may adversely affect sexual function.

For example, systemic disease may cause sexual dysfunction indirectly by causing pain or as a consequence of pain management. Chronic pain from any cause may decrease sexual activity by limiting relevant physical movement and by raising concerns regarding pain exacerbation, performance, arousal, and confidence (6). Large surveys report an increased prevalence of sexual dysfunction in those with chronic pain (6,7). Furthermore, opiates used to treat severe chronic pain can induce severe androgen deficiency (8–13). Similarly, sexual dysfunction is frequent in dialyzed men with chronic renal failure (14), but improves after successful renal transplantation (15), or even just by increasing hemoglobin with erythropoietin treatment (16–18). Hence, multiple direct and indirect mechanisms exist whereby systemic illness of any etiology can influence male sexual function.

Testosterone is a major determinant of sexual function, exerting effects predominately on libido; however, as the blood testosterone threshold for maintaining male sexual function is low (19,20), only severe impairment of testicular testosterone, such as that caused by opiate administration for chronic pain (8–13), is likely to significantly impair sexual function of men with systemic disease. In fact, most systemic diseases do not greatly suppress blood testosterone concentrations and rarely suppress to the near-castration levels required to impair sexual function. More recent evidence that exogenous testosterone enhances phosphodiesterase type 5-(PDE-5) inhibitor action on erectile mechanisms in the castrate state (21–23) suggests a possible role of endogenous testosterone in maintaining erectile function through peripheral trophic effects on penile smooth muscle and/or endothelium. The significance of these findings to the modest decline of blood testosterone concentrations in systemic disease, however, remains unclear, especially in view of results from randomized, double-blind, placebo-controlled cross-over studies that show that testosterone therapy does not improve any aspect of sexual function in non-androgen-deficient men (24,25).

In general, studies of male sexual function are encumbered with practical and ethical constraints, making reliable study unusually difficult. The primary outcome measure is neither directly observable nor quantifiable and the subjective reporting of outcome is fraught with difficulty due to reticence and unreliability in accurately disclosing intimately private activities as well as medical prudishness. These investigative handicaps make the requirements for meticulous representative sampling in observational survey research and for placebo controls and randomization in interventional studies imperative in clinical studies assessing the effects of systemic disease and its treatment on male sexual function. Considering the importance of sexual activity to men's well being and quality of life, the available literature on the effects of systemic disease on male sexual function is remarkably limited and, by the requisite standards for validity, of mostly low quality. Notably, available research focuses on heterosexuals, with little cognizance of the varieties of sexual identity, orientation, and expression, such as autoerotic, multiple, extramarital, same sex, and commercial partner sex, that abound in society.

This chapter will highlight the effect of systemic, nongonadal disease on male sexual function. It aims to highlight better quality data such as from representative population-based epidemiological studies and randomized, placebo-controlled therapeutic interventions, where available. Discussions on the various disease states that can impact male sexual function are organized by organ system; further discussion is available in other chapters: sexual dysfunction in diabetes mellitus (see Chapter 14), cardiovascular (see Chapter 36), prostate (see Chapters 16 and 39), neurological (see Chapter 15), and sexually transmitted diseases (see Chapter 21); the psychological factors that impact on male sexual function (see Chapter 12) and drug side effects (see Chapter 19). Disorders of the reproductive system, including androgen deficiency, are excluded, and indirect effects of systemic disease on blood testosterone concentrations will be reviewed only where androgen deficiency is sufficiently severe to impair male sexual function.

☐ CARDIOVASCULAR DISEASE
Risk Factors: Smoking, Hyperlipidemia, and Hypertension

Representative community-based studies have reported that important risk factors for coronary artery disease, such as cigarette smoking, hyperlipidemia, and hypertension are independently associated with erectile dysfunction (ED) even after adjusting for other key variables such as age (5,26–33). In a community-based study of 1412 men with hypertension, diabetes mellitus, or both, the prevalence of ED was 30% in men less than 50 years of age, 50% in those aged 60, and over 70% in those older than 65 (34). Furthermore, the severity of ED increased with disease duration. Studies directly assessing coronary and penile vessels by angiography show that cigarette smoking is associated with hypogastric cavernous arteriosclerosis (35), and men with more severe ED also have more extensive coronary artery disease (36). Such data are consistent with autopsy studies, which clearly show that atherosclerosis is a generalized disease process (37,38). These findings provide a theoretical framework explaining why factors that predict coronary atherosclerosis are likely to cause penile atherosclerosis and therefore ED.

Conversely, factors that protect against coronary artery disease may also be useful in reducing progression of ED. Cross-sectional multivariate analyses from representative community-based samples that include altogether over 2500 men show that the age-adjusted prevalence of ED is less in men who exercise (28,39). A randomized interventional study proved that a nine-month exercise program was superior to an organized walking program in maintaining libido and erectile function (40); however, double-blind exercise interventions are not feasible, and observational data that depend upon self-reporting may be inaccurate.

Whether interventions targeted at cardiovascular risk factors can prevent or improve ED has not been established by randomized, placebo-controlled studies. On the contrary, antihypertensive drugs worsen ED by a variety of mechanisms including lowering of blood pressure and penile perfusion pressure itself. Few other cardiovascular drug classes have been examined systematically for causing sexual dysfunction. Among lipid-lowering agents, statin therapy has been the most carefully studied since, in theory, inhibition of cholesterol biosynthesis could inhibit steroidogenesis, thereby reducing blood testosterone concentrations. However, randomized, placebo-controlled studies have shown no clinically meaningful inhibition of endogenous testosterone production (41,42).

Acute Myocardial Infarction

Sexual activity rarely precipitates acute myocardial infarction (AMI), as self-recalled sexual activity during the year prior to the first AMI in 760 men did not differ from a demographically comparable, community-based control group (43). Nevertheless, fear of precipitating exertion-induced angina or a subsequent lethal AMI may lead to voluntary reduction in sexual activity. For this reason, consensus guidelines concerning the safety of sexual activity after AMI have been developed (44). Sexual activity does decline immediately post-AMI, but then slowly returns toward previous levels. In a longitudinal (but uncontrolled) study of 462 men less than 65 years of age, frequency and satisfaction with sexual activity decreased immediately after AMI, irrespective of age and other confounders, but 80% had resumed sexual activity six months post-AMI (45). In another study of 316 men assessed after AMI or coronary artery grafting, sexual function diminished compared with a population-based control group and remained low 12 months afterwards (46). Hence, while coronary artery disease per se does not alter sexual activity, both AMI and coronary surgery are associated with sexual dysfunction for psychological and/or organic reasons that are not yet clear. Regardless of this, current oral phosphodiesterase-inhibitor therapy for ED is safe even in the presence of coronary artery disease, provided nitrate therapy is strictly avoided (44). In a retrospective analysis of data from randomized, placebo-controlled studies, sildenafil treatment was found to be safe and effective in 357 men with ED and ischemic heart disease (47).

Heart Failure

Although prevalence and other data are sparse, worsening cardiac function seems to be associated with progressively impaired sexual activity. In a study of 51 married men with advanced heart failure being evaluated for heart transplantation, three-quarters reported a marked decrease in sexual interest and coital frequency, including one-quarter who had ceased all sexual activity (48). Furthermore, worse cardiac function was associated with the greatest sexual dysfunction. These data suggest that the decrease in sexual activity was exertion- and motivation-related; however, erectile failure cannot be excluded, since it was not specifically examined.

In men with both ED and heart failure, uncontrolled open-label reports show that sildenafil is effective treatment (49). Furthermore, sildenafil may have additional beneficial cardiac effects, since exercise tolerance was improved in a single-dose, double-blind, randomized, placebo-controlled study of sildenafil therapy in 23 men (49). Although the mechanism by which this occurred and whether it is sustainable in the long term are not known, this illustrates that alleviating sexual dysfunction may also have nonsexual benefits.

☐ PSYCHIATRIC DISEASE

Evaluating the interaction of psychiatric illness and self-reported sexual function is complicated by distinctive factors. Accurate assessment is made difficult by the low motivation due to severe depression and the disorganized thought of psychotic or anxiety-related illness, all of which render self-reported sexual function unreliable. Furthermore, as the underlying psychiatric disorder improves, self-perception is likely to change independent of objective changes. Ideally, assessments from psychiatrically normal sexual partners would be more reliable, but may not be available or feasible. Interestingly, improvement in sexual function may conversely have nonsexual benefits, as

suggested by a well-controlled study of 152 untreated men with ED and incidental depressive symptoms in which sildenafil therapy improved both erectile response and depressive symptoms concomitantly when compared with placebo (50). Whether such nonsexual benefits can be replicated in men with major depression remains to be determined.

Mood Disorders

Mood disorders are relatively common, with major depression occurring in 7% and depressive symptoms in approximately 17% of a large pan-European representative community-based survey of 80,000 people (51). Representative population-based studies clearly show that depression increases the relative risk of ED twofold after age adjustment, and this effect is exacerbated according to the severity of the depression (39,52,53). In the largest community-based study, only 35% spontaneously complained of sexual dysfunction, and almost 70% reported some sexual dysfunction on questioning, although erectile function was not specifically evaluated (54). These population-based estimates are very similar to baseline data from multicenter, randomized, placebo-controlled studies of antidepressant therapy that report 59% to 65% prevalence of sexual dysfunction (55–57).

Although major depression is clearly associated with ED, the causality and mechanism of this association remains elusive. Nevertheless, the temporal relationship between ED and cardiovascular disease provides some clues. The mental effect of depression on erectile function may be mediated through the vasculature, as longitudinal data show that depression precedes cardiovascular disease. Large, longitudinal community-based representative studies of altogether over 9000 men and ranging in sample size from 409 to 2886 have consistently reported that minor depression predicts a 1.2- to 1.7-fold increase, whereas major depression predicts a larger, 3.0- to 4.5-fold increase in age-adjusted relative risk of coronary artery disease (58–63). Such effects of depression on the vasculature may arise from hypertension, as longitudinal community-based studies examining over 5000 individuals altogether have reported that men with depression are twice as likely to develop hypertension (64,65). Such data indicating that depression precedes onset of coronary artery disease, together with the observation that coinherited genetic risk factors, which predispose to depression, hypertension, and coronary artery disease, account for 60% of the variance in heart disease (66), are salient, given the possibility that ED may be considered a sentinel symptom of atherosclerotic cardiovascular disease (67). Other mechanisms of ED in the depressed may also exist.

Blood testosterone concentrations are significantly but modestly lowered in older men with dysthymia or major depression compared with nondepressed controls (68). Such small reductions in blood testosterone are unlikely to account for the prominent libidinal changes characteristic of depression. Whether a genetic polymorphism in androgen sensitivity, a shorter CAG triplet repeat in the androgen receptor that enhances androgen sensitivity, predisposes to such effects remains to be confirmed (69). Randomized, placebo-controlled trials of testosterone therapy in depressed men with low blood testosterone concentrations showed no benefit over placebo on depressed mood although sexual function improved (70). In the absence of convincing data, whether the lowered blood testosterone concentrations in depression reflect a nonspecific response to illness, an effect of depression, or an effect of lowered sexual activity itself (71) remains conjectural.

There is also convincing evidence that certain antidepressants in particular can aggravate sexual dysfunction. Cross-sectional and interventional data both conclusively show that selective serotonin reuptake inhibitors (SSRIs) or venlafaxine (a combined serotonin–norepinephrine reuptake inhibitor) have statistically more sexual side effects (particularly by decreasing libido and delaying ejaculation) than other antidepressants such as bupropion, which is comparable to placebo in terms of sexual effects (72–75). The sexual side effects of non-SSRI antidepressants have recently been comprehensively reviewed, and it appears that among non-SSRI antidepressants, sexual side effects are equivalent (76–79).

Various randomized, placebo-controlled studies have also examined the treatment of SSRI-induced sexual dysfunction (80–86). Of these approaches, only phosphodiesterase type-5 inhibitors appear to be effective, although only 200 men have been examined altogether in prospective (85) and retrospective (86) subgroup analyses.

Psychotic Disorders

Sexual dysfunction appears to be frequent (20–50%) in men with schizophrenia, from observational studies examining almost 2000 men from numerous clinic and community sources (87–91). Although apparently higher than expected for the general community, the wide prevalence estimates and inability to correct for age and other risk factors significantly limit interpretation of this data. Accurate information on the age-standardized community-based prevalence and mechanism of sexual dysfunction in schizophrenic men is not well established from population-based studies. One study has shown that treated and untreated men with schizophrenia reported more sexual dysfunction than a comparable (although not formally matched) control group (89); however, this nonrepresentative and unmatched study of only 122 men is not conclusive.

The effect of antipsychotic treatment on sexual function is also unclear. Although antipsychotic choice and dose are both reported to alter the prevalence of sexual dysfunction (87,92), the undefined population source and uncontrolled nature of these observational studies, which also show systematic demographic differences between treatment groups, are important limitations. Indeed, in the largest comparative (but not placebo controlled) clinical trial, which randomized almost 1400 men to receive haloperidol or risperidone for eight weeks (90), sexual side effects ranged from 10% to 30% and were not significantly different between antipsychotics. Nevertheless, antipsychotic agents could theoretically influence sexual function through nonspecific central nervous system actions or other peripheral effects (including α-adrenergic blockade and increased serum prolactin concentrations) (93). These peripheral effects are thought to be responsible for priapism (93). Attempts to treat presumed prolactin-related antipsychotic-induced sexual dysfunction have shown dopaminergic drugs to be ineffective, although the studies were uncontrolled (94) or underpowered (95). Whether men with adequately treated psychotic disorders remain at increased risk for sexual dysfunction is inadequately studied.

Anxiety Disorders

Severe anxiety disorders appear to be associated with sexual dysfunction. A controlled study of 42 military men with posttraumatic stress disorder and 49 reservist controls reported pervasive sexual dysfunction (ED, reduced libido) that was exacerbated by treatment with SSRIs (96). A remarkably high proportion (~80%) of such men report some sexual dysfunction (97).

Social phobia is also associated with sexual dysfunction. In a controlled study, 40 subjects (including 24 men) with social phobia exhibited more sexual performance abnormalities compared with a convenient, unmatched, but comparable, control group (98). Although more abnormalities in sexual function were noted in women, significant abnormalities particularly in sexual arousal and ease of orgasm were detected in men.

The use of anxiolytics also appears to be associated with sexual dysfunction, independent of the underlying disorder. In a representative population-based study, benzodiazepine use doubled the relative risk of ED, even after adjusting for underlying disease (99). Some anxiolytics (such as chlordiazepozide) result in significant worsening of libido compared with non-anxiolytics (such as propranolol) (100). Whether this is true for all anxiolytics is not known. Furthermore, all antidepressants used to treat anxiety disorders cause some adverse effects on sexual function (particularly ejaculatory disorders) (79). At present, the available data are inadequate to support any firm conclusions regarding the relative incidence of sexual dysfunction associated with these medications.

☐ PROSTATE DISEASE
Lower Urinary Tract Symptoms

Large representative population-based studies show that lower urinary tract symptoms (LUTS) are significantly associated with erectile and ejaculatory dysfunction, but not low sexual desire, even after adjustment for age or other important variables (2,28,33,39,101,102). Voiding as well as storage symptoms are individually associated with sexual dysfunction (102).

Both α-adrenoceptor antagonists and 5-α-reductase inhibitors are effective medical therapies for LUTS, and a combination of the two is slightly better (103). Direct comparisons in randomized, placebo-controlled studies have clearly shown that 5-α-reductase inhibitors have more sexual side effects than α-adrenoceptor antagonists, and further, that the combination has slightly more side effects on ejaculation (103–105).

Indirect comparisons also support these relationships. The randomized, placebo-controlled therapeutic trials in LUTS (106,107) and the finasteride prostate cancer chemoprevention trial (108) have confirmed that finasteride treatment decreases libido and increases ED. Similarly, randomized, placebo-controlled studies have shown that various α-adrenoceptor antagonists do not cause sexual side effects when used in men with LUTS (109,110) or hypertension (111).

Transurethral surgery for benign prostate hyperplasia may be associated with sexual dysfunction in the immediate postoperative period. In a large, but uncontrolled, cohort of 5276 men undergoing transurethral prostatectomy, up to 30% of men developed new ED and up to 70% developed retrograde ejaculation three months later (112); however, transurethral surgery was found to be no worse in effects on sexual function than watchful waiting in randomized controlled studies of 800 men followed for three years (113) or 340 men followed for 7.5 months (114). Critically, in the smaller study that assessed retrograde ejaculation separately and sooner, surgery increased the incidence of retrograde ejaculation. These data suggest that sexual function, particularly retrograde ejaculation, occurs in the immediate postoperative period, but that overall sexual function recovers over the course of three years.

Total prostatectomy has a much higher risk of postoperative ED, but this is reduced by the nerve-sparing (115) and vascular-sparing (116) surgery developed by Walsh. Furthermore, such postganglionic nerve damage significantly reduces the efficacy of oral phosphodiesterase type-5 inhibitors in restoring potency (117,118), but with the preservation of at least one neurovascular bundle, oral PDE-5 inhibitors are effective (119–121). Regardless of surgical technique, intracavernosal vasodilator injections such as prostaglandins remain effective (122).

Prostate Cancer

Adequate randomized studies comparing the effectiveness and side effect profile of surgery and radiotherapy for prostate cancer are not available. For this reason, the best available data are derived from the prostate cancer outcomes study, which is a large longitudinal observational population-based study recruiting men with prostate cancer chosen randomly from cancer registers. Analysis of 1291 such men, treated within six months of diagnosis by radical prostatectomy, revealed that sexual performance remained a problem in almost 50% even 18 months after surgery (123). In another analysis, 1156 men treated by radical prostatectomy were compared with 435 treated with external beam radiotherapy after two years of follow-up (124). These data show that erectile function is worsened with either treatment, but that surgery results in more ED (80% vs. 62%) and incontinence (10% vs. 4%). Sildenafil can effectively treat ED occurring after external beam radiotherapy (125), but its efficacy for postprostatectomy ED, in which postganglionic pelvic autonomic nerves may be severed, is more doubtful.

These data may influence the decision regarding the most appropriate therapy in the light of other factors, notably overall risk–benefit and effectiveness. For example, sexual dysfunction may be an acceptable trade-off as a life-prolonging measure in incurable metastatic prostate cancer, whereas there may not be the same justification in younger men with organ-confined curable prostate cancer.

☐ HIV/AIDS

HIV infection per se does not appear to cause sexual dysfunction in the early asymptomatic stages (126). Whether prevalence of ED is increased in men with HIV infection is not definite, since studies have been small in sample size, uncontrolled, clinic-based, and unadjusted for age. Nevertheless, sexual dysfunction does appear to be increased in small studies, given the relatively young age group being examined. Up to one-third of men had some degree of ED in a clinic study of 42 men (127). Larger estimates of up to 90% with some degree of ED and prevalence rates of 60% to 80% for low libido and ejaculatory disorders have been reported in a larger, more recent clinical study of 156 slightly older, ambulatory, HIV-positive men (128).

HIV infection is associated with androgen deficiency, particularly when the disease advances to overt AIDS (127,129,130). Indeed, in a study of 85 homosexual men, greater androgen depression in the presence of increasing gonadotropin occurred with more advanced HIV disease (129). Similar results were observed in a study of 50 homosexual men (131). These effects, which are usually modest, may represent the nonspecific effects of chronic illness rather than specific effects of HIV infection. Androgen therapy has been used, sometimes excessively, in such men, and has recently been reviewed (132); however, the effect of such therapy on sexual function has not been reported. Randomized studies examining the efficacy of sildenafil in AIDS are not available, and common antiretroviral medications may alter the pharmacokinetics of sildenafil (133).

The ethics of treating ED in a sexually transmitted disease has been discussed extensively (134).

☐ RESPIRATORY DISEASE
Chronic Pulmonary Failure

A representative population-based study examining almost 1700 men has reported that chronic airflow limitation is associated with ED, even after adjusting for age or other covariables including cigarette smoking (5). Although data are sparse and sample sizes small, it appears that ED and lung function (assessed by spirometry) worsen concurrently in men independent of age (135). Furthermore, small studies suggest that ED in men with respiratory failure may be reversed with early use of oxygen, but may subsequently become refractory if left untreated. In a sequentially allocated study in 19 men with respiratory failure and coexistent severe ED treated with oxygen therapy for one month versus one day (136), erectile function improvements were noted only in those treated for one month. Furthermore, a significant increase in serum testosterone was observed in the group treated for one month; however, in a larger study of 49 men with respiratory failure due to chronic airflow limitation already receiving long-term oxygen therapy, ED and low libido exceeded historical community-prevalence rates (137). In these men, possibly because they all had end-stage disease, no correlation between spirometry or arterial blood gases and sexual function (erectile or libido) was observed. A retrospective questionnaire survey also supported the effects of noninvasive mechanical ventilation in improving sexual activity in men with chronic respiratory failure (138).

Chronic pulmonary failure is also associated with decreased systemic testosterone concentrations, especially in men with respiratory failure, raising the possibility that sexual dysfunction may be related to consequent androgen deficiency. In the largest study, 36 men with chronic airflow limitation (but not in respiratory failure) exhibited decreased systemic testosterone concentrations (139). Men treated with glucocorticoids had lower testosterone concentrations, despite equivalent spirometry. Sexual function was not assessed. Other data suggest that hypoxia of any cause is associated with reduced systemic testosterone exposure. In a small study of eight hypoxic men with respiratory failure due to chronic airflow limitation, gonadotropin and testosterone were lower than in age-matched controls (140). In a similar study of eight hypoxic men with respiratory failure due to pulmonary fibrosis, arterial oxygen tension was positively correlated with serum testosterone concentration (141). Whether testosterone treatment would improve sexual function in these men has not been adequately assessed, although two studies have found no improvement in respiratory function or quality of life (142,143).

Obstructive Sleep Apnea

Representative, community-based studies examining the association of obstructive sleep apnea (OSA) and sexual function are not available, and spurious associations are possible since both OSA and ED increase with age. Nevertheless, ancillary data suggest that OSA is associated with ED. Disordered breathing was common in a large cohort of men ($n = 1025$) with ED (144), with severe apnea indices observed in about 10% of all men aged less than 40 years, which increased to about 30% of all men over the age of 69. Whether these estimates exceed community expectations is not known due to the absence of comparable controls. An association between OSA and ED is also suggested by another study of 25 men with OSA and without known erectile dysfunction: severe ED was subsequently detected in 11, with a total of 18 exhibiting some degree of ED (145). As expected, these relationships are attenuated when adjusted for age. In 209 men without known treated ED or risk factors for arterial disease (including hypertension, diabetes mellitus, hyperlipidemia, vascular disease), those with severe (but not mild or moderate) OSA determined by overnight laboratory sleep study had reduced erectile function. When adjusted for age, however, only level of sexual satisfaction was associated with disturbed breathing (146). Similarly, the correlation between snoring, as a marker of OSA, and ED disappeared once the effect of age was included in 285 men presenting to a urological practice of which over half presented for ED (147). For these reasons, whether OSA and ED are truly correlated still remains unclear.

Both OSA and massive obesity are associated with reduced systemic testosterone concentrations (148–150). Hence, OSA-associated sexual dysfunction could be mediated by androgen deficiency. Treatment of OSA with continuous positive airway pressure (CPAP) devices reverses these neuroendocrine abnormalities (149,151), an effect that depends on effective CPAP therapy (152) but not weight reduction (149). Overnight CPAP use, however, only inconsistently and not significantly improved laboratory-derived parameters of nocturnal penile tumescence in a small sample of 22 men with OSA and sexual dysfunction (153). More comprehensive therapeutic studies are not available.

Nevertheless, the rationale for an association between OSA and ED is strong, due to clear evidence for impaired endothelial function. Large population-based studies of over 6000 men and women clearly show that hypertension, sleep apnea, and markers of impaired vascular endothelial function are associated independently of age and obesity (154,155). Furthermore, hypoxemia may cause neuropathy, and this may lead to ED (145,156). Further investigation is required.

☐ GASTROINTESTINAL DISEASE

Gastrointestinal diseases often have endocrine consequences but usually have little major impact on sexual functioning other than from nonspecific effects of illness and the consequences of bowel surgery on erectile and ejaculatory function. Celiac disease in childhood retards puberty (157) and causes sexual dysfunction in men (158) with associated low blood dihydrotestosterone (DHT), high testosterone and luteinizing hormone levels before and after gonadotropin-releasing hormone (GnRH) stimulation (159,160). These endocrine manifestations resemble androgen insensitivity (161) and are closely related to the severity and improvement in celiac disease (as assessed by jejunal morphology) including showing reversibility after elimination of gluten (160). The precise pathophysiological mechanism linking celiac disease to biochemical and clinical manifestations of acquired androgen insensitivity remains unclear. While the antiulcer drug cimetidine, the original histamine H2 antagonist, had antiandrogenic properties, others of this class like ranitidine do not (162).

One study of patients with inflammatory bowel disease found no higher prevalence of sexual problems among patients than in controls, including a mixture of friends and patients attending the same general practitioners with other complaints (163), whereas another study of patients with irritable bowel syndrome found more complaints, particularly of loss of sexual drive, when compared with community controls (164). Whether these differences are genuinely related to the different bowel disorders or rather to control sampling bias remains to be clarified by further studies.

Colorectal cancer (by direct extension or metastasis), inflammatory bowel disease (fistulae), and diverticular disease may lead to genitourinary complications including sexual dysfunction. Abdominal or pelvic surgery for benign (165) or malignant (166) disease may injure autonomic nerves involved in erection and/or ejaculation, and the mutilating effects of these surgical interventions may damage the man's self-image as remaining sexually attractive. Laparoscopic surgery for rectal cancer may have higher rates of postoperative sexual dysfunction than that of conventional open surgery (167). Sildenafil may be effective for postsurgical ED after rectal surgery for cancer or inflammatory bowel disease (168).

□ HEPATIC DISEASE

Chronic liver disease (169) and liver transplantation (170) have prominent effects on pituitary-testicular and sexual function, although the two may not be directly linked. The androgen deficiency is related most closely to the degree of liver failure rather than underlying disease (171,172), although alcohol, a common cause of liver disease, has independent toxic effects on the testis (173) and sexual function (174). In alcohol-related liver disease, however, reduced alcohol consumption improves sexual function, whereas testosterone treatment does not (175).

Systemic iron overload, whether due to genetic hemochromatosis or acquired following blood

transfusion in supportive treatment of thalassemia and other congenital anemias, results in a high prevalence of gonadal dysfunction due to pituitary iron deposition that causes LH and androgen deficiency (176). In a minority, this can be prevented by iron chelation or reversed by iron depletion from venesection; however it is usually irreversible and requires testosterone replacement therapy (177). Men with undiagnosed or untreated iron overload may present with delayed puberty or sexual dysfunction due to androgen deficiency. These effects are usually readily and completely overcome with androgen replacement or gonadotrophin treatment if spermatogenesis and fertility (178) are required. Otherwise, hemochromatosis is rarely associated with sexual dysfunction.

The effects of systemic copper overload on reproductive function have been little studied. One study reported that among 27 men with genetic Wilson's disease, 1 reported being impotent, 6 did not want children, and 20 had a total of 28 healthy children (179). Early in the disease, personality change including sexual disinhibition and increased sexual activity is not uncommon (180). Whether these effects are due to copper deposition in neurological tissue, liver, or elsewhere requires further evaluation.

□ ENDOCRINE DISEASE

In general, endocrine diseases influence male sexual function through modifying endogenous testosterone production and androgen action. There is no evidence for nonhormonal mechanisms of sexual dysfunction associated with pituitary, thyroid, or adrenal disease, although diabetes mellitus has distinctive nonhormonal effects.

Hyperthyroidism is associated with increased blood testosterone concentrations due to concomitant increases in circulating sex hormone–binding globulin (SHBG) concentration, whereas hypothyroidism produces the reverse, with decreases in blood testosterone and SHBG concentrations. These changes are linked with concomitant gynecomastia and impaired sexual function and are usually reversed with rectification of the thyroid hormone abnormalities (181,182).

Glucocorticoid excess of either endogenous or exogenous origin may suppress testicular testosterone production due to interference at multiple levels of the hypothalamo–pituitary testicular axis (183–186). Although adrenal androgen [dehydroepiandrosterone (DHEA)] replacement improves sexual function in women with complete adrenal failure (adrenalectomy, Addison's disease) (187), no such effect is observed in men (188) presumably due to the much higher background testicular androgen production.

While growth hormone (GH) promotes sexual maturation and reproductive function (189) and GH deficiency leads to impaired quality of life including sexual function, the effects of exogenous GH on sexual functioning are subtle and involve indirect psychosocial mechanisms as well as hormonal effects on androgen action. Acromegaly may be associated with decreased sexual function attributable to concomitant androgen deficiency as well as acromegalic changes in physique and appearance that may impact adversely upon the self-image of sexual attractiveness (190).

Hyperprolactinemia in men is often associated with sexual dysfunction, sometimes as the presenting features of a microadenoma but more often with other clinical features of a macroadenoma. While hyprepro-lactinemia accounts for < 2% of cases presenting with male sexual dysfunction, most (80–90%) men with chronic hyperprolactinemia have complaints of loss of libido, impaired erections, and ejaculation (191). The mechanism causing impairment of sexual function is not well understood but may involve structural or functional inhibition of gonadotropin secretion. Dopaminergic drugs, which inhibit prolactin secretion, sometimes improve sexual function, but in the usual pituitary macroprolactinoma, testosterone replacement is generally required and effective. Additional effects, whereby neurotransmitter defects in the brain lead to both sexual dysfunction and hyperprolactinemia (192), may explain the occasional observation that sexual function is restored by prolactin suppression prior to normalization of testosterone or that testosterone alone is sometimes not fully effective. Drug-induced hyperpro-lactinemia is relatively common especially during the use of major tranquilizers as antipsychotic drugs (193), in which case it may produce gynecomastia, galactor-rhea, sexual dysfunction, and mood disturbances (194). These iatrogenic effects may be overlooked, being confused with the underlying psychological disturbances. A change of dose or drug may be considered when hyperprolactinemia causes clinically significant adverse effects including sexual dysfunction.

Diabetes Mellitus

Diabetes mellitus (DM) is the most common cause of ED in men throughout the world (195–197). As many as 28% of men presenting with ED have DM as the principal cause (195–197). Although ED may occasionally be the presenting feature, as a rule it develops progressively during the course of DM, with 50% of diabetic men experiencing ED after 10 years of DM (195–197). This risk of ED is similar in men with type 1 (198,199) and type 2 (200) diabetes and in men treated with oral hypoglycemic agents (usually type 2 DM) versus those requiring insulin treatment (195). Glycosylated hemoglobin level is a predictor of ED (200) but less predictive than age, antihypertensive medication, or alcohol intake (201). Other studies confirm that age, DM duration, and complications of DM, such as macrovascular disease (202), microangiopathy, and diabetic neuropathy, are more reliable predictors of ED (195,196,198,203,204). The pathophysiology of ED in DM may be due to a variety of factors, including endothelial dysfunction leading to impairment of smooth-muscle relaxation in the penile microvasculature

(205–208), diabetic autonomic neuropathy (196,209), particularly of the cholinergic and nonadrenergic non-cholinergic (NANC) nerves (201,210–214), reduction in nitric oxide (215–218) and in nitric oxide–induced relaxation of the corpus cavernosum smooth muscle (215–218), and disturbances in testosterone production and androgen action, although whether these represent a cause or consequences of ED remains to be clarified. Unfortunately, when patients experience erectile problems, neuropathy is already largely irreversible, and proper treatment of abnormal glucose metabolism in patients with DM has limited or no effect on ED (219). Thus, the long-term neurovascular sequelae of DM rather than its short-term control are most likely the key determinants of ED in diabetes. This highlights the need for early diagnosis and good long-term control of DM to slow complications as the best approach to prevent deterioration in sexual functioning (220–222).

☐ CHRONIC RENAL FAILURE

Sexual dysfunction is common in men with end-stage chronic renal failure (ESRF) requiring dialysis with marked improvement after successful transplantation (15,223). The prevalence of sexual dysfunction rises from approximately 9% before starting dialysis to 60% to 70% in men requiring dialysis (224,225). Comparable estimates have been found in a more recent study that reported that 86% of men on hemodialysis had some degree of ED, with 45% having severe and 25% complete ED (226). Increasing age and concomitant diabetes mellitus were both independently and directly associated with ED, whereas the use of angiotensin-converting enzyme inhibitors was inversely correlated (226,227). Vascular factors associated with ESRF are likely to be responsible for ED, and these factors include atherosclerois, hypoxia, associated changes of contractile smooth muscle, and collagen/elastin changes of erectile tissue (228). In contrast, somatic factors, which have been implicated in the etiology of sexual dysfunctions in patients with ESRF, mostly lack empirical support (15). Caloric or micronutrient malnutrition—problems in the early days of dialysis—is no longer significant (229–231), whereas accumulation of uremic toxins and "middle molecules" remains speculative. Although atherosclerosis is accelerated in ESRF, the rapid rectification of sexual function following renal transplantation makes it unlikely that this is a decisive factor and similar consideration applies to uremic neuropathy. Concomitant drug treatment such as antihypertensive drugs may also interfere with sexual functioning. In addition to somatic mechanisms, psychological factors, depression in reaction to the handicap of ESRF and a sense of loss (of job, financial security, freedom, and attractiveness), could all contribute to the sexual dysfunction in ESRF (224,232–234).

An important, carefully controlled study of the prevalence and nature of male sexual dysfunctions in men with ESRF on hemodialysis and peritoneal dialysis, and after kidney transplantation reported similar rates of ED (17–43%) between groups as well as compared with a chronic disease control (rheumatoid arthritis) (235,236). In contrast, low sexual drive was significantly more prevalent in men on dialysis compared with those after kidney transplantation or men with rheumatoid arthritis. This suggests that sexual dysfunction in men on dialysis is primarily the loss of sexual interest, subjectively ascribed to fatigue and listlessness, rather than ED. Furthermore, sexual interest can rapidly improve after kidney transplantation (235,236), although it remains impaired compared to healthy controls depending on age, time on dialysis and iterative transplants (236), and penile vascular insufficiency (237). Sildenafil is effective for ED in men on dialysis (238–241) and even more so after renal transplantation (242–244).

☐ IMMUNE, CONNECTIVE TISSUE, AND JOINT DISEASE

Autoimmune and rheumatological diseases, apart from ankylosing spondylitis, are strongly female preponderant; thus, studies of male sexual function in these disorders are very few. Nevertheless the available studies suggest a high prevalence of sexual dysfunction.

Ankylosing spondylitis is associated with impaired erectile function and lower sexual satisfaction compared with healthy controls, using a specific validated questionnaire instrument (245). These findings supplement older observations using less sensitive and specific methods (246,247). The more recent study also noted that the most striking sexual dysfunction reported by men was prolonged (> 4 hours) morning stiffness.

Scleroderma (systemic sclerosis) has a specific association with ED due to cavernosal involvement early in the natural history of the disease (248–253) and is particularly evident in men with associated Raynaud's syndrome (253). Patients with Raynaud's syndrome and scleroderma are susceptible to severe exacerbation of vasospasm by yohimbine treatment for ED (254).

Chronic rheumatoid disease, a strongly female preponderant autoimmune disorder, is characterized by episodic pain and tiredness resulting in physical deformity. Few studies of sexual function in men with chronic arthritis are available, but such men rated higher on scales of sexual avoidance and dissatisfaction than normal controls (255). The available studies suggest that physical disability, pain, and psychological factors such as self confidence and perceived attractiveness are all contributory. Inability to work or undertake activities of daily living may further exacerbate dissatisfaction, depression, and loss of self-esteem (255).

The importance of psychosexual factors in rheumatoid disease is underlined by studies showing a consistent discrepancy between the higher rates of sexual dysfunction compared with relatively lower rates of ED (246,256–258). For example, one study found 17 of 30 men experiencing a diverse range of sexual problems, whereas only 5 of 30 reported ED (256). Concerns about pain, weakness, fatigue, and limited range of motion during sexual activity explain the discrepancy between physical sexual capacity and motivation to initiate sexual behavior, most evidently among men aged 30 to 50 years (246,257,258). In addition, a long-term follow-up study of patients with juvenile idiopathic arthritis found they had fewer stable sexual relationships than unaffected siblings, presumably reflecting the consequences of disease and disability on socialization (259).

☐ NEUROLOGICAL DISEASE
Brain Injury

Following traumatic brain injury, physical disability and cognitive impairment are frequent and sexual disorders and disinhibition may become evident. Potential mechanisms include both direct effects of cerebral damage and indirect behavioral and psychosocial consequences. Decreased sexual activity, as exhibited by erectile and ejaculatory failure, is usual, although increased sexual activity is occasionally reported (260–262). Among central lesions, frontal or temporal lobe damage seems to cause more sexual problems than lesions of the parieto-occipital lobes. Bilateral anterior temporal lesions may cause the so-called Klüver-Bucy syndrome featuring indiscriminate sexual orientation including toward inappropriate and nonhuman objects (animals and inanimate objects). Uncontrolled studies suggest that either amantidine (263) or medroxyprogesterone acetate (264) may suppress inappropriate sexual behavior, but better controlled studies are needed.

Spinal Cord Injury and Disease

Spinal cord disorders are most often due to trauma, although a wide and diverse range of nontraumatic disorders of the spinal cord or cauda equina [including congenital spina bifida (265), transverse myelitis, spinal cord tumors, and prolapsed discs (266–268)] may be responsible. Regardless of etiology, the consequences for erectile and ejaculatory function are similar, depending on the site, extent, and chronology of the lesion (269), although the net effect on overall sexual function also involves the superimposition of additional important psychosocial factors.

Traumatic spinal cord injuries (SCIs) have immense psychological impact. Healthy young men typically undergo, without warning, a sudden and profound loss of body functions, including paralysis, loss of sensation and disruption of bladder, and loss of bowel and sexual function and fertility (265). Generally, more than half of the men with SCI are unable to achieve erections that permit successful sexual intercourse (270). Sexual readjustment after injury is closely and positively correlated with a young age at injury and willingness to experiment with alternative sexual expressions (271). Physical and social independence and better mood were further positive determinants. Sildenafil is beneficial in some men with SCI, improving not only sexual function but also mood (272).

Stroke

Stroke has a major impact on sexual functioning. Most (50–65%) men experience ED after a stroke (273–275) and about 75% of men who were sexually active before the stroke report an abrupt and permanent decrease in coital frequency. Orgasmic dysfunction after stroke has been reported in about 66% of men (273); however, nocturnal erections normalize in 45% by two months after stroke (276). Thus, sexual problems in poststroke patients are explained not only by the neurological condition itself but also by associated psychological factors. For example, diminished sexual initiative may be due to the patient's overwhelming feeling of sexual inadequacy. Further, cognitive impairment may diminish sexual relationships. Sexual problems occur more frequently with aphasic strokes (277) or after right, rather than left, hemisphere stroke (278), although not all studies confirm this lateralization (273,279). Lesions in the nondominant hemisphere and the parietal lobe in particular were more often associated with diminished desire. General hemihypoesthesia is associated with decreased sexual ability probably due to loss of somatic sexual stimulation.

Epilepsy

Sexual dysfunction is relatively common among patients with epilepsy, usually in the interictal period. Loss of sexual desire, reduced sexual activity, and/or inhibited sexual arousal (compared with control populations) are frequently observed in men with epilepsy (280–283), though the prevalence varies in different studies (284). Seizures may also be provoked by sexual activity (or by the associated physical stimuli or hyperventilation), and occasionally sexual manifestations such as erections, pelvic thrusts, masturbation, or ejaculation may be part of a seizure, experienced as sexual or nonsexual. Whether these sexual abnormalities are due to the underlying condition, the seizures, or antiepileptic medications requires further investigation.

Surgery for epilepsy does not have adverse effects on postoperative sexual function (285). Antiepileptic drug treatment may affect sexual desire and sexual performance via a mechanism that remains unclear, although such drugs have prominent effects on androgen metabolism and action (286–289). Psychosocial factors are likely to have complex interactions with satisfactory sexual relationships.

Parkinson's Disease and Dyskinesias

Parkinson's disease (PD) is a neurodegenerative movement disorders characterized by the progressive destruction of the dopamine-containing cells in the substantia nigra. In the early stages of PD, sexual function is normal, but in advanced PD, libido is usually low, reflex and spontaneous erections are less frequent, ED occurs in approximately 50% of men, and ejaculation and orgasm are disrupted (290–293). There is evidence of autonomic nervous system degeneration in PD that might contribute to the erectile and ejaculatory dysfunction. Muscle tremor, rigidity, and akinesia may be more pronounced during sexual arousal and activity and this can add to sexual difficulties. Depression and dementia, relatively common in later stages of PD, can also adversely affect sexual relationships (294). The pathophysiological mechanism of sexual dysfunction in patients with PD is not clear, though dopaminergic pathways are important in penile erection (295–297). A recent study suggested that elderly men with PD may be testosterone deficient (298) and that testosterone replacement may alleviate some symptoms (299). These observations warrant further replication in a controlled study particularly as the modest reduction in blood testosterone may be out of proportion to the apparent benefit. Treatment with dopaminergic compounds may rapidly normalize libido, regardless of corresponding improvement in motor function (300,301). Treatment with sildenafil improves sexual functioning in some men with PD and ED (302,303).

In the PD variant termed "Shy-Drager syndrome" or "multiple system atrophy," autonomic neuropathy is a predominant feature and impotence is almost universal (304,305); impotence may, in fact, be the presenting feature (306).

Huntington's disease (HD) is also most frequently associated with sexual inactivity due to either apathy or impotence in later stages. In the early stages, however, increased sexual activity due to sexual disinhibition, hypersexuality, and paraphilias is evident in approximately 12% of the patients, often in combination with hypomania, and promiscuity may be a presenting feature of HD (307–309). Suicide rate is particularly high in HD (310–312) compared with other neurodegenerative disorders (313), and the strongest predictor of suicide is childlessness (314). No therapeutic studies for sexual dysfunction in HD have been reported.

Tourette's syndrome is associated with sexual disinhibition and indiscriminate sexuality (315,316). Two cases have been reported to respond to the opiate blocker naltrexone (317). Further studies are required.

Multiple Sclerosis

Multiple sclerosis (MS) is an episodic demyelinating disorder of unknown etiology, resulting in progressive neural dysfunction and loss of motor control. Sexual dysfunction is rare initially but becomes common during disease progression (318). Erectile failure is the most common sexual dysfunction in men with MS, with a prevalence of 35% to 80% (319–323), and ejaculatory dysfunction is also frequent, with a prevalence of 35% to 60% (320,322). Reduced libido is also common but has not been studied in detail. The sexual dysfunction correlates most closely with location of nervous system plaques (319,324,325), with the presence of bladder and bowel dysfunction, and, to a lesser extent, with lower extremity motor and sensory function (321,326,327) but not with overall disability and disease duration (321). Depression and cognitive impairment may also play an important role. If plaques damage suprasacral parasympathetic neurons that provide cholinergic and NANC nerves to the penis, drugs acting through nitric oxide such as the phosphodiesterase inhibitors are less effective. MS symptoms such as fatigue, leg muscle spasms, sensory disturbances, voiding problems, and incontinence aids may also impact negatively on self-esteem, thereby affecting sexual function.

Motor Neuron Diseases, Peripheral Neuropathies, and Muscular Dystrophies

Early onset of the neuromuscular disease, together with rapid disease progression, results in limited psychosocial and psychosexual development and in severely reduced sexual activity (328).

Motor neuron disease (MND) is a rapidly progressive peripheral neurodegenerative disease that leads to an almost total paralysis of the whole body, including the respiratory muscles, and severe sexual difficulties might be expected. If the neurons of Onuf's nucleus in the sacral spinal cord innervating the pelvic floor muscles are spared, however, patients do not experience sensory or autonomic pelvic symptoms, and male sexual functions could therefore remain normal. Severe paralysis of all voluntary movement would eventually render intercourse impossible, but erection, ejaculation, and orgasm could continue to be experienced with the help of a partner. Yet, despite the persistence of sexual capabilities, men with MND report progressive and marked decline in sexual activity as the disease progresses, and this is mainly due to decreased libido and passivity (329).

In Kennedy's syndrome (X-linked bulbospinal muscular atrophy), a MND variant due to a CAG triplet repeat in exon 1 of the androgen receptor, mild hypogonadism featuring gynecomastia, testicular atrophy, decreased libido, and impotence occur in mid-life after normal sexual and reproductive function earlier in life (330).

Little is known systematically about sexual function in muscular dystrophies; however, hypogonadism in combination with reduced libido and ED has been described (331,332).

In addition to autonomic neuropathy in which ED is an early and prominent feature (333,334), numerous hereditary metabolic polyneuropathies are known, but very little information is available on sexual function in these conditions. Sexual dysfunctions have been reported in patients with hereditary sensory and motor neuropathy (including Charcot-Marie-Tooth syndrome) (335–337), adrenomyeloneuropathy (338,339), and primary amyloidotic polyneuropathy (340–343).

☐ CONCLUSION

Sexual dysfunction is a common accompaniment of many systemic diseases and their medical treatments, particularly illnesses that affect the cardiovascular, prostatic, neurological, and psychiatric systems. Since sexuality is an important, but often unspoken, component of overall life satisfaction, holistic medical care therefore requires cognizance of these associations. Distinguishing between the effects of underlying disease and its treatment on sexual function and satisfaction may be difficult and requires insightful knowledge of the effects on sexual function of both the natural history of the underlying disease (including its psychosocial as well as physical effects) and the drug and other medical therapies. In particular, widely consumed drugs, including certain antihypertensives, antidepressants, and anxiolytics, may adversely alter libido or penile erectile function. If recognized, substitution with other agents that have fewer such side effects may be feasible. The extent to which other drugs (such as antipsychotics) have similar undesirable effects, as distinct from the effects of the underlying diseases, requires further evaluation.

☐ REFERENCES

1. Panser LA, Rhodes T, Girman CJ, et al. Sexual function of men ages 40 to 79 years: the Olmsted County Study of urinary symptoms and health status among men. J Am Geriatr Soc 1995; 43:1107–1111.
2. Laumann EO, Paik A, Rosen RC. Sexual dysfunction in the United States: prevalence and predictors. JAMA 1999; 281:537–544.
3. Daker-White G. Reliable and valid self-report outcome measures in sexual (dys)function: a systematic review. Arch Sex Behav 2002; 31:197–209.
4. Goldstein I. Oral sildenafil in the treatment of erectile dysfunction. Sildenafil Study Group. N Engl J Med 1998; 338:933–940.
5. Blanker MH, Bohnen AM, Groeneveld FP, et al. Correlates for erectile and ejaculatory dysfunction in older Dutch men: a community-based study. J Am Geriatr Soc 2001; 49:436–442.
6. Ambler N, Williams AC, Hill P, et al. Sexual difficulties of chronic pain patients. Clin J Pain 2001; 17:138–145.
7. Monga TN, Tan G, Ostermann HJ, et al. Sexuality and sexual adjustment of patients with chronic pain. Disabil Rehabil 1998; 20:317–329.

8. Paice JA, Penn RD, Ryan WG. Altered sexual function and decreased testosterone in patients receiving intraspinal opioids. J Pain Symptom Manage 1994; 9:126–131.

9. Finch PM, Roberts LJ, Price L, et al. Hypogonadism in patients treated with intrathecal morphine. Clin J Pain 2000; 16:251–254.

10. Abs R, Verhelst J, Maeyaert J, et al. Endocrine consequences of long-term intrathecal administration of opioids. J Clin Endocrinol Metabol 2000; 85:2215–2222.

11. Roberts LJ, Finch PM, Pullan PT, et al. Sex hormone suppression by intrathecal opioids: a prospective study. Clin J Pain 2002; 18:144–148.

12. Daniell HW. Hypogonadism in men consuming sustained-action oral opioids. J Pain 2002; 3:377–384.

13. Rajagopal A, Vassilopoulou-Sellin R, Palmer JL, et al. Symptomatic hypogonadism in male survivors of cancer with chronic exposure to opioids. Cancer 2004; 100:851–858.

14. Rosas SE, Joffe M, Franklin E, et al. Prevalence and determinants of erectile dysfunction in hemodialysis patients. Kidney Int 2001; 59:2259–2266.

15. Handelsman DJ. Hypothalamic-pituitary gonadal dysfunction in chronic renal failure, dialysis, and renal transplantation. Endocrine Rev 1985; 6:151–182.

16. Trembecki J, Kokot F, Wiecek A, et al. Improvement of sexual function in hemodialyzed male patients with chronic renal failure treated with erythropoietin (rHuEPO). Przegl Lek 1995; 52:462–466.

17. Beusterien KM, Nissenson AR, Port FK, et al. The effects of recombinant human erythropoietin on functional health and well-being in chronic dialysis patients. J Am Soc Nephrol 1996; 7:763–773.

18. de Francisco AL, Fernandez Fresnedo G, Rodrigo E, et al. Past, present and future of erythropoietin use in the elderly. Int Urol Nephrol 2002; 33:187–193.

19. Buena F, Peterson MA, Swerdloff RS, et al. Sexual function does not change when serum testosterone levels are pharmacologically varied within the normal male range. Fertil Steril 1993; 59:1118–1123.

20. Bagatell CJ, Heiman JR, Rivier JE, et al. Effects of endogenous testosterone and estradiol on sexual behaviour in normal young men. J Clin Endocrinol Metabol 1994; 78:711–716.

21. Penson DF, Ng C, Cai L, et al. Androgen and pituitary control of penile nitric oxide synthase and erectile function in the rat. Biol Reprod 1996; 55:567–574.

22. Morelli A, Filippi S, Mancina R, et al. Androgens regulate phosphodiesterase type 5 expression and functional activity in corpora cavernosa. Endocrinology 2004; 145:2253–2263.

23. Aversa A, Isidori AM, Spera G, et al. Androgens improve cavernous vasodilation and response to sildenafil in patients with erectile dysfunction. Clin Endocrinol (Oxf) 2003; 58:632–638.

24. Benkert O, Witt W, Adam W, et al. Effects of testosterone undecanoate on sexual potency and the hypothalamic-pituitary-gonadal axis of impotent males. Arch Sex Behav 1979; 8:471–479.

25. Kwan M, Greenleaf WJ, Mann J, et al. The nature of androgen action on male sexuality: a combined laboratory-self-report study on hypogonadal men. J Clin Endocrinol Metab 1983; 57:557–562.

26. Mannino DM, Klevens RM, Flanders WD. Cigarette smoking: an independent risk factor for impotence? Am J Epidemiol 1994; 140:1003–1008.

27. Wei M, Macera CA, Davis DR, et al. Total cholesterol and high density lipoprotein cholesterol as important predictors of erectile dysfunction. Am J Epidemiol 1994; 140:930–937.

28. Pinnock CB, Stapleton AM, Marshall VR. Erectile dysfunction in the community: a prevalence study. Med J Aust 1999; 171:353–357.

29. Johannes CB, Araujo AB, Feldman HA, et al. Incidence of erectile dysfunction in men 40 to 69 years old: longitudinal results from the Massachusetts male aging study. J Urol 2000; 163:460–463.

30. Moreira ED Jr, Lbo CF, Diament A, et al. Incidence of erectile dysfunction in men 40 to 69 years old: results from a population-based cohort study in Brazil. Urology 2003; 61:431–436.

31. Dunn KM, Croft PR, Hackett GI. Association of sexual problems with social, psychological, and physical problems in men and women: a cross sectional population survey. J Epidemiol Community Health 1999; 53:144–148.

32. McVary KT, Carrier S, Wessells H. Smoking and erectile dysfunction: evidence based analysis. J Urol 2001; 166:1624–1632.

33. Rosen R, Altwein J, Boyle P, et al. Lower urinary tract symptoms and male sexual dysfunction: the multinational survey of the aging male (MSAM-7). Eur Urol 2003; 44:637–649.

34. Roth A, Kalter-Leibovici O, Kerbis Y, et al. Prevalence and risk factors for erectile dysfunction in men with diabetes, hypertension, or both diseases: a community survey among 1,412 Israeli men. Clin Cardiol 2003; 26:25–30.

35. Rosen MP, Greenfield AJ, Walker TG, et al. Cigarette smoking: an independent risk factor for atherosclerosis in the hypogastric-cavernous arterial bed of men with arteriogenic impotence. J Urol 1991; 145:759–763.

36. Solomon H, Man JW, Wierzbicki AS, et al. Relation of erectile dysfunction to angiographic coronary artery disease. Am J Cardiol 2003; 91:230–231.

37. Sorensen KE, Kristensen IB, Celermajer DS. Atherosclerosis in the human brachial artery. J Am Coll Cardiol 1997; 29:318–322.

38. Solberg LA, Strong JP. Risk factors and atherosclerotic lesions. A review of autopsy studies. Arteriosclerosis 1983; 3:187–198.

39. Akkus E, Kadioglu A, Esen A, et al. Prevalence and correlates of erectile dysfunction in Turkey: a population-based study. Eur Urol 2002; 41:298–304.

40. White JR, Case DA, McWhirter D, et al. Enhanced sexual behavior in exercising men. Arch Sex Behav 1990; 19:193–209.

41. Dobs AS, Miller S, Neri G, et al. Effects of simvastatin and pravastatin on gonadal function in male hypercholesterolemic patients. Metabolism 2000; 49:115–121.

42. Dobs AS, Schrott H, Davidson MH, et al. Effects of high-dose simvastatin on adrenal and gonadal steroidogenesis in men with hypercholesterolemia. Metabolism 2000; 49:1234–1238.

43. Drory Y, Kravetz S, Hirschberger G. Sexual activity of women and men one year before a first acute myocardial infarction. Cardiology 2002; 97:127–132.

44. DeBusk R, Drory Y, Goldstein I, et al. Management of sexual dysfunction in patients with cardiovascular disease: recommendations of The Princeton Consensus Panel. Am J Cardiol 2000; 86:175–181.

45. Drory Y, Kravetz S, Weingarten M. Comparison of sexual activity of women and men after a first acute myocardial infarction. Am J Cardiol 2000; 85: 1283–1287.

46. Westin L, Carlsson R, Israelsson B, et al. Quality of life in patients with ischaemic heart disease: a prospective controlled study. J Intern Med 1997; 242:239–247.

47. Conti CR, Pepine CJ, Sweeney M. Efficacy and safety of sildenafil citrate in the treatment of erectile dysfunction in patients with ischemic heart disease. Am J Cardiol 1999; 83:29C–34C.

48. Jaarsma T, Dracup K, Walden J, et al. Sexual function in patients with advanced heart failure. Heart Lung 1996; 25:262–270.

49. Bocchi EA, Guimaraes G, Mocelin A, et al. Sildenafil effects on exercise, neurohormonal activation, and erectile dysfunction in congestive heart failure: a double-blind, placebo-controlled, randomized study followed by a prospective treatment for erectile dysfunction. Circulation 2002; 106:1097–1103.

50. Seidman SN, Roose SP, Menza MA, et al. Treatment of erectile dysfunction in men with depressive symptoms: results of a placebo-controlled trial with sildenafil citrate. Am J Psychiatry 2001; 158: 1623–1630.

51. Angst J, Gamma A, Gastpar M, et al. Gender differences in depression. Epidemiological findings from the European DEPRES I and II studies. Eur Arch Psychiatry Clin Neurosci 2002; 252:2 01–209.

52. Araujo AB, Durante R, Feldman HA, et al. The relationship between depressive symptoms and male erectile dysfunction: cross-sectional results from the Massachusetts Male Aging Study. Psychosomatic Medicine 1998; 60: 458–465.

53. Moreira ED Jr, Lisboa Lobo CF, Villa M, et al. Prevalence and correlates of erectile dysfunction in Salvador, northeastern Brazil: a population-based study. Int J Impot Res 2002; 14.33–39.

54. Bonierbale M, Lancon C, Tignol J. The ELIXIR study: evaluation of sexual dysfunction in 4557 depressed patients in France. Curr Med Res Opin 2003; 19: 114–124.

55. Ekselius L, von Knorring L. Effect on sexual function of long-term treatment with selective serotonin reuptake inhibitors in depressed patients treated in primary care. J Clin Psychopharmacol 2001; 21:154–160.

56. Michelson D, Schmidt M, Lee J, et al. Changes in sexual function during acute and six-month fluoxetine therapy: a prospective assessment. J Sex Marital Ther 2001; 27:289–302.

57. Zajecka J, Dunner DL, Gelenberg AJ, et al. Sexual function and satisfaction in the treatment of chronic major depression with nefazodone, psychotherapy, and their combination. J Clin Psychiatry 2002; 63:709–716.

58. Sesso HD, Kawachi I, Vokonas PS, et al. Depression and the risk of coronary heart disease in the Normative Aging Study. Am J Cardiol 1998; 82:851–856.

59. Ferketich AK, Schwartzbaum JA, Frid DJ, et al. Depression as an antecedent to heart disease among women and men in the NHANES I study. National Health and Nutrition Examination Survey. Arch Intern Med 2000; 160:1261–1268.

60. Barefoot JC, Schroll M. Symptoms of depression, acute myocardial infarction, and total mortality in a community sample. Circulation 1996; 93:1976–1980.

61. Ariyo AA, Haan M, Tangen CM, et al. Depressive symptoms and risks of coronary heart disease and mortality in elderly Americans. Cardiovascular Health Study Collaborative Research Group. Circulation 2000; 102:1773–1779.

62. Pratt LA, Ford DE, Crum RM, et al. Depression, psychotropic medication, and risk of myocardial infarction. Prospective data from the Baltimore ECA follow-up. Circulation 1996; 94: 3123–3129.

63. Penninx BW, Beekman AT, Honig A, et al. Depression and cardiac mortality: results from a community-based longitudinal study. Arch Gen Psychiatry 2001; 58: 221–227.

64. Davidson K, Jonas BS, Dixon KE, et al. Do depression symptoms predict early hypertension incidence in young adults in the CARDIA study? Coronary artery risk development in young adults. Arch Intern Med 2000; 160:1495–1500.

65. Jonas BS, Franks P, Ingram DD. Are symptoms of anxiety and depression risk factors for hypertension? Longitudinal evidence from the National Health and Nutrition Examination Survey I Epidemiologic Follow-up Study. Arch Fam Med 1997; 6:43–49.

66. Scherrer JF, Xian H, Bucholz KK, et al. A twin study of depression symptoms, hypertension, and heart disease in middle-aged men. Psychosom Med 2003; 65:548–557.

67. Liu PY, Death AK, Handelsman DJ. Androgens and cardiovascular disease. Endocr Rev 2003; 24:313–340.

68. Seidman SN, Araujo AB, Roose SP, et al. Low testosterone levels in elderly men with dysthymic disorder. Am J Psychiatry 2002; 159:456–459.

69. Seidman SN, Araujo AB, Roose SP, et al. Testosterone level, androgen receptor polymorphism, and depressive symptoms in middle-aged men. Biological Psychiatry 2001; 50:371–376.

70. Seidman SN, Spatz E, Rizzo C, et al. Testosterone replacement therapy for hypogonadal men with major depressive disorder: a randomized, placebo-controlled clinical trial. J Clin Psychiatry 2001; 62:406–412.

71. Jannini EA, Screponi E, Carosa E, et al. Lack of sexual activity from erectile dysfunction is associated with a reversible reduction in serum testosterone. Int J Androl 1999; 22:385–392.

72. Croft H, Settle E Jr, Houser T, et al. A placebo-controlled comparison of the antidepressant efficacy and effects on sexual functioning of sustained-release bupropion and sertraline. Clin Ther 1999; 21:643–658.

73. Coleman CC, Cunningham LA, Foster VJ, et al. Sexual dysfunction associated with the treatment of depression: a placebo-controlled comparison of bupropion sustained release and sertraline treatment. Ann Clin Psychiatry 1999; 11:205–215.

74. Coleman CC, King BR, Bolden-Watson C, et al. A placebo-controlled comparison of the effects on sexual functioning of bupropion sustained release and fluoxetine. Clin Ther 2001; 23:1040–1058.

75. Settle EC, Stahl SM, Batey SR, et al. Safety profile of sustained-release bupropion in depression: results of three clinical trials. Clin Ther 1999; 21:454–463.

76. Hekimian LJ, Friedhoff AJ, Deever E. A comparison of the onset of action and therapeutic efficacy of amoxapine and amitriptyline. J Clin Psychiatry 1978; 39:633–637.

77. Kowalski A, Stanley RO, Dennerstein L, et al. The sexual side-effects of antidepressant medication: a double-blind comparison of two antidepressants in a non-psychiatric population. Br J Psychiatry 1985; 147:413–418.

78. Harrison WM, Rabkin JG, Ehrhardt AA, et al. Effects of antidepressant medication on sexual function: a controlled study. J Clin Psychopharmacol 1986; 6:144–149.

79. Montgomery SA, Baldwin DS, Riley A. Antidepressant medications: a review of the evidence for drug-induced sexual dysfunction. J Affect Disord 2002; 69:119–140.

80. Masand PS, Ashton AK, Gupta S, et al. Sustained-release bupropion for selective serotonin reuptake inhibitor-induced sexual dysfunction: a randomized, double-blind, placebo-controlled, parallel-group study. Am J Psychiatry 2001; 158:805–807.

81. Landen M, Eriksson E, Agren H, et al. Effect of buspirone on sexual dysfunction in depressed patients treated with selective serotonin reuptake inhibitors. J Clin Psychopharmacol 1999; 19:268–271.

82. Clayton AH, Warnock JK, Kornstein SG, et al. A placebo-controlled trial of bupropion SR as an antidote for selective serotonin reuptake inhibitor-induced sexual dysfunction. J Clin Psychiatry 2004; 65:62–67.

83. Nelson EB, Shah VN, Welge JA, et al. A placebo-controlled, crossover trial of granisetron in SRI-induced sexual dysfunction. J Clin Psychiatry 2001; 62: 469–473.

84. Aizenberg D, Gur S, Zemishlany Z, et al. Mianserin, a 5-HT2a/2c and alpha 2 antagonist, in the treatment of sexual dysfunction induced by serotonin reuptake inhibitors. Clin Neuropharmacol 1997; 20:210–214.

85. Nurnberg HG, Hensley PL, Gelenberg AJ, et al. Treatment of antidepressant-associated sexual dysfunction with sildenafil: a randomized controlled trial. JAMA 2003; 289:56–64.

86. Nurnberg HG, Gelenberg A, Hargreave TB, et al. Efficacy of sildenafil citrate for the treatment of erectile dysfunction in men taking serotonin reuptake inhibitors. Am J Psychiatry 2001; 158:1926–1928.

87. Bobes J, Garc APMP, Rejas J, et al. Frequency of sexual dysfunction and other reproductive side-effects in patients with schizophrenia treated with risperidone, olanzapine, quetiapine, or haloperidol: the results of the EIRE study. J Sex Marital Ther 2003; 29:125–147.

88. Wesby R, Bullmore E, Earle J, et al. A survey of psychosexual arousability in male patients on depot neuroleptic medication. European Psychiatry 1996; 11:81–86.

89. Aizenberg D, Zemishlany Z, Dorfman-Etrog P, et al. Sexual dysfunction in male schizophrenic patients. J Clin Psychiatry 1995; 56:137–141.

90. Peuskens J. Risperidone in the treatment of patients with chronic schizophrenia: a multi-national, multi-centre, double-blind, parallel-group study versus haloperidol. Risperidone Study Group. Br J Psychiatry 1995; 166:712–726; discussion:727–733.

91. Lingjaerde O, Ahlfors UG, Bech P, et al. The UKU side effect rating scale. A new comprehensive rating scale for psychotropic drugs and a cross-sectional study of side effects in neuroleptic-treated patients. Acta Psychiatr Scand Suppl 1987; 334:1–100.

92. Aizenberg D, Modai I, Landa A, et al. Comparison of sexual dysfunction in male schizophrenic patients maintained on treatment with classical antipsychotics versus clozapine. J Clin Psychiatry 2001; 62:541–544.

93. Cutler AJ. Sexual dysfunction and antipsychotic treatment. Psychoneuroendocrinology 2003; 28:69–82.

94. Weizman R, Weizman A, Levi J, et al. Sexual dysfunction associated with hyperprolactinemia in males and females undergoing hemodialysis. Psychosom Med 1983; 45:259–269.

95. Kodesh A, Weizman A, Aizenberg D, et al. Selegiline in the treatment of sexual dysfunction in schizophrenic patients maintained on neuroleptics: a pilot study. Clin Neuropharmacol 2003; 26:193–195.

96. Kotler M, Cohen H, Aizenberg D, et al. Sexual dysfunction in male posttraumatic stress disorder patients. Psychother Psychosom 2000; 69:309–315.

97. Letourneau EJ, Schewe PA, Frueh BC. Preliminary evaluation of sexual problems in combat veterans with PTSD. J Trauma Stress 1997; 10:125–132.

98. Bodinger L, Hermesh H, Aizenberg D, et al. Sexual function and behavior in social phobia. J Clin Psychiatry 2002; 63:874–879.

99. Derby CA, Barbour MM, Hume AL, et al. Drug therapy and prevalence of erectile dysfunction in the Massachusetts Male Aging Study cohort. Pharmacotherapy 2001; 21:676–683.

100. Meibach RC, Dunner D, Wilson LG, et al. Comparative efficacy of propranolol, chlordiazepoxide, and placebo

in the treatment of anxiety: a double-blind trial. J Clin Psychiatry 1987; 48:355–358.

101. Macfarlane GJ, Botto H, Sagnier PP, et al. The relationship between sexual life and urinary condition in the French community. J Clin Epidemiol 1996; 49:1171–1176.

102. Frankel SJ, Donovan JL, Peters TI, et al. Sexual dysfunction in men with lower urinary tract symptoms. J Clin Epidemiol 1998; 51:677–685.

103. McConnell JD, Roehrborn CG, Bautista OM, et al. The long-term effect of doxazosin, finasteride, and combination therapy on the clinical progression of benign prostatic hyperplasia. N Engl J Med 2003; 349:2387–2398.

104. Kirby RS, Roehrborn C, Boyle P, et al. Efficacy and tolerability of doxazosin and finasteride, alone or in combination, in treatment of symptomatic benign prostatic hyperplasia: the Prospective European Doxazosin and Combination Therapy (PREDICT) trial. Urology 2003; 61:119–126.

105. Lepor H, Williford WO, Barry MJ, et al. The efficacy of terazosin, finasteride, or both in benign prostatic hyperplasia. Veterans Affairs Cooperative Studies Benign Prostatic Hyperplasia Study Group. N Engl J Med 1996; 335:533–539.

106. Wessells H, Roy J, Bannow J, et al. Incidence and severity of sexual adverse experiences in finasteride and placebo-treated men with benign prostatic hyperplasia. Urology 2003; 61:579–584.

107. Roehrborn CG, Boyle P, Nickel JC, et al. Efficacy and safety of a dual inhibitor of 5-alpha-reductase types 1 and 2 (dutasteride) in men with benign prostatic hyperplasia. Urology 2002; 60:434–441.

108. Thompson IM, Goodman PJ, Tangen CM, et al. The influence of finasteride on the development of prostate cancer. N Engl J Med 2003; 349:215–224.

109. Roehrborn CG. Efficacy and safety of once-daily alfuzosin in the treatment of lower urinary tract symptoms and clinical benign prostatic hyperplasia: a randomized, placebo-controlled trial. Urology 2001; 58: 953–959.

110. Roehrborn CG, Van Kerrebroeck P, Nordling J. Safety and efficacy of alfuzosin 10 mg once-daily in the treatment of lower urinary tract symptoms and clinical benign prostatic hyperplasia: a pooled analysis of three double-blind, placebo-controlled studies. BJU Int 2003; 92:257–261.

111. Grimm RH Jr, Grandits GA, Prineas RJ, et al. Long-term effects on sexual function of five antihypertensive drugs and nutritional hygienic treatment in hypertensive men and women. Treatment of Mild Hypertension Study (TOMHS). Hypertension 1997; 29:8–14.

112. Emberton M, Neal DE, Black N, et al. The effect of prostatectomy on symptom severity and quality of life. Br J Urol 1996; 77:233–247.

113. Wasson JH, Reda DJ, Bruskewitz RC, et al. A comparison of transurethral surgery with watchful waiting for moderate symptoms of benign prostatic hyperplasia. The Veterans Affairs Cooperative Study Group on Transurethral Resection of the Prostate. N Engl J Med 1995; 332:75–79.

114. Brookes ST, Donovan JL, Peters TJ, et al. Sexual dysfunction in men after treatment for lower urinary tract symptoms: evidence from randomised controlled trial. BMJ 2002; 324: 1059–1061.

115. Walsh PC, Mostwin JL. Radical prostatectomy and cystoprostatectomy with preservation of potency. Results using a new nerve-sparing technique. Br J Urol 1984; 56:694–697.

116. Polascik TJ, Walsh PC. Radical retropubic prostatectomy: the influence of accessory pudendal arteries on the recovery of sexual function. J Urol 1995; 154:150–152.

117. Zippe CD, Kedia AW, Kedia K, et al. Treatment of erectile dysfunction after radical prostatectomy with sildenafil citrate (Viagra). Urology 1998; 52:963–966.

118. Zippe CD, Jhaveri FM, Klein EA, et al. Role of Viagra after radical prostatectomy. Urology 2000; 55: 241–245.

119. Lowentritt BH, Scardino PT, Miles BJ, et al. Sildenafil citrate after radical retropubic prostatectomy. J Urol 1999; 162:1614–1617.

120. Brock G, Nehra A, Lipshultz LI, et al. Safety and efficacy of vardenafil for the treatment of men with erectile dysfunction after radical retropubic prostatectomy. J Urol 2003; 170:1278–1283.

121. Montorsi F, Nathan HP, McCullough et al. Tadalafil in the treatment of erectile dysfunction following bilateral nerve sparing radical retropubic prostatectomy: a randomized, double-blind, placebo controlled trial. J Urol 2004; 172:1036–1041.

122. Montorsi F, Guazzoni G, Strambi LF, et al. Recovery of spontaneous erectile function after nerve-sparing radical retropubic prostatectomy with and without early intracavernous injections of alprostadil: results of a prospective, randomized trial. J Urol 1997; 158: 1408–1410.

123. Stanford JL, Feng Z, Hamilton AS, et al. Urinary and sexual function after radical prostatectomy for clinically localized prostate cancer: the Prostate Cancer Outcomes Study. JAMA 2000; 283:354–360.

124. Potosky AL, Legler J, Albertsen PC, et al. Health outcomes after prostatectomy or radiotherapy for prostate cancer: results from the Prostate Cancer Outcomes Study. J Natl Cancer Inst 2000; 92:1582–1592.

125. Incrocci L, Koper PC, Hop WC, et al. Sildenafil citrate (Viagra) and erectile dysfunction following external beam radiotherapy for prostate cancer: a randomized, double-blind, placebo-controlled, cross-over study. Int J Radiat Oncol Biol Phys 2001; 51:1190–1195.

126. Brown GR, Rundell JR, McManis SE, et al. Prevalence of psychiatric disorders in early stages of HIV infection. Psychosom Med 1992; 54:588–601.

127. Dobs AS, Dempsey MA, Ladenson PW, et al. Endocrine disorders in men infected with human immunodeficiency virus. Am J Med 1988; 84:611–616.

128. Lallemand F, Salhi Y, Linard F, et al. Sexual dysfunction in 156 ambulatory HIV-infected men receiving highly active antiretroviral therapy combinations with

and without protease inhibitors. J Acquir Immune Defic Syndr 2002; 30:187–190.

129. Croxson TS, Chapman WE, Miller LK, et al. Changes in the hypothalamic-pituitary gonadal axis in human immunodeficiency virus-infected homosexual men. J Clin Endocrinol Metab 1989; 68:317–321.

130. Sellmeyer DE, Grunfeld C. Endocrine and metabolic disturbances in human immunodeficiency virus infection and the acquired immune deficiency syndrome. Endocr Rev 1996; 17:518–532.

131. Newshan G, Taylor B, Gold R. Sexual functioning in ambulatory men with HIV/AIDS. Int J STD AIDS 1998; 9:672–676.

132. Liu PY, Handelsman DJ. Androgen therapy in nongonadal disease. In: Nieschlag E, Behre HM, eds. Testosterone: Action, Deficiency and Substitution. 3rd ed. Cambridge: Cambridge University Press, 2004: 445–449.

133. Muirhead GJ, Wulff MB, Fielding A, et al. Pharmacokinetic interactions between sildenafil and saquinavir/ritonavir. Br J Clin Pharmacol 2000; 50:99–107.

134. Kell P, Sadeghi-Nejad H, Price D. An ethical dilemma: erectile dysfunction in the HIV-positive patient: to treat or not to treat. Int J STD AIDS 2002; 13: 355–357.

135. Fletcher EC, Martin RJ. Sexual dysfunction and erectile impotence in chronic obstructive pulmonary disease. Chest 1982; 81:413–421.

136. Aasebo U, Gyltnes A, Bremnes RM, et al. Reversal of sexual impotence in male patients with chronic obstructive pulmonary disease and hypoxemia with long term oxygen therapy. J Steroid Biochem Mol Biol 1993; 46:799–803.

137. Ibanez M, Aguilar JJ, Maderal MA, et al. Sexuality in chronic respiratory failure: coincidences and divergences between patient and primary caregiver. Respir Med 2001; 95:975–979.

138. Schonhofer B, Von Sydow K, Bucher T, et al. Sexuality in patients with noninvasive mechanical ventilation due to chronic respiratory failure. Am J Respir Crit Care Med 2001; 164:1612–1617.

139. Kamischke A, Kemper DE, Castel MA, et al. Testosterone levels in men with chronic obstructive pulmonary disease with or without glucocorticoid therapy. Eur Respir J 1998; 11:41–45.

140. Semple PD, Beastall GH, Watson WS, et al. Hypothalamic-pituitary dysfunction in respiratory hypoxia. Thorax 1981; 36:605–609.

141. Semple PD, Beastall GH, Brown TM, et al. Sex hormone suppression and sexual impotence in hypoxic pulmonary fibrosis. Thorax 1984; 39:46–51.

142. Casaburi R, Bhasin S, Cosentino L, et al. Effects of testosterone and resistance training in men with chronic obstructive pulmonary disease. Am J Respir Crit Care Med 2004; 170:870–878.

143. Svartberg J, Aasebo U, Hjalmarsen A, et al. Testosterone treatment improves body composition and sexual function in men with COPD, in a 6-month

randomized controlled trial. Respir Med 2004; 98: 906–913.

144. Hirshkowitz M, Karacan I, Arcasoy MO, et al. Prevalence of sleep apnea in men with erectile dysfunction. Urology 1990; 36:232–234.

145. Fanfulla F, Malaguti S, Montagna T, et al. Erectile dysfunction in men with obstructive sleep apnea: an early sign of nerve involvement. Sleep 2000; 23:775–781.

146. Margel D, Cohen M, Livne PM, et al. Severe, but not mild, obstructive sleep apnea syndrome is associated with erectile dysfunction. Urology 2004; 63: 545–549.

147. Seftel AD, Strohl KP, Loye TL, et al. Erectile dysfunction and symptoms of sleep disorders. Sleep 2002; 25:643–647.

148. Glass AR, Swerdloff RS, Bray GA, et al. Low serum testosterone and sex hormone binding globulin in massively obese men. J Clin Endocrinol Metabol 1977; 45:1211–1219.

149. Grunstein RR, Handelsman DJ, Lawrence SJ, et al. Neuroendocrine dysfunction in sleep apnea: reversal by continuous positive airways pressure therapy. J Clin Endocrinol Metab 1989; 68:352–358.

150. Luboshitzky R, Aviv A, Hefetz A, et al. Decreased pituitary-gonadal secretion in men with obstructive sleep apnea. J Clin Endocrinol Metab 2002; 87: 3394–3398.

151. Brooks B, Cistulli PA, Borkman M, et al. Obstructive sleep apnea in obese noninsulin-dependent diabetic patients: effect of continuous positive airway pressure treatment on insulin responsiveness. J Clin Endocrinol Metabol 1994; 79:1681–1685.

152. Meston N, Davies RJ, Mullins R, et al. Endocrine effects of nasal continuous positive airway pressure in male patients with obstructive sleep apnoea. J Intern Med 2003; 254: 447–454.

153. Karacan I, Karatas M. Erectile dysfunction in sleep apnea and response to CPAP. J Sex Marital Ther 1995; 21:239–247.

154. Nieto FJ, Herrington DM, Redline S, et al. Sleep apnea and markers of vascular endothelial function in a large community sample of older adults. Am J Respir Crit Care Med 2004; 169:354–360.

155. Nieto FJ, Young TB, Lind BK, et al. Association of sleep-disordered breathing, sleep apnea, and hypertension in a large community-based study. Sleep Heart Health Study. JAMA 2000; 283:1829–1836.

156. Mayer P, Dematteis M, Pepin JL, et al. Peripheral neuropathy in sleep apnea. A tissue marker of the severity of nocturnal desaturation. Am J Respir Crit Care Med 1999; 159:213–219.

157. Bona G, Marinello D, Oderda G. Mechanisms of abnormal puberty in coeliac disease. Horm Res 2002; 57(suppl 2):63–65.

158. Farthing MJR, Edwards CRW, Rees LH, et al. Male gonadal dysfunction in coeliac disease: 1. Sexual dysfunction, infertility, and semen quality. Gut 1982; 23:608–614.

159. Farthing MJR, Rees LH, Edwards CRW, et al. Male gonadal dysfunction in coeliac disease: 2. Sex hormones. Gut 1983; 24:127–135.

160. Farthing MJR, Rees LH, Dawson AM. Male gonadal dysfunction in coeliac disease: 3. Pituitary regulation. Clinical Endocrinology 1983; 19:661–671.

161. Green JRB, Goble HL, Edwards CRW, et al. Reversible insensitivity to androgens in men with untreated gluten enteropathy. Lancet 1977; 1: 280–282.

162. Brock GB, Lue TF. Drug-induced male sexual dysfunction. An update. Drug Saf 1993; 8:414–426.

163. Moody GA, Mayberry JF. Perceived sexual dysfunction amongst patients with inflammatory bowel disease. Digestion 1993; 54:256–260.

164. Fass R, Fullerton S, Naliboff B, et al. Sexual dysfunction in patients with irritable bowel syndrome and non-ulcer dyspepsia. Digestion 1998; 59:79–85.

165. Bauer JJ, Gelernt IM, Salky B, et al. Sexual dysfunction following proctocolectomy for benign disease of the colon and rectum. Ann Surg 1983; 197:363–367.

166. Yeager ES, Van Heerden JA. Sexual dysfunction following proctocolectomy and abdominoperineal resection. Ann Surg 1980; 191:169–170.

167. Quah HM, Jayne DG, Eu KW, et al. Bladder and sexual dysfunction following laparoscopically assisted and conventional open mesorectal resection for cancer. Br J Surg 2002; 89:1551–1556.

168. Lindsey I, George B, Kettlewell M, et al. Randomized, double-blind, placebo-controlled trial of sildenafil (Viagra) for erectile dysfunction after rectal excision for cancer and inflammatory bowel disease. Dis Colon Rectum 2002; 45:727–732.

169. Van Thiel DH, Lester R, Sherins RJ. Hypogonadism in alcoholic liver disease: evidence for a double defect. Gastroenterology 1974; 67:1188–1199.

170. Handelsman DJ, Strasser S, McDonald JA, et al. Hypothalamic-pituitary testicular function in end-stage non-alcoholic liver disease before and after liver transplantation. Clinical Endocrinology 1995; 43:331–337.

171. Wang YJ, Wu JC, Lee SD, et al. Gonadal dysfunction and changes in sex hormones in postnecrotic cirrhotic men: a matched study with alcoholic cirrhotic men. Hepatogastroenterology 1991; 38:531–534.

172. Kaymakoglu S, Okten A, Cakaloglu Y, et al. Hypogonadism is not related to the etiology of liver cirrhosis. J Gastroenterol 1995; 30:745–750.

173. Lindholm J, Fabricius-Bjerre N, Bahnsen M, et al. Pituitary-testicular function in patients with chronic alcoholism. Eur J Clin Invest 1978; 8:269–272.

174. Schiavi RC, Stimmel BB, Mandeli J, et al. Chronic alcoholism and male sexual function. Am J Psychiatry 1995; 152:1045–1051.

175. Gluud C, Wantzin P, Eriksen J. No effect of oral testosterone treatment on sexual dysfunction in alcoholic cirrhotic men. Gastroenterology 1988; 95:1582–1587.

176. Stremmel W, Niederau C, Berger M, et al. Abnormalities in estrogen, androgen, and insulin metabolism in idiopathic hemochromatosis. Ann N Y Acad Sci 1988; 526:209–223.

177. Barton JC, McDonnell SM, Adams PC, et al. Management of hemochromatosis. Hemochromatosis Management Working Group. Ann Intern Med 1998; 129:932–939.

178. Liu PY, Gebski VJ, Turner L, et al. Predicting pregnancy and spermatogenesis by survival analysis during gonadotropin treatment of gonadotropin deficient infertile men. Human Reproduction 2002; 17:625–633.

179. Tarnacka B, Rodo M, Cichy S, et al. Procreation ability in Wilson's disease. Acta Neurol Scand 2000; 101:395–398.

180. Akil M, Brewer GJ. Psychiatric and behavioral abnormalities in Wilson's disease. Adv Neurol 1995; 65: 171–178.

181. Kidd GS, Glass AR, Vigersky RA. The hypothalamo-pituitary testicular axis in thyrotoxicosis. J Clin Endocrinol Metabol 1979; 48:798–802.

182. Donnelly P, White C. Testicular dysfunction in men with primary hypothyroidism; reversal of hypogonadotrophic hypogonadism with replacement thyroxine. Clin Endocrinol (Oxf) 2000; 52:197–201.

183. Luton JP, Thieblot P, Valcke JC, et al. Reversible gonadotropin deficiency in male Cushing's disease. J Clin Endocrinol Metabol 1977; 45:488–495.

184. Sakakura M, Takebe K, Nakagawa S. Inhibition of luteinizing hormone secretion induced by synthetic LRH by long-term treatment with glucocorticoids in human subjects. J Clin Endocrinol Metab 1975; 40:774–779.

185. MacAdams MR, White RH, Chipps BE. Reduction of serum testosterone levels during chronic glucocorticoid therapy. Ann Intern Med 1986; 104:648–651.

186. Vierhapper H, Nowotny P, Waldhausl W. production rates of testosterone in patients with Cushing's syndrome. Metabolism 2000; 49:229–231.

187. Arlt W, Callies F, van Vlijmen JC, et al. Dehydroepiandrosterone replacement in women with adrenal insufficiency N Engl J Med 1999; 341:1013–1020.

188. Hunt PJ, Gurnell EM, Huppert FA, et al. Improvement in mood and fatigue after dehydroepiandrosterone replacement in Addison's disease in a randomized, double blind trial. J Clin Endocrinol Metab 2000; 85:4650–4656.

189. Hull KL, Harvey S. Growth hormone: roles in male reproduction. Endocrine 2000; 13:243–250.

190. Ezzat S. Living with acromegaly. Endocrinol Metab Clin North Am 1992; 21:753–760.

191. Carani C, Granata AR, Fustini MF, et al. Prolactin and testosterone: their role in male sexual function. Int J Androl 1996; 19:48–54.

192. Meston CM, Frohlich PF. The neurobiology of sexual function. Arch Gen Psychiatry 2000; 57:1012–1030.

193. Kinon BJ, Gilmore JA, Liu H, et al. Prevalence of hyperprolactinemia in schizophrenic patients treated with conventional antipsychotic medications or risperidone. Psychoneuroendocrinology 2003; 28 (suppl 2): 55–68.

194. Halbreich U, Kinon BJ, Gilmore JA, et al. Elevated prolactin levels in patients with schizophrenia: mechanisms and related adverse effects. Psychoneuroendocrinology 2003; 28 (suppl 1):53–67.

195. Bacon CG, Hu FB, Giovannucci E, et al. Association of type and duration of diabetes with erectile dysfunction in a large cohort of men. Diabetes Care 2002; 25: 1458–1463.

196. Vinik AI, Freeman R, Erbas T. Diabetic autonomic neuropathy. Semin Neurol 2003; 23:365–372.

197. Sasaki K, Yoshimura N, Chancellor MB. Implications of diabetes mellitus in urology. Urol Clin North Am 2003; 30:1–12.

198. Klein R, Klein BE, Lee KE, et al. Prevalence of self-reported erectile dysfunction in people with long-term IDDM. Diabetes Care 1996; 19:135–141.

199. Metro MJ, Broderick GA. Diabetes and vascular impotence: does insulin dependence increase the relative severity? Int J Impot Res 1999; 11:87–89.

200. Romeo JH, Seftel AD, Madhun ZT, et al. Sexual function in men with diabetes type 2: association with glycemic control. J Urol 2000; 163:788–791.

201. Hakim LS, Goldstein I. Diabetic sexual dysfunction. Endocrinol Metab Clin North Am 1996; 25: 379–400.

202. Moulik PK, Hardy KJ. Hypertension, anti-hypertensive drug therapy and erectile dysfunction in diabetes. Diabet Med 2003; 20:290–293.

203. Dey J, Shepherd MD. Evaluation and treatment of erectile dysfunction in men with diabetes mellitus. Mayo Clin Proc 2002; 77:276–282.

204. McCulloch DK, Campbell IW, Wu FC, et al. The prevalence of diabetic impotence. Diabetologia 1980; 18:279–283.

205. De Angelis L, Marfella MA, Siniscalchi M, et al. Erectile and endothelial dysfunction in Type diabetes II: a possible link. Diabetologia 2001; 44:1155–1160.

206. Venkateswarlu K, Giraldi A, Zhao W, et al. Potassium channels and human corporeal smooth muscle cell tone: diabetes and relaxation of human corpus cavernosum smooth muscle by adenosine triphosphate sensitive potassium channel openers. J Urol 2002; 168:355–361.

207. Escrig A, Marin R, Abreu P, et al. Changes in mating behavior, erectile function, and nitric oxide levels in penile corpora cavernosa in streptozotocin-diabetic rats. Biol Reprod 2002; 66:185–189.

208. Podlasek CA, Zelner DJ, Bervig TR, et al. Characterization and localization of nitric oxide synthase isoforms in the BB/WOR diabetic rat. J Urol 2001; 166:746–755.

209. Bleustein CB, Eckholdt H, Arezzo JC, et al. Quantitative somatosensory testing of the penis: optimizing the clinical neurological examination. J Urol 2003; 169: 2266–2269.

210. Azadzoi KM, Saenz de Tejada I. Diabetes mellitus impairs neurogenic and endothelium-dependent relaxation of rabbit corpus cavernosum smooth muscle. J Urol 1992; 148:1587–1591.

211. Blanco R, Saenz de Tejada I, Goldstein I, et al. Dysfunctional penile cholinergic nerves in diabetic impotent men. J Urol 1990; 144:278–280.

212. Greene DA, Stevens MJ, Feldman EL. Diabetic neuropathy: scope of the syndrome. Am J Med 1999; 107:2S–8S.

213. Saenz de Tejada I, Goldstein I. Diabetic penile neuropathy. Urol Clin North Am 1988; 15:17–22.

214. Saenz de Tejada I, Goldstein I, Azadzoi K, et al. Impaired neurogenic and endothelium-mediated relaxation of penile smooth muscle from diabetic men with impotence. N Engl J Med 1989; 320:1025–1030.

215. Ari G, Vardi Y, Finberg JP. Nitric oxide and penile erection in streptozotocin-diabetic rats. Clin Sci (Lond) 1999; 96:365–371.

216. El-Sakka AI, Lin CS, Chui RM, et al. Effects of diabetes on nitric oxide synthase and growth factor genes and protein expression in an animal model. Int J Impot Res 1999; 11:123–132.

217. McVary KT, Rathnau CH, McKenna KE. Sexual dysfunction in the diabetic BB/WOR rat: a role of central neuropathy. Am J Physiol 1997; 272:R259–R267.

218. Vernet D, Cai L, Garban H, et al. Reduction of penile nitric oxide synthase in diabetic BB/WORdp (type I) and BBZ/WORdp (type II) rats with erectile dysfunction. Endocrinology 1995; 136:5709–5717.

219. Koppiker N, Boolell M, Price D. Recent advances in the treatment of erectile dysfunction in patients with diabetes mellitus. Endocr Pract 2003; 9:52–63.

220. Pirart J. Diabetes mellitus and its degenerative complications: a prospective study of 4,400 patients observed between 1947 and 1973 (3rd and last part) (author's transl). Diabete Metab 1977; 3:245–256.

221. Graf RJ, Halter JB, Pfeifer MA, et al. Glycemic control and nerve conduction abnormalities in non-insulin-dependent diabetic subjects. Ann Intern Med 1981; 94:307–311.

222. The effect of intensive diabetes therapy on the development and progression of neuropathy. The Diabetes Control and Complications Trial Research Group. Ann Intern Med 1995; 122:561–568.

223. Handelsman DJ, Dong Q. Hypothalamo-pituitary gonadal axis in chronic renal failure. Endocrinol Metabol Clin North Am 1993; 22:145–161.

224. Levy NB. Sexual adjustment to maintenance hemodialysis and renal transplantation: national survey by questionnaire: preliminary report. Trans Am Soc Artif Intern Organs 1973; 19:138–143.

225. Procci WR, Goldstein DA, Adelstein J, et al. Sexual dysfunction in the male patient with uremia: a reappraisal. Kidney Int 1981; 19:317–323.

226. Neto AF, de Freitas Rodrigues MA, Saraiva Fittipaldi JA, et al. The epidemiology of erectile dysfunction and its correlates in men with chronic renal failure on hemodialysis in Londrina, southern Brazil. Int J Impot Res 2002; 14:S19–S26.

227. Rosas SE, Joffe M, Franklin E, et al. Association of decreased quality of life and erectile dysfunction

in hemodialysis patients. Kidney Int 2003; 64: 232–238.

228. Kaufman JM, Hatzichristou DG, Mulhall JP, et al. Impotence and chronic renal failure: a study of the hemodynamic pathophysiology. J Urol 1994; 151:612–618.

229. Zetin M, Stone RA. Effects of zinc in chronic hemodialysis. Clin Nephrol 1980; 13:20–25.

230. Brook AC, Johnston DG, Ward MK, et al. Absence of a therapeutic effect of zinc in the sexual dysfunction of haemodialysed patients. Lancet 1980; 2:618–620.

231. Mahajan SK, Abbasi AA, Prasad AS, et al. Effect of oral zinc therapy on gonadal function in hemodialysis patients. A double-blind study. Ann Intern Med 1982; 97:357–361.

232. Levy NB. Sexual dysfunctions of hemodialysis patients. Clin Exp Dial Apheresis 1983; 7:275–288.

233. Abram HS, Hester LR, Sheridan WF, et al. Sexual functioning in patients with chronic renal failure. J Nerv Ment Dis 1975; 160:220–226.

234. Cerqueira J, Moraes M, Glina S. Erectile dysfunction: prevalence and associated variables in patients with chronic renal failure. Int J Impot Res 2002; 14:65–71.

235. Toorians AW, Janssen E, Laan E, et al. Chronic renal failure and sexual functioning: clinical status versus objectively assessed sexual response. Nephrol Dial Transplant 1997; 12:2654–2663.

236. Schover LR, Novick AC, Steinmuller DR, et al. Sexuality, fertility, and renal transplantation: a survey of survivors. J Sex Marital Ther 1990; 16:3–13.

237. Abdel-Hamid IA, Eraky I, Fouda MA, et al. Role of penile vascular insufficiency in erectile dysfunction in renal transplant recipients. Int J Impot Res 2002; 14:32–37.

238. Juergense PH, Botev R, Wuerth D, et al. Erectile dysfunction in chronic peritoneal dialysis patients: incidence and treatment with sildenafil. Perit Dial Int 2001; 21:355–359.

239. Chen J, Mabjeesh NJ, Greenstein A, et al. Clinical efficacy of sildenafil in patients on chronic dialysis. J Urol 2001; 165:819–821.

240. Seibel I, Poli De Figueiredo CE, Teloken C, et al. Efficacy of oral sildenafil in hemodialysis patients with erectile dysfunction. J Am Soc Nephrol 2002; 13:2770–2775.

241. YenicerioGlu Y, Kefi A, Aslan G, et al. Efficacy and safety of sildenafil for treating erectile dysfunction in patients on dialysis. BJU Int 2002; 90:442–445.

242. Prieto Castro RM, Anglada Curado FJ, Regueiro Lopez JC, et al. Treatment with sildenafil citrate in renal transplant patients with erectile dysfunction. BJU Int 2001; 88:241–243.

243. Espinoza R, Melchor JL, Gracida C. Sildenafil (Viagra) in kidney transplant recipients with erectile dysfunction. Transplant Proc 2002; 34:408–409.

244. Barrou B, Cuzin B, Malavaud B, et al. Early experience with sildenafil for the treatment of erectile dysfunction in renal transplant recipients. Nephrol Dial Transplant 2003; 18:411–417.

245. Pirildar T, Muezzinoglu T, Pirildar S. Sexual function in ankylosing spondylitis: a study of 65 men. J Urol 2004; 171:1598–1600.

246. Elst P, Sybesma T, van der Stadt RJ, et al. Sexual problems in rheumatoid arthritis and ankylosing spondylitis. Arthritis Rheum 1984; 27:217–220.

247. Gordon D, Beastall GH, Thomson JA, et al. Androgenic status and sexual function in males with rheumatoid arthritis and ankylosing spondylitis. Q J Med 1986; 60:671–679.

248. Lally EV, Jimenez SA. Impotence in progressively systemic sclerosis. Ann Intern Med 1981; 95:150–153.

249. Nowlin NS, Brick JE, Weaver DJ, et al. Impotence in scleroderma. Ann Intern Med 1986; 104:794–798.

250. Rossman B, Zorgniotti AW. Progressive systemic sclerosis (scleroderma) and impotence. Urology 1989; 33: 189–192.

251. Nehra A, Hall SJ, Basile G, et al. Systemic sclerosis and impotence: a clinicopathological correlation. J Urol 1995; 153:1140–1146.

252. Lotfi MA, Varga J, Hirsch IH. Erectile dysfunction in systemic sclerosis. Urology 1995; 45:879–881.

253. Hong P, Pope JE, Ouimet JM, et al. Erectile dysfunction associated with scleroderma: a case-control study of men with scleroderma and rheumatoid arthritis. J Rheumatol 2004; 31:508–513.

254. Johnson S, Iazzetta J, Dewar C. Severe Raynaud's phenomenon with yohimbine therapy for erectile dysfunction. J Rheumatol 2003; 30:2503–2505.

255. Schover LR, Jensen SB. Sexuality and Chronic Illness. New York: Guildford Press, 1988.

256. Ferguson K, Figley B. Sexuality and rheumatic disease. A prospective study. Sexuality Disability 1979; 2: 130–138.

257. Majerovitz SD, Revenson TA. Sexuality and rheumatic disease: the significance of gender. Arthritis Care Res 1994; 7:29–34.

258. Kraaimaat FW, Bakker AH, Janssen E, et al. Intrusiveness of rheumatoid arthritis on sexuality in male and female patients living with a spouse. Arthritis Care Res 1996; 9:120–125.

259. Packham JC, Hall MA. Long-term follow-up of 246 adults with juvenile idiopathic arthritis: social function, relationships and sexual activity. Rheumatology (Oxf) 2002; 41:1440–1443.

260. Kreutzer JS, Zasler ND. Psychosexual consequences of traumatic brain injury: methodology and preliminary findings. Brain Inj 1989; 3:177–186.

261. Sandel ME, Williams KS, Dellapietra L, et al. Sexual functioning following traumatic brain injury. Brain Inj 1996; 10:719–728.

262. Aloni A, Keren O, Cohen M, et al. Incidence of sexual dysfunction in TBI patients during the early post-traumatic in-patient rehabilitation phase. Brain Inj 1999; 13:89–97.

263. Nickels JL, Schneider WN, Dombovy ML, et al. Clinical use of amantadine in brain injury rehabilitation. Brain Inj 1994; 8:709–718.

264. Britton KR. Medroxyprogesterone in the treatment of aggressive hypersexual behavior in traumatic brain injury. Brain Inj 1998; 12:703–707.

265. Boemers TM, van Gool JD, de Jong TP. Tethered spinal cord: the effect of neurosurgery on the lower urinary tract and male sexual function. Br J Urol 1995; 76:747–751.

266. Amelar RD, Dubin L. Impotence in the low-back syndrome. JAMA 1971; 216:520.

267. Tay EC, Chacha PB. Midline prolapse of a lumbar intervertebral disc with compression of the cauda equina. J Bone Joint Surg Br 1979; 61:43–46.

268. Choy DS. Early relief of erectile dysfunction after laser decompression of herniated lumbar disc. J Clin Laser Med Surg 1999; 17:25–27.

269. Biering-Sorensen F, Sonksen J. Sexual function in spinal cord lesioned men. Spinal Cord 2001; 39:455–470.

270. Bors E, Comarr AE. Neurological disturbances of sexual function with special reference to 569 patients with spinal cord injury. Urological Survey 1960; 10:191–222.

271. Siosteen A, Lundqvist C, Blomstrand C, et al. Sexual ability, activity, attitudes and satisfaction as part of adjustment in spinal cord-injured subjects. Paraplegia 1990; 28:285–295.

272. Hultling C, Giuliano F, Quirk F, et al. Quality of life in patients with spinal cord injury receiving Viagra (sildenafil citrate) for the treatment of erectile dysfunction. Spinal Cord 2000; 38:363–370.

273. Sjogren K, Damber JE, Liliequist B. Sexuality after stroke with hemiplegia. I. Aspects of sexual function. Scand J Rehabil Med 1983; 15:55–61.

274. Monga TN, Lawson JS, Inglis J. Sexual dysfunction in stroke patients. Arch Phys Med Rehabil 1986; 67:19–22.

275. Boldrini P, Basaglia N, Calanca MC. Sexual changes in hemiparetic patients. Arch Phys Med Rehabil 1991; 72:202–207.

276. Korpelainen JT, Hiltunen P, Myllyla VV. Moclobemide-induced hypersexuality in patients with stroke and Parkinson's disease. Clin Neuropharmacol 1998; 21:251–254.

277. Wiig EH. Counselling for the adult aphasic for sexual readjustment. Rehabil Couns Bull 1973:110–119.

278. Kalliomaki JL, Markkanen TK, Mustonen VA. Sexual behavior after cerebral vascular accident. A study on patients below the age of 60 years. Fertil Steril 1961; 12:156–158.

279. Coslett HB, Heilman KM. Male sexual function. Impairment after right hemisphere stroke. Arch Neurol 1986; 43:1036–1039.

280. Saunders M, Rawson M. Sexuality in male epileptics. J Neurol Sci 1970; 10:577–583.

281. Dansky LV, Andermann E, Andermann F. Marriage and fertility in epileptic patients. Epilepsia 1980; 21:261–271.

282. Morrell MJ, Sperling MR, Stecker M, et al. Sexual dysfunction in partial epilepsy: a deficit in physiologic sexual arousal. Neurology 1994; 44:243–247.

283. Guldner GT, Morrell MJ. Nocturnal penile tumescence and rigidity evaluation in men with epilepsy. Epilepsia 1996; 37:1211–1214.

284. Jensen P, Jensen SB, Sorensen PS, et al. Sexual dysfunction in male and female patients with epilepsy: a study of 86 outpatients. Arch Sex Behav 1990; 19:1–14.

285. Christianson SA, Silfvenius H, Saisa J, et al. Life satisfaction and sexuality in patients operated for epilepsy. Acta Neurol Scand 1995; 92:1–6.

286. Herzog AG. Reproductive endocrine considerations and hormonal therapy for men with epilepsy. Epilepsia 1991; 32:S34–S37.

287. Duncan S, Blacklaw J, Beastall GH, et al. Antiepileptic drug therapy and sexual function in men with epilepsy. Epilepsia 1999; 40:197–204.

288. El-Khayat HA, Shatla HM, Ali GK, et al. Physical and hormonal profile of male sexual development in epilepsy. Epilepsia 2003; 44:447–452.

289. Rattya J, Turkka J, Pakarinen AJ, et al. Reproductive effects of valproate, carbamazepine, and oxcarbazepine in men with epilepsy. Neurology 2001; 56: 31–36.

290. Koller WC, Vetere-Overfield B, Williamson A, et al. Sexual dysfunction in Parkinson's disease. Clin Neuropharmacol 1990; 13:461–463.

291. Singer C, Weiner WJ, Sanchez-Ramos JR. Autonomic dysfunction in men with Parkinson's disease. Eur Neurol 1992; 32:134–140.

292. Wermuth L, Stenager E. Sexual problems in young patients with Parkinson's disease. Acta Neurol Scand 1995; 91:453–455.

293. Sakakibara R, Shinotoh H, Uchiyama T, et al. Questionnaire-based assessment of pelvic organ dysfunction in Parkinson's disease. Auton Neurosci 2001; 92:76–85.

294. Brown RG, Jahanshahi M, Quinn N, et al. Sexual function in patients with Parkinson's disease and their partners. J Neurol Neurosurg Psychiatry 1990; 53:480–486.

295. Andersson KE, Wagner G. Physiology of penile erection. Physiol Rev 1995; 75:191–236.

296. Nehra A, Barrett DM, Moreland RB. Pharmacotherapeutic advances in the treatment of erectile dysfunction. Mayo Clin Proc 1999; 74:709–721.

297. Moreland RB, Hsieh G, Nakane M, et al. The biochemical and neurologic basis for the treatment of male erectile dysfunction. J Pharmacol Exp Ther 2001; 296:225–234.

298. Okun MS, McDonald WM, DeLong MR. Refractory nonmotor symptoms in male patients with Parkinson disease due to testosterone deficiency: a common unrecognized comorbidity. Arch Neurol 2002; 59:807–811.

299. Okun MS, Walter BL, McDonald WM, et al. Beneficial effects of testosterone replacement for the nonmotor

symptoms of Parkinson disease. Arch Neurol 2002; 59:1750–1753.

300. Pohanka M, Kanovsky P, Bares M, et al. Pergolide mesylate can improve sexual dysfunction in patients with Parkinson's disease: the results of an open, prospective, 6-month follow-up. Eur J Neurol 2004; 11:483–488.

301. Brown E, Brown GM, Kofman O, et al. Sexual function and affect in parkinsonian men treated with L-dopa. Am J Psychiatry 1978; 135:1552–1555.

302. Zesiewicz TA, Helal M, Hauser RA. Sildenafil citrate (Viagra) for the treatment of erectile dysfunction in men with Parkinson's disease. Mov Disord 2000; 15:305–308.

303. Raffaele R, Vecchio I, Giammusso B, et al. Efficacy and safety of fixed-dose oral sildenafil in the treatment of sexual dysfunction in depressed patients with idiopathic Parkinson's disease. Eur Urol 2002; 41: 382–386.

304. Beck RO, Betts CD, Fowler CJ. Genitourinary dysfunction in multiple system atrophy: clinical features and treatment in 62 cases. J Urol 1994; 151:1336–1341.

305. Hodder J. Shy Drager syndrome. Axone 1997; 18: 75–79.

306. Kirchhof K, Apostolidis AN, Mathias CJ, et al. Erectile and urinary dysfunction may be the presenting features in patients with multiple system atrophy: a retrospective study. Int J Impot Res 2003; 15: 293–298.

307. Dewhurst K, Oliver JE, McKnight AL. Socio-psychiatric consequences of Huntington's disease. Br J Psychiatry 1970; 116:255–258.

308. Fedoroff JP, Peyser C, Franz ML, et al. Sexual disorders in Huntington's disease. J Neuropsychiatry Clin Neurosci 1994; 6:147–153.

309. Morris M. Dementia and cognitive changes in Huntington's disease. Adv Neurol 1995; 65:187–200.

310. Schoenfeld M, Myers RH, Cupples LA, Berkman B, Sax DS, Clark E. Increased rate of suicide among patients with Huntington's disease. J Neurol Neurosurg Psychiatry 1984; 47:1283–1287.

311. Di Maio L, Squitieri F, Napolitano G, et al. Suicide risk in Huntington's disease. J Med Genet 1993; 30:293–295.

312. Baliko L, Csala B, Czopf J. Suicide in Hungarian Huntington's disease patients. Neuroepidemiology 2004; 23:258–260.

313. Arciniegas DB, Anderson CA. Suicide in neurologic illness. Curr Treat Options Neurol 2002; 4:457–468.

314. Lipe H, Schultz A, Bird TD. Risk factors for suicide in Huntington's disease: a retrospective case controlled study. Am J Med Genet 1993; 48:231–233.

315. Comings DE. Role of genetic factors in human sexual behavior based on studies of Tourette syndrome and ADHD probands and their relatives. Am J Med Genet 1994; 54:227–241.

316. Lombroso PJ, Scahill LD, Chappell PB, et al. Tourette's syndrome: a multigenerational, neuropsychiatric disorder. Adv Neurol 1995; 65:305–318.

317. Sandyk R. Naltrexone suppresses abnormal sexual behavior in Tourette's syndrome. Int J Neurosci 1988; 43:107–110.

318. Bakke A, Myhr KM, Gronning M, et al. Bladder, bowel and sexual dysfunction in patients with multiple sclerosis—a cohort study. Scand J Urol Nephrol Suppl 1996; 179:61–66.

319. Lilius HG, Valtonen EJ, Wikstrom J. Sexual problems in patients suffering from multiple sclerosis. J Chronic Dis 1976; 29:643–647.

320. Minderhoud JM, Leemhuis JG, Kremer J, et al. Sexual disturbances arising from multiple sclerosis. Acta Neurol Scand 1984; 70:299–306.

321. Valleroy ML, Kraft GH. Sexual dysfunction in multiple sclerosis. Arch Phys Med Rehabil 1984; 65: 125–128.

322. Mattson D, Petrie M, Srivastava DK, et al. Multiple sclerosis. Sexual dysfunction and its response to medications. Arch Neurol 1995; 52:862–868.

323. Zorzon M, Zivadinov R, Bosco A, et al. Sexual dysfunction in multiple sclerosis: a case-control study. I. Frequency and comparison of groups. Mult Scler 1999; 5:418–427.

324. Barak Y, Achiron A, Elizur A, et al. Sexual dysfunction in relapsing-remitting multiple sclerosis: magnetic resonance imaging, clinical, and psychological correlates. J Psychiatry Neurosci 1996; 21:255–258.

325. Zivadinov R, Zorzon M, Locatelli L, et al. Sexual dysfunction in multiple sclerosis: a MRI, neurophysiological and urodynamic study. J Neurol Sci 2003; 210:73–76.

326. Goldstein I, Siroky MB, Sax DS, et al. Neurourologic abnormalities in multiple sclerosis. J Urol 1982; 128: 541–545.

327. Zivadinov R, Zorzon M, Bosco A, et al. Sexual dysfunction in multiple sclerosis: II. Correlation analysis. Mult Scler 1999; 5:428–431.

328. Anderson F, Bardach JL. Sexuality and neuromuscular disease: a pilot study. Int Rehabil Med 1983; 5: 21–26.

329. Wasner M, Bold U, Vollmer TC, et al. Sexuality in patients with amyotrophic lateral sclerosis and their partners. J Neurol 2004; 251:445–448.

330. Greenland KJ, Zajac JD. Kennedy's disease: pathogenesis and clinical approaches. Intern Med J 2004; 34:279–286.

331. Hallen O. Disturbances of potency and libido in progressive muscular dystrophy (author's transl). J Neurovisc Relat 1971; (suppl 10):573–579.

332. Zavadenko NN. Study of the hypophyseal-gonadal system in patients with hereditary muscular dystrophy. Zh Nevropatol Psikhiatr Im S S Korsakova 1990; 90:25–28.

333. McDougall AJ, McLeod JG. Autonomic neuropathy: I. Clinical features, investigation, pathophysiology, and treatment. J Neurol Sci 1996; 137:79–88.

334. McDougall AJ, McLeod JG. Autonomic neuropathy: II. Specific peripheral neuropathies. J Neurol Sci 1996; 138:1–13.

335. Nukada H, Pollock M, Haas LF. The clinical spectrum and morphology of type hereditary II sensory neuropathy. Brain 1982; 105 (Pt 4):647–665.

336. Bird TD, Lipe HP, Crabtree LD. Impotence associated with the Charcot–Marie-Tooth syndrome. Eur Neurol 1994; 34:155–157.

337. Vodusek DB, Zidar J. Pudendal nerve involvement in patients with hereditary motor and sensory neuropathy. Acta Neurol Scand 1987; 76:457–460.

338. Powers JM, Schaumburg HH. A fatal cause of sexual inadequacy in men: adreno-leukodystrophy. J Urol 1980; 124:583–585.

339. Sakakibara R, Hattori T, Fukutake T, et al. Micturitional disturbance in a patient with adrenomyeloneuropathy (AMN). Neurourol Urodyn 1998; 17:207–212.

340. Andersson R, Hofer PA. Genitourinary disturbances in familial and sporadic cases of primary amyloidosis with polyneuropathy. Acta Med Scand 1974; 195:49–58.

341. Kelly JJ Jr, Kyle RA, O'Brien PC, et al. The natural history of peripheral neuropathy in primary systemic amyloidosis. Ann Neurol 1979; 6:1–7.

342. Yamamoto T, Matsunaga K, Ohnishi A, et al. A late onset familial amyloidotic polyneuropathy (FAP) with a novel variant transthyretin characterized by a basic-for-acidic amino acid substitution (Glu61—>Lys). Rinsho Shinkeigaku 1996; 36:1065–1068.

343. Li Y, Guo Y, Ikeda S, et al. Familial amyloid polyneuropathy—clinical report of a family. Chin Med Sci J 1996; 11:113–116.

14

Sexual Dysfunction in Males with Diabetes

Michael H. Cummings and Duncan L. Browne
Academic Department of Diabetes, Queen Alexandra Hospital, Portsmouth, U.K.

□ INTRODUCTION

The prevalence of diabetes mellitus continues to increase worldwide, and it is estimated that 3% of the population suffer from this metabolic disorder (1). The majority (approximately 85–90%) have a clinical diagnosis of type 2 diabetes, characterized initially by hyperinsulinemia, insulin resistance, and finally developing into pancreatic β-cell failure. Conversely, type 1 diabetes often presents with acute metabolic upset following autoimmune destruction of pancreatic β-cells necessitating insulin replacement from diagnosis. The burden of diabetes care for the individual, caregivers, and health-care providers lies in the chronic sequelae of this condition, given the susceptibility to both macrovascular and pathognomonic microvascular complications (2). Psychological changes frequently accompany limitations imposed by diabetes following its diagnosis, treatment, or development of complications. It is not surprising, therefore, that this condition can have a profound effect upon sexual function, although until the last two decades, this was not well recognized.

This chapter will review evidence both in animal models of diabetes and in humans that contributes to our understanding of the development of sexual dysfunction in diabetic males per se. Erectile dysfunction (ED) represents the most commonly encountered sexual problem in diabetic men, but disorders of ejaculation and fertility are also recognized. Although both major forms of diabetes through chronic hyperglycemia and other metabolic abnormalities (or its treatment) may ultimately result in sexual dysfunction, the majority of research has focused upon males with type 2 diabetes. Given the insidious nature of the latter disease, it is recognized that perhaps 20% of diabetic patients may present at diagnosis with a vascular complication of the disease including ED. It is unusual, however, for type 1 diabetic patients to develop vascular complications within the first five years of diagnosis.

□ ERECTILE DYSFUNCTION
Epidemiology

The prevalence of ED in diabetic males has varied between studies and is explained in part by differing methodologies used to define the problem, the populations examined, and patient selection within that population; however, the prevalence is clearly higher in diabetic compared with nondiabetic males. Many investigators have reported an overall prevalence between a third and half of the diabetic male population studied (3–9). This compares with a prevalence of 0.1% to 18% in the nondiabetic control population (10). No difference was found in the prevalence of ED between type 1 and 2 diabetic patients (11), although assessment of the etiology suggested that vascular lesions were more common in insulin-dependent compared with non–insulin-dependent diabetic impotent men (12).

Diabetes has been implicated in the pathogenesis of 40% of patients presenting with ED (13). The frequency of new cases of diabetes, determined by a glucose tolerance test, has been reported as 11% to 12% (14,15) and impaired glucose tolerance 4.2% (14). It appears therefore that the screening tests for diabetes in all men presenting with ED would be justified.

A study of impotent males attending a diabetic clinic identified the five most important associations with development of ED: age, treatment with insulin or oral hypoglycemic agents, retinopathy, symptomatic peripheral neuropathy, and symptomatic autonomic neuropathy (6). The authors further concluded that the presence of ischemic heart disease, nephropathy, and poor glycemic control may also be associated with diabetic ED. A five-year follow-up of this diabetic population revealed an additional 28% had become impotent, whereas only 9% of impotent men had regained potency thus confirming the progressive and nonreversible nature of the problem (16). Subsequent development of ED in this group was most strongly linked to patient age, alcohol intake, initial glycemic control, intermittent claudication, and retinopathy.

Overview of the Pathophysiological Mechanisms that May Lead to ED in Diabetic Males

Part I of this textbook has identified the complex nature by which metabolic, neural, vascular, local, hormonal, psychological, and other factors act synergistically to facilitate tumescence. It is now recognized that many of these factors may be disrupted by diabetes, leading to either functional or structural changes within the tissues responsible for achieving an erection. These abnormalities are summarized in Figure 1. Commonly, diabetic patients have multiple factors that contribute to the development of ED, many of which

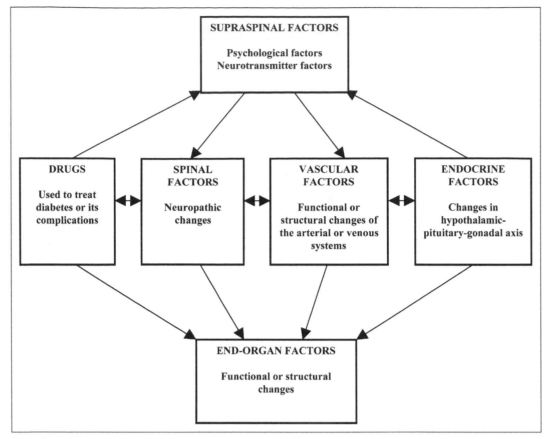

Figure 1   Factors in the diabetic male that may contribute to the development of erectile dysfunction.

may not be evident on clinical examination or from routine investigation, but it is rarely necessary to ascertain the precise organic mechanisms leading to ED, since such knowledge is unlikely to significantly affect the treatment approach for the diabetic patient (17).

Neurological Factors
Epidemiology of Neuropathic Diabetic ED

Neuropathy has been implicated in the pathogenesis of diabetic ED in up to 82% of patients (18). Conversely, the development of ED is strongly associated with the presence of neuropathy (16). In contrast to vasculopathy, neuropathy seems to predominantly cause ED in diabetic men under the age of 60 (19).

Pathophysiology of Diabetic Neuropathy

The sympathetic, parasympathetic, somatic sensory, and central nervous systems are all required for the control of male sexual function and each may be affected by diabetes. Diabetic neuropathy is a heterogeneous disease with varying pathologies (20). Metabolic abnormalities and microvascular insufficiency combine to promote disturbances of nerve function and structural changes characteristic of diabetic neuropathy. Hyperglycemia stimulates protein kinase C activity, aldose reductase pathways, and nonenzymatic glycosylation. This results in oxidative stress

and subsequent nerve damage including axonopathy and demyelination (20). In parallel with diabetic ED, diabetic neuropathy is usually progressive and related to glycemic control (21,22).

Contribution of Neuropathy to Diabetic ED

Numerous studies implicate neuropathy in the pathogenesis of diabetic ED (6,19,20); however, the extent of the neuropathic contribution depends on the tool used to assess nerve function (Table 1) (23). Studies often use indirect instead of direct measures of nerve function. Also, impotent diabetic men are compared with healthy nondiabetic subjects rather than potent

Table 1   Tools Used to Investigate the Contribution of Neuropathy to the Development of Diabetic Erectile Dysfunction

Autonomic function
Deep breathing, orthostatic hypotension, and others
Urodynamics
Thermal thresholds
Isolated nerve-fiber stimulation
Neurotransmitter level measurements
Somatic function
Conduction velocities/amplitude of dorsal nerve of penis
Somatosensory-evoked potentials of pudendal nerve
Corpus cavernous electromyography
Bulbocavernous reflex latency/sacral reflex latency
Electromyographic detection of perineal floor muscles

diabetic men. The role of altered somatic sensation in the etiology of diabetic ED is probably minimal. While somatic sensation is involved in sustaining an erection during coitus, a pure sensory neuropathic cause is unusual in diabetes. Reduced conduction velocity of the dorsal nerve of the penis has been demonstrated in diabetes, but a relationship with diabetic ED is less clear (24,25). Similarly, measurement of bulbocavernous reflex latency (BCR) has frequently been used to investigate ED, but results have been conflicting. Some studies have found that BCR discriminated between potent and impotent diabetic men (26), but one study found BCR was unaffected in 50% of men with diabetic neuropathic ED (27). Furthermore, other studies found no relationship between BCR and potency in diabetic men (28,29). Since BCR is predominantly a measure of somatic penile innervation and erections are largely controlled by the autonomic nervous system, the value of BCR in assessment of diabetic ED remains controversial. (For more information on BCR and other neurological evaluations, see Chapter 26.)

In contrast, a wealth of evidence supports the role of autonomic dysfunction in diabetic ED. Firstly, symptoms of autonomic dysfunction have been shown consistently to predict ED (6,30). Secondly, several objective neurophysiological tests have demonstrated abnormalities in autonomic function in association with diabetic ED. Diabetic patients with ED are twice as likely as potent diabetic controls to have abnormal deep breathing tests—an indicator of parasympathetic function (31). Interestingly, no difference between the two groups has been found for tests of sympathetic function. Recent work has shown a preferential involvement of small unmyelinated sensory fibers–mediating axon-reflex vasodilation in the limbs of patients with diabetic ED (27). Thermal sensation, another measure of unmyelinated nerve and autonomic function, has been found to be abnormal in association with diabetic ED (32). Studies in diabetic males have shown urinary flow rates to be a subtle test of autonomic function, that is, abnormal in 24 out of 25 diabetic impotent men, compared with 2 out of 26 diabetic potent men (29). In animal studies where diabetes was induced, although anatomical integrity of the penile autonomic system was preserved, autonomic neurotransmitter norepinephrine was found at reduced levels (33,34). Finally, rapid eye movement sleep studies in conjunction with sleep tumescence measurements suggest that central autonomic dysregulation may be a contributing factor to ED in diabetic men (35).

Vascular Factors
Role of Vascular Disease in ED

An erection is essentially a vascular event requiring an intact penile circulation (see Chapters 3 and 10). Given alterations in both the macro- and the microcirculation of diabetic men, abnormalities in the penile circulation have frequently been implicated in the pathophysiology of diabetic ED. The penile blood supply may be impaired by either diffuse atherosclerosis or isolated external iliac disease resulting in "pelvic steal" syndrome causing blood to be diverted away from the pelvis (36). Additionally, penile veno-occlusive dysfunction and resulting cavernosal fibrosis are probably secondary to arterial disease (37).

Diabetes is associated with accelerated atherosclerosis resulting in a two- to fourfold increase in cardiovascular mortality and with similar deleterious changes being observed in the peripheral circulation. Diabetic microangiopathy is characterized by the thickening of the capillary basement membrane, which is pathognomonic of diabetic retinopathy. Diabetic retinopathy has itself been linked with the development of ED (16). Moreover, vascular endothelial dysfunction, a reputed precursor of atherosclerosis, has been reported in both type 1 (38) and type 2 (39) diabetes, while abnormalities in the penile endothelial function of impotent men have also been reported (40).

Pathophysiology of Diabetic Vasculopathy

Type 2 diabetes is inexorably linked with the metabolic syndrome of insulin resistance, hypertension, and dyslipidemia, all independent vascular risk factors predisposing to atherosclerosis. Untreated hypertension per se is associated with a threefold increase of ED and may often precede the development of diabetes. The pathophysiology of vascular disease in type 1 diabetes is less clear, although hyperemic changes in response to the metabolic abnormalities (41) and other consequences of prolonged hyperglycemia—including free radicals, advanced glycosylation end-products (AGEs), and the polyol pathway—have all been implicated (42). The etiology of vascular endothelial dysfunction in the diabetic circulation is analogous to the alterations in the availability of nitric oxide (NO) and other vasoactive substances within the corporal smooth muscle as discussed earlier.

Contribution of Vascular Impairment to Diabetic ED

Wide-ranging evidence supports a role for vascular factors in the etiology of diabetic ED, but the extent of this contribution is unclear. Doppler studies have shown up to 95% of diabetic impotent men may have abnormalities in penile blood flow compared to nondiabetic healthy controls (43); however, other studies have found that penile blood flow and penile-brachial index were reduced in diabetic males irrespective of potency (26,44). Angiography has shown that stenosis of the internal pudendal artery predicts ED in the diabetic population, but a similar pattern was also demonstrated in the nondiabetic population (45). This suggests the excess of generalized arterial disease seen with diabetes is responsible for the increased ED rather than penile vascular abnormalities specific to diabetes. Thus, vascular disease per se is not as strong a predictor of ED as neuropathy in the diabetic population (6).

Factors within the Corpus Cavernosum
Functional Abnormalities

From many studies in animals and humans, several of the chemical mediators involved in smooth-muscle relaxation and contraction of the corpus cavernosum have been identified as potentially contributing to ED in the diabetic individual.

Acetylcholine (ACh) release from the parasympathetic nerve terminal (PNT) within the corpora induces smooth-muscle relaxation. It is thought that this effect is mediated principally through stimulating the release of NO from the vascular endothelium. In addition, NO is released directly from the PNT. It has been demonstrated that diabetic men with ED have impairment in both the autonomic and the endothelium-dependent mechanisms that mediate smooth-muscle relaxation of the corpus cavernosum (40,46,47). In vitro examination of penile tissue from diabetic impotent versus nondiabetic impotent men showed that autonomic-mediated smooth-muscle relaxation was less pronounced following electrical stimulation and that the degree of impairment was associated with the duration of diabetes; in addition, ACh administration induced a lower degree of muscle relaxation in the diabetic group, whereas there was no difference between groups in relaxation by papaverine or sodium nitroprusside (endothelium-dependent vasodilators) (40).

Glycated hemoglobin (GHb), which is directly correlated with the degree of chronic hyperglycemia, has been shown to significantly impair ACh-induced relaxation of isolated corpus cavernosum from Wistar rats (48). This effect was mimicked by the addition of pyrogallol, a donor of superoxide anions, while L-arginine (the precursor of NO) partially reversed this GHb-mediated defect in smooth-muscle relaxation. Moreover, the activity of NO synthase, which synthesizes NO from L-arginine, was found to be unaffected in the cavernosal tissue from streptozotocin diabetic Sprague-Dawley rats (49). These in vitro animal findings may, in part, contribute to the better understanding of ACh- and NO-mediated abnormalities observed in impotent diabetic men.

Vasoactive intestinal polypeptide (VIP) is another smooth-muscle relaxant released by the PNT. Reduced immunoreactivity of VIP has been observed both in penile tissue from streptozotocin diabetic rats (50) and in diabetic impotent men (46). While adenosine triphosphate–relaxant responses are reduced in diabetic rats, they seem unaltered in diabetic men (51). Vasoactive prostanoids are synthesized and released by the corpus cavernosum and may have some role in determining muscle tone. It has been shown that the NO pathway may become less important in determining smooth-muscle relaxation in rats with long-term diabetes (49), and it is possible that vasodilatory prostanoids assume a greater role in facilitating cavernosal muscle relaxation as they do in other diabetic vascular beds (52). The cyclooxygenase inhibitor indomethacin, however, had no effect on the GHb-mediated impaired cavernosal muscle response to ACh in rats (48).

Table 2 Possible Structural Changes Observed within the Corpus Cavernosum of Impotent Diabetic Males

Fibrosis of the penile arteries
Fibrosis of the corpus cavernosum
Reduced cavernous nerve fibers and replacement of unmyelinated axons with collagen
Fibroproliferation of erectile tissue
Altered mRNA transcript level within the corpus cavernosum
Increased apoptosis within erectile tissue

In the physiological state, the action of norepinephrine released from sympathetic nerve terminals is the dominant mechanism enabling smooth-muscle contraction within the penis. The norepinephrine content of the corpus cavernosum appears to be reduced in diabetic patients with ED (47), although the degree of smooth-muscle contraction evoked by norepinephrine appears to be similar in diabetic and nondiabetic impotent men (46). The contractile polypeptide endothelin-1 is produced by endothelial and smooth-muscle cells within the corpus cavernosum. The characteristic slow onset and prolonged contraction facilitated by endothelin-1 appear unaltered in corporal smooth-muscle strips of diabetic men (53).

Structural Abnormalities

Several structural abnormalities have been identified in diabetic penile tissue that may contribute to the development of ED (Table 2). Analysis of the ultrastructure of the corpus cavernosum from diabetic impotent humans appears to produce similar degenerative tissue responses to other medical conditions associated with this condition, such as hypertension, smoking, neurological disease, and trauma (54). Down-regulated mRNA transcript has been identified in corpus cavernosum from impotent diabetic males, suggesting that altered gene expression may play a significant role in the development of ED (55). Finally, a high rate of apoptosis has been observed in the erectile tissue of diabetic Sprague-Dawley rats (56).

Recent evidence suggests that many of the functional and structural changes within diabetic cavernosal and other tissues may be caused by AGEs, which, like GHb, are closely related to chronic hyperglycemia. AGEs affect endothelial function by reducing NO and increasing endothelin-1 availability, as well as causing irreversible cross-linking between proteins and changes in collagen structure that may affect elasticity and cell function within the penis (42). AGEs in diabetes have been shown to adversely affect NO signaling mechanisms within the corpora cavernosa (57). Alternative etiological suggestions include excessive aldose reductase activity stimulated by hyperglycemia (58).

Endocrine Factors

Table 3 summarizes the effects of diabetes upon nonglycemic endocrine factors that are implicated in the process of tumescence.

Table 3 Loss of Erectile Function in Diabetic Men

Factor	Concentrations in impotent men
LH	No change in majority of studies, or Variable response following stimulation with GnRH
Free/total testosterone	No change in majority of studies, or Reduced secretion following stimulation with HCG
Prolactin	No change, or Hyperresponsiveness following stimulation with metoclopramide
Growth hormone	No change
Thyroid axis	Not well studied, although thyroid disease more common in diabetes

Abbreviations: HCG, human chorionic gonadotropin; GnRH, gonadotropin-releasing hormone; LH, luteinizing hormone.

A number of studies have investigated the hypothalamic–pituitary–gonadal pathway with conflicting results. This is explained in part by the small sample size and variation in experimental protocols of these studies, definition of ED, and differing patient characteristics and control groups. The majority of studies have demonstrated normal luteinizing hormone (LH) concentration in diabetic males with (59–63) and without (60,61,63) ED. LH concentrations of serum (64) and urine (65) were elevated in highly selected groups of diabetic males, however, with either no obvious organic/psychological (64) or psychological (65) cause for their ED. Upon stimulating the pituitary of diabetic impotent men with gonadotropic-releasing hormone, LH release has been shown to be normal (62), reduced (61), and exaggerated (65). Similarly, most (59,60,62, 64,65), but not all (61,63), studies have shown similar circulating total or free testosterone concentration in diabetic men with ED and nondiabetic control subjects with normal sexual function. Free testosterone levels were lower in one small study of impotent diabetic men; this study also showed that three-day stimulation with human chorionic gonadotropin produced significantly lower increments of total plasma testosterone in the group of impotent diabetic men compared with diabetic and nondiabetic subjects with normal sexual function (66).

Diabetic males with ED appear to have no alterations in prolactin secretion when examined in a single venous sample (59,60), 24-hour profile (67), or following stimulation with thyrotrophin-releasing hormone (60). Stimulation of dopaminergic receptors has been shown to induce erections in animals. When metoclopramide (a dopamine antagonist) was administered to diabetic male patients with ED, there appeared to be prolactin hyperresponsiveness compared with diabetic and nondiabetic potent control subjects (68). Mean 24-hour growth hormone concentration was similar in diabetic males with and without ED (67). Both hyper- and hypothyroidism are associated with the development of ED and are more commonly encountered in the diabetic population (69). There is no evidence, however, to suggest that mean concentrations of

thyroid-stimulating hormone, thyroxine, or triiodothyronine concentrations differ in diabetic impotent versus nonimpotent men.

Psychological Factors

Although there are no robust tools to evaluate psychological factors in the etiology of ED, it would appear that a primary psychogenic or psychiatric cause is less common than an organic cause in the diabetic male. The prevalence of the former has been reported as between 9% and 39% (12,14,70–72). In a five-year longitudinal study, diabetic men with psychogenic ED were more likely to regain spontaneous potency (16). Although organic disease predominates, it is likely that performance anxiety and other psychological factors that are more commonly observed in diabetes contribute to perpetuating ED (73). Although nocturnal penile tumescence (NPT) responses have been identified as being weaker in diabetic impotent men compared with nondiabetic impotent subjects (74), the ability of NPT investigation to distinguish between organic and psychological causes of ED is much disputed (75). (NPT evaluations are discussed further in Chapter 23.)

Psychosexual evaluation of diabetic men shows an overall reduction in sexual desire; degree of coital, masturbatory, and sleep-related erections; frequency of coital activity; and sexual satisfaction (76). Anxiety and depression are more common in the diabetic population, especially in the presence of macrovascular disease and proliferative retinopathy (77) and may contribute to the development, severity, or persistence of ED. Whether there is a "central" form of autonomic neuropathy that contributes to the development of diabetic ED (35) remains uncertain. In a study of diabetic impotent men, 60% of patients reported moderate-to-severe marital strain due to their sexual dysfunction; yet, only 30% of patients ventured to discuss the problem with a health-care professional (7). Psychological influences on sexual function are discussed further in Chapter 12.

Drugs

Drug therapy accounts for up to 25% of cases of ED in the general population (78) (see Chapter 19). The diabetic male is particularly susceptible to drug-related ED, given the escalating polypharmacy required to prevent and treat diabetic complications (Table 4). Many of the medications associated with ED are frequently prescribed to patients with diabetes (79). The results of the United Kingdom Prospective Diabetes Study (80) and Heart Outcomes Prevention Evaluation (HOPE) (81) studies support aggressive treatment of blood pressure in diabetes, frequently necessitating the use of two or more antihypertensive agents, many of which have been associated with ED (79).

Type 2 diabetes is integrally related to the metabolic syndrome, thus requiring treatment for dyslipidemia to reduce the progression of atherosclerosis. Mortality benefits have been shown when treating lipid

Table 4 Typical Polypharmacy Required to Treat Diabetes

Cardiovascular drugs
  β-blockers
  Thiazide diuretics
  Angiotensin-converting enzyme inhibitors
  Angiotensin II receptor blockers
  Calcium channel blockers
  Other antihypertensive agents
  Digoxin
Lipid-lowering drugs
  Fibrates
  HMG-CoA-reductase inhibitors ("statins")
Drugs used to treat painful neuropathy
  Tricyclic antidepressants
  Carbamazepine
  Nonsteroidal anti-inflammatory agents
  Gabapentin

Abbreviation: HMG-CoA, 3-hydroxy-3methylglutaryl-coenzyme A.

abnormalities with HMG-CoA-reductase inhibitors (statins) (82) and fibrates (83). These drugs are also implicated in ED (84).

In addition, antidepressants have been associated with ED (85). Painful diabetic neuropathy is frequently treated with tricyclic antidepressant therapy, which interferes with the cholinergic component of ejaculation and has even been used to treat premature ejaculation (86).

Oral hypoglycemic agents would not appear to influence male sexual function, although there are theoretical (but not proven) inhibitory effects of glibenclamide upon potency due to its closure of potassium channels (87). Drug-induced ED is usually reversible, and it is important to consider withdrawing potential offending agents prior to labeling a patient with "diabetic impotence." Drug-related ED usually starts within two to three weeks of commencing the offending pharmacological agent.

Other Factors

Although acute deterioration in glycemic control may be associated with reversible ED, there is little evidence suggesting that improvement of chronic hyperglycemia may restore potency in diabetic impotent men.

Balanitis secondary to *Candida* is relatively common in diabetic males, particularly with poor glycemic control. The associated pain may avert the patient from attempting or achieving tumescence for intercourse.

Penile venous leakage, either as an isolated finding or in conjunction with arterial insufficiency, was found in two-thirds of diabetic males, with a vascular etiology to their ED (88). Neurophysiological investigation revealed that spontaneous cavernosal activity was frequently abnormal, implicating autonomic dysfunction in the development of venous leaks. Additionally, veno-occlusive disease has been commonly observed in impotent patients with diabetes and Peyronie's disease (89). Although these investigators concluded that there was probably a close

relationship between the two conditions, there was no evidence to suggest that diabetes was the main cause of ED in patients with Peyronie's disease.

□ DISORDERS OF EJACULATION
Premature Ejaculation

Premature ejaculation is predominantly psychogenic in origin, but there is an association between premature ejaculation and erectile failure where rigidity cannot be achieved prior to ejaculation. Therefore, in view of the high prevalence of ED in diabetes, some diabetic men may mistakenly complain of premature ejaculation during the early stages of impotence. However, there is little evidence confirming a link between premature ejaculation and diabetes in the literature.

Retrograde Ejaculation

Retrograde ejaculation occurs when the bladder neck fails to contract under sympathetic control during the preejaculatory phase. Problems with ejaculation occur in up to 32% of men with diabetes (90), and the etiology is likely due to autonomic dysfunction. Unrecognized retrograde ejaculation may account for the reduced seminal volume seen with diabetes (91). Alpha-blockers and some antidepressants have also been implicated in retrograde ejaculation (92). Novel techniques of spermatozoa harvesting have been developed to aid fertility in patients with retrograde ejaculation (93).

□ INFERTILITY

While reduced fertility in the male diabetic population is recognized, it is largely attributed to erectile and ejaculatory failure; however, there is evidence of reduced fertility per se in diabetes with quantitative and qualitative seminal abnormalities being reported. In BBWOR diabetic rats, sustained hyperglycemia leads to structural testicular abnormalities associated with reduced fertility (94), while diabetic mice suffer from oligozoospermia (95). Comparative human sperm studies have reported elevated sperm production in diabetic subjects but as much as a 60% reduction in seminal volume (96,97). Sperm motility in diabetic subjects has been reported as both normal (98) and impaired (96,97,99). Furthermore, abnormalities in sperm morphology have been noted in diabetic patients (96,97,100), and spermatozoa from diabetic patients are less able to penetrate hamster eggs (99). In addition, abnormalities in seminal amino acid concentrations have been detected in diabetic patients (101), and diabetic seminal fluid has been found to contain significantly elevated levels of prostaglandins (99). Some investigators have also noted reduced testicular volume in diabetic patients, but this may be a consequence of reduced semen production rather than a structural defect of testicular tissue (97).

□ SUMMARY

Sexual dysfunction in diabetic males, particularly ED, is more commonly seen than in the nondiabetic population. The development of a sexual problem is often underrecognized and may present additionalhazards in the diabetic patient with the potential to lead to demotivation with worsening of glycemic control, and, ultimately, the development or worsening of vascular complications. Attempts to improve glycemic control have been associated with a reduction in vascular complications in both type 1 (102) and type 2 (103) diabetes, but whether the sexual problems discussed in this chapter can be prevented by better metabolic control remains undetermined.

□ REFERENCES

1. Amos AF, McCarty DJ, Zimmet P. The rising global burden of diabetes and its complications: estimates and projections to the year 2010. Diabet Med 1997; 14(suppl 5):S1–S85.
2. Baxter H, Bottomley J, Burns E, et al. CODE-2 UK—The annual direct costs of care for people with type 2 diabetes in Great Britain. Diabet Med 2000; 17(S1):A42.
3. Rubin A, Babbott D. Impotence and diabetes mellitus. J Am Med Assoc 1958; 168(5):498–500.
4. Faerman I, Vilar O, Rivarola MA, et al. Impotence and diabetes. Studies of androgenic function in diabetic impotent males. Diabetes 1972; 21(1):23–30.
5. Kolodny RC, Kahn CB, Goldstein HH, et al. Sexual dysfunction in diabetic men. Diabetes 1974; 23(4): 306–309.
6. McCulloch DK, Campbell IW, Wu FC, et al. The prevalence of diabetic impotence. Diabetologia 1980; 18(4):279–283.
7. Cummings MH, Meeking DR, Warburton F, et al. The diabetic male's perception of erectile dysfunction. Pract Diabetes Intern 1997; 14(4):100–102.
8. Alonso Sandoica E, Sanchez Sanchez MD, Benito Fernandez M, et al. Impotence in diabetic patients: detection of prevalence and social-health implications. Aten Primaria 1997; 20(8):435–439.
9. Zweifler J, Padilla A, Schafer S. Barriers to recognition of erectile dysfunction among diabetic Mexican-American men. J Am Board Fam Pract 1998; 11(4): 259–263.
10. Kinsey AC, Pomeroy WB, Martin CE. Age and sexual outlet. In: Kinsey AC, ed. Sexual Behavior in the Human Male, Philadelphia: WB Saunders, 1948: 218–262.
11. Pointel JP, Got I, Ziegler O, et al. Impotence in the diabetic. J Mal Vasc 1989; 14(2):133–137.
12. Lehman TP, Jacobs JA. Etiology of diabetic impotence. J Urol 1983; 129(2):291–294.
13. Zonszein J. Diagnosis and management of endocrine disorders of erectile dysfunction. Urol Clin North Am 1995; 22(4):789–802.
14. Maatman TJ, Montague DK, Martin LM. Erectile dysfunction in men with diabetes mellitus. Urology 1987; 29(6):589–592.
15. Deutsch S, Sherman L. Previously unrecognized diabetes mellitus in sexually impotent men. JAMA 1980; 244(21):2430–2432.
16. McCulloch DK, Young RJ, Prescott RJ, et al. The natural history of impotence in diabetic men. Diabetologia 1984; 26(6):437–440.
17. Meeking DR, Cummings MH, Shaw KN, et al. Practical guidelines for the management of erectile dysfunction in diabetes. Pract Diabetes Int 1995; 12(5):211–214.
18. Ellenberg M. Impotence in diabetes: the neurologic factor. Ann Intern Med 1971; 75(2):213–219.
19. Yamaguchi Y, Kumamoto Y. Etiological analysis of male diabetic erectile dysfunction with particular emphasis on findings of vascular and neurological examinations. Nippon Hinyokika Gakkai Zasshi 1994; 85(10):1474–1483.
20. Vinik AI, Park TS, Stansberry KB, et al. Diabetic neuropathies. Diabetologia 2000; 43(8):957–973.
21. Watkins PJ. Progression of diabetic autonomic neuropathy. Diabet Med 1993; 10(suppl 2):77S–78S.
22. The Diabetes Control and Complications Trial Research Group. The effect of intensive diabetes therapy on the development and progression of neuropathy. Ann Intern Med 1995; 122(8):561–568.
23. Amarenco G, Kerdraon J. Electrophysiologic perineal studies in the exploration of erectile dysfunction in diabetics. Diabete Metab 1994; 20(1):60–63.
24. Kaneko S, Bradley WE. Penile electrodiagnosis: penile peripheral innervation. Urology 1987; 30(3):210–212.
25. Lin JT, Bradley WE. Penile neuropathy in insulin-dependent diabetes mellitus. J Urol 1985; 133(2): 213–215.
26. Daniels JS. Abnormal nerve conduction in impotent patients with diabetes mellitus. Diabetes Care 1989; 12(7):449–454.
27. Bird SJ, Hanno PM. Bulbocavernosus reflex studies and autonomic testing in the diagnosis of erectile dysfunction. J Neurol Sci 1998; 154(1):8–13.
28. Ho KH, Ong BK, Chong PN, et al. The bulbocavernosus reflex in the assessment of neurogenic impotence in diabetic and non-diabetic men. Ann Acad Med Singapore 1996; 25(4):558–561.
29. Buvat J, Lemaire A, Buvat-Herbaut M, et al. Comparative investigations in 26 impotent and 26 nonimpotent diabetic patients. J Urol 1985; 133(1):34–38.

30. Wellmer A, Sharief MK, Knowles CH, et al. Quantitative sensory and autonomic testing in male diabetic patients with erectile dysfunction. BJU Int 1999; 83(1):66–70.

31. Quadri R, Veglio M, Flecchia D, et al. Autonomic neuropathy and sexual impotence in diabetic patients: analysis of cardiovascular reflexes. Andrologia 1989; 21(4):346–352.

32. Fowler CJ, Ali Z, Kirby RS, et al. The value of testing for unmyelinated fibre, sensory neuropathy in diabetic impotence. Br J Urol 1988; 61(1):63–67.

33. Melman A, Henry DP, Felten DL, et al. Alteration of the penile corpora in patients with erectile impotence. Invest Urol 1980; 17(6):474–477.

34. Melman A, Henry DP, Felten DL, et al. Effect of diabetes upon penile sympathetic nerves in impotent patients. South Med J 1980; 73(3):307–309, 317.

35. Nofzinger EA, Schmidt HS. An exploration of central dysregulation of erectile function as a contributing cause of diabetic impotence. J Nerv Ment Dis 1990; 178(2):90–95.

36. Goldwasser B, Carson CC III, Braun SD, et al. Impotence due to the pelvic steal syndrome: treatment by iliac transluminal angioplasty. J Urol 1985; 133(5): 860–861.

37. Azadzoi KM, Siroky MB, Goldstein I. Study of etiologic relationship of arterial atherosclerosis to corporal veno-occlusive dysfunction in the rabbit. J Urol 1996; 155(5):1795–1800.

38. Johnstone MT, Creager SJ, Scales KM, et al. Impaired endothelium-dependent vasodilation in patients with insulin-dependent diabetes mellitus. Circulation 1993; 88(6):2510–2516.

39. McVeigh GE, Brennan GM, Johnston GD, et al. Impaired endothelium-dependent and independent vasodilation in patients with type 2 (non-insulin-dependent) diabetes mellitus. Diabetologia 1992; 35(8):771–776.

40. Saenz de Tejada I, Goldstein I, Azadzoi K, et al. Impaired neurogenic and endothelium-mediated relaxation of penile smooth muscle from diabetic men with impotence. N Engl J Med 1989; 320(16):1025–1030.

41. Tooke JE. Microvascular haemodynamics in diabetes mellitus. Clin Sci (Lond) 1986; 70(2):119–125.

42. Singh R, Barden A, Mori T, et al. Advanced glycation end-products: a review. Diabetologia 2001; 44(2): 129–146.

43. Jevtich MJ, Edson M, Jarman WD, et al. Vascular factor in erectile failure among diabetics. Urology 1982; 19(2):163–168.

44. Buvat J, Lemaire A, Buvat-Herbaut M, et al. Mechanisms of diabetic impotence. 25 cases. Presse Med 1987; 16(13):611–614.

45. Herman A, Adar R, Rubinstein Z. Vascular lesions associated with impotence in diabetic and nondiabetic arterial occlusive disease. Diabetes 1978; 27(10):975–981.

46. Kim SC, Ahn SY, Park SH, et al. A comparison of the relaxation responses of isolated cavernosal smooth muscles by endothelium-independent and endothelium-dependent vasodilators in diabetic men with impotence. J Korean Med Sci 1995; 10(1):1–6.

47. Lincoln J, Crowe R, Blacklay PF, et al. Changes in the VIPergic, cholinergic and adrenergic innervation of human penile tissue in diabetic and non-diabetic impotent males. J Urol 1987; 137(5):1053–1059.

48. Cartledge JJ, Eardley I, Morrison JFB. Impairment of corpus cavernosal smooth muscle relaxation by glycosylated human haemoglobin. BJU Int 2000; 85(6): 735–741.

49. Ari G, Vardi Y, Finberg JPM. Nitric oxide and penile erection in streptozotocin-diabetic rats. Clin Sci 1999; 96(4):365–371.

50. Crowe R, Lincoln J, Blacklay PF, et al. Vasoactive intestinal polypeptide-like immunoreactive nerves in diabetic penis. A comparison between streptozotocin-treated rats and man. Diabetes 1983; 32(11):1075–1077.

51. Gür S, Öztürk B. Altered Relaxant Responses to Adenosine and Adenosine 5′-Triphosphate in the Corpus cavernosum from Men and Rats with Diabetes. Pharmacology 2000; 60(2):105–112.

52. Meeking DR, Browne DL, Allard S, et al. Effects of cyclo-oxygenase inhibition on vasodilatory response to acetylcholine in patients with type 1 diabetes and nondiabetic subjects. Diabetes Care 2000; 23(12): 1840–1843.

53. Christ GJ, Lerner SE, Kim DC, et al. Endothelin-1 as a putative modulator of erectile dysfunction: I. Characteristics of contraction of isolated corporal tissue strips. J Urol 1995; 153(1998):2003.

54. Mersdorf A, Goldsmith PC, Diederichs W, et al. Ultrastructural changes in impotent penile tissue: a comparison of 65 patients. J Urol 1991; 145(4): 749–758.

55. Autieri MV, Melman A, Christ GJ. Identification of a down-regulated mRNA transcript in corpus cavernosum from diabetic patients with erectile dysfunction. Int J Impot Res 1996; 8(2):69–73.

56. Alici B, Gumustas MK, Ozkara H, et al. Apoptosis in the erectile tissues of diabetic and healthy rats. BJU Int 2000; 85(3):326–329.

57. Seftel AD, Vaziri ND, Ni Z, et al. Advanced glycation end products in human penis: elevation in diabetic tissue, site of deposition, and possible effect through iNOS or eNOS. Urology 1997; 50(6):1016–1026.

58. MacLeod A, Sonksen P. Diabetic neuropathy. In: Shaw KM, ed. Diabetic Complications, New York: John Wiley & Sons, 1996:123–148.

59. Fitcher M, Zuckerman M, Fishkin RE, et al. Do endocrines play an etiological role in diabetic and nondiabetic sexual dysfunctions? J Androl 1984; 5(1):8–16.

60. Zeidler A, Gelfand R, Tamagna E, et al. Pituitary gonadal function in diabetic male patients with and without impotence. Andrologia 1982; 14(1):62–68.

61. Daubresse JC, Meunier JC, Wilmotte J, et al. Pituitary-testicular axis in diabetic men with and without sexual impotence. Diabete Metab 1978; 4(4):233–237.

62. Wright AD, London DR, Holder G, et al. Luteinizing release hormone tests in impotent diabetic males. Diabetes 1976; 25(10):975–977.

63. Ando S, Rubens R, Rottiers R. Androgen plasma levels in male diabetics. J Endocrinol Invest 1984; 7(1): 21–24.

64. Levitt NS, Vinik AI, Sive AA, et al. Synthetic luteinizing hormone-releasing hormone in impotent male diabetics. S Afr Med J 1980; 57(17):701–704.

65. Murray FT. Gonadal dysfunction in diabetic men with organic impotence. J Clin Endocrinol Metab 1987; 65(1):127–135.

66. Geisthovel W, Niedergerke U, Morgner KD, et al. Androgen status of male diabetics. Total testosterone before and following stimulation with HCG, free testosterone, and testosterone binding capacity of patients with and without potency disorders. Med Klin 1975; 70(36):1417–1423.

67. Maneschi F, White MC, Porta M, et al. 24-Hour studies of prolactin and growth hormone levels in diabetic impotence. Horm Res 1981; 14(2):79–86.

68. Mainini E, Martinelli I, Scarsi G, et al. Evaluation of central dopaminergic tone in diabetes mellitus. Minerva Endocrinol 1991; 16(4):171–177.

69. Smithson MJ. Screening for thyroid dysfunction in a community population of diabetic patients. Diabete Med 1998; 15(2):148–150.

70. Ryder REJ, Facey P, Hayward MWJ, et al. Detailed investigation of the cause of impotence in 20 diabetic men. Pract Diabetes Int 1991; 8(5):174–177.

71. el-Bayoumi M, el-Sherbini O, Mostafa M. Impotence in diabetics: organic versus psychogenic factors. Urology 1984; 24(5):459–463.

72. Melman A, Tiefer L, Pedersen R. Evaluation of first 406 patients in urology department based center for male sexual dysfunction. Urology 1988; 32(1):6–10.

73. Morse WI, Morse JM. Erectile impotence precipitated by organic factors and perpetuated by performance anxiety. Can Med Assoc J 1982; 127(7):599–601.

74. Zuckerman M, Neeb M, Ficher M, et al. Nocturnal penile tumescence and penile responses in the waking state in diabetic and nondiabetic sexual dysfunctionals. Arch Sex Behav 1985; 14(2):109–129.

75. Morales A, Condra M, Reid K. The role of nocturnal penile tumescence monitoring in the diagnosis of impotence: a review. J Urol 1990; 143(3):441–446.

76. Schiavi RC, Stimmel BB, Mandeli J, et al. Diabetes mellitus and male sexual function: a controlled study. Diabetologia 1993; 36(8):745–751.

77. Ryan CM. Psychological factors and diabetes mellitus. In: Pickup JC, Williams G, eds. Textbook of Diabetes. 2nd ed. Cambridge: Blackwell, 1997: vol.2, 66.1–66.17.

78. Keene LC, Davies PH. Drug-related erectile dysfunction. Adverse Drug React Toxicol Rev 1999; 18(1): 5–24.

79. Barksdale JD, Gardner SF. The impact of first-line antihypertensive drugs on erectile dysfunction. Pharmacotherapy 1999; 19(5):573–581.

80. UK Prospective Diabetes Study Group. Tight blood pressure control and risk of macrovascular and microvascular complications in type 2 diabetes: UKPDS 38. Br Med J 1998; 317(7160):703–713.

81. Yusuf S, Sleight P, Pogue J, et al. Effects of an angiotensin-converting-enzyme inhibitor, ramipril, on cardiovascular events in high-risk patients. The Heart Outcomes Prevention Evaluation Study Investigators. N Engl J Med 2000; 342(3):145–153.

82. Pyorala K, Pedersen TR, Kjekshus J, et al. Cholesterol lowering with simvastatin improves prognosis of diabetic patients with coronary heart disease. A subgroup analysis of the Scandinavian Simvastatin Survival Study (4S). Diabetes Care 1997; 20(4): 614–620.

83. Rubins HB, Robins SJ, Collins D, et al. Gemfibrozil for the secondary prevention of coronary heart disease in men with low levels of high-density lipoprotein cholesterol. Veterans Affairs High-Density Lipoprotein Cholesterol Intervention Trial Study Group. N Engl J Med 1999; 341(6):410–418.

84. Rizvi K. Do lipid-lowering drugs cause erectile dysfunction? A systematic review. Fam Pract 2002; 19(1): 95–98.

85. Labbate LA, Croft HA, Oleshansky MA. Antidepressant-related erectile dysfunction: management via avoidance, switching antidepressants, antidotes, and adaptation. J Clin Psychiatry 2003; 64(suppl 10):11–19.

86. Hawton K. Erectile dysfunction and premature ejaculation. Br J Hosp Med 1988; 40(6):428–436.

87. Moon DG, Byun HS, Kim JJ. A KATP-channel opener as a potential treatment modality for erectile dysfunction. BJU Int 1999; 83(7):837–841.

88. Colakoglu Z, Kutluay E, Ertekin C, et al. Autonomic nerve involvement and venous leakage in diabetic men with impotence. BJU Int 1999; 83(4):453–456.

89. Culha M, Alici B, Acar O, et al. The relationship between diabetes mellitus, impotence and veno-occlusive dysfunction in Peyronie's disease patients. Urol Int 1998; 60(2):101–104.

90. Thomas AJ Jr. Ejaculatory dysfunction. Fertil Steril 1983; 39(4):445–454.

91. Klebanow D, MacLeod J. Semen quality and certain disturbances of reproduction in diabetic men. Fertil Steril 1960; 11(3):255–261.

92. Debruyne FM. Alpha blockers: are all created equal? Urology 2000; 56(5 suppl 1):20–22.

93. Fishel S, Thornton S. The use of assisted reproduction technology (ART) for achieving conception in male infertility. Br J Urol 1995; 75(1):50–56.

94. Cameron DF, Rountree J, Schultz RE, et al. Sustained hyperglycemia results in testicular dysfunction and reduced fertility potential in BBWOR diabetic rats. Am Jl Physiol Endocrinol Metab 1990; 259(6): 881–889.

95. Noguchi S, Ohba Y, Oka T. Involvement of epidermal growth factor deficiency in pathogenesis of

oligozoospermia in streptozotocin-induced diabetic mice. Endocrinology 1990; 127(5):2136–2140.

96. Handelsman DJ, Conway AJ, Boylan LM, et al. Testicular function and glycemic control in diabetic men. A controlled study. Andrologia 1985; 17(5):488–496.

97. Padron RS, Dambay A, Suarez R, et al. Semen analyses in adolescent diabetic patients. Acta Diabetol Lat 1984; 21(2):115–121.

98. Ali ST, Shaikh RN, Siddiqi NA, et al. Semen analysis in insulin-dependent/non-insulin-dependent diabetic men with/without neuropathy. Arch Androl 1993; 30(1):47–54.

99. Shrivastav P, Swann J, Jeremy JY, et al. Sperm function and structure and seminal plasma prostanoid concentrations in men with IDDM. Diabetes Care 1989; 12(10):742–744.

100. Vignon F, Le Faou A, Montagnon D, et al. Comparative study of semen in diabetic and healthy men. Diabete Metab 1991; 17(3):350–354.

101. Kaemmerer H, Mitzkat HJ. Ion-exchange chromatography of amino acids in ejaculates of diabetics. Andrologia 1985; 17(5):485–487.

102. The Diabetes Control and Complications Trial Research Group. The effect of intensive treatment of diabetes on the development and progression of long-term complications in insulin-dependent diabetes mellitus. N Engl J Med 1993; 329(14):977–986.

103. UK Prospective Diabetes Study Group. Effect of intensive blood-glucose control with metformin on complications in overweight patients with type 2 diabetes (UKPDS 34). Lancet 1998; 352(9131): 854–865.

15

Neurological Causes of Male Sexual Dysfunction and Neurological Sequelae of Sexual Activity

Per Olov Lundberg

Neurology, Department of Neuroscience, University Hospital, Uppsala, Sweden

□ INTRODUCTION

Neurosexology is a branch of neurology dealing with neurological controls of sexual physiology, as well as problems of sexual dysfunction caused by destruction or malfunction of nervous structures and altered sexual behavior in patients with neurological disorders. Neurosexology also covers neurological symptoms or lesions such as headache attacks and epileptic seizures or vascular catastrophes provoked by sexual activity.

The autonomic nervous system plays many key functions in human sexuality. (For further information on these topics, see Chapters 3 to 5.) Only rarely, however, is sexual dysfunction the result of a pure autonomic nervous failure. One example is erectile dysfunction after destruction of the cavernous nerves. Sexual function and sexual behavior are also dependent upon the rest of the nervous system, particularly hypothalamic control of the pituitary–gonadal axis. Therefore, when discussing sexuality, it is important to take a holistic view of the many neurological controls involved.

The great advances of pharmacology in recent years have yielded a number of therapeutic agents that act on the central or peripheral nervous tissues to control sexual function. There are also a number of sexual side effects associated with many neuropharmacological drugs. (For further information on this topic, see Chapter 19.) Conversely, some drugs used to treat sexual dysfunction can have adverse effects on the nervous system. These are important facts that also have to be considered during evaluation.

Patients in whom a neurological cause of sexual dysfunction is suspected should undergo a thorough physical examination, including neurological and endocrine tests (1,2). (For further information on this topic, please refer to Chapter 22.) Since the knowledge of what is actually occurring in the human brain regarding sexuality is insufficient, particular interest should be directed to sensory and motor functions related to sexual physiology. A series of clinical neurophysiology tests have been developed for such patients, the most important of which are given in Refs. 2–5.

The following is a summary of various neurological disorders of the brain, spinal cord, and periphery that can lead to sexual dysfunction in the male.

□ BRAIN DISORDERS
Hypothalamo–Pituitary Disorders

Decreased or absent sexual desire is often the first symptom in males with hypothalamo–pituitary disorders. Males rarely seek medical advice, however, due to loss of sexual desire alone. Hence, the diagnosis is usually postponed until other symptoms appear. The most important of these symptoms is usually that of visual field defect(s). In a pituitary tumor patient, it may take as long as a decade after the onset of the sexual problem before any further symptoms develop. Thus, about three-quarters of all men with hypothalamo–pituitary disorders report decreased or absent sexual desire at the time of diagnosis. Larger tumors extending into the suprasellar region leading to pressure on the hypothalamus are more often associated with sexual symptoms than are intrasellar tumors. A highly significant correlation has been found between low serum testosterone levels and a decrease in desire (6). Usually the patients also have erectile failure; this occurrence often does not present a great problem to the patient, however, due to the preexisting lack of desire. Decreased sexual desire is also the first symptom in most men with smaller pituitary tumors and hyperprolactinemia (7). Even in this group of patients, low serum testosterone is more common among those with decreased desire. Decreased testosterone levels are probably more important in causing this symptom to develop than elevated prolactin levels.

Table 1 outlines the different causes of hypothalamo–pituitary dysfunction that can lead to sexual dysfunction (1). In most instances, hypothalamo–pituitary dysfunction is caused by a hormone-secreting or non-hormone-secreting pituitary adenoma. The clinical symptomatology is dependent upon the age of onset and the rate of progression. If the tumor produces clinical symptoms before puberty, lack of sexual development is the most typical sign. More often, these disorders result in secondary hypogonadism and loss

Table 1 Hypothalamo–Pituitary Pathology Causing Male Sexual Dysfunction

Tumors of the hypothalamus and pituitary
Pituitary adenomas
Nonfunctional (several types)
Growth-hormone-producing adenomas
Prolactin-producing adenomas
Gonadotropin-producing adenomas
Thyroid-stimulating hormone-producing adenomas
Craniopharyngiomas
Meningiomas
Optic gliomas
Hypothalamic hamartomas
Metastases (kidney, prostate)
Congenital malformations
Dysplasia of the sella turcica
Dystopia of the posterior pituitary lobe
Olfactogenital dysplasia (hypogonadotropic hypogonadism
with anosmia, Kallman's syndrome)
Septo-optic dysplasia (de Morsier's syndrome)
Acquired hypothalamo–pituitary disorders
Pituitary apoplexia
Post-traumatic hypothalamic bleeding
Ruptured arterial aneurysms
Sequel of acute asphyxia
Spontaneous arrested infantile hydrocephalus
Delayed radiation necrosis
Meningoencephalitis
Sarcoidosis
Histiocytosis-X (Hand–Schüller–Christian's syndrome)
Lymphocytic hypophysitis

of sexual desire and potency. Men can be hypogonadal, however, for many different reasons. In a computed tomography (CT)/magnetic resonance imaging (MRI) study of 164 impotent males with low serum testosterone values, evidence of hypothalamo–pituitary pathology was found only in 11 men (8).

Although the loss of sexual desire and lack of sexual development are often related to hormonal insufficiency, damage to the brain center for sexual desire, which is localized in the hypothalamus can also lead to sexual dysfunction (9,10). In such a case, the hormones do not have a healthy target region in the brain, and, thus, symptomatology cannot be corrected by hormone replacement therapy.

In a number of male members of families with cerebellar atrophy and ataxia, hypogonadotropic hypogonadism was found, indicating a hypothalamo–pituitary insufficiency (11–16). This is in contrast to hypergonadotropic hypogonadism, which indicates primary testicular failure such as that found in patients with mitochondrial disorders or sex-chromosome abnormalities. The mechanism underlying the development of hypogonadotropic hypogonadism in patients with cerebellar atrophy is unknown.

In rare cases such as spontaneously arrested hydrocephalus and some hypothalamic tumors, particularly hamartomas, precocious puberty may instead be the presenting and cardinal symptom of a hypothalamo–pituitary disorder. In these cases, the boy usually shows the first signs of pubertal development

between three and seven years of age, but it may start before the first year of life. The etiology can be a gonadotropin-producing pituitary adenoma, or, more often, a gonadotropin-releasing hormone-producing hypothalamic tumor. In other cases, most often those where the lesion is in the pineal region, the mechanism involves an interruption of the nerve path to the hypothalamus that holds back normal pubertal development. Table 2 gives a list of possible causes of cerebral precocious puberty (1,17).

Traumatic Brain Injuries

Disability and cognitive impairment frequently occur after a traumatic brain injury (TBI). Sexual impairment as a consequence of cerebral lesions or psychological factors is not rare. Both decreased and increased sexual desire have been reported, as well as impotence and retarded ejaculation (18–21). Hypersexuality and altered sexual preference may also follow brain injury (22). Lesions of the septal region in particular may lead to hypersexuality (23). Lesions of the frontal and temporal lobe seem more often to lead to sexual problems than do lesions of the parieto-occipital part of the brain (24).

Sex offenses may also be a psychosocial effect of TBI (25). In Klüver–Bucy syndrome, which is caused by bilateral lesions of the anterior temporal regions, hypersexuality is a prevailing symptom (26–28). Pansexuality or sexual drive directed not only toward human beings but also toward animals and inanimate objects is often a major feature. Lesions associated with this syndrome may also be caused by viral meningoencephalitis or complications of systemic lupus erythematosus and cancer treatments.

Sexual symptoms of different types may also occur in nontraumatic encephalopathies, including

Table 2 Hypothalamo–Pituitary Disorders in Boys with Precocious Puberty

Pituitary tumors
Gonadotropin-secreting pituitary adenomas
Diencephalic tumors
Hamartoma of tuber cinereum
Hypothalamic teratoma
Hypothalamic astrocytoma
Hypothalamic spongioblastoma
Hypothalamic ependymoma
Hypothalamic choriocarcinoma
Optic glioma
Pinealoma
Teratoma of pineal gland
Neurocutaneous syndromes
Tuberous sclerosis
Neurofibromatosis
McCune–Albright syndrome
Other mid-brain processes
Hydrocephalus
Post-traumatic hypothalamic lesions
Arachnoiditis of the chiasm
Suprasellar cysts

prion diseases such as fatal familial insomnia (29) and sporadic Creutzfeldt–Jakob disease (Lundberg PO. Unpublished observation).

Stroke

An overall change in sexual life is often seen in males after experiencing a cerebrovascular event. The majority of the males (50–65%) have erectile dysfunction after stroke (30–36). Nocturnal erections were normal in only 45% of the patients two months after the stroke (36). Retarded ejaculation was reported in 15% of the men after stroke, with orgasmic dysfunction in as many as half; in fact, about three-quarters of the stroke patients who were sexually active before their stroke reported an abrupt and permanent decrease in coital frequency (31,32,34). Even in patients with mild or no disability, poststroke changes in sexual functions may occur (37).

Areas of the brain that are of importance for sexual function, such the hypothalamus and the limbic cortex, are not usually involved in the pathological process of stroke. Sexual problems in post-stroke patients are therefore most often nonspecific and not correlated to the anatomical localization. Frequently, they can be explained in terms of maladjustment attributable to psychological or interpersonal factors. Diminished sexual encounters in post-stroke patients may be due primarily to factors such as the patient's fears of inadequacy (34,38) or paralysis of movements. Cognitive impairment may also disturb the sexual part of a relationship.

Sexual problems are more often seen in cases with aphasia (39). In some studies, the prevalence of major sexual dysfunction (decrease in desire and in frequency of intercourse) was significantly greater after dominant hemisphere stroke (30,36,40,41). Other studies have not confirmed this observation (32). Lesions in the nondominant hemisphere and the parietal lobe are more often associated with declining desire. General hemihypesthesia may be associated with decreased sexual ability probably due to loss of erogenous zone sensitivity (42).

Hypersexuality in stroke patients is rare, but may be the result of a vascular lesion to the basal ganglia or limbic cortex (43–45). Rupture of an anterior communicant artery aneurysm may give rise to a hypothalamic lesion and hypogonadism (see above).

Epilepsy

Sexual function and behavior can be altered in epileptic patients, both during the interictal period and in direct relation to seizures (Table 3).

Interictal Phenomena

Loss of sexual desire, reduced sexual activity, and/or inhibited sexual arousal are seen in many men with epilepsy (46–48). Inability to maintain erection and, more rarely, ejaculatory dysfunction, decreased

Table 3 Epilepsy and Sexuality

Provocation of epileptic fits
Hyperventilation
Sexual fantasies
Masturbation
Sexual arousal
Orgasm
Sexual phenomena as a part of an epileptic fit
Pleasant sensations or paresthesia in the genitalia
Attacks of genital pain
Penile erection ("transient priapism")
Orgasm
Rhythmic contractions of pelvic muscles
Pelvic sexual movements (automatisms)
Compulsive masturbation
Undressing
Interictal phenomena
Loss of sexual desire
Low sexual activity
Impotence
Decreased orgasmic capacity
Hypersexual behavior
Changes in sexual behavior

satisfaction with sexual life, reduced sexual fantasies, and reduced sexual dreams and initiatives as well as reduced orgasmic capacity are also reported in patients with complex partial epilepsy and mesiobasal temporal lobe spike foci (49,50). The reported incidence of each of these dysfunctions varies across studies, but is generally higher than that observed in the general population.

Sexual dysfunction was more often seen in patients with partial than with primarily generalized epilepsy (51). Most patients with low sexual desire have complex partial seizures and temporal lobe lesions. Sexual interest seems to be reduced more often in patients with right rather than left temporal lobe epilepsy. Interictal hypersexual episodes are reported in a few cases (52). Life satisfaction and sexual activity are better in seizure-free patients compared to those who are not seizure-free. Surgical treatment of the epileptic focus, however, does not seem to improve sexuality (53). Epileptic male patients have a lower marriage rate compared to the general population. Social and psychological factors play an important role. It should also be noted that antiepileptic drugs, especially the older varieties (phenytoin, phenobarbital, primidone, carbamazepine, and valproate), may cause hormonal changes (particularly increased estradiol and decreased free testosterone). This may lead to decreased sexual desire and performance (54,55). In a recent large study including 200 men with epilepsy, it was found that patients with temporal lobe epilepsy had lower testosterone concentrations than patients with extratemporal focal epilepsy. In addition, treatment of temporal lobe epilepsy with carbamazepine increased the negative effects of epilepsy on serum levels of reproductive hormones and resulted in a lower T:LH ratio than that observed in patients treated with valproate (56). Thus, one has to consider both the adverse drug reactions and the occurrence of a sub-clinical hypogonadotropic hypogonadism caused by the brain damage underlying the epilepsy as an expla-nation for the sexual disorders seen in this patient population.

Seizures and Sexual Phenomena

Sexual phenomena may be a part of an epileptic seizure in itself. The patient with epilepsy may also display changes in sexual behavior that provide important insights in the sexual physiology of the human brain. Partial seizures generated from the primary sensory cortex, usually as a result of a parasagittal tumor corresponding to the genital region, may result in sen-sations, pleasant or nonpleasant, in the genital organs. Motor symptoms such as erection, ejaculation, or orgasm may also be a part of an epileptic fit. Such geni-tal events may be experienced by patients either as sexual or as nonsexual. Pelvic sexual movements as a part of epileptic automatisms or compulsive masturba-tion in front of other people may occur during or after a seizure.

Sexual phenomena (other than sensory events occurring as part of an epileptic seizure) usually pres-ent in patients with complex partial epilepsy, most often with temporal lobe lesions. Sexual automatisms may also occur with frontal lobe lesions. They are very uncommon in primary generalized epilepsy of the grand mal or petit mal type.

Deviant sexual behavior (e.g., exhibitionism, fetishism, frotteurism, sadomasochism, transvestism, violent sexual behavior, and pansexual behavior) is sometimes displayed by epileptic patients. Only a small number of such cases have been reported, but the observation that the behavior in question may occur episodically and sometimes disappears after treatment favors a causal connection between the changes in behavior and the epilepsy or the cerebral lesion behind it. In most cases, there have been partial complex epileptic seizures and lesions in one or both temporal lobes. Occasionally, the deviant behavior correlates with continuous epileptic discharges in the electroencephalogram (EEG) (psychomotor status). Paranoid delusions of being violated, abused, or seduced are not uncommon in epileptic patients. For further details on sexual phenomena and sexual behavior changes in epileptic patients, please refer to the author's review on this topic (57).

Parkinson's Disease and Other Movement Disorders

Decrease in sexual desire is common in males with Parkinson's disease (PD). Symptoms of sexual dys-function are also frequent in their healthy partners (58). Erectile dysfunction during sexual intercourse occurs in half (59–61), and nocturnal and morning erec-tions are usually absent. Many men affected by PD are also unable to ejaculate, with one study determining this proportion to be as high as 79% (62).

The mechanisms behind sexual dysfunction in PD patients are not very well understood. To some extent, it may be similar to mechanisms seen with other chronic disorders such as arthritis (63). Other types of autonomic nervous system dysfunction, however, are common (70–80%) in patients with PD (64). The high frequency of bladder detrusor hyperreflexia and para-doxical contractions of the striated sphincter muscles during defecation points to specific autonomic nerve damage in these patients (65,66). The striated pelvic floor muscles are often involved in the disease process (Table 4) (67,68).

During sexual arousal, tremor is often enhanced, which makes sexual activity more difficult. Muscle rigidity and akinesia may contribute to difficulties in performance of sexual activities. Patients with PD are often depressed and have a tendency to isolate themselves from other people. Some authors have observed a correlation between sexual dysfunction and depression (63).

Decrease of sexual desire is not directly coupled to the severity of the disease. Treatment with dopami-nergic compounds may result in an apparent increase—or, rather, a normalization of sexual desire—which may occur without corresponding improvement of the movement disorder. Indeed, increase in sexual desire has been reported as an adverse reaction to dopami-nergic drugs in PD patients (69,70).

Interestingly, the situation is quite different in Huntington's disease (HD). Here, fecundity is actually increased. Those members of an HD family who have inherited the HD gene but have not yet developed the disease tend to have significantly more children than their healthy siblings. Increased sexual activity is seen in approximately 10% of people with HD, sometimes in combination with mania or hypomania. Habitual promiscuity and marital infidelity may be noted at diagnosis of HD. HD patients, however, may have difficulty in achieving sexual arousal. Paraphilias such as sexual aggression, exhibitionism, and pedophilia have been reported in HD patients (71).

Disorders of sexual inhibition with pansex-uality (e.g., copulation with nonliving objects) are not

Table 4 Sexual Dysfunction in Men with Parkinson's Disease (PD)

Sexual problems[a]
  Decreased desire (most common)[b]
  Erectile dysfunction
  Difficulty achieving orgasm
Mechanisms
  Muscle rigidity and akinesia
  Involvement of autonomic nerve control
  High levels of sexual difficulties also present in partners of men with Parkinson's disease

[a]Sexual function not coupled to severity of disease.
[b]Treatment with dopaminergic compounds may result in an apparent increase in desire.

infrequent in patients with Tourette's syndrome (72,73). Increased sexual activity has also been reported in patients with Wilson's disease (74). Impotence is almost universal among patients with multiple system atrophy (MSA), both of the striato-nigral type and the olivo-ponto-cerebellar type. In fact, erectile dysfunction may be the presenting symptom and is of diagnostic importance (75–79). It is important to recognize that treatment with sildenafil or similar drugs may be dangerous in patients with MSA due to their difficulty in achieving acceptable blood pressure control.

Dementia

The expression of sexuality by people with dementia is an area that has been largely neglected in research, yet it is of great concern in clinical practice. A Scottish postal questionnaire study sent to residential homes for demented patients showed that most of the demented were females, as was most of the care staff. The majority of incidents involving sexual expression, however, occurred from demented males directing their attention toward the female staff or female residents (80). In a study from Israel, the sexual behavior exhibited by demented patients was mostly heterosexual, and ranged from love and caring to romance and outright eroticism (81). Another study from the same group (82) stresses that the central dilemma on the subject of sexuality in elderly or demented patients is the conflict between the staff's desire to protect the patients and maintain their dignity and the patients' desire to fulfill their sexual needs. In another postal survey, the staff reported generally positive attitudes toward the demented patients' sexuality and sexual expression (83). There was, however, a consistent tendency for administrators to be relatively more conservative than the medical staff.

☐ SPINAL CORD DISORDERS
Multiple Sclerosis

Changes in sexual functions are rare at the onset of multiple sclerosis (MS), but become very common during its evolution. Most male patients report diminished sexual desire during the course of the disease (37–86%). Some patients may only experience a temporary decrease in desire during an episode, while in others the problem is progressive. In certain cases, increased sexual desire has also been described. When this hypersexuality is transitory and concurrent with an episode of new symptoms, it is likely to have been caused by a cerebral MS lesion. The localization of such a lesion, however, has not been established. Evidence for the involvement of the ventral tegmental area in the hypersexuality of some MS patients has been demonstrated by positron emission tomography (PET) studies during sexual activity in normal men that show distinctly increased regional blood flow in this area but not in the hypothalamus or limbic cortex during orgasm/ejaculation (84).

Erectile dysfunction is the most notable sexual dysfunction in men with MS (85–90). Estimates given in the literature vary between 34% and 80% (91). There are no indications of insufficient arterial inflow or increased venous outflow in the penis. Problems with ejaculation are also frequent, ranging from 34% to 61% (91).

Sexual dysfunction in male MS patients correlates strongly with bladder and bowel sphincter dysfunction, but less with motor and sensory dysfunction in the legs (91–95). The correlation with disability scale, clinical course, or disease duration was poor. Depression and cognitive impairment play important roles. Sexual dysfunction has been correlated with MRI findings of brain stem and pyramidal abnormalities as well as with total area of lesions on MRI and lesions in the pons (95,96).

It may be difficult to determine which kinds of sexual dysfunction in MS patients are caused by the central nervous system lesions and which are caused by other factors. Changes in sexual functions in MS patients, however, usually start abruptly and correlate in time both with neurological symptoms from the sacral segments and with bladder and bowel dysfunction, as mentioned above. Neurophysiological studies may give further indications of the involvement of those parts of the nervous system controlling pelvic structures. Genital sensory-evoked potential abnormalities are common in men with MS and sexual dysfunction (97). One of the causes of sexual dysfunction in some men with MS may be due to disruption of the genital somatosensory pathway with sparing of the efferent tracts.

Symptoms related to MS, such as fatigue, muscle contractures in the lower limbs, urinary disturbances, and the use of aids to manage incontinence, as well as paroxysmal motor and sensory disturbances triggered by sexual intercourse, can indirectly exert a negative effect on sex life as well as social and physical changes.

Amyotrophic Lateral Sclerosis

Amyotrophic lateral sclerosis (ALS) is a rapidly progressive motor disease leading to an almost total paralysis of the whole body including respiratory muscles; however, the neurons of Onuf's nucleus in the sacral spinal cord innervating the pelvic floor muscles are spared, in contrast to all other motor neurons. Also, the patients do not have any sensory or autonomic symptoms. Thus, these patients usually do not have difficulty with urination or defecation and have normal sexual functions (98). The absence of bedsores is another important difference between this illness and most other paralytic disorders.

A few ALS patients report an increase in sexual desire in the early stages of the illness (99). Loss of sexual desire only occurs in later stages of the disease or not at all. Sex was still an important issue for half of the patients in need of tracheostomy ventilation for life prolongation (100). Despite the fact that the severe paralysis of all voluntary movements eventually makes intercourse impossible, erection and ejaculation can be achieved through partner masturbation and the sensation of orgasm may be experienced as normal. This illustrates that sexual function may be preserved in patients with severe chronic or life-threatening disorders if the anatomical structures and the physiological mechanisms involved remain intact.

Spinal Cord Injuries
Pathophysiological Phases Following Spinal Cord Injury

The course of spinal cord injury (SCI) is typically characterized by three pathophysiological phases: spinal shock, reflex return, and readjustment.

Spinal Shock
Immediately following a sudden and complete spinal cord transection, all voluntary movements below the level of lesion are permanently lost, all sensations below the level of lesion are abolished, and reflex functions in all segments of the isolated spinal cord are completely lost. This is called the "spinal shock" phase. Less complete lesions of the spinal cord or lesions that develop slowly may result in less pronounced or no spinal shock.

The spinal shock phase lasts from a few hours to several weeks. The tendon reflexes are abolished or profoundly diminished, as are the reflex penile erection and the genital reflexes (the bulbocavernosus, cremaster, and anal reflexes). Erectile and ejaculatory functions are lost. When the lesion is complete, a form of priapism may be evident. The penis may become enlarged and semierected due to paralytic vasodilation following the interruption of the vasoconstrictor fibers in the anterolateral tracts of the spinal cord, causing a passive engorgement of the corpora cavernosa (101). During the period of spinal shock, it is usually impossible to predict the return of erectile and ejaculatory function.

The spinal shock phase is believed to be due to the interruption of central motor neuron fiber systems. Under physiological conditions, these systems keep the spinal motor neurons in a continuous state of subliminal depolarization ready to respond (102). Without any central motor control, the motor neurons can no longer respond.

Return of Reflexes
During the next phase, reflex activity and spasticity may appear in the lower extremities. Urinary bladder and bowel function may become reflexogenic. In upper motor neuron lesions, the erection reflex becomes one of the components of the autonomic functions of the isolated cord. Thus, stimulation may result in a mass reflex response. This may appear independent of cerebral participation and thus before the reflex responses of the skeletal muscles are fully developed. Tactile stimuli of varying type and intensity, including stimuli of the penis, may result in erection (101).

Readjustment
Sexual rehabilitation after SCI is very much dependent on the wishes, experiences, and pre-SCI sexual habits of any particular person. It is also to a great extent dependent on the cooperation and helpfulness of the patient's partner (101). Sexual readjustment after injury is closely and positively correlated to a young age at injury and willingness to experiment with alternative sexual expression (103).

Levels of Lesion and Long-Term Sexual Symptoms

Much is known about long-term sexual symptoms experienced by tetraplegic and paraplegic male patients from many extensive studies, particularly in war victims. The effect of the lesion is very much dependent upon its spinal level. If there is a complete destruction of the genital reflex center in the sacral part of spinal cord, erection may be possible, but there will be a complete paresis of the striated ejaculatory muscles. Thus, ejaculation is impossible and semen appears as a dribbling from the tip of the penis. In lesions of the upper part of the spinal cord above segment T10, reflex erection—as well as seminal emission and ejaculation—may still be possible. These patients, however, have impaired sensory perception in the genital organs.

In patients with spinal cord lesions between the level of the lower thoracic segments and the conus, both cerebral and reflex erection may be possible, despite the fact that the patient cannot feel the sexual organs. This does not mean that the patients can no longer experience any type of orgasm: Although a man with a complete lesion of the spinal cord above the conus can never feel the ejaculatory contractions, a number of autonomic phenomena that occur with orgasm can be experienced. In spinal cord lesion, there is often a hyperesthetic area of the body just above or at the segment of the lesion. This is or may be trained to be a very strong erogenous zone.

A review of 24 studies (104) of more than 2500 men with spinal cord injuries showed that a median of 80% (range 54–95%) reported erections. The percentage of SCI men reporting ejaculation was much lower (median 15%, range 0–52%). Fewer of the patients with complete lower sacral lesions (26%) had erectile capacity than those with complete upper cord lesions or incomplete lesions at any level (90–99%) (105). Sexual desire is not primarily affected by SCI. Secondary to other sexual disabilities, however, sexual interest and desire may be diminished (42). A comprehensive review of erectile and ejaculatory dysfunction in patients with spinal cord disorders (particularly traumatic SCIs) and their treatment is given in a WHO International Consultation review (104).

Fertility with Therapeutic Assistance

Semen volume, sperm count, and spermatic mobility are decreased in men with SCI. This is at least partly dependent on insufficient drainage. Ejaculation can be provoked in many paraplegic men through vibratory stimulation or electrostimulation. Penile vibratory stimulation should be used as the first line of treatment for ejaculatory dysfunction of men with SCI due to its safety, efficacy, and reliability as well as its decreased invasiveness (104). It has been shown that repeated vibration-induced ejaculations result in increased semen volume, a larger number of motile sperm, and improved sperm penetration capacity. Insemination with autologous semen obtained in such a way has resulted in pregnancies. Collection of semen very early after the SCI makes it possible to store semen of good quality for future insemination.

Spinal Cord Malformations

The most important malformation that gives rise to sexual dysfunction is meningomyelocele, a congenital defect characterized by protrusion of the meninges and spinal cord through the vertebral column. Depending on the degree of the malformation, there is a more or less pronounced loss of sexual ability. Some boys will have no genital sensations at all, some have erections only, and some have both erections and emissions (106,107).

Sacral agenesis is a type of malformation of the most distal part of the spine, combined with caudal spinal cord changes. In advanced cases, the child is born with a series of malformations involving the genitourinary tract and the hindgut. In other cases, anatomical changes are not discovered at birth and instead are first manifested in adulthood as an occult form of spinal dysraphism. MRI will often disclose tethering of the spinal cord and signs of spinal stenosis (108). Sexual problems, including erectile and/or ejaculatory dysfunction, may result, in part, from sensory dysfunction in the sacral segments. Often, there have never been any ejaculations at all. Neurosurgery may correct the problems in some cases (109).

In cases of Arnold–Chiari malformation in which there is an obstruction of the foramen magnum, loss of sexual desire is very common. Some of these men are completely impotent and others have reduced potency. The onset of the sexual complaints nearly always follows the beginning of the neurological disturbances (110). This malformation is often associated with syringomyelia (111). Among these patients, about 10% have severe erectile dysfunction.

Spinal Canal Stenosis

Some patients with neurogenic intermittent claudication note that after walking a short distance, an unwanted erection may appear, unaccompanied by any sexual arousal or thoughts (112,113). Simultaneously there is often pain in the hips on walking that radiates to the thighs and legs. The legs tingle and become numb on further walking. When the patient sits down, the leg symptoms are relieved and the erection subsides over a few minutes. Erections could also appear

after kneeling for half an hour or so. Decompression by bilateral laminectomy results in complete relief of all these symptoms. The mechanism behind this type of priapism is not clear, but could be the result of a blockade of sympathetic outflow.

Myelopathies

Since both the nerve paths conveying erection, emission, and ejaculation and those leading sensory impulses from the genitalia travel through the spinal cord, myelopathies can result in a malfunction of all these mechanisms. Priapism can also be symptom of a myelopathy (114). Out of 224 consecutive male patients referred to a sexological outpatient department because of impotence, 17 patients (31–72 years old) were found to have a myelopathy (115). In most of these cases, the neurological disorder was not diagnosed at the time of referral. In those patients in whom the neurological disease was known at the time of investigation, the sexual problem had started with their falling ill, often very long ago. The etiology was unknown in seven patients; in the remaining 10, the final diagnoses were postmyelitic (five cases), spinal cord compression (three cases), posthematomyelia (one case), and vitamin B12 deficiency (one case). Morning erections, psychogenic erections, and reflex erections were disturbed in most of these men. Disturbances of ejaculation, such as retarded ejaculation, total loss of ejaculation, or dribbling ejaculation, were reported by ten patients. Seven patients reported orgasm disturbances, and in one patient, the orgasms were painful.

In one study of about 2000 patients of both sexes with injuries of the cervical spinal cord without paralysis, 85 reported sexual dysfunction (116). Thirty percent of patients with vitamin B12 deficiency reported sexual dysfunction (117). AIDS-associated vacuolar myelopathy has a striking similarity with the myelopathy of vitamin B12 deficiency (118). (For further details about sexual problems in AIDS patients, see Chapter 13.) Otherwise, myelitic processes are usually circumscribed autoimmune or more diffuse paramalignant manifestations. Infectious diseases such as neurocysticercosis may also have a similar appearance (119).

□ PERIPHERAL NERVE DISORDERS
Disorders of the Spinal Roots and Peripheral Mononeuropathies in the Sacral Region

The knowledge of sexual function in patients with spinal root disorders or sacral mononeuropathies is mostly based on single case histories or very limited material. Please refer to the author's review of such cases for further information (57).

Many patients with sacral root lesions are distressed by pain with coitus. Ejaculation may also be painful or delayed. Impotence occasionally occurs. Since bilateral loss of function is rare, some kind of sexual gratification is usually possible. Bilateral damage to all S2–S5 roots or nerves results in dribbling ejaculation. In these cases, seminal emission is preserved, but paresis of bulbo- and ischiocavernosus muscles is present. In such cases, reflex erections are also not possible, but psychogenic erection mechanisms are still active. Unilateral loss of all sacral nerves on one side results in ipsilateral genital anesthesia. Sexual function is usually not impaired, however, because the innervation of the other side is sufficient for normal genital reflex responses.

Peripheral mononeuropathies of the pudendal nerve or branches of that nerve in particular are not uncommon (120,121). These nerve lesions often result in so much pain and dyspareunia that intercourse becomes impossible or at least unpleasant.

Intrapelvic Nerve Damage

The most important intrapelvic nerves in the male from the sexual point of view are the two cavernous nerves on each side of the penis. They originate from the pelvic plexus (the inferior hypogastric plexus) and extend into the neurovascular bundle along the seminal vesicles to the posterolateral part of the prostate gland and approach the midline, traveling through the urogenital diaphragm together with the urethra. There, branches of the cavernous nerves spread to the corpora cavernosa and corpus spongiosum. The distal parts of the cavernous nerves communicate with the dorsal nerve of the penis. The autonomic erectile nerve bundles follow this somatic nerve along the penis to the cavernous bodies.

The most important risk for damage to cavernous nerves is prostatic surgery. Erectile dysfunction is a frequent complication of radical prostatectomy. It is important to consider the total course of the nerves during neural preservation techniques (122). Sildenafil has little effect in patients after radical prostatectomy (123) in contrast to patients with spinal cord injuries (124). Destruction of the postganglionic neuron (denervation of the cavernous tissues) leads to total loss of initiation of erection and thus prevents the phosphodiesterase inhibitors from facilitating erection. The observation, however, that treatment with sildenafil can be effective two years after surgery in early nonresponders (125) could indicate regeneration of the postganglionic nerves.

Polyneuropathies

Autonomic dysfunction, including sexual dysfunction, is a common complication in peripheral neuropathies (126). Polyneuropathies due to deficiencies in Vitamin B1 (127) and Vitamin B12 (117) or plasma cell dyscrasia (128) may cause erectile dysfunction. Polyneuropathies caused by intoxication from n-hexane, methyl-n-butyl-ketone, carbon disulfide, and similar substances may cause erectile dysfunction (129,130). (For further information on sexual dysfunction in patients with diabetic polyneuropathy, see Chapter 14.)

Very little has been written about sexual dysfunction in hereditary polyneuropathies. Based on pathophysiological data, however, erectile dysfunction, retarded or retrograde ejaculation, and orgasmic

difficulties are to be expected. Erectile dysfunction and ejaculation problems have been observed in patients with Guillain–Barré syndrome, Charcot–Marie–Tooth syndrome (131,132), adrenomyeloneuropathy/adrenoleukodystrophy (133,134), Refsum's disease (Lundberg PO. Unpublished observation), Friedreich's ataxia, Riley–Day syndrome, HSAN (hereditary sensory and autonomic polyneuropathy) I-IV (135), and primary amyloidotic polyneuropathy (136–141). In a study of 341 consecutive patients with erectile dysfunction, neurophysiological evaluation for polyneuropathy revealed the presence of polyneuropathy in 38% of diabetic cases and 10% of impotent cases of other etiologies (142). The adrenoleukodystrophies represent a group of patients of particular interest because of the severe prognosis of this disease, the androgen deficiency involved, and the predominance of CNS lesions (143). Involvement of the somatic nerves (pudendal nerves) does not seem to be an important underlying factor of erectile dysfunction in patients with hereditary motor and sensory neuropathies (144).

☐ OTHER NEUROLOGICAL DISORDERS
Myopathies

In certain types of progressive muscular dystrophies such as myotonic dystrophy (145–147), the Becker type (148), and particularly ocular myopathy of the autosomal progressive external ophthalmoplegia type (149,150), hypogonadism in combination with disturbances of erectile function and desire has been described. Erectile dysfunction may also occur in mitochondrial encephalomyopathies such as MERFF and MELAS syndromes (151).

Genetic Encephalo/Myelo/Neuropathies

In Kennedy's syndrome (X-linked bulbospinal muscular atrophy), gynecomastia is common, and testicular atrophy, decreased sexual desire, and erectile dysfunction may also occur (152,153). An androgen-receptor dysfunction caused by a trinucleotide repeat expansion in the androgen receptor gene has been found (154).

☐ NEUROLOGICAL DISORDERS AND DYSFUNCTION CAUSED BY SEXUAL ACTIVITY

The above discussion illustrates how sexual function can be compromised by neurological dysfunction. Just as neurological disorders can have a negative impact on sexual function, sexual activity can also sometimes cause neurological problems.

Epileptic Seizures

It is well known that hyperventilation can provoke generalized epileptic seizures. Hyperventilation during sexual intercourse may sometimes be strong enough to provoke an epileptic fit. Reflex mechanisms during sexual activity could also trigger a partial epileptic attack from the corresponding cortical area. Sexual fantasies as well as genital stimuli (masturbation) or orgasm (155,156) may be such triggers. Few cases have been published, but this phenomenon may be underreported.

Cataplexia

Cataplexia, or attacks of loss of muscular tone in situations of affect, can be provoked by sexual arousal and orgasm.

Cerebrovascular Catastrophes

Sexual activity results in an obvious increase in blood pressure, especially in certain coital positions and under certain sexual activities. (For further information on this topic, see Chapter 7.) There is a small risk that such an increase in blood pressure can cause a rupture of a preexisting intracranial arterial aneurysm. Coitus was in fact the most common circumstance that could be related to subarachnoid hemorrhage in one study (157). Intracerebral and intraspinal bleeding are less common. Transitory ischemic attacks can also be provoked by sexual activity; transitory global amnesia is one of these. These incidents are rare and usually occur in unusual and vigorous sexual circumstances such as having an affair with a new partner in a hotel room.

Headache

Since very severe headache usually is the paramount symptom of a subarachnoid hemorrhage, the term "malignant orgasmic" has been suggested in contrast to benign orgasmic cephalalgia (BOC), which is a very common and nondangerous complaint (157). BOC attacks are relatively short-lasting, from a few minutes to several hours. There should be no stiffness of the neck, blurring of consciousness, or any other neurological symptoms. The mechanisms behind these types of headache are obscure. The attacks, lasting for some hours, are very similar to migraine attacks. BOC attacks are usually recurring. Diagnosis can be a problem, however, when the patient seeks help for the first attack. A CT scan is usually sufficient to exclude bleeding. Sometimes a spinal tap is necessary. The occurrence of a new attack can often be prevented by prophylactic treatment with a β-blocker (158).

□ CONCLUSION

Sexual dysfunctions are very common among men with neurological disorders. Sexual desire, potency, ejaculation, and orgasm may be influenced. Changes in sexual behavior may also result from a brain disorder. Most important among the neurological disorders are hypothalamo–pituitary processes and temporal lobe lesions. These often occur in conjunction with epilepsy, MS, PD, and spinal cord disorders—notably, spinal cord injuries and diabetic polyneuropathy. Sexual activity can also provoke migraine attacks and epileptic fits and result in a cerebrovascular catastrophe.

□ REFERENCES

1. Lundberg PO. Neurological disorders in andrology. In: Bain J, Hafez EFE, eds. Diagnosis in Andrology. The Hague: Nijhoff Publishers, 1980:195–213.
2. Lundberg PO, Ertekin C, Ghezzi A, et al. Neurosexology. Guidelines for neurologists. European federation of neurological societies task force on neurosexology. Eur J Neurol 2001; 8(suppl 3):2–24.
3. Podnar S, Oblak C, Vodusek DB. Sexual function in men with cauda equina lesions: a clinical and electromyographic study. J Neurol Neurosurg Psychiatry 2002; 73(6):715–720.
4. Vodusek DB. Neurophysiological tests in erectile dysfunction. Scand J Sexol 1998; 1:81–95.
5. Vodusek DB, Fowler CJ. Clinical neurophysiology. In: Fowler CJ, ed. Neurology of Bladder, Bowel, and Sexual Dysfunction. Boston: Butterworth-Heinemann, 1999:109–143.
6. Lundberg PO, Wide L. Sexual function in males with pituitary tumors. Fertil Steril 1978; 29(2):175–179.
7. Muhr C, Hulting A-L, Lundberg PO, et al. Pituitary adenomas with hyperprolactinaemia in males. In: Auer LM, Leb G, Tscherne G, et al., eds. Prolactinomas: An Interdisciplinary Approach. Berlin: Walter de Gruyter Inc, 1985:169–178.
8. Citron JT, Ettinger B, Rubinoff H, et al. Prevalence of hypothalamic-pituitary imaging abnormalities in impotent men with secondary hypogonadism. J Urol 1996; 155(2):529–533.
9. Roeder FD. Stereotaxic lesion of the tuber cinereum in sexual deviation. Confin Neurol 1966; 27:162–163.
10. Dieckmann G, Hassler R. Unilateral hypothalamotomy in sexual delinquents. Report on six cases. Confin Neurol 1975; 37:177–186.
11. Berciano J, Amado JA, Freijanes J, et al. Familial cerebellar ataxia and hypogonadotropic hypogonadism: evidence for hypothalamic LHRH deficiency. J Neurol Neurosurg Psychiatry 1982; 45(8):747–751.
12. Neuhäuser G, Opitz JM. Autosomal recessive syndrome of cerebellar ataxia and hypogonadotropic hypogonadism. Clin Genet 1975; 7(5):426–434.

13. Fok AC, Wong MC, Cheah JS. Syndrome of cerebellar ataxia and hypogonadotropic hypogonadism: evidence for pituitary gonadotrophin deficiency. J Neurol Neurosurg Psychiatry 1989; 52:407–409.

14. Limber ER, Bresnick GH, Lebovitz RM, et al. Spinocerebellar ataxia, hypogonadotropic hypogonadism, and choroidal dystrophy (Boucher-Neuhäuser syndrome). Am J Med Genet 1989; 33(3): 409–414.

15. Abs R, Van Vleyman E, Parizel PM, et al. Congenital cerebellar hypoplasia and hypogonadal hypogonadism. J Neurol Sci 1990; 98(2–3):259–265.

16. Baroncini A, Franco N, Forabosco A. A new family with chorioretinal dystrophy, spinocerebellar ataxia and hypogonadotropic hypogonadism (Boucher-Neuhäuser syndrome). Clin Genet 1991; 39(4):274–277.

17. Wheeler MD, Styne DM. Drug treatment in precocious puberty. Drugs 1991; 41(5):717–728.

18. Meyer JE. Die sexuellen Störungen der Hirnverletzten. Arch Psychiatr Nervenkr Z Gesamte Neurol Psychiatr 1955; 193:449–469.

19. Kreutzer JS, Zasler ND. Psychosexual consequences of traumatic brain injury: methodology and preliminary findings. Brain Inj 1989; 3(2):177–186.

20. Hibbard MR, Gordon WA, Flanagan S, et al. Sexual dysfunction after traumatic brain injury. Neuro Rehabil 2000; 15(2):107–120.

21. Aloni R, Katz S. Sexual Difficulties After Traumatic Brain injury and Ways to Deal With It. Springfield, IL: Thomas, 2003:1–207.

22. Miller BL, Cummings JL, McIntyre H, et al. Hypersexuality or altered sexual preference following brain injury. J Neurol Neurosurg Psychiatry 1986; 49(8):867–873.

23. Gorman DG, Cummings JL. Hypersexuality following septal injury. Arch Neurol 1992; 49(3):308–310.

24. de Morsier G, Gronek B. Sur 92 cas de troubles sexual post-traumatiques. Ann Med Psychol (Paris) 1972; 2:653–670.

25. Simpson G, Blaszczynski A, Hodgkinson A. Sex offending as a psychosocial sequela of traumatic brain injury. J Head Trauma Rehabil 1999; 14(6):567–580.

26. Gerstenbrand F, Lücking CH. Hypersexualität im Rahmen der Klüver-Bucy-Symptomatik nach traumatischem apallischem Syndrom. J Neurovisc Relat 1971; (suppl 10):524–537.

27. Oliveira V, Ferro JM, Foreid JP, et al. Klüver-Bucy syndrome in systemic lupus erythematosus. J Neurol 1989; 236:55–56.

28. Hayman LA, Rexer JL, Pavol MA, et al. Klüver-Bucy syndrome after bilateral selective damage of amygdala and its cortical connections. J Neuropsychiatry Clin Neurosci 1998; 10:354–358.

29. Montagna P. Fatal familial insomnia: clinical, laboratory and pathological features [abstract]. Rev Neurol 1999; 29:1006–1009.

30. Kalliomäki JL, Markkanen TK, Mustonen KA. Sexual behavior after cerebral vascular accident. A study on patients below the age of 60 years. Fertil Steril 1961; 12:156–158.

31. Sjögren K. Sexuality after stroke with hemiplegia. II. With special regard to partnership adjustment and to fulfillment. Scand J Rehabil Med 1983; 15:63–69.

32. Sjögren K, Damber J-E, Liliequist B. Sexuality after stroke with hemiplegia. I. Aspects of sexual function. Scand J Rehabil Med 1983; 15:55–61.

33. Monga TN, Lawson JS, Inglis J. Sexual dysfunction in stroke patients. Arch Phys Med Rehabil 1986; 67(1):19–22.

34. Boldrini P, Basaglia N, Calanca MC. Sexual changes in hemiparetic patients. Arch Phys Med Rehabil 1991; 72(3):202–207.

35. Aloni R, Ring H, Rosenthul N, et al. Sexual function in male patients after stroke: a follow up study. Sex Disabil 1993; 11:121–128.

36. Korpelainen JT, Kauhanen ML, Kemola H, et al. Sexual dysfunction in stroke patients. Acta Neurol Scand 1998; 98(6):400–405.

37. Cheung RT. Sexual functioning in Chinese stroke patients with mild or no disability. Cerebrovasc Dis 2002; 14(2):122–128.

38. Korpelainen JT, Nieminen P, Myllylä VV. Sexual functioning among stroke patients and their spouses. Stroke 1999; 30(4):715–719.

39. Wiig EH. Counselling the adult aphasic for sexual readjustment. Rehabil Couns Bull 1973; 110–119.

40. Godess ED, Wagner NN, Silvermann DR. Post-stroke sexual activity of CVA disorders. Med Aspects Hum Sex 1979; 13:16–30.

41. Coslett HB, Heilman KM. Male sexual function. Impairment after right hemisphere stroke. Arch Neurol 1986; 43(10):1036–1039.

42. Fugl-Meyer AR, Fugl-Meyer K, Lundberg PO. Sexual rehabilitation. In: Frommelt P, Grötzbach H, eds. NeuroRehabilitation. Berlin: Blackwell, 1999: 370–388.

43. Monga TN, Monga M, Raina MS, et al. Hypersexuality in stroke. Arch Phys Med Rehabil 1986; 67(6): 415–417.

44. Donnet A, Schmitt A, Poncet M, et al. Hallucinations of supernumerary limbs, left hemineglect and hypersexuality in a case of right capsulo-lenticular hematoma. [Article in French]. Rev Neurol (Paris) 1997; 153(10):587–590.

45. Absher JR, Vogt BA, Clark DG, et al. Hypersexuality and hemiballism due to subthalamic infarction. Neuropsychiatry Neuropsychol Behav Neurol 2000; 13(3):220–229.

46. Saunders M, Rawson M. Sexuality in male epileptics. J Neurol Sci 1970; 10(6):577–583.

47. Dansky LV, Andermann E, Andermann F. Marriage and fertility in epileptic patients. Epilepsia 1980; 21(3):261–271.

48. Guldner GT, Morrell MJ. Nocturnal penile tumescence and rigidity evaluation in men with epilepsy. Epilepsia 1996; 37(12):1211–1214.

49. Taylor DC. Sexual behavior and temporal lobe epilepsy. Arch Neurol 1969; 21(5):510–516.

50. Shukla GD, Srivastava ON, Katiyar BC. Sexual disturbances in temporal lobe epilepsy: a controlled study. Br J Psychiatry 1979; 134:288–292.

51. Morrell MJ, Sperling MR, Stecker M, et al. Sexual dysfunction in partial epilepsy: a deficit in physiological arousal. Neurology 1994; 44(2):243–247.

52. Blumer D. Hypersexual episodes in the temporal lobe epilepsy. Am J Psychiatry 1970; 126(8): 1099–1106.

53. Christianson SA, Silfvenius H, Saisa J, et al. Life satisfaction and sexuality in patients operated for epilepsy. Acta Neurol Scand 1995; 92(1):1–6.

54. Isojarvi JI, Repo M, Pakarinen AJ, et al. Carbamazepine, phenytoin, sex hormones, and sexual function in men with epilepsy. Epilepsia 1995; 36(4):366–370.

55. Duncan S, Blacklaw J, Beastall GH, et al. Antiepileptic drug therapy and sexual function in men with epilepsy. Epilepsia 1999; 40(2):197–204.

56. Bauer J, Blumenthal S, Reuber M, et al. Epilepsy syndrome, focus location, and treatment choice affect testicular function in men with epilepsy. Neurology 2004; 62(2):243–246.

57. Lundberg PO. Sexual dysfunction in patients with neurological disorders. Annu Rev Sex Res 1992; 3:121–150.

58. Brown RG, Jahanshahi M, Quinn N, et al. Sexual function in patients with Parkinson's disease and their partners. J Neurol Neurosurg Psychiatry 1990; 53(6):480–486.

59. Koller WC, Vetere-Overfield B, Williamson A, et al. Sexual dysfunction in Parkinson's disease. Clin Neuropharmacol 1990; 13(5):461–463.

60. Takahashi A. Autonomic nervous system disorders in Parkinson's disease. Eur Neurol 1991; 31(suppl 1):41–47.

61. Wermuth L, Stenager E. Sexual problems in young patients with Parkinson's disease. Acta Neurol Scand 1995; 91:453–455.

62. Sakakibara R, Shinotoh H, Uchiyama T, et al. Questionnaire-based assessment of pelvic organ dysfunction in Parkinson's disease. Auton Neurosci 2001; 92(1–2):76–85.

63. Lipe H, Longstreth WT, Bird TD, et al. Sexual function in married men with Parkinson's disease compared to married men with arthritis. Neurology 1990; 40(9):1347–1349.

64. Zesiewicz TA, Baker MJ, Wahba M, et al. Autonomic nervous system dysfunction in Parkinson's disease. Curr Treat Options Neurol 2003; 5(2):149–160.

65. Berger Y, Blaivas JG, DeLaRocha ER, et al. Urodynamic findings in Parkinson's disease. J Urol 1987; 138(4):836–838.

66. Singer C, Weiner WJ, Sanchez-Ramos JR. Autonomic dysfunction in men with Parkinson's disease. Eur Neurol 1992; 32(3):134–140.

67. Mathers SE, Kempster PA, Swash M, et al. Constipation and paradoxical puborectalis contraction in anismus

68. and Parkinson's disease: a dystonic phenomenon? J Neurol Neurosurg Psychiatry 1988; 51(12):1503–1507.

68. Ashraf W, Pfeiffer RF, Quigley EM. Anorectal manometry in the assessment of anorectal function in Parkinson's disease: a comparison with chronic idiopathic constipation. Mov Disord 1994; 9(6):655–663.

69. Hyyppa MT, Falck SC, Rinne UR. Is L-DOPA an aphrodisiac in patients with Parkinson's disease? In: Sandler M, Gessa GL, eds. Sexual Behavior: Pharmacology and Biochemistry. New York: Raven Press, 1975:315–327.

70. Uitti RJ, Tanner CM, Rajput AH, et al. Hypersexuality with antiparkinsonian therapy. Clin Neuropharmacol 1989; 12(5):375–383.

71. Morris M. Dementia and cognitive changes in Huntington's disease. Adv Neurol 1995; 65:187–200.

72. Comings DE. Role of genetic factors in human sexual behavior based on studies of Tourette syndrome and ADHD probands and their relatives. Am J Med Genet 1994; 54(3):227–241.

73. Lombroso PJ, Scahill LD, Chappell PB, et al. Tourette's syndrome: a multigenerational, neuropsychiatric disorder. Adv Neurol 1995; 65:305–318.

74. Akil M, Brewer GJ. Psychiatric and behavioral abnormalities in Wilson's disease. Adv Neurol 1995; 65:171–178.

75. Beck RO, Betts CD, Fowler CJ. Genitourinary dysfunction in multiple system atrophy: clinical features and treatment in 62 cases. J Urol 1994; 151(5):1336–1341.

76. Hodder J. Shy Drager syndrome. Axone 1997; 18(4):75–79.

77. Palace J, Chandiramani VA, Fowler CJ. Value of sphincter electromyography in the diagnosis of multiple system atrophy. Muscle Nerve 1997; 20(11): 1396–1403.

78. Peterson T, Mathias CJ, Alam M, et al. Simultaneous arterial and urinary bladder pressure recordings in multiple system atrophy and in spinal disorders with detrusor hyperreflexia. Clin Auton Res 1997; 7(6): 299–304.

79. Pellegrinetti A, Moscato G, Siciliano G, et al. Electrophysiological evaluation of genito-sphincteric dysfunction in multiple system atrophy. Int J Neurosci 2003; 113(10):1353–1369.

80. Archibald C. Sexuality, dementias and residential care: managers report and response. Health Soc Care Community 1998; 6(2):95–101.

81. Ehrenfeld M, Bronner G, Tabak N, et al. Sexuality among institutionalized elderly patients with dementia. Nurs Ethics 1999; 6(2):144–149.

82. Ehrenfeld M, Tabak N, Bronner G, et al. Ethical dilemmas concerning sexuality of elderly patients suffering from dementia. Int J Nurs Pract 1997; 3(4):255–259.

83. Holmes D, Reingold J, Teresi J. Sexual expression and dementia. Views of caregivers: a pilot study. Int J Geriatr Psychiatry 1997; 12(7):695–701.

84. Holstege G, Georgiadis JR, Paans AM, et al. Brain activation during human male ejaculation. J Neurosci 2003; 23(27):9185–9193.

85. Valleroy ML, Kraft G. Sexual dysfunction in multiple sclerosis. Arch Phys Med Rehabil 1984; 65(3): 125–128.

86. Kirkeby HJ, Poulsen EU, Petersen T, et al. Erectile dysfunction in multiple sclerosis. Neurology 1988; 38(9): 1366–1371.

87. Minderhoud JM, Leemhuis JG, Kremer J, et al. Sexual disturbances arising from multiple sclerosis. Acta Neurol Scand 1984; 70(4):299–306.

88. Betts CD, Jones SJ, Fowler CG, et al. Erectile dysfunction in multiple sclerosis. Associated neurological and neurophysiological deficits, and treatment of the condition. Brain 1994; 117(Pt 6):1303–1310.

89. Mattson D, Petrie M, Srivastava DK, et al. Multiple sclerosis. Sexual dysfunction and its response to medications. Arch Neurol 1995; 52(9):862–868.

90. Ghezzi A, Malvestiti GM, Baldini S, et al. Erectile impotence in multiple sclerosis patients: a neurophysiological study. J Neurol 1995; 242(3):123–126.

91. Ghezzi A. Sexuality and multiple sclerosis. Scand J Sexol 1999; 2:125–140.

92. Ghezzi A, Zaffaroni M, Baldini S, et al. Sexual dysfunction in male multiple sclerosis patients in relation to clinical findings. Eur J Neurol 1996; 3:462–466.

93. Zorzon M, Zivadinov R, Bosco A, et al. Sexual dysfunction in multiple sclerosis: a case-control study. I. Frequency and comparison of groups. Mult Scler 1999; 5(6):418–427.

94. Zivadinov R, Zorzon M, Bosco A, et al. Sexual dysfunction in multiple sclerosis: II. Correlation analysis. Mult Scler 1999; 5(6):428–431.

95. Zivadinov R, Zorzon M, Locatelli L, et al. Sexual dysfunction in multiple sclerosis: a MRI, neurophysiological and urodynamic study. J Neurol Sci 2003; 210(1–2):73–76.

96. Barak Y, Achiron A, Elizur A, et al. Sexual dysfunction in relapsing-remitting multiple sclerosis: magnetic resonance imaging, clinical, and psychological correlates. J Psychiatry Neurosci 1996; 21(4):255–258.

97. Yang CC, Bowen JD, Kraft GH, et al. Physiologic studies of male sexual dysfunction in multiple sclerosis. Mult Scler 2001; 7(4):249–254.

98. Jokelainen M, Palo J. Letter: amyotrophic lateral sclerosis and autonomic nervous system. Lancet 1976; 1(7971):1246.

99. Jokelainen M. Sexual function in amyotrophic lateral sclerosis. Med Aspects Hum Sex 1981; 15:56.

100. Kaub-Wittemer D, Steinbüchel N, Wasner M, et al. Quality of life and psychosocial issues in ventilated patients with amyotrophic lateral sclerosis and their caregivers. J Pain Symptom Manage 2003; 26(4): 890–896.

101. Guttmann L. The sexual problem. In: Guttmann L, ed. Spinal Cord Injuries: Comprehensive Management and Research. 2nd ed. Oxford: Blackwell, 1976: 474–505.

102. Adams DB, Victor M, Ropper AH. Diseases of the spinal cord. In: Adams DB, Victor M, eds. Principles of Neurology. 6th ed. New York: McGraw Hill, 1981: 1227–1277.

103. Siosteen A, Lundqvist C, Blomstrand C, et al. Sexual ability, activity, attitudes and satisfaction as part of adjustment in spinal cord-injured subjects. Paraplegia 1990; 28(5):285–295.

104. Lundberg PO, Brackett NL, Denys P, et al. Neurological disorders: erectile and ejaculatory dysfunction. In: Jardin A, Wagner G, Khoury S, et al., eds. Erectile Dysfunction. Plymouth: Plymbridge Distributors Ltd, 2000:591–646.

105. Bors EH, Comarr AE. Neurological disturbances of sexual function with special reference to 529 patients with spinal cord injury. Urol Surv 1960; 10:191–222.

106. Wabrek AJ, Wabrek CJ, Burchell RC. The human tragedy of spina bifida: spinal myelomeningocele. Sex Disabil 1978; 1:210–217.

107. Sawyer SM, Roberts KV. Sexual and reproductive health in young people with spina bifida. Dev Med Child Neurol 1999; 41(10):671–675.

108. Pang D. Sacral agenesis and caudal spinal cord malformations. Neurosurgery 1993; 32(5):755–779.

109. Boemers TM, van Gool JD, de Jong TP. Tethered spinal cord: the effect of neurosurgery on the lower urinary tract and male sexual function. Br J Urol 1995; 76(6): 747–751.

110. Caetano De Barros M, Farias Da Silva W, De Azevedo Filho HC, et al. Disturbances of sexual potency in patients with basilar impression and Arnold-Chiari malformation. J Neurol Neurosurg Psychiatry 1975; 38(6):598–600.

111. Aghakhani N, Parker F, Tadie M. Syringomyelia and Chiari abnormality in the adult. Analysis of the results of a cooperative series of 285 cases. [Article in French]. Neurochirurgie 1999; 45(suppl 1):23–36.

112. Laha RK, Dujovny M, Huang PS. Intermittent erection in spinal canal stenosis. J Urol 1979; 121(1): 123–124.

113. Hopkins A, Clarke C, Brindley G. Erections on walking as a symptom of spinal canal stenosis. J Neurol Neurosurg Psychiatry 1987; 50(10):1371–1374.

114. Lundberg PO. Priapism: review. Scand J Sexol 2000; 3:13–24.

115. Lundberg PO, Brattberg A. Sexual dysfunction in selected neurological disorders: hypothalamopituitary disorders, epilepsy, myelopathies, polyneuropathies, and sacral nerve lesions. Semin Neurol 1992; 12(2):115–119.

116. Perese MD, Prezio LA, Perese EF. Sexual dysfunction caused by injuries of the spinal cord without paralysis. Spine 1976; 1:149–154.

117. Kunze K, Leitenmaier K. Vitamin B12 deficiency and subacute combined degeneration of the spinal cord. In: Vinken PJ, Bruyn GW, eds. Handbook of Clinical Neurology. Vol. 28. Amsterdam: Elsevier, 1976:141–198.

118. Di Rocco A, Simpson DM. AIDS-associated vacuolar myelopathy. AIDS Patient Care STDS 1998; 12(6): 457–461.

119. Singh NN, Verma R, Pankaj BK, et al. Cauda-conus syndrome resulting from neurocysticercosis. Neurol India 2003; 51(1):118–120.

120. Hofmann A, Jones R, Schoenvogel R. Pudendal-nerve neurapraxia as a result of traction on the fracture table. A report of four cases. J Bone Joint Surg Am 1982; 64(1):136–138.

121. Amarenco G, Lanoe Y, Ghnassia RT, et al. Syndrome du canal d'Alcock et névralgie périnéale. Rev Neurol (Paris) 1988; 144:523–526.

122. Mauroy B, Demondion X, Drizenko A, et al. The inferior hypogastric plexus (pelvic plexus): its importance in neural preservation techniques. Surg Radiol Anat 2003; 25(1):6–15.

123. Blander DS, Sanchez-Ortiz RF, Wein AJ, et al. Efficacy of sildenafil in erectile dysfunction after radical prostatectomy. Int J Impot Res 2000; 12(3):165–168.

124. Derry F, Hultling C, Seftel AD, et al. Efficacy and safety of sildenafil citrate (Viagra) in men with erectile dysfunction and spinal cord injury: a review. Urology 2002; 60(suppl 2):49–57.

125. Hong EK, Lepor H, McCullough AR. Time dependent patient satisfaction with sildenafil for erectile dysfunction (ED) after nerve-sparing radical retropubic prostatectomy (RRP). Int J Impot Res 1999; 11(suppl 1): S15–S22.

126. McDougall AJ, McLeod JG. Autonomic neuropathy, I. Clinical features, investigation, pathophysiology, and treatment. J Neurol Sci 1996; 137(2):79–88.

127. Tjandra BS, Janknegt RA. Neurogenic impotence and lower urinary tract symptoms due to vitamin B1 deficiency in chronic alcoholism. J Urol 1997; 157(3): 954–955.

128. Takatsuki K, Sanada I. Plasma cell dyscrasia with polyneuropathy and endocrine disorder: clinical and laboratory features of 109 reported cases. Jpn J Clin Oncol 1983; 13(3):543–555.

129. Windebank AJ. Neuropathies. In: Mathews WB, ed. Handbook of Clinical Neurology. Vol. 51, Amsterdam: Elsevier, 1976:263–293.

130. Frumkin H. Multiple system atrophy following chronic carbon disulfide exposure. Environ Health Perspect 1998; 106(9):611–613.

131. Bird TD, Lipe HP, Crabtree LD. Impotence associated with Charcot-Marie-Tooth syndrome. Eur Neurol 1994; 34(3):155–157.

132. Crabtree L. Charcot-Marie-Tooth disease: sex, sexuality and self-esteem. Sex Disabil 1997; 15(4):293–306.

133. Sakakibara R, Hatteri T, Fukutake T, et al. Micturitional disturbance in a patient with adrenomyeloneuropathy (AMN). Neurourol Urodyn 1998; 17(3):207–212.

134. Garside S, Rosebush PI, Levinson AJ, et al. Late-onset adrenoleukodystrophy associated with long-standing psychiatric symptoms. J Clin Psychiatry 1999; 60(7): 460–468.

135. Nukada H, Pollock M, Haas LF. The clinical spectrum and morphology of type II hereditary sensory neuropathy. Brain 1982; 105(Pt 4):647–665.

136. Kelly JJ Jr, Kyle RA, O'Brien PC, et al. The natural history of peripheral neuropathy in primary system amyloidosis. Ann Neurol 1979; 6(1):1–7.

137. Obayashi K, Ando Y, Terazaki H, et al. Effect of sildenafil citrate (Viagra) on erectile dysfunction in a patient with familial amyloidotic polyneuropathy ATTR Val30Met. J Auton Nerv Syst 2000; 80(1–2):89–92.

138. Andersson R, Hofer PA. Genitourinary disturbances in familial and sporadic cases of primary amyloidosis with polyneuropathy. Acta Med Scand 1974; 195(1–2):49–58.

139. Yamamoto T, Matsunaga K, Ohnishi A, et al. A late onset familial amyloidotic polyneuropathy (FAP) with a novel variant transthyretin characterized by a basic-for-acidic amino acid substitution (Glu61->Lys). [Article in Japanese]. Rinsho Shinkeigaku 1996; 36(9):1065–1068.

140. Li Y, Guo Y, Ikeda S, et al. Familial amyloid polyneuropathy—clinical report of a family. Chin Med Sci J 1996; 11(2):113–116.

141. Hita Villaplana G, Hita Rosino E, Lopez Cubillana P, et al. Corino-Andrade disease (familial amyloiditic polineuropathy type I) in Spain: urological and andrological disorders. Neurourol Urodyn 1997; 16(1):55–61.

142. Vardi Y, Sprecher E, Kanter Y, et al. Polyneuropathy in impotence. Int J Impot Res 1996; 8(2):65–68.

143. Powers JM, Schaumburg HH. A fatal cause of sexual inadequacy in men: adreno-leukodystrophy. J Urol 1980; 124(5):583–585.

144. Vodusek DB, Zidar J. Pudendal nerve involvement in patients with hereditary motor and sensory neuropathy. Acta Neurol Scand 1997; 76(6):457–460.

145. Marinkovic Z, Prelevic G, Würzburger M, et al. Gonadal dysfunction in patients with myotonic dystrophy. Exp Clin Endocrinol 1990; 96(1):37–44.

146. Olsson T, Olofsson B-O, Hagg E, et al. Adrenocortical and gonadal abnormalities in dystrophia myotonica—a common enzyme defect? Eur J Intern Med 1996; 7:29–33.

147. Mastrogiacomo I, Pagani E, Novelli G, et al. Male hypogonadism in myotonic dystrophy is related to (CTG)n triplet mutation. J Endocrinol Invest 1994; 17(5):381–383.

148. Hallen O. Über Potenz- und Libidostörungen bei der progressiven Muskeldystrophie. J Neurovisc Relat 1971; 10(suppl 10):573–579.

149. Lundberg PO. Observations on endocrine function in ocular myopathy. Acta Neurol Scand 1966; 42:39–61.

150. Melberg A, Arnell H, Dahl N, et al. Anticipation of autosomal dominant progressive external ophthalmoplegia with hypogonadism. Muscle Nerve 1996; 19(12): 1561–1569.

151. Chen CM, Huang CC. Gonadal dysfunction in mitochondrial encephalomyopathies. Eur Neurol 1995; 35(5):281–286.

152. Ertekin C, Sirin H. X-linked bulbospinal muscular atrophy (Kennedy's syndrome): a report of three cases. Acta Neurol Scand 1993; 87(1):56–61.

153. Hokezu Y, Yanai S, Nagai M, et al. A case of Kennedy-Alter-Sung (KAS) syndrome presenting as hypersexuality and elevated serum CK: usefulness of genetic analysis. [Article in Japanese]. Rinsho Shinkeigaku 1996; 36(3):471–474.

154. MacLean HE, Warne GL, Zajac JD. Spinal and bulbar muscular atrophy: androgen receptor dysfunction caused by a trinucleotide repeat expansion. J Neurol Sci 1996; 135(2):149–157.

155. Berthier M, Starkstein S, Leiguarda R. Seizures induced by orgasm. Ann Neurol 1987; 22(3): 394–395.

156. Calleja J, Carpizo R, Berciano J. Orgasmic epilepsy. Epilepsia 1988; 29(5):635–639.

157. Lundberg PO, Osterman PO. The benign and malignant forms of orgasmic cephalgia. Headache 1974; 14(3):164–165.

158. Lundberg PO, Osterman PO. Intercourse and headache. In: Genazzani AR, Nappi G, Facchinetti F, et al., eds. Pain and Reproduction. Carnforth: Parthenon Publishing Group, 1988:149–153.

16

Cancer and Sexual Dysfunction

Raymond A. Costabile
Department of Urology, University of Virginia, Charlottesville, Virginia, U.S.A.

□ INTRODUCTION

Over 1,200,000 new cases of invasive cancer will be diagnosed in the United States each year (1–3). A discussion of the effects of cancer and cancer therapy on erectile function is relevant as more than half of these patients are men-many of whom are of reproductive age and almost all will be interested in continuing sexual function. In published studies using quality of life (QOL) questionnaires, over 80% of men afflicted with cancer consider future reproductive and sexual function to be a principal concern (4). Additionally, female sexual dysfunction is currently being studied, with a new focus on the physiologic events of female sexual function. Unfortunately, the majority of cancer care providers do not appreciate the significant effects that cancer and cancer therapy have on sexual function. The surgical, chemotherapeutic, and ionizing radiation therapy used to treat cancer can adversely influence erectile, sexual, and reproductive function (5–8). As discussed in earlier chapters (see Chapters 3, 4, and 5). significant basic science and clinical research performed in the past decade has led to a better understanding of the mechanism of erection and sexual function at the organ, cellular, and molecular level. Research into centrally mediated mechanisms of sexual function has also shed new light into sexual physiology of both men and women. New directed developments in clinical research have led to effective local and systemic treatments for erectile dysfunction (ED). This directed approach to the evaluation and treatment of sexual dysfunction should be extended to treat sexual and erectile dysfunction in patients with cancer.

The pathophysiology of sexual dysfunction in cancer patients is often multifactorial, involving both psychogenic and physiologic mechanisms. In order to treat ED effectively in cancer patients, providers must understand the mechanism of erection and be familiar with a variety of treatment regimens. Cancer care providers must also be familiar with the complex psychological mechanisms associated with sexual dysfunction in cancer patients. Effective prophylactic care to preserve sexual function must often be initiated before or concurrently with surgery, chemotherapy, or radiation therapy. With this understanding, a majority of patients may be able to resume a satisfying sexual relationship after treatment of their malignancy.

Sexual dysfunction in cancer patients is principally the result of cancer therapy and the subsequent injury to the neurologic, vascular, and hormonal mechanisms responsible for normal sexual function (Fig. 1). Sexual and erectile dysfunction is not cancer-specific—i.e., there is little difference in ED in patients with hematological malignancies as opposed to solid tumors. The presence of comorbid disorders (e.g., age, diabetes mellitus, and smoking) that are associated with certain malignancies can increase the incidence of ED, as well as the relative response to therapy. Complex psychological factors that involve dealing with the diagnosis of cancer, as well as the side effects of cancer therapy, will further interrupt normal intimacy and libido.

This chapter will provide an overview of the pathophysiology of erectile and sexual dysfunction in patients with cancer. Specific cancer treatment effects on male sexual function, particularly in patients with prostate cancer, will be addressed as they relate to the pathophysiology of ED.

□ PATHOPHYSIOLOGY OF ED IN CANCER PATIENTS

It is important to understand that ED and sexual dysfunction are symptoms of many different disease states, not disease processes in themselves. This concept of "ED as a symptom" is important in evaluating the multifactorial nature of ED in cancer patients, as well as utilizing different treatment regimens to treat ED effectively in a variety of different patients.

Several pathophysiologic mechanisms influence sexual function in male patients with cancer as well as those who have received therapy for cancer. The mechanisms of sexual function will be broken down into their component parts in order to provide a better understanding of the pathophysiology of ED in cancer patients.

Neurologic Mechanism

The neurologic mechanism to attain or maintain an erection has been discussed previously (see Chapters 2, 3, 4, and 5). Based on external or internal input to

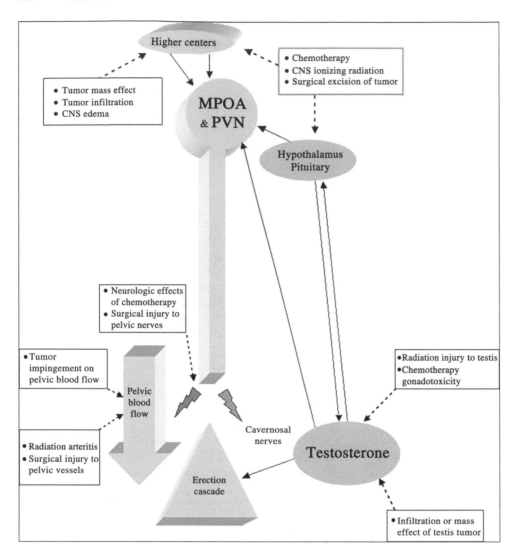

Figure 1 The effects of cancer and cancer therapy on sexual and erectile function. *Abbreviations*: CNS, central nervous system; MPOA, median preoptic area; PVN, paraventricular nucleus.

the erotic centers in the median preoptic area (MPOA) or paraventricular nucleus (PVN), impulses are sent down the spinal cord to the sacral plexus (S2–S4). These impulses are further relayed through pelvic nerves to the cavernosal nerves, where the local erectogenic cascade is initiated thorough the nonadrenergic, noncholinergic system principally mediated by nitric oxide (NO). This neurologic cascade can be adversely affected by cancer or cancer therapy, thus causing sexual dysfunction. Central nervous system (CNS) disease (tumors, infiltrative processes, or radiation effect), either focal or diffuse, can alter the initiation of erection by inhibiting the erotic or erectogenic centers located in the MPOA or PVN. Furthermore, these centers receive diffuse input from other areas in the brain that may subsequently inhibit the erectile mechanism. Complex interplay between dopamine (excitatory) and serotonin (inhibitory) may also alter sexual dysfunction and libido in cancer patients. What has previously been considered "psychogenic" ED in cancer patients may really be a disturbance in the complex CNS pathways influencing sexual function. Chemotherapeutic agents that cause permanent neurologic injury (Vinca alkaloids, platinum, etc.) may

adversely affect the neurologic mechanism responsible for sexual function.

Spinal cord impingement or peripheral nerve or nerve root involvement with cancer can interrupt the transmission of a neural impulse to initiate the erectogenic cascade. The most common neurologic cause of ED in men with cancer is surgical therapy, with subsequent neural injury. Extirpative surgery—e.g., radical prostatectomy (RP) or abdominal-perineal resection for colon cancer—can damage the cavernosal nerves as they course across the surface of the prostate (9–11). In patients who have had extirpative pelvic surgery, the neural mechanism to the penis has been injured and the local (penile) mechanism for erection is intact. Unfortunately, due to pelvic neural injury, nerve impulses from higher neural centers (CNS) are blocked prior to arriving at the corpora cavernosa preventing the local release of NO.

There are important therapeutic implications to understanding neurologic mechanisms of injury in cancer patients. The best way to treat neurologic injury in patients with cancer is to alter the surgical treatment in order to preserve neurologic function. This "nerve-sparing approach" has been undertaken in patients with severe malignancies, including prostate and colon cancer.

Pharmacotherapeutic agents that rely on an intact neural mechanism (i.e., sildenafil or apomorphine) will be far less effective in patients in whom the pelvic nerves have been injured. Locally acting agents that do not need neural input to initiate an erection, such as intracavernosal injections or transurethral therapy, can be highly effective in cancer patients with neural injury. For further information on this topic, see Chapter 30.

Vascular Mechanism

Erection is principally a vascular event. Disease processes that adversely affect penile blood flow are the most common causes of ED. Arteriogenic ED is usually due to small-vessel disease (atherosclerosis) or cavernosal smooth muscle/endothelial dysfunction, but a large pelvic tumor surrounding the common iliac artery or hypogastric artery can also significantly inhibit penile blood flow. Many disease processes have combined negative effects on erectile function. Diabetes mellitus is associated with ED by causing small-vessel disease as well as local neuropathy. For further information on diabetes and ED, see Chapter 14. In a similar manner, cancer and cancer therapy can adversely influence the vascular and neurologic mechanisms initiating erection.

Cancer therapy can cause vasculogenic ED by limiting penile blood flow and damaging the pudendal or penile arteries. The cavernosal arteries are less than 1 mm in diameter and can be easily injured by pelvic or perineal surgery. Ligation of one or both hypogastric arteries during extensive pelvic exenterative surgery will almost always lead to erectile dysfunction through reduced penile blood flow. Ligation of a solitary penile or pudendal artery may also lead to ED in older patients with preexisting arterial disease. Younger men with excellent collateral circulation can often remain potent with unilateral circulation to the corpora cavernosum.

Arteriosclerosis and cavernosal smooth muscle/endothelial injury is accelerated by ionizing radiation therapy. Patients may not manifest neurovascular injury from ionizing radiation for many years after receiving treatment. In general, these effects frequently occur three to five years following therapy. ED can occur in 85% of patients receiving pelvic irradiation (12–15).

Veno-occlusive dysfunction is a descriptive term for failure of the passive venous outflow obstructive mechanism. Patients with veno-occlusive dysfunction have adequate arterial inflow, but fail to "trap" blood in the corporal sinusoids. It is uncertain what effect pelvic surgery or radiation therapy has on the penile veno-occlusive mechanism.

Endocrine

Androgens are essential to maintain an adequate libido in males. Evidence in animal models demonstrates androgen-dependent cavernosal smooth muscle

receptors that subsequently reduce cavernosal smooth muscle response to NO in the castrated state. NO synthase levels are also decreased in castrated males. Isolated hormonal ED is rare, occurring in 6% of patients (16). Men with germ cell malignancies frequently have abnormalities in their hypothalamic pituitary–gonadal axis that lead to hypogonadism and sexual dysfunction. Varied rates of sexual dysfunction have been reported in these men. Testosterone replacement may be required to restore normal libido and sexual function.

Psychogenic

Every man with ED has, to some degree, a psychogenic component to his disease. In fact, many disease entities have psychological manifestations of physical maladies. Coexisting psychological anxiety/influence is frequently evident in men with ED. This psychogenic dysfunction rarely manifests itself as a DSM IV, Axis 1 diagnosis, but more often as a more subtle decrease in libido or sexual activity.

Depression is a significant risk factor for ED. Anxiety and fatigue may also severely inhibit sexual function in cancer patients and lead to ED. Studies of pharmacotherapeutic intervention in men treated for prostate cancer with RP have shown a high response rate when patients are challenged with the agent in a clinic setting. Despite this high clinical response rate, successful attempts at intercourse in the home environment were lower for patients with prostate cancer than for patients with other etiologies causing ED. Fear of resuming intercourse and intimacy after treatment for prostate cancer contributed to sexual dysfunction in these patients.

Counseling

For details of the medical approaches to the treatment of sexual dysfunction in males with cancer, see Chapters 37 and 39. A brief note will be made about counseling here, however.

Counseling is essential for most cancer patients in order for them to preserve or restore normal sexual function. Genitourinary cancer has a significant psychological component associated with the physiologic injury. Cancer care providers need to be aware of the particular needs of these patients with regards to psychosocial support. It is also important to remember that the ability to have an erection does not necessarily translate to the ability to have normal sexual function. Sexual counseling is a useful adjunct for many cancer patients with ED. In individuals with primarily psychogenic ED that is secondary to cancer-related depression or anxiety, counseling may be the sole treatment needed. The services of a psychologist, psychiatrist, or family/sexual counselor can restore or improve sexual function in many cancer patients. A multifaceted approach utilizing pharmacological therapy to improve erections and sexual and family counseling, however, is often successful.

☐ SEXUAL DYSFUNCTION IN MEN WITH PROSTATE CANCER

Prostate cancer is the most common invasive cancer in men and thus deserves special mention in this chapter. In 2002, over 179,000 new cases of prostate cancer were diagnosed in the United States (1–3). Unfortunately, the surgical therapy, surgical or medical castration, or ionizing radiation used to treat prostate cancer causes a significant number of men to have sexual dysfunction after therapy. The lifetime probability of developing prostate cancer is one in six, and most men diagnosed with prostate cancer in the United States will elect treatment. With treatment, however, comes the significant risk of sexual dysfunction.

Complications of prostate cancer therapy include ED, incontinence, and bowel dysfunction. These complications may significantly diminish a patient's QOL. Forty-five percent of patients receiving therapy list the maintenance of QOL as a principal concern in selecting prostate cancer therapy, and the maintenance of sexual function often comprises a primary component of QOL for these men. Treatment selection is often made after the consideration of treatment-related side effects and their subsequent impact on QOL. ED will affect 16% to 82% of men following RP, and 2% to 85% of men receiving external beam radiation therapy (ionizing radiation) (17). The use of anatomical nerve-sparing RP technique is no guarantee that erectile function will be preserved, however. Early studies suggested a lower incidence in the development of ED in patients treated with ionizing radiation, but these involved small numbers of patients with a follow-up period of less than 24 months (12,18,19).

The ability to preserve potency after prostate cancer surgery is controversial. Conflicting clinical evidence suggests that ED occurs after prostatectomy in 10% to 90% of patients (9,10,17). This disparity in the ability to preserve potency can be attributed to differences in the methods used to document and evaluate ED, surgical technique during prostatectomy, academic- or community-based surgical practice, and prospective or retrospective data collection.

A similar disparity is noted in studies looking at the preservation of potency after external beam radiotherapy. Potency rates have been documented after ionizing radiation in 20% to 80% of patients (12,17–19).

A significant factor confounding the development of ED in patients with prostate cancer is the incidence of ED in the aging male population. The risk of ED is estimated at 26 cases per 1000 men annually, and increases with age, lower educational status, and the presence of diabetes, heart disease, and hypertension. Therefore, ascribing causality to a symptom (ED) with multiple risk factors may be difficult.

The incidence of ED in some studies was highly dependent on whether a patient selected therapy for prostate cancer or was observed. No significant difference was noted in the high rate of developing ED in patients selecting prostatectomy or external beam radiation therapy. Other studies have reported a lower impact on sexual relationships with patients receiving ionizing radiation (17). Unlike surgical therapy, with which ED is immediately apparent postoperatively, ionizing radiation patients experience a more gradual decline in sexual function over a longer follow-up period. Ionizing radiation is thought to initiate ED by accelerating microvascular angiopathy, causing cavernosal fibrosis and smooth muscle/endothelial dysfunction. This process of progressive vascular injury may take years to cause clinically significant ED.

Prostatectomy, on the other hand, causes ED due to intraoperative damage to the neurovascular mechanism initiating erections. ED occurs immediately after prostatectomy, with a return of function in a variable fashion. Due to the differing time frame of onset of ED in patients after ionizing radiation or RP, it may be easier to document ED in patients after prostatectomy.

Studies on potency following prostatectomy differ with respect to the significance of age, stage, or grade on resumption of sexual function. The ability of the surgeon to preserve one or both neurovascular bundles also influences the subsequent return of erectile function.

Patients selecting "watchful waiting" have the greatest chance at preserving potency after the diagnosis of prostate cancer. Some patients will elect to forego therapy, with the risk of possible progression and death, in order to preserve sexual function (17–21). QOL studies performed on men treated for prostate cancer demonstrate high sexual bother and sexual dysfunction scores. With ED treatment, a majority of these men will show significant improvement in their QOL scores in the sexual function domain.

Patients suffering from ED following prostatectomy will frequently elect to try systemic therapy. Unfortunately, response rates to sildenafil are significantly lower than other groups (40%), and local therapy or penile implant surgery is often needed to achieve a consistent erection adequate for intercourse.

☐ CONCLUSION

Cancer care providers must be familiar with the incidence of sexual dysfunction following cancer therapy and integrate treatment methods to preserve or restore sexual function. Sexual function in cancer patients is primarily mediated by treatment effect. A multifactorial approach is often beneficial for cancer patients to resume intercourse. With this treatment approach, a majority of cancer patients will continue to enjoy a satisfying sexual life.

☐ REFERENCES

1. Landis SH, Murray T, Bolden S, et al. Cancer statistics, 1999. CA Cancer J Clin 1999; 49(1):8–31.
2. Denmeade SR, Isaacs JT. Prostate cancer: where are we and where are we going? Br J Urol 1997; 79(1):2–7.
3. SEER Cancer Statistics Review. Bethesda, MD: U.S. Department of Health and Human Services, Public Health Service, National Institute of Health, National Cancer Institute, 1996.
4. Berthelson JG. Testicular cancer and infertility. Int J Androl 1987; 10:371.
5. Litwin M, Hays R, Fink A, et al. Quality-of-life outcomes in men treated for localized prostate cancer. JAMA 1995; 273(2):129–135.
6. Geary E, Dendinger T, Freiha F, et al. Nerve sparing radical prostatectomy: a different view. J Urol 1995; 154(1):145–149.
7. Fowler F, Barry M, Lu-Yao G, et al. Patent-reported complications and follow-up treatment after radical prostatectomy: the national medicare experience. Urology 1993; 42(6):622–629.
8. Nguyen L, Pollack A, Zagars G. Late effects after radiotherapy for prostate cancer in a randomized dose-response study: results of a self-assessment questionnaire. Urology 1998; 51(6):991–997.
9. Walsh P, Donker P. Impotence following radical prostatectomy: insight into etiology and prevention. 1982. J Urol 2002; 167(2 Pt 2):1005–1010.
10. Walsh P, Partin A, Epstein J. Cancer control and quality of life following anatomical radical retropubic prostatectomy: results at 10 years. J Urol 1994; 152(5 Pt 2): 1831–1836.
11. Walsh P. Anatomic radical prostatectomy: evolution of the surgical technique. J Urol 1998; 160(6 Pt 2): 2418–2424.
12. Mantz C, Song P, Farhangi E, et al. Potency probability following conformal megavoltage radiotherapy. Int J Radiat Oncol Biol Phys 1997; 37(3):551–557.
13. Robinson J, Dufour M, Fung T. Erectile functioning of men treated for prostate carcinoma. Cancer 1997; 79(3): 538–544.
14. Lilleby W, Fossa S, Waehre H, et al. Long-term morbidity and quality of life in patients with localized prostate cancer undergoing definitive radiotherapy of radical prostatectomy. Int J Radiat Oncol Biol Phys 1999; 43(4): 735–743.
15. McCammon KA, Kolm P, Main B, Schellhammer PF. Comparative quality-of-life analysis after radical prostatectomy or external beam radiation for localized prostate cancer. Urology 1999; 54(3):509–516.
16. Jarow JP. Endocrine causes of male infertility. Urol Clin North Am 2003; 30(1):83–90.
17. Siegel T, Moul JW, Spevak M, et al. The development of erectile dysfunction in men with prostate cancer. J Urol 2001; 165(2):430.
18. Lubech D, Litwin M, Stoddard M, et al. Changes in health-related quality of life in the first year after treatment for prostate cancer: results from CaPSure. Urology 1999; 53(1):180–186.
19. Lubeck DP, Litwin MS, Henning JM, et al. Measurement of health-related quality of life in men with prostate cancer: CaPSure™ database. Qual Life Res 1997; 6(5): 385–392.
20. Thompson IM. Counseling patients with newly diagnosed prostate cancer. Oncology 2000; 14:119–136.
21. Litwin MS, Flanders SC, Pasta DJ, et al. Sexual function and bother after radical prostatectomy or radiation for prostate cancer: multivariate quality-of-life analysis from CaPSURE. Cancer of the prostate strategic urologic research endeavor. Urology 1999; 54(3): 503–508.

17

Peyronie's Disease and Trabecular Smooth Muscle Dysfunction

Danielle N. Dienert
Department of Urology, University of Pittsburgh, Pittsburgh, Pennsylvania, U.S.A.

Wayne J. G. Hellstrom
Department of Urology, Tulane University Health Sciences Center, New Orleans, Louisiana, U.S.A.

☐ PEYRONIE'S DISEASE
Introduction

Peyronie's disease is a localized connective tissue disorder that primarily affects the tunica albuginea and surrounding vascular tissue of the corpus cavernosum (1). The end result is a fibrous plaque that contains an excessive amount of collagen, alterations in the elastin framework, and fibroblastic proliferation, all of which consequently alter penile anatomy and may cause bending, narrowing, and/or shortening of the penis. These anatomical changes may dramatically affect erectile function. Penile deviation alone may cause difficulty with coital penetration; however, approximately 40% of Peyronie's patients have coexistent erectile dysfunction (ED) (2,3). Since the first well-characterized clinical series on penile curvature was reported in 1743 by Francois Gigot de la Peyronie, the etiology and mechanism of this well-recognized symptom complex have remained undetermined.

Peyronie's disease usually affects Caucasian males between the ages of 40 and 70, with a reported 0.39% to 3.2% incidence; however, there are numerous reports of cases in younger individuals (1,4–6). The actual prevalence of this disease may be higher due to patient embarrassment and limited reporting of this disorder by physicians. The disease process that takes place in Peyronie's disease is very similar to other conditions such as Dupuytren's contracture, Ledderhose's disease, tympanosclerosis of the middle ear, and scarring of the palmar fascia. In some series, up to 30% of patients with Peyronie's also suffer from Dupuytren's contracture (7).

The tunica albuginea plays a vital role in erection because of its essential properties that allow for penile elasticity, rigidity, compliance, and veno-occlusion (8). ED is known to occur in approximately 40% of men with Peyronie's disease and is recognized to affect quality of life, with 77% of Peyronie's men demonstrating significant psychological effects (1,6,9). Interestingly, a number of clinicians have noted an increased number of Peyronie's patients since the advent of oral sildenafil (Viagra, Pfizer, New York, New York, U.S.A.).

Men with Peyronie's disease may complain of any one (or a combination of) the following symptoms: penile pain, penile angulation, palpable plaque, and decreased erectile function. The rigid plaque, which is the cause of the aforementioned symptoms, is found on the side of the corpus cavernosum to which the curvature is directed. The characteristic Peyronie's plaque is most commonly located on the dorsal aspect of the penis, causing an upward curvature during erection. Plaques that are found on the ventral aspect will cause a downward curvature (Fig. 1), while plaques located on the lateral side of the penis will cause a lateral curvature. Plaques that wrap concentrically around the penile shaft will cause severe narrowing, or a phenomenon known as "bottlenecking."

Pathophysiology

The cause of Peyronie's disease is not completely understood. Several theories have been developed and proposed over the years, including vitamin E deficiency, the use of β-blocking agents, increased levels of serotonin, as in carcinoid syndrome, genetic disorders, and repetitive vascular trauma inciting a low-level autoimmune response with fibrosis and plaque formation (10–14). A number of systemic fibrosing conditions are known to occur concomitantly with Peyronie's disease (15). Peyronie's patients may have a genetic predisposition, as witnessed by the disease's association with Dupuytren's contracture and HLA-B7 antigens (7,16). More recent proposals suggest that fibrosis and collagen changes of the tunica albuginea are the result of an inflammatory process triggered by vascular trauma (9,13). Following trauma or other injury to the penis, the release of cytokines activates fibroblast proliferation and the production of collagen, the main extracellular matrix component of a Peyronie's plaque. Therefore, Peyronie's disease has been defined by some authorities as a wound-healing disorder, much like the dermatologic conditions of keloid formation, hypertrophic scarring, and Dupuytren's contracture (17). Despite many etiological theories and the myriad of medical and surgical treatments proposed for men

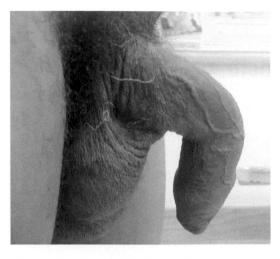

Figure 1 Erect penis demonstrating ventral curvature in a man suffering from Peyronie's disease.

with Peyronie's disease, there has been a limited number of advances and scientific understanding about its pathophysiology.

Current theories as to the origin of Peyronie's disease suggest that fibrosis and collagen changes in the tunica albuginea are the result of an inflammatory process following vascular trauma (13,17,18). Elastic fibers located within the tunica albuginea of the penis form an irregular latticed framework upon which collagen rests. These elastic fibers are important in maintaining the structure of the collagen bundles. These two structural components are essential to penile erection because they permit both an increase in girth and length during tumescence (8,19). Any defect of the tunical collagen or elastic fiber network may lead to significant alterations in the hemodynamics of erection.

The histopathology of Peyronie's disease reveals an inflammatory process, characterized by chronic lymphocytic and plasmacytic infiltration of the tunica albuginea and the surrounding erectile tissues. The origin of the initial inflammatory process that leads to fibrosis, calcification, and plaque formation in the tunica albuginea is unknown.

Devine et al. have postulated that minor penile trauma can occur during sexual intercourse, whereby the corpora cavernosa bend and stretch, resulting in a delamination injury of the tunica albuginea predominantly at the dorsal midline septum (20). This process incites further inflammation, induration, and fibrin deposition between the layers of the tunica albuginea, thereby activating the proliferation of local fibroblasts and leukocytes. Levine et al. have postulated that following injury to the penis, an anomalous process of wound healing occurs, with fibroblast proliferation and extracellular matrix deposition (21). It is suggested that at this juncture of the wound-healing process, the balance between extracellular matrix and scar tissue formation exceeds that of degradation of both collagen and extracellular matrix because of abnormal

fibroblast activity. Fibrin residues stimulate an amplification of histocytes and increased collagen deposition, which infiltrate the tunica albuginea.

There have been reports of changes in the collagen content of the tunica albuginea of patients with Peyronie's disease (22,23). Types I and III collagen expression are commonly present in penile scar tissue, while type III collagen is found more abundantly in Peyronie's plaques. Moreover, the demonstration of increased type III collagen in the "normal" penile tissue adjacent to the plaque tissue suggests that this disease is not specific to the plaque but may be more generalized throughout the corporal tissues (23–26). Of particular interest is the observation of increased type III collagen expression in patients with venogenic impotence; type III collagen fibers are found abundantly in the tunica, while this finding is rare in the tunica albuginea of potent men (25).

Elastic fiber concentrations in the tunica are also significantly decreased in Peyronie's patients, and are significantly lower in impotent men with Peyronie's compared to Peyronie's patients who maintain potency. Although antibodies to elastin are present in all individuals, Peyronie's patients exhibit increased levels of antitropoelastin (reflecting elastin synthesis) and anti–α-elastin (reflecting elastin destruction) (27). This supports the theory that an autoimmune mechanism affecting the elastin framework is involved in the pathogenesis of Peyronie's disease.

Collagen synthesis in adult tissues is subject to regulation by a variety of endogenous and exogenous factors. Biologically active peptides, such as interleukin-1, tumor necrosis factor, epidermal growth factor, and transforming growth factor (TGF)-β, have been implicated in normal collagen synthesis and fibrosis (28–30). Among them, TGF-β has been shown to be involved in many chronic fibrotic conditions, in addition to being involved in numerous vital processes such as inflammation, stimulation of extracellular matrix, and the normal healing process (28). TGF-β is a cytokine that is vital to tissue repair; however, its excess may induce tissue damage and scarring as witnessed in a variety of connective tissue diseases such as pulmonary fibrosis, fibrotic liver disease, and systemic sclerosis (28). Furthermore, TGF-β is the isoform most often implicated in tissue fibrosis and is upregulated in response to tissue injury. Recently, El-Sakka et al. have demonstrated an upregulation of TGF-β in the tunica albuginea of patients with Peyronie's disease when compared to the tunical tissue of men without Peyronie's disease (31). The expression of TGF-β mRNA and protein in the tunica albuginea of the male penis as well as the induction of collagen synthesis in cell culture suggests a role for TGF-β in corpus cavernosum tissue synthesis (31,32).

El-Sakka et al. have also proposed a rat animal model for Peyronie's disease in order to investigate the pathophysiology of this disorder. Their studies demonstrated an increase in TGF-β protein expression, as well as histological and ultrastructural alterations in the tunica albuginea of the rat, all findings consistent with those observed in human Peyronie's disease (31,33). This animal model has the potential for further investigation into the mechanisms of Peyronie's disease.

Management

A definitive medical therapy for Peyronie's disease has not yet been established, as witnessed by the plethora of therapies in the medical literature. Oral therapy for Peyronie's disease has been utilized since the 1940s, and numerous studies have shown that the Peyronie's patients most likely to benefit from medical therapy for their symptoms are those with early-stage disease (20). Peyronie's disease is classified into two phases: (*i*) an acute inflammatory phase, in which patients present with pain, slight penile curvature, and nodule formation, which lasts for 6 to 18 months; and (*ii*) a chronic phase, in which patients present with stable plaque size, penile curvature, and, in some instances, ED. Although it has been reported that up to 13% of patients with Peyronie's disease had complete resolution of their plaques with time, most experts suggest that medical therapy should be implemented early, as symptoms will most likely not resolve spontaneously (1). In most instances, patients with mild curvature, relatively little penile pain, or minimal ED require no further therapy and can be followed up conservatively.

Some of the reported medical treatment options for patients with Peyronie's disease include oral therapy with vitamin E, potassium aminobenzoate (Potaba), tamoxifen, or colchicines, as well as intralesional injection therapy with collagenase, steroids, calcium channel blockers, or interferon α-2b (10,21,34–38) (Figs. 2 and 3). When a patient has failed medical therapy, or when the deformity of the disease precludes sexual intercourse and progression has stabilized, surgery may be the only alternative. In order for surgery to be an option, the disease should not be in the acute

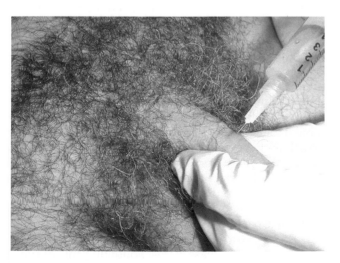

Figure 2 Intralesional injection into Peyronie's plaque.

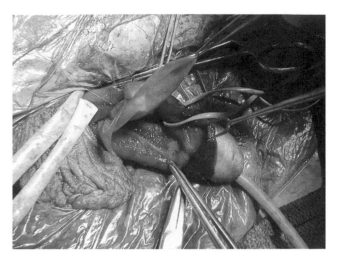

Figure 3 (*See color insert.*) Intraoperative depiction of pericardial graft material being sewn in area where Peyronie's plaque has been excised.

inflammatory phase, which usually translates into the disease being present for a minimum of one year. Exceptions include the presence of a calcified plaque; disease activity (progression of deformity, sexual dysfunction, or both) that has been stable and unchanged for at least three months; and difficulty with coitus or intromission despite the use of oral or intracavernosal vasoactive agents. (For further details on the medical and surgical management of Peyronie's disease, see Chapter 34.)

☐ TRABECULAR SMOOTH MUSCLE DYSFUNCTION
Introduction

ED is known to affect approximately 20 to 30 million men in the United States (39,40). With more men being successfully treated for ED, an increasing number of impotence cases are becoming manifest and presenting for evaluation. ED is defined as the inability to achieve and maintain an erection sufficient to permit satisfactory intercourse (41,42). Although the causes are numerous, i.e., hormonal, neurogenic, arterial, cavernosal, or psychological, this section will concentrate primarily on trabecular smooth muscle dysfunction—which, like Peyronie's disease, is a disorder of the penile tissues.

Pathophysiology and Future Therapeutic Goals

Briefly, penile erection is controlled by neurologic and vascular events; however, hormonal and psychological factors figure in to this physiological process. The cavernous nerve terminals are activated following sexual stimulation, releasing neurotransmitters such as nitric oxide (NO) (Fig. 4) (41). These neurotransmitters induce relaxation of the smooth muscle in the arteries and arterioles supplying the corpus cavernosum as well as an increase in the overall penile blood supply. As this occurs, trabecular smooth muscle

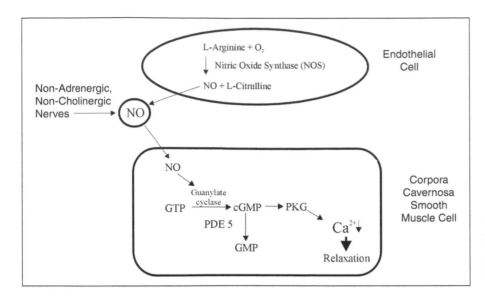

Figure 4 Nitric oxide pathway for inducing cavernosal smooth muscle relaxation. *Abbreviations*: NO, nitric oxide; GTP, guanosine triphosphate; PDE-5, Phosphodiesterase 5; GMP, guanosine monophosphate; cGMP, cyclic guanosine monophosphate; PKG, protein kinase G; NOS, nitric oxide synthase.

relaxes, allowing the sinusoids to expand and rapidly fill with blood (41). The subtunical venules are compressed between the trabeculae and tunica albuginea, occluding venous outflow and causing the penis to become erect (41,43,44). When certain physiological or structural systems are not in balance, ED secondary to trabecular smooth muscle dysfunction can occur.

Structurally, the normal aging process contributes to the loss of trabecular smooth muscle in the corpus cavernosum. From puberty until age 50, the ratio of trabecular smooth muscle to connective tissue in the corpora remains relatively constant at 50% (45). At age 50 and beyond, however, the percentage of trabecular smooth muscle in the corpora progressively decreases to 25% to 30%, with a matching relative increase in connective tissue (45). Wespes et al. used histomorphometric analysis to analyze and determine the trabecular smooth muscle composition in potent men aged 18 to 33 years and impotent men aged 25 to 70 years (46). They concluded that the percentage of trabecular smooth muscle ranged from 40% to 52% in normal men and 10% to 36% in patients experiencing impotence secondary to trabecular smooth muscle dysfunction (46). This property has also been similarly demonstrated in men who became impotent following penile irradiation treatments for pain from Peyronie's disease. Radiation injury to the corpora causes widespread fibrosis and internal structural changes within the corpus cavernosum smooth muscle structure, which leads to eventual structural ED (47).

From a physiological standpoint, Kim et al. have demonstrated that hypoxemia has a significant effect on the function of trabecular smooth muscle (48). Their study concluded that oxygen tension plays an active role in the regulation of penile erections, and hypoxia alters the erectile and contractile response of the penis. When oxygen tensions are low, inhibition of the synthesis of NO occurs in the corpus cavernosum, ultimately affecting the relaxation of trabecular smooth muscle tissue (48). These studies hypothesize that men with low oxygen tension in the corpora cavernosa secondary to vasculogenic dysfunction will not adequately activate NO synthesis to induce full trabecular smooth muscle relaxation (48,49). In severe cases of hypoxemia, metabolic acidosis may occur, which further inhibits the relaxation of the trabecular smooth muscle complex (49). The oxygen-dependent changes in the penis alter smooth muscle metabolism and connective tissue synthesis, eventually altering the structural components of the penis (50).

Moreland has proposed two theories of ED based upon both physiological and structural properties:

■ The oxygen-tension-dependent changes in the penis during erection impact the structure of the corpus cavernosum by the induction of various cytokines, vasoactive factors, and growth factors, which in turn alter smooth muscle metabolism and connective tissue synthesis (50). Decreases in the corpus cavernosum trabecular smooth muscle along with the connective tissue ratio increases the likelihood of a diffuse venous leak and dysfunction in the veno-occlusive erectile mechanism (50).

■ ED is the result of a metabolic imbalance between relaxatory and contractile processes within the trabecular smooth muscles such that trabecular smooth muscle contraction predominates (50).

In the first hypothesis, Moreland states that ED is the result of structural changes that affect penile function (50). Since the percentage of trabecular smooth muscle within the corpus cavernosum is integral to its function, an increase in connective tissue within the corpora will lead to an imbalance. To achieve this functional balance, vasoactive factors that regulate the growth and control of trabecular smooth muscle cells, such as TGF-β1 and prostaglandin E, must be regulated (51,52). Disease states such as diabetes, peripheral vascular disease, hypertension, and hypercholesterolemia decrease the smooth muscle:connective tissue ratio, via the vasoactive factors in the corpus cavernosum (51). These factors are altered during the course of the aforementioned disease states. Following this hypothesis, therapeutic strategies that alter trabecular smooth muscle structure could theoretically be viable treatment options.

Moreland addresses the second hypothesis as a metabolic imbalance that affects the contractile and relaxation forces within the corpus cavernosum (50). In this model, either the overexpression of contractile forces predominates or there is an inhibition of the relaxatory factors such that the trabecular smooth muscle remains contracted and the penis remains flaccid (50). This state can be attributed to increased adrenergic tone in the central nervous system. This theory suggests that ED occurs regardless of the trabecular smooth muscle structure in the corpus cavernosum. The therapeutic goal in this model is to develop an agent that fully relaxes the smooth muscle within the corpora so that erection will occur.

Both theories allow for future development of treatment modalities in a variety of ways, and Moreland emphasizes that the true answer lies somewhere in both theories. Although the first theory highlights the structural imbalances that affect function, he notes that these structural conditions can easily lead to a metabolic imbalance within the corpora, as suggested by the second theory. Moreland proposes that penile function is a balance between functional smooth muscle and connective tissue as well as contractile and relaxing factors (50). With this integrated model approach of trabecular smooth muscle dysfunction and how it relates to ED, the development of therapeutic models that can be adapted to a wide variety of patients may soon become feasible. Promising results in the area of tissue engineering have allowed researchers to use human corpus cavernosum smooth muscle cells and endothelium, with the hopes of replacing defective corpora with tissue grafts. With the proven effectiveness of Sildenafil and other pharmacotherapeutics,

however, effective management with oral medication demonstrates promise and gives many patients additional options before pursuing surgical avenues. (For further information on the oral treatment of ED, see Chapters 29, 30, and 31.)

□ CONCLUSION

Despite being recognized more than 250 years ago, Peyronie's disease remains an enigma for clinicians in regard to both its diagnosis and management. Studies that focus on the basic sciences of wound healing will likely open new avenues for research. Current concepts center on fibrosis and collagen changes in the tunica albuginea that are the result of an undefined inflammatory process following vascular trauma. Animal models (e.g., rat erection model) allow researchers to study different hypotheses. Most authorities believe these laboratory investigations will unlock the key to the effective treatment and possibly even the prevention of Peyronie's disease.

The penis is composed predominantly of smooth muscle. Certain disease states (e.g., diabetes) and aging are recognized to reduce the smooth muscle content of the penis with the consequence of ED. Identification of the NO-cyclic guanosine monophosphate pathway and the development of concepts regarding oxygenation of cavernosal smooth muscle have enabled scientists to explore new avenues of research in this important area. An important finding is that diseases of the cavernosal smooth muscle may reflect pathologies occurring in other sites of the body—i.e., the vascular endothelium. The study of penile physiology will continue to provide new insights into disease states in the years to come.

□ REFERENCES

1. Gelbard MK, Dorey F, James K. The natural history of Peyronie's disease. J Urol 1990; 144(6):1376–1380.
2. Pryor J. Peyronie's disease and impotence. Acta Urol Belg 1988; 56(2):317–321.
3. Schwarzer U, Klotz T, Braun M, et al. Prevalence of Peyronie's disease results of an 8,000-man survey. J Urol 2000; 163(suppl):A742.
4. Carson CC. Francois Gigot de la Peyronie. Invest Urol 1981; 19(1):62–63.
5. Lindsay MB, Schain DM, Grambsch P, et al. The incidence of Peyronie's disease in Rochester, Minnesota, 1950 through 1984. J Urol 1991; 146(4):1007–1009.
6. Shaw K, Puri K, Ruiz-Deya G, et al. Racial considerations in Peyronie's disease. Podium presentation at 2002 South-central AVA annual meeting.
7. Nyberg LM, Bias WB, Hochberg MC, et al. Identification of an inherited form of Peyronie's disease with autosomal dominant inheritance and association with Dupuytren's contracture and histocompatibility B7 cross-reacting antigens. J Urol 1982; 128(1):48–51.
8. Aboseif SR, Lue TF. Fundamentals and hemodynamics of penile erection. Cardiovasc Intervent Radiol 1988; 11(4):185–190.
9. Carson CC. Peyronie's disease: medical and surgical management. In: Hellstrom WJG, ed. Handbook of Sexual Dysfunction. San Francisco: American Society of Andrology, 1999:93–98.
10. Scardino PL, Scott WW. The use of tocopherols in the treatment of Peyronie's disease. Ann N Y Acad Sci 1949; 52:390–401.
11. Yudkin JS. Peyronie's disease is association with metoprolol. Lancet 1977; 2(8052–8053):1355.

12. Van de Berg JS, Devine CJ, Horton CE, et al. Mechanisms in calcification in Peyronie's disease. J Urol 1982; 127(1):52–56.

13. Jarow JP, Lowe FC. Penile trauma: an etiologic factor in Peyronie's disease and erectile dysfunction. J Urol 1997; 158:1388–1390.

14. Somers KD, Winters PA, Dawson DM. Chromosomal abnormalities in Peyronie's disease. J Urol 1987; 137(4):672–676.

15. Ordi J, Selva A, Fonollosa V, et al. Peyronie's disease in systemic sclerosis. Ann Rheum Dis 1990; 49(2): 134–135.

16. Chilton CP, Castle WM, Westwood CA, et al. Factors associated in the aetiology of Peyronie's disease. Br J Urol 1982; 54(6):748–750.

17. Devine CJ, Somers KD, Jordan SG, et al. Proposal: trauma as the cause of the Peyronie's lesion. J Urol 1997; 157:285–290.

18. Hellstrom WJ, Bivalacqua TJ. Peyronie's disease: etiology, medical, and surgical therapy. J Androl 2000; 21(3):347–354.

19. Hsu GL, Brock G, von Heyden B, et al. The distribution of elastic fibrous elements within the human penis. Br J Urol 1994; 37:566–571.

20. Devine CJ, Somers KD, Ladaga LE. Peyronie's disease: pathophysiology. Prog Clin Biol Res 1991; 370: 355–358.

21. Levine LA, Merrick PF, Lee RC. Intralesional verapamil injection for the treatment of Peyronie's disease. J Urol 1994; 151(6):1522–1524.

22. Somers KD, Sismour EN, Wright GL. Isolation and characterization of collagen in Peyronie's disease. J Urol 1989; 141(3):629–635.

23. Luangkhot R, Rutchik S, Agarwal V, et al. Collagen alterations in the corpus cavernosum of men with sexual dysfunction. J Urol 1992; 148(2 Pt 1):467–471.

24. Mersdorf A, Goldsmith PC, Diedrichs W. Ultrastructural changes in impotent penile tissue comparison of 65 patients. J Urol 1991; 145(4):749–754.

25. Chiang PH, Chiang CP, Shen MR, et al. Study of the changes in collagen of the tunica albuginea in venogenic impotence in Peyronie's disease. Eur Urol 1992; 21(1):48–51.

26. Iacono F, Barra S, De Rosa G, et al. Microstructural disorders of the tunica albuginea in patients affected by Peyronie's disease with or without erectile dysfunction. J Urol 1993; 150:1806–1809.

27. Stewart S, Malto M, Sandberg L, et al. Increased serum levels of anti-elastin antibodies in patients with Peyronie's disease. J Urol 1994; 152(1):l05–l06.

28. Border WA, Noble NA. Transforming growth factor beta in tissue fibrosis. N Engl J Med 1994; 331(19): 1286–1292.

29. Zhang K, Phan SH. Cytokines and pulmonary fibrosis. Biol Signals 1996; 5:232–239.

30. Nikolic-Paterson DJ, Main IW, Tesch GH, et al. Interleukin-1 in renal fibrosis. Kidney Int Suppl 1996; 54:588–590.

31. El-Sakka AI, Hassoba HM, Chui RM, et al. An animal model of Peyronie's like condition associated with an increase of transforming growth factor-β mRNA and protein expression. J Urol 1997; 158:2284–2290.

32. Moreland RB, Traish A, McMillin MA, et al. PGE 1 suppresses the induction of collagen synthesis by transforming growth factor-β in human corpus cavernosum smooth muscle. J Urol 1995; 153:826–834.

33. El-Sakka AI, Selph CA, Yen TS, et al. The effect of surgical trauma on rat tunica albuginea. J Urol 1998; 159(5):1700–1707.

34. Akkus E, Carier S, Rehman J, et al. Is colchicine effective in Peyronie's disease? A pilot study. Urology 1994; 44(2):291–295.

35. Hasche-Klunder R. Treatment of Peyronie's disease using para-aminobenzoate potassium (Potaba), para-aminobenzoic acid potassium. Urologea 1978; 17: 224–227.

36. Ralph DJ, Brooks MD, Botazzi GF. The treatment of Peyronie's disease with tamoxifen. Br J Urol 1992; 70(6):648–661.

37. Gelbard MK, James K, Reich P, et al. Collagenase versus placebo in the treatment of Peyronie's disease: a double-blind study. J Urol 1993; 149(1):56–58.

38. Ahuja S, Bivalacqua TJ, Case J, et al. A pilot study demonstrating clinical benefit from intralesional interferon alpha 2B in the treatment of Peyronie's disease. J Androl 1999; 20(4):444–448.

39. Lue TF. Erectile dysfunction. N Engl J Med 2000; 342(24):1802–1813.

40. Benet AK, Melman A. The epidemiology of erectile dysfunction. Urol Clin North Am 1995; 22(4): 699–709.

41. Feldman HA, Goldstein I, Hatzichristou DG, et al. Impotence and its medical and pyschosocial correlates: results of the Massachusetts male aging study. J Urol 1994; 151:54–61.

42. NIH Consensus Conference. Impotence. NIH Consensus Development Panel on Impotence. JAMA 1993; 270(1):83–90.

43. Fournier GR Jr, Junemann KP, Lue TF, et al. Mechanisms of venous occlusion during canine penile erection: an anatomic demonstration. J Urol 1987; 137(1):163–167.

44. Banya Y, Ushiki T, Takagane H. Two circulatory routes within the human corpus cavernosum penis; a scanning electron microscopic study of corrosion casts. J Urol 1989; 142(3):879–883.

45. Conti G, Virag R. Human penile erection and organic impotence: normal histology and histopathology. Urol Int 1989; 44(5):303.

46. Wespes E, Goes PM, Schiffmann S, et al. Computerized analysis of smooth muscle fibers in potent and impotent patients. J Urol 1991; 146(4):1015.

47. Hall S, Guido B, Bertero E, et al. Extensive corporeal fibrosis after penile irradiation. J Urol 1995; 153(2): 372–377.

48. Kim N, Vardi Y, Padma-Nathan H, et al. Oxygen tension regulates the nitric oxide pathway. Physiological role in penile erection. J Clin Invest 1993; 91(2): 437–442.

49. Moon DG, Lee DS, Kim JJ. Altered contractile response of penis under hypoxia with metabolic acidosis. Int J Impot Res 1999; 11(5):265–271.

50. Moreland RB. Pathophysiology of erectile dysfunction: the contributions of trabecular structure to function and the role of functional antagonism. Int J Impot Res 2000; 12(suppl 4):S39–S46.

51. Moreland RB. Is there a role of hypoxemia in penile fibrosis: a viewpoint presented to the Society for the Study of Impotence. Int J Impot Res 1998; 10(2): 113–120.

52. Nehra A. Mechanisms of venous leakage: a prospective clinicopathological correlation of corporeal function and structure. J Urol 1996; 156(4): 1320–1329.

18

Priapism

Ricardo Munarriz
Department of Urology, Boston University School of Medicine, Boston, Massachusetts, U.S.A.

Irwin Goldstein
Department of Sexual Medicine, Alvarado Hospital, San Diego, California, U.S.A.

□ INTRODUCTION

The term "priapism" is derived from the name of the ancient Greek mythological figure, Priapus, who was remarkable for being the god of seduction, fertility, and sexual love, as well as having a giant phallus (1). In the modern era, priapism is defined as a pathological condition of penile erection that persists after sexual stimulation has ceased or is unrelated to sexual stimulation entirely (for further information on this definition, see below "Definition and Classification"). Priapism is an important medical condition that may cause permanent, irreversible erectile dysfunction, as well as devastating psychological consequences that may develop as a result of the initial dysfunction; as such, the occurrence of priapism requires immediate evaluation and possible emergency management. Yet, since the first reported case of priapism in 1824 by Callaway (2), limited attention has been given to the study of the incidence, etiology, pathophysiology, diagnosis, and timely treatment of this disorder.

□ INCIDENCE

Well-designed, random-sample, community-based epidemiologic studies of men with priapism are limited. Current data reveal that the incidence of priapism in the general population is low. A Finnish study, based on hospital discharge data, established the incidence of priapism between 0.3 and 0.5 cases per 100,000 person-years, with a peak incidence of 1.1 cases per 100,000 person-years in the final years of the study. This peak was attributed to the new use of intracavernosal vasoactive agents introduced for the treatment of erectile dysfunction (3). More recently, Eland et al. conducted a population-based retrospective cohort study using the Integrated Primary Care Information database, a longitudinal computer-based record of all patients seen by general practitioners in the Netherlands (4). This study demonstrated a slightly higher incidence of noniatrogenic priapism (0.9 cases per 100,000 person-years) and a similar incidence of iatrogenic priapism. The incidence of priapism in the United States may be greater than that previously reported due to a higher incidence of hemoglobinopathies such as sickle cell.

□ DEFINITION AND CLASSIFICATION

The American Foundation for Urologic Disease Thought Leader Panel on Evaluation and Treatment of Priapism was developed in 2001 with input from a multidisciplinary panel that included 19 experts in pediatrics, hematology–oncology, psychiatry, and urology. This panel established the following definition and classification for priapism (5).

Priapism

Priapism is a pathological condition of a penile erection that persists beyond or is unrelated to sexual stimulation. Priapism is an important medical condition that requires evaluation and may require emergency management.

Ischemic Priapism (Veno-Occlusive)

Ischemic priapism (veno-occlusive) is the most common form of priapism; it is usually a painful, rigid erection characterized clinically by absent cavernous blood flow. Ischemic priapism beyond four hours is a compartment syndrome requiring emergent medical intervention. Potential consequences are irreversible, including corporal fibrosis and permanent erectile dysfunction.

Arterial (Nonischemic) Priapism

Arterial (nonischemic) priapism is a less common form of priapism caused by unregulated cavernous inflow. The erection is usually painless and not fully rigid. Nonischemic priapism requires evaluation, but is neither a compartment syndrome nor a medical emergency.

☐ ETIOLOGY
Ischemic Priapism (Veno-Occlusive)
Drugs

Drugs are responsible for up to 80% of cases of ischemic priapism of the veno-occlusive type (6). Intracavernosal injection of vasoactive drugs for the management of erectile dysfunction has become the most common cause of drug-induced priapism (7). The risk of priapism after intracavernosal injection of vasoactive agents such as papaverine, prostaglandin E1, or a combination of these agents is higher in men with psychogenic, neurogenic, or pure cavernosal arterial insufficiency.

Antihypertensive drugs such as phenoxybenzamine (7), labetalol (8), and prazosin (9,10) are thought to induce priapism through an α-adrenergic blocking activity, which may delay physiologic detumescence or directly cause relaxation of the smooth muscle of the corpus cavernosum (11).

Duggan et al. first reported the association between heparin and priapism after four patients developed ischemic priapism while on heparin for the management of myocardial infarction (12). This association was further studied by Singhan et al. in 17 of 3337 hemodialysis patients who received heparin and experienced an episode of priapism during or shortly after hemodialysis (13). Although the mechanism by which heparin induces priapism is unclear, it is hypothesized that a relatively hypercoagulable state may develop after heparin therapy is discontinued (14). In addition, hemodialysis patients may have a defect of von Willebrand's factor, a platelet adherence molecule. Thus, they may be more susceptible to priapism (15). The use of warfarin has also been associated with priapism (16).

Although tricyclic antidepressants have rarely been associated with priapism, trazodone, a widely used antidepressant and hypnotic, is commonly associated with prolonged erections and priapism. The most likely mechanism is thought to be mediated by an α-adrenergic blockade, which interferes with the normal detumescence mechanism.

Antipsychotic drugs such as phenothiazines have also been associated with ischemic priapism. This is most likely due to the blocking of dopamine D_1 receptors, although antihistaminic, antiserotonergic, anticholinergic, and α-blocking properties may participate to a lesser degree (17,18).

Cocaine administered either intranasally or topically has also become a common cause of ischemic priapism (19–21). The pathophysiologic mechanism of this process is complex and multifactorial; on one hand, cocaine is a potent norepinephrine reuptake inhibitor, which may deplete neuronal norepinephrine stores and prevent detumescence (22), while on the other hand, it is a potent serotonin reuptake inhibitor, which may cause central nervous system stimulation and peripheral vasodilation (23,24). The use of marijuana has also been associated with priapism (11,25,26).

In the past, when parenteral hyperalimentation contained high fat emulsions, ischemic priapism was frequently reported. Several pathophysiologic mechanisms such as hypercoagulability, fat embolism, capillary thrombosis, and decreased capillary blood flow have been hypothesized to be responsible for the development of parenteral hyperalimentation-induced ischemic priapism (26–28).

Finally, toxins such as black widow spider venom (29) and the administration of several hormones including testosterone (30) or antiestrogens such as tamoxifen (31) have been associated with ischemic priapism.

Hematologic Disorders

Hematologic disorders—particularly hemoglobinopathies—are the most common cause of priapism in the pediatric population (32). The incidence of sickle cell disease in African Americans is estimated to be 8.2% (33), and approximately 10% to 89% of patients with sickle cell disease will experience priapism (34,35). The vast majority of sickle cell priapism occurs during nocturnal erections. It is possible that the combination of erythrocyte functional and structural abnormalities, low oxygen tension, and decreased corporal pH during prolonged nocturnal erections may induce the formation of irreversible sickle cell erythrocytes, preventing venous outflow and normal penile detumescence. Sickle cell is probably the most common cause of stuttering priapism, a rare and poorly described syndrome characterized by multiple or recurrent episodes of ischemic priapism (36).

Other hyperviscosity states such as leukemia and polycythemia have also been associated with priapism. The pathophysiology is probably similar to that of the sickle cell anemia (37,38). Other hematologic disorders associated with priapism are listed in Table 1.

Metabolic Disorders

Metabolic disorders such as amyloidosis (6), nephritic syndrome (39), and Fabry's disease (40) are rare causes of priapism, and the literature is limited to single-case reports of these occurrences. The most likely pathophysiologic mechanism is due to the obstruction of the outflow pathway.

Neurologic Disorders

Spinal cord injury (41), spinal stenosis (42), and other neurologic conditions are rare causes of priapism and generally resolve spontaneously or require minimal intervention.

Idiopathic Disorders

The etiology of ischemic priapism is unknown in approximately 30% to 50% of cases (43). A comprehensive and extensive evaluation is mandatory to exclude reversible or life-threatening causes.

Table 1 Etiology of Priapism

ISCHEMIC PRIAPISM	*Drugs*	Intracavernosal agents	Papaverine Prostaglandin E1 Phenoxybenzamine
		CNS-active drugs antihypertensives	Trazodone benzodiazepines
			Phenothiazines Prazosin Phenoxybenzamine Labetalol Calcium channel blockers β-blockers Hydralazine
		Anticoagulants	Heparin Warfarin
		Hormonal agents	Testosterone Gonadotropin-releasing hormone Antiestrogens (tamoxifen)
		Illegal drugs	Cocaine Marijuana
		Other	Parenteral nutrition Carbon monoxide Black widow spider venom Alcohol
	Hematologic disorders	Hyperviscosity states	Polycythemia
		Hemoglobinopathies	Sickle cell anemia Thalassemia
	Immunological disorders		Lupus Protein C deficiency
	Metabolic disorders		Gout Diabetes Nephritic syndrome Renal failure Amyloidosis Fabry's disease
	Neurologic disorders		Spinal cord lesions Autonomic neuropathy Spinal stenosis
	Malignancies		Leukemia Prostate cancer Urethral cancer Metastatic renal cancer Multiple myeloma
	Idiopathic		—
ARTERIAL PRIAPISM	*Blunt perineal trauma*		
	Penetrating perineal trauma		Cavernosal artery laceration Intracavernosal administration of vasoactive agents
	Idiopathic		Unrecognized trauma

Abbreviation: CNS, central nervous system.

Pathophysiology of Ischemic Priapism

Ischemic priapism results from an imbalance of the vasoconstrictive and vasorelaxatory mechanisms, leading to a penile closed compartment syndrome that is biochemically characterized by hypoxia, hypercapnia, and acidosis. Prolonged corporal smooth muscle exposure to these conditions results in irreversible damage to erectile tissue with subsequent corporal fibrosis (Figs. 1 and 2). Acidosis attenuates trabecular smooth muscle contractility to α-adrenergic agonists (44). In consequence, higher doses of adrenergic agonists may be required to overcome the decreased receptor affinity in order to achieve detumescence (45).

In addition, hypoxemia activates endothelial cells, leading to a cascade of reactions characterized by increased neutrophil adhesion, decreased mitochondrial respiratory chain activity, and an increase in intracellular calcium.

Reestablishing corporal blood flow during the management of ischemic priapism is associated with the reperfusion of ischemic tissues. This drastic increase in corporal oxygen tension generates reactive oxygen species (ROS) that may cause tissue damage. Based on

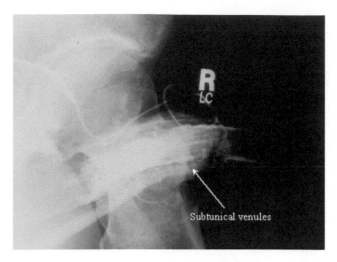

Figure 1 Cavernosography. Severe corporal fibrosis due to prolonged ischemic priapism (seven days). Subtunical venules are visualized throughout the entire penis. *Abbreviation*: LC, left corpus cavernosum.

the cardiac reperfusion model described by Goldhaber and Weiss (46), the authors propose that several events take place during penile ischemia and reperfusion in the management of priapism: (*i*) endogenous scavengers of oxygen free radicals may decrease during ischemia, resulting in reduced levels of antioxidant effects; (*ii*) decreased mitochondria aerobic metabolism results in the production of ROS; (*iii*) increased adenosine triphosphate hydrolysis results in the accumulation of hypoxanthine, which is subsequently converted to uric acid, another source of ROS; (*iv*) the nitric oxide (NO) pathway generates peroxynitrite, peroxynitrite anion, and hydroxyl radical (free radicals); and (*v*) lipid peroxidation and infiltration of the vasculature with neutrophils produces several oxygen free radicals (oxygen free radicals, hydrogen peroxide, hydroxyl radical,

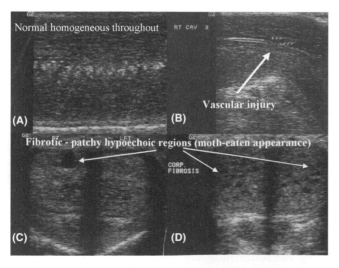

Figure 2 Penile damage documented by penile ultrasound gray scale scanning. (**A**) Normal cavernosal tissue appearance by ultrasound. (**B**) Vascular injury after 36-hour episode of ischemic priapism. (**C** and **D**) Ultrasonographic appearance of corporal fibrosis after priapism.

and hypochlorous anion) that are released in response to ischemia/reperfusion.

Arterial (Nonischemic Priapism)

High-flow priapism results from unregulated cavernous arterial flow as a result of an acute perineal trauma, which leads to the formation of an arterial-lacunar fistula (47). Turbulent arterial flow into the fistula causes unregulated release of endothelial NO, a potent vasodilator and anticoagulant, that prevents penile detumescence and clotting of the arterial-lacunar fistula. Arterial priapism is characterized by a permanent, painless partial erection that is almost always associated with normal penile axial rigidity during sexual activity. If, however, this type of priapism is associated with persistently inadequate penile erection during intercourse, one must suspect that the traumatic event that resulted in a lacerated cavernosal artery was also severe enough to cause endothelial injury, leading to arterial obstructive pathology. Alternatively, the traumatic event may also have caused corporal tissue injury that resulted in corporal veno-occlusive dysfunction. In such cases, vascular testing (duplex Doppler ultrasound and dynamic infusion cavernosometry and cavernosography) is indicated to differentiate cavernosal artery insufficiency from venous leak and to determine if vascular reconstruction is appropriate to reestablish potency. (For more information on vascular imaging of the penis, please refer to Chapter 25).

□ MANAGEMENT
Ischemic Priapism (Compartment Syndrome of the Corpora Cavernosa)

The diagnosis of priapism is usually made by history and physical examination, but some general diagnostic tests complete blood count (CBC) platelets, differential, reticulocyte count, hemoglobin electrophoresis, prostate specific antigen (PSA), urine analysis, and urine screening for metabolites of cocaine or for psychoactive drugs) should be considered when attempting to identify the etiologic factor. Assessment of corporal blood flow status must be carried out in all patients, either by corporal aspirate (color, consistency, and corporal blood gas) or by penile duplex Doppler ultrasound (Fig. 3). Corporal blood flow should be reassessed after treatment has been performed in order to evaluate the status of cavernosal arterial blood inflow continuously.

Should ischemic priapism be diagnosed and treatment initiated to reestablish cavernosal arterial blood flow, management should proceed as follows: first, penile anesthesia (dorsal nerve, subcutaneous local penile shaft block, or circumferential penile block) and/or systemic analgesia should be considered before therapeutic efforts are carried out. Pharmacologic agent administration with or without corporal aspiration, using cardiopulmonary monitoring if needed, is simply performed and is effective in many cases. Phenylephrine has been suggested as the drug of choice because of its

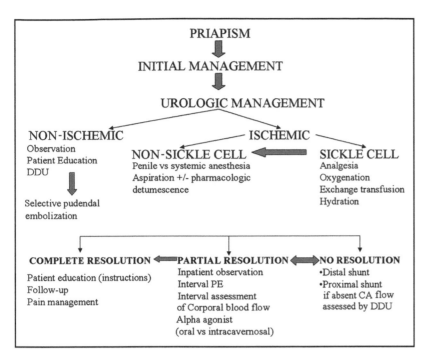

Figure 3 Algorithm for the management of priapism. *Abbreviations*: DDU, duplex Doppler ultrasound; CA, cavernosal arterial (flow); PE, physical examination.

pure α1-agonist and low β1-agonist activity (48). The recommended dose is 200 to 300 µg intracavernosally every 5 to 10 minutes, up to a maximal dose of 1.5 mg of phenylephrine. Recently, in order to overcome the decreased affinity of α-adrenergic receptors observed in the presence of the acidosis in ischemic priapism, Munarriz et al. successfully used high-dose phenylephrine (1000 µg/mL every 10 minutes as needed for 7–10 doses) without significant complications (45). Other adrenergic agents may also be used (Table 2).

If pharmacologic agent administration fails, corporal irrigation with saline, with or without pharmacologic agents to induce detumescence, should be the next logical step. In addition, appropriate analgesia, hydration, and oxygenation with or without exchange transfusion are indicated in the sickle cell patient.

Successful treatment outcome should be assessed by physical examination of the penis, and, in cases of partial resolution, interval assessment of corporal blood flow status by corporal aspirate or penile duplex Doppler ultrasound is mandatory. If the episode of priapism has been successfully resolved, the patient

may be discharged home with detailed instructions, a follow-up plan, and oral analgesics. In the case of partial resolution, however, or if the original pathology was the result of ischemic edema, persistent partial erection, or persistent pain, in-patient observation is recommended. Interval physical examination of the penis and/or interval assessment of corporal blood flow status by corporal aspirate or penile duplex Doppler ultrasound remain mandatory for these patients, as well. Adrenergic agonists may be administered (intracavernosally and/or orally) on an interval basis to induce complete detumescence. If no resolution of the ischemic priapism can be achieved after repeated first-line interventions over several hours,

Table 2 Adrenergic Agents Used in the Treatment of Ischemic Priapism

	α	β1	β2	Dose
Ephedrine	+	++	++	—
Epinephrine	+++	+++	+++	(10–20 mg/mL); 1-mL increments every 5 min
Norepinephrine	+++	++	++	—
Phenylephrine	+++	Minimal or none	Minimal or none	(1000 mg/mL); 0.3–0.5 mL every 5 min

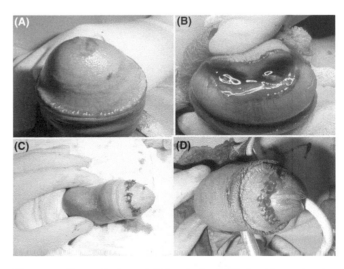

Figure 4 (*See color insert.*) Al Gorab shunt. (**A**) Semilunar glanular incision exposing tips of corporal bodies. (**B**) Removal of distal tunica albugineal exposing cavernosal tissue and allowing easy blood drainage. (**C**) Water-tight wound closure. (**D**) Assessment of cavernosal flow using Doppler.

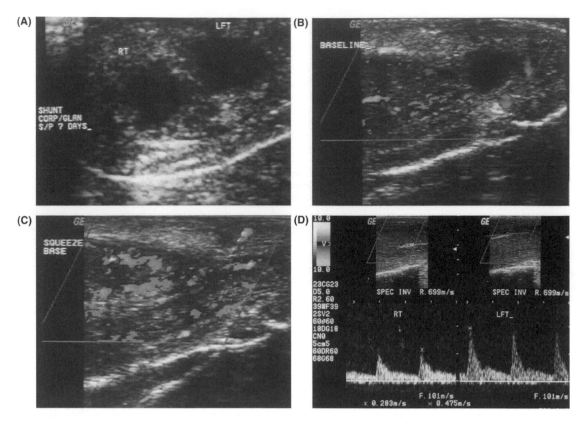

Figure 5   (*See color insert.*) Duplex Doppler ultrasound after Al Gorab shunt. (**A**) Gray scale scanning shows surgically removed distal tunical albuginea. (**B**) Color duplex ultrasound demonstrating minimal corporal drainage into the corpus spongiosum. (**C**) Excellent corporal drainage through shunt after manual compression at the base of the penile shaft. (**D**) Duplex Doppler ultrasound documenting reestablishment of cavernosal arterial blood flow.

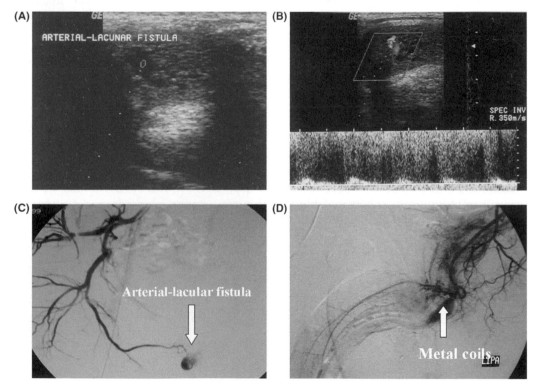

Figure 6   (*See color insert.*) Arterial priapism. (**A**) Perineal duplex Doppler ultrasound showing arterial-lacunar fistula. (**B**) Perineal duplex Doppler ultrasound showing arterial-lacunar fistula. (**C**) Selective internal pudendal arteriogram documenting arterial-lacunar fistula. (**D**) Selective internal pudendal arteriogram of an impotent man who developed cavernosal artery insufficiency after coil embolization of high-flow priapism.

advancement to surgical shunts is indicated. In the vast majority of cases, distal shunts are effective (Figs. 4 and 5). Proximal shunts are not more efficacious than distal shunts and, in addition, have a higher complication rate. Thus, proximal shunts should be avoided as a first-line surgical intervention.

The most important predictor of a return to premorbid erectile function is the duration of the priapism; therefore, rapid intervention is a necessity. Kulmala et al. reported that men with less than 24 hours of priapism have a 92% probability of achieving the restoration of premorbid level of erectile function versus only 22% if the episode of priapism extends for more than seven days (49).

Arterial Priapism Management

The diagnosis of high-flow priapism is usually made by history (perineal trauma is almost always reported by patients) and by physical examination (partial and nonpainful erection). Duplex Doppler ultrasound is a noninvasive modality that allows easy visualization and localization of the arterial-lacunar fistula (Fig. 6A and B). It is important to note that this form of priapism is not a compartment syndrome and thus is not a medical emergency. Selective internal pudendal arteriography and embolization (Fig. 6C) should only be carried out after extensive counseling. In addition, the author recommends the use of autologous clot injection. Autologous clots will temporarily occlude the lacerated artery, allowing the injured vessel to heal without causing permanent and irreversible occlusion of the cavernosal arteries, which may lead to erectile dysfunction (Fig. 6D).

□ CONCLUSION

Ischemic priapism is a rare urologic condition that requires evaluation and may require emergency urologic management to prevent corporal damage and permanent and irreversible erectile dysfunction.

□ REFERENCES

1. Papadopoulos I, Kelami A. Priapus and priapism. From mythology to medicine. Urology 1988; 32(4):385–386.
2. Callaway T. Unusual case of priapism. London Med Repository 1824; 1:286.
3. Kulmala RV, Lehtonen TA, Tammela TL. Priapism, its incidence and seasonal distribution in Finland. Scand J Urol Nephrol 1995; 29(1):93–96.
4. Eland IA, van der Lei J, Stricker BH, et al. Incidence of priapism in the general population. Urology 2001; 57(5):970–972.
5. Banos JE, Bosch F, Farre M. Drug-induced priapism. Its aetiology, incidence, and treatment. Med Toxicol Adverse Drug Exp 1989; 4(1):46–58.
6. Junemann K, Alken P. Pharmacotherapy of erectile dysfunction: a review. Int J Impot Res 1989; 1:71–89.
7. Funderburk SJ, Philippart M, Dale G, et al. Priapism after phenoxybenzamine in a patient with Fabry's disease. N Engl J Med 1974; 290(11):630–631.
8. Law MR, Copland RF, Armitstead JG, et al. Labetalol and priapism. Br Med J 1980; 280(6207):115.
9. Adams JW, Soucheray JA. Prazosin-induced priapism in a diabetic. J Urol 1984; 132(6):1208.
10. Bullock N. Prazosin-induced priapism. Br J Urol 1988; 62(5):487–488.
11. Rubin SO. Priapism as a probable sequel to medication. Scand J Urol Nephrol 1968; 2(2):81–85.
12. Duggan ML, Morgan C Jr. Heparin: a cause of priapism? South Med J 1970; 63(10):1131–1134.
13. Singhal PC, Lynn RI, Scharschmidt LA. Priapism and dialysis. Am J Nephrol 1986; 6(5):358–361.
14. Burke BJ, Scott GL, Smith PJ, et al. Heparin-associated priapism. Postgrad Med J 1983; 59(691):332–333.
15. Gralnick HR, McKeown LP, Williams SB, et al. Plasma and platelet von Willebrand factor defects in uremia. Am J Med 1988; 85(6):806–810.
16. Eadie DG, Brock TP. Corpus saphenous by-pass in the treatment of priapism. Br J Surg 1970; 57(3): 172–174.
17. Hyttel J, Larsen JJ, Christensen AV, et al. Receptor-binding profiles of neuroleptics. Psychopharmacology Suppl 1985; 2:9–18.
18. Van Rossum JM. The significance of dopamine-receptor blockade for the mechanism of action of neuroleptic drugs. Arch Int Pharmacodyn Ther 1966; 160(2):492–494.
19. Fiorelli RL, Manfrey SJ, Belkoff LH, et al. Priapism associated with intranasal cocaine abuse. J Urol 1990; 143(3):584–585.
20. Rodriguez-Blasquez HM, Cardona PE, Rivera-Herrera JL. Priapism associated with the use of topical cocaine. J Urol 1981; 143(2):358.
21. Munarriz R, Hwang J, Goldstein I, et al. Cocaine and ephedrine-induced priapism: case reports and investigation of potential adrenergic mechanisms. Urology 2003; 62(1):187–192.
22. Lakoski JM, Cunningham KA. The interaction of cocaine with central serotonergic neuronal systems: cellular electrophysiologic approaches. NIDA Res Monogr 1988; 88:78–91.
23. Cocores JA, Dackis CA, Gold MS. Sexual dysfunction secondary to cocaine abuse in two patients. J Clin Psychiatry 1986; 47(7):384–385.

24. Forsberg L, Mattiasson A, Olsson AM. Priapism: conservative treatment versus surgical procedures. Br J Urol 1981; 53(4):374–377.

25. Winter CC. Priapism. J Urol 1981; 125(2):212.

26. Klein EA, Montague DK, Steiger E. Priapism associated with the use intravenous fat emulsion: case reports and postulated pathogenesis. J Urol 1985; 133(5): 857–859.

27. Amris CJ, Brockner J, Larsen V. Changes in the coagulability of blood during the infusion of intralipid. Acta Chir Scand 1964; 86(suppl 325):70–74.

28. Brockner J, Amris CJ, Larsen V. Fat infusions and blood coagulation. Effect of various fat emulsions on blood coagulability. A comparative study. Acta Chir Scand 1965; 343:48–55.

29. Stiles AD. Priapism following a black widow spider bite. Clin Pediatr (Phila) 1982; 21(3):174–175.

30. Zelissen PM, Stricker BH. Severe priapism as a complication of testosterone substitution therapy. Am J Med 1988; 85(2):273–274.

31. Fernando IN, Tobias JS. Priapism in patient on tamoxifen. Lancet 1989; 1(8635):436.

32. Hamre MR, Harmon EP, Kirkpatrick DV, et al. Priapism as a complication of sickle cell disease. J Urol 1991; 145(1):1–5.

33. Tarry WF, Duckett JW Jr, Snyder HM III. Urological complications of sickle cell disease in a pediatric population. J Urol 1987; 138(3):592–594.

34. Fowler JE Jr, Koshy M, Strub M, et al. Priapism associated with the sickle cell hemoglobinopathies: prevalence, natural history and sequelae. J Urol 1991; 145(1):65–68.

35. Mantadakis E, Cavender JD, Rogers ZR, et al. Prevalence of priapism in children and adolescents with sickle cell anemia. J Pediatr Hematol Oncol 1999; 21(6):518–522.

36. Jackson N, Franlin IM, Hughes MA. Recurrent priapism following splenectomy for thalassaemia intermedia. Br J Surg 1986; 73(8):678.

37. Leifer W, Leifer G. Priapism caused by primary thrombocythemia. J Urol 1979; 121(2):254–255.

38. Winter CC, McDowell G. Experience with 105 patients with priapism: update review of all aspects. J Urol 1988; 140(5):980–983.

39. Witt MA, Goldstein I, Saenz de Tejada I, et al. Traumatic laceration of the intracavernosal arteries: the pathophysiology of non-ischemic, high flow, arterial priapism. J Urol 1990; 143(1):129–132.

40. Garcia-Consuegra J, Padron M, Jaureguizar E, et al. Priapism and Fabry disease: a case report. Eur J Pediatr 1990; 149(7):500–501.

41. Bedbrook GM. The Care and Management of Spinal Cord Injuries. New York: Springer Verlag, 1981.

42. Baba H, Maezawa Y, Furusawa N, et al. Lumbar spinal stenosis causing intermittent priapism. Paraplegia 1995; 33(6):338–345.

43. Pohl J, Pott B, Kleinhans G. Priapism: a three phase concept of management according to aetiology and prognosis. Br J Urol 1986; 58(2):113–118.

44. Saenz de Tejada I, Kim NN, Daley JT, et al. Acidosis impairs rabbit smooth muscle contractility. J Urol 1997; 157(2):722–726.

45. Munarriz R, Wen C, McAuley I, et al. Management of ischemic priapism with high-dose intracavernosal phenylephrine. J Sex Med 2006; 3(5):918–922.

46. Goldhaber JI, Weiss JN. Oxygen free radicals and cardiac reperfusion abnormalities. Hypertension 1992; 20(1):118–127.

47. Hakim LS, Kulaksizoglu H, Mulligan R, et al. Evolving concepts in the diagnosis and treatment of arterial high flow priapism. J Urol 1996; 155(2):541–548.

48. Bodner DR, Lindan R, Leffler E, et al. The application of intracavernous injection of vasoactive medications for erection in men with spinal cord injury. J Urol 1987; 138(2):310–311.

49. Kulmala RV, Letonen TA, Tammela TL. Preservation of potency after treatment for priapism. Scand J Urol Nephrol 1996; 30(4):313–316.

19

Pharmacological Agents Causing Male Sexual Dysfunction

William W. Finger
Mountain Home Veterans Affairs Medical Center, James H. Quillen School of Medicine, East Tennessee State University, Johnson City, Tennessee, U.S.A.

Mark A. Slagle
Department of Veterans Affairs MidSouth Healthcare Network, Nashville, Tennessee, U.S.A.

☐ INTRODUCTION

According to RxList.com, over 2.5 billion prescriptions were written for the top 300 medications in 2005 (1). Although most are effective at controlling or treating diseases states, many also have undesired side effects including sexual side effects. Over 200 medications have been cited in case reports, in prescribing literature, or in controlled studies as possibly having an impact on sexual function (2).

Certain patient trends suggest that the demands for accurate information on sexual side effects and effective treatment are emerging and will increase in the future. Longevity is increasing worldwide, and with it is the proportion of older patients who are more likely to require medication management of chronic illnesses. In addition, beliefs about aging are changing. Quality of life (QOL) is a central theme in older patient health care, and sexual health is considered an important component of QOL. While patients may have grudgingly accepted loss of sexual function in the past, they are much less willing to do so today.

Possible sexual side effects of medications are many and varied. Common sexual problems associated with medication in men include decreased desire for sex, difficulty in obtaining or maintaining erections, and delayed or absent orgasm (3). Less common side effects of medications include priapism (a sustained erection in the absence of sexual stimulation), retrograde ejaculation, painful ejaculation, spontaneous orgasm, and increased desire. All of these problems are likely to be of concern to patients, although patients may not attribute the problem to the medication and may not discuss it with their physician. Physicians should be aware of the potential for such side effects, monitor and evaluate accordingly, and treat appropriately.

Recognizing and treating these side effects is important for patient medication adherence and overall quality of care. Patients may stop taking medications without informing the prescribing physician because of bothersome side effects, resulting in serious health problems. For example, blood pressure medications are well known to impact sexual function; however, patients who stop taking these medications because of side effects run the risk of a heart attack or stroke. It is imperative that the physician addresses these issues proactively. It is likely that the patient will not voluntarily report sexual side effects to his doctor, out of discomfort in discussing such a sensitive issue. Physicians may also have some discomfort in discussing sexual issues, and may have received little or no training on evaluating and treating sexual side effects of medication. As a result, sexual side effects may be ignored or overlooked.

☐ MEDICATIONS AFFECTING SEXUAL FUNCTION

While medications in a variety of classes have been implicated in sexual disorders, certain classes have higher rates because of their mechanisms of action. The most common of these are medications used to treat hypertension and psychiatric disorders. Several classes of medications with sexual side effects are reviewed below. It should be noted that if a particular medication is not listed in the information that follows, this does not necessarily mean that a sexual side effect is not possible. In particular, newer agents may have sexual side effects that have not yet been characterized or reported. It is possible to estimate the potential sexual side effects of new or unlisted medications by comparing them to the classes of medications listed in the tables below. The final sections in this chapter outline the assessment and treatment of drug-induced changes in male sexual function.

Antihypertensive Medications

Antihypertensive medications are widely available in developed nations. In 2005, eight of the top 30 medications prescribed in the United States were for hypertension (1). The prescribing pattern of antihypertensive medications has changed significantly over the last ten years. Medications with significant side effects, including sexual side effects (e.g., hydrochlorothiazide and atenolol), have lost favor to medications with kinder side effect profiles (e.g., amlodipine and furosemide). This trend reflects an increased recognition of the importance of identifying and avoiding adverse side effects of antihypertensive medications.

Table 1 lists antihypertensive medications with known sexual side effects in men, and a more detailed discussion of these agents follows.

Diuretics

While diuretics are still prescribed widely, either alone or in combination with other antihypertensive medications, most pose substantial risk to sexual function.

Table 1 Antihypertensive Medications and Sexual Side Effects in Men

Diuretics	
Amiloride	Minimal or no sexual side effects reported
Chlorthalidone	Erectile dysfunction (high)
Furosemide	Minimal or no sexual side effects reported
Hydrochlorothiazide	Decreased sexual desire, erectile dysfunction (moderate to low)
Indapamide	Minimal or no sexual side effects reported
Spironolactone	Decreased sexual desire, erectile dysfunction, gynecomastia (high)
Triamterene	Minimal or no sexual side effects reported
β-Blockers	
Atenolol	Decreased sexual desire, erectile dysfunction (moderate to low)
Betaxolol	Minimal or no sexual side effects reported
Bisoprolol	Minimal or no sexual side effects reported
Carvedilol	Erectile dysfunction
Labetalol	Erectile dysfunction, ejaculatory dysfunction (moderate)
Metoprolol	Decreased sexual desire, erectile dysfunction (moderate to low)
Pindolol	Minimal or no sexual side effects reported
Propranolol	Decreased sexual desire, erectile dysfunction (high)
Timolol	Decreased sexual desire, erectile dysfunction (high)
Central antiadrenergic agents	
Clonidine	Decreased sexual desire, erectile dysfunction, ejaculatory dysfunction (moderate)
Guanabenz	Decreased sexual desire, erectile dysfunction, ejaculatory dysfunction (high)
Guanadrel	Decreased sexual desire, erectile dysfunction, ejaculatory dysfunction (high)
Guanethidine	Decreased sexual desire, erectile dysfunction, ejaculatory dysfunction (high)
Methyldopa	Decreased sexual desire, erectile dysfunction, ejaculatory dysfunction, gynecomastia (high)
Reserpine	Decreased sexual desire, erectile dysfunction, ejaculatory dysfunction (high)
Calcium channel antagonists (generally considered to have a low incidence of sexual side effects)	
Amlodipine	Decreased sexual desire, erectile dysfunction, ejaculatory dysfunction, gynecomastia (low)
Diltiazem	Decreased sexual desire, erectile dysfunction, ejaculatory dysfunction, gynecomastia (low)
Felodipine	Decreased sexual desire, erectile dysfunction, ejaculatory dysfunction, gynecomastia (low)
Isradipine	Decreased sexual desire, erectile dysfunction, ejaculatory dysfunction, gynecomastia (low)
Nicardipine	Decreased sexual desire, erectile dysfunction, ejaculatory dysfunction, gynecomastia (low)
Nifedipine	Decreased sexual desire, erectile dysfunction, ejaculatory dysfunction, gynecomastia (low)
Verapamil	Decreased sexual desire, erectile dysfunction, ejaculatory dysfunction, gynecomastia (low)
ACE inhibitors (generally considered free of sexual side effects)	
Benazepril	Erectile dysfunction (low)
Captopril	Erectile dysfunction (low)
Enalapril	Erectile dysfunction (low)
Lisinopril	Erectile dysfunction (low)
α-Blockers (generally considered free of sexual side effects)	
Doxazosin	Minimal or no sexual side effects reported
Prazosin	Erectile dysfunction (low), priapism (moderate)
Terazosin	Minimal or no sexual side effects reported
Angiotensin II receptor blockers (generally considered free of sexual side effects)	
Candesartan	Minimal or no sexual side effects reported
Irbesartan	Minimal or no sexual side effects reported
Losartan	Minimal or no sexual side effects reported
Telmisartan	Minimal or no sexual side effects reported
Valsartan	Minimal or no sexual side effects reported
Miscellaneous	
Hydralazine	Erectile dysfunction (low)
Mecamylamine	Erectile dysfunction, desire disorder (low)
Metyrosine	Minimal or no sexual side effects reported
Minoxidil	Minimal or no sexual side effects reported

Abbreviation: ACE, angiotensin-converting enzyme.

While exact mechanisms for these adverse sexual effects are not clear, it has been postulated that the use of diuretics may result in increased estrogens, increased prolactin, and/or decreased zinc, any one of which could contribute to changes in sexual function. In addition, diuretics cause vasodilation of vascular smooth muscles and a reduction of extracellular fluid, resulting in lowered blood pressure that may affect a man's ability to achieve and maintain an erection (4,5).

Of the thiazide diuretics, chlorthalidone may be the worst offender, perhaps because of its long duration of action. A number of studies have shown a significant rate of sexual problems, primarily erectile dysfunction in men, with the intake of therapeutic doses of chlorthalidone (6,7). Spironolactone has also been associated with significant sexual problems—primarily, changes in sexual desire in both sexes, erectile dysfunction and gynecomastia in men, and decreased vaginal lubrication in women (8–13). These effects are thought to be a direct result of the antiandrogenic effect of spironolactone and are extremely dose-dependent (14,15). Hydrochlorothiazide has been considered a reasonable alternative to chlorthalidone and spironolactone, but recent studies have questioned the sexual safety of this diuretic. In fact, hydrochlorothiazide may cause erectile dysfunction and decreased desire at a rate comparable to that of chlorthalidone (16); however, this effect may be dose-dependent, and the most common doses for mild hypertension (12.5–25 mg) may have substantially less effect on sexual function than other thiazide diuretics.

When possible, diuretics with no known effect on sexual function should be prescribed. Indapamide, furosemide, and triamterene, while somewhat less effective as antihypertensives than the thiazide diuretics, have been shown to have few if any sexual side effects and often result in an alleviation of sexual problems when substituted for other antihypertensive medications (17,18).

β-Blockers

Although they are losing some ground to newer antihypertensive medications, β-blockers are still prescribed commonly. Through their primary mechanism of action (i.e., decreasing β-adrenergic activity), β-blockers may negatively impact sexual function. Possible mechanisms through which this may occur include shunting of blood away from the penis secondary to increased α-sympathetic tone, central nervous system (CNS)-mediated sedation and depression, and decreased CNS sympathetic outflow (13,19,20). Some β-blockers may also impact sexual function indirectly through increasing serotonin or affecting serotonin nerve receptors (21). The first β-blocker commercially available, propranolol, may negatively impact sexual function through both antiadrenergic activity and changes in serotonin activity. Propranolol has been associated with a high incidence of erectile dysfunction in men and may be associated with changes in sexual desire in both sexes (13,22–28). Sexual side effects may be lower with β-blockers that have higher specificity, such as atenolol and metoprolol, but erection problems and decreased desire are reported with these medications as well (8,12,13). Bisoprolol, a newer β-blocker, has not been shown to have significant effects on sexual function, but these side effects may be revealed as clinical experience with this medication increases (29). Carvedilol has been shown to reduce frequency of sexual intercourse in men as well as increase the frequency of erectile dysfunction (30).

Timolol, an eye drop used to treat glaucoma, has a surprisingly high rate of associated sexual disorders, including erectile dysfunction in men and decreased sexual desire in men and women (31). These side effects may be alleviated if timolol is switched to a newer ophthalmic β-blocker, betaxolol (32). Labetalol, which has both β- and α-blocking effects, has sometimes been reported to cause less sexual side effects than the traditional β-blockers; however, sexual problems, primarily erection problems and blocked ejaculation, have been reported at moderate levels in a number of studies (33,34).

Central Antiadrenergic Agents

Reserpine, a rauwolfia alkaloid, has lost considerable popularity because of severe side effects, but is still used in the elderly in the United States and is relatively common in developing countries. Sexual side effects from reserpine are common and may result from decreased dopaminergic and adrenergic activity and increased prolactin. Sexual side effects include decreased desire, erection problems, and ejaculatory and orgasmic disorders. These side effects may take weeks to develop and estimated incidence varies widely, from 1% to 36% in reported studies (6,11–13,35). In addition to the direct side effects of reserpine on sexual function, depletion of catecholamine and serotonin levels often results in severe depression in patients taking reserpine, indirectly contributing to changes in sexual desire and response.

Methyldopa, a centrally acting sympatholytic, was initially reported to have few sexual side effects (36,37), but these low reported incidences might have been due to inconsistent study methodologies. Later studies that questioned patients directly found a high rate of sexual problems, including erectile dysfunction (14–36%), ejaculatory disorders (7–19%), desire disorders (7–14%), and gynecomastia (4,8,10–12,26,38–44). Methyldopa-induced desire disorders and erectile dysfunctions can be attributed to increased prolactin levels (45), and ejaculatory difficulties are due to sympatholytic activity. Erectile difficulties and low desire may also be due to general sedation and depression often seen in patients taking methyldopa (36,37,39–41). Clonidine is another centrally acting sympatholytic, with a similar therapeutic action and sexual side effect profile to methyldopa. Erectile dysfunction, delayed orgasm, and decreased sexual desire have been reported with clonidine at rates similar to those found with methyldopa (13,27,46); however, while these studies showed rates of sexual disorders as high as 24%, other studies using lower doses and transdermal systems have found relatively low levels of sexual problems with clonidine (13,46–49). Guanabenz, guanadrel, and guanethidine, while having different mechanisms of action, have all been associated with high rates of desire disorders, erectile dysfunction, and ejaculatory dysfunction (13,38,42,50–53).

Calcium Channel Antagonists

As a class, calcium channel antagonists or calcium channel blockers have few sexual side effects compared to other classes of antihypertensive medications. Nifedipine, a dihydropyridine calcium channel blocker, has been reported to cause ejaculatory problems (54), possibly due to blockage of the urethra through interaction with the skeletal muscle of the bulbocavernosus and the smooth muscle of the vas deferens and seminal vesicles (5). Other medications in this subclass, including amlodipine, felodipine, isradipine, and nicardipine, may have a similar effect, although no research has reported this finding. In addition, nifedipine has been associated with decreased erections (55,56) and gynecomastia (57). Because of the potential increase of prolactin and decrease of dopamine with all calcium channel blockers, gynecomastia and decreased sexual desire may be possible with any of these medications (58).

Angiotensin-Converting Enzyme Inhibitors

Angiotensin-converting enzyme (ACE) inhibitors have relatively little impact on sexual function. ACE inhibitors, including captopril, enalapril, and lisinopril, do not appear to cause any significant change in sexual desire or response, although a low incidence of erectile dysfunction has been reported in some studies (59).

α-Blockers

α-Blockers, including prazosin, terazosin, and doxazosin, have rarely been reported to cause erectile dysfunction (60,61); however, one study found a higher rate of erection problems when prazosin was combined with a diuretic than when hydralazine was combined with a diuretic (62). On the other hand, prazosin has been linked to numerous cases of priapism (13).

Angiotensin II Receptor Blockers

Angiotensin II receptor blockers, including valsartan, losartan, irbesartan, candesartan, and telmisartan, are relatively new medications, with few sexual side effects reported to date. Prescribing literature indicates a rate of decreased desire disorder and erection problems comparable to the rate reported with placebo, but no causation has been established. Recent placebo-controlled studies suggest that valsartan has no negative effect on sexual function, does not decrease testosterone level, and may actually improve overall sexual function when compared to β-blockers (atenolol and carvedilol) or placebo (30,63).

Antidepressant Medications

In 1995, only one antidepressant was in the top 30 prescribed medications; in 2005, this has increased to four (1). Use of antidepressants is on the rise for many reasons. While early antidepressant medications were potentially toxic, more recent ones are much less so. There has also been increased recognition and treatment of psychiatric concerns. In addition, antidepressants are being prescribed for a wider range of symptoms and disorders, including anxiety, panic attacks, obsessive-compulsive disorder, post-traumatic stress disorder, and even premenstrual symptoms. As a result, the use of these medications is widespread, and their potential side effects take on added importance.

Of the psychiatric medications, antidepressants are most commonly implicated as causing sexual dysfunction; however, the diagnostic picture is often clouded by the psychiatric disorder itself. Decreased sexual desire, and, to a lesser extent, disorders of arousal and orgasm, may be diagnosed as a symptom of depression rather than a side effect of treatment. It is assumed that treatment of the psychiatric disturbance will result in alleviation of the sexual problem. Unfortunately, disruption of sexual function secondary to psychotropic medication can lead to lowered self-esteem, consequently worsening depression. Thus, sexual side effects should be carefully considered when prescribing antidepressant medications, and monitoring for possible side effects during treatment can help to avoid or minimize this problem. In Table 2 and the sections that follow, various antidepressants and their sexual side effects in men are described.

Tricyclics

Tricyclic antidepressants were one of the first classes of antidepressants developed and had many sexual side effects. The negative effects of the tricyclics on sexual function may be related to decreased cholinergic and β-adrenergic activity, decreased histamine and oxytocin, and increased prolactin and serotonin (64,65). Commonly reported side effects in men include decreased sexual desire, erectile difficulties, decreased ejaculatory volume, and delayed or absent orgasm (66–69). Sexual side effects may develop many weeks after the initiation of tricyclic therapy (70). In addition, patients may not consider the side effect to be a problem; for example, a delay in orgasm and a decrease in ejaculatory volume may not be distressing to the patient.

Of the tricyclics, clomipramine, doxepin, amitriptyline, and imipramine may have the highest rate of sexual side effects. Sexual side effects of clomipramine are especially common, even at relatively low doses and may be attributed to its large serotonergic effect (71) and a subsequent increase in prolactin levels. Lack of orgasm and ejaculation can occur at a rate as high as 70%, delayed orgasm as high as 92%, and erectile

Table 2 Antidepressant Medications and Sexual Side Effects in Men

Tricyclics	
Amitriptyline	Decreased sexual desire, erectile dysfunction, ejaculatory dysfunction, orgasmic dysfunction (high)
Amoxapine	Decreased sexual desire, erectile dysfunction, ejaculatory dysfunction, orgasmic dysfunction (high)
Clomipramine	Decreased sexual desire, erectile dysfunction, ejaculatory dysfunction, orgasmic dysfunction (high)
Desipramine	Decreased sexual desire, erectile dysfunction, ejaculatory dysfunction, orgasmic dysfunction (low)
Doxepin	Decreased sexual desire, erectile dysfunction, ejaculatory dysfunction, orgasmic dysfunction (high)
Imipramine	Decreased sexual desire, erectile dysfunction, ejaculatory dysfunction, orgasmic dysfunction (moderate)
Nortriptyline	Decreased sexual desire, erectile dysfunction, ejaculatory dysfunction, orgasmic dysfunction (low)
Protriptyline	Decreased sexual desire, erectile dysfunction, ejaculatory dysfunction, orgasmic dysfunction (moderate)
Trimipramine	Decreased sexual desire, erectile dysfunction, ejaculatory dysfunction, orgasmic dysfunction (moderate)
Selective serotonin reuptake inhibitors	
Citalopram	Minimal or no sexual side effects reported
Fluoxetine	Orgasmic disorder (high), erectile dysfunction, desire disorder (low)
Fluvoxamine	Orgasmic disorder (high), erectile dysfunction, desire disorder (low)
Paroxetine	Orgasmic disorder (high), erectile dysfunction, desire disorder (low)
Sertraline	Orgasmic disorder (high), erectile dysfunction, desire disorder (low)
Monoamine oxidase inhibitors	
Isocarboxazid	Decreased sexual desire, erectile dysfunction, orgasmic dysfunction (moderate)
Phenelzine	Decreased sexual desire, erectile dysfunction, orgasmic dysfunction (moderate)
Tranylcypromine	Decreased sexual desire, erectile dysfunction, orgasmic dysfunction (moderate)
Moclobemide	Decreased sexual desire, erectile dysfunction, orgasmic dysfunction (moderate)
Phenylpiperazines	
Nefazodone	Minimal or no sexual side effects reported
Trazodone	Priapism (low)
Miscellaneous antidepressants and mood stabilizers	
Bupropion	Minimal or no sexual side effects reported
Lithium	Desire disorder, erectile dysfunction (moderate)
Maprotiline	Minimal or no sexual side effects reported
Mirtazapine	Minimal or no sexual side effects reported
Venlafaxine	Orgasmic disorder (high)
Duloxetine	Minimal or no sexual side effects reported

difficulties as high as 15% (68,72). Tricyclics having a relatively lower incidence of sexual side effects include desipramine and nortriptyline.

Serotonin and Norepinephrine Reuptake Inhibitors

Selective serotonin reuptake inhibitors (SSRIs) have replaced tricyclics as the most commonly prescribed antidepressant medications. Initially, these medications were thought to have fewer sexual side effects than the tricyclics. Because levels of serotonin, prolactin, and cortisol are increased by SSRIs, other sexual side effects are common, with delayed or absent orgasm being the most commonly reported (73–75). Reports of delayed orgasm range from the single digits to as high as 75%, depending on the method of data collection (76). Although spontaneous reporting of this side effect is low, higher rates of ejaculatory delay were reported by studies that specifically asked about these changes. This trend suggests that delays in orgasm or ejaculation may be underreported because men do not consider the delay a problem or are too embarrassed to report it unless specifically asked. One of the earliest SSRIs, fluoxetine, did note possible orgasmic delay in the prescribing literature, but it was not until this medication had been used for a number of years that the extent of this problem became apparent. Sertraline and paroxetine were expected to have less impact on orgasm than fluoxetine, but also a high rate of orgasmic delay (77,78).

The newer SSRIs, including citalopram and fluvoxamine, and serotonin/norepinephrine reuptake inhibitors (SNRIs) such as venlafaxine may have a lower occurrence of sexual side effects, although recent evidence suggests that the rate may still be substantial (77–80). The new SNRI duloxetine has not been shown to have significant sexual side effects, but research is limited to date (81,82).

In addition to the high incidence of ejaculatory and orgasmic changes, erectile dysfunction with SSRIs has also been noted (79). Decreased sexual desire has been associated with these agents, but, as mentioned previously, this may be hard to differentiate from the decreased sexual desire often resulting directly from depression.

Other Antidepressants

Monamine oxidase inhibitors (MAOIs) may impair sexual desire, erectile function, and orgasmic function (83,84) through decreased cholinergic and β-adrenergic activity, increased prolactin and serotonin, and decreased testosterone. Lithium has also been reported to cause impaired sexual desire and problems with erections (85,86). The phenylpiperazine class of antidepressants (e.g., trazodone and nefazodone) is less likely to impair desire, erection, or orgasmic response, although cases of priapism have been reported with trazodone (87–89). Trazodone can decrease α-1 adrenergic activity and increase cortisol and serotonin. Bupropion and mirtazapine also seem to have limited or absent effects on sexual function, although delayed orgasm has been observed in case reports with mirtazapine (90).

Other Psychotropic Medications

Many antipsychotic medications, especially the phenothiazines (e.g., thioridazine, chlorpromazine, and fluphenazine) (91), have been reported to cause erectile dysfunction and delay of ejaculation and orgasm. Disorders of desire and cases of priapism have also been reported (92,93). Mechanisms implicated in producing these sexual side effects include α-1 peripheral adrenergic blockade, decreased dopamine and testosterone secretion, and increased prolactin secretion (11,12,94). Priapism has also been reported with antipsychotics, including chlorpromazine, thioridazine, flupenthixol, fluphenazine, mesoridazine, haloperidol, molindone, trifluoperazine, perphenazine, and chlorprothixene (92,95,96). While these sexual side effects have been observed, controlled studies are lacking and specific incidences of sexual disorders for these various medications are not available. Antipsychotic medications with fewer effects on sexual function include risperidone, olanzapine, and quetiapine. Approximately 5% of patients taking risperidone experience erectile dysfunction and ejaculatory dysfunction; this is a greater number than those taking a placebo, but nevertheless considerably lower than those taking phenothiazines. Priapism has been reported with olanzapine and quetiapine use, although no causative link has been found.

Benzodiazepines may interfere with sexual desire and the ability to attain orgasm (97–99) through their effects of increased γ-aminobutyric acid, increased progesterone, decreased α-1 adrenergic activity, decreased luteinizing hormone–releasing hormone, decreased substance P, and decreased testosterone. There is some evidence that three-ring benzodiazepines (e.g., flurazepam and temazepam) have fewer sexual side effects than the older two-ring benzodiazepines. Because studies of the sexual side effects of benzodiazepines are lacking, the exact association of these medications with sexual disorders is not clearly understood. Other psychiatric medications include buspirone, an anxiolytic unrelated to the benzodiazepines, and zolpidem, an imidazopyridine sedative-hypnotic. A single case report of anorgasmia has been reported when buspirone has been added to fluoxetine, although the anorgasmia could not be definitely attributed directly to buspirone (100). To date, there are no reports of sexual side effects with zolpidem. Table 3 identifies antipsychotic, antianxiety, and sedative/hypnotic agents with known sexual side effects in men.

Miscellaneous Medications

While antihypertensives, antidepressants, and various psychiatric medications are most frequently reported to cause sexual side effects, many other medications have been implicated in causing similar effects. For example, cimetidine has long been associated with

Table 3 Other Psychotropic Medications and Sexual Side Effects in Men

Antipsychotic medications	
Chlorpromazine	Desire disorder, erectile dysfunction, orgasmic disorder, priapism (high)
Chlorprothixene	Desire disorder, erectile dysfunction, orgasmic disorder, priapism (high)
Clozapine	Desire disorder, erectile dysfunction, orgasmic disorder, priapism (high)
Fluphenazine	Desire disorder, erectile dysfunction, orgasmic disorder, priapism (low)
Haloperidol	Desire disorder, erectile dysfunction, orgasmic disorder, priapism (low)
Mesoridazine	Desire disorder, erectile dysfunction, orgasmic disorder, priapism (high)
Molindone	Desire disorder, erectile dysfunction, orgasmic disorder, priapism (high)
Olanzapine	Minimal or no sexual side effects reported
Quetiapine	Minimal or no sexual side effects reported
Perphenazine	Desire disorder, erectile dysfunction, orgasmic disorder, priapism (high)
Pimozide	Erectile dysfunction, ejaculatory dysfunction (low)
Risperidone	Erectile dysfunction, ejaculatory dysfunction (low)
Thioridazine	Desire disorder, erectile dysfunction, orgasmic disorder, priapism (high)
Thiothixene	Erectile dysfunction, ejaculatory dysfunction (high)
Trifluoperazine	Desire disorder, erectile dysfunction, orgasmic disorder, priapism (high)
Antianxiety and sedative/hypnotic medications	
Alprazolam	Desire disorder, orgasmic disorder (low)
Buspirone	Minimal or no sexual side effects reported
Clorazepate	Desire disorder, orgasmic disorder (low)
Chlordiazepoxide	Desire disorder, orgasmic disorder (low)
Clonazepam	Desire disorder, orgasmic disorder (low)
Diazepam	Desire disorder, orgasmic disorder (low)
Flurazepam	Minimal or no sexual side effects reported
Nitrazepam	Desire disorder, orgasmic disorder (low)
Oxazepam	Desire disorder, orgasmic disorder (low)
Temazepam	Minimal or no sexual side effects reported
Triazolam	Desire disorder, orgasmic disorder (low)
Zolpidem	Minimal or no sexual side effects reported

erectile dysfunction and disorders of desire. While the mechanism through which this occurs is not clear, it may be due to lowered serum testosterone secretion secondary to hyperprolactinemia known to occur in patients taking cimetidine (8,11,12,101). Ranitidine, famotidine, and nizatidine are much less likely to cause sexual side effects (102). While medications in various miscellaneous classes have been cited as causing sexual side effects, many of the reports are based on single cases and the mechanism through which these side effects occur is often not known. Nonetheless, physicians should be aware of the potential for these problems. Table 4 lists many of these miscellaneous medications reported to cause sexual side effects.

□ ASSESSMENT OF SEXUAL SIDE EFFECTS

Given the large number of medications likely to cause sexual side effects and the variety of problems caused, the assessment of these concerns may seem daunting; however, providers can easily identify and address

Table 4   Miscellaneous Medications with Sexual Side Effects in Men

Acetazolamide	Erectile dysfunction
Aminocaproic acid	Orgasmic disorder, retrograde ejaculation
Amiodarone	Erectile dysfunction, decreased desire
Atropine	Erectile dysfunction
Baclofen	Erectile dysfunction, orgasmic disorder
Benztropine	Erectile dysfunction
Biperiden	Erectile dysfunction
Bromocriptine	Erectile dysfunction
Carbamazepine	Erectile dysfunction, desire disorder
Cimetidine	Erectile dysfunction, desire disorder, gynecomastia
Clidinium	Erectile dysfunction
Clofibrate	Erectile dysfunction, decreased desire
Cyclobenzaprine	Erectile dysfunction, desire disorder, gynecomastia
Danazol	Desire disorder
Dichlorphenamide	Erectile dysfunction
Dicyclomine	Erectile dysfunction
Digoxin	Erectile dysfunction, desire disorder, gynecomastia
Disopyramide	Erectile dysfunction
Disulfiram	Erectile dysfunction
Ethinyl estradiol	Desire disorder
Ethionamide	Erectile dysfunction
Etretinate	Erectile dysfunction
Famotidine	Erectile dysfunction
Fenfluramine	Erectile dysfunction, desire disorder
Furazolidone	Erectile dysfunction
Gemfibrozil	Erectile dysfunction, desire disorder
Glycopyrrolate	Desire disorder
Heparin	Priapism
Homatropine methylbromide	Erectile dysfunction
Hydroxyzine	Erectile dysfunction, decreased desire
Indomethacin	Erectile dysfunction
Interferon	Erectile dysfunction, desire disorder
Isotretinoin	Orgasmic disorder
Ketoconazole	Erectile dysfunction, desire disorder
Mazindol	Erectile dysfunction
Meclizine	Erectile dysfunction
Medroxyprogesterone	Erectile dysfunction, desire disorder
Methadone	Erectile dysfunction, desire disorder, orgasmic disorder
Methazolamide	Erectile dysfunction, desire disorder
Methotrexate	Erectile dysfunction, orgasmic disorder
Methysergide	Erectile dysfunction
Metoclopramide	Erectile dysfunction, desire disorder
Metronidazole	Desire disorder
Mexiletine	Erectile dysfunction, desire disorder
Morphine	Erectile dysfunction, desire disorder
Naproxen	Erectile dysfunction, orgasmic disorder
Niacin	Desire disorder
Nizatidine	Erectile dysfunction
Norethindrone	Erectile dysfunction, desire disorder
Omeprazole	Erectile dysfunction, gynecomastia, priapism
Orphenadrine	Erectile dysfunction
Oxybutynin	Erectile dysfunction
Phendimetrazine	Erectile dysfunction, desire disorder, orgasmic disorder
Phenobarbital	Erectile dysfunction, desire disorder
Phentermine	Erectile dysfunction, orgasmic disorder
Phentolamine	Erectile dysfunction
Phenytoin	Erectile dysfunction, desire disorder
Primidone	Erectile dysfunction, desire disorder
Probucol	Erectile dysfunction, gynecomastia
Procarbazine	Erectile dysfunction
Prochlorperazine	Erectile dysfunction, desire disorder, orgasmic disorder, priapism
Procyclidine	Erectile dysfunction
Propantheline bromide	Erectile dysfunction
Ranitidine	Erectile dysfunction, desire disorder
Scopolamine	Erectile dysfunction
Sulfasalazine	Erectile dysfunction
Tamoxifen	Priapism
Testosterone	Priapism
Thiabendazole	Erectile dysfunction
Trihexyphenidyl	Erectile dysfunction
Trimeprazine	Erectile dysfunction, decreased desire, orgasmic disorder

medication side effects if they are willing to ask frequently and directly about sexual function. Baseline assessment of sexual function is often a key to later identifying a medication side effect. Taking a baseline sexual history is useful for comparison at a later date and also gives patients permission to discuss any sexual concerns that might arise.

Temporal Considerations

Generally, sexual side effects will become obvious shortly after the medication is initiated. Some medications may have sexual side effects that may take weeks to present, especially those that can alter hormone secretion or action. Once established, most side effects are fairly constant as long as the medication is taken regularly and other factors (e.g., progression of disease or development of psychological issues) do not interfere. For a few medications, recovery of sexual function can occur despite the continuation of intake of inciting drugs, but this is not common as only 10% of patients with SSRI-induced anorgasmia reportedly recover their orgasmic function (103).

For men with pre-existing medical problems, a sexual side effect may not appear during the initial periods of drug intake, but may develop later as the sexual function is further compromised by disease progression. For example, a patient with diabetes may have no sexual side effects from his blood pressure medication initially. After 5 to 10 years, however, he may develop erection problems as the effect of the diabetes on vascular and neurological function becomes more significant. While not directly attributable to the medication, the medication may be a complicating or exacerbating factor. Finally, medication effects may be dose-dependent and may not occur at initially low doses of drug intake.

Consistency

Medication side effects also tend to be quite consistent. For example, if a man cannot obtain an erection with a partner because he is taking a β-blocker, he probably will not be able to obtain an erection alone through masturbation and probably will not report regular morning erections. It is important to keep in mind, however, that there are some exceptions; for example, a man who is experiencing some difficulty in obtaining erections may develop considerable performance anxiety and as a result will not obtain erections with his partner. He may still be able to obtain erections with masturbation, although this may require considerably more time and stimulation. He may also report less rigidity and more difficulty in maintaining erection. Similar consistency should be expected with other sexual problems including anorgasmia. While not foolproof, lack of nocturnal penile tumescence (NPT) has been used as an indication of organic or pharmacologic involvement. A reduction in NPT has been documented for various drugs including tricyclics antidepressants and cimetidine (83,104) and has been used for years to differentiate

between psychogenic and nonpsychogenic erectile dysfunction. Various methods for determining NPT have been developed (see Chapter 23). For clinicians who may lack access to such evaluations, patient self-reports of morning erections have been shown to be the best predictor of NPT findings (105).

☐ TREATMENT OF SEXUAL SIDE EFFECTS

The treatment of pharmacologically induced sexual disorders must be approached with caution. It is not wise to ignore these concerns, as a patient who suspects that his medication is disrupting sexual function is likely to stop taking it (106). On the other hand, simply suggesting to a patient that a medication may be the cause of a sexual dysfunction without addressing the problem may contribute to nonadherence as well. The physician should review the benefits of taking the medication and the risks of abruptly stopping it and reassure the patient that steps will be taken to correct the problem.

A number of approaches for dealing with sexual side effects of medications exist. The easiest is to wait for these side effects to dissipate; however, while this will work for a few patients, it will not for most. Also, patient adherence may be threatened if this accommodation takes a long time. Discontinuing the medication completely may be an option for a few patients. For example, a man with high blood pressure who has begun exercising, dieting, and/or reducing his weight may be able to stop antihypertensive medication completely. Sexual side effects often provide great motivation for men to alter their lifestyles and get off of medication. Some men may also choose to do nothing about the sexual side effect. Just knowing that the medication is the cause of the sexual side effect may be a relief, even if nothing is done about it. For most men, however, doing nothing about the problem or stopping the medication will not be options, and the problem will require intervention.

One choice may be to try a lower dosage of the same medication, if possible. Many sexual side effects are dose related, and lowering the dose may resolve the sexual problem while maintaining therapeutic effectiveness. If therapeutic effectiveness is lost, an additional medication may be added. Often, two medications at low doses are less likely to cause sexual side effects than one medication at a higher dose.

If reducing the dose is not an option or is ineffective, a different dosing schedule can be tried. Another option is the use of "drug holidays," or the discontinuation of medication for a day or two. This has been shown to restore sexual function effectively in patients taking SSRIs without eliciting a relapse of depression (75,76). Unfortunately, this approach requires significant planning and eliminates any spontaneity as the medication must be discontinued a day or two prior to sexual activity. It is also not an option for most medications that require daily administration to maintain therapeutic effectiveness and should not be used in patients in whom adherence is already a problem.

When these options are ineffective or impractical and it appears that the medication needs to be changed, the first choice should be to stay within the same therapeutic class to minimize disruption to the patient's therapy. While many medications within the same class may have similar sexual side effects, this is not always the case. For example, a patient on propranolol may experience less sexual disruption on atenolol because of lower lipid solubility and higher cardioselectivity. This is also true of SSRIs; although paroxetine has been reported to have a high incidence of delayed orgasm, the same side effect has been reported much less frequently with citalopram (107).

If changing medications within a class does not alleviate the concern, switching to a medication class less likely to cause a problem with sexual function may be unavoidable. In these cases, many options exist for choosing a less sexually toxic medication. For example, switching from a β-blocker to an ACE inhibitor for hypertension can often alleviate sexual problems. For treating depression, changing from an SSRI to a phenylpiperazine (e.g., trazodone and nefazodone) or other antidepressant may alleviate the problem. For example, one study found that men experiencing sexual side effects on fluoxetine reported significant improvement when switched to bupropion (108).

In some cases, changing therapeutic classes may not be possible. In these cases, adding another medication may help. With SSRI-induced anorgasmia, 2 to 4 mg of cyproheptadine taken two hours prior to sexual activity may help due to its antiserotonergic effects (76,109,110) and may help alleviate the same

side effect due to tricyclics or MAOIs (111,112). Yohimbine (an α-2 antagonist), amantadine, bupropion, buspirone, and bethanechol have also been used effectively in this manner (77,103,113–115). Sildenafil has also been used in SSRI-induced anorgasmia with some success, although placebo-controlled studies are lacking (116). Sildenafil is clearly effective for medication-induced erectile dysfunction, as are other treatments for organic erectile dysfunction, including external vacuum devices, penile injections (Caverject®, Pfizer, Inc.), and penile suppositories (MUSE®, Vivus, Inc.). (For further information on these individual forms of treatment, see Part IV of this volume.)

If a sexual disorder persists over time even after following the above suggestions, it is unlikely that the medication is still the primary cause. While many medications can cause sexual side effects it is unlikely that different medications will cause identical problems in the same patient (117,118). In these cases, further evaluation of organic or psychological factors is required.

☐ CONCLUSION

The rising use of medication to treat a multitude of problems, coupled with an increased focus on QOL issues, is evidence that the issue of sexual side effects will not disappear. Fortunately, newer medications hold the promise of having less sexual adverse effects. Providers must recognize the importance of sexual function to their patients, develop the comfort and expertise to address these issues, and provide an environment in which the patient can discuss sexual concerns.

☐ REFERENCES

1. http://rxlist.com/top200.htm [accessed Sept 2006.]
2. Finger WW, Lund M, Slagle MA. Medications that may contribute to sexual disorders. A guide to assessment and treatment in family practice. J Fam Pract 1997; 44(1):33–43.
3. Crenshaw TL, Goldberg JP. Sexual Pharmacology: Drugs that Affect Sexual Functioning. New York: Norton, 1996.
4. Duncan L, Bateman DN. Sexual function in women. Do antihypertensive drugs have an impact? Drug Saf 1993; 8(3):225–234.
5. Barksdale JD, Gardner SF. The impact of first-line antihypertensive drugs on erectile dysfunction. Pharmacotherapy 1999; 19(5):573–581.
6. Geissler AH, Turnlund JR, Cohen RD. Effect of chlorthalidone on zinc levels, testosterone, and sexual function in man. Drug Nutr Interact 1986; 4(3):275–283.
7. Wassertheil-Smoller S, Blaufox MD, Oberman A, et al. Effect of antihypertensives on sexual function and

quality of life: the TAIM Study. Ann Intern Med 1991; 114(8):613–620.
8. Horowitz JD, Goble AJ. Drugs and impaired male sexual function. Drugs 1979; 18(3):206–217.
9. Greenblatt DJ, Koch-Weser J. Gynecomastia and impotence: complications of spironolactone therapy. JAMA 1973; 223(1):82.
10. Papadopoulos C. Cardiovascular drugs and sexuality: a cardiologist's review. Arch Intern Med 1980; 140(10): 1341–1345.
11. Aldridge SA. Drug-induced sexual dysfunction. Clin Pharm 1982; 1(2):141–147.
12. Buffum J. Pharmacosexology: the effects of drugs on sexual function a review. J Psychoactive Drugs 1982; 14(1–2):5–44.
13. Stevenson JG, Umstead GS. Sexual dysfunction due to antihypertensive agents. Drug Intell Clin Pharm 1984; 18(2):113–121.
14. Spark RF, Melby JC. Aldosteronism in hypertension. The spironolactone response test. Ann Intern Med 1968; 69(4):685–691.

15. Brown JJ, Davies DL, Ferriss JB, et al. Comparison of surgery and prolonged spironolactone therapy in patients with hypertension, aldosterone excess, and low plasma renin. Br Med J 1972; 2(5816):729–734.

16. Chang SW, Fine R, Siegel D, et al. The impact of diuretic therapy on reported sexual function. Arch Intern Med 1991; 151(12):2402–2408.

17. Lacourciere Y. Analysis of well-being and 24-hour blood pressure recording in a comparative study between indapamide and captopril. Am J Med 1988; 84(1B):47–52.

18. Werning C, Weitz T, Ludwig B. Assessment of indapamide in elderly hypertensive patients with special emphasis on well-being. Am J Med 1988; 84(1B):104–108.

19. Khan A, Camel G, Perry HM Jr. Clonidine (Catapres): a new antihypertensive agent. Curr Ther Res Clin Exp 1970; 12(1):10–18.

20. Forsberg L, Gustavii B, Hojerback T, et al. Impotence, smoking, and beta-blocking drugs. Fertil Steril 1979; 31(5):589–591.

21. Oksenberg D, Peroutka SJ. Antagonism of 5-hydroxy-tryptamine1A (5-HT1A) receptor-mediated modulation of adenylate cyclase activity by pindolol and propranolol isomers. Biochem Pharmacol 1988; 37(18):3429–3433.

22. Miller RA. Propranolol and impotence. Ann Intern Med 1976; 85(5):682–683.

23. Bathen J. Propranolol erectile dysfunction relieved. Ann Intern Med 1978; 88(5):716–717.

24. Warren SC, Warren SG. Propranolol and sexual impotence. Ann Intern Med 1977; 86(1):112.

25. Knarr JW. Impotence from propranolol? [Letter]. Ann Intern Med 1976; 85(2):259.

26. Hogan MJ, Wallin JD, Baer RM. Antihypertensive therapy and male sexual dysfunction. Psychosomatics 1980; 21(3):234.

27. Smith PJ, Talbert RL. Sexual dysfunction with antihypertensive and antipsychotic agents. Clin Pharm 1986; 5(5):373–384.

28. Due DL, Giguere GC, Plachetka JR. Postmarketing comparison of labetalol and propranolol in hypertensive patients. Clin Ther 1986; 8(6):624–631.

29. Broekman CP, Haensel SM, Van de Ven LL, et al. Bisoprolol and hypertension: effects on sexual functioning in men. J Sex Marital Ther 1992; 18(4):325–331.

30. Fogari R, Zoppi A, Poletti L, et al. Sexual activity in hypertensive men treated with valsartan or carvedilol: a crossover study. Am J Hypertens 2001; 14(1):27–31.

31. Shore JH, Fraunfelder FT, Meyer SM. Psychiatric side effects from topical ocular timolol, a beta-adrenergic blocker. J Clin Psychopharmacol 1987; 7(4):264–267.

32. Lynch MG, Whitson JT, Brown RH, et al. Topical beta-blocker therapy and central nervous system side effects. A preliminary study comparing betaxolol and timolol. Arch Ophthalmol 1988; 106(7):908–911.

33. Michelson EL, Frishman WH, Lewis JE, et al. Multicenter clinical evaluation of long-term efficacy and safety of labetalol in treatment of hypertension. Am J Med 1983; 75(4A):68–80.

34. Ohman KP, Asplund J. Labetalol in primary hypertension: a long-term effect and tolerance study. Curr Ther Res 1984; 35(2):277–285.

35. Boyden TW, Nugent CA, Ogihara T, et al. Reserpine, hydrochlorothiazide and pituitary-gonadal hormones in hypertensive patients. Eur J Clin Pharmacol 1980; 17(5):329–332.

36. Gollery CT, Harington M. Methyldopa in hypertension. Clinical and pharmacological studies. Lancet 1962; 1:759–763.

37. Johnson P, Kitchin AH, Lowther CP, et al. Treatment of hypertension with methyldopa. Br Med J 1966; 1(5480):133–137.

38. Bulpitt CJ, Dollery CT. Side effects of hypotensive agents evaluated by a self-administered questionnaire. Br Med J 1973; 3(5878):485–490.

39. Alexander WD, Evans JI. Letter: side effects of methyldopa. Br Med J 1975; 2(5969):501.

40. Pillay VK. Some side-effects of alpha-methyldopa. S Afr Med J 1976; 50(16):625–626.

41. Newman RJ, Salerno HR. Letter: sexual dysfunction due to methyldopa. Br Med J 1974; 4(5936):106.

42. Bauer GE, Hull RD, Stokes GS, et al. The reversibility of side effects of guanethidine therapy. Med J Aust 1973; 1(19):930–933.

43. Laganiere S, Biron P, Robert P. Opinion of 679 general practitioners on subjective side effects of antihypertensive drugs. Curr Ther Res 1986; 39(6):970–978.

44. Wartman SA. Sexual side effects of antihypertensive drugs. Treatment strategies and strictures. Postgrad Med 1983; 73(2):133–138.

45. Lamberts SWJ. Neuroendocrine aspects of centrally active hypotensive drugs. Br J Clin Pharm 1983; 15:5255–5285.

46. Onesti G, Bock KD, Heimsoth V, et al. Clonidine: a new antihypertensive agent. Am J Cardiol 1971; 28(1):74–83.

47. Langley MS, Heel RC. Transdermal clonidine. A preliminary review of its pharmacodynamic properties and therapeutic efficacy. Drugs 1988; 35(2):123–142.

48. McMahon FG, Jain AK, Vargas R, et al. A double-blind comparison of transdermal clonidine and oral captopril in essential hypertension. Clin Ther 1990; 12(2):88–100.

49. Planitz V. Comparison of moxonidine and clonidine HCl in treating patients with hypertension. J Clin Pharmacol 1987; 27(1):46–51.

50. Holland OB, Fairchild C, Gomez-Sanchez CE. Effect of guanabenz and hydrochlorothiazide on blood pressure and plasma renin activity. J Clin Pharmacol 1981; 21(4):133–139.

51. Palmer JD, Nugent CA. Guanadrel sulfate: a postganglionic sympathetic inhibitor for the treatment of mild to moderate hypertension. Pharmacotherapy 1983; 3(4):220–229.

52. Dunn MI, Dunlap JL. Guanadrel. A new antihypertensive drug. JAMA 1981; 245(16):1639–1642.

53. Hansson L, Pascual A, Julius S. Comparison of guanadrel and guanethidine. Clin Pharmacol Ther 1973; 14(2):204–208.

54. Suzuki H, Tominaga T, Kumagai H, et al. Effects of first-line antihypertensive agents on sexual function

and sex hormones. J Hypertens 1988; 6(suppl 4): S649–S651.

55. Morrissette DL, Skinner MH, Hoffman BB, et al. Effects of antihypertensive drugs atenolol and nifedipine on sexual function in older men: a placebo-controlled, crossover study. Arch Sex Behav 1993; 22(2):99–109.

56. Muller SC, el-Damanhoury H, Ruth J, et al. Hypertension and impotence. Eur Urol 1991; 19(1): 29–34.

57. Tanner LA, Bosco LA. Gynecomastia associated with calcium channel blocker therapy. Arch Intern Med 1988; 148(2):379–380.

58. Clyne CA. Unilateral gynecomastia and nifedipine. Br Med J 1986; 292:380.

59. Croog SH, Levine S, Testa MA, et al. The effects of antihypertensive therapy on the quality of life. N Engl J Med 1986; 314(26):1657–1664.

60. Pitts NE. The clinical evaluation of prazosin, a new antihypertensive agent. Postgrad Med 1975; 58:117–127.

61. Verhiest W, Croonenberghs J, Devos P, et al. Double blind cross-over study comparing prazosin and methyldopa in the treatment of mild hypertension. Acta Cardiol 1974; 29(3):217–233.

62. Comparison of prazosin with hydralazine in patients receiving hydrochlorothiazide. A randomized, double-blind clinical trial. Circulation 1981; 64(4):772–779.

63. Fogari R, Preti P, Derosa G, et al. Effect of antihypertensive treatment with valsartan or atenolol on sexual activity and plasma testosterone in hypertensive men. Eur J Clin Pharmacol 2002; 58(3):177–180.

64. Shen WW, Mallya AR. Psychotropic-induced sexual inhibition. Am J Psychiatry 1983; 140(4):514–515.

65. Shen WW, Sata LS. Neuropharmacology of the male sexual function. J Clin Psychopharmacol 1983; 3(4): 265–266.

66. Mitchell JE, Popkin MK. Antipsychotic drug therapy and sexual dysfunction in men. Am J Psychiatry 1982; 139(5):633–637.

67. Harrison WM, Rabkin JG, Ehrhardt AA, et al. Effects of antidepressant medication on sexual function: a controlled study. J Clin Psychopharmacol 1986; 6(3): 144–149.

68. Monteiro WO, Noshirvani HF, Marks IM, et al. Anorgasmia from clomipramine in obsessive-compulsive disorder. A controlled trial. Br J Psychiatry 1987; 151(1):107–112.

69. Balon R, Yeragani VK, Pohl R, et al. Sexual dysfunction during antidepressant treatment. J Clin Psychiatry 1993; 54(6):209–212.

70. Harrison WM. Response to Dr. Cooper: antidepressant medication and sexual function [Letter to the editor]. J Clin Psychopharmacol 1987; 7(2):120–121.

71. Golden RN, Hsiao J, Lane E, et al. The effects of intravenous clomipramine on neurohormones in normal subjects. J Clin Endocrinol Metab 1989; 68(3):632–637.

72. DeVeaugh-Geiss J, Landau P, Katz R. Preliminary results from a multicenter trial of clomipramine in obsessive-compulsive disorder. Psychopharmacol Bull 1989; 25(1):36–40.

73. Patterson WM. Fluoxetine-induced sexual dysfunction. J Clin Psychiatry 1993; 54(2):71.

74. Dorevitch A, Davis H. Fluvoxamine-associated sexual dysfunction. Ann Pharmacother 1994; 28(7–8):872–874.

75. Lane RM. A critical review of selective serotonin reuptake inhibitor-related sexual dysfunction; incidence, possible aetiology and implications for management. J Psychopharmacol 1997; 11(1):72–82.

76. Hirschfeld RM. Management of sexual side effects of antidepressant therapy. J Clin Psychiatry 1999; 60(suppl 14):27–30.

77. Kennedy SH, Eisfeld BS, Dickens SE, et al. Antidepressant-induced sexual dysfunction during treatment with moclobemide, paroxetine, sertraline, and venlafaxine. J Clin Psychiatry 2000; 61(4): 276–281.

78. Rothschild AJ. New directions in the treatment of antidepressant-induced sexual dysfunction. Clin Ther 2000; 22(suppl A):A42–A57.

79. Montejo AL, Llorca G, Izquierdo JA, et al. Incidence of sexual dysfunction associated with antidepressant agents: a prospective multicenter study of 1022 outpatients. Spanish Working Group for the Study of Psychotropic-Related Sexual Dysfunction. J Clin Psychiatry 2001; 62(suppl 3):10–21.

80. Clayton AH, Pradko JF, Croft HA, et al. Prevalence of sexual dysfunction among newer antidepressants. J Clin Psychiatry 2002; 63(4):357–366.

81. Goldstein DJ, Mallinckrodt C, Lu Y, et al. Duloxetine in the treatment of major depressive disorder: a double-blind clinical trial. J Clin Psychiatry 2002; 63(3):225–231.

82. Detke MJ, Lu Y, Goldstein DJ, et al. Duloxetine 60 mg once daily dosing versus placebo in the acute treatment of major depression. J Psychiatr Res 2002; 36(6):383–390.

83. Kowalski A, Stanley RO, Dennerstein L, et al. The sexual side-effects of antidepressant medication: a double-blind comparison of two antidepressants in a non-psychiatric population. Br J Psychiatry 1985; 147(4):413–418.

84. Ghadirian AM, Annable L, Belanger MC. Lithium, benzodiazepines, and sexual function in bipolar patients. Am J Psychiatry 1992; 149(6):801–805.

85. Vinarova E, Uhlir O, Stika L, et al. Side effects of lithium administration. Act Nerv Super (Praha) 1972; 14(2):105–107.

86. Blay SL, Ferraz MP, Calil HM. Lithium-induced male sexual impairment: two case reports. J Clin Psychiatry 1982; 43(12):497–498.

87. Priapism with trazodone (Desyrel). Med Lett Drugs Ther 1984; 26(658):35.

88. Coates NE. Priapism associated with buspar. South Med J 1990; 83(8):983.

89. Saenz de Tejada I, Ware JC, Blanco R, et al. Pathophysiology of prolonged penile erection associated with trazodone use. J Urol 1991; 145(1):60–64.

90. Berigan TR, Harazin JS. Sexual dysfunction associated with mirtazapine: a case report. J Clin Psychiatry 1998; 59(6):319–320.

91. Segraves RT. Sexual side-effects of psychiatric drugs. Int J Psychiatry Med 1988; 18(3):243–252.

92. Drug induced sexual dysfunction. In: DRUGDEX™ System [Internet database]. Greenwood Village, CO: Thomson Micromedex, 2006.

93. Griffith SR, Zil JS. Priapism in a patient receiving antipsychotic therapy. Psychosomatics 1984; 25(8):629–631.

94. Dorman BW, Schmidt JD. Association of priapism in phenothiazine therapy. J Urol 1976; 116(1):51–53.

95. Winter CC, McDowell G. Experience with 105 patients with priapism: update review of all aspects. J Urol 1988; 140(5):980–983.

96. Fabian JL. Psychotropic medications and priapism. Am J Psychiatry 1993; 150(2):349–350.

97. Munjack DJ, Crocker B. Alprazolam-induced ejaculatory inhibition. J Clin Psychopharmacol 1986; 6(1): 57–58.

98. Lydiard RB, Howell EF, Laraia MT, et al. Sexual side effects of alprazolam. Am J Psychiatry 1987; 144(2): 254–255.

99. Uhde TW, Tancer ME, Shea CA. Sexual dysfunction related to alprazolam treatment of social phobia. Am J Psychiatry 1988; 145(4):531–532.

100. Jenike MA, Baer L, Buttolph L. Buspirone augmentation of fluoxetine in patients with obsessive compulsive disorder. J Clin Psychiatry 1991; 52(1): 13–14.

101. Lardinois CK, Mazzaferri EL. Cimetidine blocks testosterone synthesis. Arch Intern Med 1985; 145(5):920–922.

102. Corinaldesi R, Pasquali R, Paternico A, et al. Effects of short- and long-term administrations of famotidine and ranitidine on some pituitary, sexual and thyroid hormones. Drugs Exp Clin Res 1987; 13(10): 647–654.

103. Rosen RC, Lane RM, Menza M. Effects of SSRIs on sexual function: a critical review. J Clin Psychopharmacol 1999; 19(1):67–85.

104. Jensen RT, Collen MJ, Pandol SJ, et al. Cimetidine-induced impotence and breast changes in patients with gastric hypersecretory states. N Engl J Med 1983; 308(15):883–887.

105. Ackerman MD, D'Attilio JP, Antoni MH, et al. The predictive significance of patient-reported sexual functioning in RigiScan sleep evaluations. J Urol 1991; 146(6):1559–1563.

106. Watts RJ. Sexual functioning, health beliefs, and compliance with high blood pressure medications. Nurs Res 1982; 31(5):278–283.

107. Waldinger MD, Zwinderman AH, Olivier B. SSRIs and ejaculation: a double-blind, randomized, fixed-dose study with paroxetine and citalopram. J Clin Psychopharmacol 2001; 21(6):556–560.

108. Walker PW, Cole JO, Gardner EA, et al. Improvement in fluoxetine-associated sexual dysfunction in patients switched to bupropion. J Clin Psychiatry 1993; 54(12):459–465.

109. Woodrum ST, Brown CS. Management of SSRI-induced sexual dysfunction. Ann Pharmacother 1998; 32(11):1209–1215.

110. Aizenberg D, Zemishlany Z, Weizman A. Cyproheptadine treatment of sexual dysfunction induced by serotonin reuptake inhibitors. Clin Neuropharmacol 1995; 18(4):320–324.

111. Decastro RM. Reversal of MAOI-induced anorgasmia with cyproheptadine. Am J Psychiatry 1985; 142(6):783.

112. Riley AJ, Riley EJ. Cyproheptadine and antidepressant-induced anorgasmia. Br J Psychiatry 1986; 148(2): 217–218.

113. Yager J. Bethanechol chloride can reverse erectile and ejaculatory dysfunction induced by tricyclic antidepressants and mazindol: case report. J Clin Psychiatry 1986; 47(4):210–211.

114. Segraves RT. Reversal by bethanechol of imipramine-induced ejaculatory dysfunction. Am J Psychiatry 1987; 144(9):1243–1244.

115. Ashton AK, Rosen RC. Bupropion as an antidote for serotonin reuptake inhibitor-induced sexual dysfunction. J Clin Psychiatry 1998; 59(3):112–115.

116. Nurnberg HG, Lauriello J, Hensley PL, et al. Sildenafil for iatrogenic serotonergic antidepressant medication-induced sexual dysfunction in 4 patients. J Clin Psychiatry 1999; 60(1):33–35.

117. Drugs that cause sexual dysfunction. Med Lett Drugs Ther 1983; 25(641):73–76.

118. Drugs that cause sexual dysfunction: an update. Med Lett Drugs Ther 1992; 34(876):73–78.

20

Effects of Chemotherapy and Radiotherapy on Male Sexual Function

Ratna Chatterjee

Reproductive Medicine Unit, University College London Hospital, London, U.K.

□ INTRODUCTION

Sexual dysfunction (SD) is a common problem encountered in recipients of chemotherapy (CT), radiotherapy (RT), and chemo–radiotherapy (CRT) (1). CT (2) and RT (3) are commonly used for cancer of the pelvis, abdominal, and genital organs such as germ- and non–germ-cell tumors of testis, prostate, colorectal, and anal renal cancers (2). Other malignancies of the hematological system (lymphoma, leukemia, and myeloma), sarcoma, and bone tumors also constitute a large group of the recipients of CT, RT, and CRT (3).

The exact incidence of SD is unknown, and the magnitude of the problem has not been appreciated fully. It must be recognized that cancer patients are often too embarrassed to discuss with their oncologists and primary care physicians the stigmatizing and often emotional issue of sexual relationships, which may appear trivial in comparison to their life-threatening illnesses. Thus, these patients often suffer from sexual problems in silence, which, in turn, adversely impacts quality of life.

It should be noted that patients with nonmalignant conditions, including connective tissue, immunologic, and various hematological disorders, may also require pulsatile, cyclical, or continuous CT and localized or systemic RT (4). These, however, constitute a small proportion of CT, RT, and CRT recipients. Therefore, for practical purposes, this chapter will mainly focus on SD in male patients resulting from cancer CT and RT. As the management of SD interfaces with cancer care, this chapter will first outline cancer care pathways, including the principles and pharmacology of cancer CT and RT. This will be followed by the epidemiology, pathophysiology, and molecular biology of SD of the cancer patients.

□ BACKGROUND

The survival rate for children, adolescents, and adults with hematological and other cancers has improved dramatically in recent years, such that young cancer survivors represent about 1 in 900 people aged 15 to 44 years (5) in both Europe (6) and the United States (7). This may be attributable to significant advances in modern cancer care, from better patient selection for each treatment modality to the development of novel chemoradiotherapeutic regimens such as the use of multiagent CT, CRT, brachyradiotherapy, and high-dose chemotherapy (HDC) with stem-cell transplantation (SCT). In consideration of this newfound potential for greater longevity and preservation of quality of life, attention has now been drawn to the long-term side effects of these therapeutic regimes (1,8), which include multiple endocrinopathies (9,10), metabolic syndrome (11,12), hypogonadism with compensated or uncompensated Leydig cell insufficiency (LCI) (13–17), premature andropause, infertility (13–17), and SD (18), all of which are often interrelated, representing parts of a heterogeneous, complex syndrome of multiorgan damage (19).

Although SD typically presents during or after treatment for malignancy in up to 90% of patients (20,21), the exact incidence of CT, RT, and CRT-induced SD is unknown. This may be due to a number of factors, which include a lack of standardization of the diagnostic criteria of gonadal failure or SD, the absence of a national or international registry of patients with SD, the widely variable chemotherapeutic regimens used for different cancers, and the failure of patients to report to the appropriate specialists. The diagnosis of SD in these studies is often based on a conventional questionnaire method (21), similar to what has been used by the author (22,23) or on a scale-based method such as The International Index of Erectile Function (19,24).

SD in a young adult male can cause physical, emotional, and endocrine disability (19,25). Although erectile dysfunction (ED) is the most frequently reported form of male SD overall, it should be remembered that diminished or absent libido is also common (18,20,26), followed by ejaculatory dysfunction (premature ejaculation, anejaculation, and painful ejaculation) and orgasmic dysfunction. (For further details on these individual conditions, see Chapter 10.)

In a large series of 117 recipients of high-dose CT/CRT for hematological malignancy (15), the author

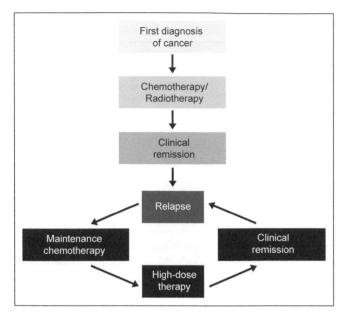

Figure 1 The cancer care pathways. Sexual dysfunction can present at any stage in cancer care.

reported that 80% have altered body image, poor self-esteem, and relationship problems. Sixty percent of patients in the series had SD, of which diminished libido and ED were the most common problems; 10% had ejaculatory disturbances with dysfunctional orgasm. Psychological components of fatigue, anxiety, mood disturbance, and depression are also common in these patients.

Figure 1 shows the care pathways in the basic plan of management of a cancer patient. Note that the patient can present with SD at any stage of the disease from initial presentation to ongoing cancer management.

□ PATHOPHYSIOLOGY OF SD IN RECIPIENTS OF CANCER CT AND/OR RT

In general, SD in cancer patients is iatrogenic in origin and is largely due to the gonadotoxic, vascular, and neurotoxic insult from CT, RT, and/or CRT. SD may also result from the presence of the malignant disease itself, particularly when there is primary or secondary involvement of the gonads (lymphoma, leukemia, and testicular tumors), or when the tumor infiltrates sexual organs (14).

It is well-known that all cytotoxic CT and RT share two properties: an ability to kill tumor cells by arresting cell division and sometimes inducing apoptosis, and an inability to distinguish between normal and abnormal cells (2). Thus, all cytotoxic drugs are potentially damaging to the normal cells, especially those with high proliferative indices such as the germ cells. Thus, hypogonadism is an invariable side effect of CT/RT (14,19). CT/RT can additionally damage

neurogenic or vasculogenic structures responsible for the functional integrity of the sexual apparatus (19).

It is well established that the adult testis is extremely vulnerable to external radiation (27). The testicular irradiation dose of 0.1 to 6 Gy causes germ-cell damage. Higher doses of direct testicular irradiation, such as those used for acute lymphoblastic leukemia or germ-cell tumors, cause hypogonadism with germ-cell and LC damage; 20 to 24 Gy causes severe LCI (28). Brachytherapy and radical prostatectomy used as prostatic cancer treatment can also cause hypogonadism and SD (29–31). CT causes gonadal damage in a dose-dependent and cumulative fashion (19). Alkylating chemotherapies are extremely damaging, especially when given in combination, such as Busulfan and cyclophosphamide (32). Cisplatin, given as monotherapy (32) or in combination with etoposide and bleomycin for germ-cell tumors, is damaging to germ cell and Leydig cells and can cause LCI, infertility, and SD (33).

Endocrine Causes

Cancer CT and RT are powerful gonadotoxins (34) and act by interrupting the biological processes of gametogenesis or steroidogenesis directly by inhibiting spermatogenesis and/or testicular androgen production (17,34) or indirectly by altering the physiological control system at the level of the hypothalamic–pituitary–testicular (H–P–T) axis (34). RT and total body irradiation (TBI) are major causes of partial hypopituitarism with growth hormone and other pituitary hormone deficiencies and can occasionally cause hyperprolactinemia (9,17). Adrenal, thyroid, and other endocrine glandular dysfunction may also occur, especially in high-dose CT and RT patients (10). Most of the toxic effects of the drugs on the endocrine system are due to normal or exaggerated pharmacological responses, classified as a type-A reaction (34).

The onset of toxic effects of CT or RT may be classified as immediate (hours to days), early (days to weeks), or delayed (weeks and months) (35). Conventionally, gonadal damage resulting from standard or high-dose therapy in adults is considered a late sequela (35,36); however, in a prospective study, the author has shown that testicular damage in adults can occur as an acute and instantaneous effect of the SCT conditioning regimen (14). The author has also shown (14) that high-dose CRT causes acute functional castration in patients with hematological malignancies within 72 hours of TBI, with a 50% loss of testicular volume. The author and others (13–15) have shown germ-cell damage, as well as LCI (low basal and human chorionic gonadotropin-stimulated testosterone levels) in such patients (17). In contrast to these acute effects, some patients may present with premature andropause (10,13,14,17,37) and SD (13–15,37,38). Gonadal damage is not an "all or none" phenomenon, but rather a heterogeneous syndrome ranging from gonadal insufficiency (GI) to full-blown premature gonadal failure

(PGF), as highlighted in the review by Chatterjee and Kottaridis (19). Even normal basal gonadotropin and sex steroid levels may not exclude gonadal damage, as PGF is a common occurrence in bone marrow transplant (BMT) recipients (9,39). Multiple doses of potentially gonadotoxic antecedent therapy can cause cumulative, dose-dependent damage, especially in females (17). Males, however, typically suffer more damage than females (16). Factors aggravating gonadal damage include old age; local therapy (testicular or pelvic irradiation) may also contribute to gonadal insult (14).

Aging may aggravate hypotestosteronemia and diminished LC reserve in CT/RT recipients (14,28,40). LC sufficiency is an important requisite for normotestosteronemia, which in turn determines libido, the herald of the cascade of events in sexual intercourse. Thus, it is understandable why hypogonadism with LCI during physiological aging or premature andropause can interfere with sexual function, especially in older men. Testosterone deficiency, however, even if severe, is compatible with normal erection in response to an erotic stimulus. Heim et al. (41) have shown that 50% of castrated mature young men were able to sustain erection, although that capacity declined with age. Importantly, many older men presenting with ED, especially with diminished nocturnal penile tumescence, will have hypogonadism with diminished bioactive testosterone levels.

Secondary hypogonadism due to hypothalamic–pituitary–gonadal axis dysfunction with hyperprolactinemia is also a common scenario in BMT recipients (10). Other drugs like corticosteroids and cimetidine may also contribute to the suppression of adrenal and sex steroid pharmacokinetics by preventing the synthesis and delivery of hormones or by blocking target organ sensitivity (42). Thus, in CT/RT recipients of cancer with hypogonadism and symptomatic LCI (diminished libido and SD/ED), testosterone replacement therapy may improve libido and also erectile performance, especially nocturnal tumescence.

In summary, patients at high risk of gonadal damage include those who are (*i*) aged greater than 30 years at transplant or time of treatment; (*ii*) recipients of local inverted Y (used to treat nodes along spine/groin area in the shape of an upside-down Y) and pelvic RT; (*iii*) recipients of multiple doses of potentially gonadotoxic antecedent conventional CT, especially alkylating agents prior to SCT; (*iv*) recipients of alkylating CT in the conditioning regimen for SCT; and (*v*) recipients of TBI.

Psychogenic and Psychosomatic Causes

Patients with cancer who receive CT/RT often suffer from multiple problems, including severe depression, poor self-esteem, altered body image from hair loss, dysmorphic physical appearance with shrunken testes (especially BMT recipients), sexual inhibition, performance anxiety, generalized malaise and fatigue, fear/anxiety of relapse of cancer, permanent infertility, the possibility of fetal abnormalities from cytotoxic spermatogenic DNA genetic damage (43), and the fear of transmission of sexually transmitted infections due to immmunosuppression. All these factors contribute to relationship problems and may cause reduced libido and SD (19). The psychological dysfunction theory of cancer is elucidated in a comprehensive descriptive survey by Litwin et al. (44), who evaluated sexual comorbidity in a large series of men with prostatic cancer presenting with ED in the University of California, Los Angeles. General and disease-specific measures were used to study the health-related quality of life (HRQOL) scores and the marital interaction scale from the Cancer Rehabilitation Evaluation System Short Form to assess each patient's relationship with his sexual partner. This study showed that 67% men had severe impairment of HRQOL scores. The emotional domains of the Medical Outcomes Study 36-item Short Form, a widely used measure of HRQOL, were associated with more profound impairment than were the physical domains in men with ED. ED and the distress it caused were discrete domains of HRQOL and distinct from each other in these patients.

Medical Diseases Associated with CT/RT or BMT

The metabolic syndrome (X syndrome) has been recently recognized in long-term cancer survivors who have received CT/RT or BMT (45). This includes hormonal deficiencies, cardiovascular disease, diabetes, insulin resistance, hypertension, hyperlipidemia, and endothelial dysfunction. Since diabetes, renal disease, and hypertension are common causes of SD (46), these metabolic diseases in cancer survivors may also cause neurogenic/vasculogenic SD and reduced libido.

Cavernosal Vasculopathy Associated with Cancer Therapy

Because it is a superficial structure, the penis is ideally suited to ultrasound imaging. Furthermore, dynamic assessment of the cavernosal arterial changes after pharmacostimulation allows for the diagnosis of arterial and venogenic causes of ED. (For further details on these assessments, see Chapter 25.) Little information is available, however, regarding the cavernosal vascular parameters in patients who have received CT/RT or BMT. The author measured penile color-flow Doppler vascular parameters in recipients of HDC/TBI for hematological cancer presenting with SD (22,23). Evidence for cavernosal arterial insufficiency in RT- as well as CT-treated patients who also had BMT for hematological malignancy was obtained. Arterial causes, a possible paradigm shift from the conventional theory of psychological dysfunction of ED, have become especially important, considering that phosphodiesterase-5 inhibitors are now available to treat vasculogenic ED.

Molecular Mechanism of SD in CT and RT Recipients

Recent findings have now highlighted the role of reactive oxygen species, ischemia/perfusion, and inflammation/repair mechanisms in the multistep endothelial-platelet molecular dynamics of vasculogenesis and vasculogenic disorders (11). It is suggested that cytokines and growth factors, including prostaglandins (PGs), nitric oxide (NO), endothelin (ET), and vascular endothelial growth factor, may all play important roles in the maintenance of cavernosal smooth muscle tone. Changes in these pathways may contribute to ED in various patient subgroups, for example, diabetes and vascular diseases (11). Neurogenic NO is still considered the most important factor for the immediate relaxation of penile vessels and corpus cavernosum; however, endothelially generated NO seems essential for maintaining erection. Endothelial dysfunction can contribute to ED in several patient subgroups (47). The intricate balance between vasoconstriction and vasodilatation of the cavernosal smooth muscle and vessels is likely to be disturbed in CT/RT-induced SD (22,23). Late vascular toxicity is reported after CT (11). The increased fibrosis and reduced NO formation may further impair penile contraction, producing additional ischemic change in the corpora. Pelvic RT may cause fibrosis to the genital organs and contribute to vasculogenic SD (3). Children and adults who receive RT involving the brain frequently experience a progressive cognitive decline due to neurovasculopathy (3). The mechanisms of radiation injury, such as white matter necrosis or vasculopathy, are the obvious responsible pathologies. Similarly, cytotoxic drugs like anthracycline, cisplatin, and the Vinca alkaloids used for germ-cell and solid tumors can induce cardiovascular, small-vessel, or generalized vasculopathy (3). Various cytostatic drugs, including bleomycin, can induce endothelial injury by generating free radicals and oxidative insult (3). Also, apart from the extrinsic neurogenic pathway of erection, spinal arc damage, NO and other cytokines involved in the paracrine and autocrine mechanisms of neurovascular control of sexual function may be perturbed (48). It is possible that the cytokine cascades involved in the nonadrenergic, noncholinergic pathway, including the neuromodulators vasoactive intestinal polypeptide and ET1, may also be disturbed by CT–RT injury. Neuroanatomical damage to penile ultrastructure by cytotoxic or radiotherapeutic drugs can induce vasculopathy with interference in release of PGs, prostanoids, and vasodilators, which are all critical in the local control of neurovascular erectile dynamics. Fibroelastic damage induced by CT/RT to the trabeculae may cause loss of compliance, compounded by aging, and altered synthesis of collagen due to hypercholesterolemia. Hypoxia can also induce increased cross-linking of collagen fibers (11). Figure 2

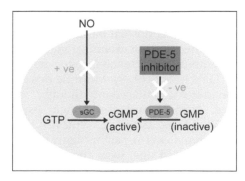

Figure 2 Potential sites of CT/RT interference with the molecular dynamics of erection. The NO/cGMP pathway in corporal smooth muscle is illustrated. The crosses indicate the possible sites of action of CT/RT. *Abbreviations*: NO, nitric oxide; GTP, guanosine triphosphate; GMP, guanosine monophosphate; cGMP, cyclic guanosine monophosphate; sGC, soluble guanylate cyclase; CT, chemotherapy; RT, radiotherapy; PDE-5, phosphodiesterase-5.

shows the proposed sites of damage by CT/RT on the molecular pathway of SD.

□ FUTURE DIRECTIONS AND RESEARCH ISSUES

SD in CT/RT recipients is not a symptom, but a manifestation of a multisystem disease—the pathophysiology of which needs better understanding at a basic science, as well as a clinical science, level. ED may be the result of metabolic disturbance (X syndrome), resulting in an imbalance between the contractile and the relaxation processes within the trabecular smooth muscle. Free radical, oxidative stress and NO liberated during CT/RT treatment or due to the cancer itself may affect erectile performance, causing hypoxia via interference in cytokines, vasoactive factors, and growth factors at two different oxygen tensions (flaccidity and erection). Further investigation of the cavernosal vascular insufficiency theory is needed at a molecular level to understand the autocrine and paracrine control of ED in CT/RT recipients. A drug shifting the balance toward vasodilatation or gene therapy approaches to supplement the deficient components favoring smooth muscle relaxation is an interesting approach. NO-related therapeutics might prove to be useful in the future. The physiologic regulation of the testes and the pathophysiology of hypogonadism may have bearing in nocturnal tumescence and libido. Hormonal suppression of the H–P–T axis by gonadotropin-releasing hormone may have a future in reducing cytotoxic gonadotoxicity of CT/RT. Future CT/RT treatment strategies must also aim to minimize testicular and cavernosal vasculopathy by using less-aggressive protocols for cancer without compromising cancer care.

☐ REFERENCES

1. Gotay CC, Muraoka MY. Quality of life in long-term survivors of adult-onset cancers. J Natl Cancer Inst 1998; 90(9):656–667.

2. Page R, Takimoto C. Principles of chemotherapy. In: Pazdur R, Coia LR, Hoskins WJ, Wagman LD, eds. Cancer Management: A Multidisciplinary Approach. Medical, Surgical and Radiation Oncology. 7th ed. New York: The Oncology Group, 2003:21–37.

3. Gazda MJ, Coia LR. Principles of radiation therapy. In: Pazdur R, Coia LR, Hoskins WJ, Wagman LD, eds. Cancer Management: A Multidisciplinary Approach. Medical, Surgical and Radiation Oncology. 7th ed. New York: The Oncology Group, 2003.

4. Jandl JH. Blood Text book of Hematology. Boston: Little Brown and Company, 1996.

5. Bleyer WA. The impact of childhood cancer on the United States and the world. CA Cancer J Clin 1990; 40(6):355–367.

6. Coebergh JW, Capocaccia R, Gatta G, et al. Childhood cancer survival in Europe, 1978–1992: the EUROCARE study. Eur J Cancer 2001; 37(6):671–672.

7. Ries LAG, Smith MA, Gurney JG, et al, eds. Cancer incidence and survival among children and adolescents: United States SEER Program 1975–1995. Bethesda, MD: National Cancer Institute, 1999.

8. Neitzert CS, Ritvo P, Dancey J, et al. The psychosocial impact of bone marrow transplantation: a review of the literature. Bone Marrow Transplant 1998; 22(5):409–422.

9. Mills W, Chatterjee R, McGarrigle HH, et al. Partial hypopituitarism following total body irradiation in adult patients with hematological malignancy. Bone Marrow Transplant 1994; 14(3): 471–473.

10. Kauppila M, Viikari J, Irjala K, et al. The hypothalamus-pituitary-gonad axis and testicular function in male patients after treatment for hematological malignancies. J Intern Med 1998; 244(5): 411–416.

11. Nuver J, Smit AJ, Postma A, et al. The metabolic syndrome in long-term cancer survivors, an important target for secondary preventive measures. Cancer Treat Rev 2002; 28(4):195–214.

12. Taskinen M, Saarinen-Pihkala UM, Hovi L, et al. Impaired glucose tolerance and dyslipidaemia as late effects after bone-marrow transplantation in childhood. Lancet 2000; 356(9234):993–997.

13. Chatterjee R, Mills W, Katz M, et al. Germ cell failure and Leydig cell insufficiency in post-pubertal males after autologous bone marrow transplantation with BEAM for lymphoma. Bone Marrow Transplant 1994; 13(5):519–512.

14. Chatterjee R, Goldstone AH. Gonadal damage and effects on fertility in adult patients with hematological malignancy undergoing stem cell transplantation. Bone Marrow Transplant 1996; 17(1):5–11.

15. Chatterjee R, Kottaridis PD, McGarrigle HH, et al. Patterns of Leydig cell insufficiency in adult males following bone marrow transplantation for hematological malignancies. Bone Marrow Transplant 2001; 28(5): 497–502.

16. Kyriacou C, Kottaridis PD, Eliahoo J, et al. Germ cell damage and Leydig cell insufficiency in recipients of non-myeloablative transplantation for hematological malignancies. Bone Marrow Transplant 2003; 31(1): 45–50.

17. Howell S, Shalet SM. Gonadal damage from chemotherapy and radiotherapy. Endocrinol Metab Clin North Am 1998; 27(4):927–943.

18. Costabile RA. Cancer and male sexual function. Oncology (Williston Park, NY) 2000; 14(2):195–200.

19. Chatterjee R, Kottaridis PD. Treatment of gonadal damage in recipients of allogeneic or autologous transplantation for hematological malignancies. Bone Marrow Transplant 2002; 30(10):629–635.

20. Steers WD. Rehabilitation of the impotent patient: an update. Mol Urol 1999; 3(3):323–326.

21. Benson CB, Aruny JE, Vickers MA Jr. Correlation of duplex sonography with arteriography in patients with erectile dysfunction. AJR Am J Roentgenol 1992; 160(1):71–73.

22. Chatterjee R, Kottaridis PD, Lees WR, et al. Cavernosal arterial insufficiency and erectile dysfunction in recipients of high-dose chemotherapy and total body irradiation for multiple myeloma. Lancet 2000; 355(9212): 1335–1336.

23. Chatterjee R, Andrews HO, McGarrigle HH, et al. Cavernosal arterial insufficiency is a major component of erectile dysfunction in some recipients of high-dose chemotherapy/chemo-radiotherapy for hematological malignancies. Bone Marrow Transplant 2000; 25(11): 1185–1189.

24. Cappelleri JC, Rosen RC. Reply to the sexual health inventory for men (IIEF-5) by JA Vroege (Letter to the editor). Int J Impot Res 1999; 11(6):353–354.

25. Kassabian VS. Erectile dysfunction in the cancer patient. Cancer Control 2000; 7(2):177–180.

26. Kolb HJ, Socie G, Duell T, et al. Malignant neoplasms in long-term survivors of bone marrow transplantation. Late effects working party of the European cooperative group for blood and marrow transplantation and the European late effect project group. Ann Intern Med 1999; 131(10):738–4429.

27. Rowley MJ, Leach DR, Warner GA, et al. Effect of graded doses of ionizing radiation on the human testis. Radiat Res 1974; 59(3):665–678.

28. Shalet SM, Tsatsoulis A, Whitehead E, et al. Vulnerability of the human Leydig cell to radiation damage is dependent upon age. J Endocrinol 1989; 120(1):161–165.

29. Lindner H. Erectile function after treatment of prostatic carcinoma [German]. Strahlenther Onkol 1999; 175(1): 44–45.

30. Mulcahy JJ. Erectile function after radical prostatectomy. Semin Urol Oncol 2000; 18(1):71–75.

31. Walsh PC, Marschke P, Ricker D, et al. Patient-reported urinary continence and sexual function after anatomic radical prostatectomy. Urology 2000; 55(1): 58–61.

32. Klein C, Glode M. Gonadal complications. In: Armitage JO, Antman KH, eds. High-Dose Cancer Therapy: Pharmacology, Hematopoietins, Stem Cells. 1st ed. Baltimore: Williams and Wilkins, 1992:555–556.

33. Brennemann W, Stoffel-Wagner B, Helmers A, Mezger J, Jager N, Klingmuller D. Gonadal function of patients treated with cisplatin based chemotherapy for germ cell cancer. J Urol 1997; 158(3 Pt 1):844–850.

34. Chatterjee R, Ralph DJ. Toxic effects on testicular function. Europ Urology Update series 1998; 7:661.

35. Coleman N, Langer M. Late complications of cancer therapy. In: Moosa AR, Schimpoff SC, Robson MC, eds. Comprehensive Textbook of Oncology. Vol. 2. 2nd ed. Baltimore: Williams and Wilkins, 1992:1802–1807.

36. Perry MC. Complications of chemotherapy. In: Mossa AR, Schimpff SC, Robson MC, eds. Comprehensive Textbook of Oncology. Vol. 2. 2nd ed. Baltimore: Williams and Wilkins, 1992:1706–1719.

37. Willemse PH, Sleijfer DT, Sluiter WJ, et al. Altered Leydig cell function in patients with testicular cancer: evidence for bilateral testicular defect. Acta Endocrinol (Copenh) 1983; 102(4):616–624.

38. Howell SJ, Shalet SM. Testicular function following chemotherapy. Hum Reprod Update 2001; 7(4): 363–369.

39. Chatterjee R, Mills W, Katz M, et al. Prospective study of pituitary-gonadal function to evaluate short-term effects of ablative chemotherapy or total body irradiation with autologous or allogenic marrow transplantation in post-menarcheal female patients. Bone Marrow Transplant 1994; 13(5):511–517.

40. Kim YC. Testosterone supplementation in the aging male. Int J Impot Res 1999; 11(6):343–352.

41. Heim N. Sexual behaviour of castrated sex offenders. Arch Sex Behav 1981; 10(1):11–19.

42. Vanderpump MP, Tunbridge WM. The effects of drugs on endocrine function. Clin Endocrinol (Oxf) 1993; 39(4):389–397.

43. Chatterjee R, Haines GA, Perera DM, et al. Testicular and sperm DNA damage after treatment with fludarabine for chronic lymphocytic leukemia. Hum Reprod 2000; 15(4):762–766.

44. Litwin MS, Lubeck DP, Stoddard ML, et al. Quality of life before death for men with prostate cancer: results from the CaPSURE database. J Urol 2001; 165(3): 871–875.

45. Socie G. Is syndrome "X" another late complication of bone-marrow transplantation? [Comment]. Lancet 2000; 356(9234):957–958.

46. Korenman SG. Advances in the understanding and management of erectile dysfunction. J Clin Endocrinol Metab 1995; 80(7):1985–1988.

47. Andersson KE. Erectile physiological and pathophysiological pathways involved in erectile dysfunction. J Urol 2003; 170(2 Pt 2):S6–S13.

48. Lue T, Goldstein I, Traish A. Comparison of oral and intracavernosal vasoactive agents in penile erection. Int J Impot Res 2000; 12(S1):S81–S88.

21

The Effect of Genital Tract Infections and Sexually Transmitted Infections on Male Sexual Function

Daniel Richardson
Royal County Sussex Hospital, Brighton and Sussex University Hospitals NHS Trust, Brighton, U.K.

David Goldmeier
Jane Wadsworth Sexual Function Clinic, The Jefferiss Wing, St. Mary's Hospital, Paddington, London, U.K.

☐ INTRODUCTION

Despite the dramatic appearance of human immunodeficiency virus (HIV) in the early 1980s, the incidence of sexually transmitted infections (STIs) continues to increase in both the developing and the developed world. The early HIV epidemic caused previously undescribed morbidity and mortality in young sexually active people in the United States and Western Europe. This coincided with a reduction in the transmission of STIs due to a reactive increase in the use of barrier contraception and so-called "safe sex." Unfortunately, since the advent of effective HIV treatment [highly active antiretroviral therapy (HAART)], sexual behaviour has changed and the incidence of STIs has increased again; even among those who are HIV infected (1). In developing countries, the incidence of HIV is explosive, and, without effective treatment and STI prevention measures, the outlook seems potentially devastating.

Logically, men with sexual problems (including erectile dysfunction, low sexual desire, and ejaculatory disorders) should not be at significant risk of STIs. Similarly, young, sexually active people who are at greatest risk of STIs should not experience sexual problems. In reality, these paradoxical situations are common in clinical practice. In the United States and the United Kingdom, the incidence of sexual dysfunction in adult men is increasing (1–4). As populations in developed society continue to increase in age, it seems that sexual dysfunction is more frequently reported (5). There is also an increase in interest among physicians in the management of sexual dysfunction.

This chapter will systematically review common STIs, nonvenereal infections of the genital tract, and chronic viral infections potentially acquired and transmitted via sexual exposure, and discuss their impact on sexual dysfunction.

☐ COMMON STIs

As the term implies, "STIs" include any infection that can be transferred from one person to another through sexual contact (vaginal, anal, and oral). The following is a review of common STIs. Table 1 provides a summary of the infective organisms and the local and systemic manifestations of the major STIs.

Syphilis

Syphilis is a bacterial infection caused by *Treponema pallidum*, a fragile motile spirochete. At the infectious stage, it rarely causes life-threatening or serious illness. Natural history studies in Oslo (1890–1910) (6) and Tuskegee in the United States (1932) (7) suggest that up to 35% of patients with early syphilis will develop serious cardiovascular, neurological, or gummatous sequelae if untreated. Organisms almost similar to *T. pallidum*, including *T. pertenue* and *T. carateum*, cause yaws and Pinta, respectively. Many accept that syphilis was imported into Europe from China after 1492; however, skeletal remains from archaeological sites in the United Kingdom that predates the discovery of the new world by 100 years show changes suggestions of syphilitic osteitis (7,8). A surge in incidence was seen in the 1950s and 1970s, and currently is seen among men who have sex with men, male and female sex workers, and crack users in Western Europe and the United States (9). Syphilis is thought to be endemic in Eastern Europe, the former Soviet states, and parts of North Africa (10).

A great stigma has arisen around the diagnosis of syphilis. Disfiguring tertiary disease, an unsightly rash (secondary syphilis), and an association with prostitute contact, especially among men in the Armed Forces, have contributed to this stigmatization. Congenital syphilis is also a factor, as many couples were unaware of their infection until the birth of a child who showed signs of infection or congenital malformation.

Syphilis is a systemic disease from the onset. Despite this, the primary stage usually produces an ulcer (chancre) between 9 and 91 days (mean 21 days) after sexual contact. Common sites are the external genitalia, including the perianal region, as well as the oral cavity, breast, cervix, rectum, and pharynx. Secondary syphilis occurs 4 to 10 weeks following the appearance of the chancre, but the two stages can be concurrent. Clinical features of secondary syphilis are a maculopapular rash affecting the entire trunk and in particular the palms and soles. Patchy alopecia,

Table 1 Major STIs: Causative Organisms and Local and Systemic Manifestations

STI	Organism	Local manifestation	Systemic manifestation
Syphilis	*Treponema pallidum*	Genital/nongenital ulceration Maculopapular rash Balanitis	Fever Meningoencephalitis Uveitis Renal impairment Lymphadenopathy Periosteitis Hepatitis Cardiovascular lesions Neurovascular lesions Gumma formation
Gonorrhea	*Neisseria gonorrhoeae*	Urethral discharge Epididymitis Tysonitis	Septicemia Arthritis Rash
Chlamydia	*Chlamydia trachomatis*: serovars B, D-K	Urethral discharge Epididymo-orchitis	Reiter's syndrome Conjunctivitis
Non-gonococcal urethritis	Multiple, including *Chlamydia, Mycoplasma, Trichomoniasis, Neisseria meningitidis*, Herpes simplex, *Candida*	Urethral discharge	Dependent upon causative agent
Genital warts	Human papilloma virus	Local papilloma Squamous cell neoplasms	
Genital herpes	Herpes simplex virus 1 and 2	Localized ulceration Neuropathy	Meningoencephalitis Radiculopathy
Scabies/pubic lice	*Sarcoptes scabiei / Phthirus pubis*	Infestation rash Itch	
HIV/AIDS	Human immunodeficiency virus	Marked, impaired cellular-mediated immune response leading to opportunistic infections	
Hepatitis B	Hepatitis B virus	Acute/chronic hepatitis Cirrhosis Hepatocellular carcinoma	Polyarteritis nodosa Membranous glomerulonephritis Cryoglobulinemia
Hepatitis C	Hepatitis C virus	Acute/chronic hepatitis Cirrhosis Hepatocellular carcinoma	Membranous glomerulonephritis Cryoglobulinemia

Abbreviation: STIs, sexually transmitted infections.

mucosal ulcers (snail track ulcers), wart-like lesions (*Condylomata lata*), asthenia, weight loss, sore throat, fever, myalgia, meningoencephalitis, uveitis, and nephrotic syndrome are also seen. There is often generalized lymphadenopathy and there may be bone pain due to periosteitis. About 20% of cases have subclinical hepatitis. Even without treatment, all of the clinical manifestations of secondary syphilis resolve spontaneously in 3 to 12 weeks (11,12).

If left untreated, patients enter the latent stage, in which no clinical symptoms or signs are present. Tertiary syphilis develops in one-third of those untreated a number of years after the primary infection (6,7). Tertiary syphilis has three clinical entities that can coexist: cardiovascular syphilis, neurosyphilis, and gummatous-syphilis. Cardiovascular syphilis essentially involves the ascending aorta, causing syphilitic aortitis. Neurosyphilis is tabes dorsalis, or involvement of the spinal cord and general paresis of the insane (6,7).

The cornerstones for the management of syphilis include education about safer sexual practices, reminding physicians of the symptoms and signs of the disease, and rapid investigation and treatment of patients and their sexual contacts (7). Treatment of syphilis varies throughout the world, and ideally patients should be referred to specialist clinics. High-dose, injectable long-acting penicillins are the mainstays of treatment in the United Kingdom and United States (12,13).

Social stigma, fear of transmission, fear of a potentially fatal or physically stigmatizing disease, and painful prolonged treatment are aspects of syphilis that affect sexual functioning in those inflicted. General pareses of the insane (GPI), psychiatric sequelae, and tabes dorsalis are rare, but, when they occur, they have devastating effects upon sexual function. The psychiatric and sexual sequelae of GPI in men with tabes are mania (sexual disinhibition), depression (low desire), and erectile dysfunction. All of these are very rare causes of sexual dysfunction in men.

Gonorrhea

Neisseria gonorrhoeae was described in 1879 by Albert Neisser, who observed the organism in smears of exudates from urethritis, cervicitis, and ophthalmia neonatorum (11). Gonorrhea is of worldwide importance and was the most commonly reported infectious disease in the United States between 1977 and 1994 (11). There is estimated to be one unreported case for each reported case. Gonorrhea is exclusively sexually transmitted. Individuals under 25 years of age who have had multiple sexual partners are at greatest risk (11). Transmission efficiency is estimated to be 50% to 60% from an infected man to an uninfected woman, and 20% from an infected woman to an uninfected man. More than 90% of men with urethral gonorrhoea develop symptoms within five days. Most men with symptomatic gonorrheal infection seek health care. Infections at other anatomical sites are less likely to produce symptoms. The evolution of antimicrobial resistance to *N. gonorrhoeae* infections has, in both developed and developing countries, potential negative implications for the control of gonorrhea.

In the majority of cases, gonorrheal infections are limited to mucosal surfaces. Infection occurs in areas of columnar epithelium, including the cervix, urethra, rectum, pharynx, and conjunctiva. The most common symptom of gonorrhea in men is urethral discharge that may range from scanty clear or cloudy fluid to one that is copious and purulent. There are few data on the similarities and differences between a syphilitic pharyngeal infection and the signs and symptoms of an ordinary sore throat or tonsillitis.

Complications of genital gonorrhea infection in men include epididymitis, tysonitis, seminal vesiculitis, and disseminated gonorrhea, and pelvic inflammatory disease in women (11).

Treatment strategies need to be based on local current epidemiological resistance data. Ceftriaxone 250 mg intramuscular injection or cefixime is the current recommendation in the author's clinical practice. As coinfections with *Chlamydia trachomatis* are common (10–50%), empirical treatment for chlamydia is recommended. Contact tracing and subsequent treatment of sexual partners is essential (13,14). The presence of a copious unsightly discharge and/or discomfort on passing urine are likely to have detrimental psychological effects on some patients causing varying degrees of sexual dysfunction.

Chlamydia

C. trachomatis genital infection is caused by serovars B, D-K, and is a common STI. The U.S. Public Health Service estimates that 3 to 5 million new cases occur each year (15). *Chlamydia* is an obligate intracellular parasite that infects columnar epithelial surfaces, causing cellular damage via immunopathological mechanisms. It accounts for 40% of non–gonococcal urethritis in developed countries. Fifty percent of men and 80% of women are asymptomatic, creating a major public health issue (11,15,16). Urethral discharge and dysuria are common presentations. Risk for infection is high in those under the age of 25 years. Other risk factors include new and multiple sexual partners, lack of barrier contraception, use of oral contraceptives, and abortion (16). Rectal infections and pharyngeal infections are usually asymptomatic, and seen in homosexual men. Complications in men include epididymo-orchitis, adult conjunctivitis, and sexually acquired reactive arthritis (16).

Treatment for genital chlamydial infections is straightforward as this organism is susceptible to many antibiotics, and acquired resistance to antimicrobials has not yet been recognized. Tetracyclines (e.g., doxycycline) and macrolides are the currently recommended choices for proven infection (15,16). Azithromycin has the advantage of being a single-dose treatment, improving compliance and reducing partner reinfection (16).

There is significant psychological morbidity associated with urethral discharge, dysuria, and a diagnosis of an STI (17–19). Low sexual desire due to fear of future infection or infectivity of sexual partners may be a problem. It is feasible that psychogenic erectile dysfunction can be caused from similar fears. Morbidity caused by Reiter's syndrome can be significant and debilitating.

Female partners suffer physical problems from sequelae of genital chlamydial infections. Deep dyspareunia and chronic pelvic pain lead to sexual avoidance and potentially to relationship and sexual problems in couples.

Nongonococcal Urethritis

Urethritis is a multifactorial condition that is primarily acquired via sexual transmission. *C. trachomatis* (already described) accounts for 30% to 50% of cases (11,20). The diagnosis of urethritis is confirmed by demonstrating an excess of polymorphonuclear leukocytes in the anterior urethra. *Ureaplasma urealyticum* and *Mycoplasma hominis* can both cause urethritis, and account for 10% to 20% of cases, respectively (20). *Trichomonas vaginalis* has been reported in 1% to 17% of cases (20). *Neisseria meningitidis*, herpes simplex virus (HSV), *Candida* species, bacterial urinary tract infections, urethral strictures, and foreign bodies account for only a small proportion of cases (>10%). There is also a possible association with bacterial vaginosis. Between 20% and 30% of men with nongonococcal urethritis will have no organism detected (20). Clinical symptoms of nongonococcal urethritis are urethral discharge, dysuria, and penile irritation, although some men are asymptomatic. Examination may reveal a urethral discharge. All patients should be screened for other STIs, and laboratory investigation of a midstream specimen of urine to exclude a bacterial urinary tract infection. Treatment should include antimicrobials that are effective against *C. trachomatis* (13,20). Painful urination and a visible discharge have a potential effect on sexual function. The uncertainty around causation at the time of diagnosis may also lead to stress.

Acute Prostatitis

Acute prostatitis is caused by gram-negative uropathogens (*Escherichia coli, Klebsiella* species, *Pseudomonas* species, *Enterococci*, and *Staphylococcus aureus*), and rarely anaerobes (*Bacteroides* species) (21). The clinical presentation may include symptoms of a urinary tract infection such as dysuria, frequency, and urgency; symptoms of prostatitis such as lower back pain, perineal, penile, and rectal pain; and symptoms of bacteremia such as fever and rigors as well as arthralgia and myalgia (11,21). Patients can present with acute urinary retention due to prostatic edema. Midstream urine cultures and blood cultures are the methods for diagnosis. Hydration, appropriate antimicrobial therapy, and analgesics are commonly prescribed therapy. Empirical treatment with high-dose, broad-spectrum cephalosporins for parenteral therapy is recommended in the first instance. Ciprofloxacin or ofloxacin is recommended for oral therapy, until treatment according to sensitivities from an identified organism can be determined (11,21).

Chronic Prostatitis

Chronic bacterial prostatitis is characterized by the identification of pathogenic bacteria in significant numbers from prostatitic fluid in the absence of concomitant urinary tract infection (21). Usual causative organisms are those that also produce acute prostatitis—most commonly, *E. coli*. Some Gram-positive bacteria such as *S. aureus*, *Streptococcus faecalis*, and *Enterococci* can cause chronic bacterial prostatitis (21). The roles of other Gram-positive bacteria, such as coagulase-negative *Staphylococci*, non-group D *Streptococci*, and *diphtheroids* remain controversial. Most evidence suggests that *Ureaplasma urealyticum* and *M. hominis* are common in healthy asymptomatic individuals (21). Evidence that they are major causes of chronic bacterial prostatitis is lacking. Most evidence also suggests that *C. trachomatis* is not a significant cause of chronic bacterial prostatitis (21). Chronic abacterial prostatitis is of unknown etiology and probably results from non-infective, inflammatory pathology.

Clinical features of chronic bacterial prostatitis are perineal pain, lower abdominal pain, penile pain, testicular pain, ejaculatory discomfort, rectal and lower back pain, and dysuria. Symptoms should have been present for at least six months. Stamey's prostatic massage localization procedure is the gold standard for diagnosis. This involves sequential collection and microbiological examination and culture of urine and pre- and postdigital massage of the prostate (22). Expressed prostatic secretions can often be collected for examination and culture. Many antimicrobials penetrate the prostate gland poorly, and this must be taken into account in the choice of agent. First-line treatment is the quinolone class (ciprofloxacin, ofloxacin, or norfloxacin) (11,21).

The impact of chronic prostatitis on sexual function is most likely related to discomfort caused by the condition. Pain on ejaculation leads to sexual avoidance (23). Lower abdominal pain, a fear of cancer, and lower urinary tract symptoms have also been shown to have an adverse effect on sexual function (19). Premature ejaculation is seen in some men with chronic prostatitis (24). Prostatic inflammation was found in 56.6% and chronic bacterial prostatitis in 47.8% of men with premature ejaculation in one series (25).

Human Papilloma Infection

The human papilloma virus (HPV) is a 55-nm DNA virus that belongs to the parvovirus family (11,26). It infects skin and mucosal membranes and replicates in the nuclei of infected epithelial cells. HPV consists of 70 distinct types, of which 34 are associated with anogenital lesions. Specific subtypes are associated with specific genital lesions (Table 1) (11,26). Prevalence of HPV varies dramatically depending upon the population; in the United States, rates of over 50% have been cited in men and women attending sexual health services (11).

Condylomata acuminata, or genital warts, are papillomatous, pedunculated, or sessile growths that can grow anywhere on anogenital skin. Single lesions are usually 1 to 4 mm in diameter. Condylomata are usually flesh-colored, but may be pigmented or erythematous. Intraepithelial neoplasia occurs on the vulva (vulvar intraepithelial neoplasia), vagina (vaginal intraepithelial neoplasia), cervix (cervical epithelial neoplasia), or penis (penile intraepithelial neoplasia, also called bowenoid papulosis). Bowenoid papulosis occurs more frequently in hyperpigmented lesions and may be interspersed with multiple condylomata. Progression to invasive squamous cell carcinoma can occur, particularly in immunosuppressed individuals. Large lesions are called giant condylomata of Buschke and Löwenstein (11,26).

Diagnosis is usually by careful clinical examination. Biopsy is recommended for any suspicious lesions. Histopathological features are papillomatosis and acanthosis of the Malpighian layer. The dermal papillae are usually elongated, narrow, and branching, forming a pattern of pseudoepitheliomatous hyperplasia. Koilocytosis occurs in the upper stratum of the malpighii, stratum granulosum, and stratum corneum (11). Treatment is either with liquid nitrogen (cryotherapy), podophylotoxin, or surgical removal. There are now newer immunomodulatory agents used in clinical practice, such as imiquimod (11,13,26).

Warts are essentially a cosmetic problem, except for oncogenic HPV strains. Their main effect on sex is to alter sexual self-image, and can thus cause low sexual desire or erectile dysfunction because of fear of infectivity. Unsightly warty lesions, social stigma, potentially painful treatment, the possibility of untreatable lesions, surgical intervention, and multiple visits to the sexual health clinic are also factors that could contribute to sexual dysfunction in men with warts (17,18,27,28). Sexual avoidance is common among young men with HPV infection.

Herpes Simplex Virus

Genital herpes is commonly seen at sexually transmitted disease (STD) clinics in the United Kingdom and the United States (11,29,30). Herpes simplex is a double-stranded DNA virus that is classified into types 1 and 2.

The nucleotide sequences of HSV-1 and HSV-2 are 50% identical, and their encoded proteins almost identical. HSV-1 is responsible for up to 90% of orolabial herpes, while HSV-2 causes the majority of genital cases (11). There is a widely held belief that the prevalence of genital herpes increased dramatically in the 1960s and 1970s. Data from the Centers for Disease Control and Prevention (CDC) support this hypothesis (29). In developed countries, symptomatic genital herpes is more prevalent among economically advantaged individuals. This contrasts to gonorrhea, which is more prevalent in the economically disadvantaged (11). Spread of HSV infection occurs when viral particles enter the skin or mucous membranes through microscopic traumatic lesions. The infected epidermal cells are destroyed. The virus enters the peripheral sensory or autonomic nerve endings and ascends to sensory or autonomic root ganglia, where it becomes latent. Subsequent viral reactivation causes the virus to descend to the involved root dermatome. Clinically, this is termed a recurrence. Commonly found factors that tend to increase the rate of recurrence are lack of sleep, adverse life events, and often presence of the infection itself (29,31,32). Recurrences may be asymptomatic. In fact, transmission occurs most commonly from partners asymptomatically shedding virus rather than from partners with active lesions. This observation is not surprising, as individuals are less likely to be sexually active while active herpetic lesions are present (11,29,30).

Acyclovir is a highly effective antiviral for the treatment of acute herpes infections. Suppressive treatment with long-term valacyclovir is effective (31,33). Saline bathing and topical anesthetic gels may be useful in providing symptomatic relief (30).

Primary and symptomatic recurrent genital herpes is distressing, not only because of the physical symptoms, but also because of the grief reaction that can follow the realization of a future with a chronic, painful, and sometimes frequently occurring genital infection that can be passed on to sexual partners (32). This can result in a tarnished self-image or loss of self-esteem that will adversely affect sexual function. The most common emotional responses are depression, anguish, anger, diminution in self-esteem, and hostility toward the person believed to be the source of infection. These emotional reactions seem to be more severe in women than in men (34,35). Long-term acyclovir suppression reduces psychological morbidity associated with recurrent genital herpes, at least during the period of treatment (35). A recent quality of life survey concluded that the burden of recurrent genital herpes has a major impact on the quality of life and is associated with marked impairment of markers of mental health and effectiveness in the workplace (36).

Varicella zoster

Reactivation of *Varicella zoster,* or shingles, within the genital area is uncommon. When it occurs, it causes painful vesicular lesions within a genital dermatome. Genital *V. zoster* recurrences are more common in immunosuppressed individuals. Treatment should be offered in the acute phase with high-dose oral acyclovir, ganciclovir, or famciclovir. Adequate analgesia and skin care are essential. There are reports of a transient radiculopathy causing erectile dysfunction in men with acute reactivated zoster (37).

Scabies and Pubic Lice

Scabies and pubic lice are conditions caused by insects that live on or within the skin. Scabies is caused by *Sarcoptes scabiei*, and pubic lice are caused by *Phthirus pubis*. These common, often sexually acquired infestations are associated with minimal morbidity and are easily treatable (11,37,38). They do, however, invoke varying psychological responses in those affected. The discovery of mobile, visible, and itch-inducing organisms on affected skin is distressing. Worry over disclosure and embarrassment may induce stress states, sexual avoidance, and subsequent sexual dysfunction in those affected.

HIV/AIDS

HIV infection was first described in the United States in 1981 as an unknown cause of immunodeficiency in homosexual men. There are currently over one million people infected with HIV in the United States (39). This compares with over 30 million in sub-Saharan Africa (39). Transmission occurs via unprotected vaginal and anal sex (11). HIV infects T-helper cells (CD4+), which have a pivotal role in cell-mediated immunity. HIV induces a steady decline in total CD4+ cells, resulting in a state of global immunodeficiency. The resulting immunodeficiency has been termed "acquired immunodeficiency syndrome" (AIDS). Affected individuals are susceptible to lethal opportunistic infections and direct organ damage from the HIV itself. Recently, mortality rates in Western countries match those seen presently in Africa. The issue of sexual functioning did not arise in those becoming rapidly terminally ill.

Unfortunately, there is currently no cure for HIV/AIDS; however, HAART, a combination of antiretroviral drugs, has been shown to increase levels of CD4+ cells, decrease incidence of opportunistic infections, and increase individual survival and longevity in those infected. Discontinuation of HAART is associated with clinical deterioration (40).

Increased survival of generally young, sexually active individuals who wish to function normally poses new challenges. HIV carries significant psychological morbidity. Early studies before the advent of HAART suggest that HIV-infected individuals have sexual difficulties (41,42). Erectile dysfunction, delayed ejaculation, and loss of desire were more frequent in HIV-infected men than matched non-HIV-infected men (43). Moreover, HIV-infected individuals are more likely to report an adverse effect on their sex life. Another group showed that patients with a decreased CD4 count reported more sexual problems over time, while patients with higher CD4 counts reported fewer sexual problems (42). Testosterone replacement of men infected with HIV is associated with improvement in both erectile dysfunction and low sexual desire, which raises the question whether there is an organic component to sexual dysfunction in HIV (44). Low serum testosterone is seen in HIV-infected men, but the pathogenesis and mechanism of this state remains unclear (45).

Men in developed countries now have ready accessibility to HAART. The influence of HAART on sexual function has yet to be established; however, a high prevalence of sexual dysfunction (including loss of libido and erectile dysfunction) has been well documented in HIV-infected men (46–52). An increased level of serum 17-β estradiol has been reported in men on HAART (53–55). A causal relationship between HAART and altered hormone levels has not yet been established. Although both protease inhibitors and nonnucleoside reverse transcriptase inhibitors are associated with sexual dysfunction and altered hormone levels (46,49,50,52), most studies have been retrospective and have not specifically shown a temporal link between introduction of HAART and abnormal estradiol levels.

Lipodystrophy is a recognized side effect of HAART (56). Lipodystrophy is a pathological fat redistribution problem manifesting in central obesity and peripheral, including facial, fat atrophy. Lipodystrophy is associated with protease inhibitors (56); however, the exact physiological mechanism is unknown. The psychological effects of lipodystrophy are potentially devastating. Patients fear disclosure and often exhibit features of depression, which can affect sexual function. Self-image and self-esteem are compromised.

Aromatization of testosterone to estrogen in pathological lipodystrophic tissue has been muted as a biological mechanism for increased estradiol levels in HIV-infected men (57). Clinical trials demonstrating the role of aromatase inhibitors in preventing raised estradiol levels in lipodystrophic individuals are currently awaiting completion.

Hepatitis B

Hepatitis B virus (HBV) is a DNA virus with an outer envelope consisting of hepatitis B surface antigen and an inner core of hepatitis B core antigen double-stranded DNA and DNA polymerise (11). HBV is present in high titers in blood and exudates (e.g., skin lesions) of acutely and chronically infected persons. Moderate viral titers are found in semen, vaginal secretions, and saliva. Thus, the principal modes of HBV transmission are percutaneous (intravenous drug use and blood or body fluid exposures among health care),

unprotected sexual contact including oral sexual contact, and perinatal (58).

Hepatitis B infection occurs worldwide. Approximately 45% of the world's population live in geographical areas with HBV endemicity (> 8% of the general population are chronically infected), 43% in areas of moderate endemicity (3–7% infected), and 1% in areas of low endemicity (< 2% infected) (11). Overall, an estimated 300 million persons worldwide are HBV-infected. Changes in sexual practices and other risk behaviors in response to the HIV/AIDS epidemic have resulted in substantial changes in the distribution of HBV, likely due to increased condom use among men who have sex with men and needle exchange programs initiated for the prevention of transmission of HIV infection in developed nations (11). The distribution has shifted to transmission via the vertical route and higher prevalence in developing countries lacking in the above intervention programs. After correcting for underreporting and asymptomatic infections, an estimated 200,000 to 300,000 new HBV infections occur annually in the United States (59,60).

The incubation of HBV ranges from two to six months. The onset of symptoms is gradual and may include skin rashes and arthralgia, in addition to the usual symptoms of viral hepatitis. Symptoms of acute hepatitis last two to four weeks, but fatigue and other symptoms may persist for several months. Acute HBV infection usually resolves with the production of protective antibodies, but may develop into the carrier state. Chronic HBV is associated with cirrhosis and hepatocellular carcinoma. Other clinical features of chronic HBV include polyarteritis nodosa, membranous glomerulonephritis, and cryoglobulinemia. Development of chronic infection is age-dependent. Children less than five years old have a 20% to 50% chance of becoming chronically infected, whereas in older children and adults, the risk is 5% to 10% (11). Treatment of chronic HBV should be performed within a specialist center. Treatment options include nucleoside/nucleotide reverse transcriptase inhibitors, lamivudine, tenofovir, and adefovir with or without interferon (61).

Hepatitis C

Hepatitis C virus (HCV) is an RNA flavivirus with similar transmission characteristics to HBV (see above), but is less common and has a lower infectivity profile. Although HCV can be transmitted sexually, studies examining the risk of sexual transmission have been limited by small sample size, variable types of serological testing, and methodological problems usually relating to a lack of appropriate control groups. As a result, the available information is conflicting. An estimated 16% of acute viral hepatitides are caused by HCV. Results from the Third National Health and Nutrition Examination Survey indicate that the prevalence of HCV in the United States is 1.4% (62). HCV-infected persons are at risk of developing cirrhosis and hepatocellular carcinoma. An estimated 8000 to 10,000 persons die annually in the United States from chronic consequences of HCV (62,63).

Acute HCV is generally mild, with 25% or fewer of infected persons having a recognized illness. The symptoms are indistinguishable from other forms of viral hepatitis. The most important feature of HCV is the frequency with which acute disease progresses to chronic infection. Most treatment strategies include the use of α-2b interferon and ribavirin. Response is dependant upon viral subtype. No effective vaccine is currently available.

The psychological burden of hepatitis B and C, particularly in those coinfected with HIV, can be devastating as these conditions carry poor prognosis. The prospect of developing cancer is also a factor. Interferon treatment for HCV makes people feel terrible and can lead to total loss of sexual desire. Ribavirin can cause profound autonomic and peripheral neuropathy and associated erectile dysfunction (64,65). Many patients infected with these blood-borne viruses are current or previous intravenous drug users and lead erratic and chaotic lives, which must also be taken into account when considering sexual dysfunction.

Balanitis

Balanitis is defined as inflammation of the glans penis often involving the prepuce (balanoposthitis) (66,67). Incidence of balanitis may be increased in uncircumcised men. Infectious causes include *Candida albicans, T. vaginalis, Streptococci* group A and B, anaerobic bacteria, *Gardnerella vaginalis, S. aureus, Mycobacterium, Entamoeba histolytica, Syphilis,* herpes simplex, and HPV (66,67). Presenting symptoms include local rashes, which may be scaly or ulcerated, soreness, itch, odor, inability to retract foreskin, and a discharge from the glans or the foreskin. Subprepucial swab for candidia and bacterial culture, urinalysis for glucose, herpes simplex culture, syphilis serology, and screening for other STIs are required to make a diagnosis. A biopsy is required if the diagnosis is uncertain and the condition persists. General advice regarding hygiene and soap avoidance is necessary. Treatment is based upon the laboratory results of the initial investigation.

Most men with balanitis assume that they have an STI despite the fact that most cases are caused by *C. albicans*, a single-celled fungal organism responsible for most vaginal yeast infections. Some men with candidal or bacterial balanitis experience severe soreness and pain. This leads to sexual avoidance and erectile dysfunction. (For further information on balanitis, see Chapter 9.)

Tuberculosis

There has been an unexpected resurgence of tuberculosis (TB) in the United States and Europe, most likely due to a combination of HIV/AIDS and increasing migration from areas where *Mycobacterium tuberculosis* is common, such as sub-Saharan Africa and the Asian subcontinent (11). TB rarely affects the genital tract, but there are increasing reports in the literature and anecdotal experience of tuberculous orchitis and cutaneous manifestations, particularly in HIV-infected individuals. In addition to carrying the stigma of TB, infected individuals often face the prospect of surgery to remove one or both testicles. TB should be treated within a specialist unit by physicians experienced in TB management. Low sexual desire is associated with the stressful state and depression from such an ordeal. Diminished testosterone levels and "loss of masculinity" as the result of testicular surgery, including orchiectomy, may also have a detrimental effect on sexual function.

Cellulitis

Cutaneous bacterial infections of the external genitalia are often secondary to genital dermatological conditions such as eczema, psoriasis, or insect bites. Streptococcal and staphylococcal species are the most likely organisms. *Streptococcal cellulitis* often requires hospital admission for intravenous antibiotics. *Streptococcal folliculitis* and impetigo can be very painful and may require potent opiate analgesia.

Venereophobia

Physicians who manage patients with STIs commonly see patients who have a fear of venereal diseases. This is a form of "health anxiety" that can manifest as pure anxiety or as sexual phobia (e.g., fear of acquiring an STI such that a person panics at the mere thought of sex). In most instances, this phenomenon is transient, being relieved by examination and reassurance. This condition is associated with depression and paranoid states, including drug use and schizophrenia. The term venereophobia is used only for those patients who persist in this mistaken belief, which is more of a delusion than a phobia (68,69). They may attend several clinics insisting that their belief will eventually be shown to be true. Others have, in fact, had an STI, but refuse to believe it has been cured. Not surprisingly, this condition is associated with sexual dysfunction (68). Most patients with venereophobia have few or no sexual experiences and do not gain sexual satisfaction. The venereophobia might have arisen during a period of sexual inadequacy and serve as an excuse for curtailing further sexual activity. If there is obvious anxiety or depression, it will require appropriate management. Unfortunately, the condition is often intractable, but the patient may learn to live with his myth. Treatment of venereophobia usually involves cognitive behavioral therapy and antidepressants and is best undertaken by a psychologist or psychiatrist.

☐ CONCLUSION

Sexual dysfunction is a multidimensional phenomenon affecting not only the individual presenting to the physician but also their sexual partners and other associates. The symptomatology of STIs ranges from asymptomatic disease to painful genital ulcers, debilitating neurological disease, and immmunosuppression. It seems logical that a patient with painful genital ulcers will not have sexual desires, but the physician must think more laterally to appreciate the patient whose partner has an STI that has induced low sexual desire in his/her partner. This can be explained by either fear of transmission or feelings of rejection. Inflammation and infection of the organs controlling sexual function potentially result in sexual dysfunction. Systemic STIs, particularly those with neurological sequelae, may cause disturbances in neural pathways controlling normal sexual function. Whatever the cause, the complexity of this problem is evident.

The psychological and emotional impacts of STIs and HIV are varied and complex. There are many aspects of having and treating STIs that may potentially have adverse effects on the psychological well-being of patients, including visiting a sexual health clinic, discussing sexual practices and exposing one's genitalia to a stranger (health care worker), or experiencing uncomfortable specimen-taking (17,18). In addition, the need to inform current sexual partners about STIs that may involve revealing other sexual partners outside a recognized relationship can be harrowing for those involved. Many patients, when diagnosed with an STI, worry or presume that they have other undiagnosed infections, such as HIV. Even patients with mild symptoms (such as genital itch) may assume the worst. These factors contribute to the psychological stress surrounding STIs, which can indirectly and adversely affect sexual function.

There are little published data on the relationship between sexual function, STIs, and infections of the genital tract; however, there are data detailing the adverse psychological impact of STDs. Extrapolation of this information and clinical experience suggest that the adverse psychological impact of STIs can result in sexual dysfunction.

☐ REFERENCES

1. Johnson AM, Mercer CH, Erens B, et al. Sexual behaviours in Britain: partnerships, practices, and HIV risk behaviours. Lancet 2001; 358(9296):1835–1842.
2. Laumann EO, Paik A, Rosen RC. Sexual dysfunction in the United States: prevalence and predictors. JAMA 1999; 281(6):537–544.
3. Nazareth I, Boynton P, King M. Problems with sexual function in people attending London general practitioners: cross sectional study. BMJ 2003; 327 (7412):423.
4. Mercer CH, Fenton KA, Johnson AM, et al. Sexual function problems and help seeking behaviour in Britain national probability sample survey. BMJ 2003; 327(7412): 426–427.
5. Araujo AB, Durante R, Feldman HA, et al. The relationship between depressive symptoms and male erectile dysfunction: cross sectional results from the Massachusetts male aging study. Psychosom Med 1998; 60(4):458–465.
6. Clarke EG, Dunbolt N. The Oslo study of the natural course of untreated syphilis: an epidemiologic investigation based on re-study of the Boeck-Bruusgaard material. Med Clin North Am 1964; 48:613.
7. Goldmeier D, Guallar C. Syphilis: an update. Clin Med 2003; 3(3):209–211.
8. Morton RS, Rashid S. 'The syphilis Enigma' the riddle resolved? Sex Transm Infect 2001; 77(5):322–324.
9. PHLS website: www.phls.co.uk.
10. Tichonova L, Borisenko K, Ward H, et al. Epidemics of syphilis in the Russian Federation: trends, origins, and priorities for control. Lancet 1997; 350(9072): 210–213.
11. Morse SA, Moreland A, Holmes K. Atlas of Sexually Transmitted Diseases and AIDS. 2nd ed. London: Mosby-Wolfe, 1996:22–266, 305–318.
12. National Guidelines for The Management of Early Syphilis. London: Association for Genitourinary Medicine (AGUM), Medical Society for the Study of Venereal Disease (MSSVD), 2002.
13. Centers for Disease Control and Prevention. Sexually transmitted disease treatment guidelines. MMWR Recomm Rep 1993; 42:1–101.
14. Clinical Effectiveness Group (Association of Genitourinary Medicine and the Medical Society for the study of Venereal Diseases). National guidelines for the management of gonorrhea in adults. Sex Transm Infect 1999; 75(suppl 1):S13–S15.
15. Centers for Disease Control and Prevention. Recommendations or the prevention and management of Chlamydia trachomatis infection. MMWR Recomm Rep 1993; 42:1–39.
16. Clinical Effectiveness Group (Association of Genitourinary Medicine and the Medical Society for the Study of Venereal Diseases). National guidelines for the management of Chlamydia trachomatis genital tract infection. Sex Transm Infect 1999; 75(suppl 1):S4–S8.
17. Goldmeier D, Keane FE, Carter P, et al. Prevalence of sexual dysfunction in heterosexual patients attending a central London genitourinary medicine clinic. Int J STD AIDS 1997; 8(5):303–306.
18. Mayou R. Psychological morbidity in a clinic for sexually transmitted disease. Br J Vener Dis 1975; 51(1): 57–60.

19. Brookes ST, Donovan JL, Peters TJ, et al. Sexual dysfunction in men after treatment for lower urinary tract symptoms: evidence from randomised control trial. BMJ 2002; 324(7345):1059–1061.

20. Clinical Effectiveness Group (Association of Genitourinary Medicine and the Medical Society for the Study of Venereal Diseases). National guidelines for the management of non-gonococcal urethritis. Sex Transm Infect 1999; 75(suppl 1):S9–S12.

21. Clinical Effectiveness Group (Association of Genitourinary Medicine and the Medical Society for the study of Venereal Diseases). National guidelines for the management of prostatitis. Sex Transm Infect 1999; 75(suppl 1):S46–S50.

22. Meares EM, Stamey TA. Bacterial localization patterns in bacterial prostatitis and urethritis. Invest Urol 1968; 5(5):492–518.

23. Kaplan HS. Post-ejaculatory pain syndrome. J Sex Marital Ther 1993; 19(2):91–103.

24. Brown AJ. Ciprofloxacin as a cure for premature ejaculation. J Sex Marital Ther 2000; 26(4):351–352.

25. Screponi E, Carosa E, Di Stasi SM, et al. Prevalence of chronic prostatitis in men with premature ejaculation. Urology 2001; 58(2):198–202.

26. Clinical Effectiveness Group (Association of Genitourinary Medicine and the Medical Society for the Study of Venereal Diseases). National guidelines for the management of HPV. www.mssvd.org.uk.

27. Conaglen HM, Hughes R, Conaglen JV, et al. A prospective study of the psychological impact on patients of first diagnosis of human papillomavirus. Int J STD AIDS 2001; 12(10):651–658.

28. Filiberti A, Tamburini M, Stefanon B, et al. Psychological aspects of genital human papillomavirus infection: a preliminary report. J Psychosom Obstet Gynaecol 1993; 14(2):145–152.

29. Genital Herpes Infection—United States, 1966–1979. Morb Mortal Wkly Rep 1982; 31:137–139.

30. Clinical Effectiveness Group (Association of Genitourinary Medicine and the Medical Society for the Study of Venereal Diseases). National guidelines for the management of genital herpes. Sex Transm Infect 1999; 75(suppl 1):S24–S25.

31. Mindel A. Psychological and psychosexual implications of herpes simplex virus infections. Scand J Infect Dis Suppl 1996; 100:27–32.

32. Mindel A. Long-term clinical and psychological management of genital herpes. J Med Virol 1993; (suppl 1): 39–44.

33. Goldmeier D, Johnson A, Jeffries D, et al. Psychological aspects of recurrences of genital herpes. J Psychosom Res 1986; 30(5):601 608.

34. Reitano M, Tyring S, Lang W, et al. Valaciclovir for the suppression of recurrent genital herpes simplex virus infection: a large-scale dose range-finding study. International Valaciclovir HSV Study Group. J Infect Dis 1998; 178:603–610.

35. Griffiths PD. Tomorrow's challenges for herpesvirus management: potential applications of valacyclovir. J Infect Dis 2002; 186(suppl 1):S131–S137.

36. Patel R, Boselli F, Cairo I, et al. Patients' perspectives on the burden of recurrent genital herpes. Int J STD AIDS 2001; 12(10):640–645.

37. Rix GH, Carroll DN, MacFarlane JR. Herpes zoster producing temporary erectile dysfunction. Int J Impot Res 2001; 13(6):352–353.

38. Clinical Effectiveness Group (Association of Genitourinary Medicine and the Medical Society for the Study of Venereal Diseases). National guidelines for the management of Phthirus pubis. Sex Transm Infect 1999; 75(suppl 1):S78–S79.

39. Clinical Effectiveness Group (Association of Genitourinary Medicine and the Medical Society for the Study of Venereal Diseases). National guidelines for the management of scabies. Sex Transm Infect 1999; 75(suppl 1):S76–S77.

40. The CASCADE Collaboration. Survival after introduction of HAART in people with known duration of HIV1 infection: concerted action on seroconversion to AIDS and death in Europe. Lancet 2000; 355:1158–1159.

41. Joint United Nations Programme on HIV/AIDS (UNAIDS). Report on the global HIV/AIDS epidemic 2002. http://www.unaids.org.

42. Jones M, Klimes I, Catalan J. Psychosexual problems in people with HIV infection: controlled study of gay men and men with haemophilia. AIDS Care 1994; 6(5):587–593.

43. Tindall B, Forde S, Goldstein D, et al. Sexual dysfunction in advanced HIV disease. AIDS Care 1994; 6(1): 105–107.

44. Catalan J, Klimes I, Bond A, et al. The psychosocial impact of HIV infection in men with haemophilia: controlled investigation and factors associated with psychiatric morbidity. J Psychosom Res 1992; 36(5): 409–416.

45. Mylonakis E, Koutkia P, Grinspoon S. Diagnosis and treatment of androgen deficiency in human immunodeficiency virus-infected men and women. Clin Infect Dis 2001; 33(6):857–864.

46. Rabkin JG, Rabkin R, Wagner GJ. Testosterone treatment of clinical hypogonadism in patients with HIV/AIDS. Int J STD AIDS 1997; 8(9):537–545.

47. Lamba H, Goldmeier D, Mackie NE, et al. Antiretroviral therapy is associated with sexual dysfunction and with increased serum oestradiol levels in men. Int J STD AIDS 2004; 15(11):234–237.

48. Sollima S, Osio M, Muscia R, et al. Protease inhibitors and erectile dysfunction. AIDS 2001; 15(17): 2331–2333.

49. Newshan G, Taylor B, Gold R. Sexual functioning in ambulatory men with HIV/AIDS. Int J STD AIDS 1998; 9:672–676.

50. Collazos J, Mayo J, Martinez E, et al. Association between sexual disturbances and sexual hormones with

specific antiretroviral drugs. AIDS 2002; 16(9): 1294–1295.

51. Collazos J, Martinez E, Mayo J, et al. Sexual Dysfunction in HIV-infected patients treated with highly active antiretroviral therapy. J Acquir Immune Defic Syndr 2002; 31(3):322–326.

52. Collazos J, Martinez E, Mayo J, et al. Sexual hormones in HIV-infected patients: the influence of antiretroviral therapy. AIDS 2002; 16(6):934–937.

53. Schrooten W, Colebunders R, Youle M, et al. Sexual dysfunction associated with protease inhibitor containing antiretroviral treatment. AIDS 2001; 15(8): 1019–1023.

54. Teichmann J, Stephan E, Lange U, et al. Evaluation of serum and urinary estrogen levels in male patients with HIV-infection. Eur J Med Res 1998; 3(11): 533–537.

55. Goldmeier D, Lamba H. Sexual dysfunction in HIV-positive individuals. Int J STD AIDS 2003; 14(1): 63–64.

56. Colson AE, Keller MJ, Sax PE, et al. Male sexual dysfunction associated with antiretroviral therapy. J Acquir Immune Defic Syndr 2002; 30(1):27–32.

57. Carr A, Samaras K, Chisholm D, et al. Pathogenesis of HIV-1-protease inhibitor-associated peripheral lipodystrophy, hyperlipidaemia, and insulin resistance. Lancet 1998; 351(9119):1881–1883.

58. Goldmeier D, Scullard G, Kapembwa M, et al. Does increased aromatase activity in adipose fibroblasts cause low sexual desire in patients with HIV lipodystrophy? Sex Transm Infect 2002; 78(1):64–66.

59. Alter MJ, Margolis HS. The emergence of hepatitis B as a sexually transmitted disease. Med Clin North Am 1990; 74(6):1529–1541.

60. Centers for Disease Control and Prevention. Hepatitis Surveillance Report No. 55. Atlanta, GA: U.S. Department of Health and Human Services, Centers for Disease Control and Prevention, 1994:36.

61. Hui CK, Zhang HY, Lau GK. Management of chronic hepatitis B in treatment-experienced patients. Gastroenterol Clin North Am 2004; 33(3):601–616.

62. Alter MJ, Margolis HS, Krawczynski K, et al. The natural history of community-acquired hepatitis C in the United States. The Sentinel Counties Chronic non-A, non-B Hepatitis Study Team. N Engl J Med 1992; 327(27):1899–1905.

63. McQuillan GM, Townsend TR, Fields HA, et al. Seroepidemiology of hepatitis B virus in the United States. 1976–1980. Am J Med 1989; 87(3A):S5–S10.

64. Fattovich G, Giustina G, Favarato S, et al. A survey of adverse events in 11,241 patients with chronic viral hepatitis treated with alfa interferon. J Hepatol 1996; 24(1):38–47.

65. Fleischer R, Boxwell D, Sherman KE. Nucleoside analogues and mitochondrial toxicity. Clin Infect Dis 2004; 38(8):79–80.

66. Alter MJ, Hadler SC, Judson FN, et al. Risk factors for acute non-A, non-B hepatitis in the United States and association of hepatitis C virus infection. JAMA 1990; 264(17):2231–2235.

67. Edwards S. Balanitis and balanoposthitis: a review. Genitourin Med 1996; 72(3):155–159.

68. Clinical Effectiveness Group (Association of Genitourinary Medicine and the Medical Society for the Study of Venereal Diseases). National guidelines for the management of balanitis. Sex Transm Infect 1999; 75(suppl 1):S85–S88.

69. Rodin P, Goldmeier D. Sexual problems seen by venereologists. In: Crown S, ed. Psychosexual Problems. London/New York: Academic press and Grune & Stratton, 1976:403–421.

Part III

Investigation of Male Sexual Dysfunction

The correct and efficient assessment of male patients presenting with sexual dysfunction depends upon a thorough understanding of the anatomical and the physiologic bases of human male sexual function and dysfunction, as described in Parts I and II. The next step in the evaluation process requires the physician to substantiate all theoretical assumptions of any potential diagnoses, both with hard data obtained via laboratory testing and through communicated data from the patient that will be interpreted on the basis of clinical experience, including information obtained from other health care providers such as diabetologists, cardiologists, oncologists, and psychologists that may be involved in the patient's care. Due to the particularly sensitive and personal nature of sexual dysfunction for many men, adroitness and compassion must be exercised during these next crucial proceedings. It must be emphasized that a detailed medical history and physical exam, elicited in a thorough and sympathetic manner, are extremely helpful in targeting the underlying cause of the sexual dysfunction, as these will reduce the need to subject the patient to additional stressful, invasive, and costly investigations, particularly when a high index of suspicion has already been raised due to the presence of preexisting comorbid conditions (e.g., elderly patients or those with established diabetes, neurologic disorders, hypertension, and hypercholesterolemia). Questions targeted toward elucidating past psychological and sexual histories can further delineate the need for specific therapeutic interventions. Similarly, portions of the physical exam may provide readily obtained, invaluable information, such as the visual and tactile examination of the genitals and the assessment of the penile-brachial index and bulbocavernosus reflex.

Generally, erectile dysfunction (ED) is the most common presenting complaint, and this may be classified as having a psychogenic, organic, or a mixed etiology. Of the organic pathologies, these are most often related to vascular or neurological defects, although a combination of these may occur in the same patient—particularly in the presence of other concomitant systemic diseases, in which case endocrine factors may also be causative. The widespread availability and efficacy of agents specifically targeted to the erectogenic mechanism, such as intrapenile vasoactive drugs (e.g., prostaglandin E_1) and oral phosphodiesterase-5 (PDE-5) inhibitors, however, tempts many treating physicians to use them as primary therapeutic modalities without necessarily determining the specific nature of an individual's sexual dysfunction.

Although this approach may be suitable for the majority of patients who indeed have defects limited to the vascular components of the erectile mechanism, it must be remembered that the potential complications of using erectogenic drugs when contraindicated could be life-threatening, such as when PDE-5 inhibitors are inadvertently administered with nitrates. Further indicating the need to perform the appropriate investigations is the existence of the subset of men with potentially correctable disorders (e.g., psychosexual problems, hypogonadism, treatable chronic illness, and/or correctable vascular insufficiency), as well as those who have a high risk for complications or cannot tolerate the side effects of erectogenic agents (e.g., with PDE-5: headache, dyspepsia, changes in vision hue or sudden decrease or loss of vision; with intraurethral prostaglandin: systemic symptoms; with intrapenile vasoactive injections: penile priapism, pain, or fibrosis). The chapters in Part III detail the methods of history-taking, conducting an appropriate physical exam, and the various office, laboratory, and other special investigations that may be performed in order to elucidate the particular nature of the sexual dysfunction.

Real-time penile tumescence monitoring can be achieved in the clinic with the use of a electrobioimpedance device, with or without concomitant administration of cavernosal vasodilatory agents or audio-visual sexual stimulation, and may be helpful in establishing or ruling out psychogenic etiology. Nocturnal penile tumescence monitoring can also be performed, but since the advent of daytime, office-based monitoring, the high level of time involvement and the cost associated with performing sleep studies often make them prohibitive for a typical patient workup.

Pharmaco-penile duplex ultrasound (PPDU) is a method that is capable of defining the arterial tree, measuring the diameter of the cavernosal arteries, and determining peak systolic flow, as well as revealing any abnormalities of the tunica albuginea. Intracorporeal injection of the vasodilator, papaverine, with or without alpha-adrenergic blockers (phentolamine or phenoxybenzamine) during PPDU may serve as an adjunct in helping to distinguish arterial from non-arterial causes of impotence. If needed, the exact location and extent of the vascular lesion can then be defined with more invasive tests. Penile arteriography is the definitive diagnostic procedure for assessing obstructive penile arterial flow. Cavernosography, on the other hand, is most helpful in assessing cavernosal body morphology and penile venous system drainage. Radioisotope techniques for assessing penile blood flow have also been developed. Available data suggest their usefulness in evaluating overall organ blood flow, particularly postoperatively. It must be noted, however, that the most invasive of these methods should not be considered as part of the routine investigation of the ED patient, and their use must be restricted to well-defined indications.

Patients suspected of having neurologic impairment after the results of non-invasive office-based testing such as vibratory stimulation or thermal sensitivity have been obtained, or those with documented abnormal NPT, may be evaluated for pudendal nerve (somatic) conduction. More invasive testing of penile innervation includes perineal electromyography, sacral latency, and genital cerebral evoked response studies. These specialized tests have the advantage of localizing the specific site of neurologic sensory impairments. Currently, there is no direct objective procedure for evaluation of the parasympathetic innervation to corporeal blood vessels; however, cystometrography and bethanechol supersensitivity testing, via assessment of the vesical parasympathetic innervation, provide indirect information and are useful in patients with a concomitant voiding dysfunction. Similarly, indirect tests of the sympathetic nervous system, such as darkness pupil-size adaptation, sympathetic skin response, histamine/acetylcholine skin tests, or electromyography of the corpus cavernosum, may be useful in selected patients.

Clinical Assessment of the Male Presenting with Sexual Dysfunction

Chakriya D. Anunta
Department of Diabetes, Endocrinology and Metabolism, City of Hope National Medical Center, Duarte, California, U.S.A.

Fouad R. Kandeel
Department of Diabetes, Endocrinology and Metabolism, City of Hope National Medical Center, Duarte, California and David Geffen School of Medicine, University of California, Los Angeles, California, U.S.A.

☐ INTRODUCTION

The evaluation of male patients presenting with sexual dysfunction depends not only on the thorough understanding of the anatomical and physiologic bases of human male sexual function, but also on the ability of the physician to collect and interpret the patient's history, physical findings, and all pertinent data from carefully selected special investigations. Due to the particularly sensitive nature of sexual dysfunction, many patients will avoid discussing their concerns with their doctors. One study found that 44% of patients being treated at a urologic clinic for unrelated conditions were suffering from some degree of erectile dysfunction (ED) but had failed to report it to their doctors (1); 74% of these patients cited embarrassment as the primary rationale for not broaching the subject. Ignorance, misinformation, and lack of affordability are other common reasons men do not seek treatment for sexual matters (2). Therefore, it is important to encourage patient disclosure of these problems routinely in order to facilitate their potential medical treatment. Once a detailed history and physical examination are completed, the focus of the medical investigation can then be shifted toward confirming the underlying pathophysiologic abnormalities and devising an appropriate treatment plan.

☐ HISTORY

Sympathetically elicited medical histories are extremely helpful in targeting the underlying cause of the sexual dysfunction. If successfully obtained, these reduce the need for expensive investigations, particularly when a high index of suspicion has already been raised due to the presence of preexisting comorbid conditions (e.g., elderly patients or those with established diabetes, neurologic disorders, hypertension, and hypercholesterolemia). Psychological and sexual histories can further direct the path of medical evaluation and the

development of appropriate therapeutic interventions. This type of approach has been advocated by many physicians in the field of sexual medicine (3–10). Because sexual dysfunction is intimately related to the responses of the patient's sexual partner(s), it is mandatory to inquire tactfully about previous and ongoing relationships; underlying relationship problems are major factors in the development of ED—the most common subset of male sexual dysfunction—and the possibility of their existence must be explored in all cases.

Medical History

Because intact sexual function requires the intricate coordination of the vascular, neurological, endocrinologic, and psychological systems, any medical disturbances in one or more of these arenas may predispose the patient to sexual dysfunction. Thus, it is very important to identify historical events related to the presence of chronic disease (e.g., hepatic failure, renal failure, and advanced pulmonary disease). If there is a current or family history of cardiovascular disease, cerebrovascular accident, hypercholesterolemia, hypertension, or diabetes, a vascular etiology should be highly suspected. Potentially irreversible pathology should be anticipated in patients who demonstrate evidence of microvascular disease elsewhere in the body (peripheral neuropathy, retinopathy, and nephropathy). (For further information on this topic, see Chapter 13.)

Any potential sources for the disruption of the neural pathways that operate the erectile mechanism should be questioned, such as prior pelvic surgeries (e.g., prostatectomy, proctectomy, and vascular surgery) or radiation, and traumatic injury (temporal lobe and spinal cord lesions, blunt pelvic trauma, scarring or fibrosis due to Peyronie's disease). Patients with neurologic disease (multiple sclerosis and tabes dorsalis) should be questioned about the temporal relationship between the development of the sexual dysfunction and that of the neurologic disorder. (For further information on this topic, see Chapter 15.)

Underlying endocrine disorders such as gonadal failure or pituitary tumors may be responsible. Patients suspected of having hypogonadism should be assessed specifically for a family history of the disease, deviation of adolescence from normality, recent changes in secondary sexual characteristics, symptoms of pituitary dysfunction, thyroid, and adrenal diseases, and a history of orchitis, testicular trauma, infertility, or exposure to radiation or cytotoxic agents.

A meticulous drug history is also essential, as a considerable number of pharmacologic agents are associated with the development of ED. Frequently implicated drugs in common use are the antihypertensives (particularly β-blockers and thiazide diuretics), antihistamines, anticholinergics, antipsychotics, and antidepressants (especially monoamine oxidase inhibitors, tricyclic compounds, and selective serotonin reuptake inhibitors; the last may not only cause ED but also retard ejaculation). The most potent pharmacologic executors in this regard are the anticancer agents (such as those used in the treatment of prostate cancer), which often cause both ED and the loss of libido. The questions of cigarette smoking, alcohol intake, and illicit substance abuse should not be neglected. (For further information on this topic, see Chapter 19.)

Psychological History

Psychological factors associated with male sexual dysfunction have been assembled into a three-tiered paradigm consisting of predisposing factors, precipitating factors, and maintaining factors (11,12). Predisposing factors include biologically and psychosocially determined vulnerabilities that render individuals more susceptible to the development of sexual dysfunction, such as disturbed family relationships, a restrictive upbringing, traumatic early sexual experiences, inadequate sexual information, and insecurity in the psychosexual role. Precipitating factors promote the onset of sexual dysfunction and may be thought of as triggering events that serve to initiate the condition; unreasonable expectations, random failure, discord in the relationship, dysfunction in the partner, infidelity, reaction to organic disease, depression, or anxiety are some of the most commonly encountered factors. Perpetuating factors sustain illness; they maintain, exacerbate, or prolong sexual dysfunction. These may include performance anxiety, guilt, poor communication, loss of attraction between partners, and impaired self-image. Affective disorders or character pathology can lead to both precipitation and maintenance of sexual problems. Appropriate intervention will involve identifying and addressing all relevant predisposing, precipitating, and perpetuating factors, and thus evidence for the presence of any of these psychological or situational conditions should be carefully assessed. Moreover, it should not be forgotten that the presence of an organic disease does not preclude the possibility of a coexisting psychogenic factor, and vice versa. Such omissions could lead to diagnostic difficulties as well as to therapeutic failures. (For further information on this topic, see Chapter 12.)

Sexual History

To obtain a clear history, it is important that the patient himself understands the characteristics that distinguish the most common sexual complaints: loss of libido, ED, and ejaculatory disturbance (13). Often, this will require some preliminary explanation on the part of the practitioner. The time and manner of onset and the consistency and severity of the course all require establishment. The development of self-administered symptom scores such as the International Index of Erectile Function (IIEF) by Rosen et al. (Appendix 1) (14) has greatly facilitated quantitative history-taking for sexual dysfunction. Further information on the use of questionnaires is given later in this chapter.

Decreased libido should alert the clinician to three probable causes: endocrinopathy, affective disorder, or relationship discord. A history of frequent strong erections under any circumstances (during foreplay, fantasy, masturbation, or upon awakening) likely indicates that the endocrine, vascular, and neurological systems are intact, and that the ED is predominantly psychogenic. Conversely, historical data relating to the presence of decreased erectile turgidity during noncoital activities are highly suggestive of an organic etiology. A report of firm sustained erections during foreplay that are lost after intromission or upon initiation of pelvic movements, however, might suggest either a psychogenic etiology or a vascular problem (pelvic steal syndrome). A history of delayed or retrograde ejaculation may imply a neuropathy or an adverse drug effect. Premature ejaculation, on the other hand, is more compatible with a psychogenic dysfunction. Finally, it must be remembered that the absence of orgasmic sensations in patients with normal erectile and ejaculatory functions is almost always due to psychogenic etiology, whereas failure of detumescence is usually organic in nature; the latter should direct investigations toward ruling out local penile neurological and hematological etiologies. Table 1 lists other historical events that are useful in differentiating predominantly psychogenic from predominantly organic EDs.

Use of Questionnaires in Evaluation of Male Sexual Dysfunction

Several well-established and validated self-administered questionnaires have been developed and used to assess the frequency and nature of sexual dysfunction in men, and some have been used to assess the adequacy of response to therapeutic modalities. Questionnaires can be a useful and time-saving way to initiate discussion on sexual dysfunction in the clinical setting. Although valuable in detecting the presence of sexual problems and in distinguishing between psychogenic and organic etiologies, questionnaires do not usually yield information that is sufficient for determining the underlying pathophysiology. Thus, the data gathered from questionnaires should be used to direct the appropriate diagnostic investigations effectively. The most

Table 1 Features Differentiating Predominantly Psychogenic from Predominantly Organic Erectile Dysfunction

Parameter	Psychogenic	Organic
Onset of disorder	Situational with defined onset	Insidious
Precipitating event	Psychogenic condition	Debilitating disease, vascular insufficiency, central nervous system abnormality, penile trauma, or interfering drugs
Erectile function before intromission	May be present	Usually absent except in patients with pelvic steal phenomenon
Erectile function after intromission	Variable with different partners	Usually absent
Erectile response to other sexual stimuli	Usually present	Usually absent
Nocturnal or morning erections	Initially present and full, lost in long-standing dysfunction	Absent or reduced in frequency and intensity
Course of disorder	Episodic or transient loss of erection	Persistent and progressive erectile dysfunction
Associated ejaculatory disorder	Premature ejaculation and intermittent loss of ejaculation	Retrograde or absent ejaculation
Nocturnal penile tumescence		
Total time	> 90–180 min/night	< 60 min/night
Circumferential change	> 2 cm	< 2 cm
Penile brachial index	> 0.70	< 0.60
Bulbocavernosus reflex latency	< 35 msec	> 40 msec

applicable questionnaire for clinical practice is the IIEF (Appendix 1); the Derogatis Interview for Sexual Functioning-Self Report (DISF-SR) (see Appendix 3) is also sometimes used. Since the development of the IIEF, however, most other types of questionnaires have largely fallen out of favor.

International Index of Erectile Function

The IIEF (Appendix 1) is a 15-item multidimensional questionnaire used for the clinical assessment of ED and treatment outcome. Responses are scored using a six-point Likert scale, with "0" indicating a total lack of function or activity and "5" being the highest possible response. The questions cover the following specific domains: erectile function, orgasmic function, sexual desire, intercourse satisfaction, and overall satisfaction (14). A high degree of internal consistency was observed for each of the five domains and for the total scale (Cronbach's α values of 0.73 and higher and 0.91 and higher, respectively) in the populations studied. Test-retest repeatability correlation coefficients for the five domains showed a high degree of sensitivity and specificity for detecting treatment-related changes in patients with ED. This questionnaire has gained widespread use as evidenced by its having been translated into many different languages (14). It has been suggested, however, that the questions are not always fully comprehended by non–English-speaking patients, raising doubts about the universal applicability of the IIEF across cultures (15).

The Sexual Health Inventory for Men (SHIM) (Appendix 2) is an abbreviated version of the IIEF. This concise, five-question assessment can be easily completed in the waiting room, and, as such, it may represent an effective means of screening for ED in order to open the door for discussion between physician and patient. The SHIM was found to detect ED in 72% of urological patients who had not initiated discussion of their sexual problems in the clinic (16).

DISF-SR

The DISF-SR is a brief testing inventory (Appendix 3) that is also designed to provide an estimate of the quality of an individual's current sexual functioning in quantitative terms. The DISF-SR consists of 25 items arranged into five domains of sexual functioning that parallel, to some degree, the phases of the sexual response cycle described by Masters and Johnson (17), i.e., sexual cognition/fantasy, sexual arousal, sexual behavior/experience, orgasm, and sexual drive/relationship. The DISF-SR has distinct, gender-keyed versions for men and women that require between 10 and 15 minutes to complete. This test can also be administered as a semistructured interview (DISF) with the same quantitative estimation for sexual functioning parameters. The DISF-SR total score summarizes the quality of sexual functioning across the five primary domains. Gender-specific norms have been developed for the DISF-SR based on several hundred non-patient community respondents, and, as in the case of DISF, they are represented as standardized area T-scores. Reported internal consistency coefficients range from 0.74 to 0.80, and test–retest coefficients ranged from 0.80 to 0.90 (18).

Other Sexual Questionnaires

The Florida Sexual History Questionnaire consists of 20 multiple-choice items, each having six ordinally scaled response categories. The questions cover areas such as the interest and desire for sexual activity, sexual development, current sexual behavior, and satisfaction with current sexual functioning. A 21st question requests the subject to list prior interventions for his sexual dysfunction. The questionnaire was shown to have high reliability in terms of internal consistency and has been found to differentiate diabetic subjects with ED from nondiabetic controls without ED (19). In a subsequent study, the same group of investigators examined the ability of the questionnaire to discriminate between men with primary psychogenic and primary organic impotence in 53 patients with type 2 diabetes and ED and in 119 non-diabetic men with ED. The correct rate of diagnosis in the diabetic sample was 81% using an eight-item discriminant function and 70% using the total questionnaire score. The rates in the larger nondiabetic sample were lower, but remained significant (73% and 66%, respectively) (20).

Most questionnaires such as those described above tend to focus more on the functional components of ED rather than on the emotional impact on the patient's personal life; Wagner et al. (21) have addressed this issue by creating a scored quality of life questionnaire (Appendix 4). Questionnaires have also been developed to specifically assess other forms of sexual dysfunction such as premature ejaculation and androgen deficiency. A 12-item quality of life self-report was developed to assess the effects of premature ejaculation on an individual in order to provide an alternative measure of improvement other than measuring stopwatch latency (22). This Premature Ejaculation Questionnaire shows potential for use as a diagnostic tool, but still requires further validation. The Androgen Deficiency in Aging Males Questionnaire is a survey that has been shown to correlate with bioavailable testosterone levels with a sensitivity of 88% and a specificity of 60% in patients over 40 years of age (23). Several other questionnaires exist that examine the psychological aspects of sexual dysfunction. (For further information on this topic, see Chapter 24.)

□ PHYSICAL EXAMINATION

Every effort should be made to elicit physical signs of pathology that may be suspected based on information obtained during the clinical history. Evidence of chronic, systemic diseases (hepatic, renal, cardiovascular, endocrine, granulomatous, and neoplastic) must be ruled out, and, if present, the current state of disease control should be determined. For example, if there is a history of diabetes, the patient should be examined for the presence of peripheral neuropathy, autonomic neuropathy, and macro- and microvascular complications. In addition to the general and systemic evaluations, a detailed assessment of gonadal function, vascular competence, neurological integrity, and genital organ normalcy should be performed on every patient. Table 2 lists some common physical signs associated with hypogonadism, vascular, neurological, and local penile disorders.

Endocrine Assessment

Hypogonadism, either primary or secondary, is a major endocrinologic cause of sexual dysfunction. Figure 1 illustrates an algorithmic approach to the work-up and treatment of patients with hypogonadism. Patients with a history of decreased libido, diminished secondary sexual characteristics, developmental disorder, anosmia, headache, visual disturbance, and drug ingestion, or patients with physical signs consistent with hypogonadism or androgen resistance such as abnormal secondary sexual characteristics, decreased testicular size, or abnormal testicular consistency should have bioavailable serum testosterone and luteinizing hormone (LH) measured.

Circulating blood testosterone exists in three states: free, albumin-bound, and sex hormone-binding globulin (SHBG)-bound (25). While it is generally considered that SHBG-bound testosterone is not available for uptake by tissues, opinion is mixed as to whether the biologically active testosterone is restricted to the small quantity of the hormone that is free (approximately 2%) or includes the larger amount of albumin-bound hormone (20–80%). Several investigations suggest that both free and albumin-bound testosterone are biologically available (26–28). The albumin-bound testosterone appears to dissociate freely at the capillary endothelium and liberated testosterone freely enters the interstitial and tissue spaces. It is estimated that approximately 60% to 100% of albumin-bound testosterone is available for tissue uptake (26,29). Measurement of non–SHBG-bound serum testosterone appears to reflect the hormone fraction that is biologically available more accurately than free-testosterone (26,30,31). Under relatively normal conditions, when the only physiological variable is a change in SHBG, free-testosterone concentrations parallel that of albumin-bound; thus, measurement of free-testosterone can adequately reflect androgen action. In some disease states, however (e.g., patients with suspected plasma protein abnormalities such as nephrotic syndrome and cirrhosis of the liver, or those who are undergoing current glucocorticoid administration), free- and albumin-bound testosterone levels do not parallel one another, and the serum free-testosterone concentration may not accurately reflect the endogenous androgen action (26). Therefore, measurement of total testosterone levels should be performed only if the patient is free of conditions that influence serum SHBG and/or albumin concentration or binding activities.

Technically, measurement of bioavailable testosterone is not difficult, since SHBG-bound testosterone is readily precipitated with half-saturation with ammonium sulfate (final concentration, 50%), leaving the non–SHBG-bound testosterone fraction in the supernatant (32); however, this procedure dilutes the concentration of testosterone in the supernatant. A tracer dose of ^{3}H-testosterone can correct the situation (30). The non–SHBG-bound testosterone can then be measured by an immunometric assay with or without solvent extraction and/or chromatography. The free-testosterone level calculated from the total testosterone level and the level of SHBG is an alternative approach, and the correlations are high among this calculated index of bioavailable testosterone, the measured free-testosterone by equilibrium dialysis, and the fractional serum testosterone not precipitated by 50% ammonium sulfate concentration (33).

Patients with primary hypogonadism may provide a history of orchitis, exposure to radiation, or toxins or may exhibit phenotypic signs of inherited disorders. These patients will have high LH and low bioavailable testosterone concentrations (34). Patients with androgen resistance will present with varying degrees of hypoplastic genitalia, lack of secondary sexual characteristics, and/or gynecomastia and feminization. Such conditions are heralded by an elevation in both total (or bioavailable) testosterone and LH (34). In subtle cases of androgen resistance, genital skin biopsy for assessment of receptor number and enzyme activities (5-α-reductase and 3-α-ketoreductase) may be required in order to establish the diagnosis (35).

Patients with secondary hypogonadism, as well as some men with obesity (Fig. 2), advanced age (Fig. 3), or reduced testosterone binding to carrying proteins, may have low total testosterone and LH serum concentrations (36). Normal or slightly depressed bioavailable serum testosterone and LH concentrations are usually found in most subjects with obesity, advanced age, or abnormal sex-hormone–binding proteins (37–44). Aging, growth hormone deficiency, hyperthyroidism, liver disease, and human immunodeficiency virus can all be associated with an increase in SHBG, and consequently a greater reduction in bioavailable than in total testosterone (38,45,46). On the other hand, obesity, hyperinsulinemia, hypercortisolemia, hypothyroidism, or familial disorders of abnormal binding proteins may be associated with decreased SHBG and thus more suppression in total testosterone than in bioavailable testosterone (47). Thus, measurement of bioavailable testosterone is likely to provide a more accurate measure of tissue exposure to testosterone under a variety of physiological and pathophysiologic conditions.

Table 2 Physical Signs that Could Be Found in Men with Sexual Dysfunction

ENDOCRINE	Hypogonadism	Primary	Genital	Small penis and testes, lack of scrotal pigmentation/rugae, small prostate, female escutcheon
			Body build	Delayed bone age, eunuchoid habitus, female fat distribution, decreased muscle mass, cross-hatching of lateral epicanthus skin
			Facial	Absence of terminal hair and temporal hair recession, possible midline defects, hyposmia
			Voice	High-pitched voice
		Secondary	Genital	Normal phallus length, soft testes, small prostate, sparse but normal pubic hair distribution
			Body build	Normal habitus but decreased muscle mass and strength, gynecomastia
			Facial	Decreased rate of beard growth
			Voice	Normal voice tone
	Pituitary tumors			In addition to those under secondary hypogonadism, patient may have: headache, visual field defects, papilledema, acromegalic features, abnormal water metabolism
	Hypothyroidism			Dry skin, puffy face and hands, hoarse/husky voice, loss of the lateral one-third of eye brows, thyroid goiter, delayed relaxation of deep tendon reflexes, myxedema of lower extremities, yellowish-colored skin
	Diabetes mellitus			Retinopathy (background/proliferative), neuropathy (see below), vascular insufficiency (see below)
	Hyperlipidemia			Xanthomas (tendon, tuberous, eruptive, plantar, subperiosteal), xanthelasma, arcus cornea, lipemic retinalis, hepatomegaly
NEUROLOGICAL	Neuropathy			Decreased sensation, motor deficits, changes in deep tendon reflexes, decreased rectal sphincter tone, abnormal bulbocavernosus reflex, orthostasis, neuropathic ulcers, Charcot foot, diabetic amyotrophy, neuropathic cachexia
	Parkinson's disease			Stooped posture, festinating gait, fixed facial expression, rhythmic tremor of limbs that improves with action, cogwheel rigidity of limbs
	Other central nervous system disease			Signs of previous stroke, encephalopathy, spinal cord injury, Alzheimer's disease or Shy–Drager syndrome
VASCULAR				Hypertension, silver-wiring of retinal arteries, signs of carotid/coronary artery disease, decreased femoral, ankle, and penile pulses, reduced penile brachial index to < 0.7, dependent venous rubor, delayed venous filling, change in hair or skin in lower extremities, thickened nails
LOCAL PENILE DISEASE				Hypospadias or other congenital anomalies including tight nonretractable foreskin, short ventral skin due to excessive skin resection during circumcision, phimosis, Plaques or fibrosis in corpora cavernosa, intermittent or persistent priapism (with or without pain), phimosis

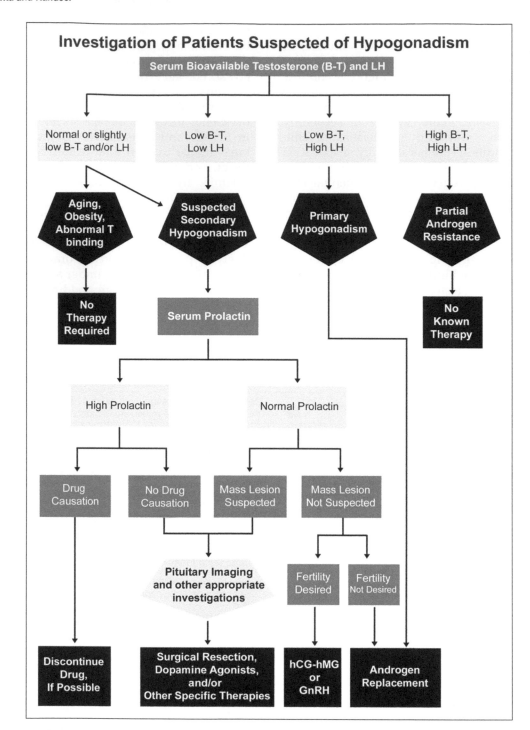

Figure 1 Algorithmic approach for the investigation and treatment of male patients with suspected hypogonadism. Elevated levels of serum B-T and LH concentrations identify patients with androgen resistance, whereas elevated LH and suppressed B-T identify patients with primary hypogonadism. Low-normal or slightly suppressed levels of B-T and/or LH may be found in many subjects with obesity, aging, and/or abnormal T-binding. Clearly suppressed B-T and LH concentrations identify patients with secondary hypogonadism. In such cases, measurement of serum prolactin should be obtained to identify patients with hyperprolactinemia. Treatment option should be selected based on the underlying pathology and the subject's need, as outlined. *Abbreviations*: B-T, bioavailable testosterone; GnRH, gonadotropin-releasing hormone; hCG, human chorionic gonadotropin; hMG, human menopausal gonadotropin; LH, luteinizing hormone; T, testosterone; *Source*: From Ref. 24.

Androgen replacement therapy is usually not required in conditions associated with normal bioavailable or free (but depressed) total testosterone. History, physical signs, and the additional measurement of serum prolactin will help to differentiate many of the subgroups of patients with secondary hypogonadism (low total and bioavailable testosterone and low to normal LH concentrations). Presentation of functional disturbances of the hypothalamic–pituitary unit depends on whether the disorder develops before or after puberty, or closure of the epiphyseal plates of long bones. Congenital defects present with midline facial

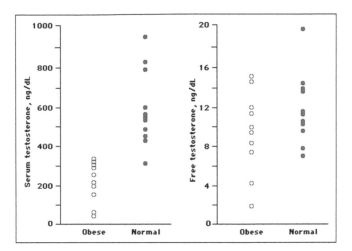

Figure 2 Serum testosterone concentrations in obesity. Obesity is characterized by a reduction in serum total testosterone concentration (*left panel*) but a normal serum free-testosterone concentration (*right panel*) due to diminished protein binding. *Source*: From Ref. 36.

defects, anosmia or hyposmia, sexual immaturity, and/ or linear growth abnormality. Disorders that develop after sexual maturation may present with a subtle change in physical well-being, such as change in the rate of facial hair growth, gynecomastia, fatigue and lack of stamina, or the mere decrease in sexual desire. Patients with mass lesions usually present with a history of headache, visual field disturbances, previous

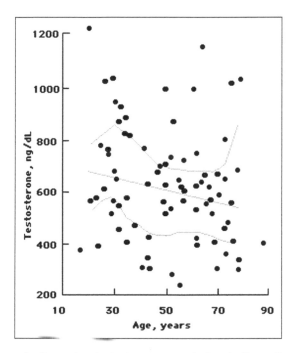

Figure 3 Serum free-testosterone concentration declines with age. The decline in serum free-testosterone with age is more marked than that of the total testosterone concentration. In this study, the serum free-testosterone concentrations of men aged 70 to 80 years were less than half that of men who were 20 to 30 years old. To convert serum free-testosterone values to pmol/L, multiply by 3.47. *Source*: From Ref. 36.

irradiation to the hypothalamus or the pituitary, or with physical signs of other neurological deficits.

Serum prolactin concentration differentiates between hyperprolactinemia and other disorders of the hypothalamic–pituitary axis. In the latter cases, prolactin is normal or low, but both testosterone (total or non-SHBG-bound) and LH are usually below their respective normal ranges. Patients with hyperprolactinemia have low-normal to suppressed levels of total and bioavailable testosterone, as well as LH concentrations. The hallmark of this condition is the elevation of serum prolactin concentration. Prolactin concentrations in excess of 100 ng/mL are frequently associated with prolactin-producing adenomas (the most common mass lesion abnormality of the pituitary), whereas lower concentrations may be seen in drug-induced or in idiopathic hyperprolactinemia (34). Patients with high prolactin levels without a history of drug intake should have imaging studies of the sella turcica performed to assess for the presence and size of an adenoma. Computerized axial tomography and magnetic resonance imaging are probably the best available techniques. Other conditions of secondary hypogonadism are characterized by normal or low serum prolactin concentration. Further work-up of these patients should be directed toward identification of the primary site of deficiency (pituitary vs. hypothalamus), since this may influence the selection of treatment modality. A recent study reviewed the reproductive hormone parameters in 508 men with sexual dysfunction (48). Serum testosterone data were available for 268 patients and prolactin for 170 patients. Hypogonadism, defined as two total testosterone levels below the lower limit of normal range of the laboratory used (below 300 ng/dL), was found in 42 of 268 patients (15.6%). A history of decreased libido by patient questionnaire and/or physical examination did not predict these cases. A normal free fraction of testosterone saved an unnecessary endocrine evaluation in 50% of patients with low total testosterone. Hyperprolactinemia was noted in only 3 of 170 patients (1.8%). Thus, this study supports the contention that endocrine screening is a necessary part of the evaluation for sexual dysfunction, that the measurement of free fraction (or biologically available) testosterone is helpful in lessening the unnecessary endocrine evaluation in about 50% of patients with reduced total testosterone (due to obesity, aging, or abnormal protein binding of sex hormones, but not due to true hypogonadism), and that measurement of prolactin is only required in some patients with hypogonadism and/or clear history of decreased libido.

Vascular Assessment

A careful vascular assessment should include the palpation of ankle, femoral, and dorsal penile arteries. Penile systolic blood pressure should be determined with a 3 cm blood pressure cuff placed around the base of the penis and a Doppler stethoscope positioned over

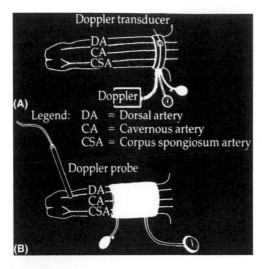

Figure 4 Techniques of penile blood pressure measurement. Schematic diagram for the measurement of penile blood pressure using a Doppler probe and a penile cuff with sphygmomanometer. *Abbreviations*: CA, cavernous artery; CSA, corpus spongiosum artery; DA, dorsal artery.

each cavernosal artery (Fig. 4) (3,4,9,49,50). The penile systolic occlusion pressure is then obtained and compared with that of a brachial artery, and thus a penile brachial index (PBI) is derived (51–54). Values greater than 0.7 are considered normal (52–54). Studies by Chiu et al. (54) suggested that PBI is highly diagnostic in patients with evidence for peripheral vascular disease but no other risk factors such as the presence of diabetes or the current intake of medications with potential adverse effects on erectile function. Further, PBI is less predictive in patients with peripheral vascular disease and diabetes, and least predictive in those without peripheral vascular disease, diabetes, or current drug intake. Repeating the measurements after three to five minutes of gluteal muscle exercise (9,55) may enhance the sensitivity of the test. Reduction in PBI by more than 0.15 is suggestive of redistribution of the blood supply due to shunting away from the arterial penile bed to the gluteal region. Such a phenomenon is characteristic of patients with pelvic steal syndrome (55). Further, the significance of a low PBI may surpass its role in aiding the diagnosis of vasculogenic ED. This is suggested by a prospective study in 130 impotent patients who were followed for 24 to 36 months in which a low PBI (0.65 or less) was shown to predict the occurrence of a future major vascular event (myocardial infarction or cerebrovascular accident) (56). Physical signs of muscular atrophy, pallor, and/or loss of hair growth of the lower extremities are also consistent with vascular pathology. (For further information on vascular investigations of male sexual dysfunction, see Chapter 25.)

Neurological Assessment

Neurologically, the patient should be evaluated for the presence of motor deficits, changes in deep tendon reflexes, loss of sphincter tone, or a decrease in light touch or pinprick sensations, particularly in the genital area. Penile temperature sensation testing could also be done with the use of alcohol swabs (57). In addition, the bulbocavernosus reflex should be elicited by squeezing the glans penis and assessing the evoked contractions of the external anal sphincter or bulbocavernosus muscles (9,58). This reflex response is clinically detectable in 70% of normal males (9). The more sensitive method of penile vibration perception threshold testing (4,9,57,59–61) may confirm results of the bulbocavernosus reflex. Testing of the penile vibration perception threshold is performed by sequentially placing a tuning fork on the glans and bilaterally on the mid-shaft of the penis. Vibration amplitude is then increased until the patient perceives the stimulus. The penis should also be examined for evidence of masses or plaque formation, angulation, unprovoked persistent erection, or tight, unretractable foreskin. (For further details on the neurological evaluations available for male sexual dysfunction, see Chapter 26.)

□ SPECIAL CONSIDERATIONS

Patients with desire disorder, premature ejaculation, and/or postejaculatory pain require a careful assessment of drug use, possible underlying hypogonadism, or the presence of psychological or psychiatric conditions. Patients with hypoactive sexual desire, absent or retarded emission, or anorgasmia may need to be evaluated for the presence of central nervous system disease. Patients with prolonged or painful erection should be evaluated for the possibility of primary penile disease, hematological disorders, or other systemic diseases associated with penile complication, or the intake of pharmacological agents or drugs of addiction that could potentially cause failure of detumescence.

Selective Investigations for Male Sexual Dysfunction

The majority of male patients presenting with sexual dysfunction have problems related to erectile insufficiency. The widespread availability of erectogenic agents such as intrapenile vasoactive drugs (e.g., prostaglandin E1) or oral phosphodiesterase-5 (PDE-5) inhibitors tempts many treating physicians to use them as primary therapeutic modalities without conducting any additional specialized investigations. Although this approach may be suitable for the significant fraction of patients with solely erectile insufficiency, it should be remembered that the potential complications of using erectogenic drugs when contraindicated could be life-threatening, such as when PDE-5 inhibitors are inadvertently administered with nitrates. Further indicating the need to perform the appropriate investigations is the existence of the subset of men with potentially correctable disorders (e.g., psychosexual problems, hypogonadism, treatable chronic illness,

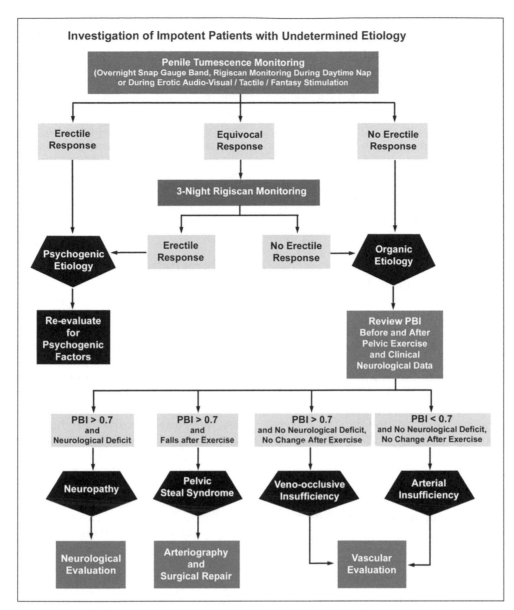

Figure 5 Investigation of erectile dysfunction with undetermined etiology. Algorithmic approach to the investigation of impotent men without hypogonadism or a clear indication for other underlying etiologies. Penile tumescence monitoring with an overnight snap gauge band, or tumescence monitoring during daytime nap or during erotic audio-visual, tactile, and/or fantasy stimulation may be cost-effective screening methods of distinguishing between a primarily organic and a primarily psychogenic dysfunction. Adequate normative data for these procedures are needed and should be established for each individual laboratory. A formal three-night Rigiscan monitoring of nocturnal penile tumescence should be reserved for patients with inconclusive screening test results. Subjects suspected of organic impotence should have the PBI measured before and after pelvic exercise, and neurological history and physical examination findings reviewed. Normal PBI before (>0.7) but not after pelvic exercise suggests a pelvic steal syndrome, a phenomenon that could be treated with surgical revascularization. Abnormally low PBI (<0.7) before and after pelvic exercise suggests arterial insufficiency. Normal PBI before and after exercise argues against arterial insufficiency and instead suggests venous leakage/smooth muscle dysfunction or neuropathy as the underlying cause(s) for impotence. Patients suspected of vascular insufficiency should undergo the appropriate vascular investigations. Presence of neurological deficits by history or on physical examination may help to identify subjects suitable for further neurological evaluation. *Abbreviation*: PBI, penile brachial index. *Source*: From Ref. 24.

and/or correctable vascular insufficiency), as well as those who have a high risk for complications or cannot tolerate the side effects of erectogenic agents (e.g., PDE-5: headache, dyspepsia, changes in vision hue; intraurethral prostaglandin: systemic symptoms; and intrapenile vasoactive injections: penile priapism or fibrosis).

Prior to the commencement of such detailed investigations, however, patients exhibiting clear evidence of chronic organic disease should be evaluated and treated for their primary illness. Those on drug therapy that is likely causing their ED should have these medications changed or discontinued for a trial period while assessing for the return of potency. Discontinuation of substance abuse prior to a full diagnostic work-up is also required. The remaining patients, in whom a history and physical examination are not helpful in identifying any specific etiology, will require an organized multidisciplinary approach involving psychological, endocrine, vascular, and neurological investigations to search for treatable etiologic factors (e.g., psychogenic or psychiatric conditions, hypogonadism, or certain vascular insufficiencies). The investigation may also help in counseling patients with uncorrectable etiologies such as microvascular disease or neurologic deficits. Figure 5 illustrates an algorithmic approach to the investigation of patients presenting with sexual dysfunction of undetermined etiology.

A brief office-based investigation with an assessment of PBI and real-time penile tumescence may be sufficient to corroborate the nature of the sexual deficit with the elicited patient history and physical exam, and thus may be capable of defining an etiologic basis for most male patients with sexual dysfunction and providing the means for treatment. Real-time penile tumescence monitoring can be achieved with the use of a Rigiscan or electrobioimpedance device while the patient is subjected to audio–visual sexual stimulation. This technique may also be helpful in establishing or ruling out psychogenic etiology.

The above view of goal-directed patient work-up is supported by a retrospective correlation study of patient history, nocturnal penile tumescence (NPT), color duplex Doppler ultrasound, and dynamic cavernosometry and cavernosography in 207 patients with ED (62). In this study, 85 out of 207 men (41%) had normal and 122 (59%) had abnormal NPT monitoring. The mean duration of ED was 3.1 months in patients with normal and 15.6 months in patients with abnormal NPT monitoring. Patients with either diabetes mellitus or a history of cigarette smoking were 2.9 times more likely to have organic dysfunction than those without history of diabetes or tobacco use. The presence of positive vascular risk factors increased the likelihood of organic dysfunction by 4.4. NPT monitoring showed normal patterns in 93% of patients with psychogenic etiology, but in only 18% of patients with arteriogenic and 3% of patients with veno-occlusive

disease. Subjective reports of waking and masturbatory erections, however, were poor predictors of outcome in NPT monitoring in men with psychogenic ED. In addition, waking and masturbatory erections were reported in 15% and 7% of men with organic ED (62). Further, normal cavernosal artery peak systolic velocity was observed in 29% of patients with abnormal NPT monitoring. Thus, a single specific modality may not be sufficient for differentiating the various etiologies of ED in a given patient, and the results of more than one modality of investigation may need to be considered if an accurate etiologic diagnosis is to be reached. (For further information on this topic, see Chapter 23.)

□ CONCLUSION

A complete history and physical evaluation remain paramount in the diagnostic work-up of male patients with sexual dysfunction, as symptoms and signs of underlying and correctable endocrine problems may be elicited. Similarly, temporal relationships between the intake of medication and the manifestation of the sexual problem, physical evidence for neurological/ vascular etiologies, and/or indicators of psychiatric/ psychological disorders may be found. Although the availability of effective erectogenic oral drugs such as PDE-5 inhibitors makes it easy for the primary-care physician to institute therapy upon presentation of the problem without adequate consideration of the underlying pathophysiology, such practices should be discouraged. A limited work-up that consists of detailed history-taking and a complete physical examination should always be conducted prior to initiation of treatment. Based on the results of the history-taking and physical exam, specialized investigations may be indicated. Patients refractory to treatment with oral erectogenic drugs may require a more thorough work-up before instituting multiagent, multimodality, or irreversible treatment options.

□ REFERENCES

1. Ginsberg PC, Harkaway RC. Underreporting of erectile dysfunction among men with unrelated urologic conditions. American Urological Association 95th Annual Meeting, Atlanta, GA, April 29–May 4, 2000.

2. Ansong KS, Lewis C, Jenkins P, et al. Help-seeking decisions among men with impotence. Urology 1998; 52(5):834–837.

3. Myer JK. Disorders of sexual function. In: Wilson JD, Foster DW, eds. Williams Textbook of Endocrinology. 7th ed. Philadelphia: WB Saunders Company, 1985:476–491.

4. Krane RJ. Sexual function and dysfunction. In: Walsh PC, Gittes RF, Perfmutter AD, et al., eds. Campbell's Urology. 5th ed. Philadelphia: WB Saunders Company, 1986:700–735.

5. Krane RJ, Goldstein I, Saenz de Tejada I. Impotence. N Engl J Med 1989; 321:1648–1659.

6. Walsh PC, Wilson JD. Impotence and infertility in men. In: Braunwald E, Isselbacher KJ, Petersdorf RS, et al., eds. Harrison's Principals of Internal Medicine. 11th ed. New York: Mc Graw-Hill Book Company, 1987:217–220.

7. NIH Consensus Conference. Impotence. NIH Consensus Development Panel on Impotence. JAMA 1993; 270(1):83–90.

8. O'Keefe M, Hunt DK. Assessment and treatment of impotence. Med Clin North Am 1995; 79(2):415–434.

9. Goldstein I. Impotence. In: Taylor B, ed. Difficult Diagnosis. Philadelphia: WB Saunders Company, 1985: 300–309.

10. Swerdloff RS, Kandeel FR. Approach to sexual dysfunction in the male. In: Kelly WN, ed. Textbook of Internal Medicine. Vol. 2. 2nd ed. Philadelphia: Lippincott Company, 1992:2098–2100.

11. Hawton K. Sex Therapy: A Practical Guide. Oxford, New York: Oxford University Press, 1985.

12. Tiefer L, Schuetz-Mueller D. Psychological issues in diagnosis and treatment of erectile disorders. Urol Clin North Am 1995; 22(4):767–773.

13. Kirby RS. An Atlas of Erectile Dysfunction: An Illustrated Textbook And Reference For Clinicians. New York: The Parthenon Publishing Group, 1998.

14. Rosen RC, Riley A, Wagner G, et al. The international index of erectile function (IIEF): a multidimensional scale for assessment of erectile dysfunction. Urology 1997; 49(6):822–830.

15. Glina S, Mello L, Martins F, et al. International index of erectile function (IIEF): is it a universal tool? Program and abstracts of the 96th Annual Meeting of the American Urological Association, Anaheim, CA, June 2–7, 2001.

16. Diamond SM, Baccarini C, Marmar JL, et al. Erectile dysfunction screening using the sexual health inventory for men questionnaire (SHIM): a novel screening tool. Program and abstracts of the 96th Annual Meeting of the American Urological Association, Anaheim, CA, June 2–7, 2001.

17. Masters WH, Johnson VE. Male sexual response. In: Little Ba C, ed. Human Sexual Response. Boston, 1966:171–220.

18. Derogatis LR. The Derogatis interview for sexual functioning (DISF/DISF-SR): an introductory report. J Sex Marital Ther 1997; 23(4):291–304.

19. Geisser ME, Jefferson TW, Spevack M, et al. Reliability and validity of the Florida sexual history questionnaire. J Clin Psychol 1991; 47(4):519–528.

20. Geisser ME, Murray FT, Cohen MS, et al. Use of the Florida Sexual History Questionnaire to differentiate primary organic from primary psychogenic impotence. J Androl 1993; 14(4):298–303.

21. Wagner TH, Patrick DL, McKenna SP, et al. Cross-cultural development of a quality of life measure for men with erectile difficulties. Qual Life Res 1996; 5(4):443–449.

22. Rosa KR, Rosen RC, Thor KB. Validation of the premature ejaculation questionnaire. Program and abstracts of the 96th Annual Meeting of the American Urological Association, Anaheim, CA, June 2–7, 2001.

23. Morley J, Charlton E, Patrick P, et al. Validation of screening questionnaire for androgen deficiency in aging males. Metabolism 2000; 49(9):1239–1242.

24. Kandeel FR, Koussa VT, Swerdloff RS. Male sexual function and its disorders: physiology, pathophysiology, clinical investigation, and treatment. Endocr Rev 2001; 22(3):342–388.

25. Westphal U. Steroid-Protein Interactions. New York: Springer-Verlag, 1971.

26. Pardridge WM. Serum bioavailability of sex steroid hormones. Clin Endocrinol Metab 1986; 15(2):259–278.

27. Vermeulen A. Transport and distribution of androgens at different ages. In: Martinin L, Motta M, eds. Androgens and Antiandrogens. New York: Raven Press, 1977:53–65.

28. Giorgi E, Moses TF. Dissociation of testosterone from plasma protein during superfusion of slices from human prostate. J Endocrinol 1975; 65(2):279–280.

29. Manni A, Pardridge WM, Cefalu W, et al. Bioavailability of albumin-bound testosterone. J Clin Endocrinol Metab 1985; 61(4):705–710.

30. Cumming DC, Wall SR. Non-sex hormone-binding globulin-bound testosterone as a marker for hyperandrogenism. J Clin Endocrinol Metab 1985; 61(5):873–876.

31. Korenman SG, Stanik-Davis S, Mooradian AD, et al. Evidence for a high prevalence of hypogonadotropic hypogonadism in sexually dysfunctional older men. Clin Res 1987; 35:182A.

32. Tremblay RR, Dube JY. Plasma concentrations of free and non-TeBG bound testosterone in women on oral contraceptives. Contraception 1974; 10(6):599–605.

33. Vermeulen A, Verdonck L, Kaufman JM. A critical evaluation of simple methods for the estimation of free testosterone in serum. J Clin Endocrinol Metab 1999; 84(10):3666–3672.

34. Handelsman DJ, Swerdloff RS. Male gonadal dysfunction. Clin Endocrinol Metab 1985; 14(1):89–124.

35. Price P, Wass JA, Griffin JE, et al. High dose androgen therapy in male pseudohermaphroditism due to 5 alpha-reductase deficiency and disorders of the androgen receptor. J Clin Invest 1984; 74(4):1496–1508.

36. Snyder PJ. Clinical features and diagnosis of male hypogonadism. www.uptodate.com, 2006.

37. Davidson JM, Chen JJ, Crapo L, et al. Hormonal changes and sexual function in aging men. J Clin Endocrinol Metab 1983; 57(1):71–77.

38. Gray A, Feldman HA, McKinlay JB, et al. Age, disease, and changing sex hormone levels in middle-aged men: results of the Massachusetts male aging study. J Clin Endocrinol Metab 1991; 73(5):1016–1025.

39. Erfurth EM, Hagmar LE. Decreased serum testosterone and free triiodothyronine levels in healthy middle-aged men indicate an age effect at the pituitary level. Eur J Endocrinol 1995; 132(6):663–667.

40. Vermeulen A. Decreased androgen levels and obesity in men. Ann Med 1996; 28:13–15.

41. Sternbach H. Age-associated testosterone decline in men: clinical issues for psychiatry. Am J Psychiatry 1998; 155(10):1310–1318.

42. Glass AR, Swerdloff RS, Bray GA, et al. Low serum testosterone and sex-hormone-binding-globulin in massively obese men. J Clin Endocrinol Metab 1977; 45(6):1211–1219.

43. Tenover JS, Matsumoto AM, Plymate SR, et al. The effects of aging in normal men on bioavailable testosterone and luteinizing hormone secretion: response to clomiphene citrate. J Clin Endocrinol Metab 1987; 65(6):1118–1126.

44. Nahoul K, Roger M. Age-related decline of plasma bioavailable testosterone in adult men. J Steroid Biochem 1990; 35(2):293–299.

45. Korenman SG, Morley JE, Mooradian AD, et al. Secondary hypogonadism in older men: its relation to impotence. J Clin Endocrinol Metab 1990; 71(4): 963–969.

46. Morley JE, Kaiser F, Raum WJ, et al. Potentially predictive and manipulable blood serum correlates of aging in the healthy human male: Progressive decreases in bioavailable testosterone, dehydroepiandrosterone sulfate, and the ratio of insulin-like growth factor 1 to growth hormone. Proc Natl Acad Sci 1997; 94:7537–7542.

47. Giagulli VA, Kaufman JM, Vermeulen A. Pathogenesis of the decreased androgen levels in obese men. J Clin Endocrinol Metab 1994; 79(4):997–1000.

48. Govier FE, McClure RD, Kramer-Levien D. Endocrine screening for sexual dysfunction using free testosterone determinations. J Urol 1996; 156(2 Pt 1):405–408.

49. Benet AE, Melman A. The epidemiology of erectile dysfunction. Urol Clin North Am 1995; 22(4):699–709.

50. Leriche R, Morel A. The syndrome of thrombotic obliteration of the aortic bifurcation. Ann Surg 1948; 127:193–206.

51. Abelson D. Diagnostic value of the penile pulse and blood pressure: a Doppler study of impotence in diabetics. J Urol 1975; 113(5):636–639.

52. Engel G, Burnham SJ, Carter MF. Penile blood pressure in the evaluation of erectile impotence. Fertil Steril 1978; 30(6):687–690.

53. Davis SS, Viosca SP, Guralnik M, et al. Evaluation of impotence in older men. West J Med 1985; 142(4): 499–505.

54. Chiu RC, Lidstone D, Blundell PE. Predictive power of penile/brachial index in diagnosing male sexual impotence. J Vasc Surg 1986; 4(3):251–256.

55. Goldstein I, Siroky MB, Nath RL, et al. Vasculogenic impotence: role of the pelvic steal test. J Urol 1982; 128(2):300–306.

56. Morley JE, Korenman SG, Kaiser FE, et al. Relationship of penile brachial pressure index to myocardial infarction and cerebrovascular accidents in older men. Am J Med 1988; 84:445–448.

57. Goldstein I. Evaluation of penile nerves. In: Tanagho EA, Lue TF, McClure RD, eds. Contemporary Management of Impotence and Infertility. Baltimore: Williams & Wilkins, 1988:70–83.

58. Steers WD. Current perspectives in the neural control of penile erection. In: Lue TF, ed. World Book of Impotence. London/Niigata-Shi: Smith-Gordon/Nishimura, 1992:23–32.

59. Goldstein I. Neurologic impotence. In: Krane RJ, Siroky MB, Goldstein I, eds. Male Sexual Dysfunction. Boston: Little, Brown and Company, 1983:193–201.

60. Padma-Nathan H, Goldstein I, Krane RJ. Evaluation of the impotent patient. Semin Urol 1986; 4(4): 225–232.

61. Padma-Nathan H. Neurologic evaluation of erectile dysfunction. Urol Clin North Am 1988; 15(1):77–80.

62. McMahon CG, Touma K. Predictive value of patient history and correlation of nocturnal penile tumescence, colour duplex Doppler ultrasonography and dynamic cavernosometry and cavernosography in the evaluation of erectile dysfunction. Int J Impot Res 1999; 11(1):47–51.

☐ APPENDIX 1
Individual Items from the International Index of Erectile Function (IIEF) Questionnaire and Response Options (US Version)[a]

Question	Response options
(All questions are preceded by "Over the past 4 weeks")	
1. How often were you able to get an erection during sexual activity?	0 = No sexual activity 1 = Almost never/never 2 = A few times (much less than half the time) 3 = Sometimes (about half the time) 4 = Most times (much more than half the time) 5 = Almost always/always
2. When you had erections with sexual stimulation, how often were your erections hard enough for penetration?	0 = No sexual activity 1 = Almost never/never 2 = A few times (much less than half the time) 3 = Sometimes (about half the time) 4 = Most times (much more than half the time) 5 = Almost always/always
3. When you attempted sexual intercourse, how often were you able to penetrate (enter) your partner?	0 = Did not attempt intercourse 1 = Almost never/never 2 = A few times (much less than half the time) 3 = Sometimes (about half the time) 4 = Most times (much more than half the time) 5 = Almost always/always
4. During sexual intercourse, how often were you able to maintain your erection after you had penetrated (entered) your partner?	0 = Did not attempt intercourse 1 = Almost never/never 2 = A few times (much less than half the time) 3 = Sometimes (about half the time) 4 = Most times (much more than half the time) 5 = Almost always/always
5. During sexual intercourse, how difficult was it to maintain your erection to completion of intercourse?	0 = Did not attempt intercourse 1 = Extremely difficult 2 = Very difficult 3 = Difficult 4 = Slightly difficult 5 = Not difficult
6. How many times have you attempted sexual intercourse?	0 = No attempts 1 = One to two attempts 2 = Three to four attempts 3 = Five to six attempts 4 = Seven to ten attempts 5 = Eleven + attempts
7. When you attempted sexual intercourse, how often was it satisfactory for you?	0 = Did not attempt intercourse 1 = Almost never/never 2 = A few times (much less than half the time) 3 = Sometimes (about half the time) 4 = Most times (much more than half the time) 5 = Almost always/always
8. How much have you enjoyed sexual intercourse?	0 = No intercourse 1 = No enjoyment 2 = Not very enjoyable 3 = Fairly enjoyable 4 = Highly enjoyable 5 = Very highly enjoyable

[a]*Source*: Reproduced with permission from Rosen et al., 1997.

9. When you had sexual stimulation or intercourse, how often did you ejaculate?

0 = No sexual stimulation/intercourse
1 = Almost never/never
2 = A few times (much less than half the time)
3 = Sometimes (about half the time)
4 = Most times (much more than half the time)
5 = Almost always/always

10. When you had sexual stimulation or intercourse, how often did you have the feeling of orgasm or climax?

1 = Almost never/never
2 = A few times (much less than half the time)
3 = Sometimes (about half the time)
4 = Most times (much more than half the time)
5 = Almost always/always

11. How often have you felt sexual desire?

1 = Very low/none at all
2 = Low
3 = Moderate
4 = High
5 = Very high

12. How would you rate your level of sexual desire?

1 = Very dissatisfied
2 = Moderately dissatisfied
3 = About equally satisfied and dissatisfied
4 = Moderately satisfied
5 = Very satisfied

13. How satisfied have you been with your overall sex life?

1 = Very low
2 = Low
3 = Moderate
4 = High
5 = Very high

14. How satisfied have you been with your sexual relationship with your partner?

I = Very low
2 = Low
3 = Moderate
4 = High
5 = Very high

15. How do you rate your confidence that you could get and keep an erection?

1 = Very low
2 = Low
3 = Moderate
4 = High
5 = Very high

☐ **APPENDIX 2ᵃ**

SEXUAL HEALTH INVENTORY FOR MEN

Patient Instructions

Sexual health is an important part of an individual's overall physical and emotional well-being. Erectile dysfunction, also known as impotence, is one type of very common medical condition affecting sexual health. Fortunately, there are many different treatment options for erectile dysfunction. This questionnaire is designed to help you and your doctor identify if you may be experiencing erectile dysfunction. If you are, you may choose to discuss treatment options with your doctor.

Each question has several possible responses. Circle the number of the response that **best describes** your own situation. Please be sure that you select one and only one response for **each question**.

Over the Past 6 Months:

1. How do you rate your <u>confidence</u> that you could get and keep an erection?

Very low	Low	Moderate	High	Very high
1	2	3	4	5

2. When you had erections with sexual stimulation, <u>how often</u> were your erections hard enough for penetration (entering your partner)?

No sexual activity	Almost never or never	A few times (much less than half the time)	Sometimes (about half the time)	Most times (much more than half the time)	Almost always or always
0	1	2	3	4	5

3. During sexual intercourse, <u>how often</u> were you able to maintain your erection after you had penetrated (entered) your partner?

Did not attempt intercourse	Almost never or never	A few times (much less than half the time)	Sometimes (about half the time)	Most times (much more than half the time)	Almost always or always
0	1	2	3	4	5

4. During sexual intercourse, <u>how difficult</u> was it to maintain your erection to completion of intercourse?

Did not attempt intercourse	Extremely difficult	Very difficult	Difficult	Slightly difficult	Not difficult
0	1	2	3	4	5

5. When you attempted sexual intercourse, <u>how often</u> was it satisfactory for you?

Did not attempt intercourse	Almost never or never	A few times (much less than half the time)	Sometimes (about half the time)	Most times (much more than half the time)	Almost always or always
0	1	2	3	4	5

Score _____

Add the numbers corresponding to questions 1–5. If your score is 21 or less, you may want to speak with your doctor.

ᵃ*Source*: Copyright © 1998, Pfizer Inc.

□ APPENDIX 3

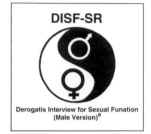

DISF-SR

Derogatis Interview for Sexual Funation (Male Version)[a]

DISF-SR (M)

NAME: _____

DATE: _____

LOCATION: _____

AGE: _____

EDUCATION: _____

ID NO: _____

VISIT NO: _____

Instructions

Below you will find a brief set of questions about your sexual activities. The questions are divided into different sections that ask about different aspects of your sexual experiences. One section asks about <u>sexual fantasies</u> or day-dreams, while another inquires about the kinds of <u>sexual experiences</u> that you have. You are also asked about the nature of your <u>sexual arousal</u> and the quality of your <u>orgasm.</u> There are also a few other questions about different areas of your sexual relationship.

On some questions you are asked to respond in terms of a frequency scale, that is "how often" do you perform the sexual activities asked about in that section. Some frequency scales go from "**0 = not at all**" to "**8 = four or more times a day.**" Other frequency scales range from "**0 = never**" to "**4 = always.**" With other questions, you will be asked to respond in terms of a satisfaction scale. This type of scale tells how much you enjoyed, or were satisfied by the sexual activity being asked about. Some satisfaction scales range from "**0 = could not be worse**" to "**8 = could not be better.**" Other satisfaction scales go from "**0 = not at all satisfied**," to "**4 = extremely satisfied.**"

In every section of the inventory the scales required for that section are printed just above the questions so it will be easy to follow. Although it is brief, take your time with the inventory. **For each item, please circle the scale number that best describes your personal experience.** If you have any questions, please ask the person who gave you the inventory for help.

Section I - Sexual Cognition/Fantasy

During the past **30 days,** or since the last time you filled out this inventory, **how often have you had thoughts, dreams or fantasies about:**

1.1	A sexually attractive person	0	1	2	3	4	5	6	7	8
1.2	Erotic parts of a woman's body (e.g., face, genitals, legs)	0	1	2	3	4	5	6	7	8
1.3	Erotic or romantic situations	0	1	2	3	4	5	6	7	8
1.4	Caressing, touching, undressing, or foreplay	0	1	2	3	4	5	6	7	8
1.5	Sexual intercourse, oral sex, touching to orgasm	0	1	2	3	4	5	6	7	8

Select one: 8 = 4 or more per day, 7 = 2 or 3 per day, 6 = 1 per day, 5 = 4 to 6 per week, 4 = 2 or 3 per week, 3 = 1 per week, 2 = 1 or 2 per month, 1 = less than 1 per month, 0 = Not at all.

Section II - Sexual Arousal

During the past 30 days, or since the last time you filled out this inventory, how often did you have the **following experiences?**

2.1	A full erection upon awakening	0 1 2 3 4 5 6 7 8
2.2	A full erection during a sexual fantasy or daydream	0 1 2 3 4 5 6 7 8
2.3	A full erection while looking at a sexually arousing person, movie or picture	0 1 2 3 4 5 6 7 8
2.4	A full erection during masturbation	0 1 2 3 4 5 6 7 8
2.5	A full erection throughout the phases of a normal sexual response cycle, that is from undressing and foreplay, through intercourse and orgasm	0 1 2 3 4 5 6 7 8

Select one: 8 = 4 or more per day, 7 = 2 or 3 per day, 6 = 1 per day, 5 = 4 to 6 per week, 4 = 2 or 3 per week, 3 = 1 per week, 2 = 1 or 2 per month, 1 = less than 1 per month, 0 = not at all.

Section III - Sexual Behavior/Experiences

During the past 30 days, or since the last time you filled out this inventory, how often did you engage in the **following sexual activities?**

3.1	Reading or viewing romantic or erotic books or stories	0 1 2 3 4 5 6 7 8
3.2	Masturbation	0 1 2 3 4 5 6 7 8
3.3	Casual kissing and petting	0 1 2 3 4 5 6 7 8
3.4	Sexual foreplay	0 1 2 3 4 5 6 7 8
3.5	Sexual intercourse, oral sex, etc.	0 1 2 3 4 5 6 7 8

Select one: 8 = 4 or more per day, 7 = 2 or 3 per day, 6 = 1 per day, 5 = 4 to 6 per week, 4 = 2 or 3 per week, 3 = 1 per week, 2 = 1 or 2 per month, 1 = less than 1 per month, 0 = not at all.

Section IV - Orgasm

During the past 30 days, or since the last time you filled out this inventory, **how <u>satisfied</u> have you been with the following?**

4.1	Your ability to have an orgasm	0 1 2 3 4
4.2	The intensity of your orgasm	0 1 2 3 4
4.3	The length or duration of your orgasm	0 1 2 3 4
4.4	The amount of seminal fluid that you ejaculate	0 1 2 3 4
4.5	Your sense of control (timing) of your orgasm	0 1 2 3 4
4.6	Feeling a sense of relaxation and well-being after orgasm	0 1 2 3 4

Select one: 4 = extremely, 3 = highly, 2 = moderately, 1 = slightly, 0 = not at all.

Section V - Drive/Relationship

5.1 With the partner of your choice, what would be your <u>Ideal</u> frequency of sexual intercourse?

0 1 2 3 4 5 6 7 8

Select one: 8 = 4 or more per day, 7 = 2 or 3 per day, 6 = 1 per day, 5 = 4 to 6 per week, 4 = 2 or 3 per week, 3 = 1 per week, 2 = 1 or 2 per month, 1 = less than 1 per month, 0 = not at all.

5.2 During this period, how interested have you been in sex?

0 1 2 3 4

Select one: 4 = extremely, 3 = highly, 2 = moderately, 1 = slightly, 0 = not at all.

5.3 During this period, how satisfied have you been with your personal relationship with your sexual partner?

0 1 2 3 4

Select one: 4 = extremely, 3 = highly, 2 = moderately, 1 = slightly, 0 = not at all.

5.4 In general, what would represent the best description of the quality of your current sexual functioning?

0 1 2 3 4 5 6 7 8

Select one: 8 = 4 or more per day, 7 = 2 or 3 per day, 6 = 1 per day, 5 = 4 to 6 per week, 4 = 2 or 3 per week, 3 = 1 per week, 2 = 1 or 2 per month, 1 = less than 1 per month, 0 = not at all.

□ APPENDIX 4
Quality of Life and Erectile Dysfunction[a]

Item list

1. I feel frustrated because of my erection problem
2. My erection problem makes me feel depressed
3. I feel like less of a man because of my erection problem
4. I have lost confidence in my sexual ability
5. I worry that I won't be able to get or keep an erection
6. My erection problem is always on my mind
7. I feel that I have lost control over my erections
8. I blame myself for my erection problem
9. I feel angry because of my erection problem
10. I worry about the future of my sex life
11. I have lost pleasure in sex because of my erection problem
12. I am embarrassed about my problem
13. I worry about being humiliated because of my problem
14. I try to avoid having sex
15. I feel different from other men because of my erection problem
16. I get less enjoyment out of life because of my erection problem
17. I feel guilty about my erection problem
18. I am afraid to "make the first move*" towards sex
19. I worry that my partner blames herself for my erection problem
20. I worry about letting her down because of my erection problem
21. I worry that I'm not satisfying her because of my erection problem
22. I worry that we are growing apart because of my erection problem
23. I worry that she is looking for someone else because of my erection problem
24. I feel that she blames me for my erection problem
25. I worry that she thinks I don't want her because of my erection problem
26. I have trouble talking to her about my erection problem
27. My erection problem interferes with my daily activities

---

[a]*Source*: Reproduced with permission from Wagner et al., 1996.

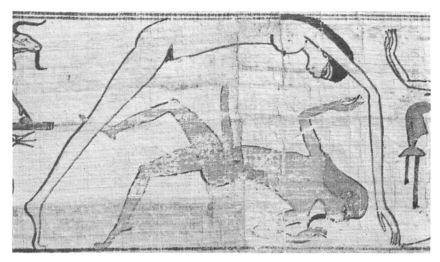

Figure 1.2 Ancient Egypt. God Neb (earth) and goddess Neb (sky).

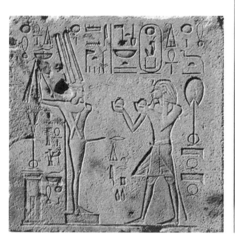

Figure 1.3 Ancient Egypt. Min, god of fertility.

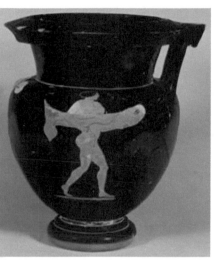

Figure 1.6 Ancient Greece. Hetera (prostitute) carrying large phallus.

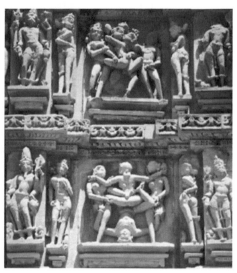

Figure 1.7 India. Erotic reliefs from Indian temple.

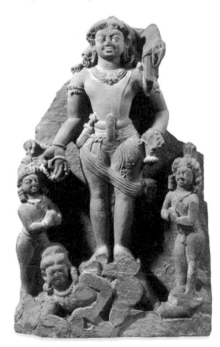

Figure 1.8 India. Male aspect of Shiva.

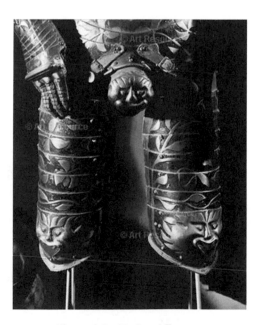

Figure 1.9 Medieval Europe. Elaborate codpiece.

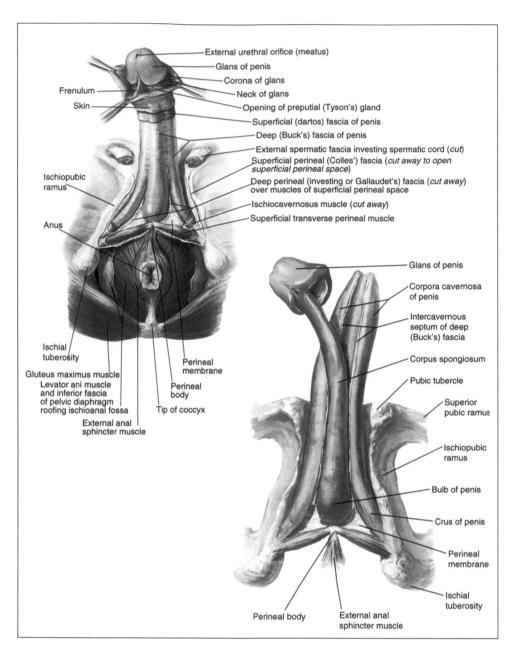

Figure 2.1 Perineum and external male genitalia: deep dissection. *Source*: From Ref. 11. Netter medical illustration used with permission of Elsevier. All rights reserved.

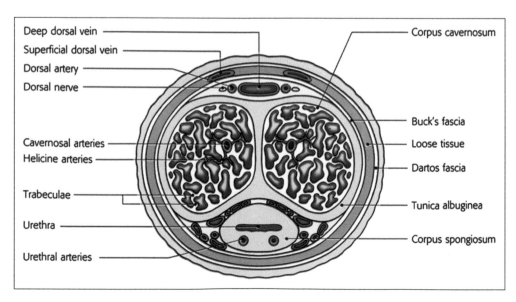

Figure 2.2 Each corpus cavernosum comprises a thick fibrous sheath, the tunica albuginea, which surrounds the erectile tissue. Each corpus has a centrally running cavernosal artery, which supplies blood to the multiple lacunar spaces, which are interconnected and lined by vascular endothelium. *Source*: From Ref. 10.

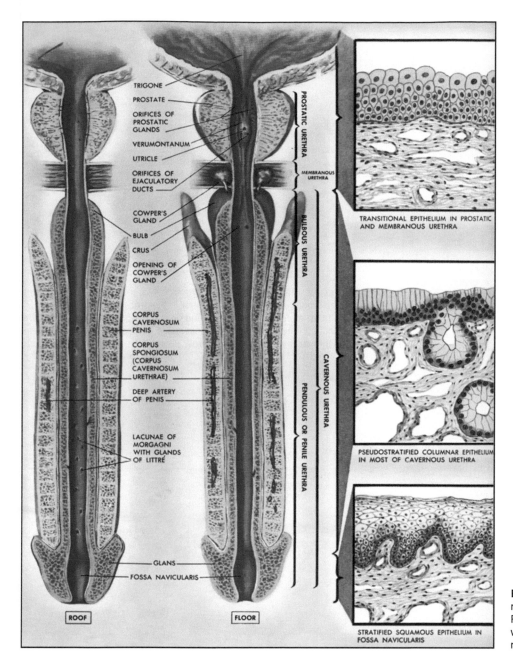

TRIGONE
PROSTATE
ORIFICES OF PROSTATIC GLANDS
VERUMONTANUM
UTRICLE
ORIFICES OF EJACULATORY DUCTS
COWPER'S GLAND
BULB
CRUS
OPENING OF COWPER'S GLAND
CORPUS CAVERNOSUM PENIS
CORPUS SPONGIOSUM (CORPUS CAVERNOSUM URETHRAE)
DEEP ARTERY OF PENIS
LACUNAE OF MORGAGNI WITH GLANDS OF LITTRÉ
GLANS
FOSSA NAVICULARIS

ROOF

FLOOR

PROSTATIC URETHRA

MEMBRANOUS URETHRA

BULBOUS URETHRA

CAVERNOUS URETHRA

PENDULOUS OR PENILE URETHRA

TRANSITIONAL EPITHELIUM IN PROSTATIC AND MEMBRANOUS URETHRA

PSEUDOSTRATIFIED COLUMNAR EPITHELIUM IN MOST OF CAVERNOUS URETHRA

STRATIFIED SQUAMOUS EPITHELIUM IN FOSSA NAVICULARIS

Figure 2.3 Cross-section of the penis: roof and floor views. *Source*: From Ref. 11. Netter medical illustration used with permission of Elsevier.

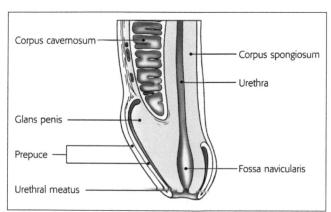

Corpus cavernosum

Corpus spongiosum

Urethra

Glans penis

Prepuce

Fossa navicularis

Urethral meatus

Figure 2.4 Skin overlying the penis is exceptionally mobile and expandable to accommodate the considerable increase in length and girth that occurs during erection. Distally, the penile skin is reflected forward over the glans penis to form the prepuce before folding back on itself to attach to the corona of the glans penis. *Source*: From Ref. 11.

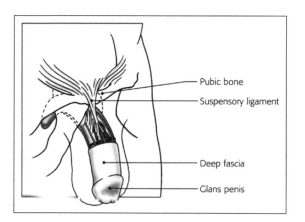

Pubic bone

Suspensory ligament

Deep fascia

Glans penis

Figure 2.5 The pendulous portion of the penis is supported by the suspensory ligament, a fibrous condensation that supports and stabilizes the erect penis. Division of this structure makes the penis appear longer in its flaccid state but does not enhance the proportions of the organ when erect. *Source*: From Ref. 10.

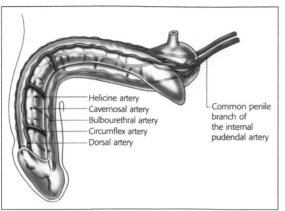

Figure 2.7 Paired dorsal arteries run along the dorsal aspect of the corpora beneath Buck's fascia, giving off multiple circumflex branches and, eventually, supplying blood to the glans penis. The cavernosal arteries run along the middle of each corpus cavernosum, giving off multiple helicine branches that supply blood to the lacunar spaces. *Source*: From Ref. 10.

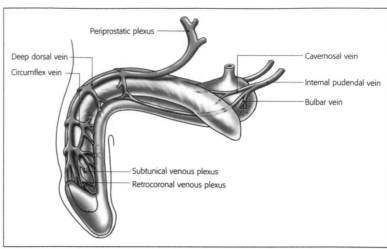

Figure 2.9 Venous drainage from the corpora cavernosa takes place mainly through the deep dorsal vein, which lies dorsally in the groove between the corpora and passes beneath the pubic arch to join the dorsal venous complex at the urethroprostatic junction. The less surgically accessible bulbar and cavernosal veins join to form the internal pudendal vein. *Source*: From Ref. 10.

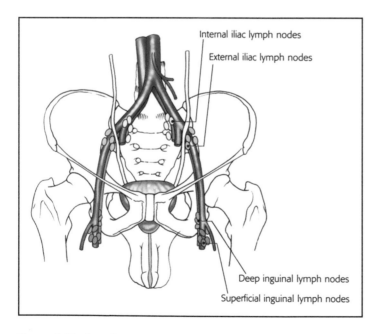

Figure 2.10 Lymphatic drainage of the penis is accomplished by the superficial and deep inguinal nodes, which, in turn, drain into the iliac and para-aortic nodes. *Source*: From Ref. 10.

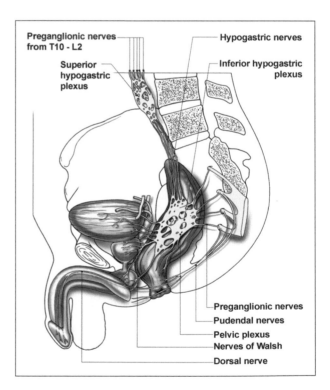

Figure 2.11 The hypogastric nerves are vulnerable during retroperitoneal lymph-node dissection. Both sympathetic and parasympathetic nerves merge in the pelvic plexus and pass posterolaterally to the prostate gland in the so-called bundles of Walsh, where they may be damaged during radical prostatectomy and cystoprostatectomy. *Source*: From Ref. 10.

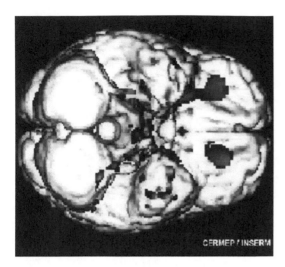

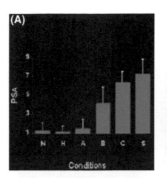

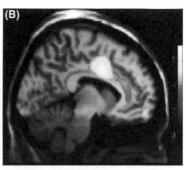

Figure 4.3 View of the inferior surface of the brain showing orbitofrontal activations in both hemispheres. Clusters of voxels with higher regional cerebral blood flow in the sexual condition than in the humor condition. *Source*: From Ref. 8.

Figure 4.4 PSA and rCBF in left anterior cingulate gyrus Means and Standard Deviations of PSA in each condition. Parasagittal section (4 mm left of midline) showing the positive correlation between rCBF in the left anterior cingulate gyrus (Brodmann area 24) and PSA. Height threshold: $z = 3.71$, $p < 0.0001$, uncorrected. Anterior is to the right. *Abbreviations*: PSA, perceived sexual arousal; rCBF, regional cerebral blood flow; N, neutral clips; H, humor clips; S, sexual clips; A, neutral photographs; B, moderately arousing photographs; C, highly arousing photographs. *Source*: From Ref. 8.

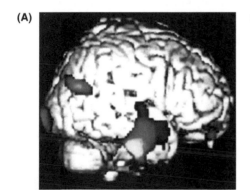

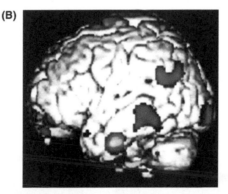

Figure 4.5 Deactivations in temporal regions and in medial orbitofrontal cortex. (A) Left view; anterior is to the right. (B) Right view; anterior is to the left. The most anterior cluster corresponds to the deactivated medial orbitofrontal cortex.

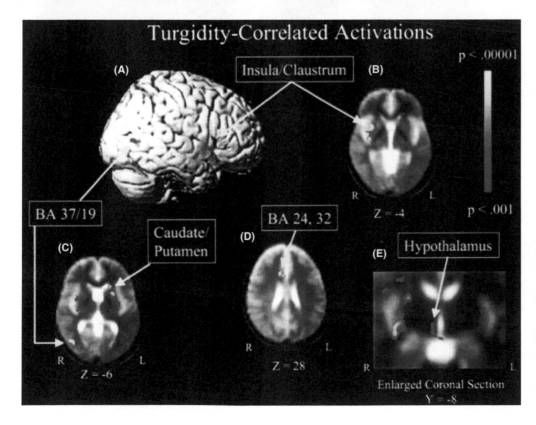

Figure 4.6 Brain regions where activation was correlated with penile tumescence in a group of 11 healthy male volunteers. (A) SPM99 surface reconstruction depicting projections of activation on the right side of the brain. (B) Axial section showing right insula and claustrum activation. (C) Axial section showing left caudate/putamen activation. (D) Right cingulate cortex activation. (E) Right hypothalamus activation. *Source*: From Ref. 10.

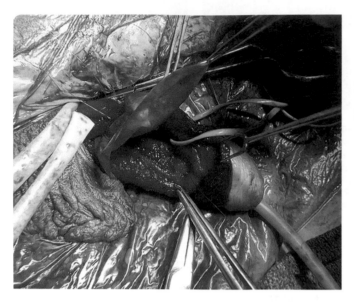

Figure 17.3 Intraoperative depiction of pericardial graft material being sewn in area where Peyronie's plaque has been excised.

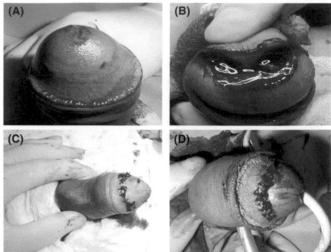

Figure 18.4 Al Gorab shunt. (**A**) Semilunar glanular incision exposing tips of corporal bodies. (**B**) Removal of distal tunica albugineal exposing cavernosal tissue and allowing easy blood drainage. (**C**) Water-tight wound closure. (**D**) Assessment of cavernosal flow using Doppler.

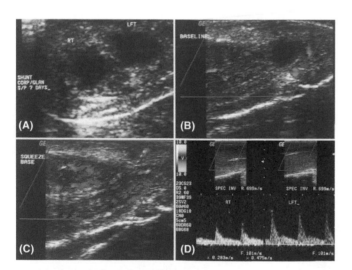

Figure 18.5 Duplex Doppler ultrasound after Al Gorab shunt. (**A**) Gray scale scanning shows surgically removed distal tunical albuginea. (**B**) Color duplex ultrasound demonstrating minimal corporal drainage into the corpus spongiosum. (**C**) Excellent corporal drainage through shunt after manual compression at the base of the penile shaft. (**D**) Duplex Doppler ultrasound documenting reestablishment of cavernosal arterial blood flow.

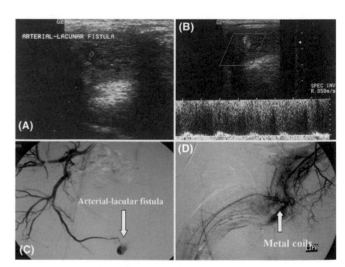

Figure 18.6 Arterial priapism. (**A**) Perineal duplex Doppler ultrasound showing arterial-lacunar fistula. (**B**) Perineal duplex Doppler ultrasound showing arterial-lacunar fistula. (**C**) Selective internal pudendal arteriogram documenting arterial-lacunar fistula. (**D**) Selective internal pudendal arteriogram of an impotent man who developed cavernosal artery insufficiency after coil embolization of high-flow priapism.

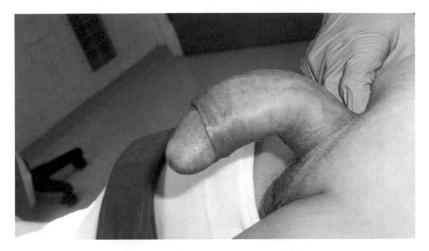

Figure 34.1 Lateral curvature with waist.

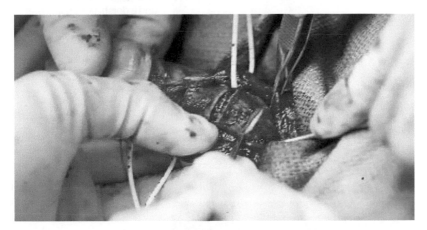

Figure 34.3 Incision of plaque with neurovascular bundle dissected laterally in preparation for graft placement.

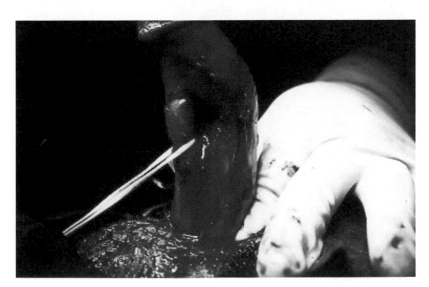

Figure 34.4 Ventral curvature with the urethra dissected.

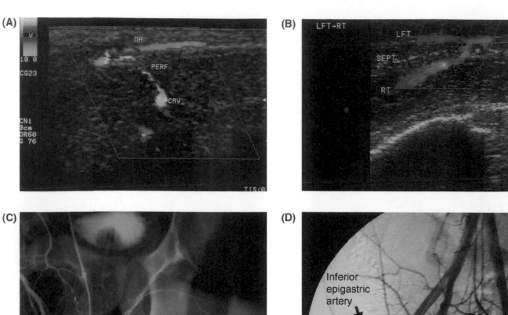

Figure 40.1 Communicating branches from the dorsal artery to the cavernosal artery (**A**) and septal communication (**B**), documented by Penile DDU. Selective internal pudendal arteriogram documenting the obstruction of cavernosal artery and a dorsal perforating branch (**C**) and inferior epigastric artery with good length and no branches (**D**).

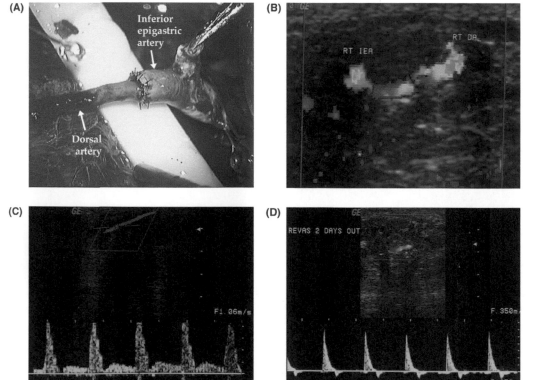

Figure 40.2 (**A**) Microsurgical anastomosis between the inferior epigastric artery and the dorsal artery using an end-to-end technique. Penile duplex Doppler color ultrasound documenting anastomotic patency (**B**) and high peak systolic velocities at anastomosis (**C**, **D**).

Use of Nocturnal and Daytime Penile Tumescence and Rigidity Monitoring for Evaluation of Male Sexual Dysfunction

Robert J. Dimitriou

Michigan Institute of Urology, P.C. Oakwood Hospital, Dearborn, Michigan and Providence Hospital, Novi/Southfield, Michigan, U.S.A.

Carlos R. Estrada

Department of Urology, Children's Hospital Boston and Harvard Medical School, Boston, Massachusetts, U.S.A.

Laurence A. Levine

Department of Urology, Rush-Presbyterian-St. Luke's Medical Center, Chicago, Illinois, U.S.A.

Fouad R. Kandeel

Department of Diabetes, Endocrinology and Metabolism, City of Hope National Medical Center, Duarte, California and David Geffen School of Medicine, University of California, Los Angeles, California, U.S.A.

□ NOCTURNAL PENILE TUMESCENCE

Introduction

Nocturnal penile tumescence (NPT) was first described by Halverson in 1940, and it was Ohlmeyer who suggested in 1944 that abnormalities of this presumed reflex were important factors in erectile dysfunction (ED) (1,2). Normal NPT occurs three to five times per night, and 80% of these erections occur during REM sleep (3,4). The association between NPT and REM stage of sleep was first elucidated in the 1950s, and in 1965, it was suggested that the monitoring of nocturnal erections could aid in the assessment of ED (1,2,5–14). In 1970, Karacan suggested that NPT testing may be useful in distinguishing between organic and psychogenic causes of ED (11). He argued that NPT would be diminished or absent in males with ED due to organic causes such as neurological or vascular factors, since these mechanisms would be present during sleep in normal individuals. He further suggested that psychological factors that inhibit sexually induced erections would be absent during sleep. Nocturnal erections would therefore be present in men with psychogenic causes of ED. Some authors have asserted that NPT testing is the best method to distinguish between organic and psychogenic causes of ED, while others are more cautious and warn that NPT values used alone can be misleading (15,16).

Despite these disparate opinions, nocturnal penile tumescence and rigidity (NPTR) monitoring remains a valuable tool in the evaluation and management of ED. NPTR is an objective, noninvasive measure of erectile activity that can be helpful in differentiating between organic and psychogenic causes of ED. NPTR testing also plays an important role in the assessment of pharmacological therapies and technological advances in the analysis and treatment of ED.

In this chapter, NPT and NPTR testing and results from such tests in normal and impotent men are described. The limitations of NPTR testing are considered, such as the difficulty in establishing the validity of results and normal criteria for sufficient erection. Finally, current recommendations for the use of NPTR testing are given.

NPT and NPTR Testing

Recent investigations into the physiology of nocturnal erections have demonstrated the important role of the locus coeruleus, a nucleus situated in the brainstem that is responsible for physiological responses to stress and panic. During the REM stages of sleep, sympathetic adrenergic tone from the locus coeruleus is diminished. When this occurs, proerectile stimuli from the hypothalamus predominate and NPT occurs (17). A better overall understanding of central nervous system proerectile and inhibitory function will allow better understanding of the pathophysiology of ED and possibly provide information pertinent to future treatments. (For further information on the relationship between the nervous system and erectile function, see chapters 3 and 5.)

NPT testing involves the continuous measurement of penile circumference during sleep and repeated measurements of penile axial rigidity near the time of maximum tumescence. Initially, the change in penile circumference was the sole measurement used to assess the adequacy of an erection: In 1978, Karacan determined that a 20 mm increase in penile circumference represented a full erection and that a 16 mm increase (80% of a full erection) would be sufficient for penetration (12). Several studies have since established, however, that in addition to changes in penile circumference, direct measurement of penile rigidity is also necessary. Earl et al. found that there is a significant disparity between what is considered to be an "adequate erection" depending if the definition is based on changes in measured circumference or the subject's perception of a sufficient erection for penetration during visual sexual stimulation (18). In addition, changes in circumference associated with a full erection are substantially different between patients, further contributing to the need for direct rigidity monitoring.

NPTR testing is often performed in a sleep laboratory with simultaneous monitoring by electroencephalogram, electrooculogram, and electromyogram. Historically, rigidity was measured by applying an external device at the time of full erection, which measured buckling pressure. Karacan suggested that a buckling pressure of 100 mmHg represented a sufficient erection for vaginal penetration and that a pressure of less than 60 mmHg was inadequate for penetration (13). Several limitations and disadvantages to this method have been described. First, buckling pressure is measured as a single isolated event during which detumescence may occur. Second, measurements are subject to observer error. Finally, the use of a sleep laboratory is costly and time-consuming, and the unnatural setting and procedures can cause anxiety, potentially compromising rigidity.

The limitations in NPTR testing have fueled the development of several other methods of monitoring. The practice of placing postal stamps around the base of the penis to examine nocturnal tumescent activity was described by Barry et al. in 1980 (19). In 1982, the snap gauge band device was introduced. This consisted of three preset snap-release fasteners with constant release forces placed around the base of the penis available from Timm Medical Technologies (Eden Prairie, Minnesota, U.S.A.). This method of NPT testing was modified by replacing the fasteners with plastic elements designed to break at 10, 15, and 20 ounces of pressure (20). The snap gauge band devices as well as portable strain-gauge monitors have been shown to correlate well with the results of sleep laboratory NPTR testing (1,21–24).

A limitation of all of these tests, however, is that they do not provide descriptive details of erectile activity such as frequency, duration, and degree of rigidity. This led to the development of small portable monitors, which measure rigidity continuously while recording the number and duration of nocturnal erections. The RigiScan (Timm Medical Technologies) is a home-monitoring device that continuously records penile circumference and rigidity throughout the night (25). It consists of two loops, one placed around the base of the penis and the other at the tip of the penis, proximal to the coronal sulcus, as well as a recording unit that is strapped to the patient's thigh (Fig. 1, *upper panel*). Several measurements occur at prescribed intervals: every 15 seconds, the penile circumference is measured and compared to the patient's baseline reading; every three minutes, rigidity is measured by the application of 2.8 N of radial compression to each loop (determined to be a safe compression force). When the circumference increases by more than 10 mm, rigidity monitoring is increased to every 30 seconds. Rigidity data are expressed as a function of displacement when the loop is tightened around the penis. When no linear displacement occurs, rigidity is 100%; for each 0.5 mm of loop shortening that occurs, the rigidity measurement is decreased by 2.3%. Data can be collected and stored in the RigiScan for three monitoring sessions, each of 10 hours duration. During these sessions, the tumescence, rigidity, and duration of each event are recorded. These data can then be downloaded and printed in graphical and numerical form. The pattern of base and tip tumescence and rigidity over time can then be compiled.

The data collected from the RigiScan are often interpreted through visual analysis of graphic printouts. In an effort to make analysis more objective, Burris et al. developed a quantitative approach using a study of 47 normal men (27). They described an integrated measure of erectile amplitude and duration using area under the curve, which was a highly reproducible method to quantify tumescence and rigidity ($p < 0.001$) and with good correlation between tip and base measurements ($p < 0.001$).

Another method of quantifying RigiScan tumescence and rigidity data was described by Levine and Carroll in 1994 (28). Using an updated version of the RigiScan summary analysis software, the number of erectile events, the cumulative duration of erectile events, the average tumescence and rigidity during each event, and the integrated time-dependent measures of tumescence [tumescence activity units (TAU)] and rigidity [rigidity activity units (RAU)] were analyzed. An erectile event was defined as a 20% increase in base circumference lasting for at least three minutes. To calculate RAU, the minutes spent at a given rigidity level are multiplied by that rigidity level and then summed for the entire erectile event. TAU is calculated similarly, with the duration of an erectile event multiplied by the increase of circumference and then divided by the estimated baseline tumescence. Both base and tip RAU and TAU measurements are collected and evaluated separately. These parameters can then be compared to the percentile distributions of a normal population. NPTR has been frequently used for the evaluation of response to therapeutic interventions for ED (29,30).

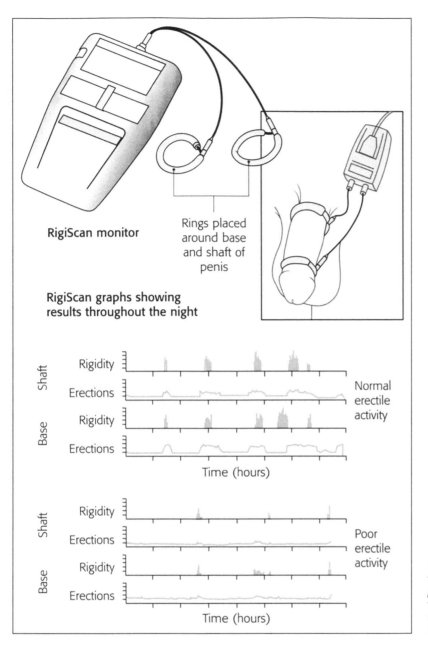

Figure 1 (*Upper panel*) RigiScan ambulatory penile tumescence and rigidity-monitoring device. (*Middle panel*) normal trace of rigidity ("Rigidity") and circumferential expansion ("Erections"). (*Lower panel*) abnormal trace shows poor erectile activity. *Source*: From Ref. 26.

NPTR Monitoring in a Normal Population of Men

The Dacomed Corporation studied over 500 men with ED at the Uro-Center of San Diego in order to provide the first normal criteria for NPTR testing using the RigiScan device (31). Normal results (Fig. 1, *middle panel*) are considered to be three to six erections per eight hours, or an average of 0.375 erections per hour lasting an average of 10 minutes. A normal increase in tumescence for an erectile event was described as a minimum increase of 3 cm at the base and 2 cm at the tip of the penis. Greater than 70% rigidity was considered adequate for vaginal penetration, while less than 40% rigidity represented a flaccid penis. Measures between 40% and 70% correlated with various degrees of penile stiffness and may not predict penile rigidity sufficient for vaginal penetration.

The consideration of 70% rigidity for normalcy of erection and its ability for vaginal penetration proposed by these findings, however, may actually be an overestimate of the necessary amount, as suggested by several later studies. Bain and Guay found that in over 1000 patients with ED, the minimal penile rigidity necessary for vaginal penetration was 60% base rigidity and 50% tip rigidity (32). Ogrinc and Linet found that decreasing the minimal "necessary" tip rigidity from 70% to 60% increased the sensitivity of RigiScan testing from 53.8% to 70.8% (33). In addition, Licht et al. compared RigiScan measurements to the assessment of adequate rigidity by a trained observer in the same evening and concluded that a base rigidity of 55% correlated best with normal rigidity (34). Clearly, further studies are necessary to define "adequate" rigidity for intromission.

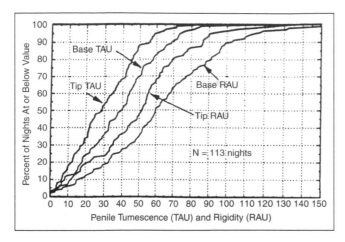

Figure 2 Cumulative distribution of penile tumescence activity (TAU) and rigidity (RAU) from 44 potent men. $N = 113$ nights. Useful for comparison of nocturnal penile tumescence and rigidity results from impotent subjects. *Abbreviations*: RAU, rigidity activity units; TAU, tumescence activity units. *Source*: From Ref. 28.

A nomogram was developed from the 1994 data of Levine and Carroll, which allowed a rapid comparison of NPTR findings (Fig. 2) (28). Data were collected from 44 normal men for three consecutive nights of monitoring, and although there was a high degree of uniformity in the population as a whole, individual responses were varied during the three nights. Six of the 144 men had little or no tip rigidity on at least three nights, suggesting that at least two nights of testing are required for adequate characterization. These results also suggested that significant erectile activity during a single night might be sufficient to demonstrate normal erectile function. Unfortunately, no simple minimal criteria for normal functioning were identified in this study. Parameters such as the minimum number of events, duration of erections, or percentage of rigidity, as previously described, could not provide evidence of normal erectile activity. In this normal patient population, however, tumescence highly correlated with rigidity, and these data were highly reproducible when studied in the same patient over time (27). The initial NPTR pattern was reproducible in 15 of 17 patients, with the two nonreproducible cases being explained by illness and alcohol ingestion.

Erectile activity in aging men has been the subject of numerous studies. Total sleep time and, in particular, the duration of REM sleep have been shown to remain constant in men between the ages of 20 and 50 years. Rigidity, as measured by buckling force, has also been shown to remain constant in men aged 30 to 60 years (35). In contrast, total tumescence time and the average number of erectile episodes have been shown to decrease with age (10,13,14,35–37); however in a study of normal potent men, Levine and Carroll found an increase in the number of nocturnal erectile events with increasing age with an apparent concomitant decrease in the duration of each event with age (28). The discrepancy between

these findings and others may be explained by the definition of a nocturnal erectile event. Levine and Carroll defined an erectile episode as an event lasting for a minimum of three minutes, whereas other studies used five minutes. A slight, but significant, trend toward decreasing tip rigidity with increasing age was also identified, but considerable variability between individual subject responses was noted. Despite these variable findings in aging men, an overall negative trend in nocturnal erectile activity appears to occur with increasing age (Fig. 3).

NPTR Monitoring in Men with ED

NPTR has been named as one of the best available methods to objectively differentiate between organic and psychogenic ED (39–46). Based on history, physical examination, biothesiometry, plethysmography, and psychological testing, a high degree of correlation was found between NPTR results and final diagnosis in a study by Davis-Joseph et al. (47). Data analysis of RigiScan monitoring, however, may be difficult for practicing physicians to interpret. Instead, a visual review of results based on a graphic printout or an assessment of the single best erectile event over the monitoring sessions may be utilized. Kaneko and Bradley have described several NPTR patterns that have been associated with impotence (48). These include dissociation of rigidity between the tip and base of the penis, uncoupling of rigidity and tumescence, a shortened duration of rigidity, low-amplitude rigidity, and lack of rigidity or tumescence. These patterns can be visually recognized (Fig. 1, *lower panel*), but are not easily compared to the results of normal control populations. Dissociation among measurements recorded for penile base and tip appears to be a common occurrence in ED.

Several investigators have suggested that selecting the "best erection" recorded during monitoring may be another method of quantitative classification of ED (7,8,49,50). Sohn et al. have identified a strong

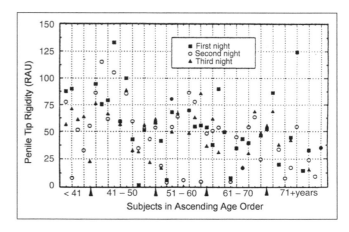

Figure 3 Penile tip rigidity measured by RAU arranged by age in 44 potent men. Note intraindividual variation on a nightly basis, but only slight downward trend of rigidity with increasing age. Abbreviation: RAU, rigidity activity units. *Source*: From Ref. 38.

correlation between NPTR and severity of ED based on the definition of the "best erection" as the erectile event with the highest rigidity and greatest tumescence (50). Another approach selects the best night of erectile activity and uses the tip RAU value to determine the percentile ranking of that patient based on known normal values (41).

The etiology of ED in a given patient can be complex, with combinations of psychogenic and organic causes present. NPTR testing has been extensively studied in the hopes of its application in defining specific subtypes of ED in more detail with mixed results. Shabsigh et al. compared NPT monitoring in 50 patients with ED to results obtained from penile duplex ultrasonography with intracavernous injection of vasoactive drugs (51). Although abnormal NPT results were found in men with vasculogenic impotence and arterial and venous causes were more readily differentiated by ultrasonography with vasoactive injection. NPT testing was more sensitive than duplex ultrasonography, however, in the evaluation of neurogenic causes of impotence. In diabetic men, Bax et al. found a high degree of correlation between penile base tumescence with abnormal cardiovascular tests, somatic tests (vibration perception threshold), and diabetic neuropathy score. NPTR was thus considered to be a useful noninvasive marker in studying parasympathetic damage of the penile region (52).

In contrast, Kirkeby found that NPTR results were normal in 11 of 26 patients with known neurological disorders that affect erectile function (i.e., multiple sclerosis) (53). This study also noted that the absence of sufficient nocturnal erections occurs over several sessions even in normal men, and that the presence of sufficient nocturnal erections proves the capability of having awake erections only in the absence of neurological disorders. When strict criteria were used for a nocturnal event (rigidity greater than 80% and duration greater than 30 minutes), Staerman et al. found that ED in men with multiple sclerosis was not always the result of neurological impairment. They concluded that the differentiation between psychogenic and organic causes of ED was difficult to make in their population of men with multiple sclerosis (54).

McMahon and Touma evaluated the predictive value of patient history and compared RigiScan NPTR with the results of color duplex ultrasonography and dynamic cavernosometry and cavernosography in a retrospective study of men with ED. Normal NPT appeared to correlate well with normal peak systolic velocity (PSV), resistive index (RI), and maintenance flow rate (Q_m). Abnormal NPTR correlated well with abnormal PSV, RI, and Q_m, and had a low false-positive rate of 4% (55).

Montague et al. compared infusion pharmacocavernosometry with NPTR monitoring in 50 patients with ED and concluded that neither method by itself appeared sufficient to make a specific diagnosis of ED (56). Intracorporeal pharmacological (ICP) erection testing has also been compared to NPT in several studies. Allen and Brendler found in their population of 37 men with ED that the response to ICP testing did not distinguish psychogenic from organic ED (57). A thorough NPT evaluation provided an accurate prediction of ICP results; the reverse, however, was not true. Based on these data, they suggested that NPT testing be performed before ICP erection testing to avoid unnecessary and inappropriate treatment of psychogenic impotence. Notably, as with ICP testing, duplex ultrasound also proved unreliable in men with a history of psychogenic illness (58). In a study of 40 men, Allen et al. compared duplex ultrasound to NPT testing and found that anxiety and increased sympathetic stimulation resulted in inaccurate responses to pharmacological stimulation and duplex ultrasound measurements. They concluded that NPT testing should be the preferred testing modality in patients suspected of having a psychogenic cause of ED.

Recently, Montorsi et al. demonstrated that NPT may be enhanced by the oral administration of sildenafil citrate (SC) taken at bedtime (59). Dimitriou, Estrada, and Levine have also demonstrated this in a series of men studied with the RigiScan device for suspected psychogenic ED, in which 77% of men showed a marked increase in NPTR parameters, including RAU, TAU, amplitude, and duration. Neither Dimitriou nor Montorsi's studies demonstrated an increase in the number of erectile events. These findings suggest that if NPTR parameters are enhanced following the administration of SC, then this could be a possible treatment to prevent ED in men at risk of developing the disorder before it manifests. Dimitriou et al. have recently employed this strategy in sexually active men under the age of 60 who have undergone radical prostatectomy and subsequent penile straightening procedure for Peyronie's disease. Theoretically, by enhancing NPT, one would expect better nocturnal oxygenation of erectile tissues, and, therefore, a decreased likelihood of corporeal fibrosis. In addition, the use of SC with NPTR may aid in differentiating between men with psychogenic versus neurogenic ED. Since SC requires intact cavernous nerve function to enhance erections by inhibiting enzymatic degradation of cyclic guanosine monophosphate, those men who demonstrate no change in RAU and TAU parameters when given SC at bedtime would be more likely to have a neurogenic etiology for their ED. On the other hand, men who demonstrate a marked improvement in parameters (especially those who have no neurovascular risk factors for ED) would be thought to have psychogenic factors influencing their ability to have sexually induced erections. Clearly, further investigation is necessary to confirm these hypotheses. (For further information on SC and phosphodiesterase-5 inhibitors, see Chapter 29.)

Limitations of NPT and NPTR Testing

Several fundamental assumptions have been made in the historical use of NPTR testing for the evaluation of

ED. First, it is assumed that the presence of a nocturnal erection indicates the capacity to have an erection while awake. Second, the physiological mechanisms responsible for nocturnal erection are assumed to be similar to those responsible for sexually stimulated erections. Although the latter assumption has been questioned, Krane has suggested that these two types of erections occur through a similar mechanism (60). Third, it is assumed that psychogenic causes of impotence do not interfere with the ability to have a nocturnal erection. It has been demonstrated, however, that dreams containing anxiety, aggression, and other "negative" content are associated with abnormal NPT results (2,6). Depression has also been shown to affect NPT parameters adversely, but these can be restored following successful treatment of the mood disorder (61–63). Furthermore, abnormal NPT results have been found in 15% to 20% of men with no identifiable organic causes of impotence (13). Because of these assumptions, several investigators have questioned the usefulness of NPT testing. Wasserman et al. have stressed that although NPT testing may be useful in differentiating organic from psychogenic causes of ED, NPT testing has never been validated independently of the NPT measurements themselves (64). Other investigators have cautioned that erectile potential in erotic circumstances may not be adequately assessed by NPT testing (16,65).

Additional assumptions required for the validity of NPT testing are that the quality of sleep experienced and the method of testing itself do not impact nocturnal erectile activity. The concept of a "first-night effect" was suggested by a decrease in the number of tumescence episodes, total tumescence time, and quality of erections on the first night of laboratory testing (66). Although it is conceivable that abnormal results could be obtained due to the discomfort associated with the unnatural NPT device, no first-night effect was found in two studies of normal, healthy volunteers using the RigiScan device (27,28). Sleep conditions such as sleep apnea, periodic leg movements, and nocturnal myoclonus can also impact NPT negatively. In these situations, diminished NPT results would most likely not reflect abnormal erectile function (67,68), as it has been suggested that disturbed sleep can inhibit the appearance of spontaneous erections (69). Schiavi et al. has demonstrated, however, that even in normal males with normal sleep patterns, full erections may not occur (70). Because NPT monitoring in a sleep laboratory is expensive and time-consuming and because home-monitoring devices cannot record the quality of sleep, several studies have investigated the potential of monitoring NPT during daytime naps (see below).

Another major difficulty with NPTR testing is the lack of accepted criteria for sufficient rigidity for vaginal penetration. Kirkeby and others have observed that in normal potent males, nocturnal erections fluctuated in rigidity and that at least half were judged to be insufficient for penetration (31). This is in agreement with other studies documenting that only 23% to 48% of nocturnal erections in normal men have sufficient rigidity for intromission (71–73). The difficulty in standardizing the concept of adequate rigidity for vaginal penetration is compounded by variability in the subject's particular partner and situation (i.e., vaginal size, lubrication, and partner receptivity) (74).

A final and important criticism of NPT monitoring is the potential inaccuracy of rigidity measurements. Early methods used parameters such as buckling pressure, which is a measure of applied axial force. In contrast, devices such as the RigiScan measure rigidity as a function of applied radial pressure. Whether radial measures of rigidity are accurate when compared with axial measurements is a matter of debate. Frohib et al. have compared measurements of axial and radial rigidity at constant intracorporeal pressures and found that they were functionally related (75). Further, they correlated with intracavernous pressure, the physiologic event considered responsible for penile rigidity. On the other hand, Munoz et al. found in a study of 17 men with ED that the RigiScan appears to underestimate rigidity at low levels (46). This underestimation could result in men with psychogenic ED being diagnosed with organic ED. In contrast, Allen et al. have found that the RigiScan did not correlate with axial rigidity at high levels (76). This overestimation could result in men with organic ED being assigned a psychogenic cause. A strong correlation between base rigidity and buckling pressure, however, has been found by Licht et al. (34). In that study, it was also noted that tip rigidity correlated poorly with axial measurements. Since it has been found that tip and base rigidity may be dissociated in impotent men, this poor correlation may merely reflect the disease state (48). Udelson et al. further examined the correlation of axial and radial rigidity. In this prospective study, axial buckling force correlated to radial rigidity measured with the RigiScan device during simultaneous pharmacocavernosometry (77). In this study, the axial buckling measurement in an individual was not predicted by RigiScan radial deformation measurement (i.e., rigidity). It was concluded that axial and radial rigidity increased with elevating of intracorporeal pressures at different rates. The explanation for this finding may be related to the fact that axial rigidity is a function of erectile tissue mechanical properties and penile geometry, whereas radial rigidity is a function of tunical surface wall tension.

It is important to bear in mind that, to date, no accepted measures of "intromission pressure" have been accepted, and measurements of axial rigidity continue to be difficult to perform. Since these studies attempted to correlate axial and radial rigidity in populations of men with ED, further studies in normal male populations are needed to determine if these conflicting results are inherent to the RigiScan device or, rather, indicative of ED.

Recommended Use of NPTR Testing

The use of NPT monitoring in all men with ED is subject to debate. In the authors' opinion, NPT testing is most likely not necessary in men with significant organic risk factors associated with ED, such as diabetes mellitus, hypertension, smoking, hyperlipidemia, or vascular disease. On the other hand, men with no known neurovascular disease or men whose history suggests a psychogenic etiology are most likely to benefit from NPTR testing. As an objective measure of erectile function, NPTR should confirm the diagnosis and aid the physician in choosing appropriate therapy. NPTR evaluation may also be helpful in men with Peyronie's disease, who may complain of a poor quality of erections or a softening of erections distal to the plaque—i.e., the penis is less rigid distal to the plaque than it is proximally. (For further information on the history and treatment of Peyronie's disease, see Chapters 17 and 34.)

Since office ICP injection provides quick, inexpensive, and conclusive evidence that a patient is capable of achieving an erection, some have argued that the use of NPTR testing should be limited (78). The injection of a drug to demonstrate that an erection can be induced, however, does not address the patient's concern as to why the problem exists. Therefore, NPT monitoring is recommended to determine the cause of a patient's erectile problems with the view of potentially identifying the most appropriate treatment.

Currently, the authors' approach includes a complete medical history and focused physical examination. NPTR is recommended when a clear psychogenic etiology is present or when neurovascular risk factors are absent. In general, duplex ultrasonography with pharmacological stimulation is performed first in men who present with a more complex history. The possibility of excessive adrenergic tone is suspected in men who present with the following ultrasound pattern: suboptimal mean PSV (less than 30 cm/sec), normal mean end-diastolic flow velocity (less than 5 cm/sec), and a full erectile response to pharmacologic stimulation (79,80). NPTR is also far less invasive and expensive than phalloarteriography or infusion cavernosometry. In addition, NPTR offers more objective evidence to support a recommendation for psychosexual rehabilitation therapy.

In the authors' opinion, the entire pattern of erectile activity, as recorded on one or more nights of study using the RigiScan device, provides a more complete assessment of that individual's nocturnal erectile capacity as compared to the use of the "best erection" criteria. The use of TAU and RAU cumulative data allows comparison. Highest tip RAU on the best night of erectile activity as a percentile ranking of normal data provides the most useful impression of nocturnal erectile function.

Although home monitoring with the RigiScan is simple and less expensive, hospital or sleep laboratory monitoring is suggested in certain circumstances—e.g., when manual dexterity may prevent some patients from properly applying the device or when validity in an unmonitored outpatient setting may be a concern, particularly during medicolegal testing when there is suspicion of either sleep disturbance or malingering.

Conclusion

The authors agree that no single test exists that enables the physician to identify the etiology and degree of ED. NPTR, however, is a valuable resource in differentiating between psychogenic and organic causes of ED. The ultimate goal for the practicing physician in evaluating ED is to provide useful information and to direct that patient to the most appropriate therapeutic options. For many patients, NPTR provides this information in a noninvasive manner.

□ DAYTIME PENILE TUMESCENCE
Introduction

The preceding section clearly illustrates the usefulness of NPT monitoring in the diagnosis of ED. Although NPT monitoring is a reliable means of distinguishing between organic and psychogenic etiologies of ED, the relatively high cost and time-consuming nature of this procedure limits its use in a clinical setting. Several adaptations for NPT monitoring have been developed to reduce the cost of nocturnal sleep laboratory testing and/or to improve the diagnostic efficiency of tumescence monitoring. These include monitoring during (*i*) morning naps preceded by modest sleep deprivation (81,82); (*ii*) audio–visual and/or fantasy stimulation (45,83–89); (*iii*) erectile response to intracavernous vasoactive drug administration with or without audio–visual enhancement (90–92); (*iv*) pulse Doppler analysis of penile arteries with audio–visual enhancement of the erectile response (90,91,93); (*v*) erotic audio–visual enhancement of the erectile response to vibrotactile stimulation (94); and (*vi*) affective and cognitive response to erotic audio and fantasy stimulation (95). These adaptations are outlined below.

Penile Tumescence Monitoring During Morning Naps

At least two preliminary studies in normal healthy men have been reported on penile tumescence monitoring during morning naps preceded by modest sleep deprivation. One study reported sleep efficiency of 92.8% and at least one sleep erection in all seven subjects studied, with a mean penile circumference change of 37.3 mm during three-hour nap monitoring performed after abbreviated night sleep (96). The second study also used three-hour nap monitoring, but performed the penile tumescence twice in 30 healthy men (82). REM sleep was documented in 80% and penile tumescence in 73% of the subjects. Another study compared daytime napping with formal sleep studies in

18 impotent subjects (81). Sixteen subjects had REM sleep during formal sleep studies performed on two nights. Of these, 12 (88%) had documented nocturnal tumescence, and nine of the 12 patients (75%) had nap-time erection. The four patients who failed to have REM-associated NPT also failed to do so during the daytime napping.

Penile Tumescence Monitoring During Audio–Visual and/or Fantasy Stimulation

Real-time tumescence monitoring during audio–visual sexual stimulation has been evaluated for its diagnostic yield in a number of studies. Bancroft et al. (83) employed five periods of sexual stimulation, each lasting for three minutes: two periods of self-recruited sexual fantasy and three periods of video watching of material with explicit sexual content. There was a three-minute recovery separating each two consecutive stimulation periods. Over the experimental period, penile shaft circumference, brachial blood pressure, and dorsal penile artery pulse were monitored in diabetic and nondiabetic impotent men and in nonimpotent controls. The degree of erectile response to viewing of erotic films distinguished between organic and psychogenic etiologies. Severe autonomic neuropathy in the diabetic patients was associated with impaired erectile and penile pulse amplitude responses. Severe retinopathy was associated with smaller baseline penile amplitude as well as smaller amplitude response. Blood pressure response to erotic stimuli did not differ between the three groups. Some of these results were further corroborated by the study of Ali et al. (84) who used the same experimental paradigm in 100 insulin-dependent diabetics and 314 non–insulin-dependent diabetics with and without objective evidence of neuropathy. In this latter study, patients with neuropathy from both groups exhibited a highly significant decrease in penile diameter, length, and penile arterial pulse amplitude compared to nondiabetic controls. The results were at variance with the results of Bancroft et al., however: both systolic and diastolic blood pressure and heart rate also exhibited a significant fall during sexual fantasy and erotic film stimulation. Further, diabetic patients without neuropathy did not differ from controls in all measured parameters. Earl et al. (18) examined the effects of visual sexual stimulation (i.e., 13 minutes of erotic videotape viewing) in 19 normal men. They found 37% of subjects unable to achieve a full erection during visual sexual stimulation under the laboratory conditions. Further, in all but one case, maximal tumescence was recorded polygraphically before the subjects signaled sufficiency of erection for vaginal penetration. Interestingly, there was a considerable delay between the subjects' perception of sufficiency and the perception of full erection despite the fact that there were no changes in tumescence monitoring detected during this latency.

Slob et al. (85) evaluated real-time tumescence monitoring in 58 impotent men during the viewing of an erotic videotape. Forty-one patients (71%) had partial or full penile tumescence, and 15 of these patients had coexisting physical disease commonly implicated in causing erectile insufficiency. Further, in 28 patients who had both NPT and erotic visual stimulation performed, 18 had subjective real-time tumescence comparable to ratings obtained with NPT monitoring; however, five of seven patients who did not respond to visual stimuli had normal NPT recordings, suggesting that a negative response to visual sexual stimulation is not a reliable indicator of sexual dysfunction. In addition, out of 14 patients with negative history for spontaneous morning or nighttime erections, six responded to erotic stimuli, and all seven patients who were monitored for NPT showed a positive response, suggesting that a negative history for NPT may not be a reliable indicator of organic disease. Moreover, six of the patients with a clear-cut increase in penile circumference had no subjective feeling of tumescence, underscoring the complexity of the subject's perception of his erectile capacity.

A much lower rate of positive response to visual sexual stimulation among impotent men was reported in two other studies by Fouda et al. (86) and Djamilian et al. (45), in which more stringent criteria for tumescence and rigidity were used. Fouda et al. (86) reported that only 31 (9%) of 331 patients with erectile insufficiency had an increase in penile circumference greater than 50% when exposed to 10 minutes of erotic visual stimulation. Similarly, Djamilian et al. (45) found only 12 of 160 patients (7.5%) to have a penile rigidity of 70% or greater, lasting for more than five minutes by RigiScan monitoring, when exposed to 30 minutes of audio–visual stimulation. In the latter study, the response rate of penile rigidity was increased to 60% when visual sexual stimulation was preceded by an intracavernous injection of 3 mg papaverine and 0.1 mg phentolamine mixture. Of the 12 subjects with normal real-time RigiScan monitoring before and after the intracavernous drug injection, six had abnormal single potential analysis of cavernous electrical (SPACE) activity, registered with a frequency range between 0.5 and 100 Hz. Of the patients who showed penile rigidity in the postinjection visual stimulation exam, 34 out of 96 (35%) had an abnormal SPACE evaluation, and 18 out of 27 (67%) had an abnormal pharmacocavernosometry evaluation. Of the nonresponders to the visual stimulation before and after the intracavernous injection, 43 out of 52 patients (83%) had abnormal SPACE testing and 19 out of 24 patients (79%) had abnormal pharmacocavernosometry testing.

Based on these results, Djamilian et al. (45) concluded that positive penile rigidity in response to visual stimulation before or after intracavernous injection of vasoactive drugs has a low predictive value for the underlying pathophysiologic abnormality, but may help to assess the therapeutic response to intracavernous injections. Visual sexual testing was also used to evaluate the effect of hypogonadism on the erectile response to erotic stimulation. Although testosterone depletion in young hypogonadal men leads to a decrease in sexual interest and activity (87), the erectile response to visual erotic stimulation was maintained within normal limits and is not further improved with testosterone replacement (97,98). Further, in another small study of 16 patients with prostate cancer, 25% maintained the ability to achieve a functional erection with visual erotic stimulation after orchiectomy (88). Despite the fact that these men had free testosterone levels in the hypogonadal range, their serum free testosterone concentration on average was higher than in other surgically and/or hormonally castrated patients who failed to respond to visual erotic stimulation (88). Collectively, these data tend to suggest that the brain requires exposure to a higher amount of free testosterone to maintain normal sexual desire than that required, if any, for the maintenance of erectile responsiveness to visual erotic stimulation.

One important criticism of visual erotic stimulation testing is the variable preference of different individuals to the nature of erotic material shown and the effect of this on the erectile response. A recent study by Martins and Reis (89) circumvented this concern by asking the patient to select three explicit or semiexplicit erotic videotape segments, each of approximately five minutes length, according to their preference. Various types of sexual stimuli and preferences were represented in the videotape materials used to evaluate 76 impotent men and 20 potent controls. The results of the visual erotic stimulation were related to the clinical diagnosis, intracavernous pharmacological stimulation with 10 µg prostaglandin E_1 (PGE_1), and penile Doppler ultrasound. Visual sexual stimulation test results confirmed the clinical diagnosis in 10 of 14 patients (71%) with psychogenic impotence (71% sensitivity and 96% specificity). The diagnosis of organic dysfunction was correctly related to the results of the RigiScan monitoring in 97% of the cases (97% sensitivity and 71% specificity). Characterization of the etiologic factor underlying the organic dysfunction by the visual erotic stimulation, however, was poor.

Audio–Visual Enhancement of the Erectile Response During Pulse Doppler Analysis of Penile Arteries

Audio–visual sexual stimulation improved vasoactive drug-induced erection in 13 of 25 (52%) patients suspected of having a vascular etiology for their ED, and this was accompanied by a modest increase in peak arterial systolic flow (3.97 cm/sec) and a modest reduction in end-diastolic flow (0.39 cm/sec) of the cavernosal arteries (99). Three of these patients would have been classified as intracorporeal drug nonresponders had they not been subjected to audio–visual stimulation. Similar results were reported in another study in which patients with ED were investigated with visual sexual stimulation alone, intracavernosal vasoactive drug mixture (7.5 mg papaverine and

0.25 mg phentolamine) injection alone, and the combination of erotic visual and intracavernous injection stimulation (90). Of the 90 total patients, 17 (19%) showed adequate erection to visual stimulation, 10 (11%) to intracavernous injection, and 60 (67%) to the combined stimulation. At least two other studies examined the additive effects of audio–visual erotic stimulation to multiple dose intracorporeal vasoactive injections. In the first study, multidose vasoactive drug mix (papaverine HCL, phentolamine mesylate, and PGE-1) induced erectile response in 17 of 33 patients with suspected vascular impotence. When erotic visual stimulation was added, five more patients became responders and seven others improved their erectile response (91). In the second study, multiphasic color Doppler sonography of the cavernous arteries was performed in 50 patients with ED before and after each of two intracavernous injections given alternately with genital stimulation and audio–visual sexual stimulation until an erectile response was obtained, or all phases of testing were completed (93). Genital and audio–visual stimulation improved erectile response to the first vasoactive injection in 41 patients (82%). Genital and audio–visual stimulation also improved the erectile response to the second injection in 11 patients (22%). After the first injection and first erotic stimulation, impotence was presumed to be due to arterial insufficiency in nine (18%), venous incompetence in 17 (34%), mixed arteriovenous disease in 10 (20%), and nonvascular etiology in 14 (28%). After the second injection and erotic stimulation, these diagnoses were cumulatively presumed in 9 (18%), 13 (26%), 10 (20%), and 18 (36%) patients, respectively. Thus, four false-positive cases (8%) of venous insufficiency were identified with the sequential paradigm of testing. It has been postulated that the additive effect of erotic stimulation to that of intracavernosal injection could result from a decrease in the sympathetic discharge to the penis, an increase in the parasympathetic tone, and/or an increase in pelvic skeletal muscle tension (93). (For further information on penile pulse Doppler ultrasound evaluations, see Chapter 25.)

Erotic Audio–Visual Enhancement of the Erectile Response to Vibrotactile Stimulation

Janssen et al. (94) studied the erectile response to penile vibrotactile stimulation at a frequency of 50 Hz, with and without audio–visual stimulation, in 50 men with psychogenic ED, 45 men with organic ED, and 50 sexually functional men. All subjects were assigned to diagnostic groups based on independent clinical criteria. The study was performed to test the hypothesis that patients with psychogenic impotence have a centrally mediated inhibition (due to feelings of guilt, hostility, or other nonsexual thoughts) of the erectile response to local genital stimulation, and that such inhibition could be overcome with erotic audio–visual stimulation. Each subject was studied with vibrotactile (two minutes) and erotic film (three minutes) stimulation separately and in combination. Sexually functioning men had higher tumescence changes in response to vibrotactile stimulation than the two patient groups, with the latter groups achieving results that were similar to each other. Patients with organic impotence responded less to visual stimulation alone and to the combined visual and tactile stimulation than the other two groups of subjects. Patients with psychogenic impotence responded less than normally functioning men to combined, but not to erotic-film-only, stimulation. These data support the contention that in neurologically intact men, local reflexogenic and central psychogenic mechanisms act synergistically in the control of penile erections (100–102), and that patients with psychogenic impotence have reduced erectile response to local tactile stimulation and to a lesser degree to audio–visual erotic stimulation. Further, an intense combined stimulation may be required to overcome such inhibition (94).

Affective and Cognitive Response to Erotic Audio and Fantasy Stimulation

Affective and cognitive responses to erotic stimulation were studied in sexually dysfunctional men before and after participation in a sex-therapy program, and their responses were compared to that of a group of functional men (95). A pool of 34 numerically scored (Likert-scaled) items assessing cognition, affect, and perception were administered during a baseline period, and repeated after listening to two erotic audiotapes (seven minutes each) and a self-generated sexual fantasy. Five aggregate indices (sexual arousal, physicality, sensuality, negative affect, and positive affect) differentiated dysfunctional men from controls, and some of the abnormal ratings normalized after therapy (95).

Summary

Daytime tumescence and rigidity monitoring during daytime naps or during audio or audio–visual erotic stimulation offers a low-cost and time-saving testing procedure compared to the lengthy and cumbersome formal laboratory sleep studies. Combining daytime monitoring with other testing modalities, including self-generated sexual fantasy, intracavernous vasoactive injections, vibrotactile sensory stimulation, penile pulse amplitude monitoring, and pulse Doppler analysis of cavernosal arteries with or without administration of intracavernous vasoactive drugs, may improve the diagnostic value of this testing procedure and may help with understanding the pathophysiology of a variety of sexual dysfunction states. Several pitfalls of real-time tumescence and rigidity testing in its present form exist, however, and these need to be addressed before a suitable adaptation for general screening could be recommended. These include (*i*) real-time response to erotic stimuli may be adversely influenced by the psychological factors underlying the dysfunction or those related to the testing environment itself; (*ii*) content of the audio–visual material used may not be consistent with the subject's preference, leading to a reduced or absent erectile response; and (*iii*) criteria for normal tumescence and rigidity response to real-time erotic stimulation have not been established or validated. The available data for NPT may not be applicable to real-time monitoring.

□ CONCLUSION

More uniformly accepted standards for both nighttime and day/real-time penile tumescence monitoring need to be developed. A careful medical history and physical examination with basic laboratory tests is currently the recommended initial investigation. The availability of sildenafil may also provide an inexpensive and practical first line of therapy regardless of etiology, and preclude the need to seek more elaborate testing for many males with ED. Despite the lack of these standards and the presence of other problems associated with penile tumescence monitoring described above, daytime penile tumescence monitoring techniques have a significant role in evaluating some patients with sexual dysfunction, particularly when psychological factors are suspected as the cause of the problem. Such patients could initially be evaluated with daytime nap monitoring or erotic audio–visual/tactile/fantasy stimulation monitoring. If adequate erection is obtained, then the patient may be presumed to have a significant psychogenic component contributing to his dysfunction. Patients without adequate erection and who desire the full evaluation should then have a formal three-night Rigiscan monitoring. Subjects who fail to exhibit an erection should have their information on penile-brachial index reviewed and should be considered for the appropriate vascular and/or neurological evaluations.

☐ REFERENCES

1. Halverston HM. Genital and sphincter behavior of the male infant. J Gen Psychol 1940; 56:95.
2. Ohlmeyer P, Brilmayer H, Hullstrung H. Periodishe vorgange im schlaf. Pfugers Arch 1944; 248:559.
3. Fisher C, Gross J, Zuch J. Cycle of penile erections synchronous with dreaming (REM) sleep. Arch Gen Psychiatry 1953; 12:29.
4. Karakan I, Goodenough DR, Shapiro A. Erection cycle during sleep in relation to dream anxiety. Arch Gen Psychiatry 1966; 15:183.
5. Aserinsky E, Kleitman N. Regularly occurring periods of eye motility and concomitant phenomena during sleep. 1953. J Neuropsychiatry Clin Neurosci 2003; 15(4):454–455.
6. Fisher C. Dreaming and sexuality. In: Loewenstein RM, Newman LM, Schur M, eds. Psychoanalysis—A General Psychology. New York: International University Press, 1966:537.
7. Fisher C, Schiavi P, Edwards A. Evaluation of nocturnal penile tumescence in the differential diagnosis of sexual impotence. Arch Gen Psychiatry 1979; 36(4):431.
8. Fisher C, Schiavi P, Lear H. The assessment of nocturnal REM erection in a differential diagnosis of sexual impotence. J Sex Marital Ther 1975; 1(4):277.
9. Karacan I, Williams RL, Thornby JI. Sleep related penile tumescence as a function of age. Am J Psychiatry 1975; 132(9):932.
10. Karacan I, Salis PJ, Thornby JI. The ontology of nocturnal penile tumescence. Waking Sleeping 1976; 1:27.
11. Karacan I. Clinical value of nocturnal erection in the prognosis and diagnosis of impotence. Med Aspects Hum Sex 1970; 4:27.
12. Karacan I, Salis PJ, Ware JC. Nocturnal penile tumescence and diagnosis in diabetic impotence. Am J Psychiatry 1978; 135(2):191.
13. Karacan I, Salis PJ, Williams RI. The role of the sleep laboratory in the diagnosis and treatment of impotence. In: Williams RL, Karacan I, Frazier SH, eds. Sleep Disorders, Diagnosis and Treatment. New York: Wiley, 1978.
14. Karacan I, Hursch CJ, Williams RL. Some characteristics of nocturnal penile tumescence in elderly males. J Gerontol 1972; 27:39.
15. Kessler WO. Nocturnal penile tumescence. Urol Clin North Am 1988; 15(1):81.
16. Morales A, Condra M, Reid K. The role of nocturnal penile tumescence monitoring in the diagnosis of impotence: a review. J Urol 1990; 143:441.
17. Goldstein I. Male sexual circuitry. Sci Am 2000; 70–75.
18. Earl CM, Morales A, Marshall W. Penile insufficiency; an operational definition. J Urol 1988; 139:536.
19. Barry JM, Blank B, Boileau M. Nocturnal penile tumescence monitoring with stamps. Urology 1987; 15(2):171.

20. Ek A, Bradley WE, Krane RJ. Nocturnal penile rigidity measured by the snap-gauge band. J Urol 1983; 129(5):964.
21. Allen J, Ellis D, Carrol JL. Snap gauge band versus multidisciplinary evaluation in impotence assessment. Urology 1989; 34(4):197.
22. Condra M, Fenemore J, Reid K. Screening assessment of penile tumescence and rigidity: clinical test of snap gauge. Urology 1987; 29(3):254.
23. Reid D, Glass CA, Evans CM. Screening impotence by home nocturnal tumescence self-monitoring. Br J Clin Psychol 1990; 29(Pt 4):439.
24. Kenepp D, Gonick P. Home monitoring of penile tumescence for erectile dysfunction. Initial experience. Urology 1979; 14(3):261–264.
25. Bradley WE, Timm GW, Gallagher JM. New method for continuous measurement of nocturnal penile tumescence and rigidity. Urology 1985; 26(1):4.
26. Evans CM, Kell P. Clinical Drawings For Your Patients: Erectile Dysfunction. Oxford: Health Press, 2000:10.
27. Burris AS, Banks SM, Sherins RJ. Quantitative assessment of nocturnal penile tumescence and rigidity in normal men using a home monitor. J Androl 1989; 10(6):492–497.
28. Levine LA, Carroll RA. Nocturnal penile tumescence and rigidity in men without complaints of erectile dysfunction using a new quantitative analysis software. J Urol 1994; 152(4):1103.
29. Dobs AS, Meikle AW, Arver S. Pharmacokinetics, efficacy, and safety of a permeation-enhanced testosterone transdermal system in comparison with bi-weekly injections of testosterone enanthate for the treatment of hypogonadal men. J Clin Endocrinol Metab 1999; 84(10):3469.
30. Meinhardt W, Schmitz PI, Kropman RF. Trazodone, a double-blind trial for the treatment of erectile dysfunction. Int J Impot Res 1997; 9(3):163.
31. RigiScan: Ambulatory rigidity and tumescence system document no. 750-156-0486. Dacomed Corporation, Minneapolis, MN, USA.
32. Bain CL, Guay AT. Classification of sexual dysfunction for management of intracavernous medication-induced erections. J Urol 1991; 146(5):1379.
33. Ogrinc FC, Linet OI. Evaluation of real-time RigiScan monitoring in pharmacological erection. J Urol 1995; 154(4):1356.
34. Licht MR, Lewis RW, Wollan PC. Comparison of RigiScan and sleep laboratory nocturnal penile tumescence in the diagnosis of organic impotence. J Urol 1994; 154:1740.
35. Reynolds CF, Thase ME, Jennings J. Nocturnal penile tumescence in healthy 20 to 59 year olds: a revisit. Sleep 1989; 12(4):368.
36. Kahn E, Fisher C. Amount of REM sleep erection in the healthy aged. Psychophysiology 1968; 5:226.

37. Kahn E, Fisher C. Amount of REM sleep and sexuality in the aged. J Geriatr Psychiatry 1969; 2:181.

38. Levine LA, Lenting EL. Use of nocturnal penile tumescence and rigidity in the evaluation of male erectile dysfunction. Urol Clin North Am 1995; 22(4):775–788.

39. Nofzinger EA, Reynolds CF, Jennings JF. Results of nocturnal penile tumescence studies are abnormal in sexually functional diabetic men. Arch Intern Med 1992; 152(1):114.

40. Van Neuten J, Verheyden B, Van Kamp K. Role of nocturnal penile tumescence and rigidity measurement in the diagnosis of erectile impotence. Eur Urol 1992; 22(2):119.

41. Nofzinger EA, Fasiczka AL, Thase ME. Are buckling force measurements reliable in nocturnal penile tumescence studies? Sleep 1993; 16(2):156.

42. Nofzinger EA, Thase ME, Reynolds CF. Sexual function in depressed men. Assessment by self report, behavioral, and nocturnal penile tumescence measures before and after treatment with cognitive behavior therapy. Arch Gen Psychiatry 1993; 50(1):24.

43. Thase ME, Reynolds CF, Jennings JF. Diminished nocturnal penile tumescence in depression: a replication study. Biol Psychiatry 1992; 31(11):1136.

44. Melman A. The evaluation of erectile dysfunction. Urol Radiol 1988; 10(3):119.

45. Djamilian M, Stief CG, Hartmann U. Predictive value of real-time RigiScan monitoring for the etiology of organogenic impotence. J Urol 1993; 149(5 Pt 2):1269–1271.

46. Munoz MM, Bancroft J, Marshall I. The performance of the Rigiscan in the measurement of penile tumescence and rigidity. Int J Impot Res 1993; 5(2):69–76.

47. Davis-Joseph B, Tiefer L, Melman A. Accuracy of the initial history and physical examination to establish the etiology of erectile dysfunction. Urology 1995; 45(3):498–502.

48. Kaneko S, Bradley WE. Evaluation of erectile dysfunction with continuous monitoring of penile rigidity. J Urol 1986; 136:1026–1029.

49. Wasserman MD, Pollack CP, Speilman AJ. The differential diagnosis of impotence. The measurement of nocturnal penile tumescence. JAMA 1980; 243(20):2038.

50. Sohn MH, Seeger U, Sikora R. Criteria for examiner-independent nocturnal penile tumescence and rigidity monitoring (NPTR): correlations to invasive diagnostic methods. Int J Impot Res 1993; 5(2):59–68.

51. Shabsigh R, Fishman IJ, Scott FB. Evaluation of erectile impotence. Urology 1988; 32(2):88.

52. Bax G, Marin N, Piarulli F. Rigiscan evaluation of specific nervous impairment in patients with diabetes and erectile disorders. Diabetes Care 1998; 21(7):1159.

53. Kirkeby HJ, Poulsen EU, Petersen T. Erectile dysfunction in multiple sclerosis. Neurology 1988; 38(9):1366.

54. Staerman F, Guiraud P, Coeurdacier P. Value of nocturnal penile tumescence and rigidity (NPTR) recording in impotent males with multiple sclerosis. Int J Impot Res 1996; 8(4):241.

55. McMahon CG, Touma J. Predictive value of patient history and correlation of nocturnal penile tumescence, colour duplex Doppler ultrasonography, and dynamic cavernosometry and cavernosography in the evaluation of erectile dysfunction. Int J Impot Res 1999; 11(1):47.

56. Montague DK, Lakin MM, Medendorp S. Infusion pharmacocavernosometry and nocturnal penile tumescence findings in men with erectile dysfunction. J Urol 1991; 145(4):768.

57. Allen RP, Brendler CB. Nocturnal penile tumescence predicting response to intracorporeal pharmacological erection testing. J Urol 1988; 140(3):518.

58. Allen RP, Engel RM, Smolev JK. Comparison of duplex ultrasonography and nocturnal penile tumescence in evaluation of impotence. J Urol 1994; 151(6):1525.

59. Montorsi F, Maga T, Strambi LF, et al. Sildenafil taken at bedtime significantly increases nocturnal erections: results of a placebo-controlled study. Urology 2000; 56(6):906–911.

60. Krane RJ. Sexual function and dysfunction. In: Walsh PC, Gittes RJ, Perlmutter AD, et al. eds. Campbell's Urology, 5th ed. Philadelphia: Saunders, 1986:719.

61. Rose SP, Glassman AH, Walsh BT. Reversible loss of nocturnal penile tumescence during depression: a preliminary report. Neuropsychobiology 1982; 8(6):284.

62. Thase ME, Reynolds CF, Glanz LM. Nocturnal penile tumescence in depressed men. Am J Psychiatry 1987; 144(1):89.

63. Thase ME, Reynolds CF, Jennings JR. Diagnostic performance of nocturnal penile tumescence studies in healthy, dysfunctional (impotent), and depressed men. Psychiatry Res 1988; 26(1):79.

64. Wasserman MD, Pollack CP, Spielman AJ. Theoretical and technical problems in the measurement of nocturnal penile tumescence for the differential diagnosis of impotence. Psychol Med 1980; 42(6):575.

65. Chung WS, Choi HK. Erotic erection versus nocturnal erection. J Urol 1990; 143(2):294.

66. Jovanovic UJ. Der effekt der ersten untersuchungschaft auf die erektionen im schlaf. Psychother Psychosom 1969; 17:295.

67. Pressman MR, Fry JM, DiPhillipo MA. Avoiding false-positive findings in measuring nocturnal penile tumescence. Urology 1989; 34(5):297.

68. Pressman MR, Fry JM, DiPhillipo MA. Problems in the interpretation of nocturnal penile tumescence studies: disruption by occult sleep disorders. J Urol 1986; 136(3):595.

69. Bradley WE. New techniques in evaluation of impotence. Urology 1987; 29(4):383.

70. Schiavi RC, Davis DM, Fogel M. Luteinizing hormone and testosterone during nocturnal penile tumescent cycle. Arch Sex Behav 1977; 6(2):97.

71. Weinberg JJ, Badlani GH. Utility of RigiScan and papaverine in diagnosis of erectile impotence. Urology 1988; 31(6):526.

72. Murray FT, Geisser M, Clark RV. Psychological and psychophysiological evaluation in men with diabetes

mellitus and organic impotence [abstr]. J Androl 1994; 14(suppl):55.

73. Wein AJ, Fishkin R, Carpiniello VL. Expansion without significant rigidity during penile tumescence testing: a potential source of misinterpretation. J Urol 1981; 126(3):343.

74. Karacan I, Moore C, Sahmay S. Measurement of pressure necessary for vaginal penetration [abstr]. J Sleep Res 1985; 14:269.

75. Frohib DA, Goldstein I, Peyton TR. Characterization of penile erectile states using external computer-based monitoring. J Biomech Eng 1987; 109(2):110.

76. Allen RP, Smolev JK, Engel RM. Comparison of the RigiScan and formal nocturnal penile tumescence testing in the evaluation of erectile activity. J Urol 1993; 149(5 Pt 2):1265.

77. Udelson D, Park K, Sadeghi-Najed H. Axial penile buckling forces versus RigiScan radial rigidity as a function of intracavernosal pressure: why RigiScan does not predict functional erections in individual patients. Int J Impot Res 1999; 11(6):327.

78. Rajfer J. Impotence—the quick work-up. Editorial. J Urol 1996; 156(6):1942–1946.

79. Levine LA, Carroll RA, Chapman TN. Identification of a new penile duplex ultrasound vascular flow pattern. J Urol 1995; 153:331A.

80. Tomaszewski CS, Carroll RA, Levine LA. Psychogenic impotence evaluated by penile duplex ultrasonography. Proc 69th Ann Western Section Am Urolog Assoc Meet, Palm Desert, CA, 1995.

81. Morales A, Condra M, Heaton JP, et al. Diurnal penile tumescence recording in the etiological diagnosis of erectile dysfunction. J Urol 1994; 152(4):1111–1114.

82. Gordon CM, Carey MP. Penile tumescence monitoring during morning naps to assess male erectile functioning: an initial study of healthy men of varied ages. Arch Sex Behav 1995; 24(3):291–307.

83. Bancroft J, Bell C, Ewing DJ, et al. Assessment of erectile function in diabetic and non-diabetic impotence by simultaneous recording of penile diameter and penile arterial pulse. J Psychosom Res 1985; 29(3):315–324.

84. Ali ST, Shaikh RN, Siddiqi NA, et al. Comparative studies of the induction of erectile response to film and fantasy in diabetic men with and without neuropathy. Arch Androl 1993; 30(3):137–145.

85. Slob AK, Blom JH, van der Werff ten Bosch JJ. Erection problems in medical practice: differential diagnosis with relatively simple method. J Urol 1990; 143(1):46–50.

86. Fouda A, Hassouna M, Beddoe E, et al. Priapism: an avoidable complication of pharmacologically induced erection. J Urol 1989; 142(4):995–997.

87. Luisi M, Franchi F. Double-blind group comparative study of testosterone undecanoate and mesterolone in hypogonadal male patients. J Endocrinol Invest 1980; 3(3):305–308.

88. Greenstein A, Plymate SR, Katz PG. Visually stimulated erection in castrated men. J Urol 1995; 153:650–652.

89. Martins FE, Reis JP. Visual erotic stimulation for initial screening of psychogenic erectile dysfunction: a reliable noninvasive alternative? J Urol 1997; 157(1):134–139.

90. Vruggink PA, Diemont WL, Debruyne FM, et al. Enhanced pharmacological testing in patients with erectile dysfunction. J Androl 1995; 16(2):163–168.

91. Katlowitz N, Albano GJ, Patsias G, et al. Effect of multidose intracorporeal injection and audiovisual sexual stimulation in vasculogenic impotence. Urology 1993; 42(6):695–697.

92. Mills RD, Sethia KK. Maximisation of the erectile response in the investigation of impotence. Int J Impot Res 1999; 11(1):29–32.

93. Montorsi F, Guazzoni G, Barbieri L, et al. The effect of intracorporeal injection plus genital and audiovisual sexual stimulation versus second injection on penile color Doppler sonography parameters. J Urol 1995; 155(2):536–540.

94. Janssen E, Everaerd W, van Lunsen RH, et al. Visual stimulation facilitates penile responses to vibration in men with and without erectile disorder. J Consult Clin Psychol 1994; 62(6):1222–1228.

95. Rowland DL, Cooper SE, Heiman JR. A preliminary investigation of affective and cognitive response to erotic stimulation in men before and after sex therapy. J Sex Marital Ther 1995; 21:3–20.

96. Gordon CM, Carey MP. Penile tumescence monitoring during morning naps: a pilot investigation of a cost-effective alternative to full-night sleep studies in the assessment of male erectile disorder. Behav Res Ther 1993; 31(5):503–506.

97. Bancroft J, Wu FC. Changes in erectile responsiveness during androgen replacement therapy. Arch Sex Behav 1983; 12(1):59–66.

98. Kwan M, Greenleaf WJ, Mann J, et al. The nature of androgen action on male sexuality: a combined laboratory-self-report study on hypogonadal men. J Clin Endocrinol Metab 1983; 57(3):557–562.

99. Katlowitz NM, Albano GJ, Morales P, et al. Potentiation of drug-induced erection with audiovisual sexual stimulation. Urology 1993; 41(5):431–434.

100. Krane RJ, Goldstein I, Saenz de Tejada I. Impotence. N Engl J Med 1989; 321:1648–1659.

101. deGroat WC, Steers WD. Neuroanatomy and neurophysiology of penile erection. In: Tanagho EA, Lue TF, McClure RD, eds. Contemporary Management of Impotence and Fertility. Baltimore: Williams & Wilkins, 1988:3–27.

102. Weiss D. The physiology of human penile erection. Ann Intern Med 1972; 76(5):793–799.

Evaluation of Psychological Functioning in Men with Sexual Dysfunction

Cynthia S. Osborne
Department of Psychiatry and Behavioral Sciences, Johns Hopkins School of Medicine, Baltimore, Maryland, U.S.A.

David L. Rowland
Department of Psychology, Valparaiso University, Valparaiso, Indiana, U.S.A.

□ INTRODUCTION

In this chapter, the rationale and process for carrying out a psychological evaluation on men seeking help for a sexual problem are discussed. The importance of such evaluation depends on a number of factors, including the nature of the sexual problem, the magnitude of presumed psychological concomitants, and the resources available to both the health-care practitioner and the client. Nevertheless, whether the health-care provider is a primary physician, urologist, endocrinologist, sex therapist, or other specialist dealing with sexual problems, at least minimal attention to the psychological health of the client is paramount to achieving a fully integrated approach to treatment. The interaction between psychological factors and elements of the human sexual response has been discussed in Chapter 12. In this chapter, we describe a process for psychosexual and psychological evaluation using both standardized and nonstandardized assessment procedures that can augment the clinician's insight into potential psychological factors that may impact the client's sexual functioning. Advantages and limitations of specific approaches are iterated, and we present examples for incorporating this process into a typical clinic or office visit.

□ RATIONALE

In men, sexual functioning and psychological health are often interrelated. Indeed, the two are bidirectional in nature, with each having the potential to affect the other (1). The psychological evaluation of male sexual dysfunction is based on the assumption that an ongoing process of recursive influence exists between psychological, biological, and relational factors and the sexual problem. By carrying out psychosexual and general psychological evaluations, the clinician is better able to understand whether psychological and relationship factors are causal to physiological sexual dysfunction, including whether they sustain or exacerbate the

dysfunction. Whether considering cause or effect or the mutual and reciprocal flow between the two, one of the immediate goals of psychological evaluation is to determine which factor is primary, and thus where treatment should be focused.

A general psychological evaluation enables the clinician to determine whether coexisting psychological disorders are present. A more detailed psychosexual evaluation assists in determining whether the disorder is linked to sexual functioning and in further assessing whether the psychological processes are the probable cause of the sexual dysfunction, or vice versa. Perhaps equally important, the clinician's attention to psychological and relationship factors permits the patient to explore the nonphysical, but no less salient, dimensions of his sexual response. Whatever the relationship, treatment that addresses the multiple dimensions of sexual response (e.g., physical, affective, cognitive, and relational) will more often than not result in the highest levels of sexual, personal, and relationship satisfaction (2).

Common presentations of psychological factors involved in male sexual dysfunction include distress due to failure to achieve adequate genital response, a complete lack of sexual activity, the perception of decreased excitement, frustration or anxiety secondary to a partner's disappointment, and feelings of inadequacy regarding perceived failure to please a partner. It is arguable that even when the dysfunction can be attributed to a somatic cause, at least a brief psychological evaluation is good practice for every case, based on the following criteria:

- To determine a pretreatment functional baseline
- To determine or rule out the presence or possibility of psychological or relational etiological or contributory factors
- To determine the extent of psychological or relational distress regarding the problem for the patient and/or for his partner
- To determine or rule out the potential usefulness of psychological, behavioral, or relational interventions

as a primary course of treatment or adjunct to a primary medical intervention.

☐ THE EVALUATION PROCESS

The extent to which psychological and dyadic factors (such as those discussed in Chapter 12) require exploration by the clinician will vary according to the manifest etiology of the problem. A man whose problem has a clear somatic etiology (e.g., radical prostatectomy or medication side effect), but who has a healthy, open relationship with his partner, may require a less comprehensive and "integrated" approach than one whose dysfunction is characterized by significant depression and anxiety on his part and/or distress for the partner. One of the major issues for medical staff is that of deciding within the context of an office visit how best to achieve the goals of the patient, what level of assessment is appropriate, and how to obtain relevant information efficiently.

The first task of the clinician in diagnosing a man's sexual dysfunction lies in ensuring an appropriate context for the discussion of the problem. The situation demands that a clinician be comfortable and skilled in the realm of assessing psychological processes and in establishing an atmosphere of candor. It is natural to think that good practice is to tread lightly and carefully through the process of taking a detailed sexual history; however, the clinician should take care to convey, through language and attitude, personal comfort with the subject and confidence that the information being gathered is crucial. This is best accomplished through eye contact, an empathic affect, and asking questions as directly as possible. It is equally important that the clinician convey sensitivity and acknowledge the discomfort that people—patients and clinicians alike—naturally feel when engaged in a detailed discussion of their or someone else's sexual lives. The questions required to complete the assessment inevitably take the physician into the private inner world of the patient's cognitive, affective, and relational vulnerabilities. It might be said that the primary guiding principle for conducting a sound psychological assessment of sexual dysfunction is to "convey comfort with being uncomfortable."

Psychological assessment includes identifying psychopathology. Even in psychologically healthy men with sexual dysfunction, however, assessment is inadequate if it fails to include a formulation regarding the "meaning" the patient attaches to the symptom. Therefore, psychological assessment has to do with identifying the presence or absence of comorbid psychopathology, the reciprocal influence between the problem and the effects of the problem, the cognitive and behavioral patterns associated with the problem, relational patterns—sexual and nonsexual—that contribute to the cause or maintenance of the problem, and the meaning of the problem in the patient's personal and relational life.

While various questionnaires, inventories, and formal measures of sexual and psychological functioning may be used, the assessment process centers around a sound clinical interview, whether brief or comprehensive, regarding the patient's psychosexual history and current functioning. The usefulness of any assessment procedure lies in its potential contribution to the clinician's ability to formulate a clinically useful understanding of the patient's problem and its etiology, to provide clarifying information to the patient and his spouse or partner, to determine a baseline of sexual functioning prior to treatment, and to develop a treatment plan that holds maximum likelihood of success.

We first discuss the clinical interview—both comprehensive and brief formats—as it serves a central assessment function across contexts and disciplines. Although aspects of the clinical interview have been touched upon elsewhere in this book, they are reiterated here in order to present a seamless format that includes both psychosexual and psychological assessment of the patient. Afterwards, we present several specific approaches and tools for psychological and psychosexual assessment of male sexual dysfunction. We have identified a number of questionnaires, inventories, and personality profiles that may enhance the assessment process and that will vary in relevance and potential usefulness depending on the context.

☐ THE CLINICAL INTERVIEW

Decisions regarding the extent of the assessment interview are most naturally determined by the context. While a sex therapist or mental health clinician will benefit from conducting a comprehensive interview, the physician in a primary care or specialty practice will find a brief, focused interview most useful. In either case, the ability to ask focused and direct questions in an efficient manner and the ability to convey sensitivity are essential features of the assessment interview. Furthermore, the professional must decide whether to interview the patient alone, whether to include the spouse or partner, and whether to interview them separately or together. While efficiency often dictates the form, clinicians should consider the potential usefulness of interviewing the partner, even if briefly, to assess the effect of the problem on the relationship, the partner's reaction to the problem, and any contributing factors in the relationship, as well as to provide a reality check to the patient's presentation of the problem. This information will assist the clinician in assessing to what extent it may be useful, critical, or counterproductive to engage the spouse or partner in treatment with the patient.

Several writers have described the structured interview to obtain psychosexual history. Wincze and Carey (3) described a structure—usually requiring an hour with the patient, an hour with the partner, and an hour with the couple together—that categorizes and orders information in the following way:

- Demographics
- The patient's definition of the problem
- Childhood sexual history
- Adolescent sexual history
- Adult sexual history
- Current sexual functioning

Tiefer and Melman (4) describe a similar one-hour interview with the patient and a separate interview with the spouse or partner. These interviews are intended to identify individual and interpersonal themes relevant to diagnosis. The information is gathered in a precise order so as to accumulate information logically. Tiefer and Melman's follow-up studies suggest that treatment compliance is significantly enhanced by including the spouse or partner in the assessment process in this way.

The evaluation template provided in Appendix 1 reflects the comprehensive integrated psychiatric/psychosexual interview format developed over the past 30 years at the Johns Hopkins Sexual Behaviors Consultation Unit (Baltimore, Maryland) and represents the current standard for a comprehensive psychosexual evaluation in a psychiatric setting. This interview format provides a model for the comprehensive integration of the psychiatric and the psychosexual evaluation. Following Tiefer and Melman's advice, this template follows a logical order based on the natural lifeline and the patient's developmental history. The logical ordering of the interview not only gathers data in an organized fashion, but also helps reduce patient anxiety by creating an atmosphere of anticipation as the interview progresses, with the nature of each question making obvious what is likely to be asked next. This is highly preferable to a more random style of interviewing.

In intensive psychiatric settings where comprehensive psychiatric/psychosexual evaluations are conducted for the full range of sexual disorders, the interview may be part of a three- to four-hour evaluation that includes a full patient interview, a separate full interview with the partner, a brief joint interview with the couple, and the administration of several formal measures of behavior and personality. In other settings, the partner interview may be less detailed and focused on the partner's reaction to the problem and availability to engage in treatment with the patient.

To the skilled clinician, there is nothing new in this template—rather, it represents a review of the essential topics covered in the comprehensive interview. To the mental health clinician wanting to develop interview skills, the template serves as a guide for conducting the interview and organizing the data gathered. To the nonpsychiatric physician, it serves as information regarding what might be gained through a referral for a comprehensive psychosexual evaluation. Parts II, III, and IV (i.e., "Chief Complaint,"

"History of the Present Illness," and "Sexual History") can be used as a guide for a brief, focused interview regarding the sexual problem during a medical interview. The interview is not specific to male sexual dysfunction but is applicable across sexual diagnoses, and modifications may be made to draw more detail about a specific area of sexual functioning. By including a sexual history, questions regarding childhood may reveal experiences relevant to the current problem. Eliciting such information can be crucial to an accurate diagnosis and relevant treatment intervention.

Here are two examples of taking case histories.

Case Example I

A male with erectile difficulties described his first masturbation at age 11 as dragging his penis back and forth across the sheets of his bed until he ejaculated. While he could not explain why he engaged in this particular masturbatory behavior, there was little doubt that, since it became his habitual method, by adulthood he had conditioned himself to have profound difficulty engaging in genital sex with a partner. He had difficulty becoming aroused when he experienced the more common shaft-style stimulation of his penis.

Without this information regarding the patient's early sexual history, one might mistakenly assume that a simple medication intervention is adequate. The data gathered from the history informs the clinician that this case requires a behavioral intervention.

Case Example II

A male with erectile difficulties reported that as early as adolescence, his masturbation experiences were accompanied by fantasies of being dominated and humiliated. This paraphilic fantasy, while never acted on, prohibited him from having successful marital sex. Although he could masturbate to ejaculation by engaging in the familiar fantasy, when he engaged in marital sex, he had difficulty attaining high enough levels of arousal for penetration.

Although vasocongestion-enhancing medication might well benefit this patient, psychotherapeutic intervention focusing on the development of skills in the management of sexual urges and fantasies may produce long-term positive outcomes. Further, antidepressant medication may assist this patient in reducing and managing obsessional fantasies and thoughts. Again, his history informs these treatment options.

□ THE BRIEF INTERVIEW

Schnarch (5) described a "Five-Question Evaluation" as a brief interview technique for initial sexual screening in primary-care settings (Table 1). The five questions efficiently elicit details regarding sexual functioning while allowing a gradual exploration and anxiety reduction by inviting the patient to follow the physician's line of thinking. Further, the questions open the

Table 1 Schnarch's Five-Question Evaluation

Are you satisfied with your sex life?
Are you currently active sexually with a partner? If so, what is the approximate frequency of sexual activity? How often do you have difficulty becoming sexually aroused?
Of men: How often do you have difficulty obtaining or maintaining an erection? How often do you have difficulty with control of ejaculation?
Of women: How often do you have pain during intercourse? How often do you have difficulty being orgasmic?
What questions or problems related to sex would you like to discuss?

door to an ongoing discussion, in the physician's office, regarding the patient's sexual issues. The questions are constructed to normalize problematic sexual experiences by implying that most or all people experience sexual problems some of the time. The combined knowledge that having sexual problems is more normal than abnormal and that one's physician or mental health-care provider can talk comfortably about sex can profoundly reduce anxiety in patients. The use of this simple screening tool assists physicians in maximizing the probability that patients will disclose sexual dysfunction during routine office visits. It can easily be adapted and applied in the general mental health professional's practice as well and serves as a guide for integrating questions regarding sexuality into mental health evaluations and therapeutic conversations. If a male patient discloses sexual dysfunction during the screening, it is necessary to continue interviewing the patient to elicit sufficient details for diagnosis.

As an alternative, Milsten and Slowinski (6) have designed a 20-item questionnaire that they recommend for self-evaluation. The questions are brief and focused, and provide an excellent foundation for the in-office interview by a primary-care physician or other provider wanting to quickly elicit details about a patient's sexual functioning.

☐ QUESTIONNAIRES AND PSYCHOMETRIC INSTRUMENTS

Information obtained during either a brief or an extensive evaluation may often be augmented with various paper and pencil instruments. These might be administered prior to the clinic visit if the problem is anticipated at the time of the appointment, during the office visit prior to seeing the professional, or following the visit if there is need for the additional information. Informal questionnaires may be constructed for the convenience of the health care provider to record preliminary perceptions from the patient, which might inform the visit and so make better use of the clinician's and patient's time. Standardized instruments may be administered to obtain a view of the patient's sexual and nonsexual psychological characteristics relative to similar or nonclinical populations. These latter instruments are sometimes copyrighted and therefore may require a nominal charge for use. A brief review of instruments useful in

the evaluation of men seeking help for a sexual problem is provided in the following sections.

Self-Report Questionnaires

Wincze and Carey (3) have outlined the advantages of self-report questionnaires in the assessment of sexual dysfunction. They are easily and inexpensively administered; provide a quick screening that may alert the clinician to areas deserving more detailed attention in an interview; give a dynamic, logically organized picture of the patient's condition; elicit information that might not be easily disclosed in a live interview; can validate or call into question information gathered in the interview; and can be repeated over time in order to track changes during the course of treatment. If a questionnaire has been determined to be sufficiently valid and reliable, it promotes objectivity in the assessment process through comparison of the patient's responses with established norms.

Despite these benefits, the use of questionnaires appears not to be widespread (7,8). Some questionnaires have been developed in conjunction with research projects in which dissemination of the instrument is not one of the project goals. Therefore, the average clinician seeking the use of a good, simple instrument for use in a practice setting may find them difficult to access. All instruments, no matter how valid or reliable, have limitations to their clinical utility. Nearly all are based on data gathered with heterosexual couples. While most instruments can be adapted for use with homosexual couples, it should be remembered that without normative data such assumptions remain untested. Furthermore, while assessment instruments have the advantage of providing very specific data regarding sexual behavior and functioning, there is a risk of using such data in a manner that overemphasizes the mechanical or quantitative aspects of sexual functioning. With reasonable limitations in mind, both the medical and the nonmedical practitioner can use a variety of formal and informal measures, in the domains of sexual and nonsexual functioning as well as individual and relational functioning, to supplement the clinical interview and to conduct a comprehensive and competent assessment.

Peter Fagan of the Sexual Behaviors Consultation Unit at Johns Hopkins in Baltimore, Maryland (personal communication) has devised an informal, self-report questionnaire to assist the clinician in interviewing the male with sexual dysfunction (Appendix 2). The 32 questions in the Male Sexual Dysfunction Interview (MSDI) are useful in assisting the clinician in determining an accurate diagnosis. Because it is common for patients to use inaccurate language when describing the problem, a process for accurately determining the primary problem (for example, between erectile problems and low desire) and for distinguishing between cause and effect is crucial. The MSDI can be self-administered as a brief self-report questionnaire, or the clinician can integrate the questions into the diagnostic interview. The MSDI may be reproduced with the permission of the author (Table 2).

Table 2 Questionnaires and Psychometric Instruments

Male Sexual Dysfunction Interview
Peter Fagan
Johns Hopkins Health care
6704 Cartes Ct.
Glen Burnie, MD 21060 USA
Phone: (410) 583-2688

CMSH Sexual Functioning Questionnaire
The Center for Marital and Sexual Health
3 Commerce Park Square #350
23200 Cahagrin Boulevard
Beachwood, OH 44122-5402 USA
Phone: (216) 831-2900
Fax: (216) 831-4306

Brief Symptom Inventory
National Computer Services
P.O. Box 1416
Minneapolis, MN 55440 USA
Phone: (800) 627-7271
Internet: http://assessment.ncs.com

Derogatis Interview for Sexual Functioning
Clinical Psychometric Research, Inc.
1228 Wind Spring Lane
Towson, MD 21204 USA
Phone: (410) 321-6165
Fax: (410) 321-6341

Golombok Rust Inventory of Sexual Satisfaction
City Psychometrics Ltd.
133 Lauderdale Tower
The Barbican
London EC2Y 8BY United Kingdom
Phone: (44) 207 588 7741
Internet: http://www.citypsychometrics.com

Dyadic Adjustment Scale
Multi-Health Systems, Inc.
908 Niagara Falls Boulevard
North Tonawanda, NY 14120-2060 USA
Phone: (800) 456-3003
Internet: www.mhs.com

Revised NEO-Personality Inventory
Psychological Assessment Resources, Inc
P.O. Box 998
Odessa, FL 33556 USA
Phone: (800) 331-8378

Another tool is the Center for Martial and Sexual Health (CMSH) Sexual Functioning Questionnaire (CMSH-SFQ) developed by Corty, Althof, and Kurit to measure global sexual functioning in men and their partners (9). The authors suggest that the instrument is particularly useful in the assessment of erectile functioning. This instrument is available in baseline and follow-up versions, providing a mechanism for tracking the impact of treatment over time. Only the baseline version has been validated. This 17-item self-report questionnaire is easily completed in less than 10 minutes. This instrument also includes a partner questionnaire, in both baseline and follow-up versions, although the patient version is useful on its own. The CMSH-SFQ is available through its authors (Table 2).

The Use of Formal Measures

In presenting formal screening measures, we emphasize those that are well validated, brief, and practical for the clinical office setting and assess explicit aspects of current sexual and psychological functioning. Some measures are applicable to the individual patient while others examine the patient's relational functioning.

Derogatis et al. (10) described the benefits and limitations of using formal instruments in the evaluation of sexual disorders. The principal benefit is that of quantifying aspects of sexual behavior in order to objectively evaluate the degree of variance from normal functioning. Furthermore, instruments provide adjunct information to clarify data gathered during the interview. For example, a brief, simple questionnaire completed prior to the interview may stimulate a more thorough discussion between professional and patient. For those in research settings or for clinicians who want to track treatment outcomes, formal measures provide essential baseline data and are a crucial component of evaluation.

At the same time, it should be remembered that none of the instruments described are designed to provide an explicit diagnosis. The scores inform the clinician about the patient's functioning in comparison to normative samples. Diagnosis requires a thoughtful consideration of the information gathered during the clinical interview and medical examination, as well as any instrument scores. Further, the lack of empirically determined standards for what constitutes "normal" versus "abnormal" functioning in human sexuality must be considered when interpreting scores from any instrument purporting to measure sexual symptomatology (11). Finally, all of the sexual functioning instruments described have been developed for use with heterosexual men and couples. Although they can be used with homosexual men and couples, claims to validity and reliability are based on heterosexual samples.

Psychological Symptom Measures

Brief, easily administered instruments that measure psychological symptoms provide an objective validation of data gathered in the usually more subjective clinical interview. Once again, the accurate assessment of the presence or absence of depression, anxiety, and other psychiatric symptomatology has significant bearing on the determination of primary and secondary diagnoses and on determining the recommended course of intervention.

An instrument that has been shown to be valid, applicable across a wide variety of contexts and populations is the Brief Symptom Inventory (BSI) (12,13) This is a 53-item, self-report measure of the nature and intensity of acute psychological symptoms across nine dimensions. It is easy to administer, score, and interpret. It provides an objective picture of the presence or absence of psychopathology as well as an overall picture of psychological distress. In the BSI, patients report how much discomfort each item caused them in the past week. The BSI can be self-administered in less than 10 minutes and is easily hand scored. The nine-symptom scales in the BSI include somatization, obsessive-compulsiveness, interpersonal sensitivity, depression, anxiety, hostility, phobic anxiety, paranoid ideation, and psychoticism. The BSI is available for purchase from National Computer Services (Table 2).

SemiStructured Interviews

The Derogatis Interview for Sexual Functioning (DISF) (14) is a relatively brief, gender-keyed instrument that describes the patient's current sexual functioning in five domains that roughly parallel phases of the sexual response cycle: (i) sexual cognition/fantasy, (ii) sexual arousal, (iii) sexual behavior/experience, (iv) orgasm, and (v) sexual drive/relationship. The DISF can be administered in less than 20 minutes by a physician, other clinician, or lay interviewer, and provides an objective measure of the clinical significance of the patient's symptoms compared to normative samples. This instrument is also available in a self-report version (DISF-SR), which may be more practical in some clinical settings where opportunity for a clinician–patient interview time is limited. The instruments and scoring manual can be purchased from Clinical Psychometric Research, Inc. (Table 2).

Dyadic Instruments

The Golombok Rust Inventory of Sexual Satisfaction (GRISS) (15) is a self-report inventory, with male and female versions, that assesses the quality of a heterosexual relationship and of each partner's sexual functioning within the relationship. The inventory generates a profile that assists in identifying behaviors of both partners that may be contributing to sexual dysfunction. It also provides a comparative description of each partner's sexual functioning.

There are 12 subscales in the GRISS. Two are specific to common categories of male sexual dysfunction: premature ejaculation and impotence. The remaining 10 scales target domains such as sexual avoidance, infrequency, dissatisfaction, and noncommunication. A significant benefit of this instrument lies in its exposure of interactive sexual patterns, thus assisting the clinician in developing a meaningful and multifaceted etiological formulation of the problem, emphasizing both individual and relational aspects. The exposure of interactive factors assists in determining the extent to which psychological or relational treatment components may be useful. An obvious limitation of the GRISS is that it can be used only with heterosexual couples. The GRISS can be completed in less than 10 minutes and is easily scored. It is a copyrighted instrument, however, and somewhat expensive; it can be purchased from City Psychometrics Ltd. (Table 2).

The Dyadic Adjustment Scale (DAS) (16) is a 32-item scale that assesses nonsexual interactional problem areas for married or cohabiting couples. It measures overall relationship satisfaction as well as more specific information concerning the major areas that the instrument's authors suggest comprise dyadic adjustment: dyadic consensus, satisfaction, cohesion, and affectional expression. The DAS is an excellent, easily administered instrument that complements

efforts to gather more specific data regarding sexual functioning where more comprehensive assessments are warranted. It can be completed in less than 15 minutes, is easily scored manually or using scoring software, and has been tested for validity and reliability. The DAS and related materials are available through Multi-Health Systems, Inc. (Table 2).

Personality Inventories

The Revised NEO-Personality Inventory (NEO-PI-R) (17) is a self-administered inventory providing a comprehensive assessment of adult personality. It measures five broad personality dimensions: neuroticism (N), extraversion (E), openness (O), agreeableness (A), and conscientiousness (C), and 30 significant personality traits that define those dimensions proposed by the Five Factor Model of Personality. While little has been written about the relationship of personality to sexual dysfunction, this is a highly reliable and valid 240-item instrument that provides a profile of personality factors that may be salient in formulating an understanding of an individual presenting with sexual dysfunction. Such information has the potential to reveal some of the subtle etiological or contributory factors of male sexual dysfunction, which may have significant implications for treatment. The administering of the NEO-PI-R is most likely to take place within a psychiatric setting where comprehensive psychosexual evaluations are conducted. Physicians who desire this level of sophistication in their diagnostic formulations will benefit from a referral resource that includes the option of personality profiling.

The NEO-PI-R is also available in a companion version (Form R) with 240 parallel items written in the third person for peer, spouse, or expert ratings. This can be useful as a way to validate or supplement a patient's self-reports. The NEO-PI-R and related materials can be purchased from Psychological Assessment Resources (Table 2).

☐ FINAL CONSIDERATIONS
Extensiveness of the Evaluation

The challenge to the health care provider, whether physician or therapist, is to ensure adequate assessment resulting in appropriate treatment options and referrals within the constraints of a clinic or medical visit. Fortunately, in many cases, patient self-selection by various types of clinics makes this process easier. For example, urology clinics often draw patients referred by primary physicians who suspect a somatic cause. On the other hand, sex therapy clinics are likely to draw men who view their psychological disposition and/or relationship problems as part of a larger overall problem. The different etiologies of these respective populations suggest that the assessment and treatment will in most cases match the needs and concerns of the clients; however, as sexual problems and their treatments become more medicalized through the application of new pharmacotherapies, it is increasingly probable that the first line of treatment for most men will involve a visit to their family physician or urologist without regard to etiology. As such, the need for familiarity with issues and procedures surrounding sexual response is becoming increasingly important within the medical profession.

Even when extensive evaluation is not possible within the framework of an office visit, a sufficient amount of information can usually be obtained from the patient through the aforementioned procedures to establish whether further assessment or referral is necessary. In addition, an appropriate script and language that opens possible avenues for couples to pursue beyond simple medication is critically important. Indeed, even when indicators suggest minimal or no need for counseling, partner inclusion in the choice and administration of the therapy (whether intracavernosal injection, medication, increased genital stimulation, etc.), openness and communication about sex, and exploration of alternatives to intercourse are typically associated with greater sexual enjoyment and overall satisfaction with treatment (2). Further, medical interventions, even when they lead to improved genital functioning, will be insufficient if relational factors prohibit intimacy and attribution of positive meaning to sexual interaction. Although such goals are generally included among those of counseling and therapy, preliminary inquiry about such issues can serve to destigmatize not only the sexual problem, but also the relevance of seeking counseling for what may be viewed as a further abnormality/deficiency by the patient. Although medical personnel often feel unprepared professionally to address issues regarding the overall quality of sexual interaction, they should be prepared to invite both the patient and his partner to explore a variety of treatment options, including brief individual or couples counseling, as a means of improving their sex life.

Clinical Assessment as Part of a Research Strategy

Important to the advancement of any applied field of study is the systematic collection of information relevant to understanding cause and effect. As such, responses collected as part of a psychosexual assessment procedure provide a wealth of information for understanding of etiology and cause of sexual problems as well as the effectiveness of various assessment and treatment programs. In attending to the broader relationships between information derived through clinical interviews/assessments and the sexual problem, clinicians are in the position not only to benefit from their intuitive understanding of causes of male sexual dysfunctions and their effective treatment, but also to investigate these relationships systematically and communicate them through formal research reports to colleagues in the field. For this reason, the use of standardized practices and instruments serves both to benefit the individual patient and to guide future procedures for evaluation in populations of sexually dysfunctional men.

□ REFERENCES

1. Lief HI. Sex and depression. Med Aspects Hum Sex 1986; 20:38–53.
2. Hawton K. Integration of treatments for male erectile dysfunction. Lancet 1998; 351(9095):7–8.
3. Wincze J, Carey M. Sexual Dysfunction: A Guide for Assessment and Treatment. New York: Guilford Publications, 1991.
4. Tiefer L, Melman A. Comprehensive evaluation of erectile dysfunction and medical treatments. In: Leiblum S, Rosen R, eds. Principles and Practice in Sex Therapy: Update for the 1990s. 2nd ed. New York: Guilford Press, 1989:207–236.
5. Schnarch D. Talking to patients about sex–Part II. Med Aspects Hum Sex 1988; 22:97–106.
6. Milsten R, Slowinski J. The Sexual Male: Problems and Solutions. New York: WW Norton & Co., 1999.
7. Conte HR. Development and use of self-report techniques for assessing sexual functioning: a review and critique. Arch Sex Behav 1983; 12(6):555–576.
8. Conte HR. Multivariate assessment of sexual dysfunction. J Consult Clin Psychol 1986; 54(2):149–157.
9. Corty EW, Althof SE, Kurit DM. The reliability and validity of a sexual functioning questionnaire. J Sex Marital Ther 1996; 22(1):27–34.
10. Derogatis L, Fagan P, Strand J. Sexual disorders measures. In: Rush A, ed. Handbook of Psychiatric Measures, Washington DC: American Psychiatric Publishing, 2000:616–646.
11. Derogatis LR, Conklin-Powers B. Psychological assessment measures of female sexual functioning in clinical trials. Int J Impot Res 1998; 10(suppl 2):S111–S116.
12. Derogatis LR, Melisaratos N. The Brief Symptom Inventory: an introductory report. Psychol Med 1983; 13(3):595–605.
13. Derogatis L. Brief Symptom Inventory (BSI). Administration, Scoring, and Procedural Manual, 3rd ed. Minneapolis, MN: National Computer Systems, 1993.
14. Derogatis LR. The Derogatis Interview for Sexual Functioning (DISF/DISF-SR): an introductory report. J Sex Marital Ther 1997; 23(4):291–304.
15. Rust J, Golombok S. The Golombok Rust Inventory of Sexual Satisfaction. Odessa, FL: Psychological Assessment Resources, 1986.
16. Spanier G. Measuring dyadic adjustment: new scales for assessing the quality of marriage and similar dyads. J Marriage Fam 1976; 38(1):15–28.
17. Costa P, McCrae R. NEO PI-R professional manual. Odessa, FL: Psychological Assessment Resources, 1992.

☐ **APPENDIX 1 Johns Hopkins Sexual Behaviors Consultation Unit Comprehensive Psychiatric/Psychosexual Interview**

Patient Name: _____

Evaluator: _____

Date: _____

I. Identification (age, gender, race, marital status)

II. Chief Complaint (include referral source, patient's statement of problem, goals for evaluation)

III. History of Present Illness (details of the presenting sexual problem)
- Onset/duration
- Trend/track development of problem
- Patient's self-explanation or theory about the problem
- Patient's description of the meaning the problem holds in his/her life
- Family history of the same or similar problems (e.g., for premature ejaculation, familial occurrence in father and/or brothers)

Sexual Status Exam:
- Ask the patient to recall the most recent sexual encounter in detail.
- Obtain a comprehensive report of the biological (medications, alcohol/drugs, and energy level), social (relationship to partner or spouse), psychological (cognitions and emotions about the sexual activity), and environmental (setting: time of day, place) conditions related to the encounter.
- Operationalize the encounter by identifying the specific activity, duration, and subjective level of arousal.
- Identify the effects of the sexual experience on the patient and partner or spouse.
- Typical encounter [frequency, initiator, foreplay, orgasm (self and partner), satisfaction (self and partner), pain]

IV. Sexual History
- How/when patient learned about sex
- Age of first nocturnal emission, first masturbation
- Early masturbation behaviors (style, method of masturbation), fantasies (including homoerotic), frequency, change over time
- Sex play, same/other sex encounters
- Subjection to sexual abuse
- Gender-related childhood behaviors (identify play behaviors as congruous or incongruous with patient's biologic gender)
- First sexual intercourse (When? What was it like? Hurried conditions? Fear of getting caught?)
- Number of lifetime partners including casual sex __ and significant relationships __.
- Patterns of heterosexual and homosexual attraction
- History of use (compulsive or not) of pornography, including Internet
- History of pain during sexual activities
- Current masturbation habits, style, methods, fantasies, frequency
- Current partner(s)
- Current sexual activity/frequency
- Paraphilic and related behaviors (Internet, other pornography, exhibitionism, voyeurism, cross-dressing, pedophilic experiences, fantasies, frotteurism, urophilia, coprophilia, zoophilia, masochism, sadism, other)

V. Dating/Marital History (including children—biological and adopted)

VI. Family History include deaths, illnesses, psychiatric history, substance abuse history, criminal history, frequent moves (and impact on patient, such as with military families)
- History of sexual problems in other family members [mother, father, parental relationship, siblings (include birth order), other relatives]

VII. Developmental History
- Place/date of birth:
- Developmental milestones/delays in milestones
- Childhood emotional or behavioral difficulties
- Hyperactivity
- Separation difficulties (anxiety when started kindergarten? Later separation difficulties?)
- Running away from home
- Cruelty to animals
- Enuresis
- Fire setting
- Other behavioral/discipline problems
- Childhood subjection to physical, verbal abuse (may cover sexual abuse in the Sexual History section)

VIII. Educational History
- Last grade completed
- Special education
- Failures
- School related behavioral problems
- Academic performance (poor, below average, average, above average, excellent)
- Social functioning (details about clubs, sports, activities in high school, as possible indicators of premorbid personality)
- College/professional training (include dates)

IX. Occupational History (include dates and type of military service)

X. Health History
- Chronic medical problems
- Significant acute illnesses
- Current medications
- Drug allergies
- History of seizures, loss of consciousness, head trauma
- HIV test results

XI. Psychiatric History
- Past diagnoses and review of symptoms (mood, anxiety, thought disorder, etc.)
- Past treatments (include dates, patient's perception of effectiveness)
- Suicide attempts

XII. Habit History

	Age of first use	Frequency	Last use
Alcohol			
Marijuana			
PCP			
Cocaine (route)			
Heroin (route)			
Nicotine (route)			
Other			

XIII. Religious History (including religiously informed parental attitudes about sex, patient's perception of the influence of their religious history on the problem, patient's current status regarding religion, including the meaning of the patient's descriptions of his or her self as religious, spiritual, etc.):

XIV. Legal History

XV. Mental Status Exam
- Appearance & Behavior (dress/grooming, posture/gate, physical characteristics, facial expressions, eye contact, motor activity, specific mannerisms)
- Speech (rate, pitch, volume, clarity, abnormality)
- Emotions (mood, affect, variability, intensity, lability, appropriateness/congruence)
- Thought (process, flow of ideas, quality of associations, content, distortions, delusions, ideas of reference, depersonalization, preoccupations, obsessions, phobias, somatic concerns, suicidal or homicidal ideation)
- Perceptions (illusions, hallucinations)
- Sensorium and Intellect (consciousness, orientation, concentration, memory, immediate, recent, remote, fund of knowledge, abstraction, judgment, insight, attitude toward evaluator, self-attitude)

XVI. Formulation (rationale for diagnosis)

XVII. DSM IV Multiaxial Diagnosis (to include both numeric codes and text)
- Axis I
- Axis II
- Axis III
- Axis IV
- Axis V

XVIII. Recommendations

Male Sexual Dysfunction Interview[a]

Name: _____ Date: _____ ID: _____

How frequently do you think about sex? _____

How often do you desire to have sex? _____

Do *you* think your desire/interest is lower than it could be? _____

Reasons for this response: _____

_____

_____

Have you <u>ever</u> had a full erection? _____ Yes _____ No

How old were you when you first experienced difficulty achieving or maintaining an erection? _____ years of age.

Has this difficulty been episodic in your life? _____ Yes _____ No

How many times in your life have you had problems with erections (other than a one time failure)? _____

Can you identify a cause for any of the previous episodes?

_____ injury   _____ alcohol/drugs

_____ illness   _____ divorce

_____ medication   _____ death of wife

_____ stressful life event   _____ psychological/emotional problems

_____ relationship problems with partner _____ other

                                  _____ don't know

How did the previous episode(s) resolve? (Check as many as appropriate)

_____ spontaneously   _____ major life change

_____ medicine change   _____ counseling or psychotherapy

_____ sex partner change   _____ do not recall

How long have you had the present problem with erections? (Fill in numbers) _____ years _____ months

How rapidly did the problem with erection appear? Over a period of:

_____ less than two weeks

_____ more than two weeks but less than six months

_____ more than six months but less than one year

_____ more than one year

_____ do not recall

Can you identify a cause of your current episode of erectile dysfunction?

_____ injury   _____ alcohol/drugs

_____ illness   _____ divorce

_____ medication   _____ death of wife

_____ stressful life event   _____ psychological/emotional problems

_____ relationship problems with partner _____ other

                                  _____ don't know

Compared to the fullest erection you have ever achieved, what percent fullness would you rate your best present erections? _____ %

When do you experience the most difficulty maintaining an erection?

_____ foreplay   _____ varied times

_____ as penetration is attempted   _____ never get an erection

_____ after penetration

What is the longest time you can presently maintain an erection?

(Fill in numbers) _____ minutes _____ seconds _____ not at all

_____

Do you wake up during the night or in the mornings with erections? Yes _____No _____

Compared with the fullest erection you have ever achieved, what percent fullness would you rate these night or morning erections? _____%

How many orgasms (regardless of means of achieving) have you had in the past month? _____

How long has it been since your last ejaculation under any circumstances?

(Fill in numbers) _____ year(s) _____ month(s) _____ day(s)

If you presently masturbate, compared with the fullest erection you have ever achieved, what percent fullness would you rate the best of these masturbatory erections?

_____%   _____ Do not masturbate

How long has it been since your last vaginal penetration?

(Fill in numbers)   _____ year(s) _____ month(s) _ day(s)

How long has it been since you ejaculated within the vagina?

(Fill in numbers) _____ year(s) _____ month(s) _____ day(s)

Do you experience pain during erection?   _____Yes   _____ No

If pain during erection, locate area of pain: (Check as many as appropriate)

_____ top of penis   _____ pubic area

_____ shaft of penis   _____ pelvic generalized

_____ scrotum   _____ no pain

Do you experience pain during *intercourse*?   _____ Yes   _____ No

If pain during intercourse, locate area of pain: (Check as many as appropriate)

_____ top of penis   _____ pubic area

_____ shaft of penis   _____ pelvic generalized

_____ scrotum   _____ no pain

Do you ever ejaculate before either you or your partner desire it? _____Yes   _____ No

If you do ejaculate sooner than you or your partner desire it, what percent of the time?

_____%   _____ Does not occur

On the average, how many seconds/minutes elapse after penetration before you ejaculate?

_____ seconds _____ minutes _____ ejaculate prior to penetration

_____ does not apply to me

If you ejaculate sooner than desired, when did this first occur relative to problems with erections?

_____ prior to erection problem   _____ after erection problem

_____ together with erection problem   _____ do not recall

Compared to the most pleasurable orgasm you have ever experienced, what percent satisfaction would you rate your present orgasmic pleasure?

_____%   _____ do not have orgasms

How do you achieve the most orgasmic pleasure?

_____ masturbation   _____ intercourse

_____ manual stimulation by partner   _____ oral stimulation by partner

_____ other circumstances

25

Investigation of Vascular and Structural Abnormalities of the Penis

Fouad R. Kandeel
Department of Diabetes, Endocrinology and Metabolism, City of Hope National Medical Center, Duarte, California and David Geffen School of Medicine, University of California, Los Angeles, California, U.S.A.

Mark Esensten
Division of Diagnostic Radiology, City of Hope National Medical Center, Duarte, California, U.S.A.

Lionel S. Zuckier
New Jersey Medical School, University Hospital, Newark, New Jersey, U.S.A.

□ INTRODUCTION

Advances in the understanding of the physiology of male erection have stimulated the development of new and improved diagnostic test procedures that can identify and quantify the vascular abnormalities leading to erectile failure. This chapter reviews the currently available procedures and assesses their respective utilities in defining the underlying pathophysiology of erectile dysfunction (ED) and in guiding the selection of corrective therapeutic interventions. Figure 1 provides an algorithmic approach to these investigations.

□ VASCULAR INVESTIGATIONS OF THE PENIS

Since the advent of phosphodiesterase-5 (PDE-5) inhibitors, in routine clinical practice, patients presenting with ED typically do not require further investigation beyond a thorough history, physical exam, basic hematologic and biochemical laboratory analyses, and a possible hormonal assessment (if there is reason to suspect an endocrinopathy). For further information on these general evaluations, see Chapter 22; for further information on PDE-5 inhibitors, see Chapter 29. A number of additional studies exist, however, to aid the clinician in assigning a specific cause to a patient's ED. These investigations fall into one of three categories: (*i*) vascular testing such as duplex ultrasound and dynamic infusion cavernosometry/cavernosography, (*ii*) neurological testing such as a biothesiometry, somatosensory-evoked potentials, and pudendal electromyography, and (*iii*) daytime and nocturnal penile tumescence and rigidity analysis. The indications for such adjunctive investigations have been controversial, but, in the authors' experience, these are typically reserved for the following groups of patients: (*i*) patients who are potentially curable, including young males with purely arteriogenic ED of traumatic etiology and young males with isolated crural venous leak, (*ii*) patients with penile curvature who require evaluation prior to undergoing penile reconstructive surgery, (*iii*) patients who require documented evidence of abnormalities for medicolegal purposes, and (*iv*) rare patients with unclear and difficult-to-diagnose psychogenic disorders in whom evidence for normal organic function could help the patient to focus on addressing the true underlying psychosocial problem.

This chapter will focus solely on a discussion of the currently available methods for vascular testing. For further information on neurologic testing, see Chapter 26; for further information on tumescence monitoring, see Chapter 23. Patients suspected of having vascular lesions, based on history, physical signs, abnormal penile-brachial index (PBI), or abnormal tumescence monitoring results, may undergo a more detailed evaluation of the penile vasculature. The first studies used indirect measures to infer the adequacy of arterial blood supply to the penis, such as intraurethral temperature recording during gluteal exercise (2) and simultaneous graphic tracing of finger and penis pulse volume changes (plethysmography) before and after temporary occlusion of blood flow in both organs (postocclusive reactive hyperemia) (3). More recently, several tests were developed that are capable of directly evaluating the integrity of the penile vasculatures—both inflow and outflow. These are listed in Table 1 and are detailed in the following sections.

Pharmacopenile Duplex Ultrasound

A duplex scanner with color-flow imaging capability, coupled with a spectral display system and a 7.5 MHz

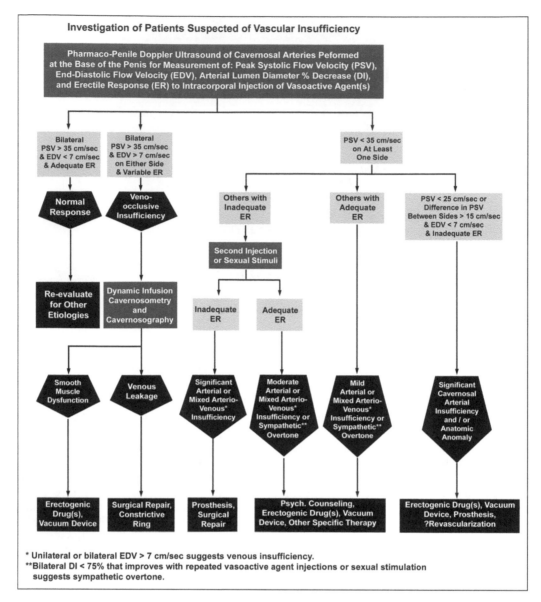

Figure 1 Investigation of patients with erectile dysfunction suspected of vascular insufficiency. Algorithmic approach to the investigation and treatment of impotent men suspected of having vascular insufficiency. Pharmacopenile Doppler ultrasound of cavernosal arteries with intracorporeal administration of 10 μg prostaglandin E_1 is suggested as the initial step of vascular investigation. Subjects with bilaterally normal response should be evaluated for other causes of impotence. Patients with normal PSV but elevated EDV are likely to have veno-occlusive dysfunction. Dynamic infusion cavernosometry and cavernosography, and, in some instances, other tests (see chapters in Part III of this book for details) may be required to identify patients with true venous leakage who may benefit from venous ligation surgery. Patients with abnormal PSV on at least one side are likely to have arterial insufficiency with or without veno-occlusive dysfunction or sympathetic overtone. The degree of abnormality in PSV in one or both cavernosal arteries, presence or absence of a normal EDV, and the degree of erectile response to one or more vasoactive drug injection(s) or other adjunct sexual stimuli may help to identify the nature and the degree of underlying pathophysiology. *Abbreviations*: PSV, peak systolic flow velocity; EDV, end-diastolic flow velocity; DI, diameter percent increase; ER, erectile response. *Source*: From Ref. 1.

linear-array transducer, is the optimal instrument for performing this study (3–7). Using B-mode ultrasonography and color-image guidance, the device can assess the penile soft tissue for the presence of structural abnormalities of the tunica albuginea, such as fibrous plaques or calcifications. It can also define the arterial tree, measure the diameter of the cavernosal arteries, and display the Doppler spectrum waveform of blood flow in the cavernosal arteries (Figs. 2 and 3). The latter is then used for determining peak systolic flow velocity (PSV), end-diastolic flow velocity (EDV),

and acceleration time or systolic rise time (time from end-diastolic to peak systolic velocity). Additional parameters derived from these data include: acceleration = (peak systolic velocity - end–diastolic velocity)/ (acceleration time), resistance index (RI) = (peak systolic velocity – peak diastolic velocity)/(peak systolic velocity), and pulsatility index (PI) = (peak systolic velocity – peak diastolic velocity)/(mean systolic velocity) (3,8–11). Cavernosal artery diameter and blood flow velocity can be measured in either the longitudinal or the transverse projection. The longitudinal

Table 1 Vascular Studies for Organic Impotence

Test	Criteria for normal response	Abnormalities	Associated diagnosis
Penile-brachial index	> 0.7	> 0.7; falls after pelvic exercise	Pelvic steal syndrome
		< 0.7; no change with pelvic exercise	Cavernosal artery insufficiency
PPDU	Bilateral PSV > 35 cm/sec, EDV < 7 cm/sec and adequate erectile response	Bilateral PSV > 35 cm/sec, EDV > 7 cm/sec on either side and variable erectile response	Venous insufficiency
		PSV > 35 cm/sec on either side with inadequate erectile response that does not improve with a second vasoactive drug injection or sexual stimulation	Significant cavernosal artery or mixed arteriovenous insufficiency[a]
		PSV > 35 cm/sec on either side with inadequate erectile response that improves with a second vasoactive drug injection or sexual stimulation	Moderate cavernosal artery, mixed arteriovenous insufficiency[a] or sympathetic overtone[b]
		PSV > 35 cm/sec on either side with adequate erectile response	Mild cavernosal artery, mixed arteriovenous insufficiency[a] or sympathetic overtone[b]
		Bilateral PSV < 25 cm/sec or differences between sides >15 cm/sec, EDV < 7 cm/sec and inadequate erectile response	Significant cavernosal artery insufficiency and/or arterial anatomical abnormalities
Dynamic cavernosometry and cavernosography	Phase I: equilibrium steady-state intracavernous pressure > 30 mm Hg (usually approximate mean arterial pressure)	Equilibrium steady-state intracavernous pressure < 30 mm Hg	Venous insufficiency
	Phase II: decline in intracavernous pressure < 45 mm Hg or to a value >105 mm Hg, over 30 sec	Decline in intracavernous pressure > 45 mm Hg or to a value < 105 mm Hg, over 30 sec	Venous insufficiency
	Phase III: gradient between systolic brachial and cavernosal artery occlusion pressure < 30 mm Hg	Gradient between systolic brachial and cavernosal artery occlusion pressure > 30 mmHg	Cavernosal artery insufficiency
	Phases II and IV: maintenance flow rate < 5 mL/min to keep intracavernosal pressure unchanged	Maintenance flow rate > 5 mL/min to keep intracavernosal pressure unchanged	Venous insufficiency
	Phase IV: normal cavernosography	Abnormal cavernosography	Venous insufficiency
Pump cavernosometry	Induction flow rate 80–120 mL/min and maintenance flow rate 20–40 mL/min	Induction flow rate > 120 mL/min and maintenance flow rate > 40 mL/min	Venous insufficiency
Gravity cavernosometry	Linear relationship between steady-state intracavernosal and infusion pressures at infusion pressures between 40 and 160 cm water, and maintenance of intracavernosal pressure higher than 110 mmHg with infusion pressure of 140 cm water	No linear relationship between steady-state intracavernosal and infusion pressures at infusion pressures between 40 and 160 cm water, and inability to maintain the intracavernosal pressure higher than 110 mm Hg with infusion pressure of 140 cm water	Venous insufficiency
Penile arteriography	Normal cavernosal artery imaging	Abnormal cavernosal artery imaging	Cavernosal artery insufficiency
Radionuclear scintigraphy Dynamic penile scintigraphy with 99mTc-labeled autologous RBCs: a) Systemic administration of 99mTc-labeled autologous RBCs	Normal background-subtracted penile time-activity curve (phallogram)	Lower rate of blood flow with rounded time-activity curve, insignificant changes in slope of radioactivity after administration of intracavernosal vasoactive drugs,	Cavernosal artery insufficiency

(Continued)

Table 1 Vascular Studies for Organic Impotence (*Continued*)

with or without intracavernosal injection of vasoactive drugs		and negligible episodic increase in penile radioactivity Normal phallogram curve, and normal flow and volume indices following systemic vasodilators, but rapid rise and fall of the phallogram curve	Venous insufficiency
b) Intrapenile injection of ^{99m}Tc-labeled autologous RBCs with or without intracavernosal injection of vasoactive drugs	Normal clearance rate of penile radioactivity	Accelerated clearance rate of penile radioactivity	Venous insufficiency
Dual isotope scintigraphy: combined intravenous ^{99m}Tc-labeled autologous RBCs time-activity, and intracavernosal Xenon wash-out curves	Normal ^{99m}Tc-labeled autologous RBCs peak cavernosal artery inflow, and Xenon peak venous outflow	Lower average ^{99m}Tc-labeled autologous RBCs peak cavernosal artery inflow	Cavernosal artery insufficiency
Cavernous oxygen tension during flaccidity and erection (during PPDU)	Normal oxygen tension at all phases	Lower oxygen tension despite normal cavernosal artery blood flow	Cavernous trabecular smooth muscle dysfunction

^{a}Unilateral or bilateral EDV > 7 suggests venous insufficiency.
^{b}Bilateral diameter increase < 75% that improves with repeated vasoactive agent injection or sexual stimulation suggests sympathetic overtone.
Abbreviations: PPDU, pharmacopenile Doppler ultrasound; PSV, peak systolic flow velocity; EDV, end-diastolic flow velocity; RBC, red blood cell.

projection (3,5,7,9,11–15) is usually performed by placing the transducer on the ventral or the dorsal aspect of the penile shaft as proximally as possible. The Doppler sample volume cursor is placed in the cavernosal artery high in the infrapubic region, and the Doppler angle correction cursor is adjusted to match the corrected axis of flow. An angle of insonation (less than 60 degrees) usually provides the optimal correction for velocity calculations. Accurate longitudinal scanning is dependent on proper angle correction. Transverse ultrasound scanning (16–20) is performed by placing the transducer across the dorsal surface at the base of the penis and angled inferiorly toward the penile root so that nontortuous segments of the cavernosal arteries proximal to any branching are imaged in longitudinal sections, vertically in the image plane. Transverse scanning as described utilizes a Doppler angle equal to zero, which does not require correction and thus eliminates the major potential source of error in measurement of blood flow velocity in the longitudinal projection (12). Figure 2 shows a normal response on pharmacopenile duplex ultrasound (PPDU) study, whereas Figure 3A and 3B represent studies of patients with significant arterial disease and significant venous leakage, respectively.

Most of the available data on PPDU utilize the intracorporeal injection of one or more of three vasoactive agents [papaverine, phentolamine, and prostaglandin E₁ (PGE₁)] (8,11–14,21–26). The use of several other vasoactive agents [(e.g., calcitonin gene-related

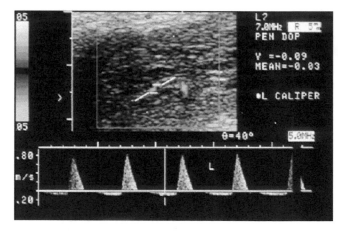

Figure 2 Normal response on PPDU study. Center inset reveals cross-section of dilated cavernosal artery lumen. PPDU study of cavernosal arteries in normal human male subject shows waveforms with good peak systolic velocity around 50 cm/sec. Venous competency (i.e., total occlusion during erection) is illustrated by reversal of flow seen during end-diastolic phase. *Abbreviation*: PPDU, pharmacopenile duplex ultrasound.

peptide, nitric oxide donors, and vasoactine intestinal polypeptide (VIP)] has also been described (27,28). Doses of papaverine used ranged from 7.5 mg to greater than 70 mg, with the lower doses being used in conjunction with phentolamine or with a phentolamine and PGE₁ mixture. Doses of PGE₁ ranged from 10 to 40 μg when used alone, and 10 μg or less when used in

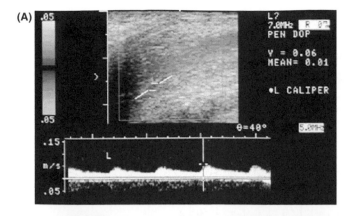

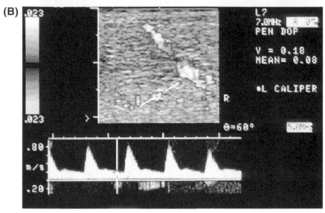

Figure 3 Arterial insufficiency and venous leakage on PPDU study. PPDU study of the cavernosal artery in a human male with erectile dysfunction demonstrates poor peak systolic velocity (< 35 cm/sec), representing arterial disease (**A**), but high end-diastolic velocity (between 10 and 20 cm/sec) suggests the presence of venous leakage (**B**). *Abbreviation*: PPDU, pharmacopenile duplex ultrasound.

combination with the other two agents. Phentolamine has always been used in conjunction with the other two agents in doses around 0.5 mg (3). PGE_1 alone (10–20 µg) was shown in a multicenter comparative study to provide the highest erection response rate (74%) and the lowest rate of priapism (0.1%) (29). The low rate of side effects to PE_1 was also confirmed in another report of literature review (E_1 2.4%, papaverine alone 9.5%, and papaverine–phentolamine 5.3%) (30). Ultrasound scanning is usually performed before and immediately after the injection, every two to five minutes for the first 10 minutes postinjection, and then every five minutes thereafter for a total scanning time of 30 minutes. Normal progression of the spectral waveform phases of blood flow within the cavernosal arteries during tumescence was described by several groups of investigators (3,5,8,12,31) and is depicted diagrammatically in Figure 4. In the flaccid state, monophasic flow is present with minimal diastolic flow. With the onset of erection or after intracorporeal vasoactive drug administration, an increase in both systolic and diastolic flow occurs. With progressively increasing intracorporeal pressure, end-diastolic flow declines to zero and then undergoes diastolic flow reversal.

When penile rigidity is attained, the systolic wave narrows and the diastolic flow disappears (5). Thus, the progression of the peak systolic and end-diastolic waveforms depends on the balance between sinusoidal relaxation and intracorporeal pressure at the given time. During latency and early tumescence when intracorporeal pressure is low, there are higher-amplitude, longer-lasting, peak systolic and end-diastolic waves. In contrast, when the full erection is attained, the peak systolic wave narrows and the end-diastolic wave reverses. With further increase in intracorporeal pressure to above systemic blood pressure subsequent to pelvic floor muscle contraction and cessation of penile venous return, all systolic blood inflow temporarily ceases. Thus, correct interpretation of peak systolic and end-diastolic velocity parameters depends on the knowledge of the spectral waveform phase in which they were taken. Similarly, the sampling location on the penile shaft influences the parameters of peak systolic and end-diastolic flow. In healthy controls, there is a mean reduction of flow velocity between the crural and distal subcoronal portions of the cavernous artery by about 20%, whereas in patients with peripheral arterial disease, velocity may be reduced by as much as 50% (3,21).

Reference values for normal PPDU parameters are variable due to differences in the selection criteria for patient groups, normal controls, dose and number of vasoactive drug injections, and the characteristics (pharmacological effectiveness and mode of action) of the vasoactive agent used. In addition, some studies have augmented the response to the injection of vasoactive agents with genital self-stimulation or with the use of tourniquet or audio–visual erotic stimulation. Reported normal ranges, using a variety of investigative protocols, include PSV > 25 to > 35 cm/sec, EDV < 5 to < 7 cm/sec, cavernosal artery diameter increase > 21% to > 75%, acceleration time < 110 to < 122 msec, acceleration > 400 cm/sec^2, and RI > 1 (>100%). Several studies have attempted to relate the results of PPDU investigation to those observed during cavernosal artery pharmacoarteriography and/or cavernosometry (4,7,11,32,33). In one of these studies, a systolic velocity < 25 cm/sec or an acceleration < 400 cm/sec^2 had sensitivities of 35% and 100%, specificities of 61% and 46%, and negative predictive values of 42% and 100% in the diagnosis of arterial insufficiency, respectively (11). In another study, the prevalence of angiographically normal cavernosal arteries increased from 0% when PSV was < 25 cm/sec to 92% with PSV > 35 cm/sec. Conversely, the prevalence of severe arterial disease decreased from 82% with PSV < 25 cm/sec to 8% with PSV > 35 cm/sec. Other angiographic correlations have shown that a systolic velocity threshold of 25 cm/sec has 92% accuracy in the diagnosis of arterial integrity (32,33). Selection bias may influence the results of these comparative studies, however, since the majority of studies report on a small number of subjects, of whom most have abnormal PSV.

SELECTED HEMODYNAMIC INVESTIGATIONS AND THEIR RELATIONSHIPS TO THE SEXUAL CYCLE: DIAGRAMATIC REPRESENTATION OF NORMAL STUDIES

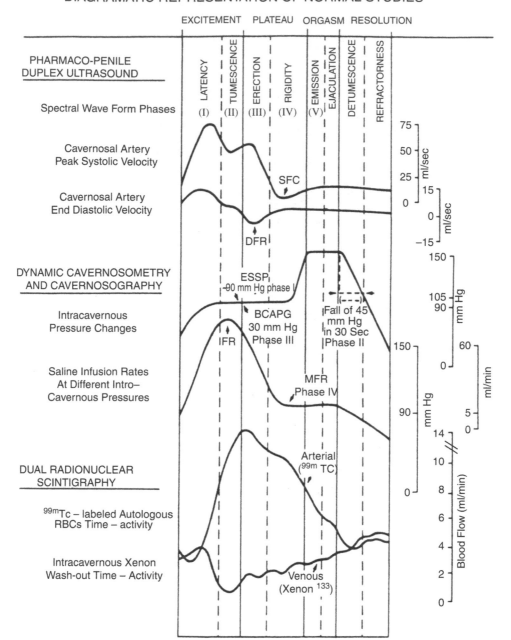

Figure 4 Graphic representation of PPDU, dynamic cavernosometry and cavernosography, and dual radionuclear scintigraphy. Drawings were made to superimpose the hemodynamic changes elicited by each of these investigations over the respective normal events of the male sexual cycle. Normal progression of the spectral waveform phases of blood flow within the cavernosal arteries in response to intracorporeal administration of vasoactive drugs (usually prostaglandin E-1, 10–20 µg), and cavernosal artery peak systolic and end-diastolic velocities are represented at the top of graph. With the onset of erection, or after intracorporeal vasoactive drug administration, both peak systolic and end-diastolic arterial velocities increase. With progressive increase in intracorporeal pressure, end-diastolic flow declines to zero and then undergoes diastolic flow reversal. When penile rigidity is attained, the systolic wave declines sharply and the diastolic flow disappears. Further elevation in intracorporeal pressure to a level above that of systemic blood pressure results in the temporary cessation of all systolic blood flow. Graphic representation of dynamic cavernosometry and associated pressure changes are depicted in the middle portion of the graph. Dynamic cavernosometry consists of four phases. In phase I, vasoactive agents are injected intracorporeally to relax the corporeal smooth muscles and to increase blood flow. Maximum equilibrium corporeal body pressure, which represents the intracorporeal pressure achieved during normal tumescence and erection, is then determined. In phase II, the corporeal body pressure is raised to 150 mmHg by infusing heparinized saline, infusion is then turned off, and the fall in pressure over 30 seconds is noted. This represents the usual rate of pressure fall during normal detumescence. In phase III, the cavernosal artery systolic pressure is determined by infusing heparinized saline intracorporeally until cavernosal artery flow ceases, then infusion is stopped and the fall in intracavernosal pressure is monitored to determine the level at which the cavernosal artery Doppler signal reappear. The difference between the cavernosal and brachial artery systolic pressures is determined. This represents the intracorporeal pressure

(Continued on opposite page)

Table 2 Pharmacopenile Duplex Ultrasound of Cavernosal Arteries in 127 Men with Erectile Dysfunction. Number and Percent of Subjects for Each Category

	Clinical response	Normal hemodynamic response	Arterial disease	Venous leakage	Mixed arterial/ venous	Structural abnormalities
Poor						
	62 (49%)	0 (0%)	39 (31%)	5 (4%)	18 (14%)	6 (5%)
Moderate						
	38 (30%)	4 (3%)	20 (16%)	9 (7%)	4 (3%)	9 (7%)
Good						
	27 (21%)	15 (12%)	8 (6%)	1 (1%)	3 (2%)	3 (2%)
Totals	127 (100%)	19 (15%)	67 (53%)	15 (12%)	25 (19%)	18 (14%)

Normal response = peak arterial flow > 35 cm/sec bilaterally.
Arterial disease = peak arterial flow < 35 cm/sec.
Venous leakage = venous flow > 7 cm/sec.
Structural abnormalities = absent cavernosal arteries, irregular vascular branching, collateral formations, dorsal thickening of tunica albuginea, penile deviations, plaques.
Source: Esensten M, Kandeel FR. Unpublished data.

Several other studies have compared the sonographic data to the physical erectile response after vasoactive drug injections. Patel et al. (7) found that in 220 impotent men, a maximal systolic velocity of 30 cm/sec identified normal penile arterial flow with 96% sensitivity and 82% specificity, using clinical response as the reference standard. When 25 cm/sec was used as the cutoff for normal PSV, the sensitivity and specificity of the test were 100% and 59%, respectively; with a cutoff of 35 cm/sec, the sensitivity and specificity were 86% and 95%. Unpublished data from 72 impotent patients at City of Hope National Medical Center (courtesy of Dr. Mark Esensten, Department of Diagnostic Radiology) showed slightly lower sensitivity and specificity values when the cutoff of 25 cm/sec (92% and 55%, respectively) or 35 cm/sec (80% and 87%, respectively) was used. The reason for the lower sensitivity and specificity rates in this group is likely related to the lack of repeating vasoactive drug administration or the lack of use of adjunctive sexual stimulation measures in patients with incomplete erectile response to a single dose PGE-1 (10 μg) (10,14,24,31,34–37). Thus, arteriogenic impotence, either due to a true structural arterial abnormality or due to a failure of arterial relaxation secondary to pharmacological resistance, can be identified with sensitivity of 82% to 100% and specificity of 64% to 96%, based on the chosen PSV threshold for normal blood flow (>25–>35 cm/sec) (Table 2).

The use of a higher cutoff value for PSV appears to improve the specificity but reduces the sensitivity for identifying adequate penile blood supply (6,7,10,11). Based on these data, a PSV of ≥35 cm/sec is recommended, with adequate erectile response (as assessed objectively by tonometry, Snap Gauge, or Rigiscan monitor) to identify the normal PPDU response. Lower PSV values in impotent patients are likely to be associated with arterial insufficiency and/or sympathetic overtone. Table 1 and Figure 1 summarize the implicated application of these reference values in clinical decision making.

Other parameters of the PPDU listed above were also used to infer arterial insufficiency. Patel et al. (7) considered an acceleration time greater than one second to be a reliable predictor of arteriogenic impotence, and a PI < 300 to be characteristic of patients with either venous leakage (see below) or arteriogenic impotence. Similarly, Oates et al. (12) found in 37 impotent men that acceleration time ≥110 msec to be the best discriminant of arterial disease with a positive predictive value of 0.92 when associated with inadequate erectile response to papaverine injections. A long systolic rise time in a papaverine responder, on the other hand, may indicate a borderline arterial supply or sinusoidal-venous abnormality (3,9,12,31). The lack of cavernous artery dilatation to >175% of baseline value in response to vasoactive drug injection, by itself,

Figure 4 (*Continued*) likely to be achieved during the erectile response of the individual, and reflects the presence or absence of arterial insufficiency. In phase IV, the infusion flow rate required for maintenance of intracavernous pressure at 90 mmHg, during cavernosography, is then determined. Again, this represents the state of blood flow during erection and reflects the presence or absence of veno-occlusive dysfunction. Dual-radioisotope (Technetium time-activity and Xenon wash-out curves) are represented in the lower portion of the diagram. This is done by the simultaneous administration of autologous ^{99m}Tc-labelled RBC's intravenously and Xe[133] intracavornously. γ ray-emission is measured before and after incorporeal administration of a vasoactive drug injection. This study provides quantitative indices of penile blood volume and flow during the erectile function and reflects the presence or absence of arterial insufficiency and/or veno-occlusive disease. *Abbreviations*: PPDU, pharmacopenile duplex ultrasonography; SFC, systolic flow cessation; DFR, diastolic flow reversal; ESSP, equilibrium steady-state pressure; BCAPG, brachial-cavernosal artery pressure gradient; IFR, induction flow rate; MFR, maintenance flow rate. *Source*: Kandeel, FR. Compiled published data in literature.

is not a reliable indicator for arterial disease (3), since it could be associated with sympathetic overtone, and the measurement of such a small diameter has a large margin of error; however, lack of arterial dilatation observed bilaterally that can be overcome by injecting an additional amount of the vasoactive drug, by genital self-stimulation, or by the exposure to audio–visual erotic stimuli may indicate the presence of sympathetic overtone (34–37).

The PPDU can also provide significant information on the competency of venous drainage. As described above, the normal spectral waveform cycle of penile erection is characterized by a progressive loss of the diastolic flow and ultimately a diastolic flow reversal. Therefore, the presence of persistent diastolic flow and elevated EDV are indirect indicators of veno-occlusive failure (5,7,9,24). Unlike PSV, which is at its highest early in the penodynamic erectile cycle, however, the nadir of EDV is observed later after full erection and rigidity have occurred, and thus may not be observed until 15 to 25 minutes after the administration of the vasoactive agent (5,7,10,15,31). The cutoff of EDV required for the diagnosis of veno-occlusive dysfunction ranges between 5 and 10 cm/sec, lasting for at least five minutes. Several studies have compared PPDU with cavernosography and cavernosometry (7,9,38–40). PPDU can diagnose veno-occlusive dysfunction with a sensitivity of 55% to 100% and a specificity of 69% to 88%, depending on the chosen threshold for normal end-diastolic velocity. For example, correlating the PPDU with the cavernosographic data in 48 patients yielded a sensitivity of 94% and a specificity of 69% when EDV >7 cm/sec was chosen for diagnosing venous incompetence. Based on this and similar studies, the use of EDV >7 cm/sec is recommended for the diagnosis of veno-occlusive dysfunction (7). It should be emphasized that the diagnosis of venous incompetence is made only if the patient has a normal peak systolic velocity, and that accurate measurement of end-diastolic velocity requires an optimal angle correction. A preliminary study by Virag and Sussman (41) used pulse Doppler ultrasound to examine the deep dorsal venous blood flow following the administration of an intravenous injection of vasoactive agents (papaverine, ifenprodil tartrate, and PGE$_1$). As expected, the administration of vasoactive agents led to cessation of venous drainage, an effect that was further modified by visual sexual stimulation (VSS). These investigators considered the early cessation of venous blood flow as a predictor of increased risk for prolonged erection with the in-home therapeutic use of intracorporeal vasoactive injections. A newly described power Doppler sonography technique appears even more promising in this regard (42).

The accuracy of diagnosing a vascular etiology based on PPDU testing is difficult in up to 20% of patients. Common causes for this difficulty include the presence of combined arteriovenous disease, suboptimal response to the pharmacological agent(s), intrinsic smooth muscle relaxation abnormality, or excessive subject anxiety resulting in sympathetic overtone. The latter can be reduced by ensuring privacy and patient comfort, as well as by the use of drug combinations, genital self-stimulation, and/or erotic audio–visual stimulation—thereby reducing any anxiety and psychic overlay (3,15). Also, quantitative analysis of waveforms, assessment of waveform evolution, and assessment of bilateral arterial compliance may aid in subclassification of individuals with borderline responses (3,5,8,11,15,31,43). Other secondary data that could be obtained from the PPDU examination may help to improve the diagnostic yield of vascular abnormalities. For example, the combination of persistent dorsal vein flow and elevated EDV resulted in 93% accuracy in diagnosing venous leakage when correlated with cavernosographic findings, even though the determination of dorsal vein flow velocity, by itself, has not proved to be useful in making such a diagnosis (5). PPDU examination may also provide significant information about the existence of significant congenital vascular anomalies and functional or structural abnormalities with the helicine arteriolar system.

Several pitfalls may influence the interpretation of PPDU data (3,7,8,15): (i) the accuracy of flow velocities calculated from Doppler shift frequencies is dependent on optimal insonation angle correction; (ii) velocity measurements at a site of arterial narrowing may not suggest the presence of disease, since artificially high blood velocity readings could be obtained at the location of stenosis; (iii) a slow blood flow may be observed in nondominant arteries (due to congenital variation), which may lead to overestimation of proximal arterial disease; (iv) blood flow may be spuriously impeded by the high intracorporeal pressure if the measurements were taken in the later phases of the waveform cycle; (v) copresence of veno-occlusive dysfunction may significantly alter the hemodynamic balance and confound the criteria for normal arterial supply; and (vi) sympathetic overtone (due to patient's anxiety) may cause marked functional alteration in the flow of the cavernous arteries that may be difficult to distinguish from reduced blood supply due to a true structural insufficiency. Some of these pitfalls could be eliminated by meticulous attention to technique, the use of color Doppler scanning, and the correlation of results with the degree of penile rigidity. Repeated vasoactive drug injections (44) or exposure to visual erotic stimuli may help to induce complete relaxation of trabecular smooth muscle, and, hence, reduce the overestimation of corporeal structural disease. Also, sufficient erectile response as assessed by a self-reporting instrument (i.e., a post-investigation questionnaire) may help to reduce the false-positive diagnosis of veno-occlusive dysfunction by as much as 50% (45).

Dynamic Infusion Cavernosometry and Cavernosography

Dynamic infusion cavernosometry and cavernosography (DICC) are widely accepted as the reference

(A) Cavernosometry

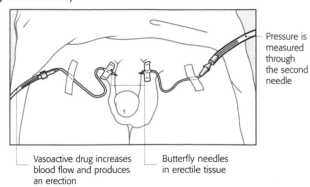

Pressure is measured through the second needle

Vasoactive drug increases blood flow and produces an erection

Butterfly needles in erectile tissue

(B) Cavernosography

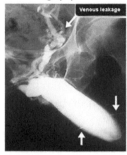

(C)

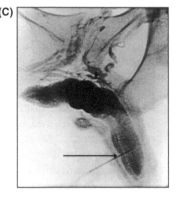

Figure 5 Venous leakage on dynamic infusion cavernosometry and cavernosography study. Cavernosometry is used to measure the blood flow rate necessary to produce and maintain an erection. While the patient is lying down, two very small (butterfly) needles are inserted into the penis (**A**). A vasodilatory drug is given to produce erection; saline is then infused, which allows the pressure to be measured at the second needle. In cavernosography, an X-ray contrast material is injected into the penis (**B,C**). X-rays are obtained to evaluate for venous leakage. If the penis is not fully rigid, venous leakage will occur, regardless. Cavernosography alone can be used to show space in the corpora following fibrosis after a prolonged erection (priapism) or removal of a penile prosthesis, and also to view plaques in Peyronie's disease. In a human male with erectile dysfunction, cavernosography demonstrates escape of dye into penile venous system (**B**, *labeled arrow, top right*). Unlabeled arrows indicate bilateral intracavernous placement of two angiocatheters for administration of vasoactive agents in phase I in order to induce erection, and then heparinized saline in phase II and contrast in phase IV. In (**C**), X-ray shows fibrosis in the penis at indicator. *Source*: From Ref. 54.

diagnostic techniques for evaluation of veno-occlusive dysfunction (Fig. 5). Commonly, the two procedures are performed consecutively as a four-phased, one-hour investigation (3,46–50). Intracavernous and systemic brachial blood pressure and penile circumference are monitored continuously throughout. After site preparation, two 21-gauge angiocatheters are introduced, one into each corpus cavernosum, to measure intracorporeal pressure and infuse fluid. In phase I, vasoactive agents (commonly 45–60 mg papaverine and 1–2.5 mg phentolamine) are injected into one corpus to relax the corporeal smooth muscle, followed by determination of the maximum equilibrium corporeal body pressure and the time required to reach the equilibrium. Intracavernosal pressure at equilibrium

represents cavernosal artery pressure, less the loss of pressure from venous drainage. In phase II, cavernosometry is performed by infusing heparinized saline to raise the corporeal body pressure to 150 mm Hg; then, the infusion pump is turned off. The fall in pressure over 30 seconds is noted. The procedure is repeated with and without perineal compression of the proximal crura. In phase III, the cavernosal artery systolic occlusion pressure is determined by locating each cavernosal artery at the base of the penis with a Doppler ultrasound probe while brachial artery pressure is continuously recorded. Heparinized saline is infused to raise intracorporeal pressure to a level higher than that required for the Doppler signal to disappear. The infusion is stopped, and, as the intracorporeal pressure falls, the level at which the cavernosal artery signal reappears is noted. The procedure is repeated several times, and an average arterial occlusion pressure for each side is determined. In phase IV, the cavernosography is performed by infusing a contrast material [diatrizoate meglumine 30% (Reno-M-Dip) or Iopamidol 41% (Isovue-M 200); Bristol-Myers Squibb Company] to raise intracorporeal pressure to 90 mmHg. Radiographs of the perineum and of the penis, including the glans and corpus spongiosum, are obtained under-fluoroscopic guidance. The flow needed to maintain intracorporeal pressure at 90 mm Hg is recorded. Following cavernosography, the corpora are aspirated, and, if veno-occlusive dysfunction is found, diluted phenylephrine (0.2–0.3 mg) is injected. It should be noted that valid DICC testing is dependent upon the complete relaxation of corporeal trabecular smooth muscle tissue in response to injected vasoactive drug administration. The presence of patient anxiety, an inadequate dose of vasoactive agent(s), or intrinsic smooth muscle dysfunction may yield false-positive results. Such relaxation can be achieved with the use of intracorporeal injection of vasoactive drugs with or without audio–VSS and is inferred when a linear relationship between three incremental infusion rates and the associated intracorporeal pressures is observed (3,47,51,52). Further, more than one vasoactive injection may be required to achieve a complete smooth muscle relaxation, which is reflected by the presence of a full, rigid, and maintained erectile response that requires intracavernous adrenergic agonist injection to resolve (53). Under the condition of complete smooth muscle relaxation, two distinct groups of steady-state intracavernous pressures have been identified and found to reflect different capacitance states (52). Pressures greater than 60 mm Hg are associated with low capacitance values, low-pressure decay, low flow to maintain erection (less than 4 mL/min), and high venous outflow resistance values (greater than 100 mm Hg/min/mL). Such hemodynamic parameters reflected the existence of substantial corporeal veno-occlusive function. In contrast, steady-state intracavernous pressures of less than 50 mm Hg were associated with extremely low venous outflow resistance (less than 29 mm Hg/min/mL), higher-to-maintain flow rates, and higher corporeal capacitance (greater than 0.049 mL/mm Hg). This latter hemodynamic group reflects the presence of severe veno-occlusive dysfunction that presumably is associated with a significant corporeal structural disease. Thus, failure to assess corporeal veno-occlusive function under the condition of complete trabecular smooth muscle relaxation is likely to overestimate the degree of corporeal structural disease (52).

False-positive results can also occur with psychogenic impotence and in normal controls. Bruising is common after DICC, but this resolves spontaneously over several days. Priapism occurs in about 1% of subjects and may require additional corporeal irrigations (48). Caution is advised in performing this study in patients with a history of contrast reaction, significant cardiac disease, or current anticoagulant use. The study is also contraindicated in patients who receive monoamine oxidase inhibitors.

Accepted diagnostic criteria for veno-occlusive dysfunction include intracorporeal pressure <30 mm Hg, at the steady state, after vasoactive drug(s) injection in phase I; a fall in intracavernosal pressure to below 105 mm Hg, or of magnitude greater than 45 mm Hg after 30 seconds from discontinuation of saline administration in phase II; the need for a saline or contrast media infusion at the rate of >5 mL/min to maintain a specific intracorporeal pressure in phases II and IV; and abnormal cavernosography in phase IV. Moreover, a gradient between brachial systolic and cavernosal artery occlusive pressures in phase III that is >30 to 35 mmHg is accepted as indicative of arterial insufficiency. The diagnosis of arterial insufficiency based on the determination of cavernosal artery occlusion pressure was validated against arteriography (3,47,48,55).

At least two other variations of cavernosometry have been described. The first is known as pump cavernosometry and involves infusion of preheated (37° C) normal saline into the penis (3,49,56,57). The flow rates required both to obtain and to maintain intracavernous pressure of 90 mm Hg are recorded. Earlier versions of this test did not employ intracorporeal vasoactive drug injections or audio–VSS, and thus adequate corporeal smooth muscle relaxation was not consistently achieved. As a result, normal induction flow rates between 80 and 120 mL/min, and maintenance flow rates between 20 and 40 mL/min were reported. These maintenance flow rates are much higher than those described above for DICC with complete smooth muscle relaxation (< 5 mL/min). Moreover, high flow rates were reported in patients with psychogenic impotence who are presumed to have normal veno-occlusive mechanisms (3,49,51), suggesting that lack of corporeal smooth muscle relaxation leads to a functional venous insufficiency and thus a high rate of false-positives. The second variant of cavernosometry is known as gravity cavernosometry (49,53,58). In this method, an intravenous infusion set is used instead of the pump, and complete corporeal

smooth muscle relaxation is induced with local vasoactive drug(s) injections with or without audio–VSS. Baseline intracorporeal pressure is then determined and followed by the infusion of heparinized normal saline at increasing pressures of 40, 80, 120, and 160 cm of water. Steady-state intracavernous pressure is determined at each infusion pressure. Linear relationship between steady-state intracavernous and infusion pressures (3), or maintenance of intracavernous pressure higher than 110 mm Hg with a constant saline infusion pressure of 140 cm of water (59,60), is suggestive of normal veno-occlusive mechanisms. Intracavernous pressure at a column of 160 cm water during gravity cavernosometry showed good correlation with the maintenance flow during pump cavernosometry, and both had the highest diagnostic value for veno-occlusive dysfunction in one study (61). Since gravity cavernosometry with complete smooth muscle relaxation by vasoactive drugs and/or audio–VSS is a pressure-controlled rather than rate-controlled cavernosometry and does not require sophisticated systems, it has been considered by several investigators to be more physiologic, safer, and cheaper than DICC or pump cavernosometry.

EDV measured by PPDU after papaverine injection was compared with DICC in 28 patients with sufficient arterial inflow (normal PSV with ultrasound) but poor erectile response to papaverine injection (40). The two methods were found to agree on the diagnosis of venous leakage in 25 (89%) patients. A second study compared PBI, PPDU, DICC, and angiography in 168 men with erectile insufficiency. Of these, 145 men had penile arterial insufficiency demonstrated by digital subtraction pharmacoangiography. PBI correctly identified 87, PSV identified 130, and cavernosal artery occlusion pressure identified 136 of these men. Cavernosal venous leakage as demonstrated by DICC was seen in 96 men. The RI calculated during PPDU determined 15 minutes after vasodilator challenge correctly identified 93 of 96 venous leakers, and 48 out of 72 nonvenous leakers; however, the RI determined five minutes after vasodilator challenge incorrectly categorized 67 nonleakers as having venous leakage. The study concluded that both PSV and cavernous artery occlusion pressure are accurate predictors of cavernosal artery insufficiency, whereas the PBI is a poor predictor. The PPDU appears reliable as angiography and is more cost-effective. The RI is an accurate predictor of cavernosal venous leakage only if determined once maximal response to vasodilator challenge has occurred (55). A third study, however, which compared PPDU and DICC in 60 impotent men with poor response to therapy with PGE$_1$ injection found PPDU parameters such as end EDV, RI, and pulsatility index to be poor predictors of venous leakage as compared to DICC (62). Further, the correlations among the results of four different methods of cavernosometry [pump, gravity, pressure-drop phase of DICC (phase II), and pharmacocavernosometry (papaverine injection followed by erotic visual stimulation)] were examined in 123 impotent subjects. Complete agreement among all methods was found to be around 50%; however, there was a considerable spectrum in the estimate of normal responses with a range of 6.5% to 64.2% depending on the method and criteria used (49).

Current techniques of cavernosometry and cavernosography have been subjected to the following criticisms: (*i*) the paucity of normative data and the lack of adjustment of data to penile size or tissue mass; (*ii*) the difficulty in relating penile outflow parameters of DICC to those of penile inflow provided by duplex ultrasonography (the first measures flow rate, while the second measures velocity); (*iii*) errors in measurement of flow rates due to inadvertent needle placement against the trabecular wall; (*iv*) the high rate of false-positives due to lack of complete relaxation of the corporeal smooth muscle fibers; (*v*) the inability of cavernosometry to distinguish accurately between true venous leakage and intrinsic smooth muscle or collagen fiber disorders; (*vi*) the presence of the same radiological cavernosography findings in some normal individuals as in patients with true veno-occlusive insufficiency; and (*vii*) the lack of correlation between hemodynamic parameters derived from DICC and penile rigidity. A recent study investigating this latter correlation in 21 impotent patients (mean age 43 years, range 24–62 years) found a poor correlation between cavernosal compliance and equilibrium intracavernosal pressure, better correlation between cavernosal compliance and expandability, and the best correlation between dimensionless compliance and the dimensionless product of expandability with equilibrium pressure. Such data implied that cavernosal compliance was dependent on multiple factors, including intracavernosal pressure, penile geometry, and erectile tissue properties. Cavernosal expandability is the most relevant tissue property for prediction of adequate penile buckling forces (63). Thus, hemodynamic indices that correlate with intracavernosal pressure alone may not predict correctly the penile buckling forces.

Penile Angiography

This study is usually performed in selected patients prior to reconstructive vascular surgery. The typical patient is a young man with a history of blunt perineal trauma that results in a blockage at the origin of the cavernosal artery. Selective pudendal angiography is helpful in defining the site of arterial block and thus in planning the appropriate surgery (64). The sensitivity of procedures for detecting arterial lesions is on the order of 95%. The value of arteriography in microvascular disease is limited, as microsurgical reconstruction is not always feasible. Further, the many variations of arterial supply to the penis and the lack of normative data may make the interpretation of the study difficult. Further, procedure-related anxiety may lead to excessive adrenergic discharge

with arterial vasoconstriction and an increased potential for false-positive results.

Radionuclide Tracer Techniques

Radionuclide methods have been applied to penile hemodynamics since the early 1970s, using a number of different combinations of radiotracers, routes of administration, and interventions (65–67). Information derived from these methods has helped to elucidate basic mechanisms of erectile physiology and by providing quantitative information regarding penile blood volume and flow (68).

Radionuclide imaging depends on the uptake of a radionuclide tracer by target tissue in an analogous manner to the usual biological process. Radionuclide methods may be subdivided into three categories: blood-pool, tracer wash-in, and tracer washout, and the simultaneous performance of blood-pool and wash-out measurements. These methods are summarized in Figure 6 and Table 3, and are discussed individually below.

Blood-Pool Methods
Techniques
The concept of studying the penile blood pool by radionuclide techniques was proposed and developed by Shirai et al. in the early 1970s (70–73). The systemic blood pool is labeled with a γ emitter such as ^{99m}Tc, and external measurements of the penile blood pool are performed. In initial blood-pool studies, erection was achieved by VSS (72,73) or systemic vasodilators (70,71, 74–76). Currently, intracavernosal injection of vasoactive drugs (77–80) is a more effective and reproducible method of achieving erection, although some authors have argued that audio–visual stimulation is more physiologic and therefore superior (81). It is important to limit the volume of vasoactive injectate, so as not to alter significantly the hematocrit of trapped blood, thereby disturbing quantitative calculations (82,83).

In the initial studies described, counts were measured in the flaccid and erect states by an external nonimaging sodium-iodide crystal, similar in design to a modern thyroid probe (70–73). In most current techniques, a γ camera is used to acquire penile counts (74,75,77–79), although a portable and inexpensive well-type scintillation crystal has also been introduced for this purpose (84). In the usual camera technique, a lead drape is used to shield surrounding background activity. Region-of-interest analysis is performed to generate time-activity curves (TACs) (Figs. 7 and 8) (69,80) from which numerical indices can be calculated (Table 4). It is also possible to generate absolute volume measurements by comparison to appropriate standards such as a measured aliquot of venous blood (73,77). These indices, and absolute measurements, have been used to assess several parameters relevant to erectile physiology, as will be reviewed below.

Oscillations in blood volume measurements have been described as a frequent finding both in flaccid

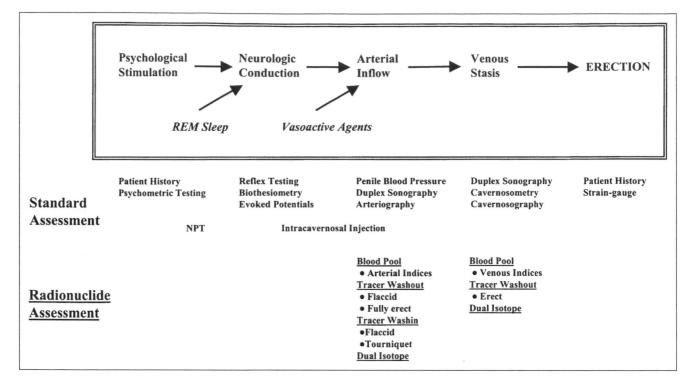

Figure 6 Flowchart illustrates normal and alternate (*italics*) pathways in the physiologic and pharmacologic development of erection (*box*). Both standard and radionuclidic (*underlined*) methods of assessment have been charted under positions corresponding to the information that they convey. *Abbreviations*: NPT, nocturnal penile tuminescence; REM, rapid eye movement. *Source*: From Ref. 69.

(87) and in tumescent (81,88,89) blood-pool TACs (Fig. 9). The interpretation of this phenomenon is debated, whether they occur in normal subjects (87,88) or psychogenic patients (81,86,89) remains unclear. Their presence could conceivably also be related to the method of erectile stimulation, sedation, or the general anxiety level of the subjects.

Arterial Assessment

Using radio-labeled blood-pool techniques, investigators have studied arterial flow after erectile stimulation, based on the absolute change, or the rate of change, of blood pool with time. This method assumes negligible concurrent venous outflow, an assumption that was ultimately confirmed by dual-isotope blood-pool/wash-out studies of Schwartz et al. (80). Shirai emphasized qualitative changes in the TACs, occurring with the development of erection (70–72). Further refinement of this method included a quantitative measure of the proportional increase of emitted radioactivity in

counts (posterection/pre-erection), as well as the absolute posterection penile volume, calculated with reference to a venous blood sample (73).

Fanous et al. (74) adopted a quantitative approach in their studies by defining a penogram index, which represented the increment in counts after erection divided

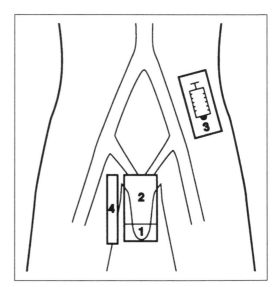

Figure 7 Idealized red blood cell blood-pool acquisition regions of interest. Schematic representation of typical field of view during blood-pool study. Numbered regions represent (**1**) glans penis, (**2**) cavernosal body, (**3**) syringe, and (**4**) background. *Source*: From Ref. 80.

Table 3 Use of Radionuclide Techniques in the Assessment of Penile Arterial and Venous Integrity

	Test	Arterial	Venous
Blood pool	Stimulated	+	+
Tracer wash-out	Erect	−	+
Tracer wash-out	Flaccid	+	−
Tracer wash-in	Post-tourniquet	+	−
Dual isotope	Combined blood pool and wash-out	+	+

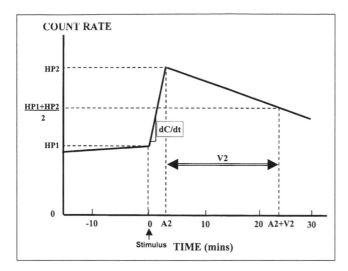

Figure 8 Idealized time-activity curve of penile blood-pool activity [after Kim et al. (79)]. To standardize terminology, time of erectile stimulation has been set at 0, with prior time points described on a negative scale. A2 has been defined as the time when peak activity after stimulation occurs (time to peak activity) Table 4 describes additional blood-pool indices based on this nomenclature, some of which are indicated in the figure. HP₁: baseline activity, HP₂: peak activity, V₂: interval between peak-counts (HP₂) and half-peak (HP₁+HP₂/2) *Source*: From Ref. 69.

This was normalized for counts in the iliac vessels, a measure of the rate of inflow, which occurs during induction of erection.

A well-considered physiologic approach has been described by Schwartz et al. (77), who calculated absolute flow rates by normalizing the change in penile counts with time to the activity of a 10 mL venous blood standard. The peak corporal flow was shown to correlate well with an angiographic index of arterial integrity. Patients with virtually normal arteries had mean peak corporal flows of 14.7 ± 4.4 mL/min, while those with severe arterial disease had calculated values of 4.8 ± 1.5 mL/min. As would be expected, no correlation was identified between peak corporal flow and intracorporeal resistance (90), a measure of venous competence. In a subsequent publication by Schwartz et al. (80), the parameter which correlated best with an angiographic scoring of arterial disease was the change in penile blood volume from one minute before to one minute after time of peak inflow ($r = 0.96$), which the authors felt reflected the ability to maintain inflow rates during the peak phase of tumescence. It is interesting to note that this methodology, although more sophisticated, is quite similar to that published by Shirai in 1976 (73).

by the baseline counts [(post-erection-pre-erection)/pre-erection] and which correlated well with the penile to brachial blood pressure index. Shen and Kao (85) have been able to show that slope and time to peak were useful in differentiating patients with arterial disease from those with venous or psychogenic dysfunction. Siraj et al. added a vasodilator response (75) or flow (78) index, which related to the relative difference in slopes of the TACs before and after vasoactive medication was given.

Venous Assessment

While the blood-pool examinations are primarily suited to evaluation of arterial sufficiency, Siraj has described the typical appearance of the TAC in venous incompetence, in which the posterection plateau in counts is not sustained (78). This appearance has been numerically quantitated by Kim et al. (79) who generated venous wash-out indices based on the fraction of activity remaining 30 minutes after peak erection and

Table 4 Described Blood-Pool Indices

Index	Full name	Description[a]	Author (Ref.)
PBV	Pooled blood volume	C(A2) normalized to venous standard	Shirai (73)
RI	Rate of increase	C(A2)/C(0)	Shirai (73)
PI	Penogram index	[C(A2) − C(0)]/C(0)	Fanous (74)
F1	Flow index 1	[C(0) − C(−7.5)]/(Σ iliac artery counts)	Siraj (75)
F2	Flow index 2	[C(+2.5) −C(+7.5)]/(Σ iliac artery counts)	Siraj (75)
VRI	Vasodilator response index	(F2 − F1)/F1	Siraj (75)
FI	Flow index	Same as VRI	Siraj (78)
PCF	Peak corporal flow	Peak dC/dt Normalized to Venous Standard	Schwartz (77)
HP1	Baseline activity	C(0)	Kim (79)
HP2	Peak activity	C(A2)	Kim (79)
A1	—	[HP2 − C(−10)]/C(−10)	Kim (79)
A2	Time to reach peak (HP2)	Fig. 8	Kim (79)
V1	—	[HP2 − C(A2 + 30)]/C(A2 + 30)	Kim (79)
V2	—	Interval between peak-counts (HP2) and half-peak (HP1 + HP2)/2	Kim (79)
WOI	Wash-out index	[C(A2) − C(90)]/C(A2)	Shen (85)
TT	Transit time	Same as A2 above	Choi (86)
EPT	Erection persistent time	Period in which activity is >75% of peak	Choi (86)
R1	Activity before stimulation	Same as HP1 above	Choi (86)
R2	Activity after stimulation	Same as HP2 above	Choi (86)
dCV	Volume change	[C(A2 + 1)−C(A2 − 1)] Normalized to venous standard	Schwartz (80)

[a]See Fig. 8 for nomenclature.
Source: From Ref. 72.

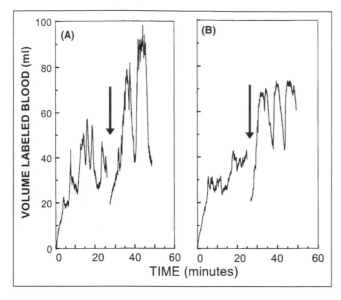

Figure 9 Oscillation in penile blood volume. Two separate studies in the same individual separated by three months, using the well-type scintillation device to assess blood-pool time activity curves (TACs). In this nervous young male, standard evaluation supported a psychogenic etiology. Beginning of stimulated segments of the curves is indicated by arrows. Note the highly reproducible oscillations in blood volume, seen on both flaccid wash-in and stimulated portion of the curves.

the time needed after peak erection to return halfway toward the baseline (Table 4). These indices were useful in differentiating patients with venous disease from those with arterial insufficiency or nonvascular disease. In contrast to the accepted utility of blood-pool studies in the evaluation of arterial etiologies of ED, the use of blood-pool indices to diagnose and quantitate venous disorders is less established.

Priapism

Priapism constitutes a special subset of ED that may be evaluated by radionuclide blood-pool studies. It may be associated with either reduced or intact inflow, categorized as stagnant or nonstagnant priapism, respectively (91). Scintigraphy has been useful in qualitatively assessing perfusion (91–94), with persistent inflow suggesting that more conservative management is appropriate, while absent inflow mandates more invasive monitoring and therapy (91). It appears that only decreased flow in both the corpus spongiosum and the corpora cavernosa predicts subsequent ED (91,94) while reduced inflow of the corpora cavernosa alone is less definitive (91).

Evaluation of Therapy

Several groups have used the blood-pool technique to evaluate patients after various methods of revascularization surgery, including three-vessel anastomosis (95–97). Drawz et al. (97), using the technique of Schwartz et al. (77), demonstrated that average corporal flow in 13 patients prior to microvascular revascularization was 1.51 ± 0.64 mL/min, ultimately

increasing by 1.21 ± 1.28 mL/min ($p = 0.01$) in 10 of the patients, in whom the anastomosis remained patent. Because the mechanism of clinical improvement following this procedure is poorly understood, the documentation of increased flow provided objective evidence for its benefit.

Quantitative blood-pool examinations have also been advocated as a means of titrating pharmacotherapy (98). Smith et al. studied a group of 48 patients with ED that was being considered for pharmacologically induced penile erection therapy by means of the blood-pool technique (99). The relative increase in penile blood volume correlated with patient satisfaction with this therapy. Thirty-eight patients who were ultimately satisfied had a mean 2.6-fold increase in blood pool (range 1.2 to 8.9), while 10 patients who were ultimately dissatisfied had a mean increase of only 1.6-fold (range 1.1 to 2.4) ($p = 0.001$). Although not directly addressed by data within the paper, the authors suggest that the blood-pool response to an initial test dose can also be used to titrate the amount of vasoactive pharmaceutical needed, thereby ensuring adequate erection but reducing the likelihood of priapism.

Dosimetry

Blood-pool studies for the investigation of impotence, using $^{99m}T_c$-labeled red blood cells (RBCs), have identical dosimetry with commonly performed cardiac and hemangioma blood-pool radionuclide examinations. Generally, accepted dosimetry values are 55 mrads to the blood and 19 mrads to the whole body per-millicurie of $^{99m}T_c$-labeled RBCs (100,101); for a 20 mCi administered dose, these values are well within the range of other diagnostic radionuclide and radiologic examinations.

Wash-in Techniques
Theory

Rather than measuring the rate of egress of activity locally deposited in the corpora cavernosa (wash-out studies) or the amount of blood present as a function of time within the penis (blood-pool studies), wash-in techniques measure the arrival of activity into the corpora cavernosa, following systemic administration. The instant introduction of a radiolabel into the systemic circulation—in this case, the rate of initial arrival of radio-labeled blood into the corpora cavernosa—is proportional to the rate of penile blood flow. An appropriate standard such as a sample of venous blood is then used to convert the TAC to a time–volume curve, and the initial slope of the curve would equal blood flow. Unfortunately, a peripheral intravenous injection of activity does not produce a well-mixed systemic blood pool prior to arrival of activity into the penile artery. Nonetheless, wash-in measurements can be used in two special circumstances, as noted below.

Cuff Method

Grech et al. (102,103) studied dynamic perfusion of the corpora cavernosa immediately after release of an inflatable cuff placed at the base of the penis, following systemic injection of radio-labeled blood. The cuff serves to isolate the penile blood pool until radioactivity is mixed within the systemic blood pool. After release, the initial slope of the blood-pool curve is proportional to blood flow. Studies were performed when flaccid, and on a different occasion, following intracavernosal injection of papaverine. The locally trapped papaverine leads to a maximal vasoactive response prior to tourniquet release. Flaccid postocclusive flow averaged 13.1 ± 4.4 mL/min/100 cc (mean ± 1 SD) in normal men, and increased to 33.5 ± 16.2 mL/min/100 cc after vasoactive stimulation. Values in patients with arterial disease were 4.3 ± 1.9, increasing to 13.2 ± 4.6 mL/min/100 cc poststimulation. In comparison to normal patients, flaccid and erect flows had *p* values of 0.001 and 0.013, respectively. There was no significant difference in flaccid and erect penile blood flow in the venous leak group compared to controls, as would be expected.

With the blood cuff method, the penis is partially ischemic upon cuff release, and it could be argued that a true flaccid blood flow is not obtained (103,104). Nonetheless, stimulated blood flow values were able to discriminate completely between patients with arterial disease and other causes of ED, making the technique potentially valuable for diagnostic purposes.

Equilibrium Method

Zuckier et al. (84,105) introduced a method of studying flaccid blood flow by measuring cavernosal activity after peripheral injection of radio-labeled blood. In this case, the ^{99m}Tc-RBC wash-in curves are used in their entirety, rather than just the initial linear portion (Fig. 10). Because of the low ratio of flow (F) to volume (V) in the corpora cavernosa, it takes between 10 and 20 minutes for penile activity to plateau and reach equilibrium after injection into the faster-equilibrating systemic compartment. Using a simple model of wash-in, this curve can be fit to an exponential equation.

$$LBV\ (t) = V \times (1 - e^{-k \times t})$$

where LBV represents the volume of labeled blood within the corpora cavernosa, and the equilibrium constant k equals the ratio of F/V. Values for flaccid blood volume and flow can be readily calculated, serving as a baseline for the subsequent stimulated measurements. Phantom studies have confirmed the assumptions underlying this method (105), and the technique has been applied to patients (105) and to laboratory animals (106,107).

Wash-out Indicators
Theory

Historically, the washout of radioactive indicators, especially ^{133}Xe, has been used to evaluate cavernosal blood flow. These measurements have been performed in the flaccid penis, after subcutaneous or intracavernosal injection, and, in the erect penis, after intracavernosal injection (69). The latter measurement is the most relevant to clinical practice because it allows for the detection of venous leak during erection.

Washout of radioactive gases is a classic physiologic tool for measuring blood flow in many organ systems. Following the deposit of a locally diffusible tracer at the site of interest, the rate of removal of activity is proportional to regional blood flow and to the relative affinity of the tracer for blood as compared to the local tissues (the partition coefficient) (108,109). External measurements over the site of radioactive deposition result in a "wash-out" TAC that reflects the rate of disappearance of activity (Fig. 11) (110). Analysis is somewhat more complicated when measuring blood flow in the corpora cavernosa, as the overall volume of distribution is variable. This simplifies when the penis is in a steady state—i.e., when arterial inflow equals venous

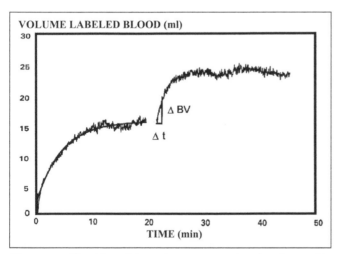

Figure 10 Flaccid wash-in and post–papaverine data from a 38-year-old man with erectile dysfunction, acquired with a scintillation probe. The initial flaccid wash-in (0–20 minutes) has been fit according to the wash-in model, yielding flaccid blood volume of 12.9 mL and flow of 2.9 mL/min. Post-papaverine data (20–45 minutes) shows a slow increase in blood volume and is consistent with described patterns of arterial insufficiency. *Source*: From Ref. 84.

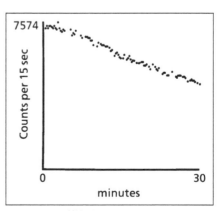

Figure 11 Washout of ^{133}Xe from the corpus cavernosum in flaccid state. Each data point represents the total count recorded by γ camera in the penile region over a 15-second time interval. Analysis of the 5- to 30-minute segment of the curve yielded a blood flow of 1.3 mL/100 g/min. *Source*: From Ref. 110.

outflow and there is a constant corporal volume. In this case, activity leaving the penis (dA/dt) is equal to the product of blood flow (F) and the concentration of activity present within the blood pool of the corpora cavernosa (A/V). In mathematical terms, dA/dt = –F × A/V, which can be solved to yield:

$$A(t) = A(0) \times e^{-(k \times t)}$$

where A(t) is the corporal activity measured at time t, and k is the ratio of blood flow divided by cavernosal volume (F/V), the inverse of the mean transit time. When corporal volume is known, then an absolute value for flow can be calculated from these tracings.

As noted, this mathematic model can only be solved when the penis is in a steady state, meaning that it is generally either flaccid or fully erect. During tumescence or detumescence, corporal volume is changing, leading to an inability to determine quantitative venous outflow and arterial inflow, although the disappearance curves can still be analyzed in a qualitative manner. For example, presence of washout of the radiotracer may be used to evaluate the veno-occlusive mechanism. After erection, there should be little egress of blood from the corpora cavernosa in a normal subject; inspection of the TAC during this period can indicate whether the veno-occlusive mechanism is operative in a given patient.

Intracavernosal ¹³³Xe in the Erect Penis

Pioneering work by Wagner and Uhrenholdt measured erect and flaccid blood flow in four normal volunteers (111). A strain-gauge plethysmograph was used to monitor circumferential size of the penis, and both flow and circumferential volumes were continuously recorded during and after attainment of erection. VSS was continued until full erection was obtained. The authors observed that penile blood flow decreased after VSS, dropping from 3 to 8 mL/100 g/min in the flaccid state to 0 to 4 mL/100 g/min while erect. During detumescence, blood flow was initially elevated (20–75 mL/100 g/min), and subsequently decreased to the flaccid levels 2.5 to 4 minutes after termination of the visual stimulation. In 1983, this group published results of intracavernosal injection of xenon in patients with Peyronie's disease (112), a disorder that is frequently accompanied by ED. In five patients with normal erectile function, normal venous closure was noted after onset of erection, similar to the finding previously noted in controls (111). In 11 of 15 patients with impotence, visually stimulated erection paradoxically resulted in insufficient venous closure. Absolute numerical values were not stated. These studies were important in that they were the first to provide objective data on blood flow during erection, thereby setting the stage for the modern concepts of erectile physiology.

More recently, Yeh studied intracavernosal penile xenon washout in patients with incomplete erectile response to the intracavernosal injection of PGE₁, both before and after administration of this vasoactive agent (113). While all six patients with nonvenous disease, as assessed by other modalities, had a decrease in ¹³³Xe corporal clearance after PGE₁ administration, 12 of 14 patients with documented venous disease had a significant increase in xenon washout.

Surprisingly, completely opposite results were obtained in an early study by Shirai (114). When intracavernosal ¹³³Xe injections were used to determine cavernosal blood flow in five subjects with complete erections after VSS, intrapenile blood flow averaged 2.0 mL/100 gm/min while flaccid and 43.0 mL/100 gm/min while erect. These anomalous results, which do not agree with other investigators, could be related to the fact that erection is a dynamic process, and measurement of flow at different times will give highly variable results. Furthermore, the erectile response is itself variable, depending on the type and effectiveness of stimulus employed. If stimulation is insufficient to adequately trigger the veno-occlusive mechanism, increased flow will result in a paradoxical increase in xenon washout.

⁹⁹ᵐTc-Based Methods

Several groups have used ⁹⁹ᵐTc-labeled tracers to measure cavernosal washout after direct introduction into the corpora cavernosa. ⁹⁹ᵐTc-colloid has the advantage of absent recirculation (81,115); upon entering the systemic circulation it becomes trapped by reticuloendothelial cells, thereby preventing reintroduction of activity by way of the arterial circulation. Groshar et al. used ⁹⁹ᵐTc-RBCs to measure rates of cavernosal washout (Fig. 12) (116). Direct intracorporeal injections of

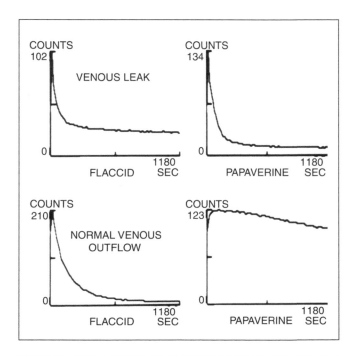

Figure 12 Time-activity curve of red blood cell corporeal clearance in representative patients with venous leak (*top panels*) and normal venous outflow (*bottom panels*). Flaccid (*left*) and post–papaverine (*right*) curves are illustrated. *Source*: From Ref. 116.

0.5 mCi of autologous ^{99m}Tc-RBCs were performed both when flaccid and erect. Although ^{99m}Tc-labeled RBCs leaving the penis would recirculate after passing through the systemic circulation, marked dilution in the systemic blood pool renders this factor negligible. Groshar et al. found that the halftime of clearance in 13 normal subjects without venous disease was significantly longer after papaverine/regitine-induced erection (2892 ± 1899 sec) as compared to that in seven patients with venous incompetence (213 ± 123 sec), while no statistically significant difference in flaccid washout was noted between these groups (halftimes of 202 ± 139 seconds vs. 92 ± 35 seconds, respectively). The approach of using ^{99m}Tc-labeled radiopharmaceuticals provides a more convenient means of determining cavernosal washout than xenon studies. While ^{99m}Tc-RBC wash-out appears to identify effectively patients with venous disease on the basis of erect halftimes of clearance, discrepancies in calculated values compared with those derived from xenon washout raise questions as to which quantitative estimates are more reliable.

Dosimetry

Radiation exposure to patients undergoing either ^{99m}Tc-RBC or ^{133}Xe wash-out studies is within the range of that encountered in other nuclear medicine studies and is considerably less than the exposure associated with pelvic angiography. Assumptions regarding the rate of transit and washout of radiopharmaceutical, which in turn depend on the quality and duration of erection, have profound implications on this dosimetry. Assuming a blood flow of 1 mL/100 mg/min, Haden et al. have calculated a radiation dose of approximately 2.1 rad/mCi to the injection site with the use of ^{133}Xe (110). The dose to the testes and entire body are similar to those of intravenous injections and are quoted as 0.065 and 0.12 mrad/mCi, respectively. Wagner has stated that a dose of 0.3 mCi of ^{133}Xe contributes 1.22 mrad, although it is unclear as to which target volume he is referring (111).

Combined Methodologies

Several groups have reported the use of combined blood-pool and xenon wash-out studies for the evaluation of penile blood flow. This method yields two simultaneous differential equations of two variables that can be iteratively solved, leading to a complete description of arterial inflow and venous outflow during erection, including non–steady-state conditions (80,117,118). This is greatly superior to the concurrent generation of arterial and venous indices alone, which also has been performed (119).

True Dual Isotope Methods

Schwartz and Graham have published a method in which blood-pool and wash-out examinations were performed on separate occasions using ^{99m}Tc-RBC and ^{133}Xe (nine patients) or simultaneously, using

^{99m}Tc-RBC and ^{127}Xe (five patients) (Fig. 13) (80). As a rule, the degree of venous outflow during time of peak inflow was shown to be negligible (80), validating the use of penile blood-pool TACs alone as an accurate measure of peak arterial inflow. Miraldi has described a slightly different method of simultaneously monitoring ^{99m}Tc-RBC blood pool and ^{133}Xe washout with erection (118,120). Based on a one-compartment model, the study included six normal subjects, three with arterial insufficiency and five with venous leak (120). Although the sample size was small, arterial insufficiency patients were notable for decreased peak arterial flow, while venous insufficiency patients had elevated peak venous flow rates.

The dual isotope approach is a major advance in the scintimetric analysis of ED as it allows the simultaneous and exact calculation of changes in both inflow and outflow of penile blood throughout the cycle or erection and detumescence (121). It is interesting to observe that the tracings obtained using this noninvasive technique (Fig. 13) are strikingly similar to the data obtained by using an invasive model for erection in monkeys (122). While a high level of technical difficulty may restrict dual-tracer examinations to a research setting, this technique affords a complete analysis of vascular factors during erection.

Limitations of Radionuclide Tracer Studies

There are several interrelated limitations applicable to all the radionuclide ED studies. First, pharmacologic stimulation, regardless of agent choice, may lead to a potentially submaximal level of erection (80). Corporal smooth muscle relaxation may also be affected by anxiety (123). Thus, data regarding either the degree of arterial inflow or adequacy of venous occlusion may be misleading. These concerns are common to all radionuclide and nonradionuclide ED examinations that rely on the injection of intracavernosal pharmacologic agents to induce erection.

A second related limitation is that scintigraphic studies, as currently performed, have not included the measurement and manipulation of intracorporeal pressures, as has been done in cavernosometry/cavernosography and rigorous color-flow Doppler protocols (80). This especially impacts on the validity of ^{133}Xe wash-out data, for which information regarding the veno-occlusive mechanism is meaningless unless the corpora have first been adequately filled. While the scintigraphic techniques are, in fact, compatible with pressure monitoring and volume augmentation, this would be at the expense of sacrificing the noninvasive benefit of scintigraphy.

An additional criticism of all diagnostic tests is their relevance. As newer pharmacologic agents have placed the treatment of ED into the hands of the general practitioner, necessity of a full diagnostic evaluation has come into question (124). It is likely that etiologic evaluation will always have a role to play in difficult-to-treat patients, as well as in research

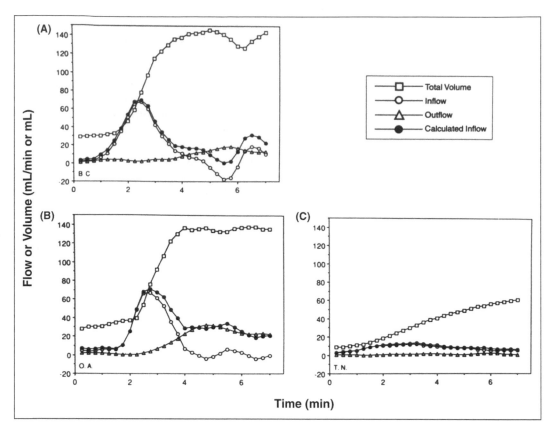

Figure 13 Dual-isotope technique showing measured and calculated values for blood volume, cavernosal inflow, outflow, and corrected inflow. (**A**) Normal study, (**B**) venous leak, and (**C**) intermediate arteries and competent veins. *Source*: From Ref. 80.

studies, for which accurate and quantitative measures of blood flow are important. Nonetheless, in spite of the stated need for objective measures of monitoring ED (125), the restricted commercial interest in these techniques has reduced the incentive for their development.

Cavernous Oxygen Tension

Measurement of oxygen tension of corporeal blood during flaccidity and during penile tumescence has been suggested as a method for the characterization of cavernous perfusion, and thus corporeal vascular dysfunction. Aoki et al. (126) reported a sudden increase in cavernous oxygen tension at the onset of penile tumescence during VSS. Others (127) have reported an increase in the corpus cavernosum oxygen tension from 25 to 40 mm Hg in the flaccid state to 90 to 100 mm Hg in the erect state of the penis. Subsequently, Vardi et al. (128) determined the changes in intracavernous oxygen tension in response to local vasoactive drug injections. More recently, Knispel and Andresen (129) correlated changes in cavernous oxygen tension during PGE_1–induced penile tumescence to PSV during Doppler ultrasonography. Some impotent men were found to have low cavernous oxygen tension (as measured by new, unbreakable, small-caliber oxygen-sensitive probes, and defined arbitrarily as <65 mm Hg) despite normal blood velocity (defined as >25 cm/

sec). Thus, a decrease in oxygen tension may occur as a result of arterial insufficiency and lead to a decrease in trabecular smooth muscle dysfunction (decrease in vascular smooth muscle cells and an increase in connective tissue formation, leading to corporeal fibrosis) in some impotent men with erectile failure. Such changes are probably mediated by an increase in transforming growth factor beta-1 (TGF-β1) with a simultaneous decrease in PGE_1 concentrations in corporeal tissue (see discussion of penile biopsy below). Substantiation of the normative data and the pathophysiologic role of cavernosal oxygen tension is emerging.

☐ STRUCTURAL INVESTIGATIONS OF THE PENIS

Several techniques are available for the evaluation of the structural and functional integrity of the penile tissue. The following is a brief description of some of these methods and their applications. It should be noted that many of these investigations remain experimental at the present time.

Penile Imaging

Structural abnormalities of the penis can be evaluated by a variety of methodologies based on the nature of the suspected lesions. Peyronie's disease and its effect on penile vascular competence can be evaluated with color duplex sonography (24,25). Arteriovenous malformations and lymphohemangiomas can be assessed for lesion extent and the involvement of adjacent structures with magnetic resonance imaging (MRI) (130). MRI can also be used to elucidate penile ruptures and tears of tunica albuginea (131,132).

Penile Biopsy

Percutaneous core biopsy, using 19- and 20-gauge coaxial automatic devices under local anesthesia, has been developed as a safe and technically easy procedure to perform (133). In addition, computerized image analysis techniques of smooth muscle and elastic fibers of the corpus cavernosum tissue samples from normal and impotent men have been developed. Ming-bo et al. (134) and Wespes et al. (135) determined the percentage of smooth muscle fibers in samples obtained from normal and impotent men. Impotent men had lower mean percentage of smooth muscle fibers as compared to normal men (10–36% compared to 40–52%, respectively). Similarly, Sattar et al. (136) determined the percentage of elastic fibers in five potent and 17 impotent men. The mean percentage of elastic fibers was 9% in normal subjects, 5.1% in 12 patients with venous leakage, and 4.3% in five patients with arterial disease. No correlation between the reduction in the amount of elastic fibers and age was observed. These data were further corroborated with the investigation of Nehra et al. (137) who measured trabecular smooth muscle content of erectile tissue in 24 impotent men with a history of vascular risk factors (age older than 50 years and a history of hypertension, diabetes, hypercholesterolemia, cigarette smoking, heart disease, or peripheral vascular disease) or exposure to a systemic or local disorder, including diffuse erectile tissue pathology (penile irradiation, connective tissue disorders, previously failed or infected implants, or veno-occlusive priapism). Histomorphologic findings were further correlated to parameters of veno-occlusive dysfunction as determined with the dynamic infusion pharmacocavernosometry. Trabecular smooth muscle content was found to correlate inversely with the intracavernosal infusion rate required for maintenance of erection as well as with the pressure decay value in 30 seconds after cessation of infusion. Trabecular muscle content correlated positively with the venous outflow resistance. Similar data were also reported by Wespes et al. (138).

Changes in oxygen tension have been shown to affect human corpus cavernosum smooth muscle cell expression of TGF-β1 and synthesis of PGE$_1$ (139). Oxygen tension consistent with blood PO$_2$ observed in flaccidity (30 mmHg) induces TGF-β1 expression and suppresses PGE$_1$ synthesis (139–141). TGF-β1 is a pleotropic cytokine that induces connective tissue synthesis and inhibits growth of vascular smooth muscle cells (141), the two principal changes observed in corporeal fibrosis (135,142). TGF-β1 alters the composition of connective tissue by inducing the expression of collagens, fibronectin, and proteoglycans while inhibiting the activity and expression of collagenases and other proteases (141), resulting in net collagen accumulation. In human corpus cavernosum smooth muscle cells in culture, TGF-β1 treatment induced a 2.5- to 4-fold increase in fibrillar collagen synthesis that was suppressed by PGE$_1$ (143). More recently, TGF-β1 treatment was also shown to produce a dose- and time-dependent decrease in the percentage of smooth muscles in the corpus cavernosum of intact rabbits, confirming that TGF-β1 is capable of inducing fibrosis in situ by altering connective tissue synthesis and structure (144). Interestingly, local administration of TGF-β1 in a rat model, using infusion pumps to provide a constant penile level, was shown to cause a threefold elevation in penile TGF-β1 levels and a corresponding decrease in penile shaft weight and androgen receptor concentration in the shaft tissue (145). These studies suggest that changes in smooth muscle and elastic fiber content may alter the relaxation properties of the cavernosal tissue and thus play a role in the development of ED. Corporeal fibrosis may develop secondary to abnormalities in the regulation of normal collagen synthesis and degradation, most likely as a result of chronic ischemia (137).

Another technique used to evaluate corporeal smooth muscle function is the patch clamp. In the study of Derouet et al. (146), application of PGE$_1$–induced smooth muscle relaxation by inhibition of voltage-dependent L-type Ca^{2+} channels. There was no difference, however, in smooth muscle fiber relaxation between samples taken from normal men and patients classified clinically as nonresponders to therapy with vasoactive intracorporeal injections.

☐ CONCLUSION

ED is increasingly recognized as an important disease in the modern male population. With the recent advances made in the understanding of the physiology of male sexual function and the development of new therapies, the diagnosis and evaluation of ED has commanded increased attention in the radiologic literature. For example, the quantitative and physiologic nature of scintigraphic studies has had considerable impact on the development of modern concepts of erectile physiology and dysfunction. Potential benefits include the ability to generate actual flow and volume measurements. It is therefore possible to assess hemodynamic consequences of anatomic lesions, to study reliably patients with variations in arterial anatomy, and to detect abnormalities of small vessels and corporal compliance beyond the capability of routine morphologic imaging techniques. In large measure, the quantitative aspects of radionuclide examinations, which are their most unique value, remain underutilized and incompletely explored. Overall, however, the methods available to evaluate penile vascular insufficiencies remain limited and are generally only semiquantitative in nature: Doppler ultrasound can illustrate the velocity of blood flow in each cavernosal artery, but it can neither ascertain the actual rate of flow itself, nor the sum total of perfusion via all collaterals to the corpora cavernosa. Even angiography, in spite of its invasive aspects, cannot always determine the hemodynamic consequence of the lesions it detects. There has been little real change in the advanced vascular evaluation of ED since the relatively successful

and well-tolerated therapy of patients with ED by primary-care physicians has reduced the incentive for thorough diagnostic evaluation. Despite the shortcomings of the existing investigations of penile vascular integrity, the tests described above can provide valuable information needed for complete patient assessment and may identify individuals with surgically correctable abnormalities. These tests could also be helpful in selecting appropriate treatment options and in determining the relative contribution of various etiologic factors in a research setting.

□ REFERENCES

1. Kandeel FR, Koussa VKT, Swerdloff RS. Male sexual function and its disorders: physiology, pathophysiology, clinical investigation, and treatment. Endocr Rev 2001; 22(3):342–388.

2. Siroky MB, Krane RJ. Neurophysiology of erection. In: Krane RJ, Goldstein I, ed. Male Sexual Dysfunction. Boston: Little, Brown and Company, 1983:9–20.

3. Meuleman EJ, Diemont WL. Investigation of erectile dysfunction. Diagnostic testing for vascular factors in erectile dysfunction. Urol Clin North Am 1995; 22(4): 803–819.

4. Lue TF, Hricak H, Marich KW, et al. Evaluation of arteriogenic impotence with intracorporeal injection of papaverine and the duplex ultrasound scanner. Semin Urol 1985; 3(1):43–48.

5. Fitzgerald SW, Erickson SJ, Foley WD, et al. Color Doppler sonography in the evaluation of erectile dysfunction. Radiographics 1992; 12(1):3–17.

6. Benson CB, Aruny JE, Vickers MA. Correlation of duplex sonography with arteriography in patients with erectile dysfunction. Am J Roentgenol 1993; 160(1):71–73.

7. Patel U, Amin Z, Friedman E, et al. Colour flow and spectral Doppler imaging after papaverine-induced penile erection in 220 impotent men: study of temporal patterns and the importance of repeated sampling, velocity asymmetry and vascular anomalies. Clin Radiol 1993; 48(1):18–24.

8. Broderick GA, Arger P. Duplex Doppler ultrasonography: noninvasive assessment of penile anatomy and function. Semin Roentgenol 1993; 28(1):43–56.

9. Montorsi F, Bergamaschi F, Guazzoni G, et al. Morphodynamic assessment of penile circulation in impotent patients: the role of duplex and color Doppler sonography. Scand J Urol Nephrol 1993; 27(3):399–408.

10. Nisen HO, Edgren J, Ruutu ML, et al. Duplex Doppler scanning with high-dose prostaglandin E1 stimulation in the diagnosis of arteriogenic impotence. Eur Urol 1993; 24(1):36–42.

11. Valji K, Bookstein JJ. Diagnosis of arteriogenic impotence: efficacy of duplex sonography as a screening tool. Am J Roentgenol 1993; 160(1):65–69.

12. Oates CP, Pickard RS, Powell PH, et al. The use of duplex ultrasound in the assessment of arterial supply to the penis in vasculogenic impotence. J Urol 1995; 153(2):354–357.

13. Wegner HE, Andresen R, Knispel HH, et al. Evaluation of penile arteries with color–coded duplex sonography: prevalence and possible therapeutic implications of connections between dorsal and cavernous arteries in impotent men. J Urol 1995; 153(5):1469–1471.

14. Mills RD, Sethia KK. Reproducibility of penile arterial colour duplex ultrasonography. Br J Urol 1996; 78(1): 109–112.

15. Hattery RR, King BF, Lewis RW, et al. Vasculogenic impotence. Duplex and color Doppler imaging. Radiol Clin North Am 1991; 29(3):629–645.

16. Gessa GL, Tagliamonte A. Role of brain monoamines in male sexual behavior. Life Sci 1974; 14(3):425–436.

17. Bowers MB, vanWoert M, Davis L. Sexual behavior during L-dopa treatment for Parkinsonism. Am J Psychiatry 1971; 127(12):1691–1693.

18. Kraemer HC, Becker HB, Brodie HK, et al. Orgasmic frequency and plasma testosterone levels in normal human males. Arch Sex Behav 1976; 5(2):125–132.

19. Brown WA, Monti PM, Corriveau DP. Serum testosterone and sexual activity and interest in men. Arch Sex Behav 1978; 7(2):97–103.

20. Armstrong EG, Villee CA. Characterization and comparison of estrogen and androgen receptors of calf anterior pituitary. J Steroid Biochem 1977; 8(4):285–292.

21. Kim SH, Paick JS, Lee SE, et al. Doppler sonography of deep cavernosal artery of the penis: variation of peak systolic velocity according to sampling location. J Ultrasound Med 1994; 13(8):591–594.

22. Mancini M, Bartolini M, Maggi M, et al. The presence of arterial anatomical variations can affect the results of duplex sonographic evaluation of penile vessels in impotent patients. J Urol 1996; 155(6): 1919–1923.

23. Wang CJ, Shen SY, Wu CC, et al. Penile blood flow study in diabetic impotence. Urol Int 1993; 50(4):209–212.

24. Amin Z, Patel U, Friedman EP, et al. Colour Doppler and duplex ultrasound assessment of Peyronie's disease in impotent men. Br J Radiol 1993; 66(785):398–402.

25. Levine LA, Coogan CL. Penile vascular assessment using color duplex sonography in men with Peyronie's disease. J Urol 1996; 155(4):1270–1273.

26. Pagani E, Puech-Leao P, Glina S, et al. The value of a second injection on the pharmaco-induced erection test. Int J Impot Res 1997; 9(3):167–168.

27. Porst H. Prostaglandin E1 and the nitric oxide donor linsidomine for erectile failure: a diagnostic comparative study of 40 patients. J Urol 1993; 149(5 Pt 2): 1280–1283.

28. Truss MC, Becker AJ, Thon WF, et al. Intracavernous calcitonin gene-related peptide plus prostaglandin E1: possible alternative to penile implants in selected patients. Eur Urol 1994; 26(1):40–45.

29. Porst H. Diagnostic use and side-effects of vasoactive drugs. A report on over 2100 patients with erectile failure. Int J Impot Res 1990; 2(suppl 2):222–223.

30. Junemann KP, Alken P. Pharmacotherapy of erectile dysfunction: a review. Int J Impot Res 1989; 1:71–93.

31. Govier FE, Asase D, Hefty TR, et al. Timing of penile color flow duplex ultrasonography using a triple drug mixture. J Urol 1995; 153(5):1472–1475.

32. Lue TF, Hricak H, Marich KW, et al. Vasculogenic impotence evaluated by high-resolution ultrasonography and pulsed Doppler spectrum analysis. Radiology 1985; 155(3):777–781.

33. Paushter DM. Role of duplex sonography in the evaluation of sexual impotence. Am J Roentgenol 1989; 153(6):1161–1163.

34. Vruggink PA, Diemont WL, Debruyne FM, et al. Enhanced pharmacological testing in patients with erectile dysfunction. J Androl 1995; 16(2):163–168.

35. Katlowitz N, Albano GJ, Patsias G, et al. Effect of multidose intracorporeal injection and audiovisual sexual stimulation in vasculogenic impotence. Urology 1993; 42(6):695–697.

36. Mills RD, Sethia KK. Maximisation of the erectile response in the investigation of impotence. Int J Impot Res 1999; 11(1):29–32.

37. Montorsi F, Guazzoni G, Barbieri L, et al. The effect of intracorporeal injection plus genital and audiovisual sexual stimulation versus second injection on penile color Doppler sonography parameters. J Urol 1995; 155(2):536–540.

38. Nisen HO, Saarinen O, Ruutu ML, et al. Duplex Doppler scanning with prostaglandin E1 in the diagnosis of cavernovenous leakage. Acta Radiol 1993; 34(4):335–337.

39. Sattar AA, Wery D, Golzarian J, et al. Correlation of nocturnal penile tumescence monitoring duplex ultrasonography and infusion cavernosometry for the diagnosis of erectile dysfunction. J Urol 1996; 155(4):1274–1276.

40. Karadeniz T, Ariman A, Topsakal M, et al. Value of color Doppler sonography in the diagnosis of venous impotence. Urol Int 1995; 55(3):143–146.

41. Virag R, Sussman H. Exploration of the deep dorsal vein of the penis using pulsed Doppler ultrasonography. Preliminary study. [Article in French]. J Mal Vasc 1998; 23(3):195–198.

42. Sarteschi LM, Montorsi F, Fabris FM, et al. Cavernous arterial and arteriolar circulation in patients with erectile dysfunction: a power Doppler study. J Urol 1998; 159(2):428–432.

43. Schwartz AN, Lowe M, Berger RE, et al. Assessment of normal and abnormal erectile function: color Doppler flow sonography versus conventional techniques. Radiology 1991; 180(1):105–109.

44. Aversa A, Rocchietti-March M, Caprio M, et al. Anxiety-induced failure in erectile response to intracorporeal prostaglandin-E1 in non-organic male impotence: a new diagnostic approach. Int J Androl 1996; 19(5):307–313.

45. Vruggink PA, Diemont WL, Meuleman EJ. The post-investigation questionnaire (PIO-R): a practical instrument to assess erectile response after intracavernous injection. Int J Impot Res 1996; 8(2):59–62.

46. Goldstein I. Vasculogenic impotence: its diagnosis and treatment. Probl Urol 1987; 1:547–563.

47. Padma-Nathan H. Dynamic infusion cavernosometry and cavernosography (DICC) and the cavernosal artery systolic occlusion pressure gradient: a complete evaluation of the hemodynamic events of a penile erection. In: Lue TF, ed. World Book of Impotence. Nishimura, London, Niigata-Shi: Smith-Gordon, 1992: 103–101.

48. Kaufman JM, Borges FD, Fitch WP, et al. Evaluation of erectile dysfunction by dynamic infusion cavernosometry and cavernosography (DICC). Multi-institutional study. Urology 1993; 41(5):445–451.

49. Glina S, Silva MF, Puech-Leao P, et al. Veno-occlusive dysfunction of corpora cavernosa: comparison of diagnostic methods. Int J Impot Res 1995; 7(1):1–10.

50. Wespes E, Schulman CC. Cavernovenous leakage: its diagnosis, treatment and importance as a cause of impotence. Probl Urol 1987; 1:487–495.

51. Puech-Leao P. Gravity cavernosometry. In: Lue TF, ed. World Book of Impotence. London/Niigata-Shi: Smith-Gordon/Nishimura, 1992:119–123.

52. Hatzichristou DG, Saenz de Tejada I, Kupferman S, et al. In vivo assessment of trabecular smooth muscle tone, its application in pharmaco-cavernosometry and analysis of intracavernous pressure determinants. J Urol 1995; 153(4):1126–1135.

53. Dickinson IK, Pryor JP. Pharmacocavernometry: a modified papaverine test. Br J Urol 1989; 63(5): 539–545.

54. Evans CM, Kell P. Clinical Drawings For Your Patients: Erectile Dysfunction. Oxford: Health Press, 2000.

55. McMahon CG. Correlation of penile duplex ultrasonography, PBI, DICC and angiography in the diagnosis of impotence. Int J Impot Res 1998; 10(3):153–158.

56. Sasso F, Gulino G, Basar M, et al. Could standardized cavernosometry be helpful in therapeutic management of veno-occlusive dysfunction? J Urol 1996; 155(1):150–154.

57. Wespes E, Schulman C. Venous impotence: pathophysiology, diagnosis and treatment. J Urol 1993; 149 (5 Pt 2):1238–1245.

58. Buvat J, Lemaire A, Dehaene JL, et al. Venous incompetence: critical study of the organic basis of high maintenance flow rates during artificial erection test. J Urol 1986; 135(5):926–928.

59. Puech-Leao P, Chao S, Glina S, et al. Gravity cavernosometry—a simple diagnostic test for cavernosal incompetence. Br J Urol 1990; 65(4):391–394.

60. de Meyer JM, Thibo P. The resistance index represents the corporeal pressure and not the cavernous wall resistance. J Urol 1997; 157(3):830–832.

61. Meuleman EJ, Wijkstra H, Doesburg WH, et al. Comparison of the diagnostic value of pump and gravity cavernosometry in the evaluation of the cavernous veno-occlusive mechanism. J Urol 1991; 146(5):1266–1270.

62. Furst G, Muller-Mattheis V, Cohnen M, et al. Venous incompetence in erectile dysfunction: evaluation with color-coded duplex sonography and cavernosometry/-graphy. Eur Radiol 1999; 9(1):35–41.

63. Udelson D, Nehra A, Hatzichristou DG, et al. Engineering analysis of penile hemodynamic and structural-dynamic relationships: Part III-Clinical considerations of penile hemodynamic and rigidity erectile responses. Int J Impot Res 1998; 10(2):89–99.

64. Mueller SC, von Wallenberg-Pachaly H, Voges GE, et al. Comparison of selective internal iliac pharmaco-angiography, penile brachial index and duplex sonography with pulsed Doppler analysis for the evaluation of vasculogenic (arteriogenic) impotence. J Urol 1990; 143(5):928–932.

65. Hilson AJ, Lewis CA. Radionuclide studies in impotence. Semin Nucl Med 1991; 21(2):159–164.

66. Zuckier LS. Use of radioactive tracers in the evaluation of penile hemodynamics: history, methodology and measurements. Int J Impot Res 1997; 9(2):99–108.

67. Zuckier LS. The scintimetric evaluation of erectile dysfunction. Nuclear Medicine Annual 1997. Philadelphia: Lippincott-Raven Publishers, 1997.

68. Beckett SD. Circulation to male reproductive organs. In: Shepherd JT, Abboud FM, eds. Handbook of Physiology. Peripheral Circulation and Organ Blood flow, Part 1. Bethesda: American Physiological Society, 1983:271–283.

69. Zuckier LS, Strober MD. Nuclear medicine in problems of fertility and impotence. Semin Nucl Med 1992; 22(2):122–137.

70. Shirai M, Nakamura M. Differential diagnosis of organic and functional impotence by the use of 131-I-human serum albumin. Tohoku J Exp Med 1970; 101(4):317–324.

71. Shirai M, Nakamura M. Radioisotope penogram by means of 113m In-microcolloid. Tohoku J Exp Med 1971; 105(2):137–140.

72. Shirai M, Nakamura M. Diagnostic discrimination between organic and functional impotence by radio-isotope penogram with 99mTcO4. Tohoku J Exp Med 1975; 116(1):9–15.

73. Shirai M, Nakamura M, Ishii N, et al. Determination of intrapenial blood volume using 99mTc-labeled autologous red blood cells. Tohoku J Exp Med 1976; 120(4): 377–383.

74. Fanous HN, Jevtich MJ, Chen DC, et al. Radioisotope penogram in diagnosis of vasculogenic impotence. Urology 1982; 20(5):499–502.

75. Siraj QH, Hilson AJ, Townell NH, et al. The role of radio-isotope phallogram in the investigation of vasculogenic impotence. Nucl Med Commun 1986; 7(3):173–182.

76. Facey P, Hayward MW, Evans WD. Radionuclide phallography in the investigation of the impotent patient. Radiogr Today 1989; 55(631):14–17.

77. Schwartz AN, Graham MM, Ferency GF, et al. Radioisotope penile plethysmography: a technique for evaluating corpora cavernosal blood flow during early tumescence. J Nucl Med 1989; 30(4):466–473.

78. Siraj QH, Bomanji J, Akhtar MA, et al. Quantitation of pharmacologically-induced penile erections: the value of radionuclide phallography in the objective evaluation of erectile haemodynamics. Nucl Med Commun 1990; 11(6):445–458.

79. Kim SC, Kim KB, Oh CH. Diagnostic value of the radioisotope erection penogram for vasculogenic impotence. J Urol 1990; 144(4):888–892.

80. Schwartz AN, Graham MM. Combined technetium radioisotope penile plethysmography and xenon washout: a technique for evaluating corpora cavernosal inflow and outflow during early tumescence. J Nucl Med 1991; 32(3):404–410.

81. Choi HK. Radioisotopic test for impotence. In: Lue TF, ed. World Book of Impotence. London/Niigata-Shi: Smith-Gordon/Nishimura, 1992:135–145.

82. Siraj QH, Bomanji J, Ahmed M. The effect of intracavernosal haemodilution on the radionuclide quantification of penile vascular changes during pharmacologically induced penile erections. Nucl Med Commun 1992; 13(7):547–552.

83. Siraj QH, Hilson AJ, Bomanji J, et al. Volume-dependent intracavernous hemodilution during pharmacologically induced penile erections. J Urol 1992; 148(5): 1441–1443.

84. Zuckier LS, Korupolu GR, Gladshteyn M, et al. A non-imaging scintillation probe to measure penile hemodynamics. J Nucl Med 1995; 36(12):2345–2351.

85. Shen YY, Kao CH. Technetium-99m–labelled RBC erection penogram to differentiate psychogenic from vasculogenic impotence. Urol Int 1998; 61(1):27–31.

86. Choi H, Kim YC. "Scroto-penogram" for combined investigation of varicocele and erectile failure. Int J Impot Res 1990; 1:73–79.

87. Siraj QH, Hilson AJ, Bomanji J, et al. A pilot study of flaccid penile blood flow patterns in normal subjects and patients with erectile dysfunction. Nucl Med Commun 1993; 14(11):976–982.

88. Siraj QH, Hilson AJ. Diagnostic value of radionuclide phallography with intravenous vasodilator stress in the evaluation of arteriogenic impotence. Eur J Nucl Med 1994; 21(7):651–657.

89. Chung WS, Choi HK. Erotic erection versus nocturnal erection. J Urol 1990; 143(2):294–297.

90. Freidenberg DH, Berger RE, Chew DE, et al. Quantitation of corporeal venous outflow resistance in man by corporeal pressure flow evaluation. J Urol 1987; 138(3):533–538.

91. Dunn EK, Miller ST, Macchia RJ, et al. Penile scintigraphy for priapism in sickle cell disease. J Nucl Med 1995; 36(8):1404–1407.

92. Schachner E, Fich A. Priapism in sickle cell anemia. Clin Nucl Med 1982; 7(4):172–173.

93. Mishkin FS, Freeman LM. Miscellaneous applications of radionuclide imaging. In: Freeman LM, ed. Freeman and Johnson's Clinical Radionuclide Imaging. 3rd ed. New York: Grune and Stratton, Inc., 1984:1365–1460.

94. Hashmat AI, Raju S, Singh I, et al. 99mTc penile scan: an investigative modality in priapism. Urol Radiol 1989; 11(1):58–60.

95. Casey WC, Zucker MI. Technetium-99 pelvic scan: use in follow-up of penile revascularization bypass operations. Urology 1979; 14(5):465–466.

96. Zumbe J, Scheidhauer K, Kieslich F, et al. Nuclear medical assessment of penile hemodynamics following revascularization surgery. Urol Int 1997; 58(1):39–42.

97. Drawz B, Drawz G, Kittner C, et al. Penile perfusion and functional scintigraphy: preliminary clinical results before and after microsurgical revascularization. Br J Urol 1998; 82(2):241–245.

98. Smith EM, Chaudhuri TK, Gladden KH. Role of nuclear penogram in the pharmacologic treatment planning of erectile dysfunction. J Nucl Med 1996; 37:288–289.

99. Smith EM, Netto IC, Gladden KH, et al. Role of radionuclide phallogram in therapeutic decision-making for erectile dysfunction. Urology 1998; 51(5A suppl):175–178.

100. Malamud H. Dosimetry of 99mTc-labeled blood pool scanning agents. Clin Nucl Med 1978; 3(11):420–421.

101. Srivastava SC, Chervu LR. Radionuclide-labeled red blood cells: current status and future prospects. Semin Nucl Med 1984; 14(2):68–82.

102. Grech P, Witherow RON. Radionuclide evaluation. In: Kirby RS, Carson CC, Webster GD, eds. Impotence: Diagnosis and Management of Male Erectile Dysfunction. London: Butterworth Heinemann, 1991:92–101.

103. Grech P, Dave S, Cunningham DA, et al. Combined papaverine test and radionuclide penile blood flow in impotence: method and preliminary results. Br J Urol 1992; 69(4):408–417.

104. Bell D, Lewis R, Kerstein MD. Hyperemic stress test in diagnosis of vasculogenic impotence. Urology 1983; 22(6):611–613.

105. Zuckier LS, Kikut JK, Benet A, et al. Quantitative analysis of Tc-99m red blood cell wash-in time-activity curves for determination of cavernosal blood volume and blood flow in the flaccid penis. J Nucl Med 1995; 36:55.

106. Buhl AE, Zuckier LS, Kappenman KE. Measurement of blood volume and flow in the flaccid and erect penis of cynomolgus monkeys. Int J Impot Res 1996; 8:185.

107. Zuckier LS, Benet A, Kikut J, et al. New radionuclidic technique for studying penile hemodynamics. Int J Impot Res 1996; 8:165.

108. Gjedde A. Compartmental analysis. In: Wagner HN Jr, ed. Principles of Nuclear Medicine. 2nd ed. Philadelphia: W B Saunders Company, 1995:451–461.

109. Lassen N, Perl W. Tracer Kinetic Methods in Medical Physiology. New York: Raven Press, 1979.

110. Haden HT, Katz PG, Mulligan T, Zasler ND. Penile blood flow by xenon-133 washout. J Nucl Med 1989; 30(6):1032–1035.

111. Wagner G, Uhrenholdt A. Blood flow measurement by the clearance method in the human corpus cavernosum in the flaccid and erect states. In: Zorgniotti AW, Rossi G, eds. Vasculogenic Impotence. Proceedings of the 1st International Conference on Corpus Cavernosum Revascularization. Springfield, IL: Charles C Thomas, 1980:41–36.

112. Metz P, Ebbehoj J, Uhrenholdt A, Wagner G. Peyronie's disease and erectile failure. J Urol 1983; 130(6):1103–1104.

113. Yeh SH, Liu RS, Chen KK, et al. Diagnosis of venous leakage by 133Xe corporeal clearance after intracavernous injection of prostaglandin E1 in poorly responding patients. Nucl Med Commun 1992; 13(1):28–32.

114. Shirai M, Ishii N, Mitsukawa S, et al. Hemodynamic mechanism of erection in the human penis. Arch Androl 1978; 1(4):345–349.

115. Nahoum CRD, Kumpinsky C. The colloid test: a new radioisotopic technique for quantitative penile wash-out measurements. Int J Impot Res 1990; 2(suppl 2):188–189.

116. Groshar D, Lidgi S, Frenkel A, et al. Radionuclide assessment of penile corporal venous leak using technetium-99m-labeled red blood cells. J Nucl Med 1992; 33(1):49–51.

117. Miraldi F, Nelson AD, Jones WT, et al. A non-invasive technique for the evaluation of male impotence. J Nucl Med 1989; 30:784.

118. Kursh ED, Jones WT, Thompson S, et al. A dynamic dual isotope radionuclear method of quantifying penile blood flow. J Urol 1992; 147(6):1524–1529.

119. Esen A, Kitapci M, Ergen A, et al. Dual radioisotopic study: a technique for the evaluation of vasculogenic impotence. J Urol 1992; 147(1):42–46.

120. Miraldi F, Nelson AD, Jones WT, et al. A dual-radioisotope technique for the evaluation of penile blood flow during tumescence. J Nucl Med 1992; 33(1):41–46.

121. Siraj QH, Hilson AJ. Penile radionuclide studies in impotence: an overview. Nucl Med Commun 1993; 14(7):517–519.

122. Lue TF. The mechanism of penile erection in the monkey. Semin Urol 1986; 4(4):217–224.

123. Seftel AD, Goldstein I. Vascular testing for impotence. J Nucl Med 1992; 33(1):46–48.

124. El-Sakka AI, Lue TF. A rational approach to investigation of the sexually dysfunctional man. In: Morales A, ed. Erectile Dysfunction. Issues in Current Pharmacotherapy. London: Martin Dunitz Ltd., 1998:50–69.

125. NIH Consensus Conference. Impotence. NIH Consensus Development Panel on Impotence. JAMA 1993; 270(1):83–90.

126. Aoki H, Takagane H, Banya Y, et al. Human penile hemodynamics studied by a polarographic method. J Urol 1986; 135(4):872–876.

127. Moreland RB. Is there a role of hypoxemia in penile fibrosis: a viewpoint presented to the society for the study of impotence. Int J Impot Res 1998; 10(2):113–120.

128. Vardi Y, Lidgi S, Levin DR. Intracavernous O_2: response to vasoactive drugs as an indicator of corporal vascular dysfunction. Int J Impot Res 1990; 2(suppl 2):242–243.

129. Knispel HH, Andresen R. Evaluation of vasculogenic impotence by monitoring of cavernous oxygen tension. J Urol 1993; 149(5 Pt 2):1276–1279.

130. Forstner R, Hricak H, Kalbhen CL, et al. Magnetic resonance imaging of vascular lesions of the scrotum and penis. Urology 1995; 46(4):581–583.

131. Rahmouni A, Hoznek A, Duron A, et al. Magnetic resonance imaging of penile rupture: aid to diagnosis. J Urol 1995; 153(6):1927–1928.

132. Fedel M, Venz S, Andreessen R, et al. The value of magnetic resonance imaging in the diagnosis of suspected penile fracture with atypical clinical findings. J Urol 1996; 155(6):1924–1927.

133. Hussain S, Nehra A, Goldstein I, et al. Percutaneous core biopsy of the penis. Int J Impot Res 1998; 10(1):57–59.

134. Ming-bo Y, Xiao-xiong W, Liu-cheng S. Computerized image analysis of smooth muscle fibers in normal Chinese men and impotence patients. Chinese Med J 1993; 106(9):679–681.

135. Wespes E, Goes PM, Schiffmann S, et al. Computerized analysis of smooth muscle fibers in potent and impotent patients. J Urol 1991; 146(4):1015–1017.

136. Sattar AA, Wespes E, Schulman CC. Computerized measurement of penile elastic fibres in potent and impotent men. Eur Urol 1994; 25(2):142–144.

137. Nehra A, Goldstein I, Pabby A, et al. Mechanisms of venous leakage: a prospective clinicopathological correlation of corporeal function and structure. J Urol 1996; 156(4):1320–1329.

138. Wespes E, Sattar AA, Golzarian J, et al. Corporeal veno-occlusive dysfunction: predominantly intracavernous muscular pathology. J Urol 1997; 157(5):1678–1680.

139. Moreland RB, Watkins MT, Nehra A, et al. Oxygen tension modulates transforming growth factor b1 expression and PGE production in human corpus cavernosum smooth muscle cells. Mol Urol 1998; 2:41–47.

140. Kim N, Vardi Y, Padma-Nathan H, et al. Oxygen tension regulates the nitric oxide pathway. Physiological role in penile erection. J Clin Invest 1993; 91(2):437–442.

141. Border WA, Noble NA. Transforming growth factor beta (in tissue fibrosis). N Engl J Med 1994; 331(19): 1286–1292.

142. Mersdorf A, Goldsmith PC, Diederichs W, et al. Ultrastructural changes in impotent penile tissue: a comparison of 65 patients. J Urol 1991; 145(4): 749–758.

143. Moreland RB, Traish AM, McMillin MA, et al. PGE1 suppresses the induction of collagen synthesis by transforming growth factor-beta 1 in human corpus cavernosum smooth muscle. J Urol 1995; 153(3 Pt 1): 826–834.

144. Nehra A, Gettman MT, Nugent M, et al. Transforming growth factor-beta1 (TGF-beta1) is sufficient to induce fibrosis of rabbit corpus cavernosum in vivo. J Urol 1999; 162(3 Pt 1):910–915.

145. Gelman J, Garban H, Shen R, et al. Transforming growth factor beta1 (TGF-beta1) in penile and prostate growth in the rat during sexual maturation. J Androl 1998; 19(1):50–57.

146. Derouet H, Eckert R, Trautwein W, et al. Muscular cavernous single cell analysis in patients with venoocclusive dysfunction. Eur Urol 1994; 25(2):145–150.

26

Neurological Investigations of Males with Sexual Dysfunction

Fouad R. Kandeel

Department of Diabetes, Endocrinology and Metabolism, City of Hope National Medical Center, Duarte, California and David Geffen School of Medicine, University of California, Los Angeles, California, U.S.A.

Nabil Koussa

H.C. Healthcare Management and Development, Inc., Long Beach, California, U.S.A.

□ INTRODUCTION

In addition to nocturnal penile tumescence (NPT) and the penile vascular assessment methods (see Chapter 25), neurological assessments can assist in the evaluation of the degree and nature of organic sexual dysfunction (Fig. 1A–D). Although the erectile process is primarily a vascular phenomenon, it is mediated by complex neural mechanisms involving the sacral reflexogenic erection center (parasympathetic) and the thoracolumbar psychogenic erection center (sympathetic) in a unique coordination of the somatic and autonomic motor nervous systems (1). Interruption of any of these pathways can result in erectile dysfunction. For example, decreased sensibility of the penis may be the sole factor causing an inability to sustain erection; similarly, impaired function of the pudendal nerve may be accountable (2). It is important to note that erectile dysfunction is commonly associated with both urologic and neurological abnormalities, and the treatment of urovascular dysfunction with, e.g., revascularization may not be sufficient or even indicated in patients with severe neurological disturbances (3).

Neurological dysfunction will remain undetected if appropriate investigations are not conducted. Several tests are available to evaluate the sensory afferent nerves from the penile skin and the motor efferent nerves to the perineum, including vibration perception sensitivity, penile thermal sensory threshold measurement, somatosensory-evoked potentials (SSEPs), the bulbocavernosus reflex, anal or urethral sphincter electromyography (EMG), and corpus cavernosum-EMG (CC-EMG) signal assessment. Many of these studies have major disadvantages, however, in that they are complex and time-consuming and do not measure autonomic function directly or correlate with the degree of erectile dysfunction (4).

A significant amount of research has been performed over the last few decades in order to define the role of neurological factors in the genesis of male sexual dysfunction. Much of the earlier work, however, was restricted to studies of the somatic innervation of the penis; only recently has significant attention been directed toward the role of autonomic disorders in the development of sexual dysfunction. As yet, many of the investigative procedures for autonomic disturbances provide only indirect evidence for their presence and may not accurately reflect genuine abnormalities in penile autonomic control. Additionally, most of the tests have not been adequately validated. Table 1 provides an overview of the currently available neurological evaluations of men with sexual dysfunction.

□ BACKGROUND

Nerves have fibers of variable diameter, with the thicker fibers having a faster conduction velocity. The fiber types are classified according to their relative size and electrophysiologic activity: type-A fibers are large-caliber and myelinated and are subdivided further into four subgroups ($A\alpha$, $A\beta$, $A\gamma$, and $A\delta$), with $A\alpha$ and $A\beta$ being the largest and fastest, respectively, and $A\delta$ the smallest and slowest. Unmyelinated type-C fibers are even smaller and slower than the $A\delta$ fibers. In general, large-caliber fibers mediate proprioception, pressure, and vibration sense, while small-caliber fibers transmit pain and temperature. Additionally, type-C fibers subserve most of the autonomic peripheral functions. Small-caliber fibers constitute approximately 70% of the peripheral nervous system. For further information on the neuroanatomy of the male genital organs, see Chapters 2 and 4.

Somatic sensory innervation is important in the development and maintenance of normal erection, and somatic motor innervation plays an important role in the control of ejaculation (Figs. 2–4). As described above, the dorsal and pudendal nerves carry the somatic sensory afferent impulses of pain, temperature, position sense, and touch-pressure sensation from the penile skin, and the pudendal

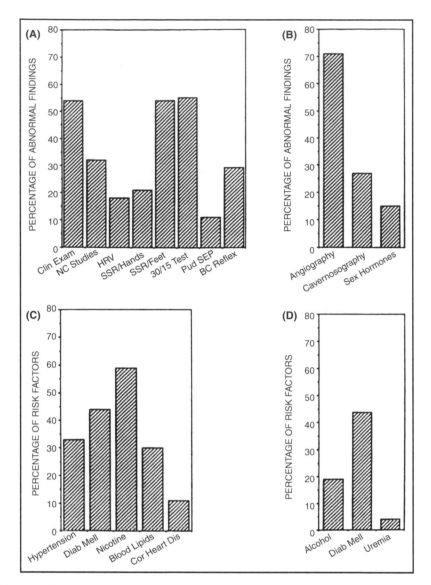

Figure 1 Percentage of abnormal findings classified according to neurological (**A**) and urovascular (**B**) investigations and risk factors for vascular disease (**C**) and polyneuropathy (**D**). Abbreviations: Clin Exam, clinical examination; NC Studies, nerve conduction studies; HRV, respiratory heart rate variation; SSR, sympathetic skin response; Pud SEP, pudendal somatosensory-evoked potentials; BC Reflex, bulbocavernosus reflex; Diab Mell, diabetes mellitus; Cor Heart Dis, coronary heart disease. *Source*: From Ref. 3.

nerve additionally supplies motor efferent fibers to the perineal and pelvic floor muscles. Both afferent and efferent somatic pathways involve the S2–S4 spinal cord segment.

Several disease processes compromise the peripheral nerves; some of these affect the entire spectrum of fibers, while others are more selective. This latter group includes metabolic diseases such as diabetes mellitus and uremia, chronic alcohol abuse, local compression of a peripheral nerve (such as carpal tunnel syndrome), and nerve injuries related to occupational injury or automobile accidents. Traditionally, the clinical assessment of neurological dysfunction consists of a clinical examination, and, if warranted, nerve conduction velocity studies and other electrophysiologic tests (see below) (8).

□ SOMATIC INNERVATION OF THE PENIS

The following provides a brief summary of each of the available methods for testing the integrity of the somatic innervations of the penis: biothesiometry, penile thermal sensory thresholds, and several electrophysiologic studies (dorsal nerve conduction velocity, bulbocavernosus reflex latency, SSEPs, and perineal EMG).

Vibration Perception Threshold (Biothesiometry)

Since large-caliber, myelinated neurons are responsible for transmitting vibratory sensation, biothesiometry

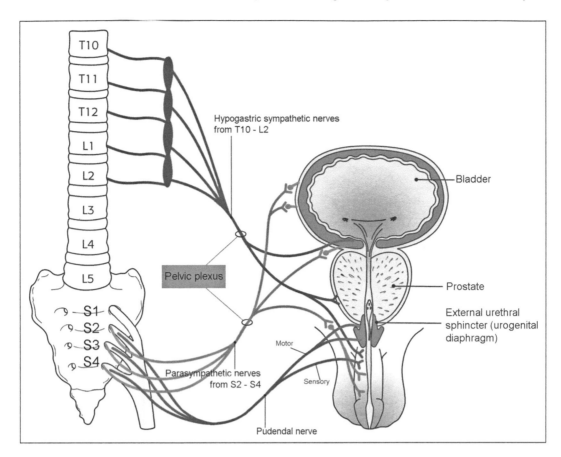

Figure 2   Illustrated overview of the neuroanatomy of the male genital tract. Three sets of peripheral nerves are involved in penile erection: two are autonomic and one is somatic. Parasympathetic nerves stem from the second to the fourth sacral segments (S2–S4) whereas sympathetic nerves have their preganglionic cell bodies in the intermediolateral cell columns of the thoracolumbar segments. Somatic fibers travel in the pudendal nerves and their cell bodies are situated in the S2–S4 segments. *Source*: From Ref. 5.

may be considered a screening method for abnormalities within the penile sensory afferent pathway (9). It is performed with a portable hand-held electromagnetic vibration device, or biothesiometer, that consists of a small, vibrating test probe that has a fixed frequency and variable amplitude of vibrations (Figs. 5 and 6) (1,10). Essentially a precisely controlled "electric tuning fork," the biothesiometer is typically placed on the following test sites: the right and left side of the penile shaft as well as on the head of the penis. The amplitude of vibrations is increased slowly, and the lowest vibration amplitude perceived by the subject is determined. An age-dependent increase in the lowest vibration amplitude perceived by normal subjects has been found and is thought to reflect Pacinian corpuscle degeneration, collagen infiltration of the skin dermis, and dermal atrophy (11).

The loss of or an abnormal decrease in vibratory sensation suggests the presence of a peripheral neuropathy. Although this procedure does not directly measure the erectile nerves, because it is easy to perform, biothesiometry serves as a reasonable screening test for possible penile sensory loss as it will indicate whether additional, more formal neurological studies

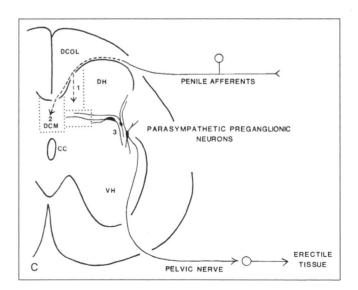

Figure 3   Diagram shows the relationship between afferent projections and efferent neurons and dendrites projecting to the penis. Abbreviations: CC, central canal; DCOL, dorsal column; DCM, dorsal commissure; DH, dorsal horn; VH, ventral horn. *Source*: From Ref. 6.

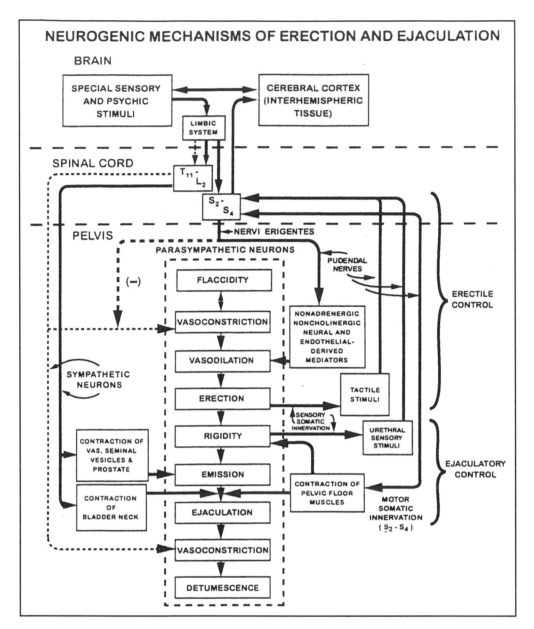

Figure 4 Neurogenic mechanisms of erection and ejaculation. Interactions between the autonomic and somatic innervations that control the male sexual cycle are diagrammed. The sensory input from the genital tract is carried by the pudendal nerve to the S2–S4 segment of the spinal cord. Ascending sensory fibers synapse in the corticomedullary junction and the thalamus, and then terminate in the contralateral primary sensory area deep in the interhemispheric tissue. The somatic motor fibers originate from sacral segments S2–S4 and supply the pelvic floor muscles and the external anal sphincter. The higher centers for the erectile function are located in the cortex, interhemispheric area, and limbic system. The descending parasympathetic innervation responsible for corporeal vasodilatation and corporeal smooth muscle relaxation (i.e., the transformation of the penis from the flaccid to the erect state) exits the spinal cord at the S2–S4 level and reaches the penis via Nervi Erigentes. Penile tactile stimuli reaching the spinal cord via the pudendal nerve generate additional reflex arcs to help initiate and/or maintain the erection. The sympathetic innervation responsible for emission and ejaculation (through the coordinated contractions of the vas deferens, ampulla, seminal vesicles, prostate, and the bladder neck) exits the spinal cord at the T11–L2 level and reaches the penis via the inferior mesenteric, hypogastric, and pelvic plexuses. Somatic-mediated contraction of the pelvic floor muscles aids in achieving maximum penile rigidity and discharging the ejaculatory fluid. Additionally, the sympathetic system mediates corporeal vasoconstriction and corporeal smooth muscle contraction, and, hence, penile detumescence after orgasmic relief. The sympathetics also maintain the flaccid state in the absence of sexual arousal. Activation of each division of the autonomic nervous system appears to occur in a reciprocal manner (i.e., activation of one division is associated with inhibition of the other). *Source*: From Ref. 7.

are warranted. In a study of 137 patients with organic erectile dysfunction tested with both biothesiometry and subsequent sensory-evoked potential testing, 80% of the 38 patients who had a normal biothesiometric examination had normal evoked potential testing (1).

This increased to 93% for those under age 60. Ninety-nine patients had an abnormal biothesiometric result, of whom 47% also had an abnormal evoked potential test. The majority of patients with erectile dysfunction related to a sensory deficit were subsequently found to

Table 1 Neurological Investigation for Organic Impotence

Test	Neural pathway	Normal criteria	Abnormal response	Associated diagnosis
I. SOMATIC INNERVATION				
Vibration perception threshold	Afferent: sensory dorsal/pudendal nerve, S_2–S_4 spinal cord segment	Ability to perceive low amplitudes of vibration	Reduced vibration perception	Sensory neuropathy
Dorsal nerve conduction velocity with and without penile stretching	Afferent: sensory dorsal/pudendal nerve	Without penile stretching, velocity: 24.4 ± 3.2 m/sec; range 21.4–29.1 m/sec	Slow nerve conduction	Peripheral neuropathy
		With penile stretching, velocity: 33.0 ± 3.8 m/sec	Slow nerve conduction	Peripheral neuropathy
Bulbocavernosum reflex latency	Afferent: sensory dorsal/pudendal nerve, efferent: motor perineal/pudendal nerve, S_2–S_4 spinal cord segment	Latency 27–42 msec; in response to pulse amplitude up to 90 V or 15 mA	Increased minimum latency to >42 msec or lost response	Sacral-cord cauda equina and conus medullaris lesion in multiple sclerosis, spinal cord lesion or tumor, herniated intervertebral discs, or diabetic or ethanol peripheral neuropathy
Pudendal nerve somatosensory-evoked potential	Afferent: sensory dorsal/pudendal and suprasacral pathway	Peripheral conduction: 12–14 msec	Prolonged peripheral conduction	Peripheral neuropathy or dorsal nerve impotence syndrome
		Central conduction: (spinal to brain): 28–30 msec	Prolonged central conduction	Transverse myelitis, cervical disc disease, tumor or trauma
			Prolonged total peripheral and central conduction	Multiple sclerosis and spinal cord trauma or tumor
Perineal electromyography	Efferent: motor perineal/pudendal pathway	Normal electromyographic action potential of individual motor units	Abnormal electromyographic action potentials, e.g., polyphase motor units, fibrillation potentials, sharp waves	Metabolic or toxic disorders (diabetes, alcoholism)
II. AUTONOMIC INNERVATION:				
Parasympathetic:				
Bulbocavernosum reflex latency with stimulation of urethrovesical junction	Afferent: autonomic pelvic plexus, efferent: lower motor neuron pathway	Normal latency values	Delayed latency	Peripheral or autonomic neuropathy
Cystometrography and bethanechol chloride super-sensitivity testing	Reflex arc involving: afferent: autonomic sensory, efferent: lower motor neuron pathway	Increase in intravesical pressure <15 cm water in response to 2.5 mg bethanechol chloride injection	Detrusor areflexia	Lower motor neuron or afferent sensory lesion (peripheral and autonomic neuropathy)
			Increased intravesical pressure >15 cm water in the absence of detrusor overactivity due to upper motor neuron lesion, spinal disease or primary bladder disorder	Spinal vascular disease of cortical or spinal regulatory tract
Pupillary light reflex latency	Parasympathetic	Normal latency	Increased latency or loss of reflex	Injury of parasympathetic innervation
Heart rate (R-R) variability (respiratory, Valsalva and/or orthostasis)	Cardiac, parasympa-thetic and sympathetic innervation, and vascular sympa-thetic innervation (Valsalva and orthostasis)	Deep breathing: increase in heart rate >15 beats, Valsalva: ratio of longest to shortest R-R intervals >1.21 standing: rapid increase in heart rate at 15th beat followed by relative decrease at 30th beat	Deep breathing: increase in heart rate <10 beats, Valsalva: ratio of longest to shortest R-R intervals <1.10 standing: gradual increase in heart rate	Autonomic neuropathy

Table 1 Neurological Investigation for Organic Impotence (*Continued*)

Test	Neural pathway	Normal criteria	Abnormal response	Associated diagnosis
Sympathetic:				
Darkness pupil size adaptation	Pupillary sympathetic control	Range for papillary constriction latencies 179–246 msec; darkness pupillary diameter increase 43–84%	Lack of or smaller changes in pupil size	Sympathetic neuropathy
Sympathetic skin response				
Penile pudendal stimulation	Afferent: somatic sensory pathway; efferent: sympathetic pathway	Palmar: 1.44 ± 0.24 sec, plantar: 2.07–2.16 ± 0.24–0.2 sec	Loss of normal response or increased latency	Sensory afferent or sympathetic efferent neuropathy
Median or tibial nerve stimulation		Hand and foot response: 1–3 sec Penile response: 1.2–1.6 sec	1.24–3.64 sec	Sensory afferent or sympathetic efferent neuropathy
Histamine and acetylcholine tests	Afferent: somatic sensory pathway; efferent: sympathetic pathway	Red flare of skin spot at site of histamine injection or dark iodine discoloration at the site of acetylcholine injection	Absent response	Sensory afferent or sympathetic efferent neuropathy

have an underlying diabetic or alcoholic neuropathy. Using this same study design with another group of more than 500 patients, abnormal biothesiometric values were seen in 23%, of whom 50% had an abnormal evoked potential test that was highly correlated with neurologic disease. A normal evoked potential test in patients with abnormal biothesiometry results suggests vascular insufficiency of the somatosensory receptor cells or collagen infiltration of the penile skin (14). These investigators concluded that penile sensation is most objectively measured by evoked potential testing; however, it may be more simply assessed by biothesiometry.

Penile Thermal Sensory Threshold

As noted above, the erectile mechanism also depends on the integrity of autonomic nerve fibers, which are

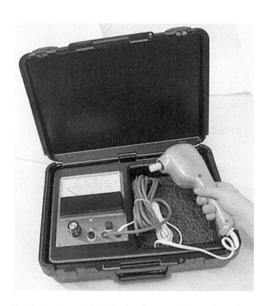

Figure 5 Typical model of biothesiometer for testing vibratory perception. *Source*: From Ref. 12.

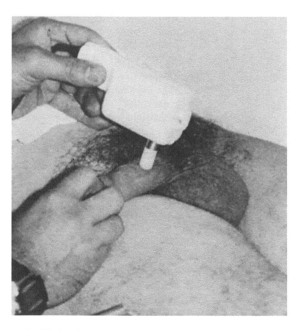

Figure 6 Biothesiometer in application. The biothesiometer is applied to the lateral aspect of the penile shaft. *Source*: From Ref. 13.

of small diameter. The small sensory fibers that are responsible for thermal sensation are similar in caliber to those in the autonomic nervous system that control sexual potency; therefore, thermal sensation could indirectly reflect autonomic function in the genitalia (8,15). Thermal somatosensory testing allows the clinician to test small nerve fibers. With this technique, the threshold for warmth or cold is quantitatively measured and then compared to age-matched normal population values. A deviation from the normal range can indicate the existence of peripheral nerve disease. Warm thermal thresholds alone, for example, offer a quick, noninvasive accurate method of evaluating penile neuropathy in an office setting (16).

This test is performed with the use of a computer-based thermal sensory analyzer (Fig. 7) by attaching a small device, called a thermode, to the patient's skin. The device is capable of heating or cooling the skin, as needed. Technically, the thermode is based on Peltier elements, and it consists of semiconductor junctions that produce a temperature gradient between the upper and lower stimulator surfaces as generated by the passage of an electric current. The patient's ability to detect small increases or decreases in temperature that are applied to the penile shaft is measured. A simple push-button response by the patient, recorded by the computer, completes each cycle of the examination. A test result printout is then provided.

Most commonly, the temperature is altered at a slow linear rate (i.e., 1°C/sec) until the patient signals his first perception of thermal sensation (method of limits). Another method of measuring thermal sensation (the method of levels) involves altering the temperature by larger increments (i.e., 2–4°C) at each

step, asking the patient if the temperature change is felt; then, according to the reply, the temperature is increased or decreased by smaller degrees until the smallest recognized change in temperature can be determined. From these measurements, the individual's thresholds for warm and cold thermal sensation can be ascertained. A high thermal threshold suggests the presence of neurogenic damage. Measuring penile thermal sensation has been shown to be effective in identifying neurogenic erectile dysfunction in patients who are post-transurethral resection of the prostate (18) as well as in patients with diabetes (8,19) and other neurogenic disorders (19).

Normative data for warm and cold sensory thresholds of the penis in a normal male population are limited, but two separate studies have had varying results: in the first, mean warm and cold threshold values were determined to be 34°C and 28.2°C, and in the second, 37.4°C and 29.9°C (8,15). The subjects' age and the size of the thermode used could be responsible for the variations found in this normative data (8).

Lefaucheur et al. (8) compared 35 impotent diabetic patients and 25 normal controls without evidence of neuropathy by evaluating their erectile dysfunction symptom scores and the results of penile warm and cold thresholds sensory testing, as well as the results from other standard electrophysiologic tests (i.e., penile sympathetic skin response, pudendal nerve SSEPs, and vibratory sensory thresholds). A significant difference between impotent diabetic males and controls was found in the erectile dysfunction symptom score ($P < 0.0001$), cold threshold ($P = 0.0007$), and warm threshold ($P = 0.0025$). Furthermore, the penile thermal testing results were found to correlate more strongly with the clinical evaluation than any other neurophysiologic test. This promising data, combined with the simplicity and sensitivity of this testing procedure, make it an important option to be considered when assessing a patient for neurogenic erectile dysfunction. Future studies are needed, however, to prove the reliability of penile thermal sensation testing in men presenting with erectile dysfunction.

Electrophysiologic Studies
Overview

In neurophysiology, an evoked potential (or "evoked response") is an electrical potential recorded following the presentation of a sensory (auditory, visual, or soamtosensory) stimulus, as distinct from the spontaneous potentials produced from electroencephalograms (EEGs) or EMG (see below). Evoked potential amplitudes tend to be low, ranging from less than a microvolt to several microvolts, compared to tens of microvolts for EEG, millivolts for EMG, and often close to a volt for electrocardiogram (EKG). To resolve these low-amplitude potentials against the background of ongoing EEG, EKG, EMG, and other biological signals and ambient noise, signal averaging is usually required.

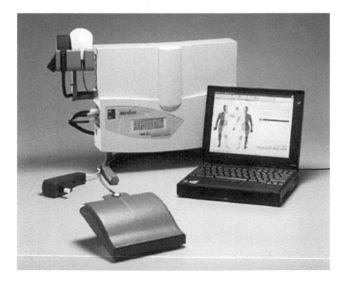

Figure 7 Model of a computer-based thermal sensory analyzer (meDoc Advanced Medical Systems, Ltd.) with two types of thermodes. *Source*: From Ref. 17.

The signal is time-locked to the stimulus and most of the noise occurs randomly, allowing the noise to be averaged out with averaging of repeated responses. Signals can be recorded from cerebral cortex, brainstem, spinal cord, and peripheral nerves. Usually, the term "evoked potential" is reserved for responses involving either the recording from or stimulation of central nervous system (CNS) structures. Thus, nerve conduction studies, which also evaluate the function (e.g., the velocity) of motor or sensory nerves, are generally not thought of as evoked potentials, although they do meet the above definition.

SSEPs consist of a series of waves that reflect sequential activation of neural structures along the somatosensory pathways. While SSEPs can be elicited by mechanical stimulation, clinical studies utilize electrical stimulation of peripheral nerves, which gives larger and more robust responses (20). For sexual dysfunction, the stimulation sites typically used for clinical diagnostic SSEP studies are the dorsum of the penis (dorsal nerve afferent pathway). Recording electrodes are then placed over the scalp, the spine, and peripheral nerves proximal to the stimulation site. The dorsal column-lemniscal system is the major anatomical substrate of the SSEPs within the CNS (Fig. 3). Several characteristics of SSEPs can be measured, including peak latencies, interpeak latencies, morphology (i.e., presence and absence of components), and dispersion. Peak latencies are the easiest SSEP features to measure and standardize. Other characteristics (i.e., morphology and dispersion) are more variable and difficult to interpret. Abnormal SSEPs can result from dysfunction at the level of the peripheral nerve, plexus, spinal root, spinal cord, brain stem, thalamocortical projections, or primary somatosensory cortex (Figs. 2–4). Since individuals have multiple parallel afferent somatosensory pathways (e.g., anterior spinothalamic tract and dorsal column tracts within the spinal cord), recordings of SSEPs can be normal even in patients with significant sensory deficits. SSEPs depend on the functional integrity of the rapidly conducting, large-diameter group IA muscle afferent fibers and group II cutaneous afferent fibers, which travel in the posterior column of the spinal cord. When a mixed peripheral nerve (with both sensory and motor components) is stimulated, both group IA muscle afferents and group II cutaneous afferents contribute to the resulting SSEP. Selective ablation of the dorsal column of the spinal cord abolishes the SSEPs generated rostral to the lesion. Diseases of the dorsal columns in which joint position sense and proprioception are impaired invariably are associated with abnormal SSEPs (20).

The development and widespread use of phosphodiesterase inhibitors and easy access to sophisticated neuroradiologic imaging, however, have had a great impact on the usage of SSEPs in clinical settings, as fewer diagnostic SSEP studies are being performed. Nevertheless, SSEPs remain a valuable diagnostic test in several clinical situations, as described below in further detail.

Dorsal Nerve Conduction Velocity

Since the maintenance of erection is thought to require continuous sensory transmission to the spinal cord and the cerebral cortex, a penile sensory deficit may reduce the ability to sustain erections during coitus. The decrease in sensory transmission from the penis is also often associated with ejaculation difficulties (1). Electrophysiological study of the lower sacral segments and their peripheral innervation is difficult due to limited external access; however, the dorsal nerve of the penis is a terminal branch of the pudendal nerve (S2-S4) and is readily accessible percutaneously as it runs parallel with the dorsal penile artery from the public symphysis to the glans penis (Fig. 8). Interruption of this nerve has produced loss of libido and ejaculatory and erectile dysfunction in laboratory animals (21). While the bulbocavernosus reflex latency (see below) and pudendal-evoked cortical response (see below) have been shown to be useful in the investigation of sexual/urinary dysfunction, abnormalities revealed during these studies may suggest either peripheral or CNS deficits. Thus, evaluating the conduction velocity of the dorsal nerve of the penis in addition to the above studies may provide aid in differentiating between central and peripheral lesions (21).

Conduction velocity in the dorsal nerve is measured by percutaneous square-wave electrical stimulation via flat surface electrodes applied to the dorsum of the penis, proximal to the glans. Additional surface recording electrodes are placed at the base of the dorsal

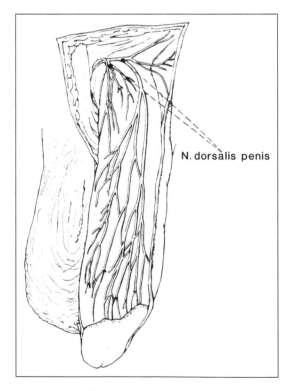

Figure 8 Anatomic illustration of the dorsal nerve of the penis. *Source*: From Ref. 22.

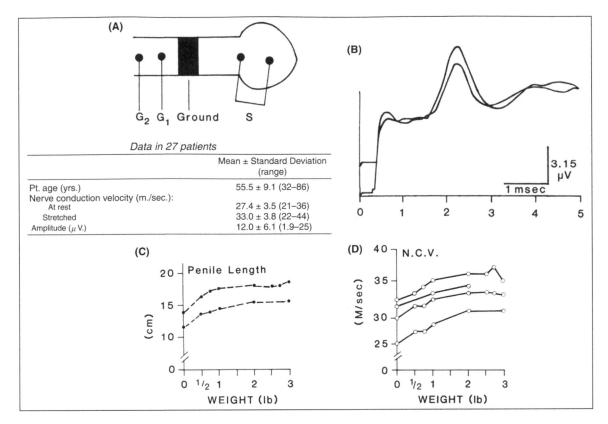

Figure 9 (**A**) Electrode placement for dorsal penile nerve conduction. Central stimulus (S) is proximal to anode. G1 is the active electrode and G2 is the reference electrode. (**B**) Tracings of compound nerve action potential after an average of 30 sweeps. (**C**) Changes of total penile length in relationship to degree of stretch. (**D**) Changes of nerve conduction velocity in relationship to degree of stretch. *Abbreviation*: NCV, nerve conduction velocity. *Source*: From Ref. 21.

penis (Fig. 9A and B). Nerve conduction velocity is calculated by dividing the distance between the stimulus and recording electrodes by the latency to either the onset of the negative voltage portion of the action potential or the peak of the negative portion of the action potential. The negative peak of the action potential is usually preferred over the onset for the measurement of latency to avoid shock artifact due to the short distance between the stimulus and the recording electrodes. Since the penis is a distensible structure and the dorsal nerve of the penis is serpiginous at rest, gentle stretching with a one-pound weight is usually performed to straighten the coiled nerve and permit the optimal and more accurate measurement of the conduction velocity (Fig. 9C and D) (22). In one study, the mean compound nerve action potential as measured in 27 normal men was $12.0 \pm 6.1\,\mu V$, with a conduction velocity of 24.4 ± 3.2 m/sec without penile stretching and 33.0 ± 3.8 m/sec with penile stretching with a one-pound weight (21). In a subsequent report, Lin and Bradley (22) reported significantly slower conduction velocity of the dorsal nerve in 20 patients with insulin-dependent diabetes as compared to normal controls. This was observed in the absence of abnormalities in bulbocavernosus reflex or pudendal-evoked response latencies. Similarly, Kaneko and Bradley (23) directly compared dorsal nerve conduction velocity and bulbo-cavernosus reflex latency and found that the average

nerve conduction velocity was 37 m/sec in diabetic men with erectile dysfunction and 45 m/sec in nondiabetic men with erectile dysfunction (Fig. 10A and B). The

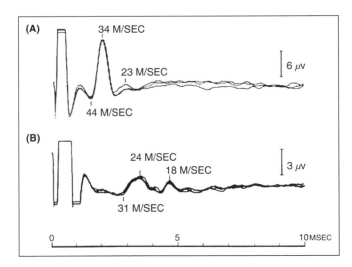

Figure 10 Sacral-evoked response. The sacral-evoked response is a crossed reflex. Stimulation on one side results in an ipsilateral and contralateral latency response. (**A**) Study in a 59-year-old man without diabetes mellitus shows two peaks. Nerve conduction velocities of the dorsal nerve were 44 m/sec (take-off) and 34 m/sec (N1). (**B**) Study in a 41-year-old man with insulin-dependent diabetes mellitus shows four waves. Nerve conduction velocities were 31 m/sec (take-off) and 24 m/sec (N1). *Source*: From Ref. 23.

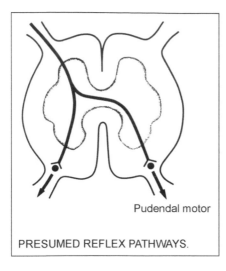

Pudendal motor

PRESUMED REFLEX PATHWAYS.

Figure 11   Sacral signal tracing. Schematic cross-section of sacral spinal cord indicates presumed reflex pathways of bulbocavernosus response. Synapses that may exist in the spinal cord are not drawn. Note that Unilateral stimulus will normally result in a bilateral response. *Source*: From Ref. 25.

latency of the bulbocavernosus reflex showed no significant difference between the groups and was within normal limits. Thus, it was concluded that the measurement of nerve conduction velocity of the dorsal nerve of the penis is a valuable test for the assessment of erectile dysfunction in patients with diabetes mellitus.

Bulbocavernosus Reflex Latency (Sacral-Evoked Response)

The sacral-evoked response is the neurophysiologic representation of the bulbocavernosus reflex (S2–S4), which refers to the crossed, polysynaptic spinal cord–mediated reflex contractions of the bulbocavernosus muscle and the external and internal anal sphincters that are classically elicited in response to a squeeze of the glans penis (Fig. 11). Thus, this reflex is a representation of both sensory and motor function (24). Since the contraction of the bulbocavernosus itself is difficult to observe clinically, however, the anal sphincter response is evaluated more commonly (25).

The clinical usefulness of this reflex is accepted widely, but there are certain deficiencies—for example, it can be demonstrated clinically in only 70% of normal male subjects (25). Further, because the reflex is graded in an extremely subjective manner from 0 to 4+, mild neuronal dysfunction cannot be detected. The application of electrophysiologic techniques allows greater accuracy and quantification of this response and is able to detect subtler degrees of neurological abnormalities.

Bulbocavernosus reflex latency testing determines the time interval required for this reflex arc, which utilizes the dorsal penile/pudendal afferent pathway, the S2-S4 spinal cord segment, and the pudendal/perineal efferent pathway. Reflex latency is defined as the time from stimulus to the first reflex

EMG response. The characteristics of this response include diminution of the minimum reflex latency with an increasing stimulus and the identification of bilateral EMG responses following unilateral nerve stimulation (13).

A bipolar block skin-stimulating electrode is taped to one side of the penile shaft and a recording concentric-needle electrode is inserted at the base of the ipsilateral bulbocavernosus muscle near the midline (Fig. 12). Square-wave stimuli are delivered at a frequency of 1/sec and duration of 1 msec, beginning at 0.01 V and increasing voltage slowly to determine the sensory threshold (first consistent bulbocavernosus muscle contraction) and the minimum latency. Several stimulations are applied and the measured latencies are averaged. Identification of the lesioned side (lateralization) is inferred from measuring the response at both sides of the perineum to stimuli applied to each side of the penile shaft (10).

Several studies have reported a normal range for the bulbocavernosus latency of 27 to 42 msec (25,26). The diagnostic sensitivity of the bulbocavernosus reflex latency measurement has been compared to other testing procedures in several studies (27–30). Neurophysiological testing of the somatic (using the bulbocavernosus reflex and the pudendal and posterior tibial nerves SSEP latencies) and the autonomic (using the urethroanal sensory response) systems revealed a high incidence of urogenital or peripheral neuropathy (85%) in impotent diabetics as compared to potent diabetics (40%) and impotent nondiabetics (44%). Furthermore, impotent diabetics had severe disease, with 33% showing three or four clearly abnormal test results. This high incidence of multiple test abnormalities was not seen in potent diabetics and only in 10% of impotent nondiabetics (30).

An abnormal bulbocavernosus reflex response is often found concomitantly with pathological conditions of the perception threshold and cortical

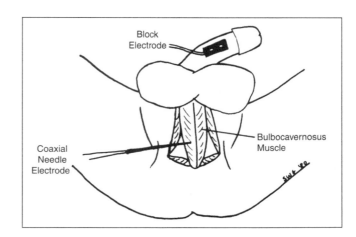

Figure 12   A schematic representation of the stimulation electrode (block electrode) location and response electrode (coaxial-needle electrode) location in the sacral-evoked response study. *Source*: From Ref. 13.

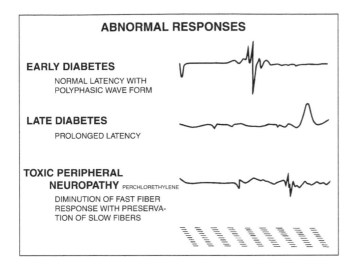

Figure 13 Examples of abnormal responses in bulbocavernosus reflex latency. Height of calibration markings, 500 μv. *Source*: From Ref. 25.

sensory response due to sensory and/or peripheral motor neuropathy of the pudendal nerve (2). Prolonged bulbocavernosus reflex latency, as the only finding, is significant for neuropathy of the motor innervation of the somatic pudendal nerve (Fig. 13). Thus, this test may be helpful in documenting suspected sacral nerve root, cauda equina, or conus medullaris lesions (S2 S4) due to diabetes, multiple sclerosis, spinal cord trauma, spinal cord tumors, and herniated intervertebral discs. Since parasympathetic sacral neurons are anatomically close to the central portion of the pudendal pathways, insults to the somatic innervation at these sites may also cause parasympathetic dysfunction (22).

Dorsal/Pudendal Nerve SSEP

This test allows the evaluation of the peripheral and suprasacral afferent pathways by stimulating the pudendal nerve at the penis and represents sensory function exclusively. The evoked waveforms are recorded at various sites within the CNS, but most typically over the conus medullaris and parietal cortex (7,31). Conventionally, the response latency is divided into the peripheral conduction time (penis to sacral cord) and the central conduction time (sacral cord to cerebral cortex). Patients with sacral lesions (distal to the sacral recording electrodes) such as multiple sclerosis, spinal cord trauma, or tumor may demonstrate prolonged peripheral and total conduction times; however, patients with suprasacral lesions (cephalic to recording electrodes) such as transverse myelitis, cervical disc disease, tumor, or trauma may have prolonged total conduction time and central conduction time, but normal peripheral conduction time (11). Further, performing both the bulbocavernosus and the pudendal nerve SSEP testing may allow the evaluation of the different components of the pudendal nerve. For example, patients having intact spinal and cortical sensory responses but an absent or delayed bulbocavernosus reflex are likely to have a peripheral motor or ventral conus medullaris lesion.

Block skin-stimulating electrodes are usually taped over the left and right sides (10,31) or the dorsum (32) of the penile shaft. The active recording electrodes are usually placed over the L1 vertebra for the sacral cord, and over the L3 and L5 vertebrae for the cauda equina. The reference electrodes are usually attached over the T4 vertebra. Cortical recording is made from the EEG recording sites C3 and C4 (approximately 2 cm back and 7 cm lateral to Cz according to the International Coding System, Fig. 14), and Fz, with the reference electrode placed at Cz. Impedance for the recording is best kept below 3000 ohm. Square-wave stimuli of 0.2 msec are delivered at a frequency of 1/sec by a constant current stimulator generally set at 6 to 15 mA sides (10,31). Responses from multiple stimuli (between 100 and 2000) applied to right, left, and bilateral penile sites are signal-averaged and latencies are determined (Fig. 15).

Normal peripheral nerve conduction as measured from the spinal-evoked response is 24 to 26 msec. The normal central conduction time, defined arbitrarily as the difference between the latencies at the spine and the scalp, is about 30 msec (10,31,32). Pickard et al. (32) studied the dorsal penile nerve cerebral-evoked response in 280 impotent patients and 34 age-matched potent men. Increased latencies or absent responses were found in 36% of impotent men; 72% of these were diabetic or had history of neurological dysfunction. Most of the abnormal results, however, could have been predicted by the presence of diabetes or preexisting neurological dysfunction or by evidence of neurological deficit on physical examination.

Perineal EMG

EMG is a technique for the measurement of muscle response to nervous stimulation by detecting the electrical potential generated by muscle cells when these cells contract. To perform perineal EMG, needle electrodes are inserted through the skin into the muscle tissue (Fig. 12). The electrical activity produced while inserting the electrode is observed, as this insertion activity provides already valuable information about the state of the muscle and its innervating nerve. Then, the electrical activity when the muscle is at rest is studied, as spontaneous activity might indicate some nerve damage. The patient is then asked to contract the muscle smoothly. The shape, size, and frequency of the resulting motor-unit potentials are judged. The electode is retracted a few millimeters, and the activity is reanalyzed until at least 10 to 20 units have been collected. Each electrode track gives only a very local picture of the activity of the whole muscle. Because skeletal muscles differ in structure, the electrode has to be placed at various locations to obtain an accurate study. A nerve conduction velocity test may often be performed at the same time as the EMG.

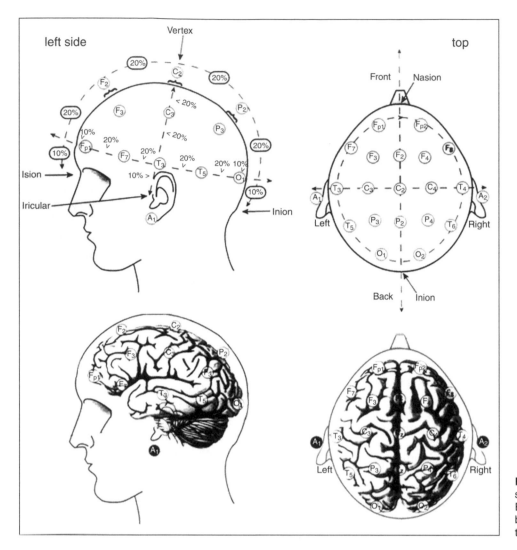

Figure 14 International 10 to 20 system of electrode placement for EEG recordings. Relationship between brain and electrode positions. *Source*: From Ref. 33.

Perineal EMG identifies disturbances in pudendal motor pathways, which may be associated with metabolic or toxic disorders such as diabetes and alcoholism (22). Structural abnormalities of the perineal striated muscles also give rise to abnormal EMG recordings. The information obtained can help in assessing the presence of neuropathic defects, the ability to contract the bulbocavernosus muscle voluntarily, and the degree of motor-unit action potential recruitment during a bulbocavernosus reflex or cough (10).

□ AUTONOMIC INNERVATION

As previously discussed elsewhere in this volume (see chapters contained within Part I), the parasympathetic efferent pathways involve the spinal S2-S4 segments and pelvic nerve (Nervi Erigentes), and the sympathetic efferent pathways involve spinal cord segment T12-L2 and the hypogastric nerve. Many of the available autonomic testing procedures provide an indirect measure of the functional state of the autonomic control of the erectile function. Further knowledge of the autonomic

parasympathetic [various forms of cystometrography, heart rate variability, and pupillary light reflex latency (34–36)], and autonomic sympathetic [pupil size adaptation and histamine and acetylcholine skin tests (37–40)] innervations show promise for the diagnosis of the various types of autonomic neuropathy that contributes to erectile dysfunction. The following section provides a brief description of available testing procedures of the autonomic nervous system function.

Parasympathetic
Bulbocavernosus Reflex Latency with Stimulation of Urethrovesical Junction

The bulbocavernosus reflex, as elicited through sensory stimulation of the urethrovesical junction (afferent through autonomic pelvic plexus) with subsequent detection of the motor response either in the anal sphincter or in the bulbocavernosus muscle, allows more accurate evaluation of the efferent autonomic nerve response. The test is performed by placing a specially designed Foley catheter into the urinary bladder. After inflation of the retaining balloon, the catheter is pulled outward gently until a pair of electrodes,

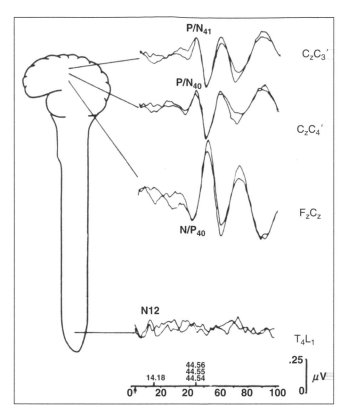

Figure 15 Cerebral and sacral waveforms in a dorsal nerve somatosensory-evoked response study. *Source*: From Ref. 13.

located proximal to the balloon, just touch the epithelium of the prostatic urethra. The sensory threshold of the urethrovesical junction is determined, and stimuli at double the threshold values are administered. The bulbocavernosus reflex is then recorded from the bulbocavernosus or the anal sphincter muscles in the usual manner. About 3 to 10 responses are averaged over an analysis time of 200 and 500 msec (41). In one study of 24 impotent diabetic men, the rate of abnormalities was 66% (vs. 12.5% when patients had the stimulus applied to the glans penis). Further, the abnormal responses correlated strongly with the presence of peripheral and autonomic neuropathy (41).

Cystometrography and Bethanechol Chloride Supersensitivity

Cystometrography is the graphic recording of the pressure exerted at varying degrees during filling of the urinary bladder. This investigation is used to evaluate for the presence of neurogenic bladder (42–44). The test is based upon the phenomenon of denervation supersensitivity (increased intrinsic sensitivity to neurohumoral transmitters when the organ is chronically deprived of its motor nerves). Cystometrography is performed by intravesical infusion of the empty bladder with 100 mL of water (1 mL/sec) through a catheter connected to the water reservoir as well as to a manometer. The intravesical pressure is then recorded and fluid infusion is

stopped. The procedure is repeated several times and the pressure measurements are averaged. Bethanechol chloride (2.5 mg) is then given subcutaneously, and the cystometric measurement is repeated 10, 20, and 30 minutes after bethanechol administration (42). In patients with normal bladder function, bethanechol administration (2.5 mg subcutaneously) does not increase the intravesical pressure by more than 15 cm water over the control value. In the absence of detrusor overactivity due to upper motor neuron lesions (e.g., stroke, Alzheimer's disease, brain tumor, and Parkinson's disease), local neurological problems (e.g., interference with spinal inhibitory pathways caused by spondylosis or metastasis in the sacral spine), or non-neurological conditions (e.g., sphincter outlet obstruction or incompetence, in situ carcinoma of the bladder, and previous radiation interstitial cystitis), a pressure response greater than 15 cm water over the control indicates that the patient has a disease involving either the lower motor neurons or the afferent sensory part of the lower reflex arc. If detrusor overactivity is found or cannot be ruled out, and a bethanechol administration induces a rise in intravesical pressure of greater than 15 cm water, then the test must be repeated on another day after administration of a spinal anesthetic or a ganglion blocker to inhibit the transmission of motor impulses from the CNS to the bladder (42).

Cystometry may also be performed through the installation of CO_2 gas and the use of continuous recording devices from isovolumetric strain gauges (45). Carbon dioxide is introduced via an indwelling catheter at an initial flow rate of up to 300 mL/min with the patient in the supine position. The cystometric examination is repeated with the patient sitting, standing, or walking in place (45). These position changes are used to evoke a detrusor reflex contraction when supine cystometry does not. The normal person can suppress the detrusor reflex contraction evoked by this procedure. Thus, the test is capable of evaluating the presence or absence of the detrusor reflex as well as the subject's ability to suppress it on command. Using this technique, two abnormalities were noted in the diabetic patients (35,46,47). The most common was detrusor areflexia due to impaired sensation of bladder fullness, which was observed in long-duration, insulin-dependent patients. The second abnormality was uninhibited detrusor hyperreflexia, most often associated with damage of the cortical or spinal regulatory tracts innervating the detrusor muscles.

Pupillary Light Reflex Latency

Assessment of the pupillary light reflex provides information on the function of both the sympathetic and the parasympathetic innervations. An increase in latency to light stimulus or a loss of pupillary light response indicates the compromise of parasympathetic innervation. The pupillary light reflex latency is measured by an iris infrared light reflex in which the retina is stimulated by a block-shaped stimulus with a fixed background and step intensity, corresponding to a retinal illumination of 1.2 and 3.7 Log Troland [1 Td of retinal illumination is produced when an eye with a pupil size of 1 mm² looks at a surface with a luminance of 1 cd/m²; (Td, Troland; cd, candela)], respectively. Latency of the pupillary constriction is averaged from at least six measurements of artifact-free responses for both eyes, with stimulus duration of 1.2 seconds each. The measurements are taken after the subject's adaptation for two minutes in darkness (34). Increased pupillary light reflex latencies are found more often than reduced darkness pupil size adaptation in diabetic patients with and without abnormal cardiovascular reflexes, suggesting that parasympathetic pupillary dysfunction precedes sympathetic pupillary denervation in diabetic autonomic neuropathy (34).

Heart Rate Variability

Several methods for the determination of respiratory-induced beat-to-beat variation in heart rate have been described (3,37,48–51). In one of these methods, respiratory-induced heart rate variation was determined by placing conventional electrocardiographic (ECG) plate electrodes on the right foot and on the left or right arm, and then connecting these to the positive and negative input terminals of a Medelec MS 20 differential preamplifier (Mystro: Medelec, Woking, U. K.). The sweep was triggered by the QRS complex, and the ECG activity was recorded with a gain of 200 or 500 mV/div, a filter band pass from 1 to 50 Hz, and a sweep duration of one to two seconds depending on the heart rate so that QRS pairs consisting of the triggering and the subsequent QRS complex were monitored on the same sweep. Using the trigger mode to capture and average interpotential differences, the variation of the time interval between consecutive QRS complexes was assessed for the duration of 50

QRS pairs taken during consecutive deep inspiration and expiration cycles at a rate of 6/min. Variation was expressed as the difference between the frequencies calculated from the shortest and the longest R-R interval found within an analysis period of approximately 45 seconds (Fig. 16) (3).

Rothschild et al. (48) assessed the effect of parasympathetic ablation with atropine on R-R variation and on the Valsalva ratio in nondiabetic subjects, and in diabetic patients with and without symptoms of autonomic neuropathy. The Valsalva ratio is believed to provide a more comprehensive cardiovascular autonomic testing procedure, since it allows the assessment of cardiac parasympathetic and sympathetic as well as vascular sympathetic innervations. The ratio is calculated by dividing maximum heart rate during the Valsalva maneuver by the slowest heart rate after the maneuver. This group, however, found the R-R variation to be more sensitive than the Valsalva ratio in detecting the decrease in parasympathetic activities.

Bennett et al. (49), on the other hand, found that a single deep breath is a more potent stimulus for heart rate change than repeated deep breaths in diabetic subjects, and that measurement of this response together with the bradycardia evoked by the Valsalva maneuver obviates the need to perform invasive investigations. Similarly, Shahani et al. (37) examined the diagnostic value of the combined testing with R-R interval variation and sympathetic skin response in patients with peripheral neuropathy. They found all patients with symptomatic autonomic neuropathy to have abnormal results in one or both tests. Further, about half of the patients with abnormality of one test result had symptoms of autonomic dysfunction. Thus, performing these two tests is likely to be helpful in assessing patients suspected for autonomic dysfunction. Similar results were reported by other investigators in

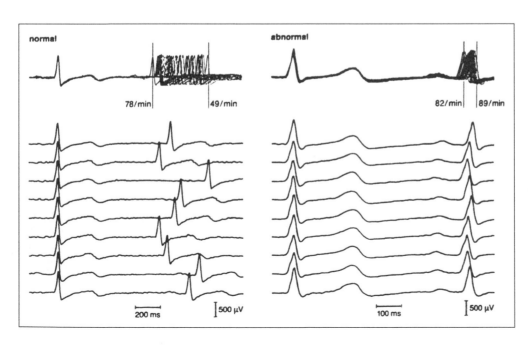

Figure 16 Respiratory heart rate variation. Examples of normal (*left panel*) and abnormal (*right panel*) heart rate variation measurements. In top traces, 50 sweeps are superimposed. Position of cursors indicate minimal and maximal RR intervals, from which heart rate/min was calculated. Nine consecutive sweeps illustrating normal variability of RR interval in left in contrast to right panel are shown below. *Source*: From Ref. 3.

patients with diabetic neuropathy using the Valsalva maneuver and hand-grip testing (52,53).

Another variant of heart rate variability testing is the determination of heart rate variation in response to orthostasis (30/15 test). This is performed by asking the subject to stand upright from the supine position as fast as possible during a continuous ECG monitoring. The R-R intervals between the 15th and 16th and between 30th and 31st QRS complexes are then measured and the ratio (30th/31st divided by 15th/16th interval) is calculated. The normal ratio is above 1.03 (3,54). The value of this technique as a diagnostic tool for the parasympathetic nervous function in patients with erectile disorders remains to be established.

Sympathetic
Darkness Pupil Size Adaptation

Failure of pupils to dilate in dim light (darkness adaptation) may suggest the loss of pupillary sympathetic control. A slit-lamp camera is used to measure the darkness adaptation of pupil size (34). After focusing the pupil and the iris with a three-stage, infrared, light-intensifier system, a photograph is taken using an electronic flashlight. Horizontal pupil diameter is then calculated as a percentage of iris-diameter from the photograph. This test has not been widely used in evaluating the sympathetic nervous function in patients with sexual disorders.

Sympathetic Skin Response

In 1890, Tarchanoff first described electrophysiologic monitoring of the peripheral autonomic nerves by means of skin response (39). Particular attention has been given to these studies as a means of evaluating diabetic patients. Nonmyelinated C fibers of the sympathetic nerves, which innervate sweat glands in the extremities, are responsible for these skin action potentials. As sympathetic fibers are also involved in sexual and voiding activity, the sympathetic skin response has the potential to assess each of these functions.

At least three methods have been described for this investigation. In the method of Park et al. (38), the biphasic skin DC-potential shifts in response to electrical shock stimuli are recorded from the volar and dorsal aspects of the hand and/or the plantar and dorsal aspects of the foot on one side of the body (Fig. 17). The electric stimuli are applied to the penile shaft using a pair of ribbon electrodes 0.5 cm wide, placed one centimeter apart. Randomly timed stimuli between 14.5 and 87.0 mA, each for 0.2 seconds, are applied at 15-second intervals. Sympathetic skin responses are recorded under the condition of a band pass of 2 to 5 Hz, with amplification sensitivity of 5 to 20 uV/cm and a sweep speed of 5 msec/cm. About 5 to 10 successive recordings are obtained (Fig. 18). Using this technique, mean palmar and plantar

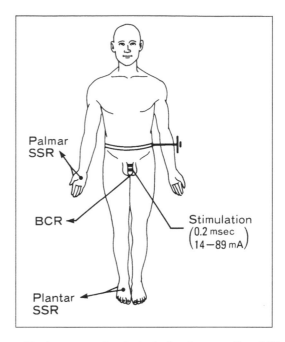

Figure 17 Arrangements of electrodes for recording SSR and BCR. *Abbreviations*: SSR, sympathetic skin response; BCR, bulbocavernosus reflex. *Source*: From Ref. 38.

sympathetic skin responses in 12 subjects with normal ejaculatory function were 1.44 ± 0.11 (SEM) and 2.07 ± 0.24 seconds, respectively. Further, 11 of 12 patients without ejaculatory function had absent plantar sympathetic skin responses (38).

Using the same method with slightly different electrical parameters, Dettmers et al. (29) studied the sympathetic skin response in 60 normal men and in 30 patients with erectile dysfunction. They were able to record the sympathetic skin response in all normal subjects with a mean lower extremity latency of 2.16 ± 0.2 seconds. Further, the sympathetic skin response was compared to the bulbocavernosus reflex and to the SSEPs of the pudendal nerve. Twenty patients were thought to have pure neurological or mixed neurological–vascular etiologies of the sexual dysfunction based on NPT, Doppler sonography, and pharmacological testing. Abnormal or absent bulbocavernosus reflex was found in 14, SSEPs in 12, and sympathetic skin responses in nine of these patients. The sensitivity of these three testing procedures was 70%, 60%, and 45%, respectively. Despite the lower sensitivity of the sympathetic skin response testing, however, it should be noted that this test demonstrated neurological abnormalities in some patients in whom all other test results were normal.

In the second method, described by Kunesch et al. (3), the recording of the response is done in the same way as described above, but supramaximal electrical shock stimuli are randomly applied at 20-second intervals to the median or tibial nerve of the contralateral side of the body. A normal response is considered to be present if clear biphasic responses are obtained at latencies of one to three seconds, consistently (Fig. 19).

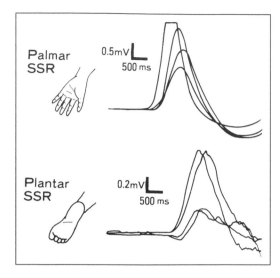

Figure 18 Reproducibility of SSR. Four successive responses were recorded from a 27-year-old normal subject. *Abbreviation*: SSR, sympathetic skin response *Source*: From Ref. 38.

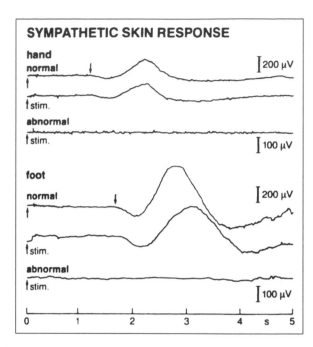

Figure 19 Sympathetic skin response. Examples of two patients with normal and absent sympathetic skin responses recorded in right hand and foot evoked by electrical stimuli applied contralaterally. For patient with absent responses, only one out of several sweeps illustrated. Stimulation and beginning of responses indicated by arrows. Note long time base. *Source*: From Ref. 3.

Using this technique in 30 patients with erectile dysfunction, abnormal sympathetic skin response in sites located on the hand and the foot was noted in about 20% and 53% of patients, respectively. The higher abnormal rate for the foot recording was thought to be related to nonspecific age-dependent abnormalities (55); however, when autonomic evaluations (the parasympathetic respiratory and 30/15 heart-rate variability tests and the sympathetic skin response in the hand test) were considered collectively, 64% of the patients had abnormal results, and this correlated well with the clinical neurological findings (53%). In contrast, the abnormalities in somatic nerve conduction (13%) and pudendal nerve SSEP testing (about 30%) were found less frequently (3).

In the third method, the electrical shocks are applied to the right median nerve at the area of the wrist, and the recording electrode is placed on the lateral aspect of the penile shaft to avoid vascular artifacts from the dorsal penile vasculatures (39).

Using this method, penile sympathetic skin response was measured in 20 normal men and in 46 patients with erectile dysfunction. Sympathetic skin responses were recorded in 80% of normal subjects, with latencies between 1.2 and 1.6 seconds. Patients with erectile dysfunction had long latencies ranging between 1.24 and 3.64 seconds. Reproducible long latencies with this technique were thought to indicate the presence of neuropathy of unmyelinated nerve fibers, which may be the first clinical sign of a general neuropathy (39). The possible correlation between urinary bladder dysfunction and other forms of autonomic dysfunction such as lost or delayed sympathetic skin response was examined in 23 diabetic patients by Ueda et al. (56). Sympathetic skin responses were lost in 12 and delayed in 11 patients. Increased residual urine and decreased detrusor contraction pressure were found in patients with lost sympathetic skin response,

whereas only the latter bladder abnormality occurred in patients with delayed sympathetic skin response.

Schurch et al. (36) examined the utility of the sympathetic skin response of the right hand and foot in the assessment of the vesicourethral autonomic nervous dysfunction in 27 spinal cord injured patients. All tetraplegic and paraplegic patients with a lesion above the T6 level who presented with bladder neck dyssynergia associated with autonomic hyperreflexia had abnormal sympathetic skin responses in the right hand and foot. All patients with lesions below the T6 and above the T12 level with abnormal sympathetic skin response in the right foot also had bladder neck dyssynergia. Thus, the absence of sympathetic skin response from upper and lower limbs may suggest an injury to the descending sympathetic spinal tract higher than the T6 level, and the presence of the response in the hand, but not the foot, localizes the lesion to a level between T6 and T12 vertebrae.

Histamine and Acetylcholine Skin Tests

This test is performed by injecting 0.1 mg of histamine phosphate (57,58) or 0.1 mL 1% acetylcholine (40) intradermally in the distribution of the L4 or L5 dermatomes, with the site of injection being examined after 10 minutes. Abnormal responses are indicated by the absence of a red flare in the histamine test or absence of uniformly distributed dark spots of iodine discoloration in the acetylcholine test (skin testing area is painted with 2% iodine in absolute alcohol followed by a thin layer of 1% thoroughly mixed fine maize starch in arachis oil) at the site of injection.

The histamine test was performed in 21 patients with erectile dysfunction. All six patients with peripheral neuropathy on physical examination had abnormal responses, but only 2 of 13 patients with normal physical examination responded abnormally (57). The acetylcholine test was performed in 24 diabetic males with erectile dysfunction, of whom 13 responded abnormally, but the agreement between the cardiovascular and sweat-spot test was found in only 17 patients (40). Although these tests have not yet been vigorously validated, they are likely to constitute an acceptable indirect means of assessing the integrity of the sympathetic supply to the genitalia, since some branches of the lumbar sympathetics accompany the lower extremity peripheral nerves and innervate the vessels of the skin.

Corpus Cavernosum Electromyography

CC-EMG is a controversial method for assessing erectile failure. The existence of electrical activity in the corpus cavernosum was first reported in 1989 (2,59). Activity was initially measured using concentric needles inserted through the skin and tunica albuginea into the center of the corpus cavernosum (59). Subsequent studies, however, have shown that surface electrodes placed on the penile skin yield similar results (60–62). Activity in the flaccid penis of normal subjects has been demonstrated to consist of continuous slow frequency firing. These bursts of activity

cease during erection induced by visual stimulation and resume again during detumescence (Fig. 20A and B) (2). It was concluded that the activity recorded during CC-EMG represented sympathetic activity in the corpus cavernosum, with increased activity causing contraction of the smooth muscle cells and penile flaccidity, whereas decreased activity allowed for smooth muscle relaxation and erection.

Unfortunately, data from CC-EMG studies are highly complex and difficult to interpret. The single potential analysis of cavernosal EMG (SPACE) was developed to simplify the cumbersome data by breaking it down into what was thought to be individual cavernosal smooth muscle potentials (63). It was never convincingly proven, however, that these recordings arose strictly from spontaneous cavernosal activity, as artifacts of systemic sympathetic activity, which could also be detected from the skin on the limbs, were also suspected of being involved (64). Due to this uncertainty, the name "SPACE" was subsequently discarded at the first international workshop on CC-EMG in 1993 (65). To further compound the issue, Colakoglu et al. (66) found that the bursts of activity measured by CC-EMG are accompanied by slow penile retractile movements, suggesting that spontaneous cavernosal activity may actually originate from normal biomechanical events in the flaccid penis. Another study (67) determined that in healthy subjects, all parameters varied extremely among individuals and were poorly reproducible at repetition; however, significant differences between healthy men and men with erectile dysfunction as defined groups were found in provocation.

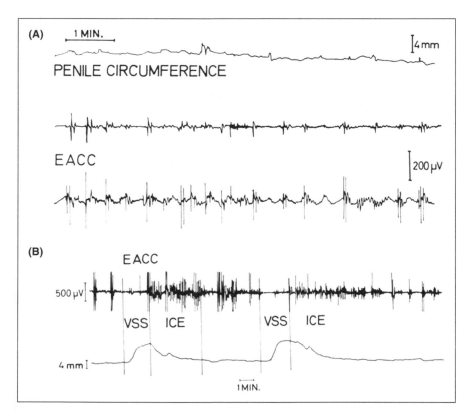

Figure 20 Corpus cavernosum electromyography. (A) Simultaneous recordings of penile circumference (upper trace) and EACC from two electrodes placed 2 cm apart (lower traces) in flaccid penis in a normal subject. Calibration for time (minutes), circumference (mm), and signal amplitude (µv) are shown. (B) Effects of VSS between vertical lines in normal subject on EACC (upper trace) and penile circumference (lower trace). Detumescence of erect penis was enhanced by ICE to thigh. Calibrations for time (minutes), signal amplitude (µv), and penile circumference (mm) are shown. *Abbreviations*: EACC, electrical activity of the corpus cavernosum; VSS, visual sexual stimulation; ICE, application of ice pack. *Source*: From Ref. 59.

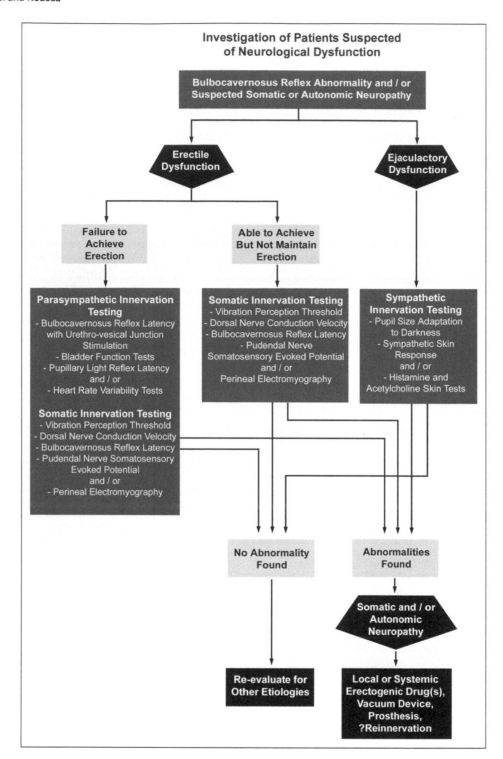

Figure 21 Algorithmic approach to the investigation and treatment of men with erectile or ejaculatory abnormality caused by neurological dysfunction. Patients with erectile dysfunction but normal ejaculatory function may have a parasympathetic and/or somatic innervation deficit(s), and, therefore, should be evaluated with the appropriate parasympathetic and/or somatic innervation testing. Patients who are able to achieve an erection, but not able to maintain it, are more likely to have somatic denervation only, and, therefore, should not be subjected to autonomic function testing. Patients with absent or retarded ejaculation, but normal erectile function, are likely to have sympathetic denervation as the underlying neurological deficit, and, therefore, should be evaluated with sympathetic pathways testing only. *Note*: ? represents data that are experimental or for which studies are not yet complete.

Although the origins of CC-EMG recordings remain unclear, their reproducibility and use in predicting neuropathology have been well documented (68,69). In subjects with normal potency, flaccidity is demonstrated by rhythmic bursts of activity and synchronous contractions of the smooth muscle cells, while erection is noted by a near or complete cessation of activity resulting in nonsynchronization of smooth muscle cell contractions followed by potentials of decreased amplitude and duration but increased frequency (2,70). Abnormal findings have been described as repeated bursts of activity during visual sexual stimulation and have been attributed to both organic (2) and psychogenic (70) causes. Similar abnormal parameters have been described in response to intracavernous injection (71). Diabetics with peripheral autonomic dysfunction tend to display desynchronization of cavernous electrical activity, while diabetics with cavernous smooth muscle degeneration often demonstrate low amplitude and slow depolarization of the potentials (70). Amplitudes of cavernous electrical activity are also low in patients with caverno-occlusive dysfunction (71). Patients with neurological lesions caused by pelvic surgeries show both normal potentials and abnormal electrical activity depending on the location and severity of the lesion.

CC-EMG is an appealing diagnostic tool because it yields results that can be categorized into distinct neuropathological categories. The fact that the data takes approximately one hour to collect and requires an experienced examiner to interpret its results, however, dramatically reduces its utility in clinical practice. A computerized program has been developed to analyze CC-EMG recordings and represents a second attempt to make cavernosal electrical activity data more manageable (72).

☐ CONCLUSION

Improvements in the understanding of the relative role of various components of the nervous system in the control of normal erectile cycle have stimulated efforts to develop new diagnostic procedures that are capable of defining the site and nature of lesion(s) contributing to erectile failure in a given patient. CNS disorders should be ruled out by clinical examination. Then, with careful assessment of the peripheral nervous system via physical signs and identification of the nature of the sexual problem (e.g., erectile vs. ejaculatory dysfunction), it is possible to narrow further the choice of required diagnostic test procedures. Figure 21 illustrates a summary of the algorithmic approach to the investigation and treatment of men with erectile or ejaculatory abnormalities caused by neurological dysfunction. Since sensorimotor polyneuropathy may often be detected clinically, as well, nerve conduction studies may not always be necessary. Currently available methods of neurological investigation, however—particularly for the autonomic systems—continue to be cumbersome and rather indirect. Thus, the need for the development of simpler and more direct testing procedures, particularly those that could be used by nonspecialists in the office setting, remains unmet. Future research should be directed toward achieving such an objective.

☐ REFERENCES

1. Padma-Nathan H. Neurologic evaluation of erectile dysfunction. Urol Clin North Am 1988; 15(1):77–80.
2. Gerstenberg TC, Nordling J, Hald T, et al. Standardized evaluation of erectile dysfunction in 95 consecutive patients. J Urol 1989; 141(4):857–862.
3. Kunesch E, Reiners K, Muller-Mattheis V, et al. Neurological risk profile in organic erectile impotence. J Neurol Neurosurg Psychiatry 1992; 55(4):275–281.
4. Bleustein CB, Arezzo JC, Eckholdt H, et al. The neuropathy of erectile dysfunction. Int J Impot Res 2002; 14(6):433–439.
5. Kirby RS. An Atlas of Erectile Dysfunction. New York: Taylor and Francis Group, 1999.
6. De Groat WC, Steers WD. Neuroanatomy and neurophysiology of penile erection. In: Tanagho EA, Lue TF, McClure RD, eds. Contemporary Management of Impotence and Infertility. Baltimore: Williams & Wilkins, 1988:3–27.
7. Kandeel FR, Koussa KT, Swerdloff RS. Male sexual function and its disorders: physiology, pathophysiology, clinical investigation, and treatment. Endocr Rev 2001; 22(3):342–388.
8. Lefaucheur JP, Yiou R, Colombel M, et al. Relationship between penile thermal sensory threshold measurement and electrophysiologic tests to assess neurogenic impotence. Urology 2001; 57(2):306–309.
9. Lue TE. Evaluation of the complex patient, additional testing, and when to refer. In: Walsh PC, ed. Campbell's Urology. 8th ed. St. Louis: W. B. Saunders Company, 2002:1638.
10. Goldstein I. Evaluation of penile nerves. In: Tanagho EA, Lue TF, McClure RD, eds. Contemporary Management of Impotence and Infertility. Baltimore: Williams & Wilkins, 1988:70–83.
11. Padma-Nathan H, Goldstein I, Krane RJ. Evaluation of the impotent patient. Semin Urol 1986; 4(4):225–232.
12. Reproduced from www.biothesiometer.com with permission by Bio-medical Instrument Company, 15764 Munn Road, Newbury, OH, USA.
13. Padma-Nathan H, Goldstein I. Neurologic assessment of the impotent patient. In: Montague DK, ed. Disorders of Male Sexual Function. Chicago: Year Book Medical Publishers, Inc., 1988:86–94.
14. Padma-Nathan H, Levine F. Vibratory testing of the penis. J Urol 1987; 137:210A.
15. Yarnitsky D, Sprecher E, Vardi Y. Penile thermal sensation. J Urol 1996; 156(2 Pt 1):391–393.
16. Bleustein CB, Eckholdt H, Arezzo JC, et al. Quantitative somatosensory testing of the penis: optimizing the clinical neurological examination. J Urol 2003; 169(6):2266–2269.

17. Reproduced from www.medoc-web.com/tsa.html with permission by: meDoc Advanced Medical Systems U.S., 1502 West Highway 54 - Suite 404, Durham, North Carolina, USA.

18. Lefaucheur JP, Yiou R, Salomon L, et al. Assessment of penile small nerve fiber damage after transurethral resection of the prostate by measurement of penile thermal sensation. J Urol 2000; 164:1416–1419.

19. Robinson LQ, Woodcock JP, Stephenson TP. Results of investigation of impotence in patients with overt or probable neuropathy. Br J Urol 1987; 60(6):583–587.

20. Legatt AD, Soliman E. Somatosensory Evoked Potentials: General Principles. E-medicine article. http://www.emedicine.com/neuro/topic640.htm. May 15, 2006.

21. Bradley WE, Lin JT, Johnson B. Measurement of the conduction velocity of the dorsal nerve of the penis. J Urol 1984; 131(6):1127–1129.

22. Lin JT, Bradley WE. Penile neuropathy in insulin-dependent diabetes mellitus. J Urol 1985; 133(2): 213–215.

23. Kaneko S, Bradley WE. Penile electrodiagnosis. Value of bulbocavernosus reflex latency versus nerve conduction velocity of the dorsal nerve of the penis in diagnosis of diabetic impotence. J Urol 1987; 137(5):933–935.

24. Shafik A, Shafik I, El-Sibai O, et al. Effect of external anal sphincter contraction on the ischiocavernosus muscle and its suggested role in the sex act. J Androl 2006; 27(1):40–44.

25. Siroky MB, Sax DS, Krane RJ. Sacral signal tracing: the electrophysiology of the bulbocavernosus reflex. J Urol 1979; 122(5):661–664.

26. Haldeman S, Bradley WE, Bhatia NN, et al. Pudendal evoked responses. Arch Neurol 1982; 39(5):280–283.

27. Mehta AJ, Viosca SP, Korenman SG, et al. Peripheral nerve conduction studies and bulbocavernosus reflex in the investigation of impotence. Arch Phys Med Rehabil 1986; 67(5):332–335.

28. Espino P. Neurogenic impotence: diagnostic value of nerve conduction studies, bulbocavernosus reflex, and heart rate variability. Electromyogr Clin Neurophysiol 1994; 34(6):373–376.

29. Dettmers C, van Ahlen H, Faust H, et al. Evaluation of erectile dysfunction with the sympathetic skin response in comparison to bulbocavernosus reflex and somatosensory evoked potentials of the pudendal nerve. Electromyogr Clin Neurophysiol 1994; 34(7):437–444.

30. Bemelmans BL, Meuleman EJ, Doesburg WH, et al. Erectile dysfunction in diabetic men: the neurological factor revisited. J Urol 1994; 151(4):884–889.

31. Goldstein I. Neurologic impotence. In: Krane RJ, Siroky MB, Goldstein I, eds. Male Sexual Dysfunction. Boston: Little, Brown and Company, 1983:193–201.

32. Pickard RS, Powell PH, Schofield IS. The clinical application of dorsal penile nerve cerebral-evoked response recording in the investigation of impotence. Br J Urol 1994; 74(2):231–235.

33. Reproduced with permission from www.heartcoherence.com by Heart Coherence Team, P.O. Box 40235, 7504 RE Enschede, The Netherlands.

34. Lanting P, Bos JE, Aartsen J, et al. Assessment of pupillary light reflex latency and darkness adapted pupil size in control subjects and in diabetic patients with and without cardiovascular autonomic neuropathy. J Neurol Neurosurg Psychiatry 1990; 53(10):912–914.

35. Bradley WE, Timm GW, Scott FB. Cystometry IV. Neuromuscular transmission in urinary bladder. Urology 1975; 6(4):520–524.

36. Schurch B, Curt A, Rossier AB. The value of sympathetic skin response recordings in the assessment of the vesicourethral autonomic nervous dysfunction in spinal cord injured patients. J Urol 1997; 157(6): 2230–2233.

37. Shahani BT, Day TJ, Cros D, et al. RR interval variation and the sympathetic skin response in the assessment of autonomic function in peripheral neuropathy. Arch Neurol 1990; 47(6):659–664.

38. Park YC, Esa A, Sugiyama T, et al. Sympathetic skin response: a new test to diagnose ejaculatory dysfunction. J Urol 1988; 139(3):539–541.

39. Derouet H, Jost WH, Osterhage J, et al. Penile sympathetic skin response in erectile dysfunction. Eur Urol 1995; 28(4):314–319.

40. Ryder RE, Marshall R, Johnson K, et al. Acetylcholine sweatspot test for autonomic denervation. Lancet 1988; 1(8598):1303–1305.

41. Sarica Y, Karacan I. Bulbocavernosus reflex to somatic and visceral nerve stimulation in normal subjects and in diabetics with erectile impotence. J Urol 1987; 138:55–58.

42. Lapides J, Friend CR, Ajemian EP, et al. Denervation supersensitivity as a test for neurogenic bladder. Surg Gynecol Obstet 1962; 114:241–244.

43. Buck AC, Reed PI, Siddiq YK, et al. Bladder dysfunction and neuropathy in diabetes. Diabetologia 1976; 12:251–258.

44. Ellenberg M. Impotence in diabetes: the neurologic factor. Ann Intern Med 1971; 75(2):213–219.

45. Bradley WE. Diagnosis of urinary bladder dysfunction in diabetes mellitus. Ann Intern Med 1980; 92(2 Pt 2): 323–326.

46. Bradley WE, Timm GW, Scott FB. Cystometry III. Cystometers. Urology 1975; 5(6):843–848.

47. Bradley WE, Timm GW. Cystometry. VI. Interpretation. Urology 1976; 7(2):231–235.

48. Rothschild AH, Weinberg CR, Halter JB, et al. Sensitivity of R-R variation and Valsalva ratio in assessment of cardiovascular diabetic autonomic neuropathy. Diabetes Care 1987; 10(6):735–741.

49. Bennett T, Farquhar IK, Hosking DJ, et al. Assessment of methods for estimating autonomic nervous control of the heart in patients with diabetes mellitus. Diabetes 1978; 27(12):1167–1174.

50. Watkins PJ, Mackay JD. Cardiac denervation in diabetic neuropathy. Ann Intern Med 1980; 92(2 Pt 2):304–307.

51. Nisen HO, Larsen A, Lindstrom BL, et al. Cardiovascular reflexes in the neurological evaluation of impotence. Br J Urol 1993; 71(2):199–203.

52. Ewing DJ, Campbell IW, Burt AA, et al. Vascular reflexes in diabetic autonomic neuropathy. Lancet 1973; 2(7842):1354–1356.

53. Ewing DJ, Campbell IW, Clarke BF. Assessment of cardiovascular effects in diabetic autonomic neuropathy and prognostic implications. Ann Intern Med 1980; 92(2 Pt 2):308–311.

54. Ewing DJ, Campbell IW, Murray A, et al. Immediate heart-rate response to standing: simple test for autonomic neuropathy in diabetes. Br Med J 1978; 1(6106): 145–147.

55. Low PA, Opfer-Gehrking TL, Proper CJ, et al. The effect of aging on cardiac autonomic and postganglionic sudomotor function. Muscle Nerve 1990; 13(2): 152–157.

56. Ueda T, Yoshimura N, Yoshida O. Diabetic cystopathy: relationship to autonomic neuropathy detected by sympathetic skin response. J Urol 1997; 157(2):580–584.

57. Grotta J, Lipshultz L, Hankins L, et al. Screening for neurologic disease in impotent patients. Tex Med 1985; 81(10):44–47.

58. DeJong RN. Examination of the autonomic nervous system. The Neurological Examination: Incorporating the Fundamentals of Neuroanatomy and Neurophysiology, 4th ed. Hagerstown, MD: Harper and Row, 1979:510–521.

59. Wagner G, Gerstenberg T, Levin RJ. Electrical activity of corpus cavernosum during flaccidity and erection of the human penis: a new diagnostic method? J Urol 1989; 142(3):723–725.

60. Stief CG, Thon WF, Djamilian M, et al. Transcutaneous registration of cavernous smooth muscle electrical activity: noninvasive diagnosis of neurogenic autonomic impotence. J Urol 1992; 147(1):47–50.

61. Merckx LA, de Bruyne RM, Keuppens FI. Electromyography of cavernous smooth muscle during flaccidity: evaluation of technique and normal values. Br J Urol 1993; 72(3):353–358.

62. Truss MC, Djamilian MH, Tan HK, et al. Single potential analysis of cavernous electrical activity. Four years' experience in more than 500 patients with erectile dysfunction. Eur Urol 1993; 24(3):358–365.

63. Stief CG, Djamilian M, Anton P, et al. Single potential analysis of cavernous electrical activity in impotent patients: a possible diagnostic method for autonomic cavernous dysfunction and cavernous smooth muscle degeneration. J Urol 1991; 146(3):771–776.

64. Yarnitsky D, Sprecher E, Barilan Y, et al. Corpus cavernosum electromyogram: spontaneous and evoked electrical activities. J Urol 1995; 153(3 Pt 1): 653–654.

65. Beck RO. Investigation of male erectile dysfunction. In: Fowler CJ, ed. Neurology of Bladder, Bowl, and Sexual Dysfunction. Boston: Butterworth Heinemann, 1999: 145–160.

66. Colakoglu Z, Kutluay E, Ertekin C. The nature of spontaneous cavernosal activity. BJU Int 1999; 83(4): 449–452.

67. Fabra M, Frieling A, Porst H, et al. Single potential analysis of corpus cavernosum electromyography for the assessment of erectile dysfunction: provocation, reproducibility and age dependence--findings in 36 healthy volunteers and 324 patients. J Urol 1997; 158(2): 444–450.

68. Sasso F, Gulino G, Alcini E. Corpus cavernosum electromyography (CC-EMG): a new technique in the diagnostic work-up of impotence. Int Urol Nephrol 1996; 28(6):805–818.

69. Sasso F, Stief CG, Gulino G, et al. Progress in corpus cavernosum electromyography (CC-EMG)-third international workshop on corpus cavernosum electromyography (CC-EMG). Int J Impot Res 1997; 9(1): 43–45.

70. Stief CG, Wetterauer U, Schaebsdau FH, et al. Calcitonin-gene-related peptide: a possible role in human penile erection and its therapeutic application in impotent patients. J Urol 1991; 146(4):1010–1014.

71. Kayigil AE. Caverno-occlusive and autonomic dysfunction: a new concept in young patients. Eur Urol 1998; 34(2):124–127.

72. Kellner B, Stief CG, Hinrichs H, et al. Computerized classification of corpus cavernosum electromyogram signals by the use of discriminant analysis and artificial neural networks to support diagnosis of erectile dysfunction. Urol Res 2000; 28(1):6–13.

Part IV

Treatment of Male Sexual Dysfunction

The treatment for male sexual dysfunction should be selected based on the particular nature of the presenting problem, as determined by the results of thorough history-taking, physical evaluation, and all pertinent laboratory and special testing procedures. As the understanding of male sexual physiology and pathophysiology has improved greatly in the last three decades, significant advances have been made in the fields of psychosexual counseling, pharmacological therapy, nonsurgical device design and availability, and operative techniques. The resulting array of treatment options can often be bewildering to the clinician. The chapters in Part IV describe in great detail each of the types of treatments available. The three tables provided here, however, function as a complete unit in providing a broad overview that will help guide the reader toward the necessary chapter depending on the particular application. The classes, agents, or modalities that are most commonly used are highlighted and compared. References are provided in parentheses to the parent chapters in which each of these treatments is described in full detail.

Table 1   Therapeutic Approaches to Male Sexual Dysfunction

Sexual disorder	Etiologic factor		Therapeutic options
I. HYPOACTIVE SEXUAL DESIRE	Psychogenic		Psychosexual counseling (27,28) Drug therapy (PDE-5 trazodone, yohimbine, bupropion) (29,31)
	Androgen deficiency	Primary or secondary hypogonadism	Testosterone replacement for primary and dopamine agonist or other appropriate (GnRH or hCG) intervention for secondary hypogonadism (29,35)
		Androgen antagonism	Change inciting agent, if possible (19,29,35)
	CNS disease		Depends on nature and extent of disease (15,38)
II. ERECTILE DYSFUNCTION	Psychogenic		Psychosexual counseling (27,28)
	Drug therapy		Discontinue drugs with parasympatholytic or sympathomimetic activities, if possible (19,29)
	Systemic disease		Treat primary disease (29–32,36)
	Arterial insufficiency	Large artery disease	Vascular reconstruction (33,40,41)
		Small artery disease	Vacuum device (32) Erectogenic drugs (PDE-5, local vasoactive agents) (29,30) Revascularization, if possible (33,40,41) Prosthesis (33,41)
	Veno-occlusive disease	True venous incompetence	Surgical ligation (33)
		Smooth muscle dysfunction — Organic	Vacuum device (32) Erectogenic drugs (primarily local vasoactive agents (29,30) Prosthesis (33,41) Tissue/molecular engineering (42)
		Functional (including sympathetic overtone)	Psychosexual counseling (27,28) Pelvic floor muscle training (28) Constrictive ring or vacuum device (32) Erectogenic drugs (local or systemic agents including alpha receptor blockers) (29,30)
	Congenital or acquired structural anomalies		Surgical reconstruction, if possible (33,40,41) Initial trial of systemic (vitamin E, Potaba, colchicine,tamoxifen) or local (collagenase, calcium channel blocker) medical therapy for Peyronie's disease (29,31,34)
	Neurogenic disorders	Neuropathy	Vacuum tumescence (32) Erectogenic drugs (PDE-5, local vasoactive agents) (29,30) Prosthesis (33,41) Surgical reinnervation, if possible (33,40,41)
		Sympathetic overtone	As per veno-occlusive dysfunction, plus: erectogenic drugs (local or systemic agents including alpha-receptor blockers) (29,30)
III. DISORDERS OF EJACULATION	Premature ejaculation	Psychogenic	Psychosexual counseling (27,28)
		Organic	Drug therapy (local or central acting agents including serotonergics, alpha-receptor blockers, and anesthetic creams) (29,30)
	Absent or retarded emission	Drug therapy	Discontinue sympatholytic drugs, if possible (19,29,30)
		Sympathetic denervation	Sympathomimetics, tricyclic antidepressants (29,30,37)
		Spinal cord injury	Vibratory stimulation (32,38)
		Androgen deficiency	Androgen replacement (29,35)
	Postejaculation pain	Psychogenic	Psychosexual counseling (27,28)
IV. ORGASMIC DYSFUNCTION	Drug therapy		Discontinue psychotropic agent, if possible (19,29)
	Psychogenic		Psychosexual counseling (27,28)
	CNS disease		Treat inciting disease, if possible (38)
V. FAILURE OF DETUMESCENCE	Primary penile disease		Surgical correction (33,40,41)
	Secondary penile disease		Treatment of inciting systemic disease (18,29,30)
	Cavernosal vasoactive drug therapy		Adjustment of agent dose Change to a different agent(s) or a different method of erection enhancement therapy (19,29–33)

General management strategies for the treatment of male sexual dysfunction are presented according to type of sexual disorder. These have been broadly classified into five main areas: (*I*) hypoactive sexual desire, (*II*) erectile dysfunction, (*III*) disorders of ejaculation, (*IV*) orgasmic dysfunction, and (*V*) failure of detumescence. These are further subdivided by the etiologic factors involved. Each of the attendant therapeutic options listed is accompanied by the chapter number in which it is discussed in further detail. Pharmacologic treatments and erectile enhancement therapies are additionally referred to in Tables 2 and 3, respectively.

Table 2 Pharmacological Agents Currently Used to Treat Erectile Failure

Drug class	Drug name	Mode of action	Dosing	Comment
PHOSPHODI-ESTERASE-TYPE 5 INHIBITORS (29)	Sildenafil	Type 5 cGMP phosphodi-esterase inhibitor	Oral agent, 25–100 mg in a single dose	Effective in up to 87% of patients with 1-yr followup. Side effects include headache, facial flush, indigestion.
	Vardenafil	Type 5 cGMP phosphodi-esterase inhibitor	Oral agent, 5–20 mg in a single dose	Very similar to sildenafil. Most common side effects reported include headache, flushing, rhinitis, dyspepsia and sinusitis.
	Tadalafil	Type 5 cGMP phosphodi-esterase inhibitor	Oral agent, 5–20 mg in a single dose	Prolonged half-life (17.5 hours) and thus prolonged mean elimination time (4.3 days). Has been shown to improve erectile functioning up to 36 hours after dosing. Affinity to PDE6 is much less than sildenafil, but affinity to PDE11 is much higher. Long-term effects of prolonged PDE11 activity still currently unknown.
INTRACORPOREAL INJECTIONS (30)	Papaverine	cAMP phosphodiesterase inhibitor and alpha-1 blocker	Intracorporeal injection, 10–80 mg	Potent local vasoactive agent produces usable erections in 30–60% of patients. Associated with a high incidence of priapism and corporeal fibrosis (up to 20%). Often supplemented with phentolamine and/or PGE$_1$ (erection rate of 60–90%).
	Prostaglandin E$_1$ (Alprostadil, Caverject, Edex/Viridal)	Prostaglandin E	Intracorporeal injection, 2.5–20 μg	Higher erectile response (74%) than papaverine, with less priapism (0.1%). Least incidence of systemic side effects or corporeal fibrosis. Often painful (20–40%). Can be supplemented with papaverine and/or phentolamine.
	Phentolamine (Regitine)	Alpha receptor blocker (mainly alpha-1 but also has alpha-2 activity)	Intracorporeal injection, 5–10 mg	Short-lived penile rigidity if used alone. Commonly used to supplement other vasoactive agents to increase effective-ness and reduce side effects. Mixtures with VIP (Invicorp—not approved in U.S.) and an oral preparation (Vasomax) were under evaluation.
INTRAURETHRAL THERAPY (30)	Prostaglandin E$_1$ (MUSE pellet)	Prostaglandin E	Intraurethral pellet, 125–1000 μg	As above for Intracorporeal injections (Prostaglandin E$_1$).
OTHER ORAL MEDICATIONS (29,31)	Yohimbine	Alpha-2 receptor blocker	Oral agent, 4.5–6 mg three times daily	Mostly ineffective except in some patients with psychogenic impotence. May increase blood pressure and sympa-thetic nervous system outflow in hypertensive patients and those taking tricyclic antidepressants. May be effective in treating sexual dysfunction induced by selective serotonin reuptake inhibitors.
	Trazodone	Triazolopyridine derivative that influences alpha-adrenergic, dopaminergic, and serotonergic functions, and indirectly stimulates corporeal smooth muscle relaxation	Oral agent, ranges from 50 mg in a single daily dose to 50 mg three times daily	Single bedtime dose of trazodone 75 mg to 150 mg may increase the frequency and quality of morning erection. May have a synergistic effect when trazodone 50 mg once daily is given with yohimbine 5 mg three times daily. Use of trazodone with PDE5 inhibitors remains to be evaluated.
	Bupropion	Inhibits the reuptake of serotonin and norepine-phrine and decreases whole body norepine-phrine turnover	Oral agent, ranges from 100 mg twice daily to 150 mg three times daily depending on response	Fluoxetine-associated sexual dysfunction was shown to improve after switching to therapy with bupropion. Dopaminergic side effects.

The most common sexual problem affecting males is erectile dysfunction; the most common drugs used in the treatment of this disorder are listed here. Also provided are details of the available trade names, mode of action, dosing, and comments from clinical experience.

Table 3   Comparison of Erectile-Enhancement Therapies

Method			Advantages	Disadvantages
ORAL ERECTION ENHANCEMENT AGENTS (29, 31)			Ease of administration.	Specific phosphodiesterase-5 inhibitors are effective, but many others are ineffective. High rate of systemic side effects.
LOCAL VASOACTIVE AGENTS (30)	**Papaverine intracorporeal injections**		Effective in >90% of neurogenic and psychogenic impotence and in 60–80% of other conditions.	Risk of infections, bruises, fibrosis, deformity, priapism, and orthostatic hypotension. Variability of dose required.
	Prostaglandin E₁ intracorporeal injections and urethral pessaries		As above for papaverine. Intraurethral application does not require self-injection.	Burning sensation, priapism.
CONSTRICTION RING AND VACUUM-INDUCED TUMESCENCE (32)			Relatively inexpensive. Constriction ring may treat venous leakage, if present. Vacuum device efficacy is comparable to papaverine injection.	Requires patient dexterity and strength to apply and remove device. Risk of injury during application or tissue ischemia with prolonged use. Not suitable for patients with primary or secondary penile disease, blood clotting disorders, or pelvic infections.
SURGICAL CORRECTION (33,40,41)	**Large-artery revascularization**		Likely to succeed if isolated lesion.	Low rate of success if associated with diffuse atherosclerosis and small-vessel disease.
	Small-artery revascularization		Possible long-term treatment effect.	Technically difficult with low rate of success.
	Venous ligation		Possible long-term treatment effect.	High rate of failure and recurrence.
	Repair of penile anomalies (congenital deformity, traumatic rupture, curvature, abnormal size)		Good surgical correction of trauma, curvature, penoscrotal webbing, or penile lymphedema, particularly in the young. Apparent gain of 1 inch with forward displacement phalloplasty, and 1–2 inches with girth-increase phalloplasty.	Peyronie's disease may have immunologic basis and could recur. Recurrent penile shortness, loss of sensation, and impotence after prolongation phalloplasty. Graft-site fat absorption, loss of sensation, and hideous appearance after dermal-fat graft.
	Penile prosthesis	Semi-rigid or nonarticulating malleable implant	Simple construction provides most straight penis in patients with curvature. Easy to insert with fewer complications. Least expensive.	Constant erection, may be difficult to conceal. Fixed, relatively small penile girth. Not suitable for patients with poor sensation or history of distal erosion.
		Self-contained articulating or inflatable implant	Relatively easy to insert. Suitable for patients with narrow phallus. Patient able to control state of erection with spring-activated and inflatable devices.	Spring-activated and inflatable devices require manual dexterity to operate. Inflatables break down more frequently than semi-rigid or malleable devices. Not suitable for patients with poor sensation or history of distal erosion.
		Two- or three-piece fully inflatable implant	Mimics natural process of rigidity and flaccidity. Patient able to control state of erection. Suitable for patients with impaired senation. Two-piece device suitable for patients with previous pelvic surgeries. Three-piece device produces maximum girth and length expansion, and thus is suitable for large phallus.	Extensive surgical procedure. Earlier versions had highest rate of mechanical failure (fluid leakage, tubing obstruction, cylinder ballooning); newer devices are more reliable. Two-piece device has limited fluid reservoir and makes it suitable only for patients with short or narrow phallus. All require high degree of dexterity to operate. Expensive.

This table provides an overview of the effective uses, advantages, and disadvantages of the most commonly used modes of therapy for male erectile dysfunction. Detailed discussions are provided in the corresponding chapters, indicated in parentheses.

27

Psychological and Behavioral Counseling in the Management of Male Sexual Dysfunction

Claudia Avina
Social Science Division, Pepperdine University, Malibu, California, U.S.A.

William T. O'Donohue
Department of Psychology, University of Nevada, Reno, Nevada, U.S.A.

Lisa Regev
Kaiser Permanente, Stockton, California, U.S.A.

□ INTRODUCTION

Sexual dysfunctions manifest themselves as impairments in the ability to achieve physical and sexual intimacy with another human being. As such, these impairments can be incredibly harmful to an individual's quality of life. Historically, society has targeted sexual prowess as the epitome of masculinity. Men suffering from sex dysfunctions must not only manage the physical problem but also struggle to maintain a favorable sexual and social identity. The delivery of effective treatments for sexual dysfunction can mitigate this potentially deleterious problem. However, effective treatments can only result from valid and expounding theories of etiology and psychometrically sound assessment instruments that do not currently exist in the area of sex dysfunction. It is essential that treatment providers have scholarly resources where information on current, empirically validated assessments and treatments available for sexual dysfunctions can be found. Although there are a great number of books, journals, and resources allocated to the subject of sexual functioning, they fail to empirically reveal any clear and valuable pathways of understanding.

The aim of this chapter is to provide up-to-date information on treatment practices for psychogenic male sexual dysfunction while elucidating the need for more rigorous research in these areas.

□ TREATMENT OF PSYCHOGENIC SEXUAL DYSFUNCTION IN THE MALE

To pursue appropriate treatment, it is essential that providers assess the patient's complete sexual functioning. This requires a thorough understanding of the nature of sexual dysfunctions, the factors involved in their development, and the means to assess sexual functioning on a variety of levels. (For further information on these topics, see Chapters 8, 10, 12, and 24.)

Informing patients about treatment options, including the option of no treatment, is an important step in the assessment process. This needs to be handled very sensitively as the clinician does not want to inordinately sway the patient toward or away from treatment. Instead, the clinician should help the client or couple rationally weigh the relevant information to make a good decision for them.

It is important to note that patients with underlying psychopathology may respond poorly to sex therapy. Possible treatment plans for patients suffering from psychopathology in conjunction with a sexual dysfunction include (*i*) initially treating the primary mental disorder followed by sex therapy, (*ii*) treating the mental disorder and the sexual dysfunction simultaneously, (*iii*) only treating the mental disorder, or (*iv*) only treating the sexual dysfunction. If the sexual dysfunction is not the primary problem, then a sexual dysfunction diagnosis is not appropriate, thus, making the fourth alternative listed above unfit.

Lobitz and Lobitz (1) suggest that the decision to treat the sexual dysfunction in light of observable psychopathology involves two criteria: (*i*) the problem does not greatly interfere with the person's everyday functioning, and (*ii*) the problems should not be likely to interfere with treatment. This first criterion is problematic considering that the Diagnostic and Statistical Manual of Mental Disorders, 4th edition, Text Revised (DSM-IV-TR) requires that a problem cause marked distress or interpersonal difficulty for it to be considered a mental disorder. The second criterion seems more relevant as it guides treatment providers in determining the severity of the psychopathology and its relevance to the sexual dysfunction (i.e., whether it is a cause or result of the other mental disorder). For example, it has been suggested that depression affects those areas that control sexual functioning and decreased activity in these areas results in sex dysfunction (2).

McConaghy (3) purports that most clinicians, regardless if they label it as such, deliver therapy that is cognitive–behavioral in nature and based on Wolpe's (4) conceptualization of sexual dysfunctions as resulting from anxiety about one's sexual performance. In their review of empirical studies investigating the validity of treatments of sexual dysfunction, Heiman and Meston (5) asserted that all of the empirically supported treatments are based on a cognitive–behavioral treatment model and the most frequent components in these treatments were sensate focus and systematic desensitization. More recently, O'Donohue et al. (6) also conducted a critical review of empirical studies evaluating the effects of psychotherapy for male sexual dysfunction. Eighty percent of the obtained publications did not meet the reviewer's inclusion criteria. They suggest that while clinicians maintain that treatments for male sexual dysfunction are efficacious, the lack of methodologically sound research in this area disallows claims regarding empirical validity.

Many studies examining the efficacy of sex therapy techniques have failed to employ control groups. Instead, they have compared treatment groups that have commonly integrated components from different techniques. For example, Everaerd and Dekker (7) compared a treatment group that included sensate focus, sexual stimulation exercises, and the squeeze technique when premature ejaculation was present against a different treatment group that involved in vivo and in vitro systematic desensitization. In this study, the majority of couples in both groups showed some improvement; however, the research design makes it difficult to make any claims about what specific treatment was effective or the appropriateness of specific treatments for particular problems. Currently, difficulties in making inferences are attributable to methodological shortcomings rather than treatment inadequacies.

Despite the paucity of rigorous empirical research, clinicians continue to deliver treatments for sexual dysfunctions. Treatments ought to be tailored to the cause of the specific problem rather than to the particular diagnosis. In other words, males suffering from similar sexual dysfunctions (i.e., meeting the same DSM diagnostic criteria) may benefit from treatments that address different causes (e.g., anxiety vs. lack of ejaculatory control). The effort to deliver appropriate treatments for sexual problems is thwarted by the fact that the detection of psychological agents that cause and maintain sexual dysfunctions remains unclear; however, because normal sexual functioning affects an individual's and couple's quality of life, mental health providers can utilize current knowledge about possible etiological variables, the few existing psychometrically sound assessment instruments, and theoretically informed treatments that are likely efficacious for valid causal pathways. These treatments that are based on a cognitive–behavioral model will be discussed below.

Sensate Focus

Sensate focus is aimed at decreasing performance demands that may interfere with sexual functioning such as premature ejaculation, male erectile disorder, and male orgasmic disorder. This treatment is appropriate for those individuals for whom the goal of reaching or sustaining an adequate erection, controlling ejaculation for a specified amount of time, and reaching or producing orgasm produces an impairment in sexual functioning. Sensate focus involves creating an environment in which the focal point is experiencing pleasure by sexual activity other than intercourse, thereby heightening sensuality and deflecting attention away from sexual performance (8).

Sensate focus is commonly carried out in three phases (7) and requires that patients complete prescribed homework exercises. Homework instructions should be tailored to the patient's knowledge and abilities, as some clients will require more specific teaching. Additionally, patients will be instructed to move from one phase to the next once they comfortably engage in the prescribed sexual activity. In the first two phases, patients are specifically instructed to not engage in intercourse. The first phase involves having the patient and his partner take turns stimulating one another by massaging, stroking, or kissing any of their partner's body except for breasts or genitals. Once the patient is able to comfortably engage in nongenital sexual activity, he is instructed to begin the next phase in which he engages in sexual activity that involves genital touching but not intercourse. These exercises provide opportunities for the individual to attend to the immediate sexual experience in an environment where they are assured that intercourse will not take place and thus, where erection, intercourse, and orgasm are not the goal. In the final phase, the patient is instructed to first engage in containment of the penis in the vagina without movement or thrusting, and later to engage in intercourse with thrusting.

Systematic Desensitization

Systematic desensitization is appropriate for individuals who experience anxiety and/or fear in response to sexual stimuli that result in an impairment of their sexual functioning. This treatment involves repeated trials of pairing relaxation to anxiety-inducing sexual situations. The first component of this treatment entails relaxation training in which a patient is taught how to quickly achieve a state of relaxation through the tensing and releasing of specific muscle groups. Once the patient has mastered this skill, he and the therapist construct a graduated hierarchy from least to most anxiety-inducing sexual stimuli. The patient is exposed to these stimuli through imaginal and/or in vivo trials and is instructed to use relaxation skills so that the sexual stimuli and relaxation are associated. Exposure begins with the least anxiety-producing stimuli and continues until the individual can be exposed to each of the conditions listed on the hierarchy without experiencing anxiety or fear.

Cognitive Restructuring

Cognitive restructuring targets the decrease of negative thoughts and dysfunctional beliefs. Negative thoughts are specific to certain situations whereas dysfunctional beliefs are assumptions that shape more negative interpretations of specific kinds of situations. Cognitive restructuring presumes that emotions result from individual's interpretations of an event rather than by the event itself and these interpretations lead to a certain type of thought or belief (9,10). In the case of males with sexual dysfunction, the interpretation of sexual stimuli as fearful or the view that sexual activity should be avoided unless the sexual partner can reach orgasm during intercourse are examples of thoughts or beliefs that could interfere with sexual functioning. Other harmful beliefs may include feeling that sexual activity is bad and shameful.

Patients who exhibit this problem are instructed to keep track of their negative attitudes and/or dysfunctional thoughts. They must identify their emotional reactions and the thought that leads to that emotional reaction. They are then instructed to challenge these attitudes or beliefs by providing evidence to support or refute them. They are also instructed in identifying the kind of cognitive distortion that they are engaging in (e.g., catastrophizing, overgeneralizing, all-or-none thinking, and emotional reasoning) and modify their negative thoughts or dysfunctional beliefs into more adaptive kinds of thinking. It is important to note that cognitive restructuring is significantly different than psychoeducation. Psychoeducation presents information in a didactic manner on physiology, myths about sexuality, and sex role stereotypes. Cognitive restructuring involves identifying the specific thoughts or beliefs of an individual and rationally evaluating their validity.

Couples Therapy

When treating couples, sometimes more general relationship variables need to be addressed prior to or in conjunction with sex therapy. According to Leiblum and Rosen (11), four primary relationship variables may develop or maintain sexual problems: status and dominance, intimacy and trust, sexual attraction and desire, and sexual scripts. They suggest that dissatisfaction with the balance of power in the relationship may result in sexual dysfunction, particularly for males. Additionally, they assert that it is difficult for couples to maintain sexual interest or receptivity to sexual advances when feeling anger and distrust. The same may be true for individuals who are not sexually attracted to their partners. Similarly, lack of attraction may result in little desire to engage in sexual activity and when engaging in these activities clients may experience low levels of arousal. Likewise, diverging sexual scripts may result in sexual dysfunction, whereby each partner is comfortable with and desires a different range of sexual behaviors. It is expected that identifying these problems and resolving them will alleviate the sexual dysfunction as well.

While sensate focus teaches couples to communicate regarding sexual issues, more general relationship skills may enhance the relationship and possibly increase the couple's desire to engage in sexual activity. This may include teaching communication and problem-solving skills (12). This treatment is based on a behavior exchange model, whereby couples are taught to increase their positive interactions with each other. Communication skills training teach couples to discuss issues in more constructive ways. For example, couples are instructed not to guess what the partner means when speaking and instead ask, not to focus on more than one issue at a time, and not to discount the other person's feelings or statements (e.g., "yes, but …"). Instead, the couple is taught to create a more validating environment that can lead to more trust and intimacy. Problem-solving skills focus on teaching couples to identify the problem to be solved and reaching an adequate solution, once each partner has communicated his or her preferences.

Jacobson and Margolin (13) provide guidelines for couples' therapists treating clients presenting with relationship and sexual problems. They suggest that the determination of which problem to treat first should depend on whether relationship problems preceded or resulted from sexual problems, the willingness and eagerness of the couple to address the identified problem, and the chosen intervention that will likely lead to the quickest and most comprehensive positive effects on the relationship.

Squeeze Technique

For males suffering from premature ejaculation, the squeeze technique is used to help gain ejaculatory control (14). This technique instructs the male to masturbate to a point just prior to ejaculation. At this time he should stop masturbating and firmly squeeze the head of his penis by placing two fingers on the bottom and his thumb on the top of the coronal ridge (Fig. 1A). He is instructed to repeat this process at least three times prior to ejaculation. Each time he is to pay attention to and attempt to enjoy the pleasurable sensations and identify the various levels of arousal that he experiences. A similar technique is the "start–stop" or "pause" technique whereby he is to stop masturbating for 10 seconds and resume without squeezing his penis. The client's partner may be incorporated into these treatments as well. If the partner is willing and able to participate, the partner can be instructed to squeeze the head of the client's penis just prior to ejaculation (Fig. 1B). This process would begin with practicing during masturbation and eventually progress to practicing during intercourse. This would be accomplished during intercourse by withdrawing or

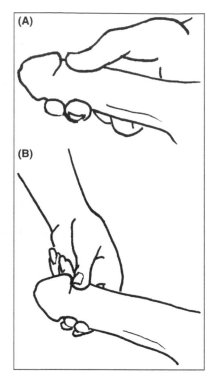

Figure 1 The squeeze technique for premature ejaculation. **(A)** Performed by a man on himself. **(B)** Performed by a willing sexual partner just prior to ejaculation to gain ejaculatory control.

pausing thrusting just prior to ejaculation. As the client continues to practice these techniques, his ejaculatory control will usually increase over the course of two to three months.

□ TREATMENT MONITORING

The clinician should always carefully monitor the impact of therapy. As discussed above, little is known about effective therapies for sexual problems. Thus, the possibility of having little effect or of even having an iatrogenic effect needs to be recognized. A very useful strategy here is to get the client or the couple to independently self-monitor both the target issue (i.e., ejaculatory latency) and any key process variables (i.e., reactions to sensate focus exercises).

□ CONCLUSION

Despite the medicalization of the field of sex therapy, it is important for new psychological theories and conceptualizations to continue being developed in the pursuit of managing psychological issues related to sex dysfunction. Leiblum and Rosen (15) assert that sexual pharmacology cannot be substituted for a thorough and comprehensive understanding of individual and couple psychology as they relate to sexual function and dysfunction. They support the close alliance between sex therapists and primary-care providers as a means for identifying and treating individuals suffering from sexual dysfunction. In order to form this partnership, both fields need to be knowledgeable about current medical and psychological technology as well as their benefits and shortcomings.

□ REFERENCES

1. Lobitz WC, Lobitz GK. Clinical assessment in the treatment of sexual dysfunctions. In: LoPiccolo J, LoPiccolo L, eds. Handbook of Sex Therapy. New York: Plenum Press, 1978:85–102.
2. Kaplan H. Disorders of Sexual Desire. New York: Brunner/Mazel, 1979:80.
3. McConaghy N. Sexual Behavior: Problems and Management. New York: Plenum Press, 1993:184–237.
4. Wolpe J. Psychotherapy by Reciprocal Inhibition. Stanford, CA: Stanford University Press, 1958:130–135.
5. Heiman JR, Meston M. Empirically validated treatment for sexual dysfunction. In: Rosen RC, Davis CM, Ruppel HJ Jr, eds. Annual Review of Sexuality. Vol. 8. Mason City, IA: Society for the Scientific Study of Sex, 1997:148–194.
6. O'Donohue WT, Swingen DN, Dopke CA, et al. Psychotherapy for male sexual dysfunction: a review. Clin Psychol Rev 1999; 19(5):591–630.
7. Everaerd W, Dekker J. Treatment of male sexual dysfunction: sex therapy compared with systematic desensitization and rational emotive therapy. Behav Res Ther 1985; 23(1):13–25.

8. Masters WH, Johnson VE. Human Sexual Inadequacy. Boston: Little, Brown, & Co., 1970:63–85.
9. Beck AT. Cognitive Therapy and the Emotional Disorders. Madison, CT: International Universities Press, 1976:47–75.
10. Beck AT, Emery G, Greenberg RL. Anxiety Disorders and Phobias: A Cognitive Perspective. New York: Basic Books, 1985:3–18.
11. Leiblum SR, Rosen RC. Couples therapy for erectile disorders: conceptual and clinical considerations. J Sex Marital Ther 1991; 17(2):147–159.
12. Jacobson NS, Margolin G. Marital therapy: Strategies Based on Social Learning and Behavior Exchange Principles. New York: Brunner/Mazel, 1979:189–261.
13. Jacobson NS, Margolin G. Marital therapy: Strategies Based on Social Learning and Behavior Exchange Principles. New York: Brunner/Mazel, 1979: 290–301.
14. Masters WH, Johnson VE. Human Sexual Inadequacy. Boston: Little Brown & Co., 1970:86–108.
15. Leiblum SR, Rosen RC. Introduction: sex therapy in the age of Viagra. In: Leiblum SR, Rosen RC, eds. Principles and Practice of Sex Therapy. 3rd ed. New York: Guilford Press, 2000:1–13.

28

Couple Therapy for Premature Ejaculation

Emmanuele A. Jannini
Department of Experimental Medicine, University of L'Aquila, L'Aquila, Italy

Andrea Lenzi
Department of Medical Pathophysiology, University of Rome "La Sapienza," Rome, Italy

☐ INTRODUCTION

In the area of male sexual dysfunctions, new pathophysiologic and therapeutic discoveries have led to renewed attention on the lack of ejaculatory control (1). In the past, rapid or premature ejaculation (PE) was typically considered to be of relational and psychological pathology. Thus, a number of behavioral and psychorelational approaches arose from the initial idea of curing sexual problems with empirical, talking therapies, including the use of behavioral and educational components, psychotherapy in the context of the relationship, and sexual timetables (2).

Recent advances in the understanding of the importance and frequency of PE, however, including insights into its organic pathophysiology and the efficacy of a growing arsenal of pharmacological therapies, have led to a treatment strategy that involves the development of integrated therapeutic alternatives from a modern holistic viewpoint. The combined application of medicine and psychology has made it possible to improve and/or restore an active sexual life to many dysfunctional couples, enhancing their overall quality of life. In this new field of medical sexology and sexual medicine, the cooperation between basic researchers (geneticists, neurophysiologists, pharmacologists, and ethologists) and a wide group of clinicians (endocrinologists, andrologists, psychologists, psychosexologists, psychiatrists, urologists, and gynecologists) is of paramount importance in order to reach the desired therapeutic goals.

☐ PREMATURE EJACULATION: SYMPTOM OR DISEASE?

As with all sexual disorders, PE is a symptom of an intrapsychic, relational, genetic, or medical pathology, rather than a disease or dysfunction in itself. From a clinical point of view, this suggests that in any case of PE, the physical and/or psychological disease/dysfunction behind the symptom must be carefully sought and addressed. This approach to therapy is usually described as etiologic, particularly when it succeeds in curing the disease. For example, bibliotherapy (with books) is an appropriate etiologic therapy for PE that is caused by ignorance of the condition on the part of the patient, while propylthiouracil is an etiologic therapy for hyperthyroidism-induced PE (3). On the other hand, a drug (such as an antidepressant) that delays the ejaculatory reflex may be considered a symptomatic type of therapy, as is the majority of psychological and medical therapies for PE that are currently available.

Conventional algorithms for the investigation and treatment of PE are based on the assumption that the condition has exclusively organic or psychogenic etiology, with the latter being considered the main cause. The distinction between psychosocial (or psychodynamic) and organic (or medical) causes of PE then produces a default corollary that psychological PE should be treated by the psychosexologist, while organic PE must be cured by the andrologist. These extreme, reductive views are dangerous for the growth of sexology and for the ultimate goal of the patient's well-being. In modern medicine, the mind–body separation has become obsolete (4). While it is clear that all psychological processes are regulated by neuronal activity (somatopsychic evidence), it is also plain that all psychogenic dysfunctions modulate organic processes (psychosomatic evidence). Psychological processes should be considered as inextricably bound with organic ejaculation function and dysfunction processes. This more holistic approach allows PE to be considered as a psychoneuroendocrine and urological disorder that affects not only the patient, but also his partner.

It should be noted, however, that the widely used adjective "psychogenic" is overtly inappropriate due to the fact that elements of psychological stress can result from the loss of ejaculatory control, irrespective of the primary cause (5). Thus, all cases of PE could become psychogenic, even if the PE originates as a symptom of an organic etiology. As couples with a sexual problem generally wait two years or more before asking for professional help, marital discomfort often develops secondary to PE. On these grounds, the treatment of PE cannot be exclusively pharmacological. In contrast, PE may be a symptom of an existing marital conflict in some couples, and, in these cases, couple therapy may not be sufficient to cure the relational PE.

History of Premature Ejaculation

During the evolution of human sexuality, the ability to control the timing of ejaculation has become one of the most important features of a couple's sexual health. In animals, sexual intercourse is usually a brief episode (6). In fact, due to an adaptive mechanism (*coitus citus*), male genitalia are designed to ejaculate quickly (7). Even during coital activity, the animal must be ready to attack or flee, thus making it essential to deposit semen with the fastest and safest technique. For example, the sequence of approach, penetration, and ejaculation in chimpanzees lasts just six seconds (7). Since one of the principal aims of human sexuality is pleasure, however, men have learned to control ejaculation in order to enhance their own and their partners' enjoyment. It can be postulated on the basis of these considerations that ejaculatory control is not natural, but cultural. For this reason, lack of ejaculatory control has a profound psychorelational basis, and its treatment is amenable to male and/or couple psychotherapy.

PE was rarely described in the literature of classic sexology. As noted by Waldinger (8), the first case report on PE was not published until 1887 (9), and the psychoanalyst K. Abraham first introduced the term *ejaculatio praecox* in 1917 (10). Even in the popular and scientific sexology texts (11,12) in circulation before and during the first half of the twentieth century [with the notable exception of Huhner's treatise (13)], PE was not included in the list of sexual disorders. As the purpose of sex was largely considered to be solely a means of reproduction until relatively recently, in consequence, PE was not thought of as pathological.

Similarly, in his historic survey on human sexuality, Kinsey rejected PE as a sexual dysfunction when he found that 75% of men ejaculated within two minutes of penetration (14). In contrast, in the same period, Shapiro argued that PE may be considered the result of the combination of a hyperanxious constitution with anatomical defects (15). It was only after reliable contraceptives became available during the sexual and feminist revolution of the mid-1960s—particularly with the "discovery" of the female orgasm—did PE become important in the cohort of symptoms connected with male sexual performance.

Definition

Even today, there is no commonly accepted definition of PE (16). Depending on the study, any ejaculation occurring within one minute (17), two to three minutes (18), or even seven minutes of penetration (19) has been defined as premature. Others specify the number of penile thrusts, considering less than 8 to 15 thrusts prior to ejaculation, as a criterion for PE (20). Both these approaches are easily quantifiable and objective, but the rationale for using these as diagnostic criteria has never been offered (21).

Other authors considered the definition of PE from a couple's point of view. Masters and Johnson suggested that a man experienced PE if he was unable to delay his ejaculation until his partner was sexually satisfied in at least 50% of their coital connections (22). As most women take longer to reach orgasm than men, the majority of men are, therefore, "precocious." Furthermore, this definition does not consider PE in homosexual couples and defines an individual pathology on the basis of the sexual responsiveness of the partner, with the 50% figure chosen by the authors appearing to be arbitrary.

The absence of a clear definition of PE has led to a "patient-dependent" definition and a "patient-decided" diagnosis. These subjective criteria consider the perceived control over the occurrence of ejaculation and the satisfaction associated with it (23). The authors recently have proposed a new definition of PE, which is diagnosed on the basis of pathological intravaginal ejaculation latency time (IELT), as measured by the stop-watch method (see below), with a feeling of loss of voluntary control and distress or relational disturbances. From this definition, two different forms of PE arise: "Objective PE" (which is defined "severe" when ejaculation occurs before penetration or with a IELT ≤ 15 seconds, "moderate" with a IELT $\leq$ one minute, and "mild" with a IELT $\leq$ two minutes), and "Subjective or Relational PE," when the loss of voluntary control is experienced with distress by the male or both partners (24). Essentially, PE is the persistent or recurrent inability to delay ejaculation voluntarily (25) upon or shortly after penetration or with minimal sexual stimulation. The "stop-watch method" proposed measures with a chronometer the exact time from intravaginal intromission to intravaginal ejaculation (26). Further, as suggested by the DSM-III-R and later editions, "the clinician must take into account factors that affect duration of the excitement phase, such as age, novelty of the sexual partner or situation, and frequency of sexual activity" (27).

Classification

The notion that men with PE are a homogeneous group is erroneous. As reported by Shapiro (15), PE should be classified into various subgroups. The dysfunction may be lifelong (i.e., from the beginning of active sexual life) or acquired (occurring after a period of normal ejaculatory control). It may also be absolute/generalized (irrespective of partners or context) or situational (relative to a partner and/or context). Ejaculation may occur before penetration (*ante portas*) or suddenly during coitus (*intra moenia*). Furthermore, it is also classified on the basis of severity (Table 1). Before any couple therapy occurs, a profound sexological anamnesis should be performed to aid classification.

Prevalence

Early ejaculation is the most frequent sexual complaint (28), but not the most frequent reason for sexual

Table 1 Analogous Comparison of the Etiologies of Premature Ejaculation

	Organic	Nonorganic/idiopathic
Affects	Anatomical and neurological constitution	Psychological constitution
Types of deficit	Acute and chronic physical illness Physical injury Pharmacological side effects	Acute psychological distress Relationship distress Psychosexual skill deficit

consultation (29). It is widespread in adolescents, young adults, and other sexually naive males, affecting from 4% up to 30% or 40% of sexually active men in an age-dependent manner (30,31). Without an accurate definition of PE, it is difficult to establish the real prevalence of this problem.

Interestingly, a familial occurrence of PE has been found. In a small, selected group of men, the calculated risk of having a first relative with PE (91%) is much higher than in the general population (32). This suggests, but does not demonstrate, a genetic influence. In fact, it can be argued that the familial environment, as for the other sexual symptoms, psychologically generates PE.

Anatomy and Physiology of Ejaculation

To understand the site of action of psychological and pharmacological PE therapies, it must be remembered that normal male copulation culminates in three psychologically and physiologically distinct events known as *emission*, *ejaculation*, and *orgasm* (33).

Emission is the coordinated contraction of smooth muscle cells of the male genital tract (MGT) involving testicular tubules, efferent ducts, the epididymis, and vasa deferentia and the secretion of seminal fluid due to rhythmic contractions of the seminal vesicles and prostate. At the time of emission, the bladder neck closes to prevent retrograde ejaculation of seminal fluid into the bladder. The seminal bolus in the prostatic urethra is thus entrapped in a loading space: a compression chamber between the distal urethra (external sphincter of the urethra), closed for erection, and the bladder neck. During emission, pressure in the seminal bolus increases due to peristaltic thrusts from the MGT and the striated muscle of the pelvic floor. Men experience the sensation of ejaculatory inevitability when the pressure within the seminal bolus exceeds the downstream resistance. Thus, any psychological mechanism delaying ejaculation must act on the emission phase, before the "point of no return."

Ejaculation is defined as the expulsion of semen from the urethra. It is a reflex response, not always requiring cerebral input, and can be triggered by the accumulation of semen in the bulbous urethra. The pelvic floor muscles (bulbospongiosus and ischiocavernosus somatic muscles, as well as the smooth musculature of the vas deferens, ejaculatory ducts, proximal urethra, and bladder neck) actively collaborate to achieve ejaculation, with three to seven contractions.

Finally, the subjective, perceptual-cognitive event of pleasure is called *orgasm* and, in normal conditions, coincides with the time of ejaculation (33).

Even though principally controlled by the same sympathetic nerves, these three elements are separate from one another and provoke different psychological perceptions (34). What information is known on central ejaculatory control mostly relates to animals. Ejaculation has been elicited in monkeys by electrical stimulation of the preoptic area, which contains fibers of the medial forebrain bundle. The serotonergic system, probably interacting with the leptinergic system (35), acts as a suppressor of the ejaculatory reflex at the hypothalamic level (36). In fact, both serotonin reuptake inhibitors (SSRIs) and serotonin agonists determine the extension of ejaculatory latency (37). In contrast, the dopaminergic pathway may act as an ejaculation stimulator (38) through D2 receptors (39). Efferent innervation is somatic through the parasympathetic sacral outflow, originates at S2-S4, and runs through the pudendal nerve (40), causing clonic contractions of the striated MGT muscles. (For more detailed information on these subjects, see Chapters 2, 3, and 5).

Psychological Pathophysiology

The psychophysiological model has been applied to the study of ejaculatory response for well over four decades. This approach illustrates the complex relationship among the cognitive, affective, and physiological components of ejaculation control. Further, the psychopathological procedures may be used systematically as a determining aid in the differential diagnosis of various PE subtypes (41).

Analytic Theories

The foundation of the analytic theory of sexual dysfunction lies in that distortions of belief and false convictions about sexuality are established in childhood as a consequence of adverse influences on sexual behavior. Destructive attitudes are usually exerted by parents, but also by other power figures within and outside the family (42). This, in a Freudian perspective, may lead to sexual dysfunction such as PE.

Classic psychoanalytic theories identify a sadistic or narcissistic behavior in PE (43). For other psychoanalysts, however, men who ejaculate prematurely are typically passive and masochistic in their marriage and obsessive-compulsive in character (44). On the strength of these ideas, the psychoanalyst Kaplan proposed that PE is thus the result of an unconscious hatred of women (45). By ejaculating quickly, a man symbolically and physically "steals" the woman's orgasm. This researcher rejected her own theory, however, when she found that men with PE do not have any particular neuroses or personality disorders (46).

Table 2 Psychosocial Factors Involved in Premature Ejaculation

Guilt (belief that the sexual activity is sinful, e.g., premarital or
   extramarital sex)
Fear (of pregnancy, sexually transmitted diseases, being
   discovered)
Anxiety (general or related to sexual performance)

Behavioral Theories

PE is a frequent, if not normal, occurrence during early sexual experiences. To this end, Masters and Johnson considered other related etiological causes that can worsen ejaculatory control that may be already physiologically poor at a young age: the risk of unwanted discovery (such as copulating in a car), experiences with prostitutes, and anxiety due to poor sexual education (e.g., absence of adequate knowledge of contraceptive methods) (Table 2) (22,47).

Kaplan's theory (see above) is also connected with the role of early experiences: the man with PE has not allowed himself to receive the sensory feedback of those sensations occurring immediately before orgasm that would enable him to bring his ejaculatory reflex under voluntary control (46). Kaplan compares this etiologic mechanism to the control of enuresis obtained when a child recognizes the sensation of a full bladder. In the same way, the lack of awareness of pre-ejaculatory sensations may lead to PE.

Varying levels of sexual activity and desire have been, in some cases, advocated in the development of PE, but this symptom is frequently characterized, or even caused, by sexual abstinence (48).

The role of anxiety over sexual performance, as well as for other, nonsexual reasons, has been frequently raised as a cause of PE (49). This is in keeping with Kaplan's theory, as anxiety may block pre-ejaculatory sensations. It should be noted, however, that anxiety may also be the effect rather than the cause of PE (Fig. 1, *Panel A*).

Finally, it should be noted that these theories have been hypothesized to explain both lifelong an acquired PE.

Critical Evaluation of Psychological Theories

Masters and Johnson's hypothesis that PE is the result of conditioning by juvenile experiences to ejaculate rapidly was not always verified when the sexual histories of patients with PE were compared with those of subjects with good ejaculatory control (50). Furthermore, Kaplan's hypothesis [that men with PE are less able than normal subjects to accurately evaluate their level of physiologically determined sexual arousal (46)] has been criticized. Two independent researchers, comparing two groups with and without PE, demonstrated that both were equally accurate in making such assessments (48,51). It is evident that the etiological approach of psychology to PE must be reconsidered.

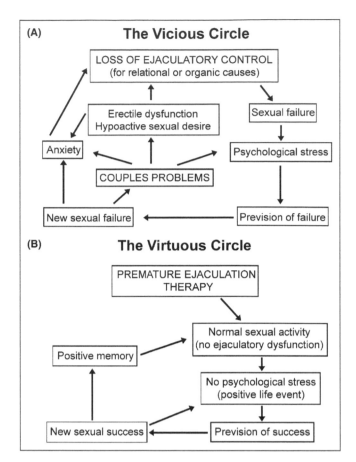

Figure 1 Pathophysiology of PE. Stress from sexual failure and subsequent anxiety exert a positive feedback during PE (*Panel A*). Pharmacological and/or psychological therapies destroy this vicious circle, transforming it into a virtuous cycle (*Panel B*). Note that, during this cycle, other couple pathologies may arise. *Abbreviation*: PE, premature ejaculation.

Medical Pathophysiology

Even if the medical causes of PE are beyond the scope of this chapter, it should be noted that their catalogue is only now becoming more evident. For more detailed information on these topics, please refer to the chapters contained in Part II: Pathophysiology of Male Sexual Dysfunction. Early ejaculation has been associated with drug consumption (52), low serum testosterone (53), and seminal plasma magnesium levels (54), hyperthyroxinemia (3,55–57), major neurological disorders (multiple sclerosis, spina bifida, tumor of the spinal cord, and traumatic brain injury) (58), and short frenum of prepuce, penile hypersensitivity, and reflex hyperexcitability (59–61). Reflex hyperexcitability in the pathophysiology of PE, however, is currently under discussion (62). The authors of this chapter have provided evidence of an intriguingly high prevalence of prostate inflammation/infections in PE, as well as a higher-than-normal prevalence of PE in patients with chronic prostatitis (63). A careful examination of the prostate should therefore be performed before any pharmacological or psychosexual treatment for PE is rendered. These results have been confirmed more recently by other independent groups (64,65). In the majority of cases, PE appears to be the result of mixed psychogenic, physiological, and organic factors, all of which may interact with each other to exacerbate the symptoms.

□ ASSESSMENT OF THE COUPLE WITH PREMATURE EJACULATION
Diagnosis

Masters and Johnson wrote that the object of the sex therapy is not the individual with the sexual problem, but the couple (22); however, most new medical and surgical therapies for erectile dysfunction, premature or delayed ejaculation, female sexual disorders, andro- or menopause, and hypoactive sexual desire are based on the symptoms of an individual, rather than the couple as a unit. The exclusive focus on the patient or on the symptom may be reductive and therapeutically dangerous.

Diagnosis of the psychological causes of PE should include extensive interviewing, possibly with standardized psychological tests such as the Chinese Index of Premature Ejaculation and Patient-Reported Outcome measures (66) in order to establish the history of the dysfunction and the circumstances under which it occurs. This must be performed alongside a thorough physical examination and medical tests to assess organ functions that may interfere with ejaculation. When medical tests are normal, a diagnosis of psychogenic PE is considered likely; however, this "diagnosis by exclusion" may lead to unreliable conclusions for various reasons: (*i*) it is impossible to demonstrate that a case of PE is generated by the mind (psychogenic), (*ii*) as stated above, all cases of PE have a psychic and/or relational aspect, and (*iii*) while research is continuously growing, there is still a severe lack of knowledge on central mechanisms of ejaculation. It can be surmised that in the near future, there will be new tests capable of discovering subjects with purely organic PE. On the basis of these arguments, the authors propose here that when the organic cause for PE (as for other sexual problems) is not identifiable, the term "idiopathic" ["denoting a disease or condition the cause of which is not known" (67)] should be used instead of the term "psychogenic."

The possibility that PE may involve marital problems should always be considered, even though it may be difficult to discern if the couple's troubles are the cause or the effect of PE. Whenever possible, sexual symptoms should be assessed in the context of the couple. Thus, it is essential to compare the male's description of the symptoms with those of his female partner. Perception of penetration time is in fact very subjective.

In the classic Masters and Johnson's setting, a dual team comprised of both a male and a female therapist treated the "marital unit" (22,47). This rarely occurs nowadays, as each individual member of the couple typically receives separate treatment by a single therapist. Structured questionnaires for PE have not been standardized, and attempts to distinguish organic versus functional sexual failure using the Minnesota Multiphasic Personality Inventory or historical data have generally proven unsuccessful (68).

As PE can be found in the absence (*primary*) or presence (*secondary*) of other sexual symptoms, the possibility of coexistence with other sexual problems should always be investigated. Hypoactive sexual desire may lead to PE, due to an unconscious desire to abbreviate the unwanted penetration. Additionally, reduced time to ejaculation is a common early manifestation of erectile dysfunction that may occur with an unstable erection due to fluctuation in penile blood flow. In these cases, the subject may ejaculate early to hide the weakness of the erection, and this type of PE will respond successfully to the appropriate treatments for impotence (24).

Finally, female sexual dysfunctions such as anorgasmia, hypoactive sexual desire, sexual aversion, sexual arousal disorders, and sexual pain disorders, including vaginismus, should also be taken into account. These may be secondary to the male PE and can be considered a frequent complication of this condition. In other cases, PE may result from hidden female arousal difficulties (69). This emphasizes the need for the diagnosis and treatment of the couple as a combined unit.

Physical Exam and Laboratory Testing

The physical examination for PE is usually normal. Penile biothesiometry, however, has been proposed as a useful method to evaluate and quantify penis sensitivity in PE (59). The biothesiometer is a vibrating device with a fixed frequency of 50 Hz and variable amplitude that is placed on the penile shaft, the glans penis, and the mid-scrotum. The patient is asked to inform the examiner of the first sensation of vibration as the amplitude is slowly increased.

A flowchart for the diagnosis and assessment of PE is proposed in Figure 2. This includes prostate evaluation by transrectal ultrasonography and standardized Meares and Stamey protocol (70). Inflammations/infections of the prostate have been found with high frequency in PE, and the presence of PE has also been demonstrated with high frequency in cases of prostate disease (63–65). These epidemiological data, together with the anatomical contiguity of nerves controlling ejaculation with prostate, as well as the role of this gland in the machinery of ejaculation, suggest a causal or concausal relationship between some subclinical prostatic pathologies and PE. Thus, urethral and midstream bladder urine, expressed prostate secretions by prostate massage, and postmassage urine samples are collected, examined microscopically, and cultured bacteriologically. Prostate inflammation is diagnosed if 10 or more white blood cells per high power field are present in the expressed prostate secretions. Nonbacterial prostatitis is defined by evidence

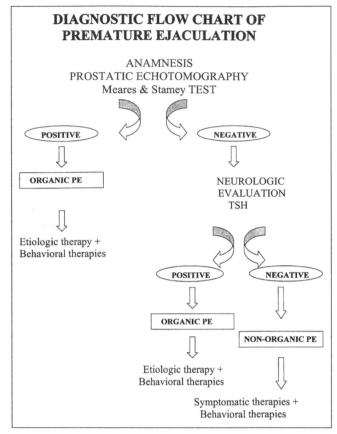

DIAGNOSTIC FLOW CHART OF PREMATURE EJACULATION

ANAMNESIS
PROSTATIC ECHOTOMOGRAPHY
Meares & Stamey TEST

POSITIVE → ORGANIC PE → Etiologic therapy + Behavioral therapies

NEGATIVE → NEUROLOGIC EVALUATION TSH

POSITIVE → ORGANIC PE → Etiologic therapy + Behavioral therapies

NEGATIVE → NON-ORGANIC PE → Symptomatic therapies + Behavioral therapies

Figure 2 Proposed flowchart of patients with PE. Before any treatment, prostate infection/inflammation should be ruled out. Selected patients can be further studied for penile sensitivity and thyroid function. Sexological (behavioral and couple) therapy should accompany both etiological and pharmacological therapies. *Abbreviations*: PE, premature ejaculation; TSH, thyroid-stimulating hormone. *Source*: From Ref. 1.

Table 3 Personality Characteristics of Men with Premature Ejaculation

Personality type	Typical behavioral characteristics
Insecure and anxious	Partner tends to be a woman of aggressive and domineering nature
Competitive	Always attempts to demonstrate virility
Young and naïve	Typically restricted to first sexual encounters

of prostate inflammation together with negative urine and prostate fluid cultures. Prostate infection is defined by a colony count 10 times greater in the expressed prostate secretion or postmassage urine sample than in the urethral urine sample. Careful screening for the presence of *Chlamydia trachomatis, Trichomonas vaginalis, Mycoplasma hominis, Candida* species, and *Ureaplasma urealyticum* should be performed.

☐ TREATMENT OF PREMATURE EJACULATION
Psychological Therapies for the Couple

The cognitive feedback from PE can lead to "performance anxiety" that may combine with other conditions to further impair ejaculatory control in a vicious cycle, as described in Figure 1, Panel A. For these reasons, a psychological approach is always useful in PE treatment.

Sexological Therapies for Premature Ejaculation

Sex therapy is a collective term, which indicates many behavioral models of short-term treatment of human sexual dysfunction (71). The common aim of these therapies is to modify the dysfunctional behavior (behavioral therapies) as directly as possible, taking into account the role of childhood conflicts, self-defeating attitudes, and the quality of the partners' relationship. The foundation of these therapies lies in the groundbreaking work of Masters and Johnson, which has been modernized with the so-called "new" sexual therapy of Kaplan, who offered a psychodynamic, or transactional, account of the dyadic causes of sexual dysfunction. While behavioral therapies can be considered as the first effective treatment of sexual symptoms, they need further research and validation.

Behavioral Therapies

The behavioral approach to treatment of sexual disorders uses the theories of learning (72). Knowing the personality characteristics (Table 3) of men with PE allows them to be corrected.

Behavioral therapy begins with the approach that it is the couple, not the individual, which is dysfunctional. Sexual counseling can be of benefit in both idiopathic and organic causes of PE (73). Involving the partner in this process can dispel misperceptions about the symptoms, decrease stress, enhance intimacy and the ability to talk about sex and PE, and increase the chances of a successful outcome. Counseling sessions are also helpful in uncovering conflicts in the relationship, other psychiatric problems, and alcohol or drug misuse (74). For these reasons, sexual homework assignments are often prescribed to the couple, such as the "sensate focus" technique, in which partners take turns in giving and receiving stimulation in nongenital body areas. This method, basically developed as a therapy for impotence and then applied to other sexual disturbances such as PE, continues with nondemanding genital stimulation, which may proceed to erection but not to orgasm. The aim of this approach is to reduce anxiety, considered a major cause of PE. To specifically approach PE, the therapist then allows the couple to perform brief intromissions with the female-on-top position. The woman inserts the penis into her vagina, thrusts a few times, and then dismounts before any anxiety is accumulated. Finally, after several weeks of these first steps, the couple is free to copulate in any position. The limitation of genital activity should reduce the pressure to "perform." In addition, the patients learn to (*i*) evaluate preorgasmic pleasure, (*ii*) be aware

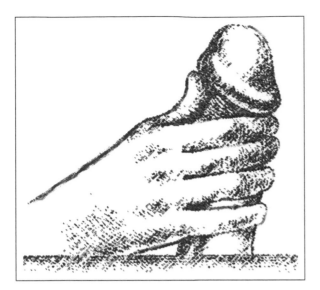

Figure 3 The squeeze technique. To treat premature ejaculation, when ejaculation seems inevitable, the man's partner applies pressure, using the thumb of the first two fingers, just below the glans penis. This pressure should inhibit ejaculation and should be performed several times before ejaculation is permitted to occur. As a step in the learning of ejaculation control, the squeeze technique is generally no longer needed after therapeutic success.

Table 4   Components of Behavioral Therapy

Assessment	Educational components	Behavioral components
General medical history	Counseling on sexual anatomy	Sensate focus
Sexual history	Counseling on sexual physiology	Squeeze
Relationship history	–	Stop-start
–	–	Kegel's exercises

of the "orgasmic point of no return," (*iii*) prolong the *plateau* phase, and (*iv*) distinguish between excitation and orgasm.

To specifically cure PE, Masters and Johnson suggested the "squeeze" technique. Upon the personal instructions of the sex therapist, the man or his partner squeezes the glans of the erect penis for about 20 seconds, just below the coronal ridge, immediately before ejaculation (Fig. 3). This prevents ejaculation, but erection may be partially lost. The first two or three sessions are performed without coitus. This is subsequently allowed in the female-on-top position, which creates less pressure to ejaculate and allows the woman to easily lift off and squeeze the penis. After some repetitions, the man should learn to tolerate higher levels of sexual stimulation without ejaculating.

The alternative stop–start method for treating PE was introduced by Kaplan, as based on the remarkable work of Semans (75). Here, during sexual stimulation or intercourse, when a man feels he is close to ejaculation, he stops and withdraws from the partner and only restarts when he feels he has regained control. The couple usually starts with simple vaginal containment, without pelvic thrusting. As the feeling of control increases, thrusting can begin, enabling the man to recognize the cues preceding his point of ejaculatory inevitability. Because the squeeze technique carries some risk of discomfort, many sex therapists prefer the stop–start method (Table 4).

Other Therapies

The cognitive and informative strategies have been considered particularly useful for single men. Whenever

possible, however, the sex therapist involves both partners, working together on the reduction of performance anxiety, strengthening of trust and confidence in the relationship between the marital partners, changing of self-defeating beliefs and attitudes, debunking of male sexual mythology, improving of sexual communication, enhancing sexual knowledge, and teaching of sexual skills. Practical suggestions and sexual counseling may be considered important steps for PE therapy. After learning insights into "natural" and "cultural" intercourse, the patient is advised to ejaculate more frequently (with the aim of decreasing the seminal bolus), to release the anal sphincter during intercourse (with the aim of decreasing intra-abdominal pressure), to favor the female-on-top position (with the aim of decreasing movement), and possibly to use special condoms (with the aim of decreasing glans sensitivity).

As PE can arise from ignorance and sexual teaching is unfortunately largely absent in schools (77), bibliotherapy with simple and clear books (78) may be a useful adjuvant treatment for PE (79,80).

Strengthening of the pubococcygeus muscles of the pelvic floor can increase ejaculatory control. These exercises, named after Arnold Kegel, the gynecologist who created them, involve the patient's identification of his pubococcygeus muscles by clenching, as if to stop urination in midstream. When the patient is more experienced, he can start the exercises with a few slow contractions of two to three seconds per day. As the muscles strengthen, the duration and number of slow contractions should gradually be extended, together with fast contractions (Table 5).

A multivariate approach to PE is based on both ejaculatory latency and perceived control (81). The coital alignment technique (CAT) is a type of couple therapy consisting of a basic physiological alignment that provides an effective stimulation for female coital orgasm (82), which may be useful in couples with PE. Reich's

Table 5   Kegel Exercises: The Rule of 5

- Contract pubococcygeus muscles for 5 seconds; release for 5 seconds. Repeat 5 times
- Contract pubococcygeus muscles 5 times as fast as possible
- In the same session, repeat steps #1 and #2 5 times
- Perform 5 sessions per day

Source: From Ref. 1.

therapy for PE is based on the use of sensate, rather than verbal, communication with the patient (83). The therapist carefully chooses the environment and atmosphere, with patients and therapists on big cushions, creating a friendly relationship on a first-name basis, and involving nonerotic massages and role-playing. Hypnosis (84), mechanotherapy (85), reeducative and supportive therapies, and the extensive training programs described in literature as alternatives to behavioral therapies all suffer from considerable methodological weaknesses, a failure to specify subject and treatment variables, inadequate or nonexistent control groups, limited follow-up, and failure to obtain the partner's validation of subject progress (86).

Treatment programs have also been designed for a group setting. The structured group treatment has been described in noncontrolled studies as a cost-efficient and effective method to overcome PE (87) for both couples and singles (88). The group treatment does not seem inferior in outcome to the classic couple format (89).

Follow-Up and Critical Evaluation of Psychological Therapies

In the last 30 years, the only change in the management of sexual symptoms has been their medical treatment. In fact, behavioral therapies are still used without substantial modification of the original definitions and format (90). Although a success rate of 60% to 95% has been claimed for behavioral approaches to sexual dysfunction (91), the field of psychosexology has only recently taken seriously the task of scientifically demonstrating the efficacy of sex therapies (92,93). There is little information on the long-term results of ejaculatory disorder treatments (94,95). Therapeutic success in sex therapy is often unpredictable (96) and is more frequent in highly motivated couples with a good relationship, in young age, in sexual dysfunction of recent onset, and in relationship of recent onset (97). Based on the limited results available from systematic analysis of the literature, it appears that behavioral therapies for PE, although revealing some immediate gains (98), remain beneficial to only a minority of men three years after treatment ends (99).

There are many reasons for therapy failure. Table 6 lists the possibilities of therapy resistance. In the authors' experience, the most important is "sticking to the symptom." This is likely to occur in couples with a long-term sexual problem (such as PE or erectile dysfunction) who have developed vicarious mechanisms to overcome the absence of sexual happiness. Even if they strongly desire recovery, they may subconsciously fear that cure might destroy their structured relationship. This is a frequent condition in which the help of sexual therapist may be decisive.

Some of these points need to be addressed by a new psychosexual research effort. For example, while the central role of couple dynamics in the genesis and continuation of many ejaculatory disorders cannot be ignored, no single theoretical approach adequately incorporates the totality of intra- and interpersonal dynamics (100). Behavioral therapies require the active participation of the partner, but often, for socioeconomic or cultural reasons, this is not possible. The experience of the past 40 years suggests that North American patients agree more easily than Europeans to behavioral treatment and its "gymnastic" aspects (101). Behavioral therapies are inappropriate for subjects in whom profound personal or relationship problems underlie sexual disorders. Furthermore, the behavioral approach is designed for the couple. These methods therefore cannot be easily proposed to single males with multiple or occasional partners, who may not cooperate with the sexologist (102). It should be noted that this is a frequent condition of young men in Western societies. Additionally, the success rate of behavioral therapies has been difficult to duplicate and verify in controlled studies (103).

Medical Therapies for the Single Man and Couple

The efficacy of talking therapies in the management of PE is not supported by convincing data from controlled clinical studies. For this reason, pharmacological treatment is now receiving increased attention from both medical sexologists and the pharmaceutical industry (104). While behavioral therapies in their original format require a couple, medical treatments may be applied to the single man.

Systemic and Local Drugs

Drugs increasing serotonin levels (such as antidepressants) and those interfering with sympathetic nervous system activation of the ejaculatory reflexes (such as α-adrenergic blockers) are widely prescribed. The effectiveness of tricyclic antidepressants (105–107) and selective SSRIs (108–112) is probably due to increasing penile threshold without changing the amplitude and latency of sacral-evoked response and cortical somatosensory-evoked potential.

Thus, the "Holy Grail" for PE treatment would have the following ideal characteristics: effective, practical (oral administration), capability of on-demand use, rapid onset, swift elimination, and low incidence of adverse effects. Meta-analysis of all drug treatment studies conducted with SSRIs and other antidepressants suggests that paroxetine exerts the strongest ejaculation delay (113).

For patients with erection weakness and PE, treatment with intracavernous medications (114) or sildenafil alone (115) or in combination with

Table 6   Causes of Resistance to Behavioral Treatment

Patient resistance	Partner resistance
Mistrust of therapist	Sex judged too "mechanical"
Mistrust of therapy	Feeling of being "used"
Mistrust of own possibilities	"Sticking to the symptom"

paroxetine (116,117) has been examined and found effective. Topical agents such as anesthetics (118) and herbal products (119) are also used, with limited efficacy (120). In patients with prostate inflammation and PE, the specific therapy for chronic prostatitis has been suggested (121,122). (For further information on drug therapy for PE, see Chapters 29 and 31.)

Follow-Up and Critical Evaluation of Medical Therapies

Current methods and measures utilized to assess treatment outcome in PE are standardized with some difficulty (123). Antidepressant drugs are generally effective in restoring ejaculatory control; however, as these drugs may significantly worsen erectile dysfunction, they are strongly contraindicated for patients suffering from both PE and impotence (124).

While pharmacological treatment of PE has been demonstrated to be reliable and efficacious, its therapeutic window is frequently localized to the period of drug consumption. In fact, after therapy, PE once more affects most patients who obtained good ejaculatory control. This is in keeping with the evidence that antidepressants are a symptomatic therapy.

The best outcome is obtained when drugs are used for a short period (60 days, in the authors' experience), during which sexual therapy with the couple is also performed. The pharmacological aid, delaying the emission phase, allows the patient to understand what is happening in his body before the point of no return. In this way, the ability to control ejaculation creates a "positive memory" of sexual success, which will help the patient overcome the problem (Fig. 1, Panel B).

□ CONCLUSION: USING THE HOLISTIC MODEL TO CURE COUPLES WITH PREMATURE EJACULATION

In the past, the aim of psychoanalysis as a tool for sexual dysfunction treatment was to recognize the deep subconscious causes of psychological diseases. Although psychoanalysis can be a powerful tool for the explanation and cure of some neurotic conflicts, the Freudian approach to sexual pathology is slow, and, very frequently, ineffective. For these reasons, Masters and Johnson pioneered a new direct behavioral approach in the 1960s, which is not necessarily focused on the cause of sexual problems, but simply on the symptoms. Behavioral therapy is still the dominant paradigm in the psychosexological approach to PE; however, medical therapies, with some limitations, are emerging, and scientific production on this front is continuously growing. This suggests three possible scenarios for the future: (i) the decline of the sexual therapist without medical training, (ii) the development of new roles for sex therapists and medical sexologists, and (iii) integration of the diagnostic and therapeutic roles of medical and nonmedical practitioners. To obtain the last possibility, a renewed effort must be made to validate psychosexological therapies.

In the interests of the patient, this complex therapeutic process should be performed not in conflict, but in harmony with behavioral approaches and with the sex therapist. Finally, considering the importance of sexual counseling in the therapy of PE and the role of prostate diseases in their pathogenesis, a policy of prevention should be focused on both the sexual and andrological education of young and adult males.

□ REFERENCES

1. Jannini EA, Simonelli C, Lenzi A. Disorders of ejaculation. J Endocrinol Invest 2002; 25(11):1006–1019.
2. Jannini EA, Simonelli C, Lenzi A. Sexological approach to ejaculatory dysfunction. Int J Androl 2002; 25(6):317–323.
3. Carani C, Isidori AM, Granata A, et al. Multicenter study on the prevalence of sexual symptoms in male hypo- and hyperthyroid patients. J Clin Endocrinol Metab 2005; 90(12):6472–6479.
4. Sachs BD. The false organic-psychogenic distinction and related problems in the classification of erectile dysfunction. Int J Impot Res 2003; 15(1):72–78.
5. Utiger RD. A pill for impotence. Editorial. N Engl J Med 1998; 338(20):1458–1459.
6. Hong J. Survival of the fastest: on the origins of premature ejaculation. J Sex Res 1984; 20:109–112.
7. Cellerino A, Jannini EA. Male reproductive physiology as a sexually selected handicap? Erectile dysfunction is correlated with general health and health prognosis and may have evolved as a marker of poor phenotypic quality. Med Hypotheses 2005; 65(1):179–184.
8. Waldinger MD. The neurobiological approach to premature ejaculation. J Urol 2002; 168(6):2359–2367.
9. Gross S. A Practical Treatise on Impotence, Sterility, and Allied Disorders of the Male Sexual Organs. 3rd ed. Edinburg, YJ: Pentland, 1887.
10. Abraham K. Über ejaculatio praecox. Zeitschr Aerztl Psychoanal 1917; 4:171–181.
11. Pierce RV. Common Sense Medical Adviser. Buffalo, NY: World Dispensary Printing Office, 1888.
12. Whitehead CS, Hoff CA. Ethical Sex Relations. Chicago: Hertel Co, 1922.
13. Huhner M. Disorders of the Sexual Function in the Male and Female. Philadelphia: F. A. Davis Co., 1916.
14. Kinsey AC, Pomeroy WB, Martin CE. Sexual Behavior in the Human Male. Philadelphia: W. B. Saunders, 1948.
15. Shapiro B. Premature ejaculation: a review of 1130 cases. J Urol 1943; 50:374–377.

16. Rowland DL, Cooper SE, Schneider M. Defining premature ejaculation for experimental and clinical investigations. Arch Sex Behav 2001; 30(3):235–253.

17. Cooper A, Magnus R. A clinical trial of the beta blocker propranolol in premature ejaculation. J Psychosom Res 1984; 28(4):331–336.

18. Strassberg DS, Mahoney JM, Schaugaard M, et al. The role of anxiety in premature ejaculation: a psychophysiological model. Arch Sex Behav 1990; 19(3):251–258.

19. Shover LR, Friedman JM, Weiler SJ, et al. Multiaxial problem-oriented system for sexual dysfunction. Arch Gen Psych 1982; 39:614–619.

20. Colpi GM, Fanciullacci F, Beretta G, et al. Evoked sacral potentials in subjects with true premature ejaculation. Andrologia 1986; 18(6):583–586.

21. Jannini EA, Lenzi A. Ejaculatory disorders: epidemiology and current approaches to definition, classification and subtyping. W J Urol 2005; 23(2): 68–75.

22. Masters WH, Johnson VE. Human Sexual Inadequacy. Boston: Little, Brown & Co, 1970.

23. Grenier G, Byers ES. The relationship among ejaculatory control, ejaculatory latency, and attempts to prolong heterosexual intercourse. Arch Sex Behav 1997; 26(1):27–47.

24. Jannini EA, Lombardo F, Lenzi A. Correlation between ejaculatory and erectile dysfunction. Int J Androl 2005; 28 suppl 2:40–45.

25. Vandereycken W. Towards a better delineation of ejaculatory disorders. Acta Psychiatr Belg 1986; 86(1): 57–63.

26. Waldinger MD, Hengeveld MW, Zwinderman AH. Paroxetine treatment of premature ejaculation: a double-blind, randomized, placebo -controlled study. Am J Psychiatr 1994; 151:1377–1379.

27. American Psychiatric Association: Diagnostic and Statistical Manual of Mental Disorders. 3rd ed. Washington: APA, 1987.

28. Laumann EO, Nicolosi A, Glasser DB, et al. GSSAB Investigators' Group. Sexual problems among women and men aged 40-80 y: prevalence and correlates identified in the Global Study of Sexual Attitudes and Behaviors. Int J Impot Res 2005; 17(1): 39–57.

29. Jannini EA, Lenzi A. Epidemiology of premature ejaculation. Curr Opin Urol 2005; 15(6):399–403.

30. Frank E, Anderson C, Rubinstein D. Frequency of sexual dysfunction in "normal" couples. N Engl J Med 1978; 299(3):111–115.

31. Schein M, Zyzanski SJ, Levine S, et al. The frequency of sexual problems among family practice patients. Fam Pract Res J 1988; 7(3):122–134.

32. Waldinger MD, Rietshel M, Nothen MM, et al. Familial occurrence of primary premature ejaculation. Psychiatr Genet 1998; 8(1):37–40.

33. Kandeel FR, Koussa VKT, Swerdloff RS. Male sexual function and its disorders: physiology, pathophysiology, clinical investigation and treatment. Endocr Rev 2001; 22(3):342–388.

34. Newman HF, Reiss H, Northrup JD. Physical basis of emission, ejaculation, and orgasm in the male. Urology 1991; 19(4):341–350.

35. Atmaca M, Kuloglu M, Tezcan E, et al. Serum leptin levels in patients with premature ejaculation before and after citalopram treatment. BJU Int 2003; 91(3): 252–254.

36. Foreman MM, Hall JL, Love RL. The role of the 5-HT2 receptor in the regulation of sexual performance of male rats. Life Sci 1989; 45(14):1263–1270.

37. Marson L, McKenna KE. Serotonergic neurotoxic lesions facilitate male sexual reflexes. Pharmacol Biochem Behav 1994; 47:883–888.

38. McIntosh TK, Barfield RJ. Brain monoaminergic control of male reproductive period. II Dopamine and post-ejaculatory refractory period. Behav Brain Res 1984; 12(3):267–273.

39. Heaton JP. Central neuropharmacological agents and mechanisms in erectile dysfunction: the role of dopamine. Neurosci Biobehav Rev 2000; 24(5):561–569.

40. Yavetz H, Yogev L, Hauser R, et al. Retrograde ejaculation. Hum Reprod 1994; 9(3):381–386.

41. Rowland DL, Slob AK. Understanding and diagnosing sexual dysfunction: a recent progress through psychophysiological and psychophysical methods. Neurosci Biobehav Rev 1995; 19(2):201–209.

42. Bieber I. The psychoanalytic treatment of sexual disorders. J Sex Marital Ther 1974; 1(1):5–15.

43. Ellis H. Studies in the Psychology of Sex. New York: Random House, 1936.

44. Finkelstein L. Awe and premature ejaculation: a case study. Psychoanal Q 1975; 44(2):232–252.

45. Kaplan HS. The New Sex Therapy: Active Treatment of Sexual Dysfunction. New York: Brunner/Mazel, 1974.

46. Kaplan HS. How to Overcome Premature Ejaculation. New York: Brunner-Mazel, 1989.

47. Masters WH, Johnson VE. Human Sexual Response. Boston: Little & Brown, 1966.

48. Spiess WF, Geer JH, O'Donohue WT. Premature ejaculation: investigation of factors in ejaculatory latency. J Abnorm Psychol 1984; 93(2):242–245.

49. Dunn KM, Croft PR, Hackett GI. Association of sexual problems with social, psychological, and physical problems in men and women: a cross sectional population survey. J Epidemiol Community Health 1999; 53(3):144–148.

50. Grenier G, Byers ES. Operationalizing premature or rapid ejaculation. J Sex Res 2001; 38:369–378.

51. Strassberg DS, Kelly MP, Carroll C, et al. The psychophysiological nature of premature ejaculation. Arch Sex Behav 1987; 16(4):327–336.

52. Buffum J. Pharmacosexology update: prescription drugs and sexual function. J Psychoact Drugs 1986; 18(2):97–106.

53. Cohen PG. The association of premature ejaculation and hypogonadotropic hypogonadism. J Sex Marital Ther 1997; 23:208–211.

54. Omu AE, Al-Baader AA, Dashti H, et al. Magnesium in human semen: possible role in premature ejaculation. Arch Androl 2001; 46(1):59–66.

55. Jannini EA, Ulisse S, D'Armiento M. Thyroid hormone and male gonadal function. Endocr Rev 1995; 16(4): 443–459.

56. Lombardo F, Gandini L, Santulli M, et al. Endocrinological diagnosis in sexology. J Endocrinol Invest 2003; 26(3 suppl):112–114.

57. Corona G, Petrone L, Mannucci E, et al. Psyco-biological correlates of rapid ejaculation in patients attending to an andrologic unit for sexual dysfunctions. Eur Urol 2004; 46:615–622.

58. Simpson G, McCann B, Lowy M. Treatment of premature ejaculation after traumatic brain injury. Brain Injury 2003; 17(8):723–729.

59. Xin ZC, Chung WS, Choi YD, et al. Penile sensitivity in patients with primary premature ejaculation. J Urol 1996; 156(3):979–981.

60. Cold CJ, Van Howe RS. Somatosensory evoked potentials in patients with primary premature ejaculation. J Urol 1998; 159(6):2103–2104.

61. Ozcan C, Ozbek E, Soylu A, et al. Auditory event-related potentials in patients with premature ejaculation. Urology 2001; 58:1025–1029.

62. Perretti A, Catalano A, Mirone V, et al. Neurophysiologic evaluation of central-peripheral sensory and motor pudendal pathways in primary premature ejaculation. Urology 2003; 61(3):623–628.

63. Screponi E, Carosa E, Di Stasi S, et al. Prevalence of chronic prostatitis in men with premature ejaculation. Urology 2001; 58(2):198–202.

64. Liang CZ, Zhang XJ, Hao ZY, et al. Prevalence of sexual dysfunction in Chinese men with chronic prostatitis. BJU Int 2004; 93(4):568–570.

65. Shamloul R, el-Nashaar A. Chronic prostatitis in premature ejaculation: a cohort study in 153 men. J Sex Med 2006; 3(1):150–154.

66. Corona G, Jannini EA, Maggi M. Inventories for male and female sexual dysfunctions. Int J Impot Res 2006; 18(3):236–250.

67. Concise Medical Dictionary. Oxford: Oxford Univ Press, 1985.

68. Kinder BN, Curtiss G. Specific components in the etiology, assessment, and treatment of male sexual dysfunctions: controlled outcome studies. J Sex Marital Ther 1988; 14(1):40–48.

69. Levine SB. Premature ejaculation: some thoughts about its pathogenesis. J Sex Marital Ther 1975; 1(4):326–334.

70. Meares EM, Stamey TA. Bacteriologic localization patterns in bacterial prostatitis and urethritis. Invest Urol 1968; 5(5):492–518.

71. Walen SR, Hauserman NM, Lavin PJ. Clinical Guide to Behavior Therapy. Baltimore: Williams & Wilkins, 1977.

72. Dengrove E. Behavior therapy for the sexual disorders. J Sex Res 1967; 3:49–61.

73. Jannini EA, Lenzi A, Wagner G. Behavioural Therapy and Counselling. In: Schill WB, Comhaire FH, Hargreave TB, eds. Andrology for the Clinician. Springer, Berlin, 2006:598–607.

74. Bhasin S, Berman J, Berman L, et al. Sexual dysfunction in men and women. In: Larsen PR, Kronenberg HM, Melmed S, et al., eds. Williams Textbook of Endocrinology. 10th ed. Philadelphia: Saunders, 2003: 771–793.

75. Semans JH. Premature ejaculation: a new approach. Southern Med J 1955; 49(4):353–358.

76. Zeiss RA. Self–direct treatment of premature ejaculation. J Consult Clin Psychol 1978; 46:1234–1241.

77. Pinchera A, Jannini EA, Lenzi A. Research and academic education in medical sexology. J Endocrinol Invest 2003; 26(3 suppl):13–14.

78. Westheimer RK. Sex for Dummies. Foster City, CA: IDG Books, 1995.

79. Lowe JC, Mikulas WL. Use of written material in learning self control of premature ejaculation. Psychol Rep 1975; 37(1):295–298.

80. Kingsberg S, Althof SE, Leiblum S. Books helpful to patients with sexual and marital problems. J Sex Marital Ther 2002; 28(3):219–228.

81. Grenier G, Byers ES. Rapid ejaculation: a review of conceptual, etiological, and treatment issues. Arch Sex Behav 1995; 24(4):447–472.

82. Pierce AP. The coital alignment technique (CAT): an overview of studies. J Sex Marital Ther 2000; 26(3): 257–268.

83. Pietikainen P. Utopianism in psychology: the case of Wilhelm Reich. J Hist Behav Sci 2002; 38(2): 157–175.

84. Austin V. Hypnosex. San Francisco: Thorsons, 1996.

85. Dengrove E. The mechanotherapy of sexual disorders. J Sex Res 1971; 7:1–12.

86. Kilmann PR, Auerbach R. Treatment of premature ejaculation and psychogenic impotence: a critical review of the literature. Arch Sex Behav 1979; 8(1): 81–100.

87. Price S, Heinrich AG, Golden JS. Structured group treatment of couples experiencing sexual dysfunctions. J Sex Marital Ther 1980; 6(4):247–257.

88. Zeiss HA, Christensen A, Levine AG. Treatment for premature ejaculation through male-only groups. J Sex Marital Ther 1978; 4(2):139–143.

89. Golden JS, Price S, Heinrich AG, et al. Group vs. couple treatment of sexual dysfunction. Arch Sex Behav 1978; 7(6):593–602.

90. Shover L, Leiblum S. The stagnation of sex therapy. J Psychol Human Sex 1994; 6(3):5–10.

91. Seftel AD, Althof SE. Premature ejaculation. In: Mulcahy JJ, ed. Diagnosis and Management of Male Sexual Dysfunction. New York: Igaku-Shoin, 1997: 196–203.

92. Bancroft J. Sexual Science in the 21st century: Where are we going? A personal note. J Sex Res 1999; 36: 226–229.

93. Heiman JR, Meston CM. Empirically validated treatment for sexual dysfunction. Ann Rev Sex Res 1999; 6: 148–194.

94. Hawton K, Catalán J, Martin P. Long-term outcome of sex therapy. Behav Res Ther 1986; 24(6):665–675.

95. LoPiccolo J, Stock WE. Treatment of sexual dysfunction. J Consult Clin Psychol 1986; 54(2):158–167.

96. Hawton K, Catalán J. Prognostic factors in sex therapy. Behav Res Ther 1986; 24(4):377–385.

97. Killman PR, Milan RJ Jr, Boland JP, et al. The treatment of secondary orgasmic dysfunction II. J Sex Marital Ther 1987; 13(2):93–105.

98. De Amicis LA, Goldberg DC, LoPiccolo J. Clinical follow-up of couples treated for sexual dysfunction. Arch Sex Behav 1985; 14(6):467–489.

99. Metz ME, Pryjor JL, Nesvacil LJ, et al. Premature ejaculation: a psychophysiological review. J Sex Marital Ther 1997; 23(1):3–23.

100. Leiblum SR, Rosen RC. Couples therapy for erectile disorders: conceptual and clinical considerations. J Sex Marital Ther 1991; 17(2):147–159.

101. Laumann EO, Paik A, Rosen RC. Sexual dysfunction in United States: prevalence, predictors, and outcomes. JAMA 1999; 281(6):537–544.

102. Stravynski A. Indirect behavioral treatment of erectile failure and premature ejaculation in a man without a partner. Arch Sex Behav 1986; 15(4):355–361.

103. McCarthy BW. Cognitive-behavioral strategies and techniques in the treatment of early ejaculation. In: Leiblum SR, Rosen RC, eds. Principles and Practice of Sex Therapy – Update for the 1990s. 2nd ed. New York: Guilford Press, 1989:141–167.

104. McMahon CG, Samali R. Pharmacological treatment of premature ejaculation. Curr Opin Urol 1999; 9(6):553–561.

105. Goodman RE. An assessment of clomipramine (Anafranil) in the treatment of premature ejaculation. J Intern Med Res 1980; 8(suppl 3):53–59.

106. Haensel SM, Rowland DL, Kallan KTHK, et al. Clomipramine and sexual function in men with premature ejaculation and controls. J Urol 1996; 156(4):1310–1315.

107. Strassberg DS, de Gouveia Brazao CA, Rowland DL, et al. Clomipramine in the treatment of rapid (premature) ejaculation. J Sex Marital Ther 1999; 25(2):89–101.

108. Kara H, Aydin S, Agargun MY, et al. The efficacy of fluoxetine in the treatment of premature ejaculation: a double-blind placebo controlled study. J Urol 1996; 156:1631–1632.

109. Kim SC, Seo KK. Efficacy and safety of fluoxetine, sertraline, and clomipramine in patients with premature ejaculation: a double-blind, placebo controlled study. J Urol 1998; 159(2):425–427.

110. McMahon CG. Treatment of premature ejaculation with sertraline hydrochloride: a single-blind placebo controlled crossover study. J Urol 1998; 159(6):1935–1938.

111. Waldinger MD, Hengeveld MW, Zwinderman AH. Ejaculation-retarding properties of paroxetine in patients with primary premature ejaculation: a double-blind, randomized, dose response study. Br J Urol 1997; 79(4):592–595.

112. Waldinger MD, Zwinderman AH, Olivier B. Antidepressants and ejaculation: a double-blind, randomized, placebo-controlled, fixed-dose study with paroxetine, sertraline, and nefazodone. J Clin Psychopharmacol 2001; 21(3):293–297.

113. Waldinger MD, Zwinderman AH, Schweitzer DH, et al. Relevance of methodological design for the interpretation of efficacy of drug treatment of premature ejaculation: a systematic review and meta-analysis. Int J Impot Res 2004; 16(4):369–381.

114. Fein RL. Intracavernous medication for treatment of premature ejaculation. Urology 1990; 35(4):301–303.

115. Abdel-Hamid IA, El Naggar EA, El Gilany AH. Assessment of as needed use of pharmacotherapy and the pause-squeeze technique in premature ejaculation. Int J Impot Res 2001; 13(1):41–45.

116. Salonia A, Maga T, Colombo R, et al. A prospective study comparing paroxetine alone versus paroxetine plus sildenafil in patients with premature ejaculation. J Urol 2002; 168(6):2486–2489.

117. Chen J, Mabjeesh NJ, Matzkin H, et al. Efficacy of sildenafil as adjuvant therapy to selective serotonin reuptake inhibitor in alleviating premature ejaculation. Urology 2003; 61(1):197–200.

118. Berkovitch M, Keresteci AG, Koren G. Efficacy of prilocaine-lidocaine cream in the treatment of premature ejaculation. J Urol 1995; 154(4):1360–1361.

119. Choi HK, Jung GW, Moon KH, et al. Clinical study of SS-cream in patients with lifelong premature ejaculation. Urology 2000; 55(2):257–261.

120. Morales A. Developmental status of topical therapies for erectile and ejaculatory dysfunction. Int J Impot Res 2000; 12(suppl 4):80–85.

121. Boneff AN. Topical treatment of chronic prostatitis and premature ejaculation. Int Urol Nephrol 1972; 4(2):183–186.

122. Brown AJ. Ciprofloxacin as cure of premature ejaculation. J Sex Marital Ther 2000; 26(4):351–352.

123. Althof SE. Evidence based assessment of rapid ejaculation. Int J Impot Res 1998; 10(suppl 2): S74–S76.

124. Rosen RC. Medical and psychological interventions for erectile dysfunction. In: Leiblum SR, Rosen RC, eds. Principles and Practice of Sex Therapy. 3rd ed. New York: Guilford Press, 2000:276–304.

Systemic Drug Therapy for Male Sexual Dysfunction

Fouad R. Kandeel

Department of Diabetes, Endocrinology and Metabolism, City of Hope National Medical Center, Duarte, California and David Geffen School of Medicine, University of California, Los Angeles, California, U.S.A.

□ INTRODUCTION

Before selecting a pharmacological agent for the treatment of any given sexual disorder, one should identify the nature of the presenting sexual problem from a detailed history-taking and thorough physical evaluation and after adequate consideration of results of all pertinent laboratory and, if necessary, special testing procedures. Moreover, if the initial investigation is suggestive of an inciting pharmacological agent or the intake of an addictive drug, a trial of the inciting pharmacological agent or discontinuation of the drug of addiction should be attempted before prescribing an additional agent for the management of the sexual problem. Identification of the presenting problem can also help in directing the subsequent physical and laboratory evaluations as well as in selection of the most suitable therapeutic intervention. For example, patients presenting with hypoactive sexual desire would need to be evaluated for possible underlying hypogonadism, hypothyroidism, or the presence of central nervous system (CNS) disease, and treatment of desire deficiency in these conditions should primarily start with the replacement of the deficient hormone(s) or treatment of the underlying CNS disorder. Similarly, patients with erectile dysfunction (ED), absent or retarded emission, anorgasmia, or painful erection should be surveyed not only for the presence of medical illnesses associated with these sexual problems but also for the adverse sexual effects of drugs used to treat these medical conditions.

The availability of oral erectogenic agents such as sildenafil tempts many treating physicians to use them as a primary therapeutic modality for patients with erectile failure without defining the underlying etiology. Although this approach may work for a significant proportion of patients, indiscriminate use of these agents could occasionally result in a life-threatening complication (e.g., refractory hypotension when sildenafil is taken with nitrates). Thus, the need to perform appropriate investigations to rule out potentially correctable disorders (e.g., psychosexual problems, hypogonadism, treatable chronic illness, and/or correctable vascular insufficiency) prior to prescribing pharmacological therapies for sexual dysfunction must be stressed. Table 1 summarizes pharmacologic agents attempted in the treatment of each form of sexual dysfunction in men (1).

Since some of the pharmacological agents that are currently being used or evaluated—particularly for treatment of desire and ejaculatory disorders—have a variety of central and peripheral effects, the term "erectogenic drugs" will occasionally be used in this chapter to more accurately reflect the varying modes of action.

□ TREATMENT OF HYPOACTIVE OR DEFICIENT SEXUAL DESIRE

The following section is limited to the discussion of systemic pharmacological agents in the treatment of hypoactive sexual desire. The role of psychosexual counseling is detailed in Chapters 8, 12, and 24.

Hormone Replacement

Several groups have examined the effect of androgen replacement on sexual responsiveness. Studies in hypogonadal men have clearly demonstrated significant improvement in libido factors (i.e., sexual motivation/interest) and spontaneous erections with testosterone replacement, even in the absence of desire deficiency disorders (7–14). The results of androgen therapy of men with desire disorder without hypogonadism, however, have been limited and inconclusive (15,16). For example, O'Carroll and Bancroft (17) compared the effects of testosterone therapy to placebo in a 12-week cross-over trial in 10 men with low sexual desire and in 10 men with ED. Higher baseline testosterone levels were found in the desire-deficient men than in impotent men, suggesting that hypogonadism was probably not the major contributing factor for desire deficiency in this patient sample. Although testosterone therapy resulted in a significant increase in sexual thoughts and fantasies in patients with desire deficiency, only three men achieved a significant clinical improvement in their sexual function. Buvat et al. (18) examined the effect of human chorionic gonadotropin (hCG) in 51 males with either ED or low sexual desire. Following one month of therapy, the frequency of sexual initiation increased significantly in both groups of sexually dysfunctional patients, which

Table 1 Pharmacological Therapy for Male Sexual Dysfunction: Drug Class and Agents Used

Sexual dysfunction	Pharmacological action		Agents
HYPOACTIVE SEXUAL DESIRE	Androgen replacement (Chapter 35) (also for erectile dysfunction due to hypogonadism)		Testosterone
	Combined α-1 adrenoreceptor antagonist and serotonin reuptake inhibitor		Trazodone, venlafaxine, and fenfluramine
	α-2 adrenoreceptor antagonists		Yohimbine (reverses SSRI-induced dysfunction)
	Cholinergic agonists		Bethanechol (reverses TCA-induced dysfunction)
	Dopaminergics	Dopamine receptor agonists	Apomorphine, bromocriptine, pergolide mesylate, and carbergoline
		Dopamine precursors	Levodopa
		Dopamine reuptake inhibitors	Amphetamine and selegiline
	Antiserotonergics (selective 5-HT-2 receptor blockers)		LY53857 and LY281067 are being evaluated
	Unknown mechanism (possibly nonadrenergic)		Bupropion
ERECTILE DYSFUNCTION	Phosphodiesterase inhibitors	cGMP phosphodiesterase (type-5) inhibitor	Sildenafil, vardenafil, and tadalafil
		cAMP phosphodiesterase inhibitor	Papaverine
	Prostaglandin (Chapters 30, 36,37)	Prostaglandin E₁ (alprostadil)	Injectable, transurethral, oral, and transcutaneous forms
		Prostaglandin E₂ (dinoprostone)	Prostin E₂
	α-1 adrenoreceptor antagonists		Papaverine, moxisylyte, ifenprodil, alfuzosin, terazosin, and doxazosin
	α-1 and -2 adrenoreceptor antagonists		Phentolamine (intracorporeal injection or oral) and Phenoxybenzamine (potent α-1 inhibitor)
	Vasoactive intestinal polypeptide (Chapter 30)		VIP alone or mixed with phentolamine
	α-2 adrenoreceptor antagonists		Yohimbine and delquamine
	β-2 adrenoreceptor antagonists		Isoxsuprine and salbutamol
	Combined α-1 adrenoreceptor antagonist and SSRI		Trazodone
	Sodium/potassium pump (membrane hyperpolarization)		Calcitonin gene-related peptide
	Nitric oxide precursors and donors		L-arginine and linsidomine chlorhydrate
	Vasodilators and smooth-muscle relaxants		Nitroglycerin (cream), naftidrofuryl, and minoxidil
	Selective serotonin reuptake inhibitor		Fluoxetine
	Combined serotonin and norepinephrine reuptake inhibitor		Venlafaxine (may increase libido)
	Antiarrhythmics (Chapters 29, 36)		Adenosine and dipyridamole
	Dopamine receptor agonists		Apomorphine
	Opioid antagonist		Naltrexone
	Xantheine derivative (improved red blood cell flexibility and vasodilatation)		Pentoxifylline
	α melanocyte-stimulating hormonal analogue		Melanotan II
	Herbal remedies (Chapter 31)		ArginMax and Korean red ginseng
EJACULATION DISORDERS	**Premature ejaculation**	Serotonergics — Combined SSRI and TCA	Clomipramine
		Serotonergics — SSRI	Paroxetine, sertraline, and fluoxetine
		α-1 adrenoreceptor antagonists	Phenoxybenzamine, alfuzosin, terazosin, moxisylyte, ifenprodil, and doxazosin
		Anesthetic creams (Chapter 30)	Lidocaine-prilocaine
	Post-ejaculation pain	Anxiolytic	Diazepam and lorazepam
ORGASMIC DYSFUNCTION	Antiserotonergics		Cyroheptadine (reverses SSRI-, TCA-, and MAOI-induced dysfunction)
	Dopamine agonist		Amantadine (reverses SSRI-induced dysfunction)
	Combined α-1 adrenoreceptor antagonists and SSRI		Trazodone
	α-2 adrenoreceptor antagonists		Yohimbine (reverses clomipramine- and SSRI-induced dysfunction)
	Unknown mechanism (possibly nonadrenergic)		Bupropion
PAINFUL ERECTION	**Functional priapism**	α-1 adrenoreceptor agonists	Pseudoephedrine, phenylephrine, noradrenaline metaraminol, terbutaline, and epinephrine
	Peyronie's disease	Systemic agents	Vitamin E, aminobenzoate potassium, colchicine, and tamoxifen
		Intralesional injections (Chapter 34)	Collagenase and calcium channel blockers (nifedipine and verapamil)

For each category of discussion, therapeutic agents are listed in descending order of their presumed efficacy.
All drug classes are described in Chapter 29, except where noted in parentheses.
Abbreviations: cAMP, cyclic adenosine monophosphate; cGMP, cyclic guanosine monophosphate; 5-HT-2, 5-hydroxytryptamine receptor-2 subtype; MAOI, monoamine oxidase inhibitors; SSRI, selective serotonin reuptake inhibitors; TCA, tricyclic antidepressants; VIP, vasoactive intestinal polypeptide.

was thought to reflect an improvement in libido. Unfortunately, results for each of the treatment groups were not analyzed separately to allow a better delineation of androgen treatment effects on desire deficiency in eugonadal men.

Male sexual dysfunction caused by insufficient androgen levels can be treated by testosterone replacement therapy. Intramuscular injection of long-acting testosterone esters in oil has been the mainstay of androgen replacement therapy in the United States for decades. The two available preparations are testosterone enanthate and testosterone cypionate. Although achieved serum testosterone levels are not physiologic (high values occur for several days after the injection and decline to low values after 10 days), most males with sexual dysfunction obtain therapeutic effects with the injection of 100 to 200 mg at two- to four-week intervals, since administration of these agents every four weeks does not maintain serum testosterone levels within normal range for the entire four-week period. Hence, other longer-acting testosterone esters, such as testosterone buciclate and microencapsulated testosterone, which potentially could provide more physiologic, long-lasting testosterone levels, continue to be evaluated. Testosterone propionate (not available in the United States) is a shorter-acting preparation that requires intramuscular injection two to three times a week (10–25 mg per injection). This may be suitable for patients who do not tolerate the large swings between the peaks and valleys of testosterone serum concentration with the longer-acting preparations (19). In addition, several transdermal testosterone preparations have become available: initially, the scrotal system (Testoderm®), followed by the nonscrotal systems (Androderm® and Testoderm-TTS®), and subsequently the approved transdermal creams AndroGel and Testim. The efficacy of these products in establishing optimal levels of testosterone in deficient males has been demonstrated (20–25). A 10% absorption rate is expected from the transdermal gel, which is recommended for use at 5- to 10-g per application. A 10-g dose of AndroGel has been shown to increase serum testosterone levels within 30 minutes, and the achieved levels remained in a steady state by the second or third day of dosing (24). Although both treatments seem to be efficacious for replacing testosterone in hypogonadal men, the more physiologic sex hormone levels and profiles associated with transdermal systems may offer possible advantages over intramuscular injections in minimizing excessive stimulation of erythropoiesis, preventing/ameliorating gynecomastia, and not oversuppressing gonadotropins (25). The direct cost of using these products is much higher than that of intramuscular testosterone ester injections unless one considers who administers the injection (patient or physician), location (home or physician's office), and time away from work if physician administered injections are required. Itching at the application site is the most common adverse effect of these transdermal systems, a problem that is not usually encountered with

the use of cream formulations. Further, the scrotal system (4- or 6-mg patch applied once daily) required skin shaving, produced a disproportionate increase in serum levels of dihydrotestosterone, and had a high rate of nonadherence to skin (26). As a result, this formulation is no longer offered.

In contrast, the nonscrotal-transdermal system (one 5.0-mg patch or two 2.5-mg patches, applied once daily to rotating sites of the back or the upper outer arms) appears to induce a higher rate of allergic dermatitis and spontaneous flaring of prior application sites (up to 12%) (27). Generally, the Testoderm-TTS system formulation produces less dermatological side effects than the Androderm formulation. Oral testosterone preparations that are alkylated at the 17-α-position are weak androgens and are known to be hepatotoxic (increased hepatic enzymes, cholestatic hepatitis, and hepatocellular carcinoma), require repeated daily dosing, and have higher potential for abuse, especially by body-building athletes. Therefore, their use is generally discouraged among testosterone-deficient males.

In 1994, the Massachusetts Male Aging Study reported an inverse correlation of serum dehydroepi androsterone (DHEA) concentrations and the incidence of ED (28). A follow-up study examined the effects of oral intake of DHEA supplement (50 mg daily for six months) in a prospective, placebo-controlled, randomized trial in 40 men with ED (29). Oral intake of dehydro epiandrosterone (DHEA) by 20 men was associated with a higher mean score in all five domains of the International Index of Erectile Function (IIEF) (reflecting an improvement in achieving and maintaining erections). Although the study reported no impact from the DHEA treatment on mean serum levels of prostatic specific antigen (PSA), prolactin, testosterone, mean prostate volume, or mean postvoid residual urine volume, the patient sample size was too small even to perform a relevant statistical analysis (29). It remains unclear, however, whether the reported DHEA therapeutic effects will be reproducible in larger-size studies, or whether DHEA exerts its effects through a direct action on the brain and/or the penile tissues or through the conversion to some other active steroid moieties. Similarly, a long-term safety profile has not been established.

Excessive androgen intake may cause a substantial rise in hematocrit levels, especially in men with chronic obstructive lung disease and heavy smokers. It also decreases the serum concentration of high-density lipoprotein cholesterol. Both these complications could increase the risk for coronary artery disease. Another potential hazard of androgen therapy is the increase in serum PSA levels and in prostate volume (30,31). It is not known whether these changes are associated with an increased risk for prostate cancer, although several cases of prostate cancer have been diagnosed after initiation of exogenous testosterone treatment (32). It is important, therefore, that patients undergoing testosterone therapy have baseline rectal examinations and baseline PSA measurements performed, and that both studies be repeated at regular intervals.

Testosterone may have a role in the treatment of male frailty (weakness, lack of physical endurance, or stamina) with hypogonadism. Sih et al. (33) investigated the yearlong effects of testosterone administration in older men with hypogonadism and age-associated physical and cognitive declines. Biweekly testosterone injections improved strength, increased hemoglobin levels, and lowered leptin level (which may reflect reduced fat mass); however, no significant changes were found in prostate-specific antigen levels or memory. Thus, with careful monitoring because of its potential risks, testosterone supplementation may be considered for improving specific outcomes in this population.

Other Pharmacological Agents

Other pharmacological approaches to the treatment of hypoactive sexual function have included the use of various centrally acting agents (Table 1) (3,4,15,34). Controlled studies on the use of these agents in the treatment of isolated hypoactive sexual desire have not been widely reported, however, and many of the currently available drugs are not selective and can alter the neurotransmission of more than one receptor type. Generally, administration of the dopamine agonists apomorphine, bromocriptine, and pergolide or the dopamine precursor levodopa (2–6,35–39) has been associated with increased libido. Cabergoline is a long-acting dopamine agonist (40–43) that is expected to have a similar effect. Also, the antidepressants bupropion and nomifensine have been shown to increase libido in some studies. For example, a significant improvement in libido and global sexual functioning was noted in a group of bupropion-treated men and women with hypoactive sexual desire as compared to placebo in a 12-week double-blind study (44). A noradrenergic mechanism of action has been advanced to explain the libido-enhancing effect of this agent (34). Studies with the serotonergic agents trazodone (45,46), venlafaxine (47), and fenfluramine (48) have also shown an increase in sexual desire, and, in the case of trazodone, there was no correlation between the improvement in libido and the changes in mood. Trazodone is an antidepressant drug with complex neurohormonal effects, including the inhibition of serotonin reuptake, the suppression of prolactin secretion, and the reduction of 5-hydroxytryptamine (5-HT) receptor-2 subtype receptor–binding activity. Other effects such as central α-adrenergic stimulation and direct α-adrenergic blockade in the corpus cavernosum have also been proposed. Venlafaxine and its metabolite O-desmethylvenlafaxine are potent inhibitors of norepinephrine and serotonin reuptake but weak inhibitors of dopamine reuptake (49). More specific serotonergic agents, however, are generally considered to have an inhibitory neurotransmitting effect in the control of sexual drive (3,4,34). As a result, agents

with serotonin receptor–blocking activity, such as methysergide, metergoline, and cyproheptadine, and agents with serotonin synthesis inhibition activity, such as parachlorophenylalanine, are expected to augment sex-seeking behavior (3). Further, selective 5-HT-2 receptor antagonists (e.g., LY53857 and LY281067) were under investigation as a treatment for hypoactive sexual dysfunction (15). Moreover, yohimbine hydrochloride, an α-2 antagonist, which also affects serotonin and dopamine transmission, has been used to restore sexual desire in depressed patients receiving serotonin reuptake inhibitors (50). Bethanechol has been reported to reverse the sexual side effects of tricyclic antidepressants, possibly through a muscarinic-agonist potentiation of adrenergic function (3).

☐ TREATMENT OF ED

This portion of the chapter will focus on the role of systemic pharmacologic therapies in the treatment of male ED. Table 1 summarizes pharmacological agents used. (For discussions on local pharmacological treatments for male sexual dysfunction, see Chapter 30, and for discussion on other treatment options, see Chapters 31, 32 and 33.)

Reproductive Hormones

Treatment of hypogonadism should depend upon its etiology and whether or not fertility is desired. Several dopamine agonists are currently available for the treatment of patients with hyperprolactinemia not caused by drug ingestion, which include the widely used and relatively short-acting bromocriptine (51,52), the short-acting pergolide mesylate (53), and the long-acting cabergoline (40–43) preparations. Patients with primary or secondary hypogonadism should be treated with androgen replacement except when fertility is desired (14,54,55). Patients with pituitary hypogonadism who desire fertility may be treated with gonadotropin replacement [hCG-hMG (human menopausal gonadotropin)] (56), whereas those with hypothalamic hypogonadism may have the option of treatment with gonadotropin-releasing hormone as well (57,58). Patients with other endocrine dysfunctions should be treated for their primary disease, as androgen therapy has no role in these conditions. (For further details on the treatment of hypogonadism, see Chapter 35.)

cGMP Phosphodiesterase Inhibitors

Comprehensive basic science research has considerably expanded the knowledge base on the biological and biochemical mechanisms of penile erection, particularly regarding attractive target enzymes and ion channels (59). The nitric oxide–guanylylcyclase–cyclic guanosine monophosphate (cGMP)–phosphodiesterase (PDE) pathway has proven itself to be of utmost interest in the development of compounds that attack the generation or cleavage of cGMP (60). PDE type-5

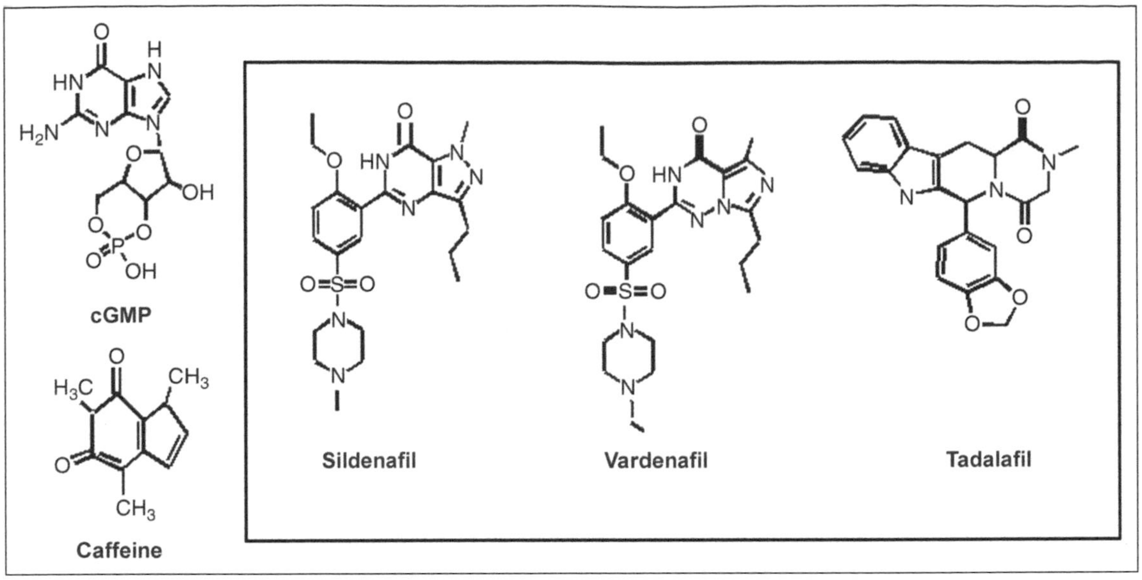

Figure 1 Phosphodiesterase-5 inhibitor molecular structures. Note similarities to cGMP and caffeine. *Abbreviation*: cGMP, cyclic guanosine monophosphate.

(PDE-5) is an enzyme that hydrolyzes cGMP in the cavernosum tissue of the penis. Inhibition of PDE-5 results in increased arterial blood flow leading to enlargement of the corpus cavernosum. Because of the increased tumescence, veins are compressed between the corpus cavernosum and the tunica albuginea, resulting in an erection (61). These general considerations are supported by the success of sildenafil, the first oral PDE-5 inhibitor in the management of ED, and subsequently by two other PDE-5 inhibitors, vardenafil and tadalafil. Over 11,000 patient-years of experience with sildenafil exist, as well as a tremendous amount of reassuring safety and efficacy data (62). This makes most physicians feel comfortable prescribing these medications as first-line therapy for ED; however, for many patients who do not have a reasonable response to sildenafil, the opportunity to try a different oral agent is a welcome option and an alternative to second-line therapy with a vacuum constriction device, an injected agent, or intraurethral alprostadil (MUSE). Tadalafil and vardenafil represent newer compounds in the PDE-5 inhibitor class (Fig. 1). Tables 2 and 3 provide information on metabolism and relative potency and selectivity of these agents toward PDE subtypes (63).

There are, at present, 11 known PDE enzymes. Selectivity is an important issue, however, because there are as yet no pure PDE-5 inhibitors (Table 3) (67). In addition to inhibiting PDE-5, both sildenafil and vardenafil also produce modest PDE-6–related effects at the upper limits of the dosage range, whereas these effects are absent with tadalafil. Sildenafil and vardenafil have no significant effects on PDEs-1 to 4 and 7 to 11. All efficacy and safety attributes are likely related to PDE-5/-6 inhibition. PDE-6 inhibition affects the cones in the retina, resulting in the "blue" vision experienced by some patients taking sildenafil. In contrast, only tadalafil has definite PDE-11 effects at therapeutic doses, although the clinical significance of this is not yet clear. PDE-11 has only recently been described and is present in the pituitary, pancreas, skeletal muscle, heart, testes, and corpus cavernosum; however, the effects on these tissues of chronic or intermittent PDE-11 inhibition are not known and require further study. In preclinical studies, tadalafil caused testicular alterations in beagle dogs characterized by degeneration of germ cell line cells in the seminiferous tubules and depressed spermatogenesis. Two studies in men who received 10 or 20 mg tadalafil daily for six months have showed that tadalafil had no adverse effects on human spermatogenesis or reproductive hormones. The effects, if any, of either prolonged or

Table 2 Pharmacokinetics of PDE-5 Inhibitors

	Sildenafil	Tadalafil	Vardenafil
Formulations	25, 50, 100 mg tablets	5, 10, 20 mg tablets	5, 10, 20 mg tablets
Bioavailability (%)	40	ND	15
C_{max} (with food) (%)	29	No change	20
T_{max} (hr)	1	2	1
$T_{1/2}$ (hr)	3–4	17.5	4–5
Metabolism	CYP3A4	CYP3A4	CYP3A4
Onset of erection (min)	30–60	16–45	25
Duration of action (hr)	4	36	4
Active metabolite	Yes	No	Yes
Excretion, urine (%)	13	36	5
Excretion, feces (%)	80	61	92

Abbreviations: C_{max}, change in maximum plasma concentration; CYP3A4, hepatic cytochrome P450 isozyme 3A4; ND, not determined; PDE-5, phosphodiesterase-5; T_{max}, time to maximum plasma concentration; T1/2, plasma half-life.
Source: From Ref. 64.

Table 3 Comparison of Sildenafil, Vardenafil, and Tadalafil Selectivity for Various PDE Subtypes

	Sildenafil	Vardenafil	Tadalafil
PDE-1	280 (80)	69 (690)	>30,000 (>4000)
PDE-2	68,000 (>19,000)	6,200 (62,000)	>30,000 (>4000)
PDE-3	16,200 (4628)	4000 (40,000)	>30,000 (>4000)
PDE-4	7200 (2,057)	4000 (40,000)	>30,000 (>4,000)
PDE-5	3.5	0.1	6.7
PDE-6 (rod)	37 (10.5)	3.5 (35)	1260 (188)
PDE-6 (cone)	34 (9.7)	0.6 (6)	1030 (153)
PDE-7	21,300 (6100)	>30,000 (>300,000)	>100,000 (>14,000)
PDE-8	29,800 (8500)	>30,000 (>300,000)	>100,000 (>14,000)
PDE-9	2610 (750)	580 (5800)	>100,000 (>14,000)
PDE-10	9800 (2800)	3000 (30,000)	>100,000 (>14,000)
PDE-11	2730 (780)	162 (1,620)	37.0 (5.5)

Top cell value represents IC$_{50}$, the concentration of drug (nM) required for 50% inhibition of the respective PDE enzyme. Bottom cell value in parentheses represents the proportional factor of increase required in drug concentration for 50% inhibition of a given PDE enzyme relative to that required for 50% inhibition of PDE-5. Higher numbers thus reflect lower selectivity. Rods and cones are the two types of photoreceptors in the retina; rods are present in larger numbers and have higher sensitivity but are not sensitive to color, while cones are receptors for color.
Abbreviation: PDE, phosphodiesterase.
Source: From Refs. 65, 66.

intermittent PDE-11 inhibition by tadalafil remain unknown (67).

PDE-5 inhibitors have become the treatment of choice for men with ED, with one study reporting up to 60% to 80% efficacy in unselected patients with ED, with approximately 73.8% of men indicating a preference for oral treatment in comparison to local injections or other forms of therapy (68,69). The characteristics of each of the three available PDE-5 inhibitors are described in further detail below.

Sildenafil (Viagra®)

Sildenafil (Viagra®) is a novel oral agent with selective inhibiting activity of PDE-isozyme-5, the major isozyme responsible for clearance of cGMP from human cavernous tissue (70). Such an effect potentiates erections during sexual stimulation. Sildenafil is rapidly absorbed, with dose-proportional peak plasma concentrations within 30 to 120 minutes of administration in the fasting state, and has an elimination half-life of three to five hours. Its absolute bioavailability is close to 40%, and it is cleared predominantly by the

hepatic microsomal isoenzyme cytochrome P450 enzyme 3A4 (CY3A4) and, to a lesser extent, by isozyme CY2C9 (71). The therapeutic dose usually ranges from 25 to 100 mg, taken one hour before intended sexual activity. Lower doses may be used in elderly patients and those with hepatic or renal impairment or those receiving CY3A4 inhibitors such as ritonavir, saquinavir, ketoconazole, erythromycin, or cimetadine (72).

The overall efficacy of sildenafil, estimated from the responses obtained in the international MALES study, which surveyed 27,838 men, found that 64% who had used sildenafil more than once reported satisfaction with this treatment (73). Sildenafil has also been used with good results in men with Peyronie's disease, with up to 70.8% of Peyronie's males able to enjoy sexual intercourse with the use of this drug (74).

Yet, although patient treatment has largely been successful, one prospective study determined the rate of abandonment of sildenafil therapy to approximate 31%, with the majority reporting that they had no opportunity or desire for sexual intercourse or that their partners had shown no sexual interest. Interestingly, few patients stated that the high cost of the medication or that adverse events were the cause of noncompliance (75). Patients with diabetes mellitus (76,77) and some of those with neurological dysfunction (77), spinal-cord injuries (78), prostatic surgery (79), and pelvic irradiation (80) may have lower response rates, between 35% and 67%. Several other studies have reported on the safety and efficacy of this agent in treating male ED (71,72,76–84). Safety and tolerability data from a series of double-blind, placebo-controlled studies and from 10 open-label extension studies of sildenafil in the treatment of ED were analyzed by Morales et al. (82). The most commonly reported adverse events (all causes) were headache (16% sildenafil, 4% placebo), flushing (10% sildenafil, 1% placebo), and dyspepsia (7% sildenafil, 2% placebo), and they were predominantly transient and mild to moderate in nature. Priapism occurs in about 3% (85), and the rate of drug discontinuation due to adverse effects was comparable to that of placebo (82). Alternately, a postmarketing surveillance study of family physicians in Korea between 1999 and 2002 reported the most frequent adverse effect being hot flushes (5.6%), followed by headache (2.6%), palpitation (1.0%), anxiety (0.5%), and elevated alanine aminotransferase (ALT) (0.5%). These side effects most likely result from the inhibition of a variety of phosphosdiesterases (86). Previous reports have demonstrated that patients with mild vasculogenic ED have a better response to sildenafil, whereas patients with severe or neurogenic ED have a lower response. No particular factor has seemed to predict absolute failure with sildenafil (77). Although the cumulative probability of achieving successful intercourse in men with ED treated with sildenafil increases with the number of attempts and reaches a plateau on the eighth attempt (87), in clinical practice, however, it is difficult to encourage patients to continue with a drug for greater than four separate trials. While doses higher than 100 mg have salvaged previous nonresponders, these attempts are limited by a significantly higher incidence of adverse effects and a subsequently high treatment discontinuation rate (88). Nevertheless, several studies have suggested that sildenafil nonresponders should be rechallenged with the drug in conjunction with proper patient education, dose titration, and additional attempts, as positive responses of 58.5% have been reported among patients who had experienced previous treatment failures (89).

Sildenafil has a potential for drug–drug interaction with nitrates and nitric oxide donors. Thus, inhibition of these PDEs by sildenafil may cause a drop in systemic vascular resistance resulting in hypotension (90,91). Significant interaction has been observed in clinical studies, with a drop in systolic pressure >25 mmHg in subjects receiving sublingual glyceryl trinitrate (500 μg) and sildenafil (25 mg, three times daily) (92). Further, in a small pilot study of men with ischemic heart disease, a 40-mg intravenous dose of sildenafil, which produces comparable plasma levels to that produced by the maximum approved oral dose (100 mg), reduced both pulmonary arterial pressure (–27% at rest and –19% during exercise) and cardiac output (–7% at rest and –11% during exercise) (93). Human platelets contain cGMP-specific PDE-5 and PDE-6, which are inhibited by sildenafil; however, while sildenafil alone was found to have no effects on human and rabbit platelet function, it was capable of potentiating the antiaggregation activity of sodium nitroprusside in vitro. It had no effects on the bleeding time (a clinical indicator of platelet aggregation) in healthy male volunteers (94). Physician-prescribing guidelines issued by the American College of Cardiology/American Heart Association have recommended extreme caution with the use of nitrates within 24 hours of sildenafil ingestion. Sildenafil should not be used within 24 hours of taking a nitroglycerine preparation, as this combination is known to cause profound hypotension in men with certain cardiovascular conditions, liver disease, or kidney disease, and in those taking medications that may prolong sildenafil's half-life (e.g., erythromycin or cimetidine) (95). Males with known or suspected coronary artery disease may benefit from an exercise test to determine whether the resumption of sexual activity with use of sildenafil is likely to be associated with an increased risk of myocardial ischemia (90). Retrospective analysis of the concomitant use of antihypertensive medications (β-blockers, α-blockers, diuretics, angiotensin-converting enzyme inhibitors, and calcium antagonists) in patients taking sildenafil, however, did not indicate an increase in the reports of adverse events or significant episodes of hypotension compared with patients treated with sildenafil alone (96). In clinical trials, the incidence of serious cardiovascular adverse events, including stroke and myocardial infarction,

was the same for patients treated with sildenafil or placebo (83). Further, the overall incidence of cardiovascular adverse events other than flushing was comparable in patients with and without ischemic heart disease for patients receiving sildenafil as compared to placebo (83). Thus, the available data support the view that oral sildenafil significantly improves erectile function and is well tolerated in appropriate patients with ED and ischemic heart disease who are not taking nitrate therapy (96). (For further information on this topic, see Chapter 36.)

Sexual activities are likely to be associated with increased cardiac risks in patients with ischemic heart disease due to the increase in cardiac workload as reflected by the increase in heart rate and blood pressure. Such an increase in cardiac workload is roughly equivalent to 5 to 6 metabolic equivalents (METs) to task on an exercise stress test (97) and is associated with increased risk for arrhythmia. Further, a relative risk of heart attack within the first two hours of intercourse was found to be 2.5 in a retrospective study evaluating men who were sexually active (98). Moreover, analysis of the adverse events related to sildenafil use posted by the Food and Drug Administration (FDA), as of early 1999, revealed that 70% of 128 patients in question had one or more risk factors for cardiovascular or cerebrovascular disease, including hypertension, hypercholesterolemia, cigarette smoking, diabetes mellitus, obesity, or previous cardiac history (85). Thus, caution should also be taken if sildenafil is to be used by patients with prior cardiac histories or patients with one or more cardiac risk factors and by those who are taking multiple antihypertensive medications (84). When appropriate, a symptom-limited maximal exercise electrocardiogram examination may be performed to predict patients at risk for ST segment depression during coitus (83). This cautious approach is warranted, particularly in view of the reported case of acute myocardial infarction that occurred 30 minutes after ingestion of sildenafil in a patient with no clear risk factors for ischemic heart disease (99).

Sildenafil also has a weak inhibiting effect on PDE-6 in the retina (about 1/10 of that for PDE-5), leading to transient color tinge, blurred vision, or increased sensitivity to light in 3% to 6% of patients (Table 3) (100). Measurement of visual acuity, visual field, intraocular pressure, and visual-evoked potentials in normal healthy volunteers immediately before and repeatedly up to six hours after ingestion of sildenafil (100 mg) remained unchanged. Measurements with an electroretinogram, however, showed a 36% reduction in a-wave amplitude and a 23% reduction in b-wave amplitude of the saturation response, with complete recovery at six hours after the intake of sildenafil (101). Caution is also recommended in prescribing this agent to patients with significant preexisting retinal abnormalities or inherited retinal disease such as retinitis pigmentosa (a portion of patients with this condition have genetic disorders of PDEs).

Sildenafil is also FDA approved in the United States for the treatment of arterial pulmonary hypertension. (PDE-5 also exists in the smooth muscles of the pulmonary vasculature.) This drug is marketed for this specific indication under the trade name Revatio™ (Pfizer, 20-mg tablets).

PDE-5 inhibitors, including sildenafil, vardenafil, and tadalafil, have been reported in a small case series to cause sudden, severe visual loss due to nonarteritic ischemic optic neuropathy (NAION). Many of the suspected cases had risk factors for NAION, including atherosclerosis, cigarette smoking, diabetes mellitus, a factor V Leiden mutation, prior intraocular surgery, previous episodes of NAION, and a small optic cup:disc ratio. The symptoms typically develop within 6 to 36 hours after the use of the drug and present as sudden, painless, unilateral diminution of visual acuity or field loss, afferent pupillary defect, or optic disc edema. The condition can sometimes be irreversible. The FDA has recently approved updated labeling for the PDE-5 drugs that advise patients of this condition (102).

Vardenafil (Levitra®)

Vardenafil (Levitra®) is a potent and highly selective oral PDE-5 inhibitor that is structurally similar to sildenafil (Fig. 1). Therefore, it is not surprising that both drugs have a similar half-life (Table 2), have an affinity to PDE-6 (mostly present in the retina and platelets) (Table 3), and can have delayed absorption with fatty meals (101). Retinal PDE-6 inhibition has not been proven to have significant long-term adverse consequences for sildenafil in chronic dose toxicology studies and in long-term patient studies (103). The long-term safety profile of vardenafil remains to be established but is expected not to be a significant issue (104).

Vardenafil improved erectile function in men with mild-to-severe ED of varying etiology (105), including ED associated with diabetes mellitus or ED after radical prostatectomy in two randomized, double-blind, multicenter, fixed-dose studies of 12 or 26 weeks' duration (104). Men receiving vardenafil 10 or 20 mg had significantly greater improvements in IIEF questionnaire erectile function domain scores than placebo recipients. Moreover, improvements in penetration and maintenance of erection (assessed using IIEF or Sexual Encounter Profile questions) were significantly greater with vardenafil 5 to 20 mg than with the placebo. Improvements in IIEF intercourse satisfaction and orgasmic function domain scores were significantly greater with vardenafil 10 or 20 mg than with placebo, and the proportion of patients with a positive response to a Global Assessment Question concerning improvement in erections after 12 or 26 weeks' therapy was significantly higher with vardenafil 5 to 20 mg than with placebo (104). Vardenafil was generally well tolerated in men with ED; treatment-emergent adverse events were of mild-to-moderate intensity and transient in nature. The most commonly reported adverse events (typical of those seen with PDE-5 inhibitors) in men receiving vardenafil (5–20 mg) included headache, flushing, rhinitis, dyspepsia, and sinusitis. There were no reports of abnormal color vision in men with ED taking vardenafil at clinically recommended doses (5–20 mg) (104). Vardenafil was also evaluated in a prospective trial in the primary care setting involving hypertensive men with ED, who were receiving at least one antihypertensive medication; vardenafil was found to improve EF significantly in hypertensive men treated with concomitant antihypertensive medication, was well tolerated, and did not significantly affect blood pressure (106).

Tadalafil (Cialis®)

Tadalafil (Cialis®) is a PDE inhibitor with a higher affinity to PDE-11 than both sildenafil and vardenafil (Table 3) and has a half-life of 17.5 hours (Table 2) (101). As a result of its long half-life, its mean elimination time is 4.3 days. Both 10- and 20-mg doses of tadalafil have been shown to improve erectile function for up to 36 hours postdosing in men with ED of varied severity (107) (see discussion below for potential implications).

Tadalafil's affinity to PDE-6 is much less than that of sildenafil, but its affinity for PDE-11 is much higher (Table 3). Although the long PDE-5 inhibition may suit some patients who desire more spontaneity in their sexual activity (108), the effects of extended inhibition of PDE-11 on the testes, pituitary, myocardium, skeletal muscle, and pancreas (organs known to have PDE-11 enzyme activity) remain unknown. Thus, the safety profile of tadalafil differs from that of sildenafil. When taken as needed, tadalafil is associated with fewer headaches and a less frequent incidence of flushing. The most common adverse effect associated with the use of tadalafil is back pain, which may arise from inhibition of PDE-11 (63,96). Dyspepsia and nasopharyngitis have also been reported (107).

Numerous studies have demonstrated that in men with mild-to-severe ED, tadalafil 20 mg significantly improves erectile function, demonstrates superior treatment satisfaction relative to placebo, and is well tolerated (63,109–115).

Comparison of Sildenafil, Vardenafil, and Tadalafil

To help select the most appropriate PDE-5 inhibitor for patients with ED, it is important to examine some of the distinguishing characteristics of these agents, including biochemical potency, biochemical selectivity, onset, duration of action, and safety and efficacy data (Tables 2 and 3). At present, there are no carefully controlled head-to-head trials with the three PDE-5 inhibitors (64).

Among the three oral agents, the most clinically significant differences are found in their durations of action. The reported half-lives of sildenafil, vardenafil, and tadalafil are 4 hours, 4 to 6 hours, and 17 to

21 hours, respectively. The duration of activity that is seen with sildenafil and vardenafil appears to be suited to the average couples' patterns of sexual interaction. In a study of sexually active men aged 40 to 69 years both with and without ED, investigators found that the average frequency of sexual intercourse was one episode per week, and that the average time for foreplay was approximately 14 minutes; the vast majority (> 70%) of men studied reported that they had sex only once in a 24-hour period (64). The duration of activity that is seen with tadalafil, however, offers ED patients a new sexual paradigm. It is possible that sexual spontaneity may be enhanced by the long half-life.

The safety of all PDE-5 inhibitors is an important concern, since many men with ED also have cardiovascular disease. A careful assessment of cardiovascular status before prescribing treatments for ED and/or advising the patient to resume sexual activity is recommended. To date, there is no evidence that any of the PDE-5 inhibitors has any direct adverse cardiovascular effects. In fact, the reverse may be true, as studies suggest that sildenafil may delay exercise-induced ischemia and angina (64).

Other safety issues specific to tadalafil also need to be considered. Because of the drug's prolonged duration of action (i.e., approximately 17 hours in a healthy man and up to 21 hours in an elderly patient), it will take up to four days for tadalafil to be completely eliminated from the body. This could potentially extend the duration of adverse effects or delay intervention with nitroglycerin during a cardiac event. In addition, because tadalafil inhibits PDE-11, additional studies examining the effects of tadalafil on cardiac function are needed (64).

In general, the PDE-5 inhibitors are well tolerated and have similar mild-to-moderate adverse effects profiles. In clinical trials, the most commonly reported adverse events were vasodilation resulting in headache, nasal congestion, facial flushing, and dyspepsia. There appears to be a greater incidence of myalgia and low back pain with tadalafil, although the etiology of the myalgia remains unclear (64).

None of the PDE-5 inhibitors has any significant drug interactions, except for an absolute contraindication for the concomitant use of organic nitrates. All agents in this class potentiate nitrate-induced vasodilation. In addition, they are all metabolized by the CY3A4 isoenzyme system, and concomitant administration of inhibitors of this pathway (e.g., cimetidine, ketoconazole, erythromycin, and protease inhibitors) will prolong duration of action and raise serum concentrations of the drugs.

Vasodilator Agents

The use of oral vasoactive agents other than PDE inhibitors in the management of ED has garnered increasing interest, and evidence for the effectiveness of these agents in patients is currently under evaluation. With the exception of yohimbine, however, most of the available studies were performed on a small number of patients, with ill-defined pathophysiology. The studies underscore the need for development of new selective receptor modulators. The following is a brief description of available agents.

Yohimbine

Yohimbine (e.g., Yocon®, Yohimex®) is an indole alkaloid obtained from the bark of the African tree, *Pausinystalia yohimbine*. Since it has an α-2 adrenoceptor blocking action, it was initially thought to facilitate erectile function via a sympatholytic effect, similar to its chemical relative, reserpine. It was suggested that yohimbine facilitates erections by blocking central α-2 adrenoceptors and produces an increase in sympathetic drive and firing rate of neurons within the brain's noradrenergic nuclei (112). It has also been suggested that yohimbine is active at other CNS receptors, including some serotonergic and dopaminergic subtypes (116,117). Several studies (118), however, have shown yohimbine to induce a rise in blood pressure and plasma norepinephrine, suggesting that it also exerts peripheral adrenergic actions. Placebo-controlled studies have suggested the effectiveness of yohimbine (usually in doses of 4.5–6 mg three times daily) in treating erectile insufficiency due to psychogenic or mild organic etiology. The return of complete or partial erections in these studies ranges from 33% to 71% (119,120). A meta-analysis study of seven therapeutic trials with yohimbine found it to be superior to placebo in treatment of ED (odds ratio 3.85, 95% confidence interval 6.67 to 2.22) (121). Poor therapeutic effects of yohimbine were reported in several other studies, however, particularly in patients with clear organic etiology (122–124). The combination of yohimbine (5 mg three times daily) with other agents such as trazodone (50 mg once daily) produced higher response rates in patients with psychogenic impotence (72% of complete and partial erections), with 56% of patients continuing to draw clinical benefit after six months of treatment (125). Some authors have advocated the intake of yohimbine on an "as needed" basis (1–3 tablets swallowed 45–60 minutes before the sexual encounter) (117). In some cases, a single oral dose of 75-mg trazodone was also added. Higher doses of yohimbine are usually not tolerated due to an increased feeling of anxiety. Even on the small repeat dosing regimen, some patients may complain of dizziness, anxiety, nervousness, insomnia, nausea, headache, and muscle cramps.

Delquamine is another agent with a selective α-2 adrenoceptor antagonist property that shows promising therapeutic effects in treating impotence. It is undergoing evaluation in multicenter trials (126).

Phentolamine

Phentolamine induces relaxation of the corpus cavernosum erectile tissue by direct antagonism of both α-1 and α-2 adrenergic receptors and by indirect functional antagonism via a nonadrenergic, endothelium-mediated effect, possibly through nitric oxide synthesis activation (127). Previously, phentolamine has mainly been used as an adjuvant to other intracavernous vasoactive agents (see Chapter 30). An oral formulation of phentolamine mesylate (Vasomax®, formerly Zonagen Inc., now Repros Therapeutics), however, is currently under development for management of erectile insufficiency. Systemic administration of phentolamine may exert a central antianxiety effect in addition to the local vasodilatation effect on the corpus cavernosum. Gwinup (128) reported 68% successful intercourse 1.5 hours after oral intake of 50-mg Vasomax by impotent patients with various etiologies. The rate of response was somewhat lower (30–50%) in a double-blind, placebo-controlled study (129). Adverse effects associated with systemic phentolamine administration include nasal congestion, dizziness, tachycardia, and nausea (130–132). Currently, regulatory approval for the marketing of oral phentolamine has been obtained in Mexico and seven other Latin American countries; however, Vasomax is on partial clinical hold in the United States until the results of a mechanistic study on brown fat proliferation in rats demonstrate that similar brown fat proliferation is not expected to occur in humans (133).

Isoxsuprine

Isoxsuprine (Vasodilan®) is a β-2 adrenoceptor agonist that causes vasodilatation by direct stimulation of vascular smooth muscle. It is commonly used as an adjuvant therapy for patients with peripheral vascular disease. Data on its use in the management of ED, however, is scant. Hanash (134) reported a 35% success rate when isoxsuprine was used together with yohimbine in treatment of 79 impotent men. Knoll et al. (135) in a randomized cross-over study using the combination of isoxsuprine and yohimbine versus pentoxifylline in 20 impotent patients with mixed vasculogenic ED failed to show any therapeutic benefit of either regimen. Safarinejad (136) reported that isoxsuprine is no better than placebo as a first-line treatment for mixed-type ED. Further studies are therefore needed to clarify the role of agents with β-2 receptor stimulation properties in the treatment of male ED.

Pentoxifylline

Pentoxifylline (Trental®) is a xanthine derivative agent that is widely used in management of intermittent claudication. Pentoxifylline has two major therapeutic effects: an increase in flexibility of red blood cells and a vasodilatation property. These effects decrease blood viscosity, improve microcirculation, and enhance tissue oxygenation. Korenman and Viosca (137) used oral pentoxifylline (400 mg three times daily) in a double-blind placebo-controlled study of 18 impotent men with mild-to-moderate penile vascular insufficiency. Fourteen men were able to

reestablish the erectile function on pentoxifylline therapy. Further, the majority of patients had significant improvement in penile-brachial index. Patients with advanced diabetes mellitus, however, did not respond to pentoxifylline. The lack of efficacy of pentoxifylline in treating impotence in diabetic patients was further supported by a subsequent study in 34 men. Similarly, a study in 20 men with mixed vasculogenic impotence was unable to show a therapeutic benefit for pentoxifylline.

Other Agents

Limited studies have attempted the use of an oral PGE_1 derivative (Limaprost®) (138) and the nitric oxide donor L-arginine (139) to treat patients with erectile insufficiency with a subjective response rate ranging from 30% to 45%. Urinary nitrite and nitrate levels were initially low, and their concentrations doubled by six weeks of oral intake of L-arginine in the nine subjects with improved sexual performance (139). In a study examining the effect of dietary supplementation of L-arginine on penile erection and penile nitric oxide synthase (NOS) content and activity in the aging rat, serum and penile levels of L-arginine were found to increase by 64% to 148% in treated animals as compared to controls. Further, penile eNOS and nNOS content remained unchanged, but penile NOS activity increased nearly 100% in the L-arginine–treated animals. The authors postulated that L-arginine in the penis is likely to be the rate-limiting factor for NOS activity and that L-arginine intake may upregulate penile NOS activity but not tissue expression (140).

A number of herbal remedies used by native healers, mostly in eastern countries, as an oral treatment for ED, have been reviewed (141). Placebo-controlled clinical trials examining the efficacy and safety of these agents are currently scarce, and much of the available evidence is unsubstantiated. For example, no placebo control arm was included in the reported 88.9% improvement in erectile capacity induced by the daily intake of ArginMax®, a natural dietary supplement, in 25 patients with mild-to-moderate sexual dysfunction (142). A controlled study in rabbits, however, examined the effect of treatment with Korean red ginseng (mixed in physiologic saline solution and given by mouth) on acetylcholine-induced relaxation of cavernosal muscle strips precontracted with phenylephrine in vitro and on electrostimulation-induced rise in the intracavernosal pressure in vivo. Korean red ginseng-treated animals showed significantly enhanced erectile capacity over that of placebo-treated animals in both experiments (143). Careful scientific studies examining the safety and efficacy of these naturally occurring remedies in animals and human subjects must be awaited before the use of any agent can be accepted. (For further information on herbal and alternative remedies for sexual dysfunction, see Chapter 31.)

Centrally Acting Drugs

The use of centrally acting agents to target specific neuronal centers responsible for regulation of the erectile function provides an attractive therapeutic option, particularly for treating patients without local vascular disease or significant peripheral neuropathy. These studies are hampered, however, by the lack of clear identification of the various receptor subtypes participating in the regulation of erectile function, the relative contribution of each to the overall functional mechanisms, agent selectivity for the receptor subtypes, and the small number of patients involved in the reported studies. The following is a brief summary of these agents.

Trazodone

Trazodone (Desyrel®) is a triazolopyridine derivative that influences α-adrenergic, dopaminergic, and serotonergic functions and indirectly stimulates corporeal smooth-muscle relaxation. A number of publications have examined the effectiveness of trazodone in the treatment of ED. Its therapeutic use for management of erectile function remains controversial, since two controlled studies have failed to show a significant improvement in erectile function above that of placebo (144,145). A retrospective study, however, suggested that trazodone produces significant improvement in the erectile ability in 78% of patients less than 60 years of age and who have no known risk factors for ED. Smokers and patients older than 60 years with a history of peripheral vascular disease respond poorly to trazodone. Further, duration of ED was found to inversely relate to the response to trazodone (146). It is likely, therefore, that major therapeutic effects of trazodone on libido and erectile function are mediated by a central effect through the inhibition of serotonin reuptake and an increase in serotonin stimulation of the 5-HT-1c receptor (147). This appears to be at variance with the loss of libido induced by serotonin interaction with other receptor subtypes (148). Additional evidence suggests that trazodone may aid erectile function through α-adrenoceptor blockade and the subsequent reduction in the sympathetic tone (149). Improved libido, improved erectile function, prolonged erection, and priapism have been reported in about 200 patients who were treated for depression with trazodone (149,150). As a single agent, trazodone may restore erectile function in up to 60% of patients and is superior to placebo (144,151). Doses of trazodone used range from 50 mg once daily to 50 mg three times daily. Also, a single bedtime dose of 75 to 150 mg may increase the frequency and quality of morning erection (150). A simultaneous use of trazodone with yohimbine has been advocated (125,126), and its use in combination with PDE inhibitors remains to be evaluated. Major adverse effects of trazodone intake are drowsiness and sedation.

Apomorphine

Apomorphine alkaloids are naturally occurring dopaminergic agonists that may have been responsible for the psychotropic effects of waterlily tubers reported by the ancient Egyptians and the Maya (116). When administered subcutaneously, apomorphine induces bouts of yawning and penile erection in animals and humans (126). It has been used to induce emesis, induce sedation, and treat refractory on–off oscillations in Parkinson's disease. Subcutaneous administration of apomorphine has been shown to induce erection in approximately 60% of men with psychogenic ED (152). Its effects on sexual function appear to be due to central dopaminergic activities that lower the response threshold for erectile and ejaculatory reflexes (116) and, at least in rats, are mediated by the sacral parasympathetic and thoracolumbar sympathetic pathways (153). The subcutaneous use of apomorphine is discussed in further detail in Chapter 30.

A sublingual controlled absorption preparation of apomorphine (Uprima®, Abbott Laboratories, Chicago, Illinois, U.S.A.) has been marketed in Europe (114,154). In one study, doses of 3 and 4 mg were shown to induce erection in about 65% of a small sample of 12 patients with erectile insufficiency not due to organic etiologies (155). In another study using 2, 4, and 6 mg, slightly lower success rates were reported, with 47% to 53% of patients able to successfully obtain and maintain sufficient erections (156). Sequential administration, however, has been shown to improve the drug's effect (157). The safety profile of sublingual apomorphine in clinical studies in over 5000 patients with over 120,000 doses (2 and 3 mg) has been shown to be associated with few side effects, with the most common including nausea, headache, and dizziness (158). These side effects seem to be neurogenic (vasovagal), rather than cardiogenic in nature, and the use of a dose-optimization schedule was successful in reducing the incidence of side effects (156). Further, unlike sildenafil, it appears that apomorphine is not contraindicated in patients taking nitrates (158). Bromocriptine, a dopamine receptor agonist, may offer another therapeutic modality for the apomorphine-responsive men (159).

Naltrexone

Naltrexone (ReVia®) is a long-acting opiate antagonist. Naltrexone (25–50 mg daily) was reported to produce a full return of erectile function in six patients (160). Further, in two other placebo-controlled studies, naltrexone (50 mg daily) was shown to increase the frequency of morning erection and successful coital attempts (161,162) and to completely restore the erectile function in 20% of patients (163). The combination of opioid receptor blockade with yohimbine may increase the rate of return of erectile function over that obtained with the use of opiate antagonists alone (164). In the absence of history of substance abuse, there are no significant side effects at stated doses. A reversible elevation in liver enzymes, however, may occur at higher doses.

Fluoxetine

Fluoxetine (Prozac®) is a highly selective serotonin reuptake inhibitor that produces sexual side effects in up to 16% of patients receiving the agent for treatment of depression (165). Case reports of priapism have been reported with the use of fluoxetine, however. Mechanisms proposed to explain the conflicting sexual stimulation and inhibition effects of fluoxetine and other selective serotonin uptake inhibitor (SSRI) class of medications include selective blockade of 5-HT receptor subtypes, partial agonist/antagonist neurotransmission, and/or receptor downregulation with subsequent activation of central serotonin release (116). As a significant lengthening of the ejaculatory reflex is commonly seen with SSRI, these agents are best suited for the treatment of premature ejaculation.

☐ TREATMENT OF DISORDERS OF EJACULATION

Table 1 outlines available therapeutic therapies for the various ejaculatory disorders.

Treatment of Premature Ejaculation
Serotonergic Antidepressants

Several scientific articles and reviews have addressed the use of serotonergic drugs in treating patients with premature ejaculation (4,166,167). Data earlier than 1995 on the use of clomipramine were reviewed by Althof (167) and by Harvey and Balon (4). These data indicate that clomipramine at doses from 25 to 50 mg is effective in prolonging the intravaginal intercourse to at least two minutes in about 70% of men, compared to a 10% improvement in patients treated with placebo. Further, a study by Segraves et al. (168) suggested that the intake of clomipramine could be limited to the day of intercourse. The minimum time between drug ingestion and maximum ejaculatory control, however, has not yet been fully established. A prospective, double-blind, placebo-controlled, cross-over design study examined the effect of 25 mg clomipramine, ingested as needed, 12 to 24 hours before anticipated sexual activity (coitus or masturbation) was evaluated in eight patients with primary premature ejaculation, six with combined premature ejaculation and ED, and eight controls (169). Significant increase in ejaculatory latency from two to eight minutes was reported by men with primary premature ejaculation but not by the other two groups of patients. Clomipramine inhibited nocturnal penile tumescence in all subjects. Moreover, the mechanism(s) by which clomipramine retards the ejaculatory latency is not totally clear. Clomipramine is a tricyclic antidepressant, which also acts centrally at the 5-HT-2 receptor to inhibit serotonin reuptake and thus promotes serotonin activities. Some

studies have suggested, however, that clomipramine increases the sensory threshold for stimuli in the genital area (170), possibly through the inhibition of the adrenergic receptors in the peripheral sympathetic system (171). The effect of clomipramine on sexual function is not always consistent, and both spontaneous orgasms and ejaculation (172) and anorgasmia (173) have been reported to occur in some patients. Painful ejaculation is another possible side effect to the intake of clomipramine (174).

SSRIs, including sertraline (Zoloft®), fluoxetine (Prozac®), and paroxetine (Paxil®), have also been used to treat premature ejaculation (174–180). Similar to clomipramine, these agents also have the potential for inducing variable effects on sexual function, including spontaneous orgasms and ejaculation, anorgasmia, or painful ejaculation (34,166,173). Further, the earlier reports on treatment of premature ejaculation with antidepressants have been criticized by Althof (167) for the following reasons: (i) relying on the subject's self-report of ejaculatory latency; (ii) inconsistent adherence to strict controls, dosages, washout periods, or investigator blindness; (iii) lack of long-term follow-up; (iv) lack of determination of drug effects on psychosocial or other sexual parameters; and (v) lack of distinction between life-long and acquired conditions. More recent reports have been placebo controlled (178–180), and one study measured penile sensory threshold, sacral-evoked response, and cortical somatosensory-evoked potential testing to gain insight into the mechanism of drug action (180). In this study, fluoxetine increased the penile sensory threshold, without changing the amplitude and latencies of sacral-evoked response and cortical somatosensory-evoked potential.

α-Adrenergic Receptor Blockers

The use of α-adrenergic receptor blockers to delay premature ejaculation is based on the understanding that the sympathetic nervous system is responsible for the peristaltic movement of the seminal fluid through the male genital tract. Shilon et al. (181) administered phenoxybenzamine to nine men with premature ejaculation, seven of whom reported an increase in their ejaculatory latencies. Cavallini (182) reported the effects of treatment with two other α-1-blockers (alphuzosin and terazosine) on premature ejaculation in 91 men who were resistant to psychological therapy. The study was a double-blind, placebo-controlled, cross-over in which each drug and placebo were administered for two months. Approximately 50% of patients and their partners reported improved ejaculatory latencies for both α-blocking agents, as compared to approximately 13% for patients on placebo. Side effects, mainly hypotension and epigastric pain, were experienced by about 5% of patients on active drug. Another side effect of α-receptor blockade reported in the above referenced study with phenoxybenzamine is dry ejaculation (ejaculation without expulsion of the seminal fluid). These preliminary studies suggest that the effectiveness of α-blockers in treating premature ejaculation is close to that seen in treatment of benign prostatic hyperplasia (183). The final assessment of the role of α-receptor blocking agents in treating premature ejaculation, however, must await the results of large well-controlled trials to examine both efficacy and safety of long-term use.

Treatment of Absent or Retarded Ejaculation

Retrograde ejaculation (RE) results from damage to the sympathetic innervation of the ejaculatory system and bladder neck. Such a condition may follow injury to the spinal cord or cauda equina, retroperitoneal lymphadenectomy, radical prostatectomy, or extensive abdominal surgery. RE can also be associated with diabetic autonomic neuropathy or with intake of α-adrenergic blocking agents. A nerve-sparing surgical technique or adequate control of hyperglycemia may guard against the development of such a complication. Moreover, patients in whom RE is traceable to the ingestion of α-adrenergic drugs may benefit from trial with alternate classes of medications. Similarly, patients with bladder neck incompetence due to injury may be considered for surgical reconstruction, although the success of this procedure is usually limited. The majority of patients with established dysfunction may not, however, have an existing modifiable condition. Such patients could be considered for therapy with either an α-adrenergic agent (e.g., ephedrine or midodrine) or an imipramine (a tricyclic antidepressant of the dibenzazepine group of compounds). Generally, restoration of successful antegrade ejaculation with these agents is possible in approximately 30% of patients with diabetic neuropathy or postretroperitoneal lymphadenectomy (184–186).

□ TREATMENT OF ABSENCE OF ORGASM

Since the most common etiology of anorgasmia is the intake of pharmacological agents (such as the SSRIs, the tricyclic antidepressants, or the monoamine oxidase inhibitors), regaining of the orgasmic sensation may be achieved with discontinuation of the inciting drug and, when possible, substitution with an alternate psychotropic. For example, fluoxetine-associated sexual dysfunction was shown to improve after switching to therapy with bupropion (an antidepressant that inhibits the reuptake of serotonin and norepinephrine and decreases whole body norepinephrine turnover in man) or nefazodone (an antidepressant known as Serzone® with multiple sites of action, including inhibition of neuronal uptake of serotonin and norepinephrine and antagonism of 5-HT-2 and α-1 adrenergic receptors) (187–189). Another therapeutic strategy is to discontinue intake of the inciting agent temporarily for one or two days of each week during which sexual activity is contemplated. Such an approach has been termed a "drug holiday" and is not associated with the exacerbation of

the underlying psychiatric condition in patients treated with sertraline or paroxetine (190). Specific pharmacological agents were also shown to be effective in counteracting the orgasmic inhibition of certain drugs (191,192). For example, cyproheptadine (an agent with both anticholinergic and antiserotonergic properties) has been reported to counteract anorgasmia induced by selective serotonin reuptake inhibitors (fluoxetine and fluvoxamine), tricyclic antidepressants (clomipramine), and monoamine oxidase inhibitors (193). The usual dosage is 4 to 16 mg taken 1 to 2 hours prior to coitus (3). Intermittent dosing of amantadine, 100 mg taken five to six hours prior to coitus, was also reported to be successful in the treatment off luoxetine-induced anorgasmia (194). Similarly, yohimbine (10 mg, orally) can reverse clomipramine-induced anorgasmia (195).

□ TREATMENT OF FAILURE OF DETUMESCENCE

Table 1 outlines the various therapeutic options for the management of failure of detumescence.

Modification of Inciting Systemic Drug Therapy

Priapism that is associated with systemic drug ingestion such as phenothiazines and trazodone should be treated with drug dose reduction, or, when possible, with drug substitution. Patients who are on illicit drugs such as cocaine should be counseled with rehabilitation programs. Cocaine-induced priapism can be a high-flow variant that is refractory to therapy (Fig. 2). In some cases, treatment of cocaine-induced priapism may require shunt placement or even partial penectomy (196).

Arterial high-flow priapism, which is caused by arterial-lacunar fistula and is characterized by delayed onset of a constant, painless, nontender erection after blunt trauma, can be treated with mechanical compression, surgical resection of the fistula and ligation of the internal pudendal or cavernous arteries, selective internal pudendal arteriography with transcatheter embolization, or watchful waiting. The latter two modalities have been reported to be associated with excellent rates of long-term resolution and restoration of erectile function (198,199). (For further information on priapism, see Chapter 18.)

Medical Treatment of Peyronie's Disease

Treatment of structural penile diseases depends upon the nature of the underlying disease. Peyronie's disease can be self-limiting in many cases and may not require therapeutic intervention. Medical treatment is suitable in the acute phase (less than 12 months) of the disease when the plaque is unstable. Oral therapeutic agents may include vitamin E, p-aminobenzoate (Potaba®), colchicine, or tamoxifen. Generally, use of these agents could be useful in patients with mild-to-moderate

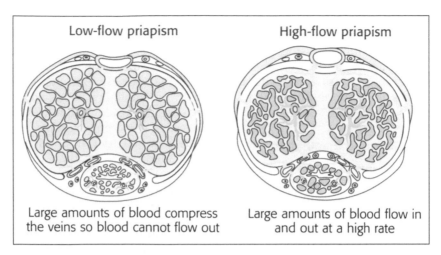

Low-flow priapism | High-flow priapism

Large amounts of blood compress the veins so blood cannot flow out | Large amounts of blood flow in and out at a high rate

Figure 2 Priapism is a painful, prolonged erection, lasting more than four hours, in the absence of sexual desire. It can be caused by intracavernosal therapy or the use of oral pharmacological agents such as trazodone, chlorpromazine, or prazosin. Conditions such as sickle-cell anemia, leukemia, metastatic cancer, and trauma can also produce priapism. There are two types of priapism: low flow, the more common type, and high flow, which is very rare and related to injury of the perineum. High-flow priapism can occur intermittently. With low-flow priapism, the erection must be relieved within 12 hours. Under local anesthetic, blood will be taken from the penis with a syringe to lower the pressure and relieve the discomfort. The corpora cavernosa are then flushed with saline to remove any blood clots. If this does not work, a drug (phenylephrine) can be given to constrict the blood vessels and reduce the blood flow to the penis. This will be repeated as necessary. If unsuccessful, surgery may be required. If the condition has persisted for 24 hours or more, surgery is likely to fail. The priapism can eventually lead to fibrosis, making recovery unlikely. *Source*: From Ref. 197.

disease and is associated with 30% to 50% reduction in plaque size and/or shaft deformity. In addition, erection-associated pain is reduced by 60% to 80% (200). Other forms of medical therapy may include local or systemic glucocorticoids and the intralesional injection of a collagenase or a calcium channel blocker (e.g., verapamil). These locally administered agents appear to have approximately the same therapeutic effects as the systemic medications. Medical therapy may help patients with moderate disease, whereas surgical correction is the treatment of choice for those with severe penile deformity. (For further details on Peyronie's, see Chapters 17 and 34.)

□ CONCLUSION

Significant advances have been made over the past three decades in the way of developing effective treatments for the various forms of male sexual dysfunction. The discovery of nitric oxide and cGMP as important neurochemicals regulating the function of the corporeal smooth-muscle cells has led to the development of the first orally administered inhibitor of penile-specific PDE isoenzyme-5 as a promising effective treatment for ED. More complete characterization of the physiologic importance of other vasoactive and neuroactive peptides and amines found in the penis will lead to the development of additional physiologically based therapeutic drug interventions that are both safe and efficacious.

Currently, several clinical trials are evaluating the efficacy of single and combined use of other oral agents in treatment of ED. These include a myriad of agents with varying peripheral and central activities, such as PDE-5 inhibitors, the α-adrenoceptor antagonists yohimbine, delquamine, and phentolamine, the β-2-receptor agonist isoxsuprine, the dopamine agonist apomorphine, the antidepressants trazodone and fluoxetine, and the opioid receptor blocker naltrexone. For instance, a synergistic effect has been reported with combined sildenafil and doxazosin oral therapy for nonorganic ED (201). The addition of an antiadrenergic drug was thought to reduce penile vasoconstrictive tone, thereby enhancing the vasoactive effects of sildenafil. Similarly, the combinations of apomorphine and sildenafil and apomorphine and α-1 adrenoreceptor antagonists may also have therapeutic potential in patients who do not respond to single-drug treatment. Thus, there is a rational for combinations of existing oral therapies. Controlled clinical trials need to be performed to optimize the potential advantages and reduce possible side effects.

Significant physiologic and pathophysiologic data are currently accumulating on the role of central neuromediators in the regulation of sexual drive, erectile control, and perception of orgasmic pleasure. It is hoped that this knowledge will lead to the development of pharmacologic agents that are highly selective in targeting these regulatory sites. For example, the development of highly selective serotonergic agonists for the 5-HT-1c receptor subtype would greatly improve the ability to treat loss of libido and erection without experiencing the untoward and often contradictory effects of serotonin interaction with other receptor subtypes. Similarly, the development of highly selective central α-2 adrenoceptor antagonists and peripheral β-2 adrenoceptor agonists will help to treat impotence without the side effects induced by excessive stimulation of peripheral α-1 adrenoceptor subtype. Moreover, studies with newer antidepressants and other psychotropics are increasingly improving our understanding of pathogenesis and consequently our ability to treat premature ejaculation and anorgasmia.

Several issues remain unresolved regarding the use of antidepressants and pharmacological agents in the treatment of male sexual dysfunction; these include the determination of the efficacy of a drug holiday (daily drug intake vs. treatment on the day of sexual encounter), the minimum required time from drug ingestion to the intended sexual activity, the effectiveness of single agent versus combination regimens, total duration of treatment required for certain types of sexual dysfunction (e.g., premature ejaculation, and orgasmic disorders), and the indications for, and methods of, combining pharmacological therapy with behavioral counseling. Similarly, the use of androgen supplementation of men with erectile difficulties and low-normal bioavailable testosterone needs critical revisiting, particularly in view of the data implicating androgens in local regulation of penile NOS production and action. Further work is needed to advance and refine the development of new therapeutic approaches such as the use of topically applied vasoactive agents, more selective PDE-5 inhibitors, and gene therapy interventions in the treatment of erectile insufficiency.

☐ REFERENCES

1. Kandeel FR, Koussa VKT, Swerdloff RS. Male sexual function and its disorders: physiology, pathophysiology, clinical investigation and treatment. Endocr Rev 2001; 22(3):343–388.

2. Hyyppa M, Rinne UK, Sonninen V. The activating effect of L-dopa treatment on sexual functions and its experimental background. Acta Neurol Scand 1970; 46(suppl 43):223.

3. Segraves RT. Effects of psychotropic drugs on human erection and ejaculation. Arch Gen Psychiatry 1989; 46(3):275–284.

4. Harvey KV, Balon R. Clinical implications of antidepressant drug effects on sexual function. Ann Clin Psychiatry 1995; 7(4):189–201.

5. Jenkins RB, Groh RH. Mental symptoms in Parkinsonian patients treated with L-dopa. Lancet 1970; 2(7665):177–179.

6. Barbeau A. L-dopa therapy in Parkinson's disease: a critical review of nine years' experience. Can Med Assoc J 1969; 101(13):59–68.

7. O'Carroll R, Shapiro C, Bancroft J. Androgens, behavior and nocturnal erection in hypogonadal men: the effects of varying the replacement dose. Clin Endocrinol 1985; 23(5):527–538.

8. Morley JE. Impotence. Am J Med 1986; 80(5):897–905.

9. Armstrong EG, Villee CA. Characterization and comparison of estrogen and androgen receptors of calf anterior pituitary. J Steroid Biochem 1977; 8(4):285–292.

10. Lloyd RV, Karavolas HJ. Uptake and conversion of progesterone and testosterone to 5alpha-reduced products by enriched gonadotropic and chromophobic rat anterior pituitary cell fractions. Endocrinology 1975; 97(3):517–526.

11. Davidson JM, Camargo CA, Smith ER. Effects of androgen on sexual behavior in hypogonadal men. J Clin Endocrinol Metab 1979; 48(6):955–958.

12. Arver S, Dobs AS, Meikle AW, et al. Improvement of sexual function in testosterone deficient men treated for 1 year with a permeation enhanced testosterone transdermal system. J Urol 1996; 155(5):1604–1608.

13. Nicholls DP, Anderson DC. Clinical aspects of androgen deficiency in men. Andrologia 1982; 14(5):379–388.

14. Wu FC, Bancroft J, Davidson DW, et al. The behavioural effects of testosterone undecanoate in adult men with Klinefelter's syndrome: a controlled study. Clin Endocrinol 1982; 16(5):489–497.

15. Rosen RC, Leiblum SR. Hypoactive sexual desire. Psychiatr Clin North Am 1995; 18(1):107–121.

16. Beck JG. Hypoactive sexual desire disorder: an overview. J Consult Clin Psychol 1995; 63(6):919–927.

17. O'Carroll R, Bancroft J. Testosterone therapy for low sexual interest and erectile dysfunction in men: a controlled study. Br J Psychiatry 1984; 145(2):146–151.

18. Buvat J, Lemaire A, Buvat-Herbaut M. Human chorionic gonadotropin treatment of nonorganic erectile failure and lack of sexual desire: a double blind study. Urology 1987; 30(3):216–219.

19. Snyder PJ, Lawrence DA. Treatment of male hypogonadism with testosterone enanthate. J Clin Endocrinol Metab 1980; 51(6):1335–1339.

20. Carani C, Granata AR, Bancroft J, et al. The effects of testosterone replacement on nocturnal penile tumescence and rigidity and erectile response to visual erotic stimuli in hypogonadal men. Psychoneuroendocrinology 1995; 20(7):743–753.

21. Medical Economics Data Production Company. Physicians' Desk Reference. 50th ed. Montvale, NY: Medical Economics Data Production Company, 1996.

22. Cofrancesco J, Dobs AS. Transdermal testosterone delivery systems. Endocrinologist 1996; 6:207–213.

23. Parker S, Armitage M. Experience with transdermal testosterone replacement for hypogonadal men. Clin Endocrinol 1999; 50(1):57–62.

24. Wang C, Berman N, Longstreth JA, et al. Pharmokinetics of transdermal testosterone gel in hypogonadal men: application of gel at one site versus four sites: a general clinical research center study. J Clin Endocrinol Metab 2000; 85(3):964–969.

25. Dobs AS, Meikle AW, Arver S, et al. Pharmokinetics, efficacy, and safety of a permeation-enhanced testosterone transdermal system in comparison with bi-weekly injections of testosterone enanthate for the treatment of hypogonal men. J Clin Endocrinol Metab 1999; 84(10):3469–3478.

26. Korenman SG, Viosca S, Garza D, et al. Androgen therapy of hypogonadal men with transscrotal testosterone systems. Am J Med 1987; 83(3):471–478.

27. Jordan WP. Allergy and topical irritation associated with transdermal testosterone administration: a comparison of scrotal and nonscrotal transdermal systems. Am J Contact Dermat 1997; 8(2):108–113.

28. Feldman HA, Goldstein I, Hatzichristou DG, et al. Impotence and its medical and psychosocial correlates: results of the Massachusetts male aging study. J Urol 1994; 151(1):54–61.

29. Reiter WJ, Pycha A, Schatzl G, et al. Dehydroepiandrosterone in the treatment of erectile dysfunction: a prospective, double-blind, randomized, placebo-controlled study. Urology 1999; 53(3):590–594.

30. Korenman SG. Androgen function after age 50 years and treatment of hypogonadism. In: Bardin CW, ed. Current Therapy in Endocrinology and Metabolism. 5th ed. St. Louis: Mosby Year Book, 1994:585–587.

31. Morales A, Johnston B, Heaton JP, et al. Testosterone supplementation for hypogonadal impotence: assessment of biochemical measures and therapeutic outcomes. J Urol 1997; 157(3):849–854.

32. Loughlin KR, Richie JP. Prostate cancer after exogenous testosterone treatment for impotence. J Urol 1997; 157(5):1845.

33. Sih R, Morley JE, Kaiser FE, et al. Testosterone replacement in older hypogonadal men: a 12-month randomized controlled trial. J Clin Endocrinol Metab 1997; 82(6):1661–1667.

34. Margolese HC, Assalian P. Sexual side effects of antidepressants: a review. J Sex Marital Ther 1996; 22(3):209–217.

35. Hull EM, Du J, Lorrain DS, et al. Testosterone, preoptic dopamine, and copulation in male rats. Brain Res Bull 1997; 44(4):327–333.

36. Gessa GL, Tagliamonte A. Role of brain monoamines in male sexual behavior. Life Sci 1974; 14(3):425–436.

37. O'Brien CP, DiGiacomo JN, Fahn S, et al. Mental effects of high-dosage levodopa. Arch Gen Psychiatry 1971; 24(1):61–64.

38. Sathananthan G, Angrist BM, Gershon S. Response threshold to L-dopa in psychiatric patients. Biol Psychiatry 1973; 7:139–146.

39. Bowers MB, vanWoert M, Davis L. Sexual behavior during L-dopa treatment for Parkinsonism. Am J Psychiatry 1971; 127(12):1691–1693.

40. Colao A, Sarno AD, Sarnacchiaro F, et al. Prolactinomas resistant to standard dopamine agonists respond to chronic cabergoline treatment. J Clin Endocrinol Metab 1997; 82(3):876–883.

41. Colao A, Sarno AD, Landi ML, et al. Long-term and low-dose treatment with cabergoline induces macroprolactinoma shrinkage. J Clin Endocrinol Metab 1997; 82(11):3574–3579.

42. DeRosa M, Colao A, Sarno AD, et al. Cabergoline treatment rapidly improves gonadal function in hyperprolactinemic males: a comparison with bromocriptine. Eur J Endocrinol 1998; 138(3):286–293.

43. Ferrari C, Paracchi A, Mattei AM, et al. Cabergoline in the long-term therapy of hyperprolactinemic disorders. Acta Endocrinol (Copenh) 1992; 126(6):489–494.

44. Crenshaw TL, Goldberg JP, Stern WC. Pharmacologic modification of psychosexual dysfunction. J Sex Marital Ther 1987; 13(4):239–252.

45. Gartrell N. Increased libido in women receiving trazodone. Am J Psychiatry 1986; 143(6):781–782.

46. Sullivan G. Increased libido in three men treated with trazodone. J Clin Psychiatry 1988; 49:202–203.

47. Michael A, Owen A. Venlafaxine-induced increased libido and spontaneous erections. Br J Psychiatry 1997; 170(2):193.

48. Stevenson RW, Solyom L. The aphrodisiac effect of fenfluramine: two case reports of a possible side effect to the use of fenfluramine in the treatment of bulimia. J Clin Psychopharmacol 1990; 10(1):69–71.

49. Medical Economics Data Production Company. Physicians' Desk Reference, 53rd ed. Montvale, NY: Medical Economics Data Production Company, 1999.

50. Hollander E, McCarley A. Yohimbine treatment of sexual side effects induced by serotonin reuptake blockers. J Clin Psychiatry 1992; 53(6):207–209.

51. Nishimura K, Matsumiya K, Tsuboniwa N, et al. Bromocriptine for infertile males with mild hyperprolactinemia: hormonal and spermatogenic effects. Arch Androl 1999; 43(3):207–213.

52. Handelsman DJ, Swerdloff RS. Male gonadal dysfunction. J Clin Endocrinol Metab 1985; 14(1):89–124.

53. Perryman RL, Rogol AD, Kaiser DL, et al. Pergolide mesylate: its effects on circulating anterior pituitary hormones in man. J Clin Endocrinol Metab 1981; 53(4):772–778.

54. McClure RD, Oses R, Ernest ML. Hypogonadal impotence treated by transdermal testosterone. Urology 1991; 37(3):224–228.

55. Nachtigall LB, Boepple PA, Pralong FP, et al. Adult-onset idiopathic hypogonadotropic hypogonadism—a treatable form of male infertility. N Engl J Med 1997; 336(6):410–415.

56. Winters SJ, Troen P. Hypogonadotropin hypogonadism: gonadotropin therapy. In: Krieger DT, Bardin CW, eds. Current Therapy in Endocrinology and Metabolism. Toronto: BC Deker Inc., 1985:152–154.

57. Zini D, Carani C, Baldini A, et al. Sexual behavior of men with isolated hypogonadotropic hypogonadism or prepubertal anterior panhypopituitarism. Horm Behav 1990; 24(2):174–185.

58. Spratt DI, Crowley WF. Hypogonadotropic hypogonadism: GnRH therapy. In: Krieger DT, Bardin CW, eds. Current Therapy in Endocrinology and Metabolism. Toronto: BC Becker, Inc., 1985:155–159.

59. McKinlay JB. The worldwide prevalence and epidemiology of erectile dysfunction. Int J Impot Res 2000; 12 (suppl 4):S6–S11.

60. Carvajal JA, Germain AM, Huidobro-Toro JP, et al. Molecular mechanism of cGMP mediated smooth muscle relaxation. J Cell Physiol 2000; 184(3):409.

61. Omrod D, Easthope SE, Figgitt DP. Vardenafil. Drugs Aging 2002; 19(3):217–227.

62. Levine LA. New oral agents for erectile dysfunction. (http://www.irwingoldsteinmd.com/PPublications. html#noaf).

63. Porst H. IC351 (tadalafil, Cialis). Update on clinical experience. Int J Impot Res 2002; 14(suppl 1):S57–S64.

64. Kuritzky L, Samraj G. How to choose among the PDE5 inhibitors for erectile dysfunction. Patient Care 2003; 37:52–61.

65. Gbekor E, Bethell S, Fawcett L, et al. Phosphodiesterase 5 inhibitor profiles against all human phosphodiesterase families: implications for use as pharmacological tools [abstr 244]. Eur Urol 2002; 1(suppl 1):63.

66. Ballard SA, Gingell CJ, Tang K, et al. Effects of sildenafil on the relaxation of human corpus cavernosum tissue in vitro and on the activities of cyclic nucleotide phoshpodiesterase isozymes. J Urol 1998; 159(6): 2164–2171.

67. Goldstein I. Current and emerging medical therapies for male erectile dysfunction. (http://www.irwin-goldsteinmd.com/PPublications.html#caem).

68. Kim NN. Phosphodiesterase type 5 inhibitors: a biochemical and clinical correlation survey. Int J Impot Res 2003; 15(suppl 5):S13–S19.

69. Montorsi F, Althof SE, Sweeney M, et al. Treatment satisfaction in patients with erectile dysfunction switching from prostaglandin E1 intracavernosal injection therapy to oral sildenafil citrate. Int J Impot Res 2003; 15(6):444–449.

70. Boolell M, Allen MJ, Ballard SA, et al. Sildenafil: an orally active type 5 cyclic GMP-specific phosphodiesterase inhibitor for the treatment of penile erectile dysfunction. Int J Impot Res 1996; 8(2):47–52.

71. Goldenberg MM. Safety and efficacy of sildenafil citrate in the treatment of male erectile dysfunction. Clin Ther 1998; 20(6):1033–1048.

72. Langtry HD, Markham A. Sildenafil: a review of its use in erectile dysfunction. Drugs 1999; 57(6):967–989.

73. Rosen RC, Fisher WA, Eardley I, et al. The multinational Men's Attitudes to Life Events and Sexuality (MALES) study: I. Prevalence of erectile dysfunction and related health concerns in the general population. Curr Med Res Opin 2004; 20(5):607–617.

74. Levine LA, Latchamsetty KC. Treatment of erectile dysfunction in patients with Peyronie's disease using sildenafil citrate. Int J Impot Res 2002; 14(6):478–482.

75. Klotz T, Mathers M, Sommer F. Preliminary report: why do patients with erectile dysfunction abandon effective therapy with sildenafil (Viagra)? Int J Impot Res 2005; 17(1):2–4.

76. Rendell MS, Rajfer J, Wicker PA, et al. Sildenafil for treatment of erectile dysfunction in men with diabetes: a randomized controlled trial. Sildenafil diabetes study group. JAMA 1999; 281(5):421–426.

77. Jarow JP, Burnett AL, Geringer AM. Clinical efficacy of sildenafil citrate based on etiology and response to prior treatment. J Urol 1999; 162(3 Pt 1):722–725.

78. Derry FA, Dinsmore WW, Fraser M, et al. Efficacy and safety of oral sildenafil (Viagra) in men with erectile dysfunction caused by spinal cord injury. Neurology 1998; 51(6):1629–1633.

79. Zippe CD, Kedia AW, Kedia K, et al. Treatment of erectile dysfunction after radical prostatectomy with sildenafil citrate (Viagra). Urology 1998; 52(6): 963–966.

80. Zelefsky MJ, McKee AB, Lee H, et al. Efficacy of oral sildenafil in patients with erectile dysfunction after radiotherapy for carcinoma of the prostate. Urology 1999; 53(4):775–778.

81. Goldstein I, Lue TF, Padma-Nathan H, et al. Oral sildenafil in the treatment of erectile dysfunction. Sildenafil study group. N Engl J Med 1998; 338(20):1397–1404.

82. Morales A, Gingell C, Collins M, et al. Clinical safety of oral sildenafil citrate (VIAGRA) in the treatment of erectile dysfunction. Int J Impot Res 1998; 10(2):69–73.

83. Conti CR, Pepine CJ, Sweeney M. Efficacy and safety of sildenafil citrate in the treatment of erectile dysfunction in patients with ischemic heart disease. Am J Cardiol 1999; 83(5A):C29–C34.

84. Cheitlin MD, Hutter AM, Brindis RG, et al. ACC/AHA expert consensus document. Use of sildenafil (Viagra) in patients with cardiovascular disease. American College of Cardiology/American Heart Association. J Am Coll Cardiol 1999; 33(1):273–282.

85. McCullough A. Sildenafil (Viagra™) one year later: a retrospective. Sex Dysfunc Med 1999; 1:2–7.

86. Sunwoo S, Kim YS, Cho BL, et al. Post-marketing surveillance study of the safety and efficacy of sildenafil prescribed in primary care to erectile dysfunction patients. Int J Impot Res 2005; 17(1):71–75.

87. McCullough AR, Barada JH, Fawzy A, et al. Achieving treatment optimization with sildenafil citrate (Viagra) in patients with erectile dysfunction. Urol 2002; 60(2 suppl 2): 28–38.

88. McMahon GG. High dose sildenafil citrate as a salvage therapy for severe erectile dysfunction. Int J Impot Res 2002; 14:533–538.

89. Jiann B.-P, Yu C.-C, Su C.-C. Rechallenge prior sildenafil nonresponders. Int J Impot Res 2004; 16(1):64–68.

90. Vallance P, Collier J, Moncada S. Effects of endothelium-derived nitric oxide on peripheral arteriolar tone in man. Lancet 1989; 2(8670):997–1000.

91. Umans JG, Levi R. Nitric oxide in the regulation of blood flow and arterial pressure. Annu Rev Physiol 1995; 57:771–790.

92. Webb DJ, Freestone S, Allen MJ, et al. Sildenafil citrate and blood-pressure-lowering drugs: results of drug interaction studies with an organic nitrate and a calcium antagonist. Am J Cardiol 1999; 83(5A): 21–28.

93. Jackson G, Benjamin N, Jackson N, et al. Effects of sildenafil citrate on human hemodynamics. Am J Cardiol 1999; 83(5A):13–20.

94. Wallis RM, Corbin JC, Francis SH, et al. Tissue distribution of phosphodiesterase families and the effects of sildenafil on tissue cyclic nucleotides, platelet function, and the contractile responses of trabeculae carneae and aortic rings in vitro. Am J Cardiol 1999; 83(5A):C3–C12.

95. Kloner RA, Zusman RM. Cardiovascular effects of sildenafil citrate and recommendations for its use. Am J Cardiol 1999; 84(5B):N11–N17.

96. Zusman RM, Morales A, Glasser DB, et al. Overall cardiovascular profile of sildenafil citrate. Am J Cardiol 1999; 83(5A):C35–C44.

97. Kloner RA. Cardiovascular risk factors and erectile dysfunction. Am J Manag Care 1999; 5(suppl):31–39.

98. Mueller JE, Mittleman MA, Maclure M. Triggering myocardial infarction by sexual activity: low absolute risk and prevention by regular physical exercise. J Am Med Assoc 1996; 275(18):1405–1409.

99. Feenstra J, van Drie-Pierick FJ, Lacle CF, et al. Acute myocardial infarction associated with sildenafil. Lancet 1998; 352:957–958.

100. Vobig MA, Klotz T, Staak M, et al. Retinal side-effects of sildenafil. Lancet 1999; 353(9162):375.

101. Patterson B, Bedding A, Jewell H, et al. The effect of intrinsic and extrinsic factors on the pharmacokinetic properties of tadalafil (IC351). 4th Biennial Congress of the European Society for Sexual and Impotence Research, Rome, Italy, Sep 30–Oct 3, 2001.

102. www.fda.gov/fdac/departs/2005/505_upd.htm.

103. Laties AM, Fraunfelder FT. Ocular safety of Viagra, (sildenafil citrate). Trans Am Ophthalmol Soc 1999; 97:115–125.

104. Keating GM, Scott LJ. Spotlight on vardenafil in erectile dysfunction. Drugs Aging 2004; 21(2):135–140.

105. Donatucci C, Eardley I, Buvat J et al. Vardenafil improves erectile function in men with erectile dysfunction irrespective of disease severity and disease classification. J Sex Med 2004; 1(3):301–309.

106. van Ahlen H, Wahle K, Kupper W. Safety and efficacy of vardenafil, a selective phosphodiesterase 5 inhibitor, in patients with erectile dysfunction and arterial hypertension treated with multiple antihypertensives. J Sex Med 2005; 2(6):856–864.

107. Young JM, Feldman RA, Auerbach SM, et al. Tadalafil improved erectile function at twenty-four and thirty-six hours after dosing in men with erectile dysfunction: US trial. J Androl 2005; 26(3):310–318.

108. Fardley I, Mirone V, Montorsi F, et al. An open-label, multicentre, randomized, crossover study comparing sildenafil citrate and tadalafil for treating erectile dysfunction in men naive to phosphodiesterase 5 inhibitor therapy. BJU Int 2005; 96(9):1323–1332.

109. Skoumal R, Chen J, Kula K, et al. Efficacy and treatment satisfaction with on-demand tadalafil (Cialis) in men with erectile dysfunction. Eur Urol 2004; 46(3): 362–369.

110. Lewis RW, Sadovsky R, Eardley I. The efficacy of tadalafil in clinical populations. J Sex Med 2005; 2(4):517–531.

111. Carson C, Shabsigh R, Segal S. Efficacy, safety, and treatment satisfaction of tadalafil versus placebo in patients with erectile dysfunction evaluated at tertiary-care academic centers. Urology 2005; 5(2):353–359.

112. Carrier S, Brock GB, Pommerville PJ. Efficacy and safety of oral tadalafil in the treatment of men in Canada with erectile dysfunction: a randomized, double-blind, parallel, placebo-controlled clinical trial. J Sex Med 2005; 2(5):685–698.

113. Seftel AD, Wilson SK, Knapp PM. The efficacy and safety of tadalafil in United States and Puerto Rican men with erectile dysfunction. J Urol 2004; 172(2): 652–657.

114. Padma-Nathan H, Giuliano F. Oral drug therapy for erectile dysfunction. Urol Clin North Am 2001; 28(2):321–334.

115. Padma-Nathan H, McMurray JG, Pullman WE, et al. On-demand IC351 (Cialis) enhances erectile function in patients with erectile dysfunction. Int J Impot Res 2001; 13(1):2–9.

116. Montorsi F, Guazzoni G, Rigatti P, et al. Pharmacological management of erectile dysfunction. Drugs 1995; 50(3):465–479.

117. Riley A. Oral treatments for erectile dysfunction. Int J STD AIDS 1996; 7(suppl 3):16–18.

118. Grossman E, Rosenthal T, Peleg E, et al. Oral yohimbine increases blood pressure and sympathetic nervous outflow in hypertensive patients. J Cardiovasc Pharmacol 1993; 22(1):22–26.

119. Reid K, Surridge DH, Morales A, et al. Double-blind trial of yohimbine in treatment of psychogenic impotence. Lancet 1987; 2(8556):421–423.

120. Vogt HJ, Brandl P, Kockott G, et al. Double-blind, placebo-controlled safety and efficacy trial with yohimbine hydrochloride in the treatment of nonorganic erectile dysfunction. Int J Impot Res 1997; 9(3):155–161.

121. Ernst E, Pittler MH. Yohimbine for erectile dysfunction: a systematic review and meta-analysis of randomized clinical trials. J Urol 1998; 159:433–436.

122. Teloken C, Rhoden EL, Sogari P, et al. Therapeutic effects of high dose yohimbine hydrochloride on organic erectile dysfunction. J Urol 1998; 159(1):122–124.

123. Morales A, Condra M, Owen JA, et al. Is yohimbine effective in the treatment of organic impotence? Results of a controlled trial. J Urol 1987; 137(6): 1168–1172.

124. Susset JG, Tessier CD, Wincze J, et al. Effect of yohimbine hydrochloride on erectile impotence: a double-blind study. J Urol 1989; 141(6):1360–1363.

125. Montorsi F, Strambi LF, Guazzoni G, et al. Effect of yohimbine-trazodone on psychogenic impotence: a randomized, double-blind, placebo-controlled study. Urology 1994; 44(5):732–736.

126. Morales A, Heaton JP, Johnston B, et al. Oral and topical treatment of erectile dysfunction. Present and future. Urol Clin North Am 1995; 22(4): 879–886.

127. Traish A, Gupta S, Gallant C, et al. Phentolamine mesylate relaxes penile corpus cavernosum tissue by adrenergic and non-adrenergic mechanisms. Int J Impot Res 1998; 10(4):215–223.

128. Gwinup G. Oral phentolamine in nonspecific erectile insufficiency. Ann Intern Med 1988; 109(2):162–163.

129. Becker AJ, Stief CG, Machtens S, et al. Oral phentolamine as treatment for erectile dysfunction. J Urol 1998; 149:1214–1216.

130. Goldstein I, Padma-Nathan H, Payton T, et al. Penile revascularization: five year experience in 225 patients [abstr 542]. J Urol 1988; 139:298A.

131. Goldstein I. Oral phentolamine: an alpha-1, alpha-2 adrenergic antagonist for the treatment of erectile dysfunction. Int J Impot Res 2000; 12(suppl 1): S75–S80.

132. Goldstein I, Carson C, Rosen R, et al. Vasomax for the treatment of male erectile dysfunction. World J Urol 2001; 19:51–56.

133. Hafez B, Hafez ES. Andropause: endocrinology, erectile dysfunction, and prostate pathophysiology. Arch Androl 2004; 50(2):45–68.

134. Hanash KA. Comparative results of goal oriented therapy for erectile dysfunction. J Urol 1997; 157(6): 2135–2138.

135. Knoll LD, Benson RC, Bilhartz DL, Minich PJ, Furlow WL. A randomized crossover study using yohimbine and isoxsuprine versus pentoxifylline in the management of vasculogenic impotence. J Urol 1996; 155: 144–146.

136. Safarinejad MR. Therapeutic effects of high-dose isoxsuprine in the management of mixed-type impotence. Urology 2001; 58(1):95–97.

137. Korenman SG, Viosca SP. Treatment of vasculogenic sexual dysfunction with pentoxifylline. J Am Geriatr Soc 1993; 41:363–366.

138. Sato Y, Horita H, Adachi H, et al. Effect of oral administration of prostaglandin E1 on erectile dysfunction. Br J Urol 1997; 80(5):772–775.

139. Chen J, Wollman Y, Chrnichovsky T, et al. Effect of oral administration of high-dose nitric oxide donor L-arginine in men with organic erectile dysfunction: results of a double-blind, randomized, placebo-controlled study. Br J Urol Int 1999; 83(3):269–273.

140. Moody JA, Vernet D, Laidlaw S, et al. Effects of long-term oral administration of L-arginine on the rat erectile response. J Urol 1997; 158(3):942–947.

141. Guirguis WR. Oral treatment of erectile dysfunction: from herbal remedies to designer drugs. J Sex Marital Ther 1998; 24(2):69–73.

142. Ito T, Kawahara K, Das A, et al. The effects of ArginMax, a natural dietary supplement for enhancement of male sexual function. J Hawaii Med 1998; 57(12):741–744.

143. Choi YD, Rha KH, Choi HK. In vitro and in vivo experimental effect of Korean Red Ginseng on erection. J Urol 1999; 162(4):1508–1511.

144. Meinhardt W, Schmitz PI, Kropman RF, et al. Trazodone, a double blind trial for treatment of erectile dysfunction. Int J Impot Res 1997; 9(3):163–165.

145. Costabile RA, Spevak M. Oral trazodone is not effective therapy for erectile dysfunction: a double-blind, placebo controlled trial. J Urol 1999; 161(6):1819–1822.

146. Lance R, Albo M, Costabile RA, et al. Oral trazodone as empirical therapy for erectile dysfunction: a retrospective review. Urology 1995; 46(1):117–120.

147. Foreman MM, Wernicke JF. Approaches for the development of oral drug therapies for erectile dysfunction. Semin Urol 1990; 8(2):107–112.

148. Broderick GA. Intracavernous pharmacotherapy: treatment for the aging erectile response. Urol Clin North Am 1996; 23(1):111–126.

149. Saenz de Tejada I, Ware JC, Blanco R, et al. Pathophysiology of prolonged penile erection associated with trazodone use. J Urol 1991; 145(1):60–64.

150. Warner MD, Peabody CA, Whiteford HA, et al. Trazodone and priapism. J Clin Psychiatry 1987; 48(6):244–245.

151. Chiang PH, Tsai EM, Chiang CP. The role of trazodone in the treatment of erectile dysfunction. Gaoxiong Yi Xue Ke Xue Za Shi 1994; 10(6):287–294.

152. Segraves RT, Bari M, Segraves K, et al. Effect of apomorphine on penile tumescence in men with psychogenic impotence. J Urol 1991; 145(6):1174–1175.

153. Paick JS, Lee SW. The neural mechanism of apomorphine-induced erection: an experimental study by comparison with electrostimulation-induced erection in the rat model. J Urol 1994; 152(6 Pt 1):2125–2128.

154. Mulhall JP, Bukofzer S, Edmonds AL, et al. An open-label, uncontrolled dose-optimization study of sublingual apomorphine in erectile dysfunction. Clin Ther 2001; 23(8):1260–1271.

155. Heaton JP, Morales A, Adams MA, et al. Recovery of erectile function by the oral administration of apomorphine. Urology 1995; 45(2):200–206.

156. Dula E, Keating W, Siami PF, et al. Efficacy and safety of fixed-dose and dose-optimization regimens of sublingual apomorphine versus placebo in men with erectile dysfunction. The apomorphine study group. Urology 2000; 56(1):130–135.

157. Heaton JP, Dean J, Sleep DJ. Sequential administration enhances the effect of apomorphine SL in men with erectile dysfunction. Int J Impot Res 2002; 14(1):61–64.

158. Bukofzer S, Livesey N. Safety and tolerability of apomorphine SL (Uprima). Int J Impot Res 2001; 13(suppl 3):S40–S44.

159. Lal S, Kiely ME, Thavundayil JX, et al. Effect of bromocriptine in patients with apomorphine-responsive erectile impotence: an open study. J Psychiatry Neurosci 1991; 16(5):262–266.

160. Goldstein JA. Erectile function and naltrexone. Ann Intern Med 1986; 105(5):799 (Letter).

161. Fabbri A, Jannini EA, Gnessi L, et al. Endorphins in male impotence: evidence for naltrexone stimulation of erectile activity in patient therapy. Psychoneuroendocrinology 1989; 14(1–2):103–111.

162. van Ahlen H, Piechota HJ, Kias HJ, et al. Opiate antagonists in erectile dysfunction: a possible new treatment option? Results of a pilot study with naltrexone. Eur Urol 1995; 28(3):246–250.

163. Brennemann W, Stitz B, vanAhlen H, et al. Treatment of idiopathic erectile dysfunction in men with the opiate antagonist naltrexone—a double-blind study. J Androl 1993; 14(6):407–410.

164. Charney DS, Heninger GR. Alpha 2-adrenergic and opiate receptor blockade. Synergistic effects on anxiety in healthy subjects. Arch Gen Psychiatry 1986; 43(11):1037–1041.

165. Smith DM, Levitte SS. Association of fluoxetine and return of sexual potency in three elderly men. J Clin Psychiatry 1993; 54(8):317–319.

166. Rosen RC, Ashton AK. Prosexual drugs: empirical status of the "new aphrodisiacs." Arch Sex Behav 1993; 22(6):521–543.

167. Althof SE. Pharmacologic treatment of rapid ejaculation. Psychiatr Clin North Am 1995; 18(1):85–94.

168. Segraves RT, Saran A, Segraves K, et al. Clomipramine versus placebo in the treatment of premature ejaculation: a pilot study. J Sex Marital Ther 1993; 19: 198–200.

169. Haensel SM, Rowland DL, Kallan KT. Clomipramine and sexual function in men with premature ejaculation and controls. J Urol 1996; 156(4):1310–1315.

170. Colpi GM, Fanciullacci F, Aydos K, et al. Effectiveness mechanism of clomipramine by neurophysiological tests in subjects with true premature ejaculation. Andrologia 1991; 23(1):45–47.

171. Assalian P. Clomipramine in the treatment of premature ejaculation. J Sex Res 1988; 24:213–215.

172. McLean JD, Forsythe RG, Kapkin IA. Unusual side effects of clomipramine associated with yawning. Can J Psychiatry 1983; 28(7):569–570.

173. Monteiro WO, Noshirvani HF, Marks IM, et al. Anorgasmia from clomipramine in obsessive-compulsive disorder. A controlled trial. Br J Psychiatry 1987; 151(1):107–112.

174. Mendels J, Camera A, Sikes C. Sertraline treatment for premature ejaculation. J Clin Psychopharmacol 1995; 15:341–346.

175. Waldinger MD, Hengeveld MW, Zwinderman AH. Paroxetine treatment of premature ejaculation: a double-blind, randomized, placebo-controlled study. Am J Psychiatry 1994; 151(9):1377–1379.

176. Lee HS, Song DH, Kim CH, et al. An open clinical trial of fluoxetine in the treatment of premature ejaculation. J Clin Psychopharmacol 1996; 16:379–382.

177. Haensel SM, Klem TM, Hop WC, et al. Fluoxetine and premature ejaculation: a double-blind, crossover, placebo-controlled study. J Clin Psychopharmacol 1998; 18:72–77.

178. Waldinger MD, Hengeveld MW, Zwinderman AH. Ejaculation-retarding properties of paroxetine in patients with primary premature ejaculation: a double-blind, randomized, dose-response study. Br J Urol 1997; 79(4):592–595.

179. McMahon C, Touma K. Treatment of premature ejaculation with paroxetine hydrochloride as needed: 2 single-blind placebo controlled crossover studies. J Urol 1999; 161:1826–1830.

180. Yilmaz U, Tatlisen A, Turan H, et al. The effects of fluoxetine on several neurophysiological variables in patients with premature ejaculation. J Urol 1999; 161(1):107–111.

181. Shilon M, Paz GF, Homonnai ZT. The use of phenoxybenzamine treatment in premature ejaculation. Fertil Steril 1984; 42(4):659–661.

182. Cavallini G. Alpha-1 blockade pharmacotherapy in primitive psychogenic premature ejaculation resistant to psychotherapy. Eur Urol 1995; 28(2):126–130.

183. Lepor H. Nonoperative management of benign prostatic hyperplasia. J Urol 1989; 141(6):1283–1289.

184. Brooks ME, Berezin M, Braf Z. Treatment of retrograde ejaculation with imipramine. Urology 1980; 15(4):353–355.

185. Stockamp K, Schreiter F, Altwein JE. Alpha-adrenergic drugs in retrograde ejaculation. Fertil Steril 1974; 25(9):817–820.

186. Jonas D, Linzbach P, Weber W. The use of midodrine in the treatment of ejaculation disorders following retroperitoneal lymphadenectomy. Eur Urol 1979; 5(3):184–187.

187. Walker PW, Cole JO, Gardner EA, et al. Improvement in fluoxetine-associated sexual dysfunction in patients switched to bupropion. J Clin Psychiatry 1993; 54(12):459–465.

188. Labbate LA, Pollack MH. Treatment of fluoxetine-induced sexual dysfunction with bupropion: a case report. Ann Clin Psychiatry 1994; 6(1):13–15.

189. Moore BE, Rothschild AJ. Treatment of antidepressant-induced sexual dysfunction. Hosp Pract 1999; 34(1):89–96.

190. Rothschild AJ. Selective serotonin reuptake inhibitor-induced sexual dysfunction: efficacy of a drug holiday. Am J Psychiatry 1995; 152(10):1514–1516.

191. Gitlin MJ. Psychotropic medications and their effects on sexual function diagnosis, biology, and treatment approaches. J Clin Psychiatry 1994; 55(9): 406–413.

192. Woodrum ST, Brown CS. Management of SSRI-induced sexual dysfunction. Ann Pharmacother 1998; 32(11):1209–1215.

193. Aizenberg D, Zemishlany Z, Weizman A. Cyproheptadine treatment of sexual dysfunction induced by serotonin reuptake inhibitors. Clin Neuropharmacol 1995; 18(4):320–324.

194. Balon R. Intermittent amantadine for fluoxetine-induced anorgasmia. J Sex Marital Ther 1996; 22(4):290–292.

195. Price J, Grunhaus LJ. Treatment of clomipramine-induced anorgasmia with yohimbine: a case report. J Clin Psychiatry 1990; 51(1):32–33.

196. Altman AL, Seftel AD, Brown SL, et al. Cocaine associated priapism. J Urol 1999; 161(6):1817–1818.

197. Evans CM, Kell P. Clinical Drawings For Your Patients: Erectile Dysfunction. Smith RJ, ed. Oxford: Health Press, 2000:31.

198. Bastuba MD, SaenzdeTejada I, Dinlenc CZ, et al. Arterial priapism: diagnosis, treatment and long-term follow up. J Urol 1994; 151(5):1231–1237.

199. Hakim LS, Kulaksizoglu H, Mulligan R, et al. Evolving concepts in the diagnosis and treatment of arterial high flow priapism. J Urol 1996; 155(2):541–548.

200. Aboseif S, Tamaddon K. Peyronie's disease: an update. Sex Dysfunct Med 1999; 1:34–41.

201. De Rose AF, Giglio M, Traverso P, et al. Combined oral therapy with sildenafil and doxazosin for the treatment of non-organic erectile dysfunction refractory to sildenafil monotherapy. Int J Impot Res 2002; 14(1):50–53.

30

Local Drug Therapy for Male Sexual Dysfunction

Fouad R. Kandeel

Department of Diabetes, Endocrinology and Metabolism, City of Hope National Medical Center, Duarte, California and
David Geffen School of Medicine, University of California, Los Angeles, California, U.S.A.

☐ INTRODUCTION

The field of sexual medicine has been revolutionized over the last two decades. Several treatment options are available today, most of which are associated with high efficacy rates and favorable safety profiles. The recent success in the use of phosphodiesterase-5 (PDE-5) inhibitors for the treatment of erectile dysfunction (ED) has made oral therapy an attractive first-line treatment. Not all patients respond adequately to such therapy, however. Further, the management of patients who fail oral therapy is often ill defined. Local vasoactive agents continue to offer an alternative therapeutic solution for these men. This chapter will describe the available local penile therapies for ED and other selected male sexual disorders (Table 1).

☐ LOCAL TREATMENT OF ED

There are several locally applied options for the treatment of ED, including intracavernous injections, topical applications, and urethral suppositories. These are described below.

Intracavernous Injections
Overview

The first reports of the ability of intracavernous injection to initiate and maintain erection used the drugs papaverine (1) and phenoxybenzamine (78), respectively. The most common medications that continue to be used for this purpose include papaverine, phentolamine, and prostaglandin E-1 (PGE-1) (alprostadil), in a variety of combinations and with good effect. While PDE-5 inhibitors have become the most prescribed medication for the treatment of ED, injection therapy still remains an important and effective therapy (2,3,14,79–83), particularly for those patients who fail to respond to PDE-5 inhibitors. In a recent study (84), oral sildenafil with audiovisual sexual stimulation led to a significant clinical response and increment in blood flow in the cavernosal arteries; however, more patients responded to intracavernosal injection of a combination of papaverine, PGE-1, and phentolamine (commonly known as "Trimix"; please see below for

further information) than to sildenafil, and the response, as measured by clinical assessment and cavernosal duplex ultrasonography, was significantly better. Generally, the use of combination agents is preferred to that of single agents to minimize side effects and maximize effectiveness. For example, Trimix has been shown to be more effective than high-dose PGE-1 alone and to be associated with a lower incidence of painful erections (due to the lower concentration of prostaglandin) (83).

In comparison to the currently available oral agents, the primary advantage of intracavernosal medications is that they induce erection even in the presence of only minimal stimulation. Oral pills, on the other hand, do not produce their intended effects if the patient is experiencing too much anxiety, not enough sexual stimulation, too low a testosterone level, or excessive venous outflow (4). The disadvantages of intracavernosal agents, however, include a more complex route of administration, a greater potential for bleeding, bruising, and penile fibrosis, and a higher incidence of priapism (albeit, all uncommon side effects). Additionally, the use of intracavernosal injections is usually limited to twice a week with a minimum of 24 hours between injections; yet, even with this low frequency of administration, the drugs may be prohibitively expensive (85). Rare complications include postinjection cavernositis and intracoporeal needle breakage (86). Intracavernosal injections are contraindicated in patients with penile deformity or predisposing conditions for priapism (e.g., sickle cell disease or trait, leukemia, multiple myeloma, polycythemia, or thrombocythemia), those with a known hypersensitivity to the injected drug, or those who have been advised for medical reasons to avoid sexual intercourse (87). These side effects and contraindications will be discussed below in further detail.

One approach to intracorporeal vasoactive drug administration was described by Cornell Urology (85). Under the guidelines of this method, detailed instructions on the use of this type of therapy and administration of the first dose in the clinic are mandatory. Each visit consists of an important combination of physician assessment, trial dose administration, and patient education. The patient is given instructions on cleaning the penis. An alcohol swab is used to cleanse the intended area of injection. An insulin-type syringe is then used to administer the medication. The injection is given at the ten o'clock or two o'clock position on the penis (away from the ventrally located urethra), away from visible veins, and never in the midline. To minimize the chance of scar formation, the site is changed with each dose. The needle is aimed at a right angle to the skin and pushed in to the hub, ensuring delivery of the medication into the center of the ipsilateral corporal cavernosal tissue. After administration of the medication, the patient holds direct pressure to the area of injection for a few minutes. Patients taking blood thinners are advised to continue pressure for a full six minutes. Typically, the staff gives the first dose with the patient watching. This will be a very low dose (which varies, depending on the choice of drug). Patients with ED due to neuropathy (e.g., prior nerve damage) are started on lower doses than those with suspected vascular ED. After intrapenile drug administration, assessment of erectile response should be performed at 5, 10, and 30 minutes, and the patient should wait in the clinic until the erection dissipates. The dose of medication is increased with each subsequent visit until a satisfactory response is obtained. The patient's role in the administration of the medication will also progressively increase. The dosage goal should be to produce an in-clinic erection of 60% maximum (barely adequate for penetration) that lasts less than one hour. It is presumed that at home with less anxiety and more appropriate stimulation, etc., the effect will be greater. Ultimately, the patient (or his partner) must also demonstrate the ability to draw up the drug and properly inject it with an aseptic technique without staff assistance. At this point, he is graduated from the clinic and given prescriptions for at-home use.

The initial acceptance of intracavernous injection therapy by patients capable of responding to it has ranged from 86% to less than 50% (3). The most commonly cited reasons for rejecting this modality of treatment include penile pain, the artificiality of erection, and the concern over long-term complications. Further, of those patients who start on a home-injection therapy program, only 50% to 80% continue to use it long-term. Most of the dropout appears to occur in the first six months of therapy. Frequently cited reasons for the dropout include loss of efficacy, loss of interest, fear of complications, lack of sexual spontaneity, resumption of spontaneous erections, and favoring other forms of therapy (3,80,81). The most likely cause for the resumption of spontaneous erection after initiation of intrapenile injection therapy is the resolution of performance anxiety. In addition, an increase in arterial peak flow velocity may occur in some patients (88). Interestingly, despite the potential side effects of this relatively invasive form of therapy, when given the choice to pursue either a transdermal, needle-free (using liquid CO_2) route of alprostadil administration or the traditional one, patients expressed a clear preference for the needle-tipped injection over the needle-free device

(89). In fact, pain produced by the needle-free injector was reported to be significantly greater than that produced by the needle-tipped injections.

Two other rather unusual permanent delivery systems for intracavernous vasoactive drug therapy have been described. In the first, a small cannula is surgically inserted at the penile scrotal junction into the corporeal tissue at a depth of 2.8 mm, and a connected reservoir is placed in a small pouch between the testes. The reservoir is filled with a mixture of phentolamine 3.3 mg/mL and verapamil 1.7 mg/mL. Pumping the reservoir four times results in the delivery of 2.2 mg phentolamine and 1.12 mg verapamil, which is sufficient for inducing erection in the majority of patients. The reservoir has an average capacity for approximately 18 erections before needing to be refilled. The system was implanted in eight patients with organic impotence and was reported to be functional in all patients after an average follow-up duration of 13.3 months. Average frequency of use was one to three times per week, and two to four pumps were needed for each erection (90). In the second system, a 1-cm square window was created in Buck's fascia and the tunica albuginea and was then covered with a piece of the deep dorsal vein of the penis. The penile skin overlying the window was marked with India ink, and the patient was instructed to apply a vasoactive drug (nitroglycerin) to this area. The procedure was performed on six patients with ED. Only two patients preferred this method to intracorporeal injections, three others used the two methods interchangeably, and the sixth patient preferred the injection as the sole therapeutic intervention (91).

The potential side effects of scarring, priapism, bleeding, and bruising can be minimized by using combination medications, carefully titrating to the correct dose in the clinic, and thoroughly educating the patient on injection technique. Scarring can manifest as the occurrence of a nodule, plaque, or penile curvature. Patients must be clearly instructed that prolonged erections constitute a medical emergency. If the patient has an erection that lasts longer than two hours and is not relieved by ejaculation, they should be instructed to call a urology answering service for advice and should be in the Emergency Department by the fourth hour. There is evidence that suggests that the risk of prolonged erection due to intracavernosal injection may be greater with ED of a psychogenic or neurogenic etiology than with a vasculogenic one (92). The standard therapy for priapism of this cause (please see below for further details) is drainage and irrigation of the corporal bodies with sympathomimetic agents. There is no established oral medication, although some reports have suggested that pseudoephedrine and terbutaline may be effective in reversing such erections (74). (For further information on priapism, see Chapter 18.)

The following is a brief summary of the pharmacological effects and the reported clinical experience with individual intracavernosal agents (Table 1).

Table 1 Local Pharmacological Therapy of Male Sexual Dysfunction

		Drug	Drug type/action	Dose	Comment	Ref.
LOCAL TREATMENT OF ERECTILE DYSFUNCTION	**Intracavernous injections**	**Agents resulting in penile rigidity and usable erection**				
		Papaverine	cAMP phosphodiesterase inhibitor	10–80 mg	Often supplemented with α-blockers like phentolamine	1–13
		PGE₁ (Alprostadil®)	Prostaglandin	5–20 μg	Least toxic, most natural, but often painful	14–26
		Linsodomine (SIN-1)	Nitric oxide donor	1 mg	Does not appear to be associated with priapism	2,14,27,28
		Phenoxybenzamine	Non-selective α-blocker	1–4 mg	Most rigid and long-lasting but toxic; some tumescence with systemic injection	2,29
		SNO-yohimbine, SNO-moxisylyte	Ntirosylated α-adrenergic receptor antagonists	10–30 mg	Less priapism and pain	30–34
		Calcitonin gene-related peptide	Acts on sodium-potassium pump to hyperpolarize cell membrane	5 mg	Can be used in conjunction with PGE₁	14,35
		Sodium nitroprusside (nitroglycerin)	Vasodilator	100–400 mg	Moderate risk of severe hypotension when used intracavernously; see below for comments on topical use	29,36
		Agents resulting in brief penile rigidity or tumescence but unusable erection				
		Phentolamine (Regitine®)	α₁ and α₂-blocker	5–10 mg	Rigid less than 10 min; some effect taken orally	37–42
		Vasoactive intestinal peptide (VIP)	Calcium-channel blocker/α₁ blocker	1–5 mg	Rigid less than 5 min	43–49
		Trazodone	Central: inhibition of serotionin uptake; peripheral: α-adrenergic blocker	20–40 mg	Much less effective in initiating penile erections than direct smooth muscle relaxants	50–53
	Topical applications	PGE₁	Prostaglandin	125–1000 μg cream	Most effective topical cream	14,54–56
		Papaverine	cAMP phosphodiesterase inhibitor	15–20% gel	Less effective topically than PGE₁	57
		Minoxidil	Vasodilator	2% solution	Less effective topically than PGE₁	58,59
		Nitroglycerin	Vasodilator	0.5 in. of 2% ointment	Less effective topically than PGE₁	60–62

(Continued)

Table 1 Local Pharmacological Therapy of Male Sexual Dysfunction (*Continued*)

	Drug	Drug type/action	Dose	Comment	Ref.
Urethral applications	Transurethral prostaglandin E₁ (MUSE®)	Prostaglandin	125–1000 μg	Most effective urethral agent	63–70
	Prostaglandin E₂ (Dinoprostone®)	Prostaglandin	20, 40 mg suppositories mixed with 2% lidocaine and surgical lubricant to form cream; 2 mL cream instilled in urethral meatus	Used more frequently prior to advent of MUSE; mild transient urethral burning with placement of cream	71
LOCAL TREATMENT OF PREMATURE EJACULATION	Lidocaine 2.5%/Prilocaine 2.5% (Emla®cream)	Topical anesthetic cream	Apply to glans penis and shaft under occlusive cover (condom) at least 30 min prior to sexual encounter	Dermal analgesia reaches its max in 2–3 hr, and persists for 1–2 hr after removal. May cause transient local blanching followed by transient erythema	72
	Lidocaine 7.5 mg/Prilocaine 2.5 mg topical spray	Topical anesthetic spray	Apply to the glans for 10–15 min, wipe off carefully prior to intercourse	May experience glandular numbness, may be difficult to maintain erection during waiting period	73
LOCAL TREATMENT OF FAILURE OF DETUMESCENCE	Pseudoephedrine	α-receptor agonist	30 mg by mouth × 1 or 2 at 30-min intervals	Indicated for mild cases of prolonged erection	2
	Terbutaline	β-receptor agonist	By mouth	Indicated for cases of prolonged erection < 4 hr in duration	2,9,74
	Phenylephrine	α-adrenergic receptor agonist	200 μg every 5 min after aspirating 10–20 mL of blood from corpora cavernosa or 500 mg every 15 min	Indicated for more severe cases of prolonged erection > 4 hr in duration	2,75,76
	Norepinephrine, ephedrine, metaraminol	Adrenergic agonists	Norepinephrine—irrigation with 1 mg/L solution; Pseudoephredrine—30 mg once or twice at 30-min intervals	All can cause significant increase in blood pressure	2,75–77

Abbreviations: cAMP, cyclic adenosine monophosphate.; PGE₁, prostaglandin E₁; SNO, nitrosylated.

Agents Resulting in Penile Rigidity and Usable Erection

Papaverine

Papaverine is an opium alkaloid that does not exhibit the clinically recognized narcotic effects of other opioids. It has a direct relaxing effect on smooth muscle tone via the nonselective inhibition of cyclic nucleotide phosphodiesterases, which results in the accumulation of cyclic adenosine monophosphate (cAMP) and cyclic guanosine monophosphate (cGMP) (5). It also blocks voltage-dependent calcium channels, reduces calcium influx, and inhibits the release of intracellular calcium stores. These effects may directly relax the corporeal arterioles, sinusoids, and veins (2,3,6). Papaverine is acidic in solution (as it may precipitate at pH > 5) and slowly cleared from the corporeal tissue, has a plasma half-life of one to two hours, and is metabolized by the liver (3,7). Injections of papaverine alone produce a full erection in about 35% to 57% of patients, depending on the dose used and the underlying pathology (3). Papaverine has been used at doses ranging from 3 mg to over 100 mg, with the onset of response occurring within 10 to 30 minutes and the duration of erection ranging from 30 minutes to over 240 minutes. Patients with underlying arterial disease tend to require higher doses and have a lower rate of erectile response. In contrast, patients with neurological disease require small amounts and experience a more prolonged erection that is more likely to require corporeal drainage (8–10).

Side effects associated with papaverine injections are both systemic and local (2,3,11,12). Systemic effects may include peripheral vasodilatation, hypotension, reflex tachycardia, and elevation in liver enzymes. Hemodynamic complications may be more pronounced in patients with veno-occlusive dysfunction and are reported to occur in 1% to 8% of patients. Local adverse effects include fibrosis and priapism. Fibrosis occurs in up to 20% of patients and is thought to result from repeated local shear trauma or repeated chemical injury from the low pH of injected solution. Priapism has been reported with more frequency in patients with neurological or psychological etiologies than in patients with vasculogenic impotence. In addition, papaverine-induced erection was found to decrease penile sensitivity as assessed by the perception of vibratory tactile stimulation at two different locations on the underside of the penis (13). Since many of these patients have reduced penile sensitivity at baseline (possibly subsequent to neuropathy), intracavernous papaverine injection may augment such an abnormality.

Prostaglandin E₁

PGE₁ (or alprostadil) is a metabolite of arachidonic acid and is found in high concentrations in the seminal vesicle and seminal plasma. Injectable PGE₁ is available as a sterile solution (Prostin VR® Pediatric) or as sterile powder (Caverject® and Edex/Viridal®) (15). Only the latter formulation has current Food and Drug Administration approval for the management of ED and is available in 10-, 20-, and 40-µg dose-level packaging. PGE₁ is a potent smooth muscle relaxant and vasodilator in man. It also has an α-2 adrenergic blocking effect and thus has the potential of reducing sympathetic overtone in patients with psychogenic ED. Local metabolism of PGE₁ within the corporeal tissue has also been suggested (16). Systemic blood levels of PGE₁ and its metabolites are significantly lower between seven and twenty minutes after its intracavernous injection in patients who exhibit an erection as compared to those who do not (17), suggesting that retention of PGE₁ and its metabolites within the corporeal tissue is an important factor in the development of erectile response. The overall erectile response to prostaglandin intracorporeal injections is about 70% (18). Pain is the most common side effect, occurring in 13% to 80% of patients, and is dose related. Possible causes of pain include the high acidity of solution, local secretion of other vasoactive substances, and/or direct activation of pain receptors by PGE₁ (14). Reduction in the perception of pain could be achieved by adding 7.5% sodium bicarbonate or procaine 20 mg to the injected solution (19,20), and via slow administration (21). Other side effects associated with PGE₁ injections include local corporeal hematoma or ecchymosis (8%), prolonged erection to between four and six hours (5%), priapism of greater than six hours' duration (1%), penile edema (2%), and fibrosis (2.3%) (22).

Long-term efficacy and safety of PGE₁ intracavernous self-injection were determined in several studies (23–26). The rate of dropout from treatment was 47% after three years (24) and 67% after four years (25). Patient satisfaction with their erections increased from approximately 23% without injections (24) to a range of 67% to 91% with injections (24,26). Reported side effects in one four-year study (26) were prolonged erection for more than six hours, occurring during the first year in 1.2% of subjects; penile pain caused by the injected agent in 29% of subjects during year one, declining to 12.1% by year four; hematomas in 33.3% of subjects in year 1 that also declined to 12.1% by year 4; and fibrotic penile alteration (nodules, plaques, deviations) in 11.7% of subjects, with spontaneous healing in 48%.

Vasoactive Drug Mixtures

The mixture of papaverine with phentolamine (see below) has been extensively used to induce therapeutic erection, since 1985 (93). The mixture is usually constituted to contain 15 to 30 mg/mL papaverine and 0.5 to 1 mg/mL phentolamine. The mixture has been shown to be superior to papaverine alone in inducing erection (65% vs. 36%), particularly in geriatric patients (83,94) and in those with organic dysfunction (93). Both of these patient populations tend to require larger quantities (50% or more) of these vasoactive agents than either younger populations or those with psychogenic or neurogenic impotence (2,3).

Another popular mixture of vasoactive drugs (Trimix®) includes papaverine (15–30 mg/mL), phentolamine (0.5–5.0 mg/mL), and PGE₁ (8.33–500 μg/mL) and is used in quantities ranging from 0.1 to 0.75 mL per injection. In some instances, atropine (3 mg/mL, see below for further details) and/or normal saline (up to 2.4 mL) is added to the tri-mixture (2,3,14,95–97). The clinical efficacy of the tri-mixture has been documented in several studies. For example, Goldstein et al. (96) used a mixture of papaverine 22.5 mg/mL, phentolamine 0.83 mg/mL, and PGE₁ 8.33 μg/mL to salvage 62% of nonresponders to either PGE₁ monotherapy or therapy with a mixture of papaverine and phentolamine. Several other studies showed rates of response ranging from 66% to 92% (2,3,14). Since a small quantity of each vasoactive agent is used in the intracavernous drug mixture, side effects related to each agent are also minimized, including the corporeal fibrosis and hepatic dysfunctions associated with papaverine and the pain associated with PGE₁. A lower incidence of prolonged erection was also reported for the tri-mixture as compared to papaverine alone and the papaverine–phentolamine combination, but not for PGE₁ monotherapy. This conclusion is supported by literature reviews in which papaverine alone was found to produce priapism in 9.5% of 213 patients, papaverine–phentolamine in 5.3% of 2914 patients, and PGE₁ in 2.4% of 1284 patients (10). In a different literature review of five studies of 765 patients by Fallon, the overall rate of priapism was found to be 1.4% (3). A time-dependent and statistically predictable increase in PCO_2 and a decrease in pH and PO_2 during pharmacologically prolonged erection have also been described (98,99). Prolonged pharmacologically induced priapism is particularly of concern because it is usually ischemic (veno-occlusive) in nature. If left untreated, it produces significant morphological damage including trabecular interstitial edema at 12 hours, destruction of sinusoidal endothelium, exposure of basement membrane and thrombocyte adherence at 24 hours, and sinusoidal space thrombosis and smooth muscle transformation to fibroblast-like cells at 48 hours after onset (100).

Several other complications have been reported in patients receiving intracavernous vasoactive drugs with varying frequency, depending on the administered agent. Fibrotic nodules seem to occur more frequently with papaverine monotherapy [5.4% of 1573 patients from different series reviewed by Junemann and Alken (10)] than with PGE₁ [ranging from occasional cases of Peyronie's-like plaque, up to 3% (101–103)], or with the tri-mixture [0–4.2% (97,104,105)]. A higher incidence of nodules with increasing duration of therapy with any vasoactive agent has also been suggested (95). Further, light microscopy studies in monkeys showed that long-term intracavernous injection of papaverine produces mild to moderate fibrotic changes with distortion of normal architecture. In contrast, only limited fibrosis and hypertrophy of smooth muscles were noted in animals treated with PGE₁ (106). In humans, however, the architectural changes in patients receiving intracavernous vasoactive agents do not appear to differ from those seen in other impotent patients without prior history of such treatment (107). The disparity between this negative observation and the penile fibrosis noted in many clinical studies has been reconciled by the suggestion that the trauma from the repeated administration of vasoactive drugs is responsible for the local fibrotic reaction of the tunica albuginea, rather than the drug causing a generalized corporeal fibrotic effect (3). This contention is further supported by the lack of penile curvature and by the dissipation of nodules upon cessation of injections for one to two months. Such complications may be minimized or prevented by varying the site of injection and the use of smaller needles. Other rare complications of intracavernous vasoactive injections include local infections (108), hepatotoxicity with the use of papaverine–phentolamine mix in patients with a history of alcohol abuse (109), penile shaft hypopigmentation with the use of PGE₁ (110), and accidental breakage of needles in the penile shaft (111).

Nitric Oxide Donors

Linsidomine. Linsidomine (SIN-1) is a metabolite of the antianginal drug molsidomine and acts by releasing NO from the endothelial cells nonenzymatically. It also hyperpolarizes the cell membrane by influencing the sodium–potassium pump, rendering it less responsive to adrenergic stimulation (2). Linsidomine injection at a dose of 1 mg produces an erection sufficient for vaginal penetration in about 70% of patients (27) and full erection in up to 50% of patients (28). Linsidomine does not appear to be associated with priapism (14).

Phenoxybenzamine, Sodium Nitroprusside, Moxisylyte

Intracavernous injection of phenoxybenzamine (nonspecific α-receptor blocker) or sodium nitroprusside (cGMP pathway activator) has been found to be associated with significant systemic side effects (e.g., phenoxybenzamine is toxic, and there is a moderate risk of severe systemic hypotension with the use of intracavernous sodium nitroprusside), rendering these agents unacceptable modalities of local treatment of ED (2,29,36). In contrast, administration of moxisylyte (Mox or Thymoxamine, a competitive postsynaptic α-1 receptor selective antagonist) in doses ranging from 10 to 30 mg was shown to produce an adequate erection in 85% of patients, with a very low incidence of side effects (30). In comparative studies, however, PGE₁ was shown to be more effective in producing a full penile rigidity than moxisylyte (31,32). Side effects reported with the use of moxisylyte were minimal and include dry mouth 2.73%, somnolence 1.9%, and sinus congestion 0.71% (33). Nitrosylated α-adrenergic receptor antagonists, SNO-moxisylyte (NMI-221) and SNO-yohimbine (NMI-187), were shown in a concentration-dependent manner to relax endothelin-induced contraction of human and rabbit corpus cavernosum strips in organ chambers to a greater extent than their respective parent compounds (34). NMI-221–induced accumulation of cGMP in rabbit corpus cavernosum tissue, and its effects were potentiated by a specific phosphodiesterase-5 inhibitor (Zaprinast) in human corpus cavernosum tissue. Further, intracavernous injection of NMI-221 in animal models induced a more long-lasting increase in intracavernous pressure than moxisylyte with no differences in effect on the systemic mean arterial pressure. Thus, nitrosylated α-adrenergic receptor antagonists may have a therapeutic role in the treatment of ED by acting as nitric oxide donors as well as α-receptor blockers (34).

Calcitonin Gene-Related Peptide

Calcitonin gene-related peptide (CGRP) acts on the sodium–potassium pump to produce hyperpolarization of the cell membrane. Local administration of CGRP leads to cavernous smooth muscle relaxation and penile erection (14,35). It has been used in 5-μg doses as an addition to other vasoactive agents such as PGE-1 to treat patients not responding to a papaverine–phentolamine combination (35).

Agents Resulting in Brief Penile Rigidity or Tumescence but Unusable Erection
Phentolamine

Phentolamine is an α-1 and α-2 adrenoceptor blocker. Some studies have shown the relative efficacy of this compound for the long-term preventive pharmacological treatment of men with mild to moderate ED (37). When used alone as a primary treatment for ED, however, it only has a weak erectile promoting effect. When used in combination with papaverine and/or PGE$_1$, it potentiates their erectile effects (38–42). By blocking α-receptors, phentolamine helps to reduce the vasoconstrictive effects of the sympathetic innervation of the corporeal arteries and thereby aids in the erectile response. There has been evidence to suggest that phentolamine relaxes the corpus cavernosum independent of an α-adrenergic blockade and instead involves the calcium-sensitive and adenosine triphosphate–regulated K+ channels that modulate corporal smooth muscle tone (37). Adverse effects related to the use of phentolamine alone include orthostatic hypotension and tachycardia.

Vasoactive Intestinal Polypeptide

Vasoactive intestinal polypeptide (VIP) is a potent vasodilator and smooth muscle relaxant. It colocalizes with NO synthase in penile nerve fibers (43,44). Its injection as monotherapy in man, however, was not shown to produce adequate erection (10). This may relate to the fact that it causes accumulation of cAMP and not cGMP (45). Combined VIP and phentolamine preparations (e.g., Invicorp, Vasopten) have been shown to be effective in treating patients with ED even after failing to respond to mixtures of papaverine, PGE$_1$, and phentolamine (46–49). In these preparations, 25 μg of VIP is combined with either 1 or 2 mg of phen-

tolamine; response rates to this drug mixture range from 66.5% to 75% compared with 12% to 18% for placebo. Major side effects reported were facial flushing 34% to 53%, truncal flushing 9%, bruising 20%, pain 11%, and priapism 0.05% (46,48,49).

Trazodone

Trazodone is an antidepressant that causes central inhibition of serotonin uptake. Peripherally, it may act as an α-adrenergic blocker (50,51). Its clinical use as an antidepressant is associated with priapism as a side effect (52). This may be related to serotonin accumulation in the brain, possibly through activation of 5-HT-1c receptor subtype (53). Intracorporeal administration of trazodone was shown, like other α-blocking agents, to be much less effective in initiating penile erections than direct smooth muscle relaxants (50). When given orally, however, trazodone increases the number and duration of nocturnal penile tumescence episodes in man (51).

Other Agents

Several other agents were evaluated for the local induction of penile erection, either alone or with one or more of the well-established drugs. These agents include atropine (112), adenosine (45,113), enprodyl tartrate (available in France as a separate agent or as a mixture with papaverine under the trade name Vadilex) (114), and α-melanocyte-stimulating hormone analogue (115). Atropine failed to augment the response to other agents, whereas α-melanocyte-stimulating hormone analogue (Melanotan-II, a superpotent, prolonged acting, enzymatically resistant melanocortin, part of a family of multifunctional peptidergic hormones) and adenosine were effective as single agents in human and canine experiments, respectively. Additional data on the clinical efficacy and safety of these compounds in humans are still lacking (116).

Topical Applications

The success in treating ED with the intracavernous injection of vasoactive drugs has generated high interest in the topical application of these substances in the hopes of providing a more spontaneous and partner-accepted means of inducing erection and circumventing problems associated with injections, such as corporeal bruising, pain, priapism, and fibrosis. Vasodilating agents used include PGE-1, papaverine, minoxidil, nitrates (nitroglycerin, isosorbide dinitrate), aminophylline, and co-dergocrine (54,55,57–62,117–119). In general, achieving a functional erection with the topical application of these agents has been limited, with more success in patients with psychogenic and neurogenic disorders than in those with vascular problems.

Prostaglandin E$_1$

As described above, PGE$_1$ (alprostadil) has appreciable efficacy in the treatment of ED when administered in the form of intracavernosal injection, but this route of administration is relatively inconvenient to use. The topical application of alprostadil cream (Al-Prox TD, NexMed Inc., Robbinsville, New Jersey, U.S.A.) has been attempted as a noninvasive first-choice treatment for patients with ED (56). The efficacy of intrameatal delivery is enhanced via a proprietary skin permeation-enhancing technology (NexACT, NexMed Inc.) (56). The cream is designed for retention in the meatus and fossa navicularis of the penis until absorption of the active ingredient, alprostadil, is achieved. The cream is simply dropped from a dispenser onto the glans meatus, where it is absorbed directly into penile tissue. The treatment appears to be safe and well tolerated, with mild adverse effects limited to the area of application (56).

Montorsi et al. (14) assessed the effects of a gel containing 500 µg PGE$_1$ applied to the shaft and glans penis of undefined subjects in a placebo-controlled study: they noted a significant increase in the peak systolic flow velocity of the cavernosal arteries and in penile tumescence and rigidity as measured by the Rigiscan device. McVary et al. (54) reported on the use of a topical gel formulation containing PGE$_1$ plus 5% SEPA (2-n-nonyl-1,3-dioxolane, a volatile compound used to enhance cutaneous absorption) in 48 men with ED due to vascular, neurogenic, psychogenic, or mixed etiologies in a single-blind, placebo-controlled trial. Application of the PGE$_1$ gel was associated with erectile response in 67% to 75% of patients, as compared to 17% when placebo (SEPA alone) was used. Another report (55) evaluated the efficacy of liposome-encapsulated PGE$_1$ in five patients with ED in a double-blind, placebo-controlled study using three different PGE$_1$ formulations. One effective formulation resulted in a sevenfold increase in mean peak systolic flow velocity in deep cavernosal arteries at 45 minutes after the application compared to baseline.

Papaverine

Kim et al. (57) examined the efficacy of 15% and 20% papaverine formulated in gel applied to the scrotum, perineum, and penis in 20 men with organic impotence in a placebo-controlled, nonblind study. Seventeen patients completed the study, 13 of whom had spinal cord injury as the cause for their impotence. Full clinical erection was observed in only three patients, with a mean duration of 38.7 minutes. The same patients developed erection after topical application of placebo, but with a mean duration of 8.0 minutes. Color flow Doppler ultrasound showed a mean increase in arterial lumen diameter of 36% and peak systolic flow velocity of 26%. Although serum papaverine levels did not change during the study, a drop in blood pressure and heart rate were observed.

Minoxidil

Low response rates were reported with minoxidil by Radomski et al. (58). In this study, 1 mL of 2% minoxidil solution was applied to the glans penis of 21 patients with ED. The etiology of the impotence was neuro-

genic in eight patients, vascular in seven, psychogenic in four, and due to other causes in two. Only two patients, however, demonstrated some improvement in their erectile function (one in rigidity, and one in duration but not rigidity).

Chancellor et al. (59) compared the effectiveness of 2% minoxidil to that of vacuum-constrictive devices and of the intracorporeal injections in 18 spinal injury patients. Minoxidil (1 mL of 2% solution) was aerosol-sprayed to the glans penis and followed by application of the vacuum device, and then the intracorporeal injection of 10 mg papaverine was administered. The erectile response was monitored with the Rigiscan device, and full detumescence was documented between each therapeutic application. Papaverine increased rigidity at the base of the penis by a median of 77% (range, 30–100%), while the vacuum device produced a median of 57% (range 30–80%). In contrast, no changes in rigidity were observed with minoxidil.

Nitroglycerin

Topical application of nitroglycerin was reviewed by Anderson and Seifert (60). Effects of topical nitroglycerin on erectile function have been studied using nitroglycerin 2% to 10% ointment, nitroglycerin patches, and sustained release nitroglycerin adhesive plasters. Owen et al. (61) compared the effects of 2% nitroglycerin ointment to placebo in 26 patients with psychogenic, organic, or mixed impotence. Placebo or 0.5-in. of 2% nitroglycerin ointment was applied to the penile shaft and followed by viewing a five-minute erotic heterosexual videotape. Eighteen of the 26 patients had a greater increase in penile circumference with nitroglycerin than with placebo, and in 20 patients who were studied with Doppler ultrasound, seven demonstrated a 50% or greater increase in arterial diameter and blood flow after nitroglycerin; however, only three patients demonstrated an increase in tumescence. Similarly, in three other studies reviewed by Anderson and Seifert (60), the rate of full erectile response to the local application of nitrates ranged between 10% and 46%. The use of slow-release patches is likely to produce a poorer result (62).

Vasoactive Mixtures

Gomaa et al. (117) investigated the utility of a cream containing three vasodilating agents—aminophylline 3%, isosorbide dinitrate 0.25%, and co-dergocrine mesylate 0.05%—in a placebo-controlled study. Upon crossing the skin, aminophylline releases theophylline, which leads to the accumulation of cAMP. Isosorbide dinitrate generates NO, while co-dergocrine blocks α-receptors and may have central facilitating actions (possibly through the actions of one of its components, dihydroergocryptine). Creams containing either the vasoactive agents or a placebo were applied to the glans and the shaft penis, each for one week's duration. Erectile response was judged on the basis of the patient's home records of having an erection and succeeding in having intercourse. In addition, penile tumescence and arterial flow were measured in the laboratory before and after each week's trial. Twenty-one patients had a full erection, and eight others had partial erection or tumescence only with the vasoactive cream. In contrast, only three patients had full erection with placebo. This study, like many others, suggests that topical vasoactive agent mixtures are most effective in patients with a psychogenic etiology for their ED. Thus, patient selection may explain why the same vasoactive combination failed to induce erectile responses in a subsequent study (118). Chiang et al. (119) developed an alternative iontophoretic transdermal drug delivery system to improve the penetration of topical vasoactive agents, meaning that administration of ionic therapeutic agents occurs through the skin by the application of a low-level electric current, and thus the drug ions are propelled through the skin to the underlying tissue. Their clinical data on the utility of the system, however, is very sparse. Moreover, the consequences of inadvertent topical contact with any transdermal vasoactive drug by female partners have not been fully evaluated.

Major side effects reported by the patient and/or his sexual partner with the topical application of vasoactive agents include headache and a drop in blood pressure and heart rate. Several precautionary measures were suggested to reduce the incidence of such adverse effects, including careful selection of patients and treatment agents, limiting the topical application to two to six hours prior to intercourse, intake of acetaminophen prior to the topical application, and the use of a latex condom to protect the partner (60).

Urethral Applications

Both PGE_1 (alprostadil) and PGE_2 (dinoprostone) have been used as intraurethral treatments of erectile insufficiency.

Transurethral Prostaglandin E₁

Transurethral alprostadil [Medicated Urethral System for Erection (MUSE®)] has been approved as a treatment for ED in the United States, and further, it has been shown to be effective for treating ED due to neurogenic, psychogenic, arteriogenic, and mixed vasculogenic etiologies, including after non–nerve-sparing radical prostatectomy (63). The results of a double-blind, placebo-controlled study of 1511 men aged 27 to 88 years, with chronic ED from various organic causes, were reported (64). The men were first tested in the clinic with up to four doses of the drug (125, 250, 500, and 1000 µg); those who had sufficient responses were randomly assigned to either the effective dose of PGE_1 or placebo for three months of home treatment program. During in-clinic testing, 996 men (65.9%) had erections sufficient for intercourse. Of these men, 961 reported the results of at least one home treatment, and 299 of 461 treated with PGE_1

(64.9%) had intercourse successfully at least once, as compared with 93 of the 500 patients who received placebo (18.6%). On average, 7 of 10 PGE_1 administrations were followed by intercourse in men responsive to treatment. The efficacy of PGE_1 was similar regardless of age or cause of ED. The most common side effect was mild penile pain, which occurred after 10.8% of PGE_1 treatments. Hypotension occurred in 3.3% of patients receiving PGE_1 in the clinic. Priapism or penile fibrosis was not observed in this multicenter trial. The observation that approximately one-third of patients responding to transurethral PGE_1 in a clinical setting fail to do so at home has been consistent among many studies (65–68). When accounting for this, the overall in-home response rate for transurethral PGE_1 use is approximately 40%. Moreover, at least two studies have reported even more disappointing results with transurethral PGE_1 (69,70).

Dinoprostone

Prior to the commercial availability of the PGE_1 transurethral preparation, Wolfson et al. (71) used Prostin E_2 vaginal suppositories as a source of dinoprostone, a naturally occurring PGE_2 with oxytocic and vasodilating effects. Dinoprostone (20 and 40 mg suppositories) were mixed with 2% lidocaine and surgical lubricant to form a cream. Using a syringe, 2 mL of the cream was instilled in the urethral meatus of 20 impotent men. Overall, 70% of patients showed a response, and 30% of these developed a full penile erection. The only adverse effect reported was a mild transient urethral burning with placement of the cream.

☐ LOCAL TREATMENT OF PREMATURE EJACULATION
Lidocaine–Prilocaine Cream (Emla)

Local (topical) anesthetic preparations have been used to treat premature ejaculation (Table 1). Very limited data are available on their use, however. An example of these preparations is Emla® cream (Astra U.S.A. Inc., Westborough, Massachusetts), which consists of a eutectic mixture of lidocaine 2.5% and prilocaine 2.5%. The onset, depth, and duration of dermal analgesia provided depend primarily on the duration of application. Generally, the topical anesthetic creams are applied to the glans penis and penile shaft under occlusive cover (condom) for at least one half-hour prior to the sexual encounter. Dermal analgesia reaches its maximum at two to three hours and persists for one to two hours after removal. Some authors, however, advocate not removing the condom during intercourse, as this practice will not only prevent the transfer of remnant anesthetics to the partner's genitalia, but also provide a physical barrier and thus help to reduce penile sensitivity. Patients should be advised that dermal application of Emla cream may cause transient, local blanching followed by a transient, local redness or erythema. A recent study by Berkovitch et al. (72) in 11 patients with premature ejaculation who used the Emla cream without the condom found a significant improvement in the ejaculatory latency in five patients, improvement in four patients, and no change in two patients.

Lidocaine–Prilocaine Spray

One small open-label pilot study has described the use of a new lidocaine–prilocaine spray that delivers 7.5 mg lidocaine and 2.5 mg prilocaine, applied using a metered-dose aerosol delivery system. The spray is applied to the glans penis, left on for 10 to 15 minutes, and then wiped off carefully before intercourse. Eleven of the 14 patients completed the study, reporting an average eightfold increase in intravaginal ejaculation latency time (IVELT) from 1 minute and 24 seconds to 11 minutes and 21 seconds ($p = 0.008$). No subjects reported a decrease in IVELT, and the average satisfaction score for both patients and partners was 1.0 (-1 = worse, 0 = same, $+1$ = better, $+2$ = much better). Thus, topical lidocaine–prilocaine spray appears to prolong ejaculation time and improve sexual satisfaction for both men with premature ejaculation and their partners. Glandular numbness, noted in two cases, was not reported to affect the quality of orgasm. Occasionally, patients reported difficulty maintaining erection while waiting the required 15 minutes between application of the spray and the initiation of intercourse (73).

☐ LOCAL TREATMENT OF FAILURE OF DETUMESCENCE

Prolonged erection is a small but significant risk in patients treated with intracorporeal injections of vasoactive drugs. Patients receiving this form of therapy should be adequately counseled on the risk of priapism and advised on the use of minimum effective dose of chosen agent(s) (Table 1). Younger individuals and patients with psychogenic and/or neurogenic impotence usually exhibit satisfactory erectile responses to small doses of vasoactive drugs, but they also have a higher risk for the development of priapism than patients with vascular insufficiency (8–10,120,121). Mild cases of prolonged erection may be treated with the oral intake of α-receptor agonists such as pseudophedrine 30 mg once or twice at 30-minute intervals. Also, the β-receptor agonist terbutaline has been used orally to treat priapism of less than four hours duration in traumatic paraplegic patients (9,74). More severe cases of priapism extending for longer than four hours usually require corporeal aspiration and irrigation with a solution containing heparin (5000 U/L) and epinephrine (1 mg/L) (3,122). Another method involves the aspiration of 10 to 20 mL of blood from the corpora with a 19-gauge needle, followed by injection of phenylephrine, beginning with doses of 200 μg every five minutes and increasing to 500 μg, if necessary. This appears to be effective in resolving

erections of less than 12 hours duration (2). Phenylephrine doses of 500 μg in 2 mL saline have also been injected into the corpus cavernosum every 15 minutes without aspiration until detumescence is achieved (75). Other adrenergic agonists such as norepinephrine, ephedrine, and metaraminol have been used to stimulate corporeal vasoconstriction and to reverse priapism. All of these agents can cause a significant increase in blood pressure, and the use of metaraminol was reported to cause death in two cases (77). Occasionally, prolonged priapism (usually of more than 36 hours' duration) due to vasoactive drug injection requires the surgical placement of an arteriovenous shunt (8–12,123). This will cause a venous leakage, however, and the possible failure of response to future vasoactive drug injections. Recently, the association of a positive erectile response to visual sexual stimulation and a penile brachial index (PBI) of more than 0.8 was identified as an indicator of a high risk for postinjection priapism, but such risk was reduced to 1% with careful adjustment of vasoactive drug doses administered (124).

Other forms of medical therapy may include local or systemic glucocorticoids and the intralesional injection of a collagenase or a calcium channel blocker (e.g., Verapamil). These locally administered agents appear to have approximately the same therapeutic effects as the systemic medications. (For further information, see Chapter 29.) Medical therapy may help patients with moderate disease, whereas surgical correction is the treatment of choice for those with severe penile deformity.

☐ CONCLUSION

Although oral pharmacotherapy represents an attractive first-line treatment option for most patients with ED, a significant number of patients are either unsuited or unresponsive to this form of therapy. For such patients, the use of local penile drug treatments continues to offer a useful alternative approach to therapy, either along or in combination with oral erectogenic drugs. Of the local drug options currently available for ED, intracavernous injections have the highest efficacy; however, the invasive nature of this form of therapy deters many patients from the long-term use of intrapenile injections. Topical agents provide an appealing method for drug delivery; however, the permeation of many agents through the penile skin is often inadequate, and further enhancement is needed to optimize the efficacy of this approach. As safer and more effective oral erectogenic drugs are developed, the use of local agents is likely to decline; however, their potential to enhance the efficacy of oral therapies may continue to be useful. New local penile pharmacotherapy for ejaculatory disorders also continues to be explored. The effort to develop oral agents is likely to offer a safe and effective approach to the management of these problems in the future.

☐ REFERENCES

1. Virag R. Intracavernous injection of papaverine for erectile failure. Lancet 1982; 2(8304):938.
2. Broderick GA. Intracavernous pharmacotherapy: treatment for the aging erectile response. Urol Clin North Am 1996; 23(1):111–126.
3. Fallon B. Intracavernous injection therapy for male erectile dysfunction. Urol Clin North Am 1995; 22(4):833–845.
4. Virag R. Comments from Ronald Virag on intracavernous injection: 25 years later. J Sex Med 2005; 2(3): 289–290.
5. Poch G, Kukovetz WR. Papaverine-induced inhibition of phosphodiesterase activity in various mammalian tissues. Life Sci 1971; 10(3):133–144.
6. Tanaka T. Papaverine hydrochloride in peripheral blood and the degree of penile erection. J Urol 1990; 143(6):1135–1137.
7. Hakenberg O, Wetterauer U, Koppermann U, et al. Systemic pharmacokinetics of papaverine and phentolamine: comparison of intravenous and intracavernous application. Int J Impot Res 1990; 2(suppl 2): 247–248.
8. Hellstrom WJG, McAninch JW, Lue TF. Priapism: physiology and treatment. Probl Urol 1987; 3:518–529.
9. Soni BM, Vaidyanathan S, Krishnan KR. Management of pharmacologically induced prolonged penile erection with oral terbutaline in traumatic paraplegics. Paraplegia 1994; 32(10):670–674.
10. Junemann KP, Alken P. Pharmacotherapy of erectile dysfunction: a review. Int J Impot Res 1989; 1:71–93.
11. Bardin ED, Krieger JN. Pharmacological priapism: comparison of trazodone- and papaverine-associated cases. Int Urol Nephrol 1990; 22(2):147–152.
12. Halsted DS, Weigel JW, Noble MJ, et al. Papaverine induced priapism: 2 case reports. J Urol 1986; 136(1):109–110.
13. Rowland DL, Leentvaar EJ, Blom JH, et al. Changes in penile sensitivity following papaverine-induced erection in sexually functional and dysfunctional men. J Urol 1991; 146(4):1018–1021.
14. Montorsi F, Guazzoni G, Rigatti P, et al. Pharmacological management of erectile dysfunction. Drugs 1995; 50(3):465–479.
15. Coker C, Bettocchi C, Pryor J. Caverject: a new licensed prostaglandin preparation for use in erectile dysfunction. J Androl 1994; 15(6 suppl):71S.
16. Roy AC, Adaikan PG, Sen DK, et al. Prostaglandin 15-hydroxydehydrogenase activity in human penile corpora cavernosa and its significance in prostaglandin-mediated penile erection. Br J Urol 1989; 64(2):180–182.
17. Cawello W, Schweer H, Dietrich B, et al. Pharmacokinetics of prostaglandin E1 and its main metabolites after intracavernous injection and short-term infusion of prostaglandin E1 in patients with erectile dysfunction. J Urol 1997; 158(4):1403–1407.
18. Porst H. The rationale for prostaglandin E1 in erectile failure: a survey of worldwide experience. J Urol 1996; 155(3):802–815.
19. Moriel EZ, Rajfer J. Sodium bicarbonate alleviates penile pain induced by intracavernous injections for erectile dysfunction. J Urol 1993; 149(5 Pt 2): 1299–1300.
20. Schramek P, Plas EG, Hubner WA, et al. Intracavernous injection of prostaglandin E1 plus procaine in the treatment of erectile dysfunction. J Urol 1994; 152(4): 1108–1110.
21. Gheorghiu D, Godschalk M, Gheorghiu S, et al. Slow injection of prostaglandin E1 decreases associated penile pain. Urology 1996; 47(6):903–904.
22. Linet OI, Ogrinc FG (The Alprostadil Study Group). Efficacy and safety of intracavernosal alprostadil in men with erectile dysfunction. N Engl J Med 1996; 334(14):873–877.
23. Lehmann K, Caselia R, Blochlinger A, et al. Reasons for discontinuing intracavernous injection therapy with prostaglandin E1 (Alprostadil). Urology 1999; 53(2):397–400.
24. Kunelius P, Lukkarinen O. Intracavernous self-injection of prostaglandin E1 in the treatment of erectile dysfunction. Int J Impot Res 1999; 11(1):21–24.
25. Parkerson GR, Wilke RJ, Hays RD. An international comparison of the reliability and responsiveness of the Duke Health Profile for measuring health-related quality of life patients treated with alprostadil for erectile dysfunction. Medical Care 1999; 37(1):56–67.
26. Porst H, Buvat J, Meuleman E, et al. Intracavernous alprostadil alfadex-an effective and well tolerated treatment for erectile dysfunction. Results of a long-term European study. Int J Impot Res 1998; 10(4): 225–231.
27. Truss MC, Becker AJ, Djamilian MH, et al. Role of the nitric oxide donor linsidomine chlorhydrate (SIN-1) in the diagnosis and treatment of erectile dysfunction. Urology 1994; 44(4):553–556.
28. Stief CG, Holmquist F, Djamilian M, et al. Preliminary results with the nitric oxide donor linsidomine chlorhydrate in the treatment of human erectile dysfunction. J Urol 1992; 148(5):1437–1440.
29. Brock G, Breza J, Lue TF. Intracavernous sodium nitroprusside: inappropriate impotence treatment. J Urol 1993; 150(3):864–867.
30. Costa P, Sarrazin B, Bressolle F, et al. Efficiency and side effects of intracavernous injections of moxisylyte in impotent patients: a dose-finding study versus placebo. J Urol 1993; 149(2):301–305.
31. Buvat J, Lemaire A, Herbaut-Buvat M. Intracavernous pharmacotherapy: comparison of moxisylyte and prostaglandin E1. Int J Impot Res 1996; 8(2):41–46.

32. Buvat J, Costa P, Morlier D, et al. Double-blind multicenter study comparing alprostadil alpha-cyclodextrin with moxisylyte chlorhydrate in patients with chronic erectile dysfunction. J Urol 1998; 159:116–119.

33. Arvis G, Rivet G, Schwent B. Prolonged use of moxisylyte chlorhydrate (Icavex) by intracavernous self-injections in the treatment of impotence. Evaluation of long-term tolerance (Article in French). J Urol (Paris) 1996; 102(4):151–156.

34. Saenz deTejada I, Garvey DS, et al. Design and evaluation of nitrosylated alpha-adrenergic receptor antagonists as potential agents for the treatment of impotence. J Pharmacol Exp Ther 1999; 290(1):121–128.

35. Truss MC, Becker AJ, Thon WF, et al. Intracavernous calcitonin gene-related peptide plus prostaglandin E1: possible alternative to penile implants in selected patients. Eur Urol 1994; 26(1):40–45.

36. Martinez-Pineiro L, Cortes R, Cuervo E, et al. Prospective comparative study with intracavernous sodium nitroprusside and prostaglandin E1 in patients with erectile dysfunction. Eur Urol 1998; 34(4):350–354.

37. Silva LFG, Nascimento NRF, Fonteles MC, et al. Phentolamine relaxes human corpus cavernosum by a nonadrenergic mechanism activating ATP-sensitive K+ channel. Int J Impot Res 2005; 17(1):27–32.

38. Meinhardt W, delaFuente RB, Lycklama A, et al. Prostaglandin E1 with phentolamine for the treatment of erectile dysfunction. Int J Impot Res 1996; 8(1):5–7.

39. Brindley GS. Pilot experiments on the actions of drugs injected into the human corpus cavernousm penis. Br J Pharmacol 1986; 87(3):495–500.

40. Kaplan SA, Reis RB, Kohn IJ, et al. Combination therapy using oral alpha-blockers and intracavernosal injection in men with erectile dysfunction. Urology 1998; 52(5):739–743.

41. Meinhardt W, Kropman RF, Vermeij P. Comparative tolerability and efficacy of treatments for impotence. Drug Saf 1999; 20(2):133–146.

42. Shmueli J, Israilov S, Segenreich E, et al. Progressive treatment of erectile dysfunction with intracorporeal injections of different combinations of vasoactive agents. Int J Impot Res 1999; 11(1):15–19.

43. Ehmke H, Junemann KP, Mayer B, et al. Nitric oxide synthase and vasoactive intestinal polypeptide colocalization in neurons innervating the human penile circulation. Int J Impot Res 1995; 7(3):147–156.

44. Tamura M, Kagawa S, Kimura K, et al. Coexistence of nitric oxide synthase, tyrosine hydroxylase and vasoactive intestinal polypeptide in human penile tissue—a triple histochemical and immunohistochemical study. J Urol 1995; 153(2):530–534.

45. Saenz de Tejada I, Moreland RB. Physiology of erection, pathophysiology of impotence, and implications of PGE1 in the control of collagen synthesis in the corpus cavernosum. In: Goldstein I, Lue TF, eds. The Role of Alprostadil in the Diagnosis and Treatment of Erectile Dysfunction. Princeton: Excerpta Medica, 1993:1–33.

46. Sandhu D, Curless E, Dean J, et al. A double blind, placebo controlled study of intracavernosal vasoactive intestinal polypeptide and phenotolamine mesylate in a novel auto-injector for the treatment of non-psychogenic erectile dysfunction. Int J Impot Res 1999; 11(2): 91–97.

47. McMahon CG. A pilot study of the role of intracavernous injection of vasoactive intestinal peptide (VIP) and phentolamine mesylate in the treatment of erectile dysfunction. Int J Impot Res 1996; 8(4):233–236.

48. Dinsmore WW, Alderdice DK. Vasoactive intestinal polypeptide and phentolamine mesylate administered by autoinjector in the treatment of patients with erectile dysfunction resistant to other intracavernosal agents. Br J Urol 1998; 81(3):437–440.

49. Dinsmore WW, Gingell C, Hackett G, et al. Treating men with predominantly nonpsychogenic erectile dysfunction with intracavernosal vasoactive intestinal polypeptide and phentolamine mesylate in a novel auto-injector system: a multicentre double-blind placebo-controlled study. Br J Urol Int 1999; 83(3): 274–279.

50. Azadzoi KM, Payton T, Krane RJ, et al. Effects of intracavernosal trazodone hydrochloride: animal and human studies. J Urol 1990; 144(5):1277–1282.

51. Saenz de Tejada I, Ware JC, Blanco R, et al. Pathophysiology of prolonged penile erection associated with trazodone use. J Urol Clin 1991; 145(1):60–64.

52. Warner MD, Peabody CA, Whiteford HA, et al. Trazodone and priapism. J Psychiatry 1987; 48(6): 244–245.

53. Foreman MM, Wernicke JF. Approaches for the development of oral drug therapies for erectile dysfunction. Semin Urol 1990; 8(2):107–112.

54. McVary KT, Polepalle S, Riggi S, et al. Topical prostaglandin E1 SEPA gel for the treatment of erectile dysfunction. J Urol 1999; 162(3 Pt 1):726–730.

55. Foldvari M, Oguejiofor C, Afridi S, et al. Liposome encapsulated prostaglandin E1 in erectile dysfunction: correlation between in vitro delivery through foreskin and efficacy in patients. Urology 1998; 52(5):838–843.

56. Yeager J, Beihn RM. Retention and migration of alprostadil cream applied topically to the glans meatus for erectile dysfunction. Int J Impot Res 2005; 17(1):91–95.

57. Kim ED, el-Rashidy R, McVary KT. Papaverine topical gel for treatment of erectile dysfunction. J Urol 1995; 153(2):361–365.

58. Radomski SB, Herschorn S, Rangaswamy S. Topical minoxidil in the treatment of male erectile dysfunction. J Urol 1994; 151(5):1225–1226.

59. Chancellor MB, Rivas DA, Panzer DE, et al. Prospective comparison of topical minoxidil to vacuum constriction device and intracorporeal papaverine injection in treatment of erectile dysfunction due to spinal cord injury. Urology 1994; 43(3):365–369.

60. Anderson DC, Seifert CF. Topical nitrate treatment of impotence. Ann Pharmacother 1993; 27(10):1203–1205.
61. Owen JA, Saunders F, Harris C, et al. Topical nitroglycerin: a potential treatment for impotence. J Urol 1989; 141(3):546–548.
62. Gramkow J, Lendorf A, Zhu J, et al. Transcutaneous nitroglycerin in the treatment of erectile dysfunction: a placebo controlled clinical trial. Int J Impot Res 1999; 11(1):35–39.
63. Raina R, Agarwal A, Ausmundson S, et al. Long-term efficacy and compliance of MUSE for erectile dysfunction following radical prostatectomy: SHIM (IIEF-5) analysis. Int J Impot Res 2005; 17(1):86–90.
64. Padma-Nathan H, Hellstrom WJ, Kaiser FE, et al. The Medicated Urethral System for Erection (MUSE) Study Group. Treatment of men with erectile dysfunction with transurethral alprostadil. N Engl J Med 1997; 336(1):1–7.
65. Hellstrom WJ, Bennett AH, Gesundheit N, et al. A double-blind, placebo-controlled evaluation of the erectile response to transurethral alprostadil. Urology 1996; 48(6):851–856.
66. Williams G, Abbou CC, Amar TE, et al. Efficacy and safety of transurethral alprostadil therapy in men with erectile dysfunction. MUSE study group. Br J Urol 1998; 81(6):889–894.
67. Engel JD, McVary KT. Transurethral alprostadil as therapy for patients who withdrew from or failed prior intracavernous injection therapy. Urology 1998; 51(5):687–692.
68. Costabile RA, Spevak M, Fishman IJ, et al. Efficacy and safety of transurethral alprostadil in patients with erectile dysfunction following radical prostatectomy. J Urol 1998; 160(4):1325–1328.
69. Werthman P, Rajfer J. MUSE therapy: preliminary clinical observations. Urology 1997; 50(5):809–811.
70. Peterson CA, Bennett AH, Hellstrom WJ, et al. Erectile response to transurethral alprostadil, prazosin and alprostadil-prazosin combinations. J Urol 1998; 159(5):1523–1527.
71. Wolfson B, Pickett S, Scott NE, et al. Intraurethral prostaglandin E-2 cream: a possible alternative treatment for erectile dysfunction. Urology 1993; 42(1):73–75.
72. Berkovitch M, Keresteci AG, Koren G. Efficacy of prilocaine-lidocaine cream in the treatment of premature ejaculation. J Urol 1995; 154(4):1360–1361.
73. Henry R, Morales A. Topical lidocaine-prilocaine spray for the treatment of premature ejaculation: a proof of concept study. Int J Impot Res 2003; 15(4): 277–281.
74. Priyadarshi S. Oral terbutaline in the management of pharmacologic prolonged erection. Int J Impot Res 2004; 16(5):424–426.
75. Muruve N, Hosking DH. Intracorporeal phenylephrine in the treatment of priapism. J Urol 1996; 155(1):141–143.
76. Kandeel FR, Koussa VKT, Swerdloff RS. Male sexual function and its disorders: physiology, pathophysiology,

clinical investigation, and treatment. Endocr Rev 2001; 22(3):342–388.
77. Stanners A, Colin-Jones D. Metaraminol for priapism [Lett]. Lancet 1984; 2(8409):978.
78. Brindley GS. Cavernosal alpha-blockade: a new technique for investigating and treating erectile impotence. Br J Psychiatry 1983; 143(4):332–337.
79. O'Sullivan JD, Hughes AJ. Apomorphine-induced penile erections in Parkinson's disease. Mov Disord 1998; 13(3):536–539.
80. Soli M, Bertaccini A, Carparelli F, et al. Vasoactive cocktails for erectile dysfunction: chemical stability of PGE1, papaverine and phentolamine. J Urol 1998; 160(2):551–555.
81. Sundaram CP, Thomas W, Pryor LE, et al. Long-term follow-up of patients receiving injection therapy for erectile dysfunction. Urology 1997; 49(6):932–935.
82. Rowland DL, Boedhoe HS, Dohle G, et al. Intracavernosal self-injection therapy in men with erectile dysfunction: satisfaction and attrition in 119 patients. Int J Impot Res 1999; 11(13):145–151.
83. Richter S, Gross R, Nissenkorn I. Cavernous injection therapy for the treatment of erectile dysfunction in elderly men. Int J Impot Res 1990; 2:43–47.
84. Copel L, Katz R, Blachar A, et al. Clinical and duplex US assessment of effects of sildenafil on cavernosal arteries of the penis: comparison with intracavernosal injection of vasoactive agents—initial experience. Radiology 2005; 237(3):986–991.
85. Cornell University, Weill Medical College, Department of Urology Sexual Medicine Program. Drug treatment of erectile dysfunction. http://www.cornellurology.com/sexualmedicine/ed/drugs.html.
86. Shamloul R, Kamel I. A broken intracavernous needle: successful ultrasound-guided removal. J Sex Med 2005; 2(1):147–148.
87. Viera AJ, Clenney TL, Shenenberger DW, et al. Newer pharmacologic alternatives for erectile dysfunction. Am Fam Phys 1999.
88. Marshall GA, Breza J, Lue TF. Improved hemodynamic response after long-term intracavernous injection for impotence. Urology 1994; 43(6):844–848.
89. Harding LM, Adeniyi A, Everson R, et al. Comparison of a needle-free high-pressure injection system with needle-tipped injection of intracavernosal alprostadil for erectile dysfunction. Int J Impot Res 2002; 14(6):498–501.
90. Carter PG, Joyce AD, Dickinson IK, et al. A drug delivery system for treating erectile impotence: a preliminary communication. J Androl 1994; 15(6 suppl):70S.
91. Borges FD. A new approach to the pharmacologic treatment of impotence. Int J Impot Res 1994; 6(3):137–143.
92. Lomas GM, Jarow JP. Risk factors for papaverine-induced prolonged erection. J Urol 1992; 147:1280–1281.
93. Zorgniotti AW, Lefleur RS. Auto-injection of the corpus cavernosum with a vasoactive drug combination for vasculogenic impotence. J Urol 1985; 133(1): 39–41.

94. Kerfoot WW, Carson CC. Pharmacologically induced erections among geriatric men. J Urol 1991; 146(4): 1022–1024.

95. Valdevenito R, Melman A. Intracavernous self-injection pharmacotherapy program: analysis of results and complications. Int J Impot Res 1994; 6(2):81–91.

96. Goldstein I, Borges FD, Fitch WP, et al. Rescuing the failed papaverine/phentolamine erection: a proposed synergistic action of papaverine, phentolamine and PGE1. J Urol 1990; 143:304A (Abstract).

97. Bennett AH, Carpenter AJ, Barada JH. An improved vasoactive drug combination for a pharmacological erection program. J Urol 1991; 146(6):1564–1565.

98. Weiske WH. Efficacy of PGE1 and SIN-1 testing under Rigiscan real-time monitoring. Int J Impot Res 6(suppl 1994; 1):D109.

99. Broderick GA, Harkaway R. Pharmacologic erection: time-dependent changes in the corporal environment. Int J Impot Res 1994; 6(1):9–16.

100. Spycher MA, Hauri D. The ultrastructure of the erectile tissue in priapism. J Urol 1986; 135(1):142–147.

101. Chen J, Godschalk M, Katz PG, et al. Peyronie's-like plaque after penile injection of prostaglandin E1. J Urol 1994; 152(3):961–962.

102. Ravnik-Oblak M, Oblak C, Vodusek DB, et al. Intracavernous injection of prostaglandin E1 in impotent diabetic men. Int J Impot Res 1990; 2:143–150.

103. Schramek P, Waldhauser M. Dose-dependent effect and side-effect of prostaglandin E1 in erectile dysfunction. Br J Clin Pharmacol 1989; 28(5):567–571.

104. Hamid S, Dhabuwala CB, Pontes EJ. Combination intracavernous pharmacotherapy in the management of male erectile dysfunction. Int J Impot Res 1992; 4:109–112.

105. Govier FE, McClure RD, Weissman RM, et al. Experience with triple-drug therapy in a pharmacological erection program. J Urol 1993; 150(6):1822–1824.

106. Hwang TI, Yang CR, Ho WL, et al. Histopathological change of corpora cavernosa after long-term intracavernous injection. Eur Urol 1991; 20(4):301–306.

107. Sidi AA, Cherwitz DL, Becker EF. The effect of intracavernous pharmacotherapy on human erectile tissue: a light microscopic analysis. Int J Impot Res 1989; 1:27–33.

108. Schwarzer JU, Hofmann R. Purulent corporeal cavernositis secondary to papaverine-induced priapism. J Urol 1991; 146(3):845–846.

109. Brown SL, Haas CA, Koehler M, et al. Hepatotoxicity related to intracavernous pharmacotherapy with papaverine. Urology 1998; 52(5):844–847.

110. English JC, King DH, Foley JP. Penile shaft hypopigmentation: lichen sclerosus occurring after the initiation of alprostadil intracavernous injections for erectile dysfunction. J Am Acad Dermatol 39 (5 Pt 1998; 1): 801–803.

111. Mark SD, Gray JM. Iatrogenic penile foreign body. Br J Urol 1991; 67(5):555–556.

112. Sogari PR, Teloken C, Souto CA. Atropine role in the pharamcological erection test: study of 228 patients. J Urol 1997; 158(5):1760–1763.

113. Takahashi Y, Ishii N, Lue TF, et al. Pharmacological effects of adenosine on canine penile erection. Tohoki J Exp Med pulsed 1991; 165(1):49–58.

114. Virag R, Sussman H. Exploration of the deep dorsal vein of the penis using Doppler ultrasonography. Preliminary study (Article in French). J Mal Vasc 1998; 23(3):195–198.

115. Wessells H, Fuciarelli K, Hansen J, et al. Synthetic melanotropic peptide initiates erections in men with psychogenic erectile dysfunction: a double-blind, placebo controlled crossover study. J Urol 1998; 160(2): 389–393.

116. Hadley ME, Dorr RT. Melanocortin peptide therapeutics: historical milestones, clinical studies and commercialization. Peptides 2006; 27(4):921–930.

117. Gomaa A, Shalaby M, Osman M, et al. Topical treatment of erectile dysfunction: randomised double blind placebo controlled trial of cream containing aminophylline, isosorbide dinitrate, and co-dergocrine mesylate. Br Med J 1996; 312(7045):1512–1515.

118. Roux PJL, Naude JH. Topical vasoactive cream in the treatment of erectile failure: a prospective, randomized placebo-controlled trial. Br J Urol Int 1999; 83(7): 810–811.

119. Chiang HS, Kao YH, Sheu MT. Papaverine and prostaglandin E1 gel applications for impotence. Ann Acad Med Singapore 1995; 24(5):767–769.

120. Weidner W, Schroeder-Printzen I, Weiske WH, et al. Sexual dysfunction in Peyronie's disease: an analysis of 222 patients without previous local plaque therapy. J Urol 1997; 157(1):325–328.

121. Bastuba MD, Saenz de Tejada I, Dinlenc CZ, et al. Arterial priapism: diagnosis, treatment and long-term follow up. J Urol 1994; 151(5):1231–1237.

122. Molina L, Bejany D, Lynne CM, et al. Diluted epinephrine solution for the treatment of priapism. J Urol 1989; 141(5):1127–1128.

123. Kulmala RV, Tamella TL. Effects of priapism lasting 24 hours or longer caused by intracavernosal injection of vasoactive drugs. Int J Impot Res 1995; 7(2): 131–136.

124. Fouda A, Hassouna M, Beddoe E, et al. Priapism: an avoidable complication of pharmacologically induced erection. J Urol 1989; 142(4):995–997.

31

The Use of Complementary or Alternative Medicine in the Treatment of Male Sexual Dysfunction

Mark A. Moyad
Department of Urology, University of Michigan Medical Center, Ann Arbor, Michigan, U.S.A.

□ INTRODUCTION

In general, overall sexual function tends to decline in healthy aging men (1). The latent time period between sexual stimulation and erection increases, erectile turgidity decreases, ejaculation is not as forceful, the volume of the ejaculate is reduced, and the interval between erections becomes longer. Testosterone levels and penile sensitivity to stimulation are reduced, and there is an increase in cavernous muscle tone. Chronic medical conditions frequently associated with aging also contribute to the rising incidence of erectile dysfunction (ED). Approximately 50% of the men with long-standing diabetes have ED (1), and chronic renal failure has also been correlated with reduced erectile function and libido. Men with coronary artery disease or heart disease, peripheral vascular disease, and stroke also have an increased risk of ED (2–4). Other factors associated with ED include smoking, hypertension, obesity, dyslipidemia, lack of physical activity, stress, and chronic alcoholism or drug abuse (5,6).

Several large epidemiological studies have suggested that the incorporation of heart-healthy lifestyle changes may impact one's overall risk of ED. For example, the frequently cited Massachusetts Male Aging Study demonstrated a fairly consistent link between cardiovascular disease and ED (7). Follow-up to this study has continued to demonstrate this correlation (8,9). Recently, the results of the Health Professionals Follow-up Study, one of the largest ongoing prospective studies in medicine, showed that physical activity was associated with a 30% reduced risk of ED and that obesity was associated with a 30% higher risk of ED. Smoking, alcohol intake, and television-viewing time were also related to an increased risk of ED. The men in this epidemiologic study with the lowest risk of ED were those without chronic medical conditions and those who regularly engaged in healthy activities (10).

Healthy lifestyle modifications initiated at any age may also have a significant impact on reducing the risk of ED, although it is likely that good practices begun earlier in life will impact the quality and duration of an individual's physical condition more significantly. This author believes that no discussion of dietary supplements, prescribed agents, or any other intervention for ED should commence without the mention of lifestyle factors that may influence the risk or progression of ED. Because of the potential synergism that may occur, the implementation of lifestyle changes should continue to be emphasized early and often throughout the course of ED treatment.

□ COMPLEMENTARY AND ALTERNATIVE MEDICINE AND ED

Complementary or alternative medicine (CAM), as defined by the National Center for Complementary and Alternative Medicine (NCCAM, a component of the National Institutes of Health), is a group of diverse medical and healthcare systems, practices, and products that are not presently considered to be part of conventional medicine (11). "Complementary medicine" is any such therapy that is used in conjunction with conventional medicine, and "alternative medicine" represents treatment used in place of conventional medicine. "Integrative medicine" combines mainstream medical therapies and CAM therapies for which there is some high-quality scientific evidence of safety and effectiveness. CAM therapies continue to enjoy tremendous popularity around the world (12,13). Approximately half of the population in the United States has used some form of CAM, and more visits to CAM practitioners occur annually compared to the total number of visits to all primary care physicians (14).

One of the most rapidly increasing areas of CAM usage is that of dietary supplements (herbs, vitamins, minerals, and other orally consumed compounds) (15). Although sales of dietary supplements have blossomed into a billion-dollar industry (16), unfortunately, studies attempting to establish the prevalence, safety, and efficacy of the use of dietary supplements for the treatment of ED are lacking (17). Even casual searches of the Internet, magazines, and national newspapers, however, will reveal a multitude of potential sources from which the public is able to obtain a wide variety of supplements for the treatment of ED. This may be partially the result of the 1994 U.S. Dietary Supplement

Health and Education Act (DSHEA) (18), which permitted almost any compound or substance to be advertised as a dietary supplement as long as no specific health claims or benefits are made on the label of the supplement container regarding the compound's ability to treat, cure, mitigate, or diagnose any disease or condition. Therefore, this act severely limits the authority of the Food and Drug Administration (FDA) to regulate manufacturers of dietary supplements. Further, the supplement industry is not currently held to the same standards as the pharmaceutical industry, which is required to supply sufficient clinical evidence that their products are safe and effective and have good or adequate quality control before they can be released to the public market. In one of the largest Internet studies ever published (19), researchers found that out of 443 web sites advertising eight of the top-selling supplements, 81% of the retail web sites made one or more health claims, and 55% actually claimed to treat, prevent, diagnose, or cure specific diseases. More than 50% of the web sites with a health claim omitted the standard federal disclaimer.

The lack of regulatory oversight of the supplement industry in the United States has led to a significant discrepancy between label information and the actual content of packaged supplements. For example, a supplement label may report a specific dosage of a compound, but there may actually be significantly higher, lower, or no amounts of the compound (20,21). Without independent and universally randomized quality-control studies, it is difficult to evaluate the actual quality and quantity of any dietary supplement sold in the United States.

An absence of clinical research into the interactions between supplements and medications is another constant source of confusion. For example, a recent study has highlighted one of the biggest selling herbal supplements for depression, St. John's Wort. This supplement is metabolized by liver cytochrome P450 3A4, as are over 50% of the available prescription drugs in the United States. There is concern that these medications may be less effective when administered to patients also using St. John's Wort (22). It is imperative for clinicians to inform patients that when a prescription drug is combined with any dietary supplement, there is potential for interaction. This is especially true prior to a surgical procedure, as numerous supplements have already demonstrated the ability to interfere with either anesthetic agents or coagulation factors (23).

Clinicians must be consistent in warning patients of the possible health risks when purchasing some dietary supplement products. Large-scale surveys suggest, however, that the American public does not believe that physicians have sufficient knowledge about dietary supplements and are actually biased against their use (15); yet, the majority of the participants surveyed were also in favor of increased governmental regulation of supplements.

The Role of the Placebo Effect in ED

ED studies generally include some subjective self-evaluations. Thus, even with the use of randomized clinical trials, the results of these studies may be dramatically influenced by the presence of placebo effect (1). For example, it has not been unique in clinical studies to observe a 25% to 40% overall placebo response when investigating medications for pain control (24), hair growth (25), or a reduction in hair loss (26) for men or women. Thus, the effect of the placebo response cannot be discounted when considering the use and efficacy of CAM therapies for ED.

□ POPULAR CAM THERAPIES FOR ED

While it is not possible to analyze comprehensively all the benefits and detriments of the hundreds of supplements that seem to exist, several procedures or compounds seem to be more common to most of these dietary supplements. These will be discussed below and summarized in Table 1. Only those dietary supplements and procedures that are currently regarded as "complementary" or "alternative" treatments will be discussed in this chapter.

Acupuncture

Acupuncture has been used in China for over 2500 years for a variety of medical conditions (27–29), and even today, this therapy represents a popular component of the modern Chinese healthcare system. Practitioners believe that there are pathways of energy flow (Qi) throughout the human body, which are necessary for maintaining adequate health; therefore, any potential disturbance of this flow is thought to be responsible for disease. A trained, licensed acupuncturist can apparently correct inadequate Qi by manipulating various subepidermal sites with the insertion of needles at a number of defined acupuncture points. For example, auricular acupuncture is regarded as having particularly good medicinal value since the ear is thought to contain a series of points that represents various anatomic positions throughout the human body. These needles may be left in the skin for a specified amount of time; additionally, depending on the condition being treated, heat or electrical stimulation may be applied through the needles.

Studies have shown there may be an actual neurophysiologic basis for the purported effectiveness of acupuncture: the placement of a needle at a specific site may stimulate the nervous system, or other similar physiologic pathways, to release a variety of endogenous compounds—e.g., opioids—in the muscles, spinal cord, and brain (29). These compounds may stimulate the production and release of other compounds and hormones that affect the body's internal homeostasis. Thus, the natural healing potential of the body may be enhanced with the use of

Table 1   A Partial Summary of Alternative Therapies and Commercially Available ED Supplements

ED alternative/supplement	Overall conclusions
Acupuncture	May favorably impact several medical conditions, but adequate trials for ED have not been completed. Could be of potential benefit in psychogenic ED.
Androstenedione/DHEA	Precursors to testosterone. Increases estradiol and possibly testosterone in men with normal testosterone levels and lowers high-density lipoprotein by an average of 10%. May increase testosterone dramatically in hypogonadal men, although direct replacement with testosterone itself would be more practical. May provide a benefit for nonorganic ED and others in men with suboptimal levels of these precursors only.
Ginkgo biloba	May have a blood-thinning effect and increase the risk of hemorrhages. Lacks any benefit thus far in a small number of studies with men with ED.
Korean Red Ginseng (Panax ginseng)	Two preliminary trials suggest a potential benefit for men with ED. It may be one of the more promising supplements because of its ability to increase NO levels in some studies; however, quality control is a serious issue with this supplement and more randomized trials are needed.
L-Arginine	Another precursor to NO and potentially promising. High daily doses may benefit a minority of men that secrete low levels of NO. May lower blood pressure and some cardiovascular risk serum markers. Needs more randomized trials.
Yohimbine	May be partially effective as a prescription drug for psychogenic ED; as a supplement, however, it lacks quality control for adequate benefit. Can cause serious side effects.
Zinc	May benefit only those with a severe zinc deficiency. Otherwise there is a lack of data and high dosages can be immunosuppresive and increase the risk of a variety of prostatic and other diseases.
Other supplements	Avena sativa and other potential cholesterol and blood pressure reducers, and *Tribulus terrestris* (precursor to DHEA?) need additional clinical trials.

Abbreviations: DHEA, dehydroepiandrosterone; ED, erectile dysfunction; NO, nitric oxide.

acupuncture. Because the compounds may also alter the perception of symptoms, the benefit of a placebo response with this treatment modality cannot be discounted.

In 1997, the National Institutes of Health issued a consensus statement on acupuncture (30,31), citing that while additional research into this treatment modality is warranted, the quality of currently available acupuncture research, particularly in regards to placebo controls, is severely limited. Additionally, the majority of published data concerns traditional needle acupuncture and has not adequately involved other synergistic acupuncture techniques such as electrostimulation (electroacupuncture), laser (laser acupuncture), external pressure (acupressure), or heat (moxibustion). While the effect of acupuncture in the treatment of psychogenic ED has been successfully evaluated in a small prospective, randomized, placebo-controlled trial (32) demonstrating a satisfactory response in 68.4% of the treatment group versus 9% of the placebo group, it should be noted that there are virtually no sound, randomized studies published to date that demonstrate the possible role of acupuncture in treating patients experiencing organic ED. Additional randomized, placebo-controlled studies utilizing large sample sizes are warranted.

The side effects of acupuncture are reportedly minimal in the hands of a well-trained or licensed practitioner; however, severe side effects are a more likely possibility when training is inadequate or improper. Forgotten needles and transient hypotension were some of the more commonly reported adverse effects (33). Pneumothorax and infection from the procedure is possible in the hands of lesser-trained practitioners (34–36).

L-ARGININE

L-arginine is a semiessential amino acid and is a precursor to nitric oxide, one of the primary neurotransmitters in the mediation of penile erection (1,37,38). Thus, it would seem theoretically plausible that an adequate amount of L-arginine would have the potential to improve ED in some men.

Nitric oxide is released during nonadrenergic, noncholinergic neurotransmission and from endothelium. Within the muscle itself, nitric oxide activates a guanylyl cyclase, which increases the intracellular levels of cyclic guanosine monophosphate (GMP). Cyclic GMP is an intracellular second messenger that mediates smooth muscle relaxation and activates specific protein kinases that phosphorylate specific proteins to cause the opening of potassium channels and the closing of calcium channels and an overall sequestration of intracellular calcium. The reduction in intracellular calcium results in smooth muscle relaxation and an increase in the flow of penile blood. (For further details on the physiology of erectile function, see Chapter 3.)

Three small pilot clinical studies of L-arginine versus placebo (39–41) have been completed with mixed results. The first study was a placebo-controlled clinical trial that used 2800 mg/day of L-arginine for only two weeks and documented that 40% of patients had improvement in their erections (39). The actual responders were younger and had better overall vascular function by hemodynamic investigation versus the nonresponders. The second pilot trial (40) included

1500 mg/day of L-arginine versus placebo for two weeks for men with mixed type ED. L-arginine at this specific dosage did not demonstrate a benefit over placebo. In the third small trial (41), patients (n = 50) were given a high dosage (5 g/day) of L-arginine or placebo for six weeks for organic ED (mostly from diabetic or arteriogenic etiologies). Approximately 31% of the men in the L-arginine group self-reported a statistically significant benefit versus 12% in the placebo group. Additionally, men who benefited were found to have low concentrations of nitric oxide in the urine. The primary side effect was primarily a decrease of systolic and/or diastolic blood pressure of approximately 10% in the L-arginine group.

Therefore, it seems possible that men secreting low levels of nitric oxide, who are willing to take fairly large daily dosages of L-arginine, may see a benefit. Larger randomized clinical trials are needed in this area, but it appears that L-arginine may be one of several possible exceptions to the rule that dietary supplements provide little to no benefit currently for men with ED. It is also of interest that recent cardiovascular studies utilizing very large oral dosages (12 g/day) of L-arginine versus placebo for short time periods (three weeks) in hypercholesterolemic men with normal blood pressures have demonstrated reductions in blood pressure and homocysteine levels (42).

It should be noted that fairly large sources of dietary L-arginine exist naturally in plant and animal proteins; however, soy protein and other plant proteins are richer in L-arginine than are animal proteins, which are richer in lysine. Small amounts of free L-arginine are found in vegetable juices and fermented foods, such as miso and yogurt. Typical dietary intake of L-arginine is 3.5 to 5 g daily (43).

Androstenedione and Dehydroepiandrosterone

Both androstenedione and dehydroepiandrosterone (dhea) are androgen precursors thought to have pharmacological effects similar to that of testosterone; however, while testosterone is a regulated by the 1990 Anabolic Steroid Control Act, loopholes in the definition of steroids permit legal, over-the-counter (OTC) sale of these two other compounds (18). It is thought that by using these supplements, one can affect endogenous testosterone levels and have an effect on sexual function. In one study, 30 healthy young men (ages 19–29) with normal testosterone levels were randomly assigned 300 mg of androstenedione or placebo over eight weeks (44). While those in the androstenedione group did experience an increase in serum levels of estrone and estradiol, no significant increase in testosterone levels occurred in either group, and there was no effect on muscle size and strength. This result suggested that more aromatization occurred with this supplement and/or from increasing testosterone levels. The ingestion of this dietary supplement was also associated with decreased serum levels of

high-density lipoproteins (HDL), or "good cholesterol," of approximately 10%.

Other clinical trials, however, have had interesting results with androstenedione dietary supplements (45–50). For example, 42 healthy men (ages 20–40) received 100 or 300 mg of androstenedione daily for seven days versus a similar group that did not receive any supplements (47). Although the men receiving no supplements or 100 mg of androstenedione demonstrated no significant mean increases in testosterone, the group receiving 300 mg did experience a mean increase in testosterone of 34%. Estradiol levels increased significantly by 42% and 128% for both the 100-mg and 300-mg groups, respectively. Another short clinical trial of 55 healthy men 30 to 56 years old utilized either a 100 mg of androstenedione or placebo three times daily for 28 days (49). Total serum testosterone and prostate-specific antigen (PSA) levels were not altered by supplementation, although increases in free testosterone (FT), estradiol, and dihydrotestosterone (DHT) were observed. Reductions in serum HDL cholesterol also occurred with the supplemented group. A final noteworthy finding was that no difference in the perception of mood, health, or libido occurred between treatment and placebo groups. This has also been documented in other studies with this and other related supplements (50).

Some studies have reported that other androgenic-anabolic steroids have demonstrated some beneficial effects on muscle size and strength with some types of resistance training (51,52). While it is highly likely that androstenedione does, in fact, promote muscle growth when higher dosages are used, trials specific to this compound have not yet been initiated. Therefore, under current federal law, companies are still allowed to market androstenedione and DHEA to the public.

Derived from such plants as the wild yam (see *Tribulus terrestris*, below), DHEA supplements belong in the same category as androstendione supplements. Because these require a laboratory conversion to produce an actual DHEA-like structure (53), many available DHEA supplements have not undergone this conversion and thus contain little to no actual DHEA-specific activity.

Orally active DHEA increases serum testosterone levels (54–58) and estradiol levels (54,55,59) in both postmenopausal women and those with panhypopituitarism. Other potentially potent DHEA supplements appear to exhibit the same estrogen-producing qualities, as demonstrated in past clinical trials with men (60). In hypogonadal men, or those receiving androgen suppression treatment for prostate cancer, a subsequent testosterone increase (flare) or transient symptomatic benefit may occur, although other associated negative effects do not currently make these supplements an attractive option (61,62).

Because testosterone replacement remains a sensible and practical form of treatment, the administration of testosterone precursors such as DHEA should not be regarded as first-line therapy. One scenario that would preclude testosterone replacement, however, involves men with normal levels of testosterone, but with low levels of serum DHEA. A small, randomized trial of men ($n = 40$) fitting this unique and specific category was completed (63). Men with DHEA sulfate levels below 1.5 μmol/L and normal serum levels of testosterone, DHT, prolactin, and PSA received 50 mg DHEA/day versus placebo for six months. All of the men in this study had initially demonstrated the ability to achieve a full erection with 10 μg of prostaglandin E_1, and patients with obvious or well-known causes of organic ED were excluded from the study. DHEA treatment was correlated with higher mean scores in all five domains of the International Index of Erectile Function (IIEF). A significant increase in serum DHEA began at eight weeks and was sustained throughout the treatment period compared to placebo. A significant initial increase in testosterone occurred and was also sustained in the DHEA group compared to placebo (at eight weeks), but estrogen levels or lipid markers were not measured in this study.

A follow-up to the above study that included more men and more definable etiologies for ED demonstrated that oral DHEA could potentially benefit men with ED due to hypertension or without an organic etiology (64). No impact of DHEA on men with diabetes or with neurological conditions was observed. Interestingly, in the widely cited Massachusetts Male Aging Study, the only hormone measured that demonstrated an inverse correlation with ED was DHEA (65). Thus, DHEA may provide some benefit in men with early organic or psychogenic ED. Larger randomized trials of greater duration are needed. Further studies should be of considerable interest, including studies that address whether or not replacement or pharmacological doses have any impact on ED (66).

Tribulus terrestris

Normally, androstenedione is produced by the gonads and adrenal glands and can be converted to testosterone (67). Androstenedione can also be produced by some plants, resulting in the harvesting and marketing of these botanical supplements as "natural" alternatives to anabolic steroid utilization for ED therapy.

Tribulus terrestris is a plant that grows in numerous countries around the world. It contains many unique compounds that have steroid-like or steroid saponin activity (68–70). A compound called "protodioscin" can be derived from some of these plants and can apparently be transformed into the compound DHEA (71).

Some initial laboratory investigations have found some activity with *Tribulus terrestris* for potentially enhancing erectile function (72,73), but this plant supplement has failed, at least in initial studies, to change body composition, enhance exercise, or impact testosterone levels in young men; however, it has

demonstrated an ability to increase levels of androstenedione and/or estradiol when combined with other DHEA-like products (46,74). It seems that somewhat similar results as with androstendione/DHEA could be expected, but specific and adequate clinical trials addressing its individual impact or other unique effects on hormonal levels in hypogonadal men and/or those with ED have not been published.

In summary, several randomized trials of androstenedione have demonstrated a dramatic correlation between dosage and estradiol levels and an inverse relationship with HDL levels. Other potential benefits such as an increase in muscle mass or improved sexual function remain unsubstantiated versus placebo. Estrogen has been associated with some favorable cardiovascular benefits (75), but in men, these increases may also raise the risk of cardiovascular disease (76), gynecomastia (77), pancreatic cancer, and other abnormal medical conditions (78). Additionally, reductions in HDL contribute negatively to cardiovascular protection (79). It is plausible that with higher intakes of androstenedione, or the use of androstenedione in men with baseline low levels of testosterone, an increase in testosterone can be observed with these supplements (47,49). The combination of negative effects associated with these supplements, however, does not make them an attractive option for most individuals. The results of past short-term clinical trials should encourage individuals to inquire about testosterone replacement itself, instead of attempting to consume a precursor to this and other hormones (80,81).

Ginkgo biloba

Due to its widespread popularity in many varied health applications, medical professionals are likely to encounter patients who are utilizing Ginkgo biloba. There is some clinical evidence that demonstrates Ginkgo extracts can improve vascular perfusion; however, most of these trials have primarily focused on its use in the treatment of dementia (82–84). Ginkgo has been approved in Germany for this condition, and there is also some limited clinical evidence that it may improve chronic cerebrovascular insufficiency (85). The results from Ginkgo biloba in sexual function applications, however, have been unimpressive. In one of these (86), 60 patients who did not respond to papaverine injections (50 mg or less) were treated with 60 mg of an extract of Ginkgo biloba for 12 to 18 months (no placebo group was included). Ultrasound techniques detected an improved blood perfusion after six to eight weeks in some patients, and after six months, 50% of these patients regained erectile function, and in a smaller number, papaverine injections were later successful. The authors' follow-up study (87) was designed as a placebo-controlled, double-blind, randomized study utilizing 240 mg daily of an extract of Ginkgo for 24 weeks versus placebo for vasculogenic ED; however, no significant difference was observed between the two groups in this case.

Another clinical study of sexual dysfunction apparently induced by the use of selective serotonin reuptake inhibitors (SSRIs) initially reported a dramatic 91% "relative success" in women ($n = 33$) and 76% in men ($n = 30$) when 209 mg/day of Ginkgo extract was taken per day for four weeks (88), but while Ginkgo was initially implicated in the resultant improvement in sexual function, including enhanced desire, excitement, orgasm, and resolution, a closer analysis of this manuscript revealed numerous problems (89). No placebo group was utilized, and the apparent overall success rate was miscalculated. The manuscript reported a success rate of 84%, when in fact it was later determined to be 68%. The authors also did not document other important details such as the potential treatment benefit of the antidepressant itself. Medications that these patients were taking for other comorbidites were also not reported in the publication. The authors concluded that the sexual side effects "appeared" to be a result of the use of the SSRIs, but since no pretreatment evaluation was reported, the authors' conclusion is unsubstantiated. Finally, the authors stated that "no adverse side effects were reported" with the use of Ginkgo, although closer analysis of the data did reveal some adverse effects (e.g., headaches) after ingesting Ginkgo.

Additional comparative studies (90,91) have found no improvement in similar patients treated with Ginkgo when examined versus placebo. It is important to emphasize that there is no current data that clearly indicates the use of Gingko biloba for patients with any type of ED. In addition, several studies have suggested that Ginkgo may increase bleeding time and the risk of hemorrhages and enhance the action of anticoagulants (92–94). Further studies need to be completed to confirm these findings, particularly in view of its widespread use in the overall population when compared with the limited number of observed adverse effects published (95).

Yohimbine

Yohimbine is an indole alkaloid extracted from the bark of West African yohim trees (96). This compound is a prescription drug (e.g., Yocon®, Yohimex®) that has obtained previous FDA approval for use in pupillary dilation. As its mechanism of action seemed to produce blood vessel dilation and increased blood flow, some researchers began to test the ability of yohimbine to improve erectile function. This compound contains some properties similar to an α-2 adrenoreceptor antagonist, with some central and peripheral effects, appearing to act primarily at receptors in brain centers associated with libido and erections. A meta-analysis of seven randomized trials of over 400 men with ED from a variety of etiologies determined that yohimbine (15–43 mg/day) was better compared to placebo for all forms of ED combined, but its most recognizable benefit occurred with

nonorganic ED (97). The most common side effects are palpitations, fine tremor, elevation of diastolic blood pressure, anxiety, and nausea.

Yohimbe is also sold as an OTC supplement, but it is questionable whether or not these forms have any value or contain any of the active ingredients found in the drug yohimbine itself (98–100). In 1995, the FDA found little or no yohimbine in the majority (11 of 18) yohimbe supplements brands that were evaluated (100). None of the other seven brands contained amounts of yohimbine that were similar to what has been used in past clinical trials. Thus, there seems no justification currently for purchasing any supplement that claims to contain yohimbine. If a patient is interested in this compound or combining this agent with other ED treatments, the potential for using the prescription drug should be discussed. Yohimbine should not be recommended for men with organic ED because of the availability of newer and more effective ED agents; further, the effectiveness of yohimbine is probably inadequate for the treatment of most ED (1).

Zinc

Zinc is found in high concentrations in seminal fluid as well as in certain accessory locations such as the prostate. The potential of zinc supplements to augment the immune system and treat benign prostatic hyperplasia (BPH). BPH and ED has been touted by numerous books on alternative medicine, but the evidence to support these claims is seriously lacking. Further, zinc supplementation in high quantities may suppress the immune system, and the limited dietary studies of BPH have found an increased risk of this condition to be associated with greater quantities of zinc (101,102).

There is little evidence that zinc can impact ED. Several previous studies have tested zinc supplements on sexual function, but these mostly included men on kidney dialysis. Some investigations demonstrated a benefit, while others did not (103,104). Patients on dialysis may have a pretreatment zinc deficiency with concomitant hyperprolactinemia, and adding supplemental zinc in these patients may serve to correct this deficiency and produce higher levels of male hormone (105,106). Thus, these studies cannot provide a proper assessment of the role, if any, zinc has in general ED treatment. Clinicians should explain to patients that the evidence is not available, and that taking zinc supplements can result in numerous side effects. One recent potential concern is that the intake of high-dose zinc supplements for long periods of time may actually increase the risk of advanced prostate cancer (107).

Korean Red Ginseng

In general, there are a variety of other popular dietary supplements, and because these have limited clinical data, it is difficult to evaluate their effect on ED. A recent exception, however, is that of Korean red ginseng (panax ginseng), which has been preliminarily investigated for its use in the treatment of HIV (108), as well as a potential agent for the reduction of severe climacteric symptoms in postmenopausal women. There have been some limited positive results in both applications (109). Other studies with this herbal product have found that it may contain numerous beneficial compounds (110)—notably, some with antiplatelet and blood thinning potential (111). Korean red ginseng may also improve vascular endothelial abnormalities in hypertensive patients by increasing the concentration of nitric oxide (112). A laboratory study of this type of ginseng on rabbit corpus cavernosal smooth muscle found that it can cause a dose-dependent relaxation by increasing the release of nitric oxide from corporal sinusoids and may increase intracellular sequestration of calcium (113). Another laboratory study has confirmed this finding and also found that this product may enhance peripheral neurophysiologic mechanisms (114). Two small clinical trials of Korean red ginseng have demonstrated some encouraging results (115,116). The older trial (published in 1995) utilized 90 patients with ED who were divided into three groups of 30 men, with each group given Korean red ginseng, placebo, or trazodone (115). No significant changes in the frequency of intercourse, premature ejaculation, and morning erections occurred after treatment in any group. The group taking Korean red ginseng experienced significant positive changes in a number of other erectile parameters such as penile rigidity, penile girth, libido, and patient satisfaction versus the other groups. Approximately 60% of the patients taking ginseng experienced a therapeutic benefit, versus 30% for the placebo and drug arms. It should be noted that there were no complete remissions of ED; only partial responses were observed. Penile hemodynamic changes did not occur after the administration of this specific type of ginseng.

In view of the available data, it is difficult to conclude whether or not Korean red ginseng had a noticeable objective effect without further investigations. The apparent ability of this compound to increase nitric oxide levels and/or reduce fatigue, insomnia, and/or depression does suggest that specific compound(s) within this herb may have some activity for some types of ED or sexual dysfunction (105,114). A new preliminary trial of Korean red ginseng has recently been published (116). A total of 45 patients with ED were enrolled in this placebo-controlled crossover study that consisted of eight weeks of treatment, a two-week washout period, followed by another eight weeks of treatment. The dose of oral ginseng was 900 mg given three times daily. The mean patient age was 54 years, and organic comorbidities (hypertension, diabetes, dylipidemia) were found in over 50% of the men. Exclusion criteria included men with a history of radical prostatectomy, neurological problems, hormonal and chemotherapy treatment, Peyronie's disease, substance abuse, and the current use of drugs

that are known to interfere with sexual function. The mean IIEF scores were significantly higher in the ginseng-treated patients, as well as the parameters of penetration and maintenance. Penile tip rigidity (RigiScan) also demonstrated significant improvement for ginseng compared to placebo; however, there was no significant difference found in orgasmic function and overall satisfaction. It was noted that with ginseng treatment, serum testosterone normalized in four of the seven patients with a decreased baseline level, so more research is needed to resolve this issue. Other potential mechanisms of action offered from animal studies include an inhibitory effect on the uptake of γ-aminobutyric acid, glutamate, dopamine, and other neurotransmitters, along with increased production of nitric oxide (117,118). These small trials suggest that ginseng may provide benefit for some subjective symptoms of ED, including enhanced penile tip rigidity, but a larger placebo trial is needed to determine its overall role in ED treatment.

Avena sativa

Avena sativa, also known as wild oats, oat bran, or oatstraw, has been demonstrated to reduce cholesterol and possibly blood pressure in numerous clinical trials (119–122). Several dietary supplements for ED tend to contain some quantity of *Avena sativa*, perhaps with the belief that reducing cholesterol levels/blood pressure or altering the male hormone environment may impact ED favorably. No specific trials of *Avena sativa* and ED have been published to date.

Numerous other OTC soluble fiber products (123–125) that also possess some limited cholesterol-lowering ability, such as psyllium, pectin, guar gum, and locust bean gum, may make up a portion of some ED supplements—possibly due to the belief that cholesterol reduction could lead to enhanced erectile function. No clinical trials, however, have used these specific compounds in the treatment of ED. Other potential cholesterol-lowering products or supplements, such as soy, may be found in some ED products, but their minimal to moderate ability to decrease cholesterol remains controversial (126–128). It seems that any product that can impact cholesterol (or weight) has the potential to become a part of some herbal blend for ED, and the limitations of this marketing decision without appropriate clinical trials should always be discussed with patients.

Other OTC Supplements

Other ED supplements such as damiana (Turnera diffusa) combined with numerous other herbals and vitamins and minerals, as well as other plants and their extracts, have demonstrated some initial sexual enhancement effects in both women and men (129,130), but larger randomized trials are needed to confirm these results and to determine their safety profiles and any potential mechanisms of action.

☐ CONCLUSION

Dietary supplements have recently come to enjoy a tremendous amount of attention and support among the general public. The large and growing market for ED treatment seems to have been a partial impetus for the development of numerous products. Due to the limited regulation of the supplement industry, the number of men utilizing complementary or alternative medicines for ED is currently unknown. While it is likely that many plants/herbs do contain compounds that could benefit ED, many OTC supplements have not been investigated in a laboratory or clinical setting prior to commercial sale. Without the demonstration of efficacy through adequate research channels, benefits cannot be advertised on product labels. Whether or not most of these supplements have merit beyond the placebo effect is questionable, and several may actually have the potential to cause harm. Thus, adequately designed clinical trials are needed. As a general rule, lifestyle changes should be emphasized before any discussion of supplements is initiated.

☐ REFERENCES

1. Lue TF. Erectile dysfunction. N Engl J Med 2000; 342(24):1802–1813.
2. Feldman HA, Johannes CB, Derby CA, et al. Erectile dysfunction and cardiovascular risk: prospective results from the Massachusetts Male Aging Study. Prev Med 2000; 30(4):328–338.
3. Michal V. Arterial disease as a cause of impotence. Clin Endocrinol Metab 1982; 11(3):725–748.
4. Agarwal A, Jain DC. Male sexual dysfunction after stroke. J Assoc Physicians India 1989; 37(8):505–507.
5. Derby CA, Mohr BA, Goldstein I, et al. Modifiable risk factors and erectile dysfunction: can lifestyle changes modify risk? Urology 2000; 56(2):302–306.
6. Levine SB. Erectile dysfunction: why drug therapy isn't always enough. Cleveland Clin J Med 2003; 70(3): 241–246.
7. Feldman HA, Goldstein I, Hatzichristou DG, et al. Impotence and its medical and psychosocial correlates: results of the Massachusetts Male Aging Study. J Urol 1994; 151(1):54–61.
8. Johannes CB, Araujo AB, Feldman HA, et al. Incidence of erectile dysfunction in men 40 to 69 years old: longitudinal results from the Massachusetts Male Aging Study. J Urol 2000; 163(2):460–463.
9. Kolodny L. Erectile function and vascular disease: what is the connection? Postgraduate Med 2003; 114(4):30–40.
10. Bacon CG, Mittleman MA, Kawachi I, et al. Sexual function in men older than 50 years of age: results from the Health Professionals Follow-up Study. Ann Intern Med 2003; 139(3):161–168.
11. Barrett B, Marchand L, Scheder J, et al. Themes of holism, empowerment, access, and legitimacy define complementary, alternative, and integrative medicine in relation to conventional biomedicine. J Altern Complement Med 2003; 9(6):937–947.
12. Crocetti E, Crotti N, Feltrin A, et al. The use of complementary therapies by breast cancer patients attending conventional treatment. Eur J Cancer 1998; 34(3): 324–328.
13. MacLennan AH, Wilson DH, Taylor AW. Prevalence and cost of alternative in Australia. Lancet 1996; 347(9001):569–573.
14. Eisenberg DM, Davis RB, Ettner SL, et al. Trends in alternative medicine use in the United States, 1990–1997. JAMA 1998; 280(18):1569–1575.
15. Blendon RJ, DesRoches CM, Benson JM, et al. Americans' views on the use and regulation of dietary supplements. Arch Int Med 2001; 161(6):805–810.
16. Seamon MJ, Clauson KA. Ephedra: yesterday, DSHEA, and tomorrow—a ten year perspective on the Dietary Supplement Health and Education Act of 1994. J Herb Pharmacother 2005; 5(3):67–86.
17. Noonan C, Noonan PW. Marketing dietary supplements in the United States: a review of the requirements for new dietary ingredients. Toxicology 2006; 221(1):4–8.
18. Yesalis CE. Medical, legal, and societal implications of androstenedione use. JAMA 1999; 281(21): 2043–2044.
19. Morris CA, Avorn J. Internet marketing of herbal products. JAMA 2003; 290(11):1505–1509.
20. Harkey MR, Henderson GL, Gershwin ME, et al. Variability in commercial ginseng products: an analysis of 25 preparations. Am J Clin Nutr 2001; 73(6): 1101–1106.
21. Parasrampuria J, Schwartz K, Petesch R. Quality control of dehydroepiandrosterone dietary supplement products. JAMA 1998; 280(18):1565.
22. Markowitz JS, Donovan JL, DeVane CL, et al. Effect of St. John's Wort on drug metabolism by induction of cytochrome P450 3A4 enzyme. JAMA 2003; 290(11): 1500–1504.
23. Ang-Lee MK, Moss J, Yuan C-S. Herbal medicines and perioperative care. JAMA 2001; 286(2):208–216.
24. Hrobjartsson A, Gotzsche PC. Is the placebo powerless? An analysis of clinical trials comparing placebo with no treatment. N Engl J Med 2001; 344(21): 1594–1602.
25. McClellan KJ, Markham A. Finasteride: a review of its use in male pattern hair loss. Drugs 1999; 57(1): 111–126.
26. Whiting DA, Jacobsen C. Treatment of female androgenetic alopecia with minoxidil 2%. Int J Derm 1992; 31(11):800–804.
27. Ernst E. A primer of complementary and alternative medicine commonly used by cancer patients. Med J Australia 2001; 174(2):88–92.

28. Avants SK, Margolin A, Holford TR, et al. A randomized controlled trial of auricular acupuncture for cocaine dependence. Arch Intern Med 2000; 160(15): 2305–2312.

29. Moyad MA, Hathaway S, Ni H-S. Traditional Chinese Medicine, acupuncture, and other alternative medicines for prostate cancer: an introduction and the need for more research. Semin Urol Oncol 1999; 17(2): 103–110.

30. NIH Consensus Development Panel on Acupuncture. Acupuncture. JAMA 1998; 280(17):1518–1524.

31. Morey SS. NIH issues consensus statement on acupuncture. Am Fam Phys 1998; 57(10):2545–2546.

32. Engelhardt PF, Daha K, Zils T, et al. Acupuncture in the treatment of erectile dysfunction: first results of a prospective randomized placebo-controlled study. Int J Impot Res 2003; 15(5):343–346.

33. Yamashita H, Tsukayama H, Tanno Y, et al. Adverse effects related to acupuncture. JAMA 1998; 280(18): 1563–1564.

34. Norheim AJ, Fonnebo V. Adverse effects of acupuncture. Lancet 1995; 345(8964):1576.

35. Rosted P. The use of acupuncture in dentistry: a review of the scientific validity of published papers. Oral Dis 1998; 4(2):100–104.

36. Peacher WG. Adverse reactions, contraindications, and complications of acupuncture and moxibustion. Am J Chin Med 1975; 3(1):35–46.

37. Saenz de Tejada I, Goldstein I, Azadzoi K, et al. Impaired neurogenic and endothelium-mediated relaxation of penile smooth muscle from diabetic men with impotence. N Engl J Med 1989; 320(16): 1025–1030.

38. Ignarro LJ, Bush PA, Buga GM, et al. Nitric oxide and cyclic GMP formation upon electrical field stimulation cause relaxation of corpus cavernosum smooth muscle. Biochem Biophys Res Commun 1990; 170(2):843–850.

39. Zorgniotti AW, Lizza AF. Effect of large doses of nitric oxide precursor l-arginine, on erectile dysfunction. Int J Impot Res 1994; 6(1):33–35.

40. Klotz T, Mathers MJ, Braun M, et al. Effectiveness of oral l-arginine in the first-line treatment of erectile dysfunction in a controlled crossover study. Urol Int 1999; 63(4):220–223.

41. Chen J, Wollman Y, Chernichovsky T, et al. Effect of oral administration of high-dose nitric oxide donor l-arginine in men with organic erectile dysfunction: results of a double-blind, randomized, placebo-controlled study. BJU Int 1999; 83(3):269–273.

42. Likos A, Mariotti F, Brown PH, et al. Oral l-arginine reduces blood pressure, cardiac output, and homocysteine levels in men with high cholesterol. Circulation 2003; 108(17):IV-784[abstr 3538].

43. Oomen CM, van Erk MJ, Feskens EJ, et al. Arginine intake and risk of coronary heart disease mortality in elderly men. Arterioscler Thromb Vasc Biol 2000; 20(9): 2134–2139.

44. King DS, Sharp RL, Vukovich MD, et al. Effect of oral androstenedione on serum testosterone and adaptations to resistance training in young men. A randomized controlled trial. JAMA 1999; 281(21): 2020–2028.

45. Ballantyne CS, Phillips SM, MacDonald JR, et al. The acute effects of androstenedione supplementation in healthy young males. Can J Appl Physiol 2000; 25(1): 68–78.

46. Brown GA, Vukovich MD, Reifenrath TA, et al. Effects of anabolic precursors on serum testosterone concentrations and adaptations to resistance training in young men. Int J Sport Nutr Exerc Metab 2000; 10(3): 340–359.

47. Leder BZ, Longcope C, Catlin DH, et al. Oral androstenedione administration and serum testosterone concentrations in young men. JAMA 2000; 283(6): 779–782.

48. Rasmussen BB, Volpi E, Gore DC, et al. Androstenedione does not stimulate muscle protein anabolism in young healthy men. J Clin Endocrinol Metab 2000; 85(1):55–59.

49. Brown GA, Vukovich MD, Martini ER, et al. Endocrine responses to chronic androstenedione intake in 30- to 56-year-old men. J Clin Endocrinol Metab 2000; 85(11): 4074–4080.

50. Wallace MB, Lim J, Cutler A, et al. Effects of dehydroepiandrosterone vs androstenedione supplementation in men. Med Sci Sports Exerc 1999; 31(12): 1788–1792.

51. Kuipers H, Wijnen JAG, Hartgens F, et al. Influence of anabolic steroids on body composition, blood pressure, lipid profile and liver functions in body builders. Int J Sports Med 1991; 12(4):413–418.

52. Bhasin S, Storer TW, Berman N, et al. The effects of supraphysiologic doses of testosterone on muscle size and strength in normal men. N Engl J Med 1996; 335(1):1–7.

53. Araghınıknam M, Chung S, Nelson-White T, et al. Antioxidant activity of dioscorea and dehydroepiandrosterone (DHEA) in older humans. Life Sci 1996; 59(11):147–157.

54. Genazzani AD, Stomati M, Strucchi C, et al. Oral dehydroepiandrosterone supplementation modulates spontaneous and growth hormone-releasing hormone-induced growth hormone and insulin-like growth factor-1 secretion in early and late postmenopausal women. Fertil Steril 2001; 76(2):241–248.

55. Stomati M, Monteleone P, Casarosa E, et al. Six-month oral dehydroepiandrosterone supplementation in early and late postmenopause. Gynecol Endocrinol 2000; 14(5):342–363.

56. Morales AJ, Haubrich RH, Hwang JY, et al. The effect of six months treatment with a 100 mg daily dose of dehydroepiandrosterone (DHEA) on circulating sex steroids, body composition and muscle strength in age-advanced men and women. Clin Endocrinol 1998; 49(4):421–432.

57. Morales AJ, Nolan JJ, Nelson JC, et al. Effects of replacement dose of dehydroepiandrosterone in men and women of advancing age. J Clin Endocrinol Metab 1994; 78(6):1360–1367.

58. Mortola JF, Yen SSC. The effects of oral dehydroepiandrosterone on endocrine-metabolic parameters in postmenopausal women. J Clin Endocrinol Metab 1990; 71(3):696–704.

59. Young J, Couzinet B, Nahoul K, et al. Panhypopituitarism as a model to study the metabolism of dehydroepiandrosterone (DHEA) in humans. J Clin Endocrinol Metab 1997; 82(8):2578–2585.

60. Arlt W, Haas J, Callies F, et al. Biotransformation of oral dehydroepiandrosterone in elderly men: significant increase in circulating estrogens. J Clin Endocrinol Metab 1999; 84(6):2170–2176.

61. Jones JA, Nguyen A, Straub M, et al. Use of DHEA in a patient with advanced prostate cancer: a case report and review. Urology 1997; 50(5):784–788.

62. Goldberg M. Dehydroepiandrosterone, insulin-like growth factor-I, and prostate cancer. Ann Intern Med 1998; 129(7):587–588.

63. Reiter WJ, Pycha A, Schatzi G, et al. Dehydroepiandrosterone in the treatment of erectile dysfunction: a prospective, double-blind, randomized, placebo-controlled study. Urology 1999; 53(3):590–595.

64. Reiter WJ, Schatzl G, Mark I, et al. Dehydroepiandrosterone in the treatment of erectile dysfunction in patients with different organic etiologies. Urol Res 2001; 29(4):278–281.

65. Feldman HA, Goldstein I, Hatzichristou DG, et al. Impotence and its medical and psychological correlates: results of the Massachusetts Male Aging Study. J Urol 1994; 151(1):54–61.

66. Dhatariya KK, Nair KS. Dehydroepiandrosterone: is there a role for replacement? Mayo Clin Proc 2003; 78:1257–1273.

67. Horton R, Tait JF. Androstenedione production and interconversion rates measured in peripheral blood and studies on the possible site of its conversion to testosterone. J Clin Invest 1966; 45:301–313.

68. Yan W, Ohtani K, Kasai R, et al. Steroidal saponins from fruits of Tribulus terrestris. Phytochemistry 1996; 42(5):1417–1422.

69. Bedir E, Khan IA. New steroidal glycosides from the fruits of Tribulus terrestris. J Nat Prod 2000; 63(12): 1699–1701.

70. Cai L, Wu Y, Zhang J, et al. Steroidal saponins from Tribulus terrestris. Planta Med 2001; 67(2):196–198.

71. Adimoelja A. Phytochemicals and the breakthrough of traditional herbs in the management of sexual dysfunctions. Int J Androl 2000; 23(suppl 2):82–84.

72. Acrasoy HB, Erenmemisoglu A, Tekol Y, et al. Effect of Tribulus terrestris L. saponin mixture on some smooth muscle preparations: a preliminary study. Boll Chim Farm 1998; 137(11):473–475.

73. Adaikan PG, Gauthaman K, Prasad RN, et al. Proerectile pharmacological effects of Tribulus terrestris extract on the rabbit corpus cavernosum. Ann Acad Med Singapore 2000; 29(1):22–26.

74. Antonio J, Uelmen J, Rodriguez R, et al. The effects of Tribulus terrestris on body composition and exercise performance in resistance-trained males. Int J Sport Nutr Exerc Metab 2000; 10(2):208–215.

75. Stevenson JC. Mechanisms whereby oestrogens influence arterial health. Eur J Obstet Gynecol Reprod Biol 1996; 65(1):39–42.

76. Phillips GB, Pinkernell BH, Jing TY. The association of hyperestrogenemia with coronary thrombosis in men. Arterioscler Thromb Vasc Biol 1996; 16(11): 1383–1387.

77. Berkovitz GD, Guerami A, Brown TR, et al. Familial gynecomastia with increased extraglandular aromatization of plasma carbon 19-steroids. J Clin Invest 1985; 75(6):1763–1769.

78. Fyssas I, Syrigos KN, Konstandoulakis MM, et al. Sex hormone levels in the serum of patients with pancreatic adenocarcinoma. Horm Metab Res 1997; 29(3): 115–118.

79. Gordon DJ, Probstfield JL, Garrison RJ, et al. High-density lipoprotein cholesterol and cardiovascular disease: four prospective American studies. Circulation 1989; 79(1):8–15.

80. Shifren JL, Braunstein GD, Simon JA, et al. Transdermal testosterone treatment in women with impaired sexual function after oophorectomy. N Engl J Med 2000; 343(10):682–688.

81. Gruenewald DA, Matsumoto AM. Testosterone supplementation therapy for older men: potential benefits and risks. J Am Geriatr Soc 2003; 51(1):101–115.

82. Kleijnen J, Knipschild P. Ginkgo biloba. Lancet 1992; 340(8828):1136–1139.

83. Mashour NH, Lin GI, Frishman WH. Herbal medicine for the treatment of cardiovascular disease: clinical considerations. Arch Intern Med 1998; 158(20): 2225–2234.

84. Le Bars PL, Katz MM, Berman N, et al. A placebo-controlled, double-blind, randomized trial of an extract of Ginkgo biloba for dementia. JAMA 1997; 278(16): 1327–1332.

85. Lin CC, Cheng WL, Hsu SH, et al. The effects of Ginkgo biloba extracts on the memory and motor functions of rats with chronic cerebral insufficiency. Neuropsychobiology 2003; 47(1):47–51.

86. Sikora R, Sohn MH, Deutz F-J, et al. Ginkgo biloba extract in the therapy of erectile dysfunction. J Urol 1989; 141:188A[abstr 73].

87. Sikora R, Sohn MH, Engelke B, et al. Randomized placebo-controlled study on the effects of oral treatment with Ginkgo biloba extract in patients with erectile dysfunction. J Urol 1998; 159:240A[abstr 917].

88. Cohen AJ, Bartlik B. Ginkgo biloba for antidepressant-induced sexual dysfunction. J Sex Marital Ther 1998; 24(2):139–143.

89. Balon R. Ginkgo biloba for antidepressant-induced sexual dysfunction? J Sex Marital Ther 1999; 25(1):1–2.

90. Kang BJ, Lee SJ, Kim MD, et al. A placebo-controlled, double-blind trial of Ginkgo biloba for antidepressant-induced sexual dysfunction. Hum Psychopharmacol 2002; 17(6):279–284.

91. Solomon PR, Adams F, Silver A, et al. Ginkgo for memory enhancement: a randomized controlled trial. JAMA 2002; 288(7):835–840.

92. Rowin J, Lewis SL. Spontaneous bilateral subdural hematoma associated with chronic Ginkgo biloba ingestion. Neurology 1996; 46(6):1775–1776.

93. Rosenblatt M, Mindel J. Spontaneous hyphema associated with ingestion of Ginkgo biloba extract. N Engl J Med 1997; 336(15):1108.

94. Fong KCS, Kinnear PE. Retrobulbar haemorrhage associated with chronic Ginkgo biloba ingestion. Postgrad Med J 2003; 79:531–532.

95. Wong AH, Smith M, Boon HS. Herbal remedies in psychiatric practice. Arch Gen Psychiatry 1998; 55(11):1033–1044.

96. Goldberg MR, Robertson D. Yohimbine, a pharmacological probe for the study of the alpha2-adrenoreceptor. Pharmacol Rev 1983; 35(3):143–180.

97. Ernst E, Pittler MH. Yohimbine for erectile dysfunction: a systematic review and meta-analysis of randomized clinical trials. J Urol 1998; 159(2):433–436.

98. Silverman E. Herbal sex pills thrive on fantasy more than fact. Newark-Star Ledger, January 30, 2000.

99. Sharlip I. Report on "Herbal sex pills thrive on fantasy more than fact". International Society for Sexual and Impotence Research News Bulletin, Summer:17, 2001.

100. Foster S, Tyler VE. Tyler's Honest Herbal. 4th ed. New York, NY: The Haworth Herbal Press, 2000:393–395.

101. Moyad MA. The ABCs of Nutrition and Supplements for Prostate Cancer. Ann Arbor, MI: JW Edwards Publishing, 2003.

102. Lagiou P, Wuu J, Trichopoulou A, et al. Diet and benign prostatic hyperplasia: a study in Greece. Urology 1999; 54(2):284–290.

103. Mahajan SK, Abbasi AA, Prasad AS, et al. Effect of oral zinc therapy on gonadal function in hemodialysis patients. A double-blind study. Ann Intern Med 1982; 97(3):357–361.

104. Brook AC, Johnston DG, Ward MK, et al. Absence of a therapeutic effect of zinc in the sexual dysfunction of haemodialysed patients. Lancet 1980; 2(8195 Pt 1):618–620.

105. Mahajan SK. Zinc in kidney disease. J Am Coll Nutr 1989; 8(4):296–304.

106. Leake A, Chrisholm GD, Busuttil A, et al. Subcellular distribution of zinc in the benign and malignant human prostate: evidence for a direct zinc androgen interaction. Acta Endocrinol (Copenh) 1984; 105(2):281–288.

107. Leitzmann MF, Stampfer MJ, Wu K, et al. Zinc supplement use and risk of prostate cancer. J Natl Cancer Inst 2003; 95(13):1004–1007.

108. Cho YK, Sung H, Lee HJ, et al. Long-term intake of Korean red ginseng in HIV-1-infected patients: development of resistance mutation to zidovudine is delayed. Int Immunopharmacol 2001; 1(7):1295–1305.

109. Tode T, Kikuchi Y, Hirata J, et al. Effect of Korean red ginseng on psychological functions in patients with severe climacteric syndromes. Int J Gynaecol Obstet 1999; 67(3):169–174.

110. Park JD, Lee YH, Kim SI. Ginsenoside Rf2, a new dammarane glycoside from Korean red ginseng (Panax ginseng). Arch Pharm Res 1998; 21(5):615–617.

111. Yun Y, Do J, Ko S, et al. Effects of Korean red ginseng and its mixed prescription on the high molecular weight dextran-induced blood stasis in rats and human platelet aggregation. J Ethnopharmacol 2001; 77(2–3):259–264.

112. Sung J, Han KH, Zo JH, et al. Effects of red ginseng upon vascular endothelial function in patients with essential hypertension. Am J Chin Med 2000; 28(2): 205–216.

113. Choi YD, Xin ZC, Choi HK. Effect of Korean red ginseng on the rabbit corpus cavernosal smooth muscle. Int J Impot Res 1998; 10(1):37–43.

114. Choi YD, Rha KH, Choi HK. In vitro and in vivo experimental effect of Korean red ginseng on erection. J Urol 1999; 162(4):1508–1511.

115. Choi HK, Seong DH, Rha KH. Clinical efficacy of Korean red ginseng for erectile dysfunction. Int J Impot Res 1995; 7(3):181–186.

116. Hong B, JI YH, Hong JH, et al. A double-blind crossover study evaluating the efficacy of Korean red ginseng in patients with erectile dysfunction: a preliminary report. J Urol 2002; 168(5):2070–2073.

117. Chen X, Lee TJ. Ginsenosides-induced nitric oxide-mediated relaxation of the rabbit corpus cavernosum. Br J Pharmacol 1995; 115(1):15–18.

118. Tsang D, Yeung HW, Tso WW, et al. Ginseng saponins: influence on neurotransmitter uptake in rat brain synaptosomes. Planta Med 1985; 3(June):221–224.

119. Bell S, Goldman VM, Bistrian BR, et al. Effect of beta-glucan from oats and yeast on serum lipids. Crit Rev Food Sci Nutr 1999; 39(2):189–202.

120. Onning G, Wallmark A, Persson M, et al. Consumption of oat milk for 5 weeks lowers serum cholesterol and LDL cholesterol in free-living men with moderate hypercholesterolemia. Ann Nutr Metab 1999; 43(5): 301–309.

121. Saltzman E, Das SK, Lichtenstein AH, et al. An oat-containing hypocaloric diet reduces systolic blood pressure and improves lipid profile beyond effects of weight loss in men and women. J Nutr 2001; 131(5): 1465–1470.

122. Zava DT, Dollbaum CM, Blen M. Estrogen and progestin bioactivity of food, herbs, and spices. Proc Soc Exp Biol Med 1998; 217(3):369–378.

123. Jensen CD, Haskell W, Whittam JH. Long-term effects of water-soluble dietary fiber in the management of hypercholesterolemia in healthy men and women. Am J Cardiol 1997; 79(1):34–37.

124. Brown L, Rosner B, Willett WW, et al. Cholesterol-lowering effects of dietary fiber: a meta-analysis. Am J Clin Nutr 1999; 69(1):30–42.

125. Anderson JW, Allgood LD, Lawrence A, et al. Cholesterol-lowering effects of psyllium intake adjunctive to diet therapy in men and women with hypercholesterolemia: meta-analysis of 8 controlled trials. Am J Clin Nutr 2000; 71(2):472–479.

126. Moyad MA. Soy, disease prevention, and prostate cancer. Semin Urol Oncol 1999; 17(2):97–102.

127. Dent SB, Peterson CT, Brace LD, et al. Soy protein intake by perimenopausal women does not affect circulating lipids and lipoproteins or coagulation and fibrinolytic factors. J Nutr 2001; 131(9):2280–2287.

128. Gerhardt AL, Gallo NB. Full-fat rice bran and oat bran similarly reduce hypercholesterolemia in humans. J Nutr 1998; 128(5):865–869.

129. Ito TY, Trant AS, Polan ML. A double-blind placebo-controlled study of ArginMax, a nutritional supplement for enhancement of female sexual function. J Sex Marital Ther 2001; 27(5):541–549.

130. Sperling H, Lorenz A, Krege S, et al. An extract from the bark of the tree Aspidosperma Quebracho Blanco inhibits human penile alpha-adrenoceptors. J Urol 2001; 165:227 [abstract 938].

Nonsurgical Devices in the Treatment of Male Sexual Dysfunction

Fouad R. Kandeel

Department of Diabetes, Endocrinology and Metabolism, City of Hope National Medical Center, Duarte, California and David Geffen School of Medicine, University of California, Los Angeles, California, U.S.A.

Nabil Koussa

H.C. Healthcare Management and Development, Inc., Long Beach, California, U.S.A.

☐ INTRODUCTION

Many reasonable nonsurgical treatment options exist for erectile dysfunction (ED), including external vacuum devices, medications (oral and topical), hormonal therapy, penile injection therapy, and intraurethral pellet therapy. This chapter will focus solely on the use of vacuum devices and constriction rings. For further information on the psychological and pharmacological avenues of treatment, see chapters in Part IV of this volume.

☐ VACUUM PUMP
Background

From the first "small exhausting pump" used to excite new activity in the blood vessels of the penis, described by John King, M.D. in 1874, vacuum erection devices, also known as vacuum constriction devices, have been utilized for the improvement of erectile rigidity for over a century (1). The first patent for such a device was issued in 1917 to Dr. Otto Lederer, but it was not well accepted by his medical peers. The modern version of that original prototype was developed in 1982 by a Georgian businessman, Geddings D. Osbon, Sr., and continues to be used today, with only some minor design modifications (Figs. 1 and 2) (3). There are three main parts: (*i*) a wide, clear plastic cylinder that is placed around the penis and sealed against the pubic region; (*ii*) a hand- or battery-operated pump that withdraws air from the cylinder; and (*iii*) one or more constrictive rubber rings, which, when placed at the base of the penis, serve to maintain the erection. The rings may be constructed as tri-rings (Fig. 3) with an additional loop on each side of the central loop for greater ease of application. Some types of constrictive rings may require positioning in advance of the vacuum placement, however, and this should be confirmed with the manufacturer's instructions prior to use.

 The vacuum erection device has been approved by the Food and Drug Administration (FDA) for use in the management of men with ED (4). There are a number of medical equipment companies that have specially designed devices that incorporate a safety valve to prevent the creation of dangerously high-pressures—approximately 200 to 250 mmHg—and, consequently, pressure-induced penile injury. In contrast, there are also non–medically approved devices available via the Internet, mail order catalogs, and erotic boutiques that have not been tested and are constructed without safety valves; these harbor the risk of exposing the penis to pressures well in excess of the recommended figures. It is important for clinicians and patients to be aware that these instruments are potentially hazardous and have no FDA clearance. Patients both with and without ED are to be discouraged from using these latter devices.

Technique

Once the decision has been made to pursue sexual relations, water-soluble jelly is applied to the base of the penis in order to prevent air from seeping into the chamber by creating a watertight seal. This helps to maintain the negative pressure within the cylinder. Some men may find that trimming the pubic hair aids in this endeavor. Once the cylinder has been placed over the penile shaft and is held firmly against the pubic bone, the pump mechanism can be activated (either by hand or battery). Slow generation of the negative pressure will prevent penile pain due to too rapid a buildup of pressure within the cylinder. The negative pressure causes a similar reduction in the pressure within the cavernous sinusoidal spaces, thus increasing the inflow of blood to the penis and producing erection. The erection obtained with a vacuum device, however, is different from one that is achieved naturally (1). There is no initial relaxation of the sinus smooth muscle; so the circumference of the corpora cavernosa does not enlarge as much as with a natural erection. Instead, all tissues of the penis are engorged with trapped blood. Because the buried portion of the corpora cavernosa does not become tumescent below the constriction band, there is usually a lack of fixation of the penis compared with a normal erection.

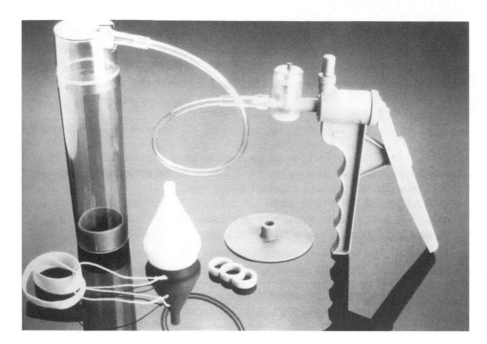

Figure 1 A hand-operated vacuum erection device, shown with three types of tension components: rubber bands, a plastic cylinder disk, and molded plastic rings. *Source*: From Ref. 1.

It should be noted that the manually operated type of pump generally requires two hands to control the device: one on the pump handle and the other to steady the cylinder on the penis itself. The battery-operated device, however, has its trigger mechanism built into the vacuum unit, which attaches to the outer end of the cylinder, and thus, one hand can activate the pump and steady the cylinder at the same time. This is an important consideration for patients with poor manual dexterity or strength, such as men with Parkinson's disease or rheumatoid arthritis.

Many men find that "double-pumping" increases their physical comfort level with the vacuum device and may result in greater penile engorgement (1,5). This technique involves the generation of negative pressure for one to two minutes, then releasing some of the negative pressure, waiting a brief period, and recommencing the generation of negative pressure with the pump for three to four minutes; the process is repeated until a full erection is achieved. Early on in a patient's experience with the vacuum device, this technique is to be encouraged until an individual tolerance level is developed for the amount of negative pressure that produces a functional erection. To achieve adequate rigidity of the penis, the vacuum pressure must exceed 90 mmHg (1).

Once the erection has been achieved, a constriction ring (band) must be applied to the base of the penis to act as an artificial valve in order to maintain the blood within the corporal bodies. The rings come in a variety of shapes, sizes, and, most importantly, tension (tightness). Trial and error is used to define which ring size is most efficient. Selection of the proper ring is critical: if it is too small, it will be

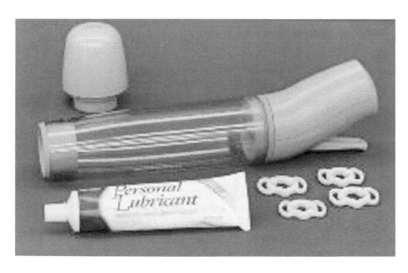

Figure 2 A modern battery-operated vacuum erection device kit, shown with lubricating jelly and constriction rings of various sizes. *Source*: From Ref. 2.

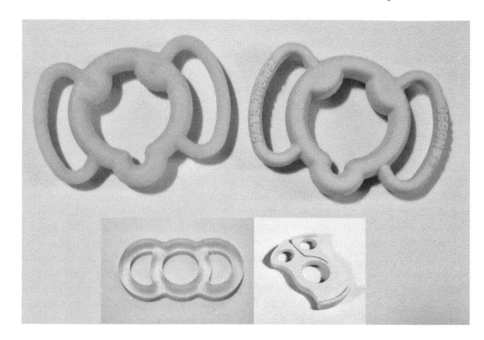

Figure 3 Various designs of constriction rings.

uncomfortable, and if it is too large, the erection may be lost. Most manufacturers suggest that the constriction ring remain in place for no longer than 30 minutes in order to prevent the occurrence of significant tissue ischemia. Once the ring is in place, the plastic cylinder can be removed and sexual relations may commence. When detumescence is desired, the ring is simply removed. Patients should be forewarned that seminal fluid will usually run or drip from the penile meatus once the band has been released (1). A schematic illustration that summarizes this process is shown in Figure 4.

Indications

The vacuum device is indicated for men with ED (5). Caution should be exercised, however, if the intended patient is (*i*) using blood-thinners or has a history of

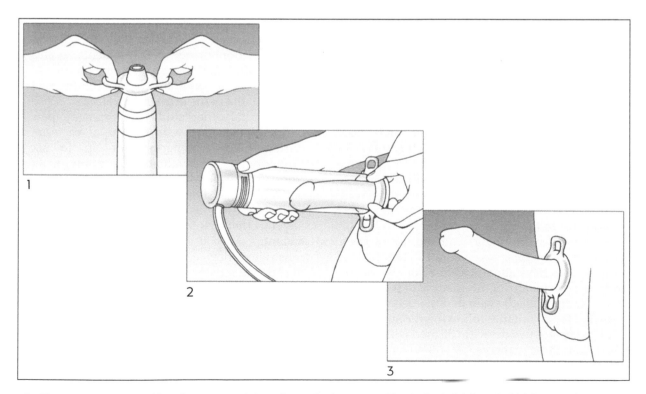

Figure 4 The vacuum device to induce tumescence is based on a simple concept. The device is lubricated with jelly around the rim to create an air-tight seal (1). A vacuum is then created, using a hand-operated or electrical pump, which draws blood into the penis, thereby inducing tumescence (2). The erection is maintained by slipping the ring off the base of the device onto the base of the penis (3). *Source*: From Ref. 6.

bleeding disorders, (ii) has diminished penile sensation, (iii) has significant penile curvature (see Chapter 17), or (iv) has a history of priapism (prolonged erection) or is at risk for its development. (For further information, see Chapter 18.) Anticoagulant therapy may cause the patient to develop bruising and swelling due to rupture of the superficial veins on the shaft of the penis as a result of the constriction ring. Similarly, patients with a history of bleeding disorders should avoid the use of vacuum erection devices. This trauma is uncommon in the absence of anticoagulant therapy, however, and if it does occur, it usually resolves of its own accord.

Patients who have reduced penile sensation, particularly men with spinal cord injury, are also at increased risk for trauma with repeated use of the constriction band. If used at all in this group, the ring should be applied for only short periods of time.

Men with significant degrees of penile curvature should also be discouraged from using a vacuum device, because the straight cylinder may exert significant stress on the curved penis, resulting in additional trauma.

Patients with hematologic forms of veno-occlusive priapism (sickle cell disease, thalassemia, or leukemia) should not use a vacuum device under any circumstances.

Efficacy and Acceptability

For the majority of men, the vacuum erection device is a simple and safe form of therapy. It typically receives good insurance coverage, and, most importantly, the mechanism for inducing or reducing erection is totally noninvasive and reversible. If the patient does not wish to continue with this therapy, it is easily stopped; if used in the proper manner, there is little likelihood of long-term negative effects. The above-mentioned patient groups who are not suited for the use of vacuum devices represent a fractional proportion of all patients presenting with erectile failure.

Generally, vacuum erection devices can be used as a first-line, noninvasive method of treatment for patients with vascular and/or neurologic ED, particularly for those who do not respond satisfactorily to phosphodiesterase inhibitors. In fact, many of the studies performed with vacuum erection devices were completed prior to the marketing of these erectogenic agents. (For further information on the use of phosphodiesterase inhibitors, see Chapter 29.) Several follow-up studies have attempted to evaluate the efficacy and the acceptability of this method of therapy for ED (7–10). Nadig et al. (7) evaluated the penodynamic effects during the 30 minutes following the application of a vacuum-constrictive device in 35 men with organic impotence. Of these patients, 27 (77%) achieved a penile longitudinal rigidity of more than 454 Gm of buckling force, the minimum criterion required for adequate rigidity by sleep laboratories (7). Circumference, measured at the penoscrotal angle, increased from 1.1 to 6.4 cm (mean 4.3 cm). The amount of vacuum applied ranged from 175 to 380 mmHg. Strain gauge plethysmography confirmed that penile blood continued to flow in all patients, even though the skin temperature decreased by an average of 0.96°C. Of the 35 men, 24 (69%) were satisfied with the device and used it regularly.

Marmar et al. (8) utilized plethysmography (pulse volume recording from a sensor cuff placed around the penis and inflated to just below the diastolic pressure) to estimate penile blood flow in 51 men with mixed etiologies of ED before, during, and after the use of a constriction ring. The constriction ring was placed on the penis after obtaining an erection with a vacuum pump. All patients demonstrated a 70% to 75% decline in the amplitude of the pulse-volume curve during constriction, but continuous blood flow was maintained in each case. Within 60 seconds after removal of the ring, the amplitude returned to baseline values for all men, including 12 patients with a penile brachial index of <0.7. Among 33 patients, there was evidence of a transient increase of amplitude following constriction release, which was consistent with the postischemic hyperemia. All investigated individuals exhibited an increase in penile length and circumference, with a mean increase in length of 3.7 cm and in circumference of 3.41 cm. Further, 37 patients had a penile buckling pressure of greater than 100 mmHg, 12 achieved a buckling pressure between 60 and 100 mmHg, and only two patients failed to achieve a buckling pressure of 60 mmHg. Analysis of blood gases immediately after the application of vacuum pump in 12 patients with ED showed that both arterial and venous blood contribute (58% and 4%, respectively) to the penile blood volume achieved during the erection induced by this method (9). In addition, Rigiscan monitoring of 26 patients evaluated six months after the start of vacuum pump use, in the same study, showed an average rigidity at the base and tip of the penis greater than 80%.

Several other studies reported on patient and partner satisfaction with the use of vacuum devices during follow-up periods of up to six years. Witherington (10) evaluated the utility of the device from 1517 responders out of a total 1700 users who obtained the system between 1974 and 1987. Of these patients, 92% either achieved an erection or an erection-like state that was satisfactory for intercourse, and 77% had intercourse at least every two weeks. The vacuum constrictive device was reportedly particularly effective in patients with partial impotence (defined as infrequent success at intercourse or achieving only a partial erection) (10). The participants in this survey did not report any serious side effects.

A few other follow-up studies, each with a much smaller number of patients, corroborated these results and suggest a stable use of the device by over 60% of patients who are able to apply it successfully (9–12). Thus, the vacuum device is likely to be an effective treatment for erectile failure in the majority of appropriately selected patients.

As expected, however, negative patient selection for vacuum pump treatment was shown to be associated with a high rate of dropout. In a study of 74 men with ED who failed sexual counseling, self-injection therapy, venous ligation surgery, or penile implant, only 20 patients (27%) were satisfied with the erections achieved, and about half of these patients objected to its regular use (13). Since other studies have reported much higher erectile response and satisfaction rates in patients with history of penile implant or severe pelvic disease (14) and in patients with venous leakage (15,16), reasons for failure of use of the vacuum device were likely due to unidentified significant psychological problems, lack of adequate patient education and training, poor patient dexterity, poor partner acceptance, or poor cavernosal structural integrity.

There are, however, a significant number of patients who find the use of vacuum erection devices clearly unacceptable because of two important factors: cosmetics and difficulty integrating this technique into lovemaking (5). In males with lighter-colored skin, the inflow of blood combined with the application of a constriction band renders the penis cooler in temperature and is accompanied by a large amount of superficial vein swelling. Thus, the use of the vacuum erection device is aesthetically unappealing, particularly to younger patients and those not currently in a stable long-term relationship (17). It has been estimated that the surface temperature of the penis during use of the vacuum erection device is about 1°C lower than the temperature prior to application of the device (7). The patient and his partner should be counseled regarding this fact prior to the initial use of the device. The typical man will take between 10 and 20 minutes to obtain an erection of penetration rigidity using the vacuum erection device. For some patients, this is a relatively long period of time, which when combined with the mechanical nature of the treatment modality, makes this option too cumbersome.

Side Effects

Although these devices are generally safe, as mentioned above, bruising and lower penile temperature can occur. Another commonly reported problem with erections achieved via the vacuum device is that the portion of the penis proximal to the ring remains soft, and only that portion of the shaft that is distal to the ring has any degree of hardness; thus, the penis may lack support during intercourse. Therefore, the ring must be applied as far toward the base of the penis as possible. Other possible side effects include skin breakdown, temporary numbness, pain associated with the inadvertent pulling of scrotal tissue into the cylinder, and penile pain associated with the application of the constriction ring. A band that is too tight may result in the failure to achieve an ejaculation, but there should be no interference with the occurrence of orgasm. Many of these side effects can be prevented or ameliorated by proper selection of the tension rings and

cylinder size, the use of adequate lubrication, adequate practice with the device, and proper technique.

Although the majority of available studies have reported no major acute or chronic adverse effects to the use of a vacuum device, some studies have underlined the potential of serious side effects such as severe penile skin erosion and cellulitis resulting from prolonged application of the constrictive ring (18), rare necrotizing inflammation and Fournier's gangrene of the penile and scrotal skin occurring even in the absence of specific risk factors (19), and Peyronie's plaques caused by a high pulling force on the penile tissue subsequent to the use of devices without safety pressure-release valves (20). Adequate measures should be taken to guard against the occurrence of such rare, but significant complications.

Constrictive Devices Alone

The use of a constrictive ring placed at the base of the penis or manually gripping the base of the penis with a hand has likely existed as a home remedy for ED for a long time. The principle of trapping blood in the penis, and thus assisting in the maintenance of penile erection and rigidity for the duration of sexual intercourse is, however, sound, and in practice, this constitutes a simple means of restricting the penile venous return. The actual efficacy of these methods in treating certain forms of ED, however, has not been subjected to scientific scrutiny. Therefore, their description has remained limited to "self-help" books on male sexuality (21), and the availability of the constrictive rings is mostly limited to so-called sex boutiques. The few medical rings available are usually sold as part of the FDA-approved vacuum erection device kit.

Without research to document the effects, it can only be intuitively surmised that the constrictive ring could suffice as the sole external device in the management of ED in patients with mild to moderate venous leakage and no coexisting significant arterial insufficiency. In these cases, given adequate sexual arousal, such patients should have enough penile arterial inflow to achieve the erect state; thus, the simple constriction of venous return after the attainment of full penile erection may be all that is needed to treat a significant number of men with isolated veno-occlusive dysfunction.

Of the available medical devices, two ring designs deserve special note here: the first consists of a rubber plate with a narrow central neck protruding approximately 0.5 in. vertically (Fig. 1). Using an application cone, the plate is placed against the male's body with the projecting neck portion wrapping around the base of the penis. The plate facilitates the removal of the ring without entangling the pubic hair. The second type of ring (Fig. 3) is constructed of soft rubber and includes a V-shaped section on the ventral segment to reduce the obstruction to the flow of semen in the urethra. In addition, this ring incorporates two internally protruding portions at the dorsolateral junctions to exert more focal pressure at these locations and consequently restrict the venous outflow more efficiently. Two outer loops are also incorporated on the lateral sides to facilitate its removal. Because of the cord-like construction, however, it is possible for pubic hair to wrap painfully around the device during its removal. It is frequently recommended, as above, that pubic hair be shaved prior to using these devices.

□ CONCLUSION

Despite the apparent drawbacks to the use of vacuum devices, it has allowed many couples to resume penetrative sexual relations successfully and easily. A number of reports have cited extremely high satisfaction rates. This treatment has been shown to result in definite improvement in the hardness of erection, the frequency of sex, and overall sexual satisfaction for both the patient and his partner. The most common reasons for discontinued use of this device include inadequate rigidity, penile pain, failure to ejaculate, and dissatisfaction with penile appearance and temperature. The vacuum device is suitable for the majority of patients with ED. Patients should be comprehensively counseled regarding the benefits and disadvantages of this treatment modality, and explicit, extensive in-office training by a health-care worker experienced in the working of the device is strongly advised, because this approach maximizes patient acceptance, satisfaction, and long-term compliance. Since the advent of effective oral therapy for ED, the vacuum erection device has often been relegated to that of a second-line therapy, but its high rates of patient/partner satisfaction and excellent safety profile recommend itself for more widespread use.

□ REFERENCES

1. Lewis RW. Vacuum devices. In: Mulcahy JJ, ed. Diagnosis and Management of Male Sexual Dysfunction. New York: Igaku-Shoin, 1997.
2. Timm Medical Technologies (online catalog), www.timmmedical.com.
3. Nadig PW. Six years' experience with the vacuum constriction device. Int J Impot Res 1989; 1:55–58.
4. Marmar JL. Vacuum constriction devices. In: Hellstrom WJG, ed. Male Infertility and Sexual Dysfunction. New York: Springer Verlag, 1997:409.
5. Cornell Sexual Medicine Program, Department of Urology. Vacuum devices for erectile dysfunction. http://cornellurology.com/sexualmedicine/ed/vacuum.shtml.
6. Kirby RS. An Atlas of Erectile Dysfunction. New York: The Parthenon Publishing Group, 1999.
7. Nadig PW, Ware JC, Blumoff R. Non-invasive device to produce and maintain an erection-like state. Urology 1986; 27(2):126–131.
8. Marmar JL, DeBenedictis TJ, Praiss DE. Penile plethysmography on impotent men using vacuum constrictor devices. Urology 1988; 32(3):198–203.
9. Bosshardt RJ, Farwerk R, Sikora R, et al. Objective measurement of the effectiveness, therapeutic success and dynamic mechanisms of the vacuum device. Br J Urol 1995; 75(6):786–791.
10. Witherington R. Vacuum constriction device for management of erectile impotence. J Urol 1989; 141(2): 320–322.
11. Baltaci S, Aydos K, Kosar A, et al. Treating erectile dysfunction with a vacuum tumescence device: a retrospective analysis of acceptance and satisfaction. Br J Urol 1995; 76(6):757–760.
12. Cookson MS, Nadig PW. Long-term results with vacuum constriction device. J Urol 1993; 149(2): 290–294.
13. Meinhardt W, Lycklama A, Nijeholt AA, et al. The negative pressure device for erectile disorders: when does it fail? J Urol 1993; 149:1285–1287.
14. Korenman SG, Viosca SP. Use of a vacuum tumescence device in the management of impotence in men with a history of penile implant or severe pelvic disease. J Am Geriatr Soc 1992; 40(1):61–64.
15. Blackard CE, Borkon WD, Lima JS, et al. Use of vacuum tumescence device for impotence secondary to venous leakage. Urology 1993; 41(3):225–230.
16. Kolettis PN, Lakin MM, Montague DK, et al. Efficacy of the vacuum constriction device in patients with corporeal venous occlusive dysfunction. Urology 1995; 46(6): 856–858.
17. Sidi AA, Becher FF, Zhang G, et al. Patient acceptance of and satisfaction with an external negative pressure device for impotence. J Urol 1990; 144(5):1154.
18. LeRoy SC, Pryor JL. Severe penile erosion after use of a vacuum suction device for management of erectile dysfunction in a spinal cord injured patient. Case report. Paraplegia 1994; 32(2):120–123.
19. Theiss M, Hofmockel G, Frohmuller HG. Fournier's gangrene in a patient with erectile dysfunction following use of a mechanical erection aid device. J Urol 1995; 153(6):1921–1922.
20. Hakim LS, Munarriz RM, Kulaksizoglu H, et al. Vacuum erection associated impotence and Peyronie's disease. J Urol 1996; 155(2):534–535.
21. Berger RE, Berger D. Biopotency: A Guide to Sexual Success. Emmaus, PA: Rodale Press, 1987.

Surgical Treatment of Male Sexual Dysfunction

Shahram S. Gholami and Tom F. Lue
Department of Urology, University of California, San Francisco, California, U.S.A.

□ INTRODUCTION

Despite the many advances in surgical therapy, medical therapy remains the standard of care for initial treatment or management of erectile dysfunction (ED). Nonsurgical treatment includes neurological, psychological, medical, and pharmacological interventions. This also includes treatment of ED with the use of sex therapy as well as external erection devices. With advances in basic science research, newer pharmacological and genetic therapies may help treat patients previously thought to be strictly operative candidates. Surgical therapy, however, remains an important arsenal in the urologist's armamentarium for the treatment of medically refractory ED.

□ HISTORY

It was not until the turn of the twentieth century when attempts were made to treat the flaccid penis with surgical interventions. Surprisingly, similar procedures are still being practiced today. In 1902, Wooten described the ligation of the dorsal vein of the penis as a method for restoring erections (1). Penile prosthesis surgery was described in the early 1930s. These early prostheses were made from bone and rib but failed due to problems with bone reabsorption, infection, and extrusion (2). Superficially placed rigid prostheses made from synthetic material soon followed. These prostheses were placed beneath Buck's fascia or subtunically; again, they had poor success due to problems with extrusion and discomfort (3). It was not until the early 1970s that satisfactory results with prostheses were seen with the introduction of modern prosthetic devices that fit into the corpora cavernosa; these provided both good functional and cosmetic results (2,4,5). The early 1970s also saw the first penile arterial bypass surgery as a treatment for ED, with many variations in the technique existing in the literature. Finally, in the early 1980s, venous leak surgery was reintroduced to treat corporal veno-occlusive dysfunction; however, to this day, prosthesis surgery is considered the standard surgical treatment of ED, except in a judiciously selected group of patients, which can be offered vascular surgical repair.

□ PATIENT EVALUATION AND SELECTION FOR SURGICAL TREATMENT OF ED

Diagnostic and treatment options should be contemplated only after assessing the needs of the patient. Consideration must be paid to the patient's physical and mental health as well as his goals and motivation. The patient's performance status and cardiovascular health also need to be evaluated in consultation with a cardiologist, if necessary, in order to assess the patient's ability to tolerate a surgical procedure. For patients who have failed medical management of ED or are dissatisfied with its result, surgical therapy may be considered; however, all nonsurgical options should be fully explored prior to embarking on a surgical course.

Young patients with congenital or traumatically acquired ED may also be candidates for curative surgical therapy (arterial bypass or venous surgery). Also, patients with generalized penile disease that are not likely to respond to medical therapy may be offered prosthesis surgery. Indications for prosthesis surgery include patients with a poor response to nonsurgical therapies. Inappropriate candidates for vascular surgery are those having generalized arterial disease or chronic systemic disease, are older, heavy smokers, drug abusers. Patients who decline vascular surgery (arterial and venous) or nonsurgical therapies may also be considered for prosthesis surgery after receiving appropriate counseling and a detailed informed consent.

Patients considering vascular surgery need a more detailed evaluation of their pelvic and perineal vasculature. Arterial revascularization will not be covered here, because it is discussed in detail in Chapter 40. Venogenic ED is the inability to achieve or maintain erection due to the inability to store blood within the corpora cavernosa. The various causes of veno-occlusive dysfunction have been broadly categorized into the following: ectopic veins, abnormalities of the tunica albuginea (e.g., Peyronie's disease), abnormalities of the cavernosal smooth muscle leading to inadequate relaxation (fibrosis secondary to priapism, aging), inadequate neurotransmitter release, and an abnormal communication between the corpus cavernosum and spongiosum or glans penis secondary to trauma or a surgical procedure to treat priapism (e.g., Winter shunt).

Venogenic dysfunction is often suspected during evaluation by the finding of a suboptimal erectile response to intracavernosal injection despite a normal arterial response on duplex Doppler sonography. The presence of persistent diastolic flow of greater than 5 cm/sec on duplex sonography has also been shown in some studies to correlate with the finding of venous leakage (6,7). The gold standard test for the diagnosis of venogenic ED remains the dynamic infusion caverno-sometry and cavernosography (DICC). Cavernosometry and cavernosography can be used to document the severity of venous leakage as well as visualize the sites of leakage (8,9). This evaluation technique is described in further detail in Chapter 25.

☐ VENOUS SURGERY

The limited long-term success of venous ligation procedures can be partially explained by the complexity of venous drainage of the penis. In the majority of patients, multiple venous leak sites can be visualized on cavernosography. Common leak sites include the superficial and deep dorsal vein, crural veins, corpus spongiosum, and glans penis. The deep dorsal, cavernosal, and crural veins are the main venous drainage of the corpora cavernosa and are the most common sites for ligation procedures. Another possible explanation for the widely varied results of venous surgery in the literature may be due to the many variations of surgical techniques developed to treat patients with veno-occlusive ED.

Deep dorsal vein ligation is the most commonly reported treatment for venogenic dysfunction. The procedure is performed through an infrapubic incision. Dissection beneath the plane of Buck's fascia allows identification of the deep dorsal venous complex at the base of the penis (Fig. 1). A variation of this technique described by Wespes et al. advocates resecting the deep dorsal vein and ligating its tributaries, as opposed to simple ligation of the vein (10). Lue further refined this technique in order to prevent leakage via the cavernosal veins by also ligating the cavernous and crural veins in addition to deep dorsal vein resection and ligation of its tributaries (11). A more radical technique to decrease venous leakage was suggested by Gilbert et al., involving ligation of the deep dorsal vein and complete spongiolysis (12). Spongiolysis is achieved by complete surgical separation of the corpora cavernosa from the glans penis and the corpus spongiosum, thus severing all venous connections between these structures.

Patient Selection

Penile venous surgery is limited to men under the age of 50 because the high incidence of penile smooth muscle atrophy in older men leads to an unacceptably high failure rate in this age group. Other relative

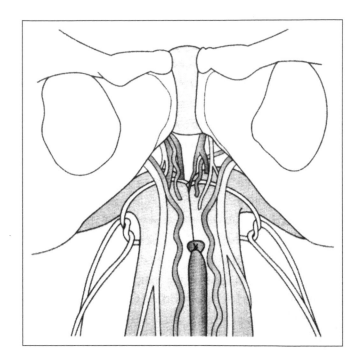

Figure 1 Deep dorsal venous ligation for correction of venogenic erectile dysfunction.

contraindications to the procedure are diabetes mellitus, generalized arterial disease, and unwillingness or inability to quit smoking. Informed consent should include the risks of possible numbness of the penile skin, shortening of penile length, penile curvature, and hematoma. Some investigators also advocate concomitant deep dorsal vein arterialization (13,14).

The ideal candidate for venous surgery is a young patient with radiographically proven veno-occlusive dysfunction or a venous shunt between the spongiosum and the cavernosum from trauma. Venous leak secondary to smooth muscle atrophy, corporal fibrosis, and nerve dysfunction will not benefit from venous surgery.

Surgical Technique

At our institution, penile venous surgery is performed through a parapenile incision from the inguinal region to the mid-scrotum. This is done in a modified low lithotomy position to allow access to the penile hilum and crura. A 3-in. vertical incision is made about 1 in. lateral to the root of the penis along the course of the spermatic cord. The root and the pendulous portion of the penis are delivered through the incision by invaginating the distal portion of the penis. The fundiform and suspensory ligaments are completely detached from the pubic bone. The dorsal vein is exposed, and with careful dissection with a sponge stick, the penile hilum is freed from the pubic bone. Using silk ties and suture ligatures, all emissary and circumflex branches of the deep dorsal vein are ligated and divided. A segment of deep dorsal vein from the lower end of the pubis to just proximal to the glans is dissected, ligated at both ends, and resected. Care is taken to visualize and stay clear of the neurovascular bundles lateral to the deep dorsal vein. With optical magnification, the cavernous vein, artery, and nerves are located. Proximal to the entrance of the cavernous artery into the corpora cavernosum, an umbilical tape is placed around each crus and tied in place. Careful attention should be given during this step to prevent ligation of the spongiosum during encircling of the crura opposite to the incision site. Crural ligation must be proximal to the cavernous artery and nerve. If significant cavernous vein leakage is noted on cavernosography, ligation of the cavernous vein is best accomplished with suture ligation with optical magnification to prevent damage to the cavernous artery and nerve. A minority of patients will have substantial cavernosal to spongiosal shunts on cavernosography. In these patients, the spongiosum can be carefully dissected off of the cavernosum and each individual venous communication suture-ligated as it is encountered. Care must be taken not to damage the urethra.

Closure is begun by approximating the tunica of the corpus cavernosum to the periosteum of the pubic bone using 0 silk sutures. This returns the penis to its anatomic position. A 7-mm Jackson-Pratt drain is placed and brought out through a separate stab incision. The layers are then closed in succession using an absorbable suture. The infrapubic space dorsal to the penis is carefully closed to prevent adhesion, which can result in shortening of the penis. A urethral catheter is placed, and a loose compressive dressing is applied to the penis and scrotum.

The compressive dressing and scrotal support are checked three to four hours after surgery to ensure that the glans is not swollen. The Jackson-Pratt drain is removed when drainage is minimal, usually the next day. The urethral catheter is removed on the first postoperative day. The patient normally remains hospitalized until the morning after surgery. Sexual intercourse may begin one month after operation.

Results

The results of surgical treatment of male sexual dysfunction, as reported in the literature, vary vastly. The authors' believe that this is due to the difficulty in establishing the proper diagnosis, improper patient selection, and a large variability in surgical technique. The reasons for failure of the procedure will vary, but include improper diagnosis, incomplete surgical resection or ligation of abnormal venous channels, the presence of an arteriogenic component, and the formation of collateral vessels. In a retrospective review of 50 patients (25 successful and 25 failures) who underwent penile venous surgery, the most important factors affecting surgical outcome were the findings on cavernosography and the consequent ease of identification and suture-ligation of the abnormal leak (11,15). Those patients with leaks into unusual sites (e.g., glans, corpus spongiosum, or crura) in combination with a large amount of drainage to the deep dorsal or cavernous vein had the highest rate of failure. If the venous

leak could be easily identified on the cavernosogram and could be suture-ligated at the tunica albuginea, success was more likely. Development of venous collaterals and persistent venous leakage appears to be a contributing factor in many patients who fail to improve following venous surgery.

Factors that may predict a poor prognosis include increasing patient age, duration of impotence, the presence of multiple leak sites, and concomitant arteriogenic insufficiency. Presently, in the authors' clinic, approximately 61% of patients with veno-occlusive dysfunction treated with venous surgery are reported as normal or improved after surgical correction at one year. The etiology of veno-occlusive incompetence remains incompletely understood. As our understanding of the cavernosal and sinusoidal function of the penis improves, treatment of venous leakage, both medical and surgical, can be directed toward treating the underlying cause rather than the symptom of the disease (16–18).

□ PROSTHESIS SURGERY

Penile prosthesis devices consist of paired malleable or inflatable cylinders, which are implanted within the cavernosal bodies. The introduction of sildenafil (Viagra®) in 1998 has significantly decreased the number of prosthesis implantations performed. Nevertheless, penile implantation remains an excellent choice in patients who have failed to respond to medical therapies or those who have penile fibrosis.

Types of Prostheses

There are two general types of prosthesis: semi-rigid and inflatable (Table 1).

Table 1 Penile Prostheses

Type	Prosthesis	Vendor
Semi-rigid	Mentor malleable	Mentor
	Acu-Form® (Fig. 2)	Mentor
	650M	American Medical Systems
	600M	American Medical Systems
	Malleable	Small-Carrion
	Dura II® Malleable	American Medical Systems (previously Timm Medical)
Inflatable		
2-piece	Ambicor® (Fig. 3)	American Medical Systems
3-piece	Alpha 1® standard	Mentor
	Alpha 1® narrow-base	Mentor
	Titan™	Mentor
	700CX™	American Medical Systems
	700CXM™	American Medical Systems
	700CXR™	American Medical Systems
	700 Ultrex® (3 connectors) (Fig. 4)	American Medical Systems
	700 Ultrex Plus (1 connector)	American Medical Systems

Semi-Rigid Prostheses

Semi-rigid prostheses consist of malleable rods that can easily be bent upwards to create an erection and bent downwards to recreate a flaccid state. The underlying construction of semi-rigid prostheses varies. Some malleable prostheses are made of silicone rubber with a central intertwined metallic core, such as the Mentor Acu-Form® Malleable Penile Prosthesis (Fig. 2). American Medical Systems (Minnetonka, Minnesota.; http://www.american-medicalsystems.com) and Mentor (Santa Barbara, California.; http://www.mentorcorp.com) are the major manufacturers of these prostheses. Other semi-rigid devices are also made of silicone rubber with interlocking rings in a column, which provide rigidity when the rings are lined up in a straight line and flaccidity when the penis is bent (please follow up with manufacturers for most recent devices). The advantages of semi-rigid devices are that they are easy to implant, have few mechanical parts with minimal mechanical failure, and generally last longer than inflatable devices. The major disadvantage of semi-rigid devices is that the penis is neither fully rigid nor fully flaccid. These devices are difficult to conceal and have a higher likelihood of device erosion.

Inflatable Prostheses

Inflatable prostheses involve two cylinders that can be inflated with fluid at will to create a more natural-looking erection. There are two types of inflatable prostheses: two-piece and three-piece prostheses.

Two-piece inflatable prostheses consist of a pair of cylinders attached to a scrotal pump/reservoir. There is a two-piece inflatable prosthesis on the market: the AMS Ambicor® (Fig. 3). The AMS Ambicor has a scrotal pump that transfers fluid from the proximal

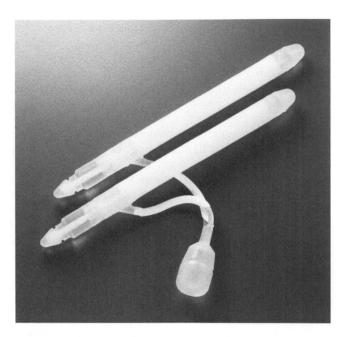

Figure 3 AMS Ambicor® Penile Prosthesis (a two-piece inflatable prosthesis).

portion of the cylinders to the distal portion to provide rigidity. The prosthesis can be deflated by bending the penis at midshaft. Two-piece prostheses have not generated a lot of excitement. When fully erect, they are not as rigid as the three-piece device and do not provide the same girth expansion. In the flaccid state, they are not as flaccid as the three-piece prosthesis and yet bear a risk similar to that of a multiple component device.

Three-piece inflatable prostheses consist of a pair of penile cylinders, a scrotal pump, and a suprapubic reservoir. They provide better rigidity when erect and a more natural appearance when flaccid. Mentor Corporation makes two three-piece inflatable prostheses (standard and narrow base) while American Medical Systems makes five three-piece devices: the AMS 700CX™, the AMS 700CXM™, the AMS 700CXR™ with InhibiZone™ (an antibiotic surface treatment), the AMS 700 Ultrex® (Fig. 4), and the AMS Ultrex Plus prostheses. The Ultrex prostheses contain distal expansion mechanisms that can give slightly longer penile length during erection.

Comparison of Prosthesis Types

Hydraulic, three-piece implants have been the most popular, accounting for 85% of the market. In our opinion, the three-piece inflatable prosthesis most closely replicates the normal erection. With the three-piece, not only does the cylinder become harder, but it also grows in size. The patient has control over the penis to produce an erection and return to flaccidity as needed.

About 15% of patients choose semi-rigid rod implants, and those with limited mental or manual

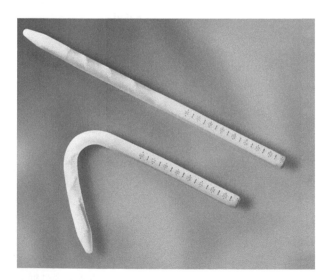

Figure 2 Mentor Acu-Form® Malleable Penis Prosthesis (a semi-rigid prosthesis).

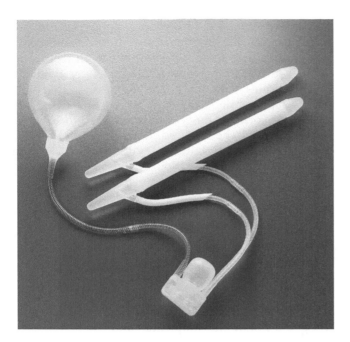

Figure 4 AMS 700 Ultrex® Penile Prosthesis (a three-piece inflatable prosthesis).

Table 2 Indications and Contraindications for Penile Prosthesis Implantation

Indications	Contraindications
Organic impotence—failed or unsatisfied with nonsurgical therapy	Temporary or reversible impotence
Psychogenic impotence—failed sex or psychosexual therapy, failed nonsurgical therapy	Unrealistic expectations
Peyronie's disease with erectile dysfunction and severe deformity	Convicted sex offenders
	Active venereal or infectious diseases

dexterity are encouraged to have this type of device. In general, the semi-rigid devices last longer than the inflatable prostheses. Most devices will need to be replaced in 10 to 15 years. When three-piece inflatable cylinders were compared, it was found that the girth-only expanding variety (AMS CX and Mentor Alpha 1®) proved more reliable and caused fewer penile deformities than those that expanded in both length and girth (Ultrex) (19). Repair rates of 5% to 20% in the first five years are realistic (20,21). Problems with device erosion and infection still occur, although they are less catastrophic. Techniques to correct these with corporoplasty and salvage have proven successful in the majority of these cases.

Patient Selection

Since nonsurgical treatments have a high success rate in improving ED, only men who fail or reject second-line therapies (i.e., intraurethral or intracavernosal vasoactive drugs, vacuum/constrictive devices) and those who are not candidates for curative surgical therapy should be considered for penile prosthesis implantation (Table 2). (For further information on local treatment or nonsurgical devices, see Chapters 30 and 32.)

We recommend three-piece inflatable prostheses to the majority of our patients. We reserve the use of semi-rigid and two-piece prostheses for patients with multiple medical problems, severe underlying systemic disease, very advanced age, or inability to use multicomponent devices due to lack of manual dexterity or understanding. In patients with congenital penile curvature or Peyronie's disease, we do not use three-piece prostheses that expand length-wise

(Ultrex-AMS). In patients with fibrotic corpora or in patients with smaller penile size, we use a narrow prosthesis. Other special circumstances may also alter prosthesis selection (Table 3). For example, for men who require repeat cystoscopy or transurethral procedures (e.g., in patients with bladder cancer), an inflatable device is the preferred choice of prosthesis.

Prior to surgery, it is important to review the risks and complications associated with prosthesis surgery. Patients should be shown a representative prosthesis and receive instructions on how it works. The risks of infection, malfunction, and erosion should be explicitly stated to the patient and he should be made aware that if complications occur, the prosthesis may need to be removed, replaced, or repaired. Fortunately, infection and erosion rates are quite low, with a 1% to 3% infection rate in healthy patients. The risk of mechanical malfunction is between 10% and 20% at five years (20).

Implantation Technique

For malleable prostheses, the most convenient incision is the penoscrotal incision, which facilitates corporeal dilation in difficult cases and, if perforation occurs, can be extended proximally or distally to correct the problem. For mechanical devices (Dura II), the best incision is a distal semi-circumcision or circumcision incision. For inflatable devices, several incisions can be used: (*i*) transverse scrotal incision, (*ii*) penoscrotal incision, and (*iii*) infrapubic incision.

Table 3 Prosthesis Selection

Profession or conditions	Preferred type of rosthesis
Athletes, teachers, swimmers	Inflatable
History of bladder cancer or urinary stone	Inflatable
History of prostatism or urethral stricture	Inflatable
Peyronie's disease	Avoid American Medical Systems Ultrex
Small or fibrotic penis	American Medical Systems CXM, Mentor narrow base
Poor manual dexterity	Semi-rigid, mechanical
High surgical risk	Semi-rigid, mechanical

After the tunica albuginea is exposed, stay sutures are placed and longitudinal corporotomies about 2 cm long are made on each corpus cavernosum. Dilation is done with Hegar dilators or the metal rod used for corporal length measurement to 14 mm distally and 16 mm proximally. A sizing instrument is used and the total corporeal length is determined from the crus to the mid-glans.

The correct length malleable or mechanical device is obtained and placed in the corpora cavernosa and the wound is closed. For inflatable prosthesis, the cylinders are implanted distally with the aid of a Furlow cylinder inserter. If any rear tip extenders are needed, they are applied at this stage, and the proximal cylinder is inserted into the proximal corpus cavernosum. The wounds are closed with preplaced sutures (2-0 Maxon or Dexon); otherwise, a needle guard should be used to avoid perforation of the inflatable portion of the device. A Dartos pouch is then created in the scrotum and the pump is placed in it. The newer devices are provided without connection between the pump and the cylinders and, therefore, the surgeon needs to determine which device (infrapubic or penoscrotal) will be used prior to surgery.

For reservoir implantation, a Foley catheter is inserted and the bladder is completely emptied. If surgery is performed through an infrapubic incision, the rectus sheath is separated and a prevesical space is created under direct vision to house the reservoir. If surgery is performed through penoscrotal or scrotal incision, long Metzenbaum scissors are used to perforate the transversalis fascia in the floor of the external ring. The scissors are placed medial to the cord structures to avoid injury. A long blade nasal speculum is then introduced into the fascial defect and is used to hold this defect open as the empty reservoir is inserted into the retropubic space. The reservoir is filled with either 65 or 100 mL of normal saline. A connection between the pump and the reservoir is made with a sutureless connector.

Continuous 3-0 Dexon is used to close the Dartos fascia over the pump. A suction drain is placed through an inguinal stab incision on the side of the reservoir and brought down into the scrotum. A second 3-0 Dexon suture is used to bury the tubing connectors and drain under the dartos fascia. The skin is closed with a running subcuticular 4-0 Monocryl or interrupted 4-0 chromic suture.

A sterile dressing is applied around the penis and the prosthesis is left semi-inflated overnight. The next morning, the Foley catheter and Jackson-Pratt drain are removed and the prosthesis is deflated. The patient is sent home with two weeks of antibiotics, typically a fluoroquinolone. Sexual intercourse may begin six weeks post-operatively following office counseling and instruction on inflation and deflation of the prosthesis.

Results

Patient and partner satisfaction with implants has been very good, in the range of 80% or higher (20).

A smaller penile size, lack of spontaneity, and unmet expectations regarding sensitivity, arousal, and enjoyment are reasons for disappointment with results. In general, the semi-rigid devices last longer than the inflatable ones. Patients should be informed that a 5% to 20% failure rate is expected in the first five years and the majority of devices will fail in 10 to 15 years and will need to be replaced. Potential complications include mechanical failures, cylinder leaks, tubing leaks, infection, perforation, persistent pain, and self-inflation.

Management of the Infected Penile Implant

In primary cases, the infection rates have been low (2–3%) but are higher in cases of implant replacement or penile reconstruction. Antibacterial medications should be used systemically prior to the induction of anesthesia and continued for at least 48 hours after surgery until the wound is sealed. The authors prefer using the antibiotics ampicillin and gentamycin, or vancomycin and gentamycin for patients allergic to penicillin. Prior to the procedure, treating urinary infections, if present, will reduce the incidence of infections.

Signs that an infection is imminent include persistent pain in the penis or over the prosthesis pump (if one is present), erythema or hyperemia, fluctuance, purulent drainage from the wound, and/or fixation of the tubing or pump to the overlying tissues. If any part of the prosthesis is exposed, it must be considered as being contaminated or infected. Once faced with infection, one has the choice of removing the device and returning at a later date for reinsertion or attempting what is known as a "salvage" procedure (22,23). When attempting to replace a new device after an infection, dilatation of the corporal bodies will be very difficult because of the scar tissue. In addition, the erect penis will be noticeably shorter due to diminished elasticity. The other option, termed the "salvage" procedure involves removing all parts of the infected prosthesis, washing the wound, and replacing the device during the same procedure (described in detail below). It is the authors' current practice to offer salvage to patients who present with an infected penile implant. Patients in whom it might be wiser to remove the prosthesis rather than salvage it are those with life-threatening systemic conditions such as septicemia or diabetic ketoacidosis or those in whom necrotizing infection with death of penile skin is occurring.

Salvage Technique

The salvage technique, as described by Mulcahy et al., involves removing the prosthesis and all foreign bodies, washing the wound, and replacing the prosthesis in the same setting (22,23). The patient presenting with an infected penile prosthesis is admitted to the hospital and placed on parenteral vancomycin and gentamycin for 72 hours. Any abscess or phlegmon should be surgically drained. Once the prosthesis, pump, reservoir, tubing, and sutures are removed, the wound is irrigated with a series of seven antibacterial solutions as described by Mulcahy (22). After wound irrigation, the entire operative team re-preps and changes all instruments, draping, gloves, gowns, aspiration devices, and cautery devices. The new prosthesis is then inserted, and the wound is closed without drains or catheters. Oral antibiotics should be continued for one month. The purpose of the salvage procedure is to cure the existing infection, while maintaining penile length, and to allow for easier reinsertion of the prosthesis. Approximately 80% of salvage procedures are successful, with no subsequent signs of infection (22).

□ CONCLUSION

As the understanding of the basic mechanisms of erectile function continues to grow, new therapies will emerge in the treatment of ED, with the eventual goal of eliminating the need for surgical therapy of the disease. In the meantime, advances in prosthesis development are needed in order to spare erectile tissue so that patients may benefit from more physiologic therapies as they become available. Different prostheses should also be designed to treat impotence of different causes (e.g., a drug-delivery system to deliver neurotransmitters for neurogenic impotence or vasodilators for arteriogenic impotence; implantable neural stimulation devices for neurogenic impotence; or venous compressive devices for venogenic impotence). Intracavernosal prostheses could then be reserved for patients with cavernosal fibrosis. Finally, as gene therapy begins to define its place in the urologist's armamentarium, we will use these therapies to help restore corporal, neural, vascular, and tunical tissues to their normal state.

□ REFERENCES

1. Wooten JS. Ligation of the dorsal vein of the penis as a cure for atonic impotence. Texas Med J 1902; 18:325–327.

2. Carson CC. Urologic Prostheses: The Complete Practical Guide to Devices, Their Implantation, and Patient Follow Up. Totowa, NJ: Humana Press, 2002.

3. Goodwin WE, Scardino PL, Scott WW. Penile prosthesis for impotence: case report. J Urol 1981; 126(3):409.

4. Scott FB, Bradley WE, Timm GW. Management of erectile impotence. Use of implantable inflatable prosthesis. Urology 1973; 2(1):80–82.

5. Small MP, Carrion HM, Gordon JA. Small-Carrion penile prosthesis. New implant for management of impotence. Urology 1975; 5(4):479–486.

6. Benson CB, Vickers MA. Sexual impotence caused by vascular disease: diagnosis with duplex sonography. Am J Roentgenol 1989; 153(6):1149–1153.

7. Fitzgerald SW, Erickson SJ, Foley WD, et al. Color Doppler sonography in the evaluation of erectile dysfunction: patterns of temporal response to papaverine. Am J Roentgenol 1991; 157(2):331–336.

8. Delcour C, Wespes E, Vandenbosch G, et al. Impotence: evaluation with cavernosography. Radiology 1986; 161(3):803–806.

9. Wespes E, Delcour C, Struyven J, et al. Pharmaco-cavernometry-cavernography in impotence. Br J Urol 1986; 58(4):429–433.

10. Wespes E, Delcour C, Preserowitz L, et al. Impotence due to corporeal veno-occlusive dysfunction: long-term follow-up of venous surgery. Eur Urol 1992; 21(2):115–119.

11. Lue TF. Penile venous surgery. Urol Clin North Am 1989; 16(3):607–611.

12. Gilbert P, Sparwasser C, Beckert R, et al. Venous surgery in erectile dysfunction. The role of dorsal-penile-vein ligation and spongiosolysis for impotence. Urol Int 1992; 49(1):40–47.

13. Virag R, Saltiel H, Floresco J, et al. Surgical treatment of vascular impotence by arterialization of the dorsal vein of the penis. Experience of 292 cases [French]. Chirurgie 1988; 114(9):703–714.

14. Virag R, Bennett AH. Arterial and venous surgery for vasculogenic impotence: a combined French and American experience. Arch Ital Urol Nefrol Androl 1991; 63(1):95–100.

15. Lue TF. Penile Venous Surgery: Factors Affecting Outcome. Annual Meeting of Western Section American Urological Association, Kauai, Hawaii, 1990.

16. Motiwala HG, Patel DD, Joshi SP, et al. Experience with penile venous surgery. Urol Int 1993; 51(1):9–14.

17. Kim ED, McVary KT. Long-term results with penile vein ligation for venogenic impotence. J Urol 1995; 153(3 Pt 1):655–658.

18. Gholami SS, Gonzalez-Cadavid NF, Lin CS, et al. Peyronie's disease: a review. J Urol 2003; 169(4):1234–1241.

19. Milbank AJ, Montague DK, Angermeier KW, et al. Mechanical failure of the American Medical Systems Ultrex inflatable penile prosthesis: before and after 1993 structural modification. J Urol 2002; 167(6):2502–2506.

20. Montague DK, Angermeier KW. Contemporary aspects of penile prosthesis implantation. Urol Int 2003; 70(2):141–146.

21. Mulhall JP, Ahmed A, Branch J, et al. Serial assessment of efficacy and satisfaction profiles following penile prosthesis surgery. J Urol 2003; 169(4):1429–1433.

22. Mulcahy JJ. Long-term experience with salvage of infected penile implants. J Urol 2000; 163(2):481–482.

23. Mulcahy JJ. Surgical management of penile prosthesis complications. Int J Impot Res 2000; 12(suppl 4):S108–S111.

34

Advances in the Treatment of Peyronie's Disease

Sherif R. Aboseif
Division of Neurology and Reconstructive Surgery, Department of Urology, Kaiser Permanente Medical Center, Los Angeles, California, U.S.A.

Gary W. Chien
Department of Urology, Kaiser Permanente Medical Center, Bellflower, California, U.S.A.

Kirk Tamaddon and Timothy F. Lesser
Department of Urology, Kaiser Permanente Medical Center, Los Angeles, California, U.S.A.

☐ INTRODUCTION

Peyronie's disease was first described by Fallopius in 1561. Most of the credit for the discovery, however, was given to Francois de la Peyronie, a French physician who named the disease nearly two centuries later in 1743. De la Peyronie described a condition in which patients have fibrous cavernositis, "preventing them from having normal ejaculation of semen" (1). He suggested that drinking the waters of Bareges, a location in southern France (2), could successfully cure the condition.

Since de la Peyronie's first description, extensive clinical and basic science research has been performed to understand the pathophysiology of this condition more clearly and to investigate various types of medical and surgical therapy. Today, Peyronie's disease is defined as a disabling deformity of the penis caused by fibrous lesions on the tunica albuginea of the corpus cavernosum. This condition is thought to affect 0.388% to 1% of adult men, typically in their fifth or sixth decade of life (3). The fibrous plaque on the tunica albuginea leads to shortening of the corpora on the affected side, which then leads to curvature or constriction of the penis during an erection (Fig. 1).

☐ ETIOLOGY AND PATHOGENESIS

The exact etiology of Peyronie's disease remains controversial despite the recent increase in knowledge and understanding of the disease. Patients with Peyronie's disease present with three main complaints: painful erection, palpable plaque, and penile curvature. The disease manifests itself in two phases: an acute inflammatory phase and a chronic phase. During the acute phase, patients present with pain, penile curvature, and nodule formation. Since the disease is evolving during this phase, the patient's pain, as well as the degree of curvature and size of the plaque, may

fluctuate. This phase usually has a self-limiting course, lasting for periods that range from 6 to 18 months (4). In the chronic phase, patients have minimal or no pain, with stable nodule size and variable degrees of penile deformity. Fibrosis is a characteristic feature of Peyronie's disease, and this results in noncompliance of the tunica albuginea.

Fibrosis occurs due to a sequence of events. Ischemia and inflammation cause a disruption in the normal tissue architecture, followed by tissue repair and subsequent accumulation of mesenchymal cells in the area of derangement. This, in turn, causes noncompliance in the tunica albuginea. Some studies have shown a genetic predisposition to the disease due to an association with Dupuytren's contracture and with human leukocyte antigen (HLA)-B7 and HLA-B27 antigens. Others have suggested an autoimmune/immunologic cause of the disease modulated by circulating antibodies (5–7). Various pharmacologic agents, including methotrexate and propanolol, have also been linked to the development of Peyronie's disease (8).

The most widely accepted theory that explains the histological changes in the tunica albuginea, however, is that of trauma. Repeated and sustained trauma to a partially or fully erect penis during sexual intercourse can cause "delamination" between the layers of the tunica albuginea, as described by Devine et al. (9). This delamination usually occurs at the junction of the midline septal strands and the dorsal/ventral circular layers of the tunica albuginea, leading to microvascular tears that cause hemorrhage in the areas of delamination. Eventually, clot resolution in this area causes fibrin (and fibroblast) aggregation, which results in an inflammatory response and cellular proliferation. The final result of this process is the deposition of collagen. Since the tunica albuginea is poorly vascularized, deposited collagen is not removed easily. Therefore, over time, collagen aggregation leads to plaque formation.

Jarow and Lowe (10) supported this theory in their retrospective study of 207 patients with

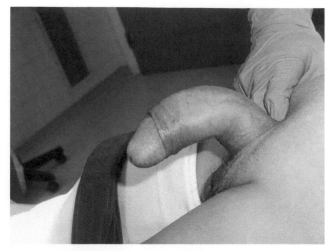

Figure 1 (*See color insert.*) Lateral curvature with waist.

Peyronie's disease. These patients were compared to a group of 250 impotent men without Peyronie's and a control group of 275 age-matched potent men. The authors found that penile trauma occurred more frequently in the patients with Peyronie's disease (40%) and in the impotent patients (37%) than in the group of age-matched potent men (11%), ($p < 0.001$).

Brock et al. (11) compared the histologic architecture of normal tunica albuginea with tissue from men with Peyronie's disease. The study included dissection of six human cadavers with normal tunica albuginea, five surgical patients with Peyronie's disease, and five patients with normal penile anatomy. Under light microscopy and scanning electron microscopy, the authors demonstrated that the normal tunica albuginea consisted of thick collagen bundles/elastic fibers, with an inner circular and outer longitudinal layer. In Peyronie's disease, however, the layers of the tunica albuginea have lost their organization, with excessive deposition of collagen and "disordered" elastic fibers within the region of the plaque. Thus, the data of Brock et al. show that the structural organization that gives the tunica albuginea its flexibility and rigidity is lost in Peyronie's disease (11). Further histologic studies have confirmed the above-mentioned findings: Davis (12) evaluated the penile lesions of patients with Peyronie's disease with hematoxyline and eosin staining. In all 19 patients examined, there was structural loss of collagen in the tunica albuginea. In 6 of these 19 patients, lymphocytic infiltration was identified. Ten of the specimens were then further evaluated using fibrinogen immunostaining to identify fibrin. Three of the 10 were found to be positive, and four were equivocal.

Research in molecular biology has also been applied to the study of fibrosis and plaque formation in Peyronie's disease. In laboratory mice, transforming growth factor-β (TGF-β) has been shown to cause fibrosis (13). These polypeptides cause inflammation and an increase in the production of extracellular matrix by fibroblasts. In another study using Hart and trichome staining, El-Sakka et al. (14) analyzed tunica albuginea

tissue from 30 patients with Peyronie's disease and six impotent patients who had penile prosthesis implants. The authors demonstrated the presence of focal and diffuse elastosis, as well as disorganization of collagen bundles, in patients with Peyronie's disease. Furthermore, Western blotting showed TGF-β1 expression in 86% of patients, TGF-β2 in 23%, and TGF-β3 in 17%. By comparison, in normal patients, only one out of six had expression of TGF-β1 and TGF-β2. The role of TGF-β1 in the fibrotic process has been elucidated by Gholami et al. (15). TGF-β1 induces the expression of collagen, proteoglycans, and fibronectin and inhibits collagenases. Additionally, TGF-β1 has been shown to induce formation of reactive oxygen species and inhibit nitric oxide synthesis. This situation has been shown to lead to fibrosis and abnormal wound healing.

Hence, although the exact etiology of the formation of Peyronie's plaques is still unknown, these studies suggest that penile trauma, or even microtrauma, is the most likely cause. Fibrin deposition and collagen disruption between the layers of the tunica albuginea with activation of fibroblasts and leukocytes result in plaque formation.

□ CLINICAL DIAGNOSIS

The evaluation of Peyronie's disease begins with a thorough history and physical examination. Details of the history should include the presence and duration of pain, the quality of erection before and after the onset of symptoms, the progression of symptoms, the presence of penile deformity, and the experience of sexual dysfunction. A prior history of any penile trauma or instrumentation should be noted. The physical examination should encompass not only a careful genital exam, but also the presence of relevant extragenital signs; e.g., the patient's hands and feet should be examined, since Peyronie's disease has been found to be associated with Dupuytren's contracture. The genital examination should include measurement of the length and the girth of the penis in its stretched state, since patients frequently complain of shortening of the penis after surgical intervention. Plaque location and dimension should be measured and noted. As part of the workup, patients are often asked to provide photographs of the side and overhead views of the erect penis. The degree and direction of the curvature is then noted from the photographs, as is the type of deformity. The quality of the erection and degree of curvature must be further evaluated in the office with intracavernosal injection of vasoactive agents and/or the use of a vacuum device.

If surgical reconstruction is anticipated, the use of penile duplex ultrasound has been recommended (16). Duplex ultrasound provides valuable information regarding the size, extent, and location of the plaque, as well as the anatomy and function of the penile arteries (dorsal and cavernous arteries and their communications, the dorsal artery perforators) and collateral arterial blood flow. These arterial branches and all of the nerves within the penis are important for the erectile process and must be identified and preserved during surgery, particularly in patients with erectile dysfunction. In addition, measuring penile blood flow and determining both the penile vascular integrity and the venous outflow can aid in the investigation of erectile dysfunction commonly associated with Peyronie's disease. In a study (17) that used duplex ultrasonography to evaluate erectile dysfunction in 222 men with Peyronie's disease, the main cause of erectile dysfunction was found to be occlusive vascular disease. Other studies (18) have confirmed these results.

□ TREATMENT

The appropriateness of treatment choice depends on the severity and the stage of the disease as well as on the quality of erectile function. Patients with Peyronie's disease usually seek help for one or more of several reasons: (*i*) pain during erection, (*ii*) cosmetic reasons (palpable nodule, penile deformity), (*iii*) difficulty with coitus, and/or (*iv*) erectile dysfunction. Nonsurgical treatment is usually the first option most physicians offer to patients with Peyronie's disease. In a study by Gelbard et al. (4), 97 patients with Peyronie's were followed from three months to eight years. Approximately 40% of the patients felt that the pain, degree of curvature, and ability to have intercourse did not change significantly during the study period. An additional 40% indicated that the degree of curvature and ability to have relations worsened during this time. Interestingly, only 6% of those in the study had worsening of pain. The authors concluded that the majority of patients with Peyronie's will have painless persistence of their curvature and plaque.

Medical Therapy

Most experts would agree that medical therapy is most suitable in the acute phase of Peyronie's disease, during which time the plaque continues to evolve—usually within the first 12 months of the onset of symptoms. Another indication for medical therapy, regardless of the duration or severity of disease, is in patients who are not surgical candidates or who do not demonstrate psychological readiness for surgery. The major agents involved in the medical management of Peyronie's disease include oral vitamin E, aminobenzoate potassium (Potaba, Glenwood-Palisades, Tenafly, New Jersey), colchicine, and tamoxifen. Intralesional injections of calcium channel blockers and collagenase have also been used, as well as vacuum therapy. All of these agents are discussed below.

Oral Therapy
Vitamin E
The rationale for using vitamin E as treatment for Peyronie's disease mainly regards its antioxidant

properties, which may prevent fibrosis. Early reports of vitamin E (19) suggest a high cure rate (78%) for penile curvature, along with a high rate of decrease (91%) in plaque size. More recent research on vitamin E, however, has challenged the early results. At a 1997 National Institute of Health conference, Devine (20) described a series of 105 patients who were treated with vitamin E. Only 13% reported a decrease in curvature. Vitamin E is now generally thought to have limited therapeutic value, but due to its low cost and relative lack of side effects, many clinicians still recommend its use.

Aminobenzoate Potassium (Potaba)
The exact mechanism of action for Potaba is unclear, but it is thought to limit collagen synthesis in fibroblast cells (21). Potaba can increase the utilization of oxygen by tissues, increase the activity of monoamine oxidase, and decrease serotonin levels. Early reports of Potaba use claimed promising results. In a literature review of 2752 patients treated with Potaba, Wagenknecht (22) showed that the median improvement rate was 60% (with a range of 10–82%). Carson (23) demonstrated similar results in a study of 32 men who were treated with daily oral Potaba for three months. These patients were then followed for 8 to 24 months. Eighteen of 32 patients (56%) had a decrease in plaque size; an equal proportion (56%) of patients also showed a decrease in penile angulation. In another study (24) involving 59 patients in a prospective, randomized, placebo-controlled trial, the efficacy of Potaba (3 g/day for one year) was analyzed. Thirty-two percent reported a decrease in plaque size and 36% had a decrease in deformity (compared to the placebo groups of 12.5% and 0%, respectively). Most recently, Weidner et al. (25) demonstrated in a randomized, double-blind, placebo-controlled trial of 103 patients in the acute phase that Potaba had a significant protective effect on the progression of curvature.

The drawbacks of Potaba, however, are not insignificant: its gastrointestinal side effects promote poor compliance, and the drug is also expensive, costing approximately one thousand dollars per patient per year.

Colchicine
Colchicine has been recommended recently as a potentially useful medication in treating Peyronie's disease. It is thought to decrease inflammation by modulating chemokine and prostanoid production and inhibiting neutrophil and endothelial cell adhesion molecules (26). In an uncontrolled study involving 24 patients treated with 0.6 to 1.2 mg of colchicine twice a day for three to five months (27), the authors reported encouraging results: 26% of the patients showed marked decrease in penile curvature, 21% reported reduction in plaque size, and 78% reported decrease in pain. Side effects experienced included gastrointestinal upset and diarrhea. In a recent randomized double-blind placebo-controlled trial, however, Safarinejad

(28) demonstrated no difference between the effectiveness of colchicine and placebo with respect to curvature, pain, or plaque size. It should be noted, though, that the mean duration of the disease for the men enrolled in the study was 15 months, indicating that most were in the chronic phase of the disease.

Tamoxifen

The therapeutic mechanism of Tamoxifen involves modification of TGF-β production, regulation of inflammation and tissue repair, and suppression of macrophage activity. Ralph et al. (29) studied 36 patients with Peyronie's disease who received oral Tamoxifen (20 mg twice daily for three months). Of these, 35% patients reported a decrease in penile curvature, and plaque size was decreased in 34% of patients. In 1999, Teloken et al. (30) compared this dosage of tamoxifen to placebo in a clinical trial and found no difference between the two with respect to the degree of curvature, pain, or plaque size. Again, with a mean pretreatment disease time of 20 months, these patients were generally in the chronic phase of the disease.

Oral Therapy: Summary

In summary, although most currently available oral agents for Peyronie's disease initially showed promising results, many of the agents have been shown to be similar to placebo for the treatment of the curvature, pain, and plaque size associated with Peyronie's. They may nonetheless help to ameliorate progression for patients in the acute phase of their disease.

Vacuum Therapy

In 1999, Lue and El-Sakka (31) first published data on vacuum constriction devices for use after plaque incision and venous grafting in four patients with Peyronie's. The authors have had excellent anecdotal results with the use of vacuum therapy during the acute phase of Peyronie's disease. Long-term data is forthcoming.

Intralesional Injections
Collagenase

Collagenase was one of the earliest forms of treatment for Peyronie's disease. Its use was based on the principle that collagen, a major extracellular matrix plaque component, is degraded by collagenase. Most work on collagenase has been reported by Gelbard et al. (32,33), who concluded that its use should be limited only for patients with mild disease.

Calcium Channel Blocker

Calcium deposits are often found in plaques, as evidenced by radiographic findings. The mechanism of action for calcium channel blockers (namely, verapamil), is thought to occur by stopping the influx of calcium through the calcium channel. This theoretically decreases collagen synthesis, since extracellular

deposition of collagen is a calcium-dependent process. Verapamil can also increase extracellular collagenase activity and decrease fibroblastic activity. An in vitro study showed that calcium channel blockers modify the expression of cytokines involved in wound healing (34). In a clinical study by Levine (35) in 1997, 38 patients with Peyronie's disease used a multiple puncture technique to inject intralesional verapamil 10 mg every two weeks for 24 weeks. All patients were evaluated using duplex ultrasonography and a standardized questionnaire both before and after treatment. The authors reported resolution of pain in 97%, improved sexual function in 72%, and an objective reduction of curvature in 54% of the patients, as measured by ultrasonography. Similar results were confirmed by Rehman et al. (36), who reported a 57% decrease in plaque size in patients who received intralesional verapamil (vs. 28% of patients who received placebo), with subjective improvement in erection in 43% of the verapamil group versus 0% for the placebo group. These promising results were confirmed in 2002 by Levine et al. (37), who followed 156 men treated with intraplaque verapamil injection. Of the 140 men who completed the treatment with a mean follow-up of 30.4 months (range of 10–81 months), 60% had an objective decrease in curvature while 62% reported a subjective decrease. Additionally, 83% reported an increase in girth, 80% reported an increase in rigidity distal to the plaque, and 71% reported improvement in sexual function.

The results of verapamil intralesional therapy are not unanimous, however. At the 1996 International Society of Impotence Research Meeting, Teloken et al. (38) presented a series of 36 patients who had intralesional injection of either saline or verapamil 10 mg for six weeks. The authors found no advantage to verapamil therapy as each group had a 30% correction of curvature.

Notwithstanding these conflicting results, it should be noted that the intralesional injection of verapamil has been found to have minimal side effects, typically limited to skin ecchymoses. In addition, no infection or episodes of hypotension or cardiac arrhythmias have been reported. The low morbidity of verapamil makes this therapy a viable option, particularly for patients who are in the acute inflammatory phase or who are not surgical candidates.

Surgery

The primary goal of the reconstructive surgical treatment of Peyronie's disease is to correct the penile deformity, allowing the resumption of sexual intercourse. In general, surgery does not lessen pain or improve penile rigidity. Thus, the reconstructive surgical treatment of Peyronie's should be considered only for patients with stable disease and a severely deformed penis that interferes with coitus. The choice of surgical therapy depends on the presurgical quality of the erection, the length of the penis, and the type of deformity. Patients with Peyronie's disease and concomitant erectile dysfunction who fail to respond to oral/intracavernous pharmacological therapy or the use of a vacuum constriction device, or those who refuse these treatment modalities, are not considered good surgical candidates for penile reconstruction. Instead, these patients will benefit more greatly from the insertion of a penile prosthesis, with or without incision of the plaque.

The four main methods of penile reconstruction are (*i*) excision and suturing, (*ii*) corporeal plication, (*iii*) incision/excision of plaque with grafting using synthetic or autologous grafts, and (*iv*) insertion of a penile implant. These methods are discussed below.

Excision and Suturing (Nesbit Procedure)

In 1965, Nesbit (39) first described a procedure for the treatment of congenital penile curvature and chordee—a downward curvature of the penis that is usually associated with hypospadias. This procedure has also been recommended in patients with Peyronie's disease. The Nesbit technique involves the excision of an ellipse of tunica albuginea on the opposite side of the curvature. Later, Yachia (40) modified this technique by making a longitudinal incision with a transverse closure. Unfortunately, the Nesbit procedure has been associated with some complications and morbidity (41), particularly recurrence of curvature, erectile dysfunction, and penile shortening and is increasingly being replaced by either simple plication or incision/excision and grafting.

Corporeal Plication

Plication techniques are considered the least complicated of all penile reconstruction procedures and can even be done on an outpatient basis under local anesthesia. The procedure involves the placement of four to six deep, parallel plicating sutures into the tunica albuginea of the corporal body on the side opposite the plaque, either 2 to 3 mm from the corpus spongiosum [in the case of dorsal curvature (Fig. 2)], or between the deep dorsal vein and the dorsal artery (in the case of ventral curvature). 2–0 Ti-Cron permanent sutures are used.

The main advantage of corporeal plication is the avoidance of the dissection of the urethra or neurovascular bundles. Additionally, the suture tightness can be adjusted to avoid over- or undercorrection of the deformity. The primary drawback of this procedure, however, is usually further shortening of the penis by 2 to 3 cm. Patients with mild to moderate curvature without erectile dysfunction and with adequate penile length are good candidates for this procedure. Mufti et al. (42) have reported better results with plication when compared with the Nesbit procedure or tunica incision with a transverse closure. Another study by Thiounn et al. (43) reported results of 29 patients who underwent corporeal plication. All patients had penile angulation of greater than 30° and

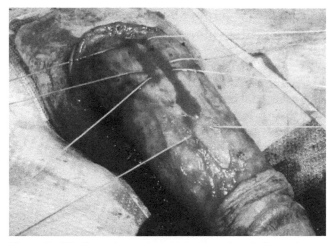

Figure 2 Plication sutures placed in a case of ventral curvature.

an inability to have intercourse initially. Of these men, 81% had satisfactory cosmetic results, and 62% had satisfactory functional results with minimal morbidity.

Plaque Excision/Incision and Grafting

This procedure has recently gained wide popularity over other techniques because penile length is preserved (an important consideration for patients with Peyronie's disease). In addition, this procedure can correct not only ventral and dorsal curvature, but also the "hourglass" deformity, which neither plication nor the Nesbit procedure can correct. Graft material can be derived from numerous sources including autologous fat (44), dura (45), vein (46), rectus fascia (47), tunica vaginalis (48), temporalis fascia (49), dermis, cadaveric pericardium (50), and synthetic Dacron (51) and Gore-Tex (52). The decision to choose an autologous versus a synthetic graft should be individualized to each patient. Synthetic grafts are readily available and do not require a second incision to harvest from a donor site; however, a synthetic graft is less elastic and may predispose the patient to postsurgical wound infection, since it is a foreign body. Consideration for synthetic graft placement should be reserved for patients who are planning to have a penile implant placement as well.

One of the more commonly used and effective nonautologous grafts is cadaveric pericardium, which provides excellent tensile strength and has the added advantages of preserving the saphenous vein for possible future use (i.e., cardiac) and negating the morbidity of a donor site incision. Levine and Estrada (50) demonstrated a 98% straightening rate in the immediate postoperative period, with 95% being able to have intercourse using cadaveric pericardial grafts.

Dermal and venous donor sites are the two most common types of autologous grafts used. The advantage of using a dermal graft is that it is readily available and can be used to repair defects of any size. The results of skin grafts have been controversial, however, since Horton and Devine (53) introduced the dermal graft technique in the early 1970s. Some authors (54) have reported promising results; others (55) have had disappointing outcomes, including the recurrence of penile curvature, as seen in 35% of a large series of patients from Austoni et al. (56). In another study, dermal graft contracture was seen in two out of five patients (57), causing progressive penile shortening that eventually required placement of a penile prosthetic. To prevent these complications, Jordan et al. (58) recommended the placement of skin grafts that are 30% larger than the corporotomy defect in all dimensions to prevent shortening of the penis when the graft contracts.

The use of venous grafts (i.e., the deep dorsal vein or saphenous vein) has been popularized by Lue and El-Sakka (59). This group theorized that venous grafts are more physiologic than other autologous tissues, since the intercorporeal space is essentially a large blood vessel. In addition, venous grafts are more elastic, less likely to contract than other autologous tissues, and relatively easy to harvest. Venous grafts also provide a strong anastomosis that prevents subsequent hematoma formation and fibrosis. Further, this group theorizes that venous endothelium offers the advantage of nitric oxide secretion, an important component in erectile physiology.

In a series of 115 patients with Peyronie's disease who had plaque incision and venous grafting, El-Sakka et al. (60) reported that 96% of the patients had a straight penis immediately following the surgery, with an overall satisfaction rate of 92%. These results were confirmed by Montorsi et al. (61). As previous experience has shown that the dorsal vein of the penis is often inadequate in size for this purpose, saphenous vein grafts are being used with increasing frequency. Saphenous vein can be harvested either at the medial malleolus or in the thigh (62).

More recently, Kalsi et al. (63) reported their results of 113 patients treated with plaque incision and saphenous vein grafting. With a mean follow-up of 12 months and a mean deformity of 64.5°, 93% reported satisfactory results, with 86% reporting a completely straightened penis. Interestingly, in the 51 patients followed for five years or longer, the penis remained straight in 80%, but erectile dysfunction developed in 22.5%. Additionally, 35% of these men experienced penile shortening of 1 cm or more.

Finally, Montorsi et al. (64) reported on their five-year data using the incision and vein grafting technique at the American Urologic Association Annual Meeting in 2004. Objective and subjective [International Index of Erectile Function (IIEF) and Erectile Dysfunction Inventory of Treatment Satisfaction (EDITS) questionnaires] data were gathered from 50 men followed for a minimum of five years. Although 60% remained satisfied, according to the EDITS survey, 41% complained of a decrease in orgasmic function, and 34% noted a decrease in erectile function, according to the IIEF questionnaire. Most notably, an objective reduction in erect penile length occurred in all patients.

Regardless of the type of graft used, the surgical procedure for plaque incision and grafting is the same. For dorsal curvatures, the neurovascular bundles are dissected and retracted laterally, exposing the plaque (Fig. 3). For ventral curvatures, the urethra is similarly dissected (Fig. 4). Routine excision of the plaque is not recommended since it causes a large corporotomy defect that requires a larger graft, increasing the risk of postoperative complications. If possible, the simple incision of the plaque leaves the plaque in place, but avoids the morbidity associated with excision. Even though some patients can still feel the plaque, it is usually of minimal clinical significance. In the case of a ventral curvature, the graft is sutured into place over the defect so as to result in a straight penis.

Plaque Incision and Grafting Vs. Plication

Recent published data evaluated 68 patients treated for Peyronie's disease using either the Lue procedure or penile plication, between 1998 and 2005 (65). Of those responding to the survey, 26 patients treated with plication were compared with 20 patients treated with plaque incision and venous grafting. Eighty-one percent of the patients treated with plication were satisfied with the quality of their erections, compared with 70% of the incision and grafting group. Additionally, two of the patients in the plication group and three patients in the graft group complained of significant penile shortening. The similarities in these results are interesting within the context of the relatively shorter operative time (65 minutes vs. 200 minutes) and the anesthetic used (local with intravenous sedation vs. general) in the plication group. Long-term comparative results have yet to be generated.

Insertion of Penile Implant

Placement of a penile implant is a good option when patients have concomitant erectile dysfunction that does not respond to available treatment modalities. Both semirigid and inflatable penile implants can be used with or without incision of the plaque. Wilson and Delk (66) recommend the modeling of the penis

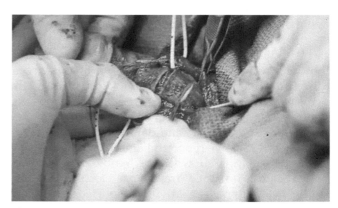

Figure 3 (*See color insert.*) Incision of plaque with neurovascular bundle dissected laterally in preparation for graft placement.

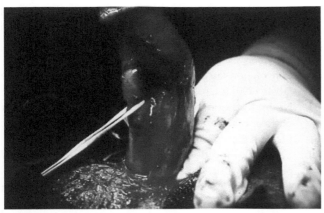

Figure 4 (*See color insert.*) Ventral curvature with the urethra dissected.

over the penile prosthesis; however, this should only be performed in patients with minimal deformity. If plaque incision is necessary, the authors have used a rectus sheath to cover the defect with excellent results and minor risk of infection. With a mean follow-up of 18 months (range 12–64 months), seven out of seven patients treated with this technique demonstrated a return to adequate sexual function in 8 to 10 weeks, with no infectious or erosive complications (47).

(For further information on phallic reconstruction, see Chapters 33 and 41.)

□ CONCLUSION

Although Peyronie's disease has been described for the last four and one-half centuries the exact cause of this disabling disease is still being debated. Current literature points to trauma as the most likely cause of the disease. The evaluation of this disease involves a careful history taking and physical examination, supplemented by duplex ultrasonography with intracavernous injection of a vasoactive agent. The choice of treatment should be tailored to the individual patient. The duration of symptoms, presence of pain, severity of penile curvature, and adequacy of erectile function must be considered before treatment is provided. Treatment options include conservative management, oral medications, intralesional injections, vacuum therapy, or reconstructive surgery. The limitations of each treatment must be explained to the patient to allow for realistic expectations. While many milestones have been achieved in the understanding and treatment of Peyronie's, much more remains to be learned about this disabling disease.

□ REFERENCES

1. de la Peyronie FG. Sur quelques obstacles qui s'opposent a l'ejaculation naturelle de la semence. Mem Acad R Chir 1743; 1:425.
2. Lindsay MB, Schain DM, Grambsch P, et al. The incidence of Peyronie's disease in Rochester, Minnesota, 1950 through 1984. J Urol 1991; 146:1007–1009.
3. Carson CC, Lue T, Levine L, et al. Symposium on Peyronie's disease, [New Orleans, Louisiana] April 12, 1997. Int J Impot Res 1998; 10(2):121–122.
4. Gelbard MK, Dorey F, James K. The natural history of Peyronie's disease. J Urol 1990; 144(6):1376–1379.
5. Somers KD, Winters BA, Dawson DM, et al. Chromosome abnormalities in Peyronie's disease. J Urol 1987; 137(4):672–675.
6. Ralph DJ, Mirakian R, Pryor JP, et al. The immunological features of Peyronie's disease. J Urol 1996; 155(1): 159–162.
7. Nachtsheim DA, Rearden A. Peyronie's disease is associated with an HLA class II antigen, HLA-DQ5, implying an autoimmune etiology. J Urol 1996; 156(4):1330–1334.
8. Phelan MJ, Riley PL, Lynch MP. Methotrexate associated Peyronie's disease in the treatment of rheumatoid arthritis. Br J Rheumatol 1992; 31(6):425–426.
9. Devine CJ Jr, Somers KD, Jordan SG, et al. Proposal: trauma as the cause of the Peyronie's lesion. J Urol 1997; 157(1):285–290.
10. Jarow JP, Lowe FC. Penile trauma: an etiologic factor in Peyronie's disease and erectile dysfunction. J Urol 1997; 158(4):1388–1390.
11. Brock G, Hsu GL, Nunes L, et al. The anatomy of the tunica albuginea in the normal penis and Peyronie's disease. J Urol 1997; 157(1):276–281.
12. Davis CJ Jr. The microscopic pathology of Peyronie's disease. J Urol 1997; 157(1):282–284.
13. Border WA, Ruoslahti E. Transforming growth factor-beta in disease: the dark side of tissue repair. J Clin Invest 1992; 90(1):1–7.
14. El-Sakka AI, Hassoba HM, Pillarisetty RJ, et al. Peyronie's disease is associated with an increase in transforming growth factor-beta protein expression. J Urol 1997; 158(4):1391–1394.
15. Gholami SS, Gonzalez-Cadavid NF, Lin CS, et al. Peyronie's disease: a review. J Urol 2003; 169(4): 1234–1241.
16. Breza J, Aboseif SR, Orvis BR, et al. Detailed anatomy of penile neurovascular structures: surgical significance. J Urol 1989; 141(2):437–443.
17. Weidner W, Schroeder-Printzen I, Weiske WH, et al. Sexual dysfunction in Peyronie's disease: an analysis of 222 patients without previous local plaque therapy. J Urol 1997; 157(1):325–328.
18. Ahmed M, Chilton CP, Munson KW, et al. The role of colour Doppler imaging in the management of Peyronie's disease. Br J Urol 1998; 81(4):604–606.

19. Scott WW, Scardino PL. A new concept in the treatment of Peyronie's disease. South Med J 1948; 41:173–177.

20. Devine CJ. International Conference on Peyronie's disease: advances in basic and clinical research, Mar 17–19, 1993. Introduction. J Urol 1997; 157(1): 272–275.

21. Levine LA. Advances in the medical therapy of Peyronie's disease: a brief review. Int J Impot Res 1998; 10(2):123–124.

22. Wagenknecht LV. Differential therapies in various stages of penile induration. Arch Esp Urol 1996; 49(3): 285–292.

23. Carson CC. Potassium para-aminobenzoate for the treatment of Peyronie's disease: is it effective? Tech Urol 1997; 3(3):135–139.

24. Levine LA. Peyronie's disease. Course presented at American Urological Association meeting, Dallas, 1999.

25. Weidner W, Hauck EW, Schnitker J. Potassium para-aminobenzoate (POTABA) in the treatment of Peyronie's disease: a prospective, placebo-controlled, randomized study. Eur Urol 2005; 47(4):530–535; discussion 535–536.

26. Molad Y. Update on colchicine and its mechanism of action. Curr Rheumatol Reports 2002; 4(3):252–256.

27. Akkus E, Carrier S, Rehman J, et al. Is colchicine effective in Peyronie's disease? A pilot study. Urology 1994; 44(2):291–295.

28. Safarinejad MR. Therapeutic effects of colchicine in the management of Peyronie's disease: a randomized double-blind, placebo-controlled study. Int J Impot Res 2004; 16(3):238–243.

29. Ralph DJ, Brooks MD, Bottazzo GF, et al. The treatment of Peyronie's disease with tamoxifen. Br J Urol 1992; 70(6):648–651.

30. Teloken C, Rhoden EL, Grazziotin TM, et al. Tamoxifen versus placebo in the treatment of Peyronie's disease. J Urol 1999; 162(6):2003–2005.

31. Lue TF, El-Sakka AI. Lengthening shortened penis caused by Peyronie's disease using circular venous grafting and daily stretching with a vacuum erection device. J Urol 1999; 161(4):1141–1144.

32. Gelbard MK, Lindner A, Kaufman JJ. The use of collagenase in the treatment of Peyronie's disease. J Urol 1985; 134(2):280–283.

33. Gelbard MK, James K, Riach P, et al. Collagenase versus placebo in the treatment of Peyronie's disease: a double-blind study. J Urol 1993; 149(1):56–58.

34. Levine LA, Merrick PF, Lee RC. Intralesional verapamil injection for the treatment of Peyronie's disease. J Urol 1994; 151(6):1522–1524.

35. Levine LA. Treatment of Peyronie's disease with intralesional verapamil injection. J Urol 1997; 158(4): 395–1399.

36. Rehman J, Benet A, Melman A. Use of intralesional verapamil to dissolve Peyronie's disease plaque: a long-term single-blind study. Urology 1998; 51(4):620–626.

37. Levine LA, Goldman KE, Greenfield JM. Experience with intraplaque injection of verapamil for Peyronie's disease. J Urol 2002; 168(2):621–625.

38. Teloken C, Vaccaro F, Da Ros C, et al. Objective evaluation of non-surgical approach for Peyronie's disease [abstr 1290]. J Urol 1996; 155(suppl):633A.

39. Nesbit RM. Congenital curvature of the phallus: report of three cases with description of corrective operation. J Urol 1965; 93:230–232.

40. Yachia D. Modified corporoplasty for the treatment of penile curvature. J Urol 1990; 143(1):80–82.

41. Andrews HO, Adeniyi AA, Ralph DJ, et al. The Nesbit operation for Peyronie's disease: an analysis of the failures over 20 years [abstr]. J Urol 1999; 161(suppl): 206,788A.

42. Mufti GR, Aitchison M, Bramwell SP, et al. Corporeal plication for surgical correction of Peyronie's disease. J Urol 1990; 144(2 Pt 1):281–288; discussion:283.

43. Thiounn N, Missirliu A, Zerbib M, et al. Corporeal plication for surgical correction of penile curvature: experience with 60 patients. Eur Urol 1998; 33(4):401–404.

44. Lowsley OS. Surgical treatment of plastic induration of the penis [Peyronie's disease]. N Y State J Med 1943; 43:2273–2278.

45. Kelami A. Surgical treatment of Peyronie's disease using human dura. Eur Urol 1977; 3(3):191–192.

46. Sachse H. Venenwandplastik bei Induratio penis plastica [Venous wall graft in Peyronie's disease]. Urologe [A] 1976; 15:131–132.

47. Pathak AS, Chang JH, Parekh AR, et al. Use of rectus fascia graft for corporeal reconstruction during placement of penile implant. Urology 2005; 65(6): 1198–201.

48. Amin M, Broghamer WL Jr, Harty JI, et al. Autogenous tunica vaginalis graft for Peyronie's disease: an experimental study and its clinical application. J Urol 1980; 124(6):815–817.

49. Bruschini H, Mitre AI. Peyronie's disease: surgical treatment with muscular aponeurosis. Urology 1979; 13:505–506.

50. Levine LA, Estrada CR. Human cadaveric pericardial graft for the surgical correction of Peyronie's disease. J Urol 2003; 170(6 Pt 1):2359–2362.

51. Ho PC, Parsons CL, Schmidt JD. Surgical treatment of Peyronie's disease with a dacron graft. Annual Meeting of the Western Section, American Urological Association, Tucson, Arizona, 1979.

52. Cohen ES, Schmidt JD, Parsons CL. Peyronie's disease: surgical experience and presentation of a proximal approach. J Urol 1989; 142(3):740–742.

53. Horton CE, Devine CJ Jr. Peyronie's disease. Plast Reconstr Surg 1973; 52:503–510.

54. Hicks CC, O'Brien DP III, Bostwick J III, et al. Experience with the Horton-Devine dermal graft in the treatment of Peyronie's disease. J Urol 1978; 119(4):504–506.

55. Fenster HN, McLoughlin MG. Surgical management of Peyronie's disease. Can J Surg 1980; 23(5):471–473.

56. Austoni E, Mantovani F, Colombo F, et al. Erectile complications after radical surgery for penile plastic induration [Article in Italian]. Arch Ital Urol Androl 1994; 66(1):19–22.

57. Rigaud G, Berger RE. Corrective procedures for penile shortening due to Peyronie's disease. J Urol 1995; 153(2):368–370.

58. Jordan GH, Schlossberg SM, Devine CJ. Surgery of the penis and urethra. In: Walsh PC, Retic AB, Vaughan ED, Wein AJ, eds. Campbell's Urology. 7th ed. Philadelphia: Saunders, 1998:3316–3394.

59. Lue TF, El-Sakka AI. Venous patch graft for Peyronie's disease. Part I: technique. J Urol 1998; 160(6 Pt 1): 2047–2049.

60. El-Sakka AI, Rashwan HM, Lue TF. Venous patch graft for Peyronie's disease. Part II: outcome analysis. J Urol 1998; 160(6 Pt 1):2050–2053.

61. Montorsi F, Maga T, Salonia A, et al. Evidence based long-term assessment of plaque incision and vein grafting for Peyronie's disease [abstr]. J Urol 1999; 161(suppl):206,790A.

62. Montorsi F, Salonia A, Maga T, et al. Evidence based assessment of long-term results of plaque incision and vein grafting for Peyronie's disease. J Urol 2000; 163(6): 1704–1708.

63. Kalsi J, Minhas S, Christopher N, et al. The results of plaque incision and venous grafting (Lue procedure) to correct the penile deformity of Peyronie's disease. BJU Int 2005; 95(7):1029–1033.

64. Montorsi F, Salonia A, Briganti A, et al. Five-year follow-up of plaque incision and vein grafting for Peyronie's disease. Annual Meeting of the American Urologic Association, San Francisco, 2004.

65. Kim D, Ree M, Kaswick J, et al. Correction of penile deformity: long-term outcomes of penile plication versus plaque incision with venous graft. J Urol 2006; 175(4).

66. Wilson SK, Delk Jr II. A new treatment for Peyronie's disease: modeling the penis over an inflatable penile prosthesis. J Urol 1994; 152(4):1121–1123.

35

Androgen Treatment of Male Hypogonadism

Alvin M. Matsumoto

Department of Medicine, University of Washington School of Medicine, and Clinical Research Unit, Seattle, Washington, U.S.A.

□ INTRODUCTION

Male hypogonadism is a common clinical condition that causes testosterone (T) deficiency and affects the health and well-being of males of all ages. For example, androgen deficiency is a major manifestation of the Klinefelter syndrome, a chromosomal disorder that is characterized classically by an XXY karyotype and affects about one in 500 males (1,2). Furthermore, low serum T levels occur commonly in a broad spectrum of common clinical conditions such as in men with chronic medical illnesses (e.g., chronic renal failure, lung disease, and liver failure), wasting syndromes (e.g., HIV infection and cancer), the use of certain medications (e.g., glucocorticoids and central nervous system-acting drugs such as opiates), and normal aging (commonly referred to as "andropause") (3). These conditions are also associated with clinical manifestations that are consistent with androgen deficiency such as decreased muscle mass and strength, low bone mineral density (BMD), sexual dysfunction, and reduced energy, well-being, and mood.

Androgen replacement therapy has proven beneficial in severely T-deficient hypogonadal men, and male hypogonadism is the main clinical indication for T treatment. Preliminary studies also suggest potential beneficial anabolic and behavioral effects of androgen therapy in T-deficient men with some chronic illnesses or wasting syndromes, those taking medications that lower T levels, and aging older men (4–11). The long-term benefits and risks of T therapy in these disorders, however, are not known.

□ THERAPEUTIC GOALS OF T TREATMENT

The therapeutic goals of T replacement therapy in male hypogonadism are to improve the clinical manifestations of androgen deficiency that vary with the stage of sexual development of the individual (3). Therefore, the specific goals of T treatment vary depending on whether the hypogonadal condition occurs in prepubertal boys or adults (12).

Males with prepubertal T deficiency usually present as adolescents or young adults with delayed puberty, manifesting varying degrees of eunuchoidism characterized by a small penis, a poorly developed scrotum, small testes (< 5 mL), and prostate, lack of male hair growth (facial, chest, axillary, pubic, perianal, and extremity hair), body habitus characterized by long arms and legs relative to height, poorly developed muscle mass, prepubertal fat distribution; reduced bone mass, high-pitched voice, poor libido (sexual interest and desire) and sexual function, reduced energy, mood alterations and lack of motivation, benign breast enlargement (gynecomastia), failure to produce an ejaculate (aspermia) and initiate spermatogenesis (azoospermia), and a relatively low hematocrit (in the female range).

Therefore, in boys with delayed puberty, the therapeutic goals of T treatment are to promote the development of secondary sexual characteristics, including growth of the penis, the scrotum, and a male hair pattern; stimulate the acquisition of peak bone mass, long bone growth, and eventual closure of epiphyses [through the aromatization of T to estradiol (E_2)] without compromising adult height; increase muscle mass and strength and reduce fat mass; induce laryngeal enlargement and deepening of the voice; stimulate libido and erections; improve energy, mood, and motivation; and increase red-blood-cell production into the normal adult male range. By stimulating accessory sex glands (seminal vesicles and prostate), T treatment stimulates seminal fluid production and an increase in ejaculate volume, but it does not stimulate sperm production sufficient for induction of fertility. Because the most common cause of delayed puberty is not pathological but rather constitutional, T therapy in boys with delayed puberty is usually intermittent and continued only until spontaneous puberty occurs (see below).

Unless severe, T deficiency in adult males is usually more difficult to diagnose because the clinical manifestations are often subtle and attributable to other causes. T-deficient men usually present with poor sexual performance manifested by reduced libido and erectile dysfunction (ED) as their major complaints, although T deficiency is not the primary etiology in the majority of men with ED. They may also manifest gynecomastia; infertility due to impaired sperm production; diminished chest, axillary, and pubic hair; decreased muscle bulk and strength; low BMD that may result in osteopenia or osteoporosis; low energy and motivation; irritability and a depressed mood; and a mild hypoproliferative anemia in the normal female range. Testis size is usually normal but may be small (< 15 mL) in men with profound reductions in sperm production. Hot flushes may occur in men with a rapid onset of severe androgen deficiency.

So, the goals of T therapy in adults with male hypogonadism are to restore libido and improve erectile function; stimulate male hair growth; increase muscle mass and strength; increase BMD, potentially reducing the risk of fractures; improve energy, mood, and motivation; and increase hematocrit into the normal adult male range. In most men with ED, T treatment alone is insufficient to restore complete erectile function and permit satisfactory intercourse. Because spermatogenesis requires high local T concentrations that cannot be achieved by exogenous androgen administration, T replacement therapy does not stimulate sperm production and testis size, nor does it restore fertility. Treatment of infertility in hypogonadal men is usually only possible in men with secondary hypogonadism and gonadotropin deficiency, using gonadotropin or gonadotropin-releasing hormone (GnRH) therapy.

The normal "physiological" range of serum T concentrations in adults is broad and usually established in healthy young men. In young hypogonadal men, T treatment produces beneficial clinical effects when serum T concentrations are increased into this normal range. With increasing age, serum T levels decline gradually and progressively, but the physiological significance of this decline is not clear (8). Initial studies in older hypogonadal men have also demonstrated some beneficial effects of T treatment that increase serum T levels into the normal range. Therefore, the goal of T treatment of male hypogonadism, irrespective of age, is to restore serum T concentrations to within the normal adult range.

An important consideration in the clinical use of T therapy is the dose–response effect of T on different target organs (13–17). Recent studies suggest that some actions of T demonstrate continuous dose-response effects as T levels are increased from below normal to within and above the physiological range—e.g., muscle mass (13–15). In contrast, other T actions exhibit threshold effects—e.g., libido—that are stimulated near maximal levels at relatively low T concentrations (16). In some patients—e.g., elderly men with severe prostate disease—low-dose T supplementation may be more prudent than full T replacement. Although not demonstrated in clinical trials, low doses of T may be sufficient to induce some beneficial effects such as the stimulation of libido and, to a limited extent, anabolic actions on muscle and bone, while minimizing adverse stimulatory effects on prostate growth.

□ DIAGNOSTIC CONSIDERATIONS PRIOR TO INITIATION OF T TREATMENT

In men with clinical manifestations of androgen deficiency (as described previously), the diagnosis of hypogonadism is confirmed by measurement of serum total or free T concentrations, preferably in the morning at the peak of the circadian variation in T levels (typically around 8 A.M.) (18). In most clinical laboratories, both total and free T are measured using automated platform-based immunoassays that utilize T analogs as standards. Most of these platform analog total T assays provide reliable and accurate measurements compared to those performed by gold standard, mass spectrometry methodologies (19,20).

The majority of T in circulation is bound to serum proteins, primarily sex hormone-binding globulin (SHBG) and albumin. Only 1% to 2% of T in blood is free of protein binding. Alterations in SHBG concentrations occur commonly, and they affect total and free T measurements by analog immunoassays that vary directly with SHBG levels. Therefore, clinical conditions that lower SHBG concentrations (e.g., moderate obesity) also reduce total and free T levels by these analog methods, potentially resulting in an incorrect diagnosis of hypogonadism. Conversely, situations that increase SHBG (e.g., aging) raise total and free T levels by analog immunoassays, mistakenly leading to an impression of eugonadism. Therefore, in clinical conditions where SHBG concentrations may be altered, or when total or free T levels by automated analog assays are in the low-normal to moderately low range (e.g., 200–350 ng/dL), the diagnosis of hypogonadism should be confirmed by using free or bioavailable (free plus albumin or weakly bound) T assays that are not affected by changes in SHBG levels. These assays include free T by equilibrium dialysis or centrifugation, bioavailable T by ammonium sulfate precipitation, and free and bioavailable T calculated from measurements of total T and SHBG (21,22).

If an initial serum T concentration is low, patients should be evaluated for transient or reversible conditions associated with low T levels (e.g., acute or chronic illnesses, medications, or malnutrition) (8,11). In these situations, serum T should be repeated after these conditions are resolved completely and offending medications are discontinued. T concentrations exhibit significant biological and measurement variation (23,24). Therefore, prior to initiating T replacement therapy, a T level should be repeated in order to confirm the diagnosis of hypogonadism.

Secondary hypogonadism, characterized by a low T in the presence of low or inappropriately normal gonadotropin [luteinizing hormone (LH) and follicle-stimulating hormone (FSH)] levels has important therapeutic implications. Therefore, serum gonadotropins should also be obtained prior to initiating T therapy in order to differentiate androgen deficiency due to testicular disease (primary hypogonadism) from that caused by hypothalamic–pituitary disease or dysfunction (secondary hypogonadism) (3,11). Gonadotropin deficiency may be caused by hypothalamic–pituitary disease that requires therapeutic interventions other than T treatment alone. For example, hypothalamic or large pituitary tumors may cause mass effects such as visual field defects or may be associated with deficiencies or excessive secretion of other pituitary hormones. In some cases, treatment of the underlying etiology of hypothalamic–pituitary dysfunction may correct T deficiency—e.g., discontinuation of a medication that causes hyperprolactinemia and gonadotropin deficiency. Finally, in men with gonadotropin deficiency but otherwise normal testes, who are interested in fathering children, sperm production and restoration of fertility, as well as T secretion, may be induced by using gonadotropin therapy. Similarly, men with hypogonadism due to hypothalamic disease may be given pulsatile GnRH treatment. Therefore, careful investigation of the cause of secondary hypogonadism is needed prior to starting T treatment.

Finally, a comprehensive clinical approach is essential for optimal management of men with hypogonadism. Thus, it is important to consider etiologies other than T deficiency that may contribute as much or more to clinical manifestations and outcomes, and to manage them appropriately (8). For example, in older hypogonadal men who complain primarily of sexual dysfunction, although T deficiency may contribute to both reduced libido and failure of erections, underlying neurovascular disease or medications are usually the major causes of ED. In these men, T therapy does not fully restore erections, and additional treatment—e.g., vacuum devices, type 5 phosphodiesterase inhibitors (sildenafil, vardenafil, or tadalafil), or prostaglandin E_1 [by penile injection (alprostadel) or by urethral suppository (Medicated Urethral System for Erection or MUSE)]—is usually needed for a satisfactory clinical outcome. In hypogonadal men with osteoporosis, it is essential to perform a comprehensive evaluation for other common causes of bone loss and treat them (e.g., vitamin D deficiency, medications, immobility or inactivity, alcohol abuse, and hyperparathyroidism) and to institute measures to prevent falls in order to decrease the risk of fractures.

☐ T FORMULATIONS

The formulations used for T replacement therapy of male hypogonadism in the United States are summarized in Table 1 (11,12). These include 17β-hydroxyl T esters that are administered by intramuscular injections, transdermal T patches and gels, and a transbuccal T tablet.

Oral 17α-alkylated T derivatives such as methyltestosterone and fluoxymesterone are weak androgens that have low bioavailability. Therefore, it is difficult to achieve full androgen replacement with these preparations (11,12). These also induce an atherogenic lipid profile [lowering high-density lipoprotein (HDL) and raising low-density lipoprotein (LDL) cholesterol], are relatively expensive, and have potential hepatotoxicity [most commonly cholestasis, but of more concern, peliosis hepatis (blood-filled cysts in the liver), and benign and malignant hepatic tumors]. Because these oral androgens offer fewer therapeutic benefits with greater potential risks compared to other T formulations, they should not be used for androgen replacement therapy.

Intramuscular T Ester Injections

Long-acting, parenteral 17β-hydroxyl T esters include T enanthate (Delatestryl®, Watson Pharmaceuticals, Corona, California, U.S.A.) and T cypionate (Depo-Testosterone®, Pharmacia & Upjohn, Kalamazoo, Michigan, U.S.A.). These are effective and relatively safe T preparations that have been used for androgen replacement for decades (12,25,26). Although transdermal T formulations provide more physiological T levels and are used more commonly than T ester injections, the latter continue to be used for androgen replacement therapy, primarily because they are the least expensive T formulation available. Some hypogonadal men prefer T ester treatment because they require less frequent administration and generally produce higher average serum T concentrations.

Esterification of the 17β-hydroxyl group of native T increases its hydrophobicity and permits the formulation of T esters within an oil vehicle—sesame oil for T enanthate and cottonseed oil for T cypionate. Following intramuscular injection, T esters are released slowly from the oil vehicle within muscle and hydrolyzed rapidly to T, which is then released into circulation, resulting in relatively high-peak serum T concentrations as well as an extended duration of release into circulation. T enanthate and T cypionate have similar pharmacokinetic profiles; hence, they are considered clinically equivalent.

In adult hypogonadal men, the usual starting dose of T enanthate or cypionate is 150 to 200 mg intramuscularly (i.m.) every two weeks. Following injection of 200 mg of T enanthate, serum T concentrations increase to the upper normal range or above for one to three days, and then decline gradually over two weeks to the lower normal range (or occasionally below normal) prior to the next injection (Fig. 1) (25,26). The extreme rise and fall of serum T levels may be associated with disturbing fluctuations in energy, mood, and sexual desire. In men who complain of reduced energy, mood, or libido prior to their next scheduled T injection, shortening the dosing interval to every 10 days may alleviate these symptoms. In order to reduce fluctuations in T concentrations and associated symptoms, T enanthate or cypionate 100 mg i.m. weekly is preferred by some patients.

Table 1 Formulations for Testosterone (T) Replacement Therapy

Formulation	Adult dosage	Cost[a]	Advantages	Disadvantages
Parenteral Testosterone Esters				
T enanthate (Delatestryl®), T cypionate (Depo-Testosterone®)	150–200 mg i.m. every 2 wk or 75–100 mg i.m. every week	$34–38/mo (200 mg/2 wk); $20–23/mo (200 mg/2 wk)	Extensive clinical experience; inexpensive; some dose flexibility	Intramuscular injections, discomfort; high T levels at 1–3 days to low T levels at nadir → fluctuations in libido, energy, mood; erythrocytosis > transdermal formulations
T undecanoated (Nebido®)	1000 mg i.m. followed by 1000 mg at 6 wk, then 1000 mg every 12 wk		Less frequent injections	Intramuscular injections, discomfort; large-volume (4 mL) injection
Transdermal Testosterone				
Testoderm®d (scrotal patch)	4 or 6 mg/day (every A.M.)	$119/mo (6 mg/day)	Physiological T levels, mid- to low-normal range, circadian variation No injections	Adequate size, clean and shaven scrotum, briefs needed Poor adhesion to scrotum (adhesive strips added) High DHT levels More expensive than T esters No dose flexibility Scrotal location unacceptable to some men
Androderm® (permeation-enhanced, corticosteroid cream)	5 or 7.5 mg/day (every P.M.)	$192/mo (5 mg/day)	Physiological T levels, mid- to low-normal range, circadian variation No injections Good adhesion Normal DHT levels	Frequent skin irritation, occasionally severe (↓ by coapplication of nonscrotal patch) More expensive than T esters Higher dose requires 2 patches/day
AndroGel® (1% T in hydroalcoholic gel)	50, 75, or 100 mg (every A.M.)	$210/mo (50 mg/day)	Steady-state T levels, low-, mid- or high-normal range No injections Little skin irritation Dose flexibility	Potential transfer of T to women and children by contact (prevented by clothing and washing after 1–6 hr) Most expensive T formulation High DHT levels
Testim® (1% T in hydroalco-holic gel)	50 or 100 mg (every A.M.)	$201/mo (50 mg/day)	Steady-state T levels, low- or mid-normal range No injections Little skin irritation Some dose flexibility Musk odor	Potential transfer of T to women and children by contact (prevented by clothing and washing after 2 hr) Less expensive than AndroGel but more expensive than Androderm High DHT levels Musk odor
Transbuccal Testosterone				
Striant® (buccal T tablet)	30 mg twice daily (every 12 hr)	$190/mo (450 mg/3 mo)	Steady-state T levels, mid-normal range	Twice-daily application

Preparation	Dose	Cost	Advantages	Disadvantages
			No injections; No patch or gel; No contact transfer of T; No covering of site or washing instructions	Buccal application unacceptable to some men, requires instruction; Pellets not easily removable; More expensive than T esters; No dose flexibility; High DHT levels
Oral Testosterone				
Testosterone undecanoated (Andriol®)	40–80 mg 2–3 times daily		Oral administration	Must be administered with food; Some formulations must be refrigerated; High DHT levels
Subcutaneous T implant				
Testopel® Pellets[d]	225–450 mg (3–6 pellets) implanted s.c. every 3–4 mo	$30/mo (450 mg/3 mo)	Longer-term, steady-state T levels	Minor surgical procedure; Extrusion, bleeding, and infection, although uncommon
Testosterone Pellets[b]	600–1200 mg (3–6 pellets) implanted s.c. every 4–6 mo			Pellets not easily removable; Large number of pellets; Very seldom used
hCG[c]				
Profasi® (urinary hCG)	1000–5000 IU s.c. 2–3x/wk	$75/mo (1000 IU qod)	Stimulates T and sperm production	Subcutaneous injections 2–3x/wk; Breast tenderness or gynecomastia secondary to higher E_2 levels
Pregnyl® (urinary hCG)		$71/mo (1000 IU qod)	Easier injection, smaller needle than T ester	More expensive than T ester injections, greater expense if high dose is needed; Requires dilution
Novarel® (urinary hCG)		$75/mo (1000 IU qod)	Less fluctuation in T levels than T ester	Occasional burning with injection
Chorex® (urinary hCG) Ovidrel® (recombinant hCG)	$26/mo (1000 IU qod) Not approved for use in men; Dose in men is unclear (only available in one-time-use vials containing 0.25 mg ≅ 5000–10,000 IU)		No patch, gel or buccal tablet	Ineffective if it is primary hypogonadism

[a]Average wholesale price (AWP) from 2005, 2003, or 2001 Drug Topics Redbook. Medical Economics Thomson Health Care, Montvale, New Jersey, U.S.A.

[b]Currently not available in the United States.

[c]Used only for men with hypogonadotropic hypogonadism.

Abbreviations: DHT, dihydrotestosterone; hCG, human chorionic gonadotropin; i.m., intramuscularly; s.c., subcutaneously.

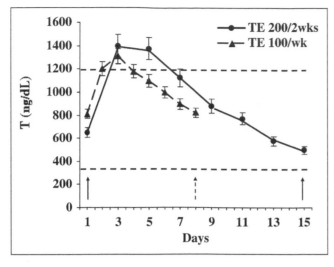

Figure 1 Mean serum T concentrations during T ester therapy in hypogonadal men. Serum T levels after the last injection of T enanthate 100 mg i.m. every week (*triangles*) or 200 mg i.m. every 2 weeks (*circles*), at the end of 12 weeks of treatment. Arrows represent the times of T enanthate injections, and dashed lines represent the normal range for T. *Abbreviation*: i.m., intramuscularly. *Source*: Adapted from Ref. 26.

Doses of T esters greater than 200 mg administered less frequently than every two weeks (e.g., 300 mg i.m. every three weeks or 400 mg i.m. every four weeks) are not recommended (Fig. 1). These doses produce extremely wide fluctuations in serum T levels, characterized by markedly supraphysiological concentrations for several days after injection and levels below normal after three weeks (26). With careful instruction, most patients are able to self-administer intramuscular T ester injections or have a family member administer them.

In men with long-standing and severe androgen deficiency, full T replacement induces profound alterations in behavior, sexuality, and physical appearance that may be distressing, both to the patients and to their sexual and life partners. In order to reduce the likelihood of serious adjustment problems associated with androgen therapy, it is important to counsel hypogonadal men and their partners prior to and during T treatment regarding the changes in behavior and body characteristics that are expected during therapy. In some men with severe hypogonadism, initiating T treatment using a low-dosage regimen—e.g., T enanthate or cypionate 100 mg every two weeks for several months—followed by an increase to full androgen replacement may result in a more gradual and less symptomatic transition from hypogonadism to eugonadism.

In some clinical situations, full androgen replacement may be ill advised, especially in older hypogonadal men with severe benign prostatic hyperplasia (BPH) in whom stimulation of sexual function or anabolic actions on muscle and bone are the therapeutic goals. In these instances, low-dose T supplementation (T enanthate or cypionate 50–100 mg i.m. every two weeks) may be sufficient to produce the desired clinical effects to a limited extent, such as increasing libido, energy, and anabolic effects on muscle and bone mass,

while minimizing potential adverse effects such as stimulation of prostate growth.

Low-dose T ester supplementation has not been evaluated fully in long-term clinical trials; however, its potential effectiveness is suggested by earlier studies of short-acting T formulations (T undecanoate and cyclodextrin) that produced anabolic effects, despite serum T levels that were not sustained within the normal range (27–29). This is analogous to the situation with glucocorticoid replacement therapy using hydrocortisone in which the duration of its biological action on tissues is not reflected by its serum concentrations. Recently, short-term administration of low-dose T enanthate (50 mg i.m. weekly) was found to increase muscle strength and power in some young men with hypogonadism induced by concomitant GnRH agonist treatment (13,15).

The use of transdermal T formulations is an alternative to low-dose T ester supplementation in clinical situations when it is not desirable to use androgen replacement that results in high-normal or transient supraphysiological T concentrations. T acts directly on the bone marrow and indirectly by increasing erythropoietin production to stimulate red-blood-cell production. In some men, T may stimulate erythropoiesis excessively. In hypogonadal men, excessive erythrocytosis was less common during T patch therapy than T enanthate injections, suggesting that physiological T levels produced by transdermal T may be associated with fewer androgenic adverse effects (30). Because of the short half-life of T in subcutaneous tissue and circulation, discontinuation of transdermal T preparations (patches or gels) results in a rapid fall in serum T concentrations and a shorter duration of action when compared to intramuscular T enanthate and cypionate. Therefore, an important advantage of transdermal T is the relatively rapid withdrawal of androgen replacement if adverse effects (e.g., excessive erythrocytosis, prostate enlargement, or growth of prostate cancer) develop. Although the short-acting 17β-hydroxyl T ester, testosterone propionate, also has a short duration of action so that androgen therapy may be withdrawn quickly, the frequent i.m. injections that are needed to maintain normal T levels (25–50 mg i.m. three times weekly) make it a much less desirable option (3). T propionate is rarely used for androgen replacement.

Constitutional delayed puberty is a common condition in which pubertal development is delayed considerably but eventually occurs spontaneously. It is indistinguishable clinically and biochemically from delayed puberty caused by permanent hypogonadotropic hypogonadism—e.g., Kallmann syndrome. Therefore, in boys with prepubertal androgen deficiency and delayed puberty, T treatment is usually withheld until approximately 14 years of age (bone age at least 10.5 years), an age when pubertal development has started in most boys (31–33). If delayed genital development and growth cause severe psychological distress in affected boys and their families, therapy is occasionally initiated at a younger age.

Treatment is initiated with a very low dose of T enanthate or cypionate, e.g., 50 to 100 mg i.m. monthly, in order to prevent the premature closure of long bone epiphyses and the compromise of adult height. Low doses of T are sufficient to stimulate long bone growth and induce some virilization without interfering with the spontaneous puberty that occurs eventually in boys with constitutional delayed puberty. Also, T treatment in boys with delayed puberty is intermittent. T is continued for three to six months and then stopped for three to six months in order to determine whether spontaneous pubertal onset occurs, as evidenced by an increase in testes size to greater than 8 mL. If spontaneous puberty does not occur, intermittent T treatment is continued. The dosage of T ester is increased gradually to 50 to 100 mg i.m. every two weeks, and then to full adult replacement doses, over the next several years. Transdermal T formulations are not approved for use in boys with delayed puberty; however, by avoiding the need for intramuscular injections, lower-dose transdermal T patches and gels can provide very useful alternatives for the treatment of prepubertal androgen deficiency. They are currently being tested for this use.

Transdermal T Patches and Gels

Two T patches and two T gels are available as safe and effective transdermal alternatives to T ester injections for androgen replacement therapy in hypogonadal men (Table 1) (12,34). These transdermal preparations are used in hypogonadal men who prefer or are unable to tolerate or administer intramuscular T ester injections. T gel has become the most frequently used formulation for treatment of male hypogonadism in the United States (35).

In contrast to T ester injections, application of either T patches or gels produces physiologic T concentrations that exhibit a normal circadian variation or steady-state T levels, respectively. All transdermal T delivery systems, however, require application daily, are more expensive than T ester injections, and have some limitations—e.g., an undesirable application site (scrotal T patch), frequent skin irritation or rash (nonscrotal T patch), poor adherence to skin and limited dose flexibility (T patches), and the potential for transfer of T to others with skin contact (T gels). Many of these limitations are a consequence of the need to deliver relatively large amounts (5–10 mg) of T through the skin. Adequate transdermal T delivery requires the use of a thin, vascular area of skin that is wide enough to accommodate the surface area of the patch when applied (such as the scrotum) and often the use of solvents (e.g., alcohol) or chemical agents to enhance skin permeation. Inherent skin sensitivity is a factor that may limit the use of transdermal T formulations in some hypogonadal men.

Scrotal T Patch

The first transdermal T delivery system that was developed by Alza (Palo Alto, California, U.S.A.) for

androgen replacement in hypogonadal men was a scrotal T patch, Testoderm® (Ortho-McNeil, Raritan, New Jersey, U.S.A.) (36–38). T is contained within the matrix of this patch. Because this patch is applied to the thin and highly vascular skin of the scrotum, adequate delivery of T does not require permeation-enhancing agents. Scrotal T patches are available in two sizes that deliver either 6 mg (60 cm²) or 4 mg (40 cm²) of T daily. When applied to the scrotum in the morning, this patch produces serum T levels in hypogonadal men that mimic the circadian variation of endogenous T in normal men. Long-term daily use of Testoderm maintains T levels in the mid- to low-normal range and improves the clinical manifestations of androgen deficiency in hypogonadal men (39–41).

For optimal skin adhesion, the Testoderm patch requires application on a clean, dry, and preferably shaven scrotum of adequate size and the use of brief-type underwear. These requirements are not acceptable to some hypogonadal men. Furthermore, in some men with long-standing, severe prepubertal androgen deficiency, the scrotum may be underdeveloped and too small to accommodate even the smaller Testoderm patch. Because of poor adherence to scrotal skin, thin adhesive strips were added as an option to this patch. Although uncommon, some men may experience skin irritation and itching.

T is converted to the more potent androgen, dihydrotestosterone (DHT) by the enzymes 5α-reductase type 1 and 2. In hypogonadal men, chronic use of the Testoderm patch increases serum DHT levels to the upper limit of normal or above the normal range as a result of the high 5α-reductase activity within scrotal skin. The clinical significance of chronic exposure of androgen-responsive organs such as the prostate gland to high serum DHT concentrations is unclear. No increase in prostate disease was observed in small, short-term trials (lasting up to three years) of older men treated with the Testoderm patch (39–41) or DHT gel formulations (42–44). These studies, however, did not address the potential long-term risks of high DHT levels. Therefore, careful monitoring of the development of adverse androgenic effects should be performed. The use of nonscrotal T patches and T gels (see below) have since supplanted the use of the Testoderm patch for androgen replacement therapy in hypogonadal men. The Testoderm patch is currently not available in the United States.

Nonscrotal T Patch

Androderm® (Watson Pharmaceuticals, Corona, California, U.S.A.) is a T patch that is applied to nonscrotal skin and has replaced scrotal T patches for androgen replacement therapy (45,46). It is composed of a central reservoir containing T and permeation-enhancers in an alcohol-based gel within an adhesive patch. This patch may be applied to the skin of the back, abdomen, upper arms, or thighs, avoiding areas over a bony prominence. When applied at night, Androderm produces serum T levels in hypogonadal men that mimic the circadian variation of endogenous T concentrations in normal men, peaking in the morning. Androderm patches are available in two sizes that deliver either 2.5 mg (37 cm²) or 5 mg (44 cm²) of T daily. Long-term daily application of a 5-mg Androderm patch maintains serum T levels within the mid- to low-normal range and improves the clinical manifestations of androgen deficiency (47–49). In order to achieve T concentrations that are consistently within the mid- to high-normal range, the application of two Androderm patches are usually necessary (i.e., one 2.5-mg patch plus one 5-mg patch or two 5-mg patches) (50).

The major limitation of the Androderm patch is that skin irritation and rash occur in at least 30% of the patients (47,51–53). The severity of skin reactions is variable. Mild-to-moderate redness and irritation is very common, and is thought to be due to a reaction to the permeation-enhancing agents and/or the adhesive. Although uncommon, severe contact dermatitis that may progress to severe burn-like reactions has been reported with Androderm use. Pretreatment of skin under the reservoir with a topical corticosteroid, e.g., triamcinolone acetonide 0.1% cream, reduces the incidence and severity of skin irritation produced by Androderm (54). In contrast to the Testoderm patch, serum DHT concentrations remain within the normal range with this nonscrotal patch. It should be noted that Androderm is more expensive than the Testoderm scrotal T delivery system.

Until recently, another nonscrotal T patch, Testoderm TTS® (Alza, Palo Alto, California, U.S.A.) was also available for T replacement therapy (55–57). It was composed of a central reservoir containing 5 mg of T in an alcohol-based gel but no permeation enhancers within a relatively large (60 cm²), slightly adhesive patch. When applied in the morning on the back, abdomen, or upper buttocks, the pharmacokinetics of this patch were similar to that of Androderm. Because it did not use permeation-enhancing agents and had less adhesive, Testoderm TTS caused much less skin irritation than the Androderm patch (58); however, the major limitations of this patch were its poor adherence to skin, especially with sweating, and the relatively low serum T concentrations achieved when using a single patch. It is no longer being marketed in the United States.

T Gels

In 2000, a transdermal formulation of T in a 1% hydro-alcoholic gel, AndroGel® (Solvay, Marietta, Georgia, U.S.A.) became available for androgen replacement therapy in hypogonadal men (59). It has rapidly become the most frequently used T formulation for the treatment of male hypogonadism in the United States (35). AndroGel is applied daily in the morning to clean, dry skin over the shoulders and upper arms and/or abdomen and flanks, but not to scrotal skin. After application, the alcohol-based gel dries rapidly and

most of the T is absorbed into the subcutaneous tissue, where it is released steadily over the remainder of the day, producing steady-state T levels over 24 hours. Some residual T remains on the surface of the skin. Therefore, application sites should be covered with clothing, and skin contact with others (especially women and children) and water (e.g., showering or bathing) should be avoided for five to six hours (or one to two hours if done infrequently), in order to avoid both transfer of T to others and impaired T absorption due to the washing off of skin residue. Similarly, care should be taken to wash hands with soap and water after the application of AndroGel.

Long-term daily application of AndroGel in hypogonadal men maintains steady-state physiological serum T concentrations and improves the clinical manifestations of androgen deficiency (24,60). The beneficial effects of AndroGel have been reported in a study for up to three years (61). AndroGel is available in foil packets of two sizes [either 2.5 g of gel (25 mg of T) per packet or 5 g of gel (50 mg of T) per packet] that deliver 2.5 or 5.0 mg of T daily, respectively (i.e., approximately 10% absorption). The usual starting dose of AndroGel is 5 g daily (50 mg of T, delivering 5 mg of T daily). Approximately two weeks after the initiation of therapy, serum T levels should be measured in order to determine if the initial dose is adequate. If the desired serum T concentration or clinical response is not achieved, the dose of AndroGel is then increased to 7.5 g (i.e., one 2.5-g packet plus one 5.0-g packet) or 10.0 g (i.e., two 5.0 g packets) daily, delivering 7.5 or 10.0 mg of T daily, respectively. After 90 days treatment

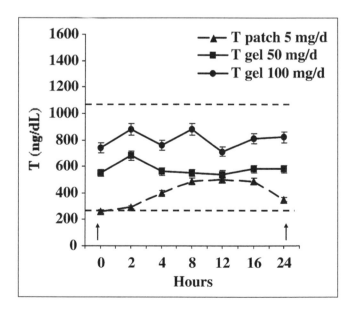

Figure 2 Mean serum T concentrations during T gel therapy in hypogonadal men. Serum T levels before and after applications of T gel (AndroGel®) 5 g (50 mg of T, *squares*) or 10 g (100 mg of T, *circles*) daily, or a T patch (Androderm®) 5 mg (*triangles*) daily, after 90 days of treatment. Arrows represent the times of transdermal T application (time 0 was 0800 hr), and dashed lines represent the normal range for T. *Source*: Adapted from Ref. 59.

in hypogonadal men, AndroGel 5 and 10 g daily produced average serum T concentrations in the mid-normal and high-normal range, respectively, compared to Androderm 5 mg daily that produced serum T levels in the low- to mid-normal range (Fig. 2) (59). Recently, a metered-dose pump that dispenses 1.25 g AndroGel (12.5 mg of T, delivery 1.25 mg of T) per actuation became available, permitting dose titration and greater dose flexibility.

AndroGel may produce serum DHT levels at the upper limit of or above the normal range in some men, probably as a result of 5α-reductase activity in the relatively large surface area of skin over which it is applied; however, local skin irritation is very uncommon, occurring in ≤ 5 of the patients. A major limitation to the use of AndroGel for androgen replacement therapy is its cost. It is currently the most expensive T formulation that is available, and if more than one packet is needed for adequate T replacement, the cost may be prohibitive for many patients who do not have third-party medication coverage.

In 2003, another 1% hydroalcoholic T gel, Testim® (Auxilium, Norristown, Pennsylvania, U.S.A.) became available for androgen replacement therapy in hypogonadal men (62,63). It is applied daily in the morning to intact, clean, dry skin over the shoulders and arms but not over the abdomen or on scrotal skin, and produces steady-state T levels over 24 hours. As with AndroGel, the potential for the transfer of residual T from the skin surface of application sites to other people exists, and similar precautions are recommended. It is also recommended that application sites should not be washed for at least two hours, in order to maintain serum T levels in the normal range.

In placebo-controlled trials, short-term daily application of Testim in hypogonadal men maintains steady-state physiological serum T concentrations and improves the clinical manifestations of androgen deficiency (62,63). No long-term efficacy and safety data have yet been published for Testim. Serum T levels after the initial application of Testim are slightly (~30%) higher than for AndroGel (64); however, a direct comparison of steady-state T levels achieved with longer-term use of the two T gels is not available. In separate clinical trials using different T assays, average serum T levels at 30 days of treatment seemed to be comparable in hypogonadal men treated with the same dosages of AndroGel and Testim: 566 ± 262 ng/dL and 365 ± 187 ng/dL, respectively, with the 5-g dosage; and 792 ± 294 ng/dL and 612 ± 286 ng/dL, respectively, with the 10-g dosage.

Testim is available in 5-g and 10-g tubes, each containing 50 and 100 mg of T, and delivering approximately 5 mg and 10 mg of T, respectively (i.e., ~10% absorption). In contrast to AndroGel, an intermediate dosage of 7.5 g and a metered-dose dispenser are not available. The starting dose of Testim is 5 g (50 mg) daily. After 90 days of treatment in hypogonadal men, this dose produced average serum T concentrations in the low-normal range, comparable to those achieved with daily application of an Androderm patch (63). Two weeks after initiating therapy, a serum T level should be checked in the morning in order to assess the adequacy of initial dose in achieving mid-normal T concentrations. If the desired serum T level or clinical response is not achieved, the dose of Testim should be increased to 10 g (100 mg). This dose typically produces average serum T levels in the mid-normal range (65).

Unlike AndroGel, which is odorless, Testim has a musk-like scent. Depending on the individual patient and his partners, this odor may be either pleasant or objectionable. Because Testim contains an emollient, it is theoretically less drying to the skin than AndroGel, but both are tolerated well with very little skin irritation, occurring in ≤ 5% of patients. Similar to AndroGel, Testim may also produce high serum DHT levels in some men. The cost of Testim is slightly less than AndroGel and is comparable to the Androderm patch.

Transbuccal T Tablet

In 2003, a novel, mucoadhesive buccal T system, Striant® (Columbia Laboratories, Livingston, New Jersey, U.S.A.), was approved and became available for the T replacement therapy of hypogonadal men (Table 1). This system is a small, self-mucoadhesive tablet that is composed of T (30 mg) in an oil–water emulsion carrier vehicle that contains polycarbophil, which remains attached to buccal epithelium until cells turn over (approximately 12–15 hours). When placed in the mouth between the inner cheek and the gum above the incisors with the monoconvex side of the tablet toward the gum (and the flat side toward the cheek), the tablet softens, swells with hydration, and becomes gelatinous and sticky, adhering to the gum. Within the tablet, T is stored in a lipophilic fraction that is in equilibrium with an aqueous fraction and is thus released at a controlled and sustained constant rate from the latter fraction into the systemic circulation, circumventing first-pass hepatic metabolism.

The recommended dosage schedule for Striant is twice daily, with application of one buccal tablet in the morning followed by its removal after 12 hours and the application of another buccal tablet in the evening on the opposite side. Alternating sides of the mouth should be used with each application. It is important to educate patients that the buccal system should be oriented with the rounded side against the gum and held firmly in place with a finger over the lip for approximately 30 seconds. If the tablet falls off or is dislodged, a new buccal system should be applied and left in place until the next regularly scheduled dosing. The buccal tablet should be removed by gently sliding it down toward the tooth to avoid scratching the gum.

Clinical pharmacokinetic studies of Striant have been published (66). Application of this buccal tablet containing 30 mg of T twice daily for three months produced average steady-state T levels in the mid-normal range, averaging 520 ± 205 ng/dL. Average T levels were consistent over two consecutive 12-hour periods of application, but absolute range of levels was broad. Although a formal study has not yet been conducted, unrestricted food and beverage (including alcohol) intake, tooth brushing, mouth washing, and gum chewing did not appear to affect the use of Striant or the absorption of T in pharmacokinetic studies.

As with transdermal T gels, Striant produced high serum DHT concentrations in some hypogonadal men. In general, therapy was tolerated well. In initial studies, approximately 9% of men had gum or mouth irritation, 4% experienced a bitter taste, and 2% to 3% developed gum pain, tenderness, or edema. Most (~94%) of the adverse gum effects were mild and transient, and only 4% of men discontinued therapy because of gum-related side effects.

The cost of Striant is comparable to Androderm and slightly less than AndroGel and Testim. Initially, patients may be aware and bothered by the tablet between their cheek and gum, and this may lead to premature discontinuation of Striant. With continued use, the unusual sensation and awareness of the buccal tablet decreases and is less bothersome. Because twice-daily application is needed to sustain physiological T levels, it is likely that patient compliance will be challenging in clinical practice and may limit its use. Patients should be made aware of these potential disadvantages prior to initiating Striant therapy in order to avoid poor compliance and premature discontinuation. Linking Striant application to a routine daily activity, such as brushing teeth in morning and evening, may help to improve and maintain compliance.

Subcutaneous T Pellets

The subcutaneous T pellets, Testopel® Pellets (Bartor Pharmacal, Rye, New York, U.S.A.) in a range of doses from 225 to 450 mg (i.e., three to six 75-mg T pellets) implanted every three to four months were, but are no longer, available in the United States for long-term androgen replacement therapy in hypogonadal men (Table 1). Although T pellets are very rarely used in the United States, they are used more commonly for T replacement in Australia and some European countries (67–69). Using a different pellet formulation, European studies have shown that subcutaneous implantation of three to six 200-mg T pellets (600–1200 mg of T) in hypogonadal men produced the nearly zero-order, sustained release of T and maintained steady-state physiological serum T levels for four to six months (67–69). T pellets are implanted using a trocar that is introduced into the subcutaneous space through a small skin incision. This minor surgical procedure to implant the T pellets is required two to three times yearly in order to maintain normal serum T levels. Although an uncommon occurrence in experienced hands, the extrusion of pellets and local side effects such as bleeding and infection do take place occasionally. A major concern is that if adverse effects develop after implantation, the subsequent removal of the T pellets is difficult, if not impossible. For these reasons, the use of T pellets for T replacement therapy is inappropriate for older patients who are predisposed to erythrocytosis and prostate disease during treatment, and it is not acceptable to many hypogonadal men and physicians.

□ GONADOTROPIN THERAPY

In men with secondary hypogonadism due to gonadotropin deficiency, endogenous T production may be stimulated by administration of LH-like activity using human chorionic gonadotropin (hCG) (3). The most commonly used preparations for gonadotropin therapy are urinary hCG preparations, e.g., Profasi® (Serono, Randolph, Massachusetts, U.S.A.), Pregnyl® (Organon, Oss, The Netherlands), Novarel (Ferring, Suffern, New York, U.S.A.), and generic Chorex (Hyrex, Memphis, Tennessee, U.S.A.) that are purified from pregnant women's urine and contain LH-like bioactivity almost exclusively. A recombinant hCG (rhCG) preparation, Ovidrel® (Serono, Randolph, Massachusetts, U.S.A.), is available for gonadotropin therapy in women (ovulation induction and assisted reproductive technologies) but not for men. It is only available in one-time use vials containing 0.25 mg, which provide the equivalent of approximately 5000 to 10,000 IU of hCG activity. Although the purity of rhCG is much higher than urinary preparations, its cost is also much greater. Because urinary hCG preparations are highly effective in treating men with hypogonadotropic hypogonadism, they remain the most commonly utilized preparations for gonadotropin therapy in this patient population.

Human CG stimulates Leydig cells of the testis to produce T, and in men with partial or postpubertally acquired gonadotropin deficiency, it may also stimulate sperm production. Because hCG preparations require multiple injections per week, T, rather than hCG, treatment is used to induce and maintain T levels in men with hypogonadotropic hypogonadism. Therapy with hCG is usually used if induction of spermatogenesis and fertility are the ultimate therapeutic goals (3). Sperm production and fertility may ultimately require the addition of FSH to hCG treatment. Some patients prefer hCG treatment to T replacement therapy because the use of hCG may increase testis size slightly due to stimulation of spermatogenesis, particularly in men with partial gonadotropin deficiency. In contrast, T treatment usually reduces testis size due to inhibition of gonadotropin secretion and consequently inhibition of spermatogenesis. With the availability of a generic preparation, the cost of hCG therapy is comparable to T replacement using T esters, and less costly than using transdermal and transbuccal T preparations.

Gonadotropin therapy is usually initiated with hCG 500 to 1000 IU subcutaneously (s.c.) two to three times weekly. Subcutaneous injections of hCG are as effective as intramuscular injections. Because they are administered using a small needle and syringe into subcutaneous fat, aqueous hCG injections are usually tolerated better than larger volume intramuscular injections of viscous T esters in oil. Because the cost is comparable to T ester therapy, some men with hypogonadotropic hypogonadism prefer hCG therapy to T treatment. Clinical evidence of androgenization and serum T levels are monitored to determine the need for dosage adjustment. The dosage of hCG is increased until serum T concentrations are within the eugonadal range. Men with gonadotropin deficiency, who also have testicular disease (e.g., cryptorchidism), i.e., combined primary and secondary hypogonadism, or severe prepubertal isolated hypogonadotropic hypogonadism, may require larger dosages of hCG up to 3000 to 5000 IU two to three times weekly. If there is severe testis damage, these patients may be completely unresponsive to hCG treatment. A recent controlled trial in older men with partial age-related androgen deficiency demonstrated that hCG 5000 IU given twice weekly for three months increased serum T levels and resulted in increased lean body mass and reduced fat mass without changes in muscle mass or strength, or physical activity, or function (69).

Because hCG stimulates aromatase activity within the testis, serum E_2 levels may rise disproportionately to T concentrations, and breast tenderness or gynecomastia may occur more frequently than with T replacement therapy. Uncommonly, some men complain of burning with subcutaneous injections of hCG.

□ ANDROGEN FORMULATIONS UNDER DEVELOPMENT

There is continuing interest in developing additional T formulations and tissue-selective androgen receptor modulators for the treatment of male hypogonadism and other clinical conditions associated with low T levels. This interest has stimulated the potential expansion of indications for androgen therapy, such as wasting syndromes, chronic illnesses, and age-related androgen deficiency ("andropause").

Short-Acting Formulations

There is substantial interest in developing short-acting T formulations—especially orally active preparations—for T replacement therapy and the low-dose androgen supplementation of hypogonadal men. Because T levels fall quickly after discontinuation of these formulations, short-acting T preparations are particularly useful in older hypogonadal men in whom rapid withdrawal of androgen action is desirable if adverse effects develop during T replacement or in whom only low-dose androgen supplementation is needed.

In many countries outside the United States, an orally administered 17β-hydroxyl ester, T undecanoate marketed as Andriol® (Organon, Oss, The Netherlands),

has been used for many years to provide safe and effective T replacement therapy in hypogonadal men (27,70). T undecanoate is formulated in oleic acid, which facilitates the absorption of T directly from the gastrointestinal tract into the lymphatics and then into the systemic circulation, bypassing first-pass hepatic inactivation. In hypogonadal men, replacement therapy using T undecanoate requires relatively high doses (80–240 mg daily), administered in divided doses (two to three times daily). Unlike oral 17α-alkylated androgens, T undecanoate is not associated with liver toxicity. The absorption of T undecanoate is dependent upon concomitant food ingestion, however, resulting in highly variable serum T levels and clinical responses. Furthermore, serum DHT levels are often very high, due to 5α-reductase activity in the gastrointestinal tract. A new formulation of T undecanoate in castor oil and propylene glycol laurate instead of oleic acid (Andriol Testocaps®, Organon, Oss, The Netherlands) is being tested for use in hypogonadal men (71,72). T undecanoate in oleic acid requires refrigeration and has a limited shelf life; in contrast, this new formulation is stable at room temperature for at least three years, yet maintains pharmacokinetic and pharmacodynamic characteristics similar to the original formulation.

T cyclodextrin is a short-acting sublingual formulation composed of 2.5 or 5 mg of T that is complexed to hydroxypropyl-β-cyclodextrin. In hypogonadal men, sublingual administration of T cyclodextrin results in a rapid increase in serum T levels that peaks in 20 to 40 minutes and decreases rapidly to baseline within two to four hours (28,29,73). Despite this unfavorable pharmacokinetic profile, T cyclodextrin improved sexual function, mood, and muscle strength and reduced markers of bone resorption, suggesting that sustained physiological T concentrations may not be necessary for some clinical effects of T.

Other transdermal and transbuccal T formulations are being developed for androgen replacement therapy in hypogonadal men (74,75). In some countries in Europe, a 2% hydroalcoholic DHT gel has been used for androgen replacement therapy of young men with hypogonadism (42), and it has been tested recently in older hypogonadal men (43,44,76); however, intraprostatic DHT and possibly estradiol (E_2) are thought to play important roles in the pathogenesis of BPH and stimulation of prostate cancer growth. Thus, a rationale for the potential use of DHT treatment in older hypogonadal men is that DHT administration will suppress circulating gonadotropin and endogenous T and E_2 levels sufficiently to lower intraprostatic T, E_2, and DHT concentrations, thereby reducing stimulation of prostate growth (77). Furthermore, because it is not aromatizable to an estrogen, DHT treatment also may not induce or worsen gynecomastia. Evidence for these potential advantages of DHT therapy in hypogonadal men, however, is lacking. Two controlled trials in older hypogonadal men of three and six months' duration each have demonstrated that DHT gel 70 and 150 mg to 250 mg daily decreased fat mass, increased lower limb muscle strength, and improved sexual function, respectively (43,44). In these short-term studies, there were no adverse effects on the prostate [symptoms, volume, or prostate-specific antigen (PSA)] or cardiovascular (lipids, vascular reactivity) safety outcomes. Longer-term randomized, controlled studies are needed to assess the clinical benefits and risks of DHT treatment in older men with hypogonadism, particularly regarding BPH and prostate cancer.

As with T gel, there is concern regarding the contact transfer of this more potent androgen from the skin of application sites to females and children. Also, because DHT is nonaromatizable and the production of endogenous gonadotropin and E_2 is suppressed, there is considerable concern regarding the potential adverse clinical consequences of estrogen deficiency induced by DHT treatment in hypogonadal men on bone, blood vessels, lipids, and the brain.

Long-Acting Formulations

A number of long-acting T formulations are being developed that produce prolonged and sustained serum T levels within the normal range, both for use in androgen replacement in young hypogonadal men and, potentially, for other novel uses such as in hormonal male contraception. In hypogonadal men, intramuscular administration of the 17β-hydroxyl esters, T undecanoate formulated in castor or tea seed oil 500 to 1000 mg (78–80) or T buciclate 200 to 600 mg (81) every 6 to 12 weeks maintains serum T concentrations within the eugonadal range (although for T buciclate, concentrations are maintained in the low-normal range). Testosterone undecanoate in castor oil (Nebido®, Schering, Berlin, Germany) is approved and used in Europe and other countries. It is being tested currently in the United States (Indevus, Lexington, Massachusetts, U.S.A.). T has also been incorporated into biodegradable polylactide co-glycolide microcapsules, and intramuscular or subcutaneous injections of 537 mg T microcapsules produce serum T levels in the normal range for 10 to 11 weeks (82,83). Although these T preparations show promise, major limitations of these long-acting formulations include the large injection volumes needed (a 4-mL intramuscular injection for 1000 mg of T undecanoate in castor oil; a 4-mL and 8-mL intramuscular injection for 500 and 1000 mg T undecanoate in tea seed oil, respectively; a 2.4-mL intramuscular injection for 600 mg of T buciclate; and two 2.5-mL intramuscular or subcutaneous injections for T microcapsules) that may require two separate injection sites that not only are often uncomfortable, but also produce highly variable T levels.

Selective Androgen Receptor Modulators

There is escalating interest in developing so-called "designer" androgens that maintain the beneficial actions of T on muscle, bone, sexual function, and mood but have reduced adverse effects on the prostate gland and reduced cardiovascular risk. Steroid hormone action on specific target organs is dependent upon interactions among the steroid hormone ligand and receptor, and tissue-specific coactivator and corepressor proteins (84). It is thought that these unique interactions may exert selective hormone actions in different target tissues. Methods analogous to those used to identify and develop selective estrogen receptor modulators (SERMs), such as raloxifene, have been utilized to identify nonsteroidal, orally active selective androgen receptor modulators (SARMs). These are currently under investigation (85,86).

SARMs are being developed that have anabolic actions in muscle and bone, but reduced stimulatory effects on the prostate gland. Although SARMs may have selective androgen actions on different target organs, they will not have intrinsic estrogen activity. Thus, if an SARM acts in the pituitary and/or hypothalamus to suppress endogenous gonadotropin, T, and E_2 secretion, administration of this compound will produce a state of relative estrogen deficiency. Therefore, in studies evaluating the clinical benefits and risks of an SARM for a specific clinical indication such as muscle wasting syndromes, careful attention must be paid to the potential adverse effects on target organs such as bone, lipids, and the brain that are also regulated by E_2.

An alternative approach to developing a "designer" androgen is the identification of an androgen that undergoes aromatization to an estrogen but does not undergo 5α-reduction to a more potent androgen. One androgen that has these properties and was synthesized over 20 years ago is 7α-methyl-19-nortestosterone or MENT (87). In castrated monkeys, MENT is 10 times more potent than T in stimulating body weight gain and suppressing gonadotropin levels but only twice as potent in stimulating prostate size (88).

In a short-term study, two subcutaneous MENT acetate implants maintained sexual function and mood in hypogonadal men for six weeks (89). In a recent, uncontrolled study, a small number of hypogonadal men were treated with one or two MENT acetate implants for 24 weeks (90). Both doses of MENT severely suppressed endogenous gonadotropins and T levels. The lower dose of MENT resulted in an increase in lean body mass but no change in fat mass; unchanged hematocrit; decreased sexual behavior and erectile function; decreased lumbar BMD; and decreased prostate volume and PSA. These findings suggest that low-dose MENT treatment results in an overall reduction in androgen action within the prostate but inadequate estrogen replacement. The higher dose of MENT resulted in an increase in lean body mass and decrease in fat mass; unchanged hematocrit; unchanged sexual function and erectile function; decreased lumbar BMD; and unchanged prostate size but decreased PSA. These findings suggest that compared to the lower dose, high-dose MENT produced greater androgen action in target tissues including the prostate and sufficient estrogen action in the brain but not in bone. These findings support the theoretical importance of estrogen in the maintenance of bone mass.

□ MONITORING OF CLINICAL RESPONSE AND T LEVELS

The clinical response to androgen replacement and serum T levels are used to monitor the adequacy of T therapy in hypogonadal men (11,12). Within the first few months of T treatment, most hypogonadal men experience improvements in libido, sexual function and activity, energy, well-being, motivation and mood, and reduced irritability. The anabolic effects of T, such as increases in body hair growth, muscle mass and strength, and BMD occur throughout the subsequent several months to years of therapy. Serum T levels should be monitored to determine the adequacy of therapy and to avoid over- or underreplacement. The goal of T replacement is to achieve serum T concentrations in the mid-normal range at the midpoint of the interval between T ester injections or at various times within the interval between applications of transdermal or transbuccal T.

In hypogonadal men on T ester injections, if the clinical response to androgen therapy is not adequate or wanes toward the end of the injection interval, measurements of blood T concentrations at various times after an injection may be useful. Serum T levels measured either at the expected peak or at the midpoint between T ester injections (one to two days and five to seven days after an injection, respectively, in men receiving injections every two weeks) may help to document an inadequate dose or absorption if levels are low, or an excessive dose if they are high. Serum T levels measured at the nadir of the injection interval (just before the next T ester injection) may help to document an inadequate dosing interval (12,91).

In order to assess the adequacy of T delivery in hypogonadal men on T patches, it is recommended that after three to four weeks of daily use, serum T levels should be measured two to four hours after morning application of the Testoderm scrotal patch and 8 to 10 hours after application of the Androderm patch on the previous evening. After two weeks of daily use of AndroGel or Testim and four to six weeks after initiating Striant, it is recommended that a morning serum T level should be measured in order to assess the adequacy of T delivery.

□ POTENTIAL RISKS OF T TREATMENT AND ADVERSE-EFFECT MONITORING
Contraindications

Androgen treatment is contraindicated in men with existing prostate cancer and breast cancer (11,12); because these are androgen-dependent malignancies, T administration may stimulate tumor growth. T treatment is especially dangerous in men with metastatic prostate cancer, in whom rapid growth of metastatic tumors may worsen severe bone pain or cause spinal cord compression. Removal of endogenous androgen production using orchiectomy or GnRH agonists and antiandrogens is the mainstay of treatment for metastatic prostate cancer. Although the effect of T in hypogonadal men with localized prostate cancer is not known, it is prudent to avoid T treatment in men with any clinical evidence of prostate cancer. The safety of T therapy is not clear in hypogonadal men who have been surgically cured of prostate cancer for several years with clinically undetectable disease and an undetectable PSA. In these patients, a careful discussion of the potential benefits and risks of T treatment should be undertaken, and T therapy should be initiated only after informed consent and with careful monitoring. For further information on the management of sexual dysfunction in men with prostate cancer, see Chapter 37.

Prior to initiating T replacement therapy, a careful breast examination for suspicious masses and a digital rectal examination (DRE) for a suspicious prostate nodule or induration should be performed in middle-aged and older men with androgen deficiency. Measurement of PSA should also be performed, especially in men at higher risk for prostate carcinoma—e.g., older men, African–American men, and men with an abnormal DRE or family history of prostate cancer. Hypogonadal men with an abnormal DRE and/or consistently elevated or rising PSA should have a urological evaluation that may include a transrectal ultrasound and biopsy of the prostate.

Relative contraindications to androgen therapy include men with untreated obstructive sleep apnea, in whom T treatment may worsen sleep apnea and its complications; patients with baseline erythrocytosis (hematocrit > 50), in whom further stimulation of erythropoiesis induced by T may result in hyperviscosity and vascular complications; men with severe edematous conditions (e.g., severe congestive heart failure), in whom the fluid retention associated with T therapy may worsen preexisting edema; and men with severe lower urinary tract symptoms (LUTS) due to BPH [e.g., men with International Prostate Symptom Score, (IPSS) > 19].

Prostate

In hypogonadal men, prostate size is reduced and T replacement increases prostate volume to that of age-matched eugonadal men, but does not cause excessive prostate enlargement (92,93). There is currently no evidence to suggest that T replacement therapy worsens symptoms of BPH, reduces urinary flow rate, causes urinary retention, or increases the need for invasive intervention for BPH, such as transurethral resection of the prostate (TURP). It should be noted, however, that long-term controlled studies have not been performed to evaluate these parameters in hypogonadal men over the age of 45 years, who are most at risk for developing clinically significant BPH. Therefore, in middle-aged and older hypogonadal men, symptoms of BPH should be monitored using the American Urological Association (AUA) Symptom Index or IPSS prior to and during T replacement (11,94–96). Concomitant therapy for BPH (e.g., α-adrenergic receptor antagonists, 5α-reductase inhibitors, or bladder outlet procedures) should be considered in hypogonadal men with bothersome moderate-to-severe symptoms.

There is no evidence that T replacement therapy of hypogonadal men causes prostate cancer. In middle-aged and older hypogonadal men, however, the most concerning potential long-term risk of T therapy is the stimulation of previously unrecognized localized or metastatic prostate cancer or the further growth of pre-existing subclinical disease into clinically apparent and significant prostate cancer (8,95). Although there is evidence that indicates T stimulates the growth of metastatic and locally invasive prostate cancer, the effect of T treatment on subclinical prostate cancer is not known. Small, short-term, controlled studies (up to three years in duration) have not found an increased incidence of prostate cancer in older men treated with T (41,97,98). Large, long-term, prospective, controlled trials are needed to determine whether T therapy will stimulate the growth and progression of subclinical prostate cancer into clinically evident and significant disease.

In hypogonadal men, serum PSA concentrations are reduced and T replacement increases PSA to levels observed in age-matched eugonadal men (92). Whether PSA levels are monitored during T therapy in older hypogonadal men depends (to some extent) on whether an individual physician feels that PSA screening is justified in eugonadal men (8,99). Yearly PSA screening in men over the age of 45 years is controversial; however, it is increasingly becoming a standard of care and many patients are demanding PSA screening. An important reason for more intensive PSA monitoring during T therapy in older hypogonadal men is that T is a potentially disease-modifying intervention that may alter the natural history of prostate cancer. Also, if T ester injections are used, serum T concentrations usually rise, albeit transiently, into the supraphysiological range. Therefore, careful monitoring of PSA levels is prudent both for clinical and for medical–legal reasons.

An argument against more intensive PSA monitoring is that abnormal PSA levels that would trigger a prostate biopsy are more likely to occur in older hypogonadal men on T therapy (100). Therefore, there is an increased likelihood of detecting localized prostate cancer for which the management is unclear. Although the diagnosis of subclinical or localized prostate cancer may not affect overall mortality, the potential medical, surgical, psychological, and socioeconomic consequences and morbidity of this diagnosis may be considerable.

Considering these important issues, recent consensus recommendations, including The Endocrine Society Clinical Practice Guidelines on Testosterone Therapy for Adult Men with Androgen Deficiency Syndromes recommend that, in older hypogonadal men, a DRE and PSA level check should be performed prior to starting T treatment, three to six months after starting therapy, and then yearly thereafter (8,11,95,101). Indications for further urological evaluation in men receiving T therapy include a verified serum PSA above 4 ng/mL; an increase in PSA above 1.4 ng/mL in any 12-month period during therapy; a PSA velocity of above 0.4 ng/mL per year with the value at three to six months as baseline (if 2 or more years of PSA values are available); an abnormal DRE; or an AUA symptom score or IPSS above 19 (11,95,96).

Erythrocytosis

In hypogonadal men, T replacement stimulates erythropoiesis, increasing the hemoglobin concentration and hematocrit from the female range into the normal adult male range (102). Occasionally, T treatment causes excessive erythrocytosis (hematocrit > 54) that may require temporary discontinuation of therapy and/or therapeutic phlebotomy. Although adverse clinical consequences of erythrocytosis induced by T are poorly documented, there is concern that a severe increase in red-cell volume and blood viscosity may cause vascular complications such as thrombosis in some patients, especially older men with underlying atherosclerotic vascular disease. Therefore, a hematocrit should be measured prior to starting T treatment, three to six months after starting therapy, and then yearly during therapy (11,96). Some hypogonadal men who develop erythrocytosis on T replacement may have an underlying predisposing condition such as hypoxia due to chronic lung disease or obstructive sleep apnea. Therefore, an evaluation of the underlying causes of erythrocytosis should be considered in hypogonadal men who develop erythrocytosis during T therapy. Compared to hypogonadal men treated with transdermal T patches that produce physiological T levels, erythrocytosis occurs more commonly in men treated with T ester injections that produce supraphysiological T levels for a few days after administration and overall higher average T concentrations (30).

Sleep Apnea

In hypogonadal men, T treatment may induce or worsen obstructive sleep apnea (103,104). The prevalence of clinically significant obstructive sleep apnea during T replacement therapy is not known but is probably low and may be dose related. In a recent report, short-term, high-dose T treatment of older hypogonadal men significantly worsened sleep apnea, increased the duration of hypoxemia, and shortened total sleep time, as assessed by polysomnography (105). In contrast, older men treated with a scrotal T patch for three years did not demonstrate a significant worsening of sleep apnea, as assessed by a portable device (41).

Sleep apnea is associated with significant morbidity and mortality and may be associated with or cause low T levels. Therefore, hypogonadal men, especially those at increased risk—namely, obese men—should be questioned about symptoms of obstructive sleep apnea (apnea or loud snoring during sleep, sleep disturbance, or daytime somnolence), both prior to and during T replacement. If symptoms are present, a formal sleep study should be performed, and if obstructive sleep apnea is confirmed, treatment should be instituted (e.g., continuous positive airway pressure) before T treatment is started or continued. If the patient is unresponsive to therapy for sleep apnea or cannot tolerate treatment, T therapy should not be instituted or it should be discontinued.

Gynecomastia

Occasionally, breast tenderness or gynecomastia develops in hypogonadal patients receiving T treatment. Gynecomastia develops most commonly in boys or young men receiving T for the induction of puberty, severely hypogonadal men receiving relatively high doses of T, and men who have a predisposing condition such as hepatic cirrhosis (12). A careful examination usually reveals some gynecomastia and increased adipose tissue surrounding the breast in hypogonadal men prior to the initiation of T therapy. Small amounts of palpable breast tissue, usually less than 2 cm, are commonly detectable in eugonadal men. Therefore, it is important to do a careful breast examination both prior to and during T therapy in order to detect gynecomastia and, more importantly, the rare occurrence of male breast cancer.

Sperm Production

T treatment reversibly suppresses endogenous gonadotropin production, which in turn suppresses spermatogenesis to varying degrees, depending on the T dosage, duration of treatment, underlying etiology of hypogonadism, and baseline sperm production (3). The suppression of spermatogenesis may further impair fertility in hypogonadal men receiving T therapy. This effect of exogenous T is only clinically relevant in men who have hypogonadotropic hypogonadism and otherwise normal testes. If men with gonadotropin deficiency wish to father children, T therapy should be discontinued and gonadotropin treatment should be started, initially with hCG alone, and then, if necessary, with combined hCG and FSH treatment (3). In the absence of coexisting testicular disease (e.g., cryptorchidism), prior T therapy does not impair the subsequent induction of spermatogenesis with gonadotropins.

Lipids and Cardiovascular Disease

In severely androgen-deficient young men, T treatment decreases HDL cholesterol concentration (106–109). The reduction in HDL cholesterol is greater in more severely androgen-deficient men and in men treated with supraphysiological T dosages or nonaromatizable oral 17α-alkylated androgens (12,106). In contrast, T treatment of older, mildly hypogonadal men does not suppress HDL cholesterol, and total and LDL cholesterol are either not affected or also suppressed (8,98). The clinical significance of lipid changes induced by T on cardiovascular risk is not known.

Because men have a higher risk of coronary artery disease than women do, there is concern that T replacement therapy of hypogonadal men will increase the risk of cardiovascular disease; however, most cross-sectional epidemiological studies have found that low (not high) T levels are associated with an increase in the risk and severity of coronary artery disease, and longitudinal studies have failed to find a relationship between T levels and development of coronary heart disease (8,99,110,111). Furthermore, short-term intervention studies suggest that T treatment improves exercise-induced coronary ischemia and angina (112–118). The effects of T therapy on major cardiovascular outcomes such as the incidence of coronary death, myocardial infarction, and stroke will require larger, long-term, randomized, controlled studies. At present, cardiovascular risks and plasma lipids should be evaluated as dictated by general practice guidelines, and more intensive monitoring in men on T therapy is not justified.

Other Systemic Effects

In general, androgen replacement therapy using any of the available T formulations is tolerated very well, and serious adverse effects are rare (12). In patients receiving T therapy for induction of puberty, acne and increased oiliness of the skin are relatively common. These complaints usually respond to local skin measures (e.g., benzoyl peroxide or retinoic acid) and antibiotics and/or a reduction in T dosage. Although not well documented in the literature, frontal balding or androgenic alopecia may develop in genetically predisposed hypogonadal men during T therapy. Mild-to-moderate weight gain usually occurs during T treatment, due to both anabolic actions of T and fluid retention. Clinically significant edema does not usually occur with T treatment, except in hypogonadal men with underlying edematous states (e.g., congestive heart failure, nephrotic syndrome, and hepatic cirrhosis).

Excessive stimulation of libido and erections are rare, occurring mostly in boys or young men with severe, long-standing androgen deficiency, who are then treated with high dosages of T. In these patients, symptoms usually resolve spontaneously or with a reduction in the dosage of T. Contrary to popular belief, T treatment in physiological or moderately supraphysiological dosages does not cause pathological aggressiveness or anger (14,24,28,119,120). Rather, T replacement therapy increases mild social aggressiveness, motivation, and initiative, and reduces irritability and anger. The behavioral and physical changes induced by T therapy in men with long-standing androgen deficiency may be distressing both to patients and to their sexual partners. Therefore, a discussion of the behavioral and physical changes that are expected should be undertaken with patients and their partners prior to and during T treatment.

Potentially serious hepatotoxicity occurs only with the use of oral 17α-alkylated androgens, and does not occur with the use of injectable T esters or transdermal or transbuccal T formulations (12). Therefore, routine liver function testing is not necessary with the use of the latter preparations for T replacement in hypogonadal men.

Local Side Effects

Local discomfort or bleeding may occur at the site of T ester injections. The use of proper intramuscular injection techniques may minimize these side effects. Inadvertent injection of T esters s.c. may cause severe local irritation and pain. Rarely, men may experience an allergic reaction to the drug carrier vehicle, which is sesame oil for T enanthate and cottonseed oil for T cypionate. As discussed previously, T patches may cause local skin irritation, itching, contact dermatitis, and, occasionally, more severe reactions. Skin reactions occur more commonly with the Androderm patch than with the Testoderm patch and uncommonly with the T gels, AndroGel or Testim. Gum and mouth irritation and a bitter taste may occur in some men who use Striant.

□ SUMMARY AND CONCLUSIONS

Male hypogonadism is a common clinical condition that causes T deficiency and affects the health and well-being of males of all ages. T replacement therapy has proven beneficial effects on body composition (muscle, bone, and fat), sexual development and function, and behavior. The goals of T replacement therapy for male hypogonadism are to improve the clinical manifestations of androgen deficiency that depend on whether hypogonadism occurs in prepubertal boys or adults.

The diagnosis of male hypogonadism is suspected when an individual presents with a clinical syndrome that is consistent with androgen deficiency, and repeatedly low serum T levels confirms the diagnosis. The clinical manifestations of androgen deficiency vary with the stage of sexual development and findings may be subtle in adults compared to prepubertal boys with hypogonadism. T levels should be measured using an accurate and reliable assay that preferably is not affected by alterations in SHBG, and it should be repeated to confirm the diagnosis of hypogonadism. Other important considerations in the management of hypogonadism include evaluation for potentially reversible causes of low T levels; concomitant measurements of gonadotropin and T levels to diagnose secondary hypogonadism that has important therapeutic implications; and consideration of other causes of clinical manifestations consistent with androgen deficiency.

Currently, T formulations that are available for androgen replacement include injections of T esters, transdermal T patches or gels, and a transbuccal T tablet. T esters are effective and relatively safe, and they provide the least expensive method of T replacement; however, they usually require intramuscular injections every one to two weeks and produce wide excursions in T levels that may cause disturbing fluctuations in symptoms. Transdermal T patches or gels or the transbuccal T tablet provide more physiological T levels, but they require daily skin or twice-daily buccal application, may cause local skin or gum irritation, and are more expensive than T esters. A number of short- and long-acting T formulations and "designer" androgens (SARMs) are currently being developed, which should greatly expand the methods available for androgen treatment in the future.

Prostate and breast cancer are absolute contraindications to T replacement therapy, and untreated obstructive sleep apnea, erythrocytosis, severe edematous states, and severe LUTS due to BPH are relative contraindications to T treatment. In general, T replacement therapy is tolerated very well and serious adverse effects are rare. Occasionally, T treatment may cause erythrocytosis or induce or worsen obstructive sleep apnea. Therefore, hematocrit and symptoms of sleep apnea should be assessed prior to and during T therapy. In middle-aged and older hypogonadal men, monitoring of DRE and PSA for prostate cancer and BPH symptoms is also recommended. The long-term risks of T treatment in older hypogonadal men, with regard to the manifestation of clinical prostate cancer and/or its severity, the need for invasive intervention for BPH, and cardiovascular outcomes such as cardiac death, myocardial infarction, and stroke, remain unknown. A large, prospective, randomized, controlled trial is needed to determine both the long-term risks and benefits of chronic T treatment in older hypogonadal men.

□ REFERENCES

1. Amory JK, Anawalt BD, Paulsen CA, et al. Klinefelter's syndrome. Lancet 2000; 356(9226): 333–335.
2. Lanfranco F, Kamischke A, Zitzmann M, et al. Klinefelter's syndrome. Lancet 2004; 364(9430): 273–283.
3. Matsumoto AM. The testis. In: Felig P, Frohman LA, eds. Endocrinology and Metabolism. 4th Ed. New York, NY: McGraw-Hill, 2001:635–705.
4. Bhasin S, Storer TW, Asbel-Sethi N, et al. Effects of testosterone replacement with a nongenital, transdermal system, Androderm, in human immunodeficiency virus-infected men with low testosterone levels. J Clin Endocrinol Metab 1998; 83(9): 3155–3162.
5. Grinspoon S, Corcoran C, Askari H, et al. Effects of androgen administration in men with the AIDS wasting syndrome. A randomized, double-blind, placebo-controlled trial. Ann Intern Med 1998; 129(1): 18–26.

6. Grinspoon S, Corcoran C, Stanley T, et al. Effects of hypogonadism and testosterone administration on depression indices in HIV-infected men. J Clin Endocrinol Metab 2000; 85(1): 60–65.

7. Handelsman DJ, Liu PY. Androgen therapy in chronic renal failure. Baillieres Clin Endocrinol Metab 1998; 12(3):485–500.

8. Matsumoto AM. Andropause: clinical implications of the decline in serum testosterone levels with aging in men. J Gerontol A Biol Sci Med Sci 2002; 57(2): M76–M99.

9. Reid IR, Wattie DJ, Evans MC, et al. Testosterone therapy in glucocorticoid-treated men. Arch Intern Med 1996; 156(11):1173–1177.

10. Crawford BA, Liu PY, Kean MT, et al. Randomized placebo-controlled trial of androgen effects on muscle and bone in men requiring long-term systemic glucocorticoid treatment. J Clin Endocrinol Metab 2003; 88(7):3167–3176.

11. Bhasin S, Cunningham GR, Hayes FJ, et al. Testosterone therapy in adult men with androgen deficiency syndromes: an Endocrine Society clinical practice guideline. J Clin Endocrinol Metab 2006; 91(6): 1995–2010.

12. Matsumoto AM. Clinical use and abuse of androgens and antiandrogens. In Becker KL, ed. Principles and Practice of Endocrinology and Metabolism. 3rd Ed. Philadelphia, PA: Lippincott Williams & Wilkins, 2001: 1181–1200.

13. Bhasin S, Storer TW, Berman N, et al. The effects of supraphysiologic doses of testosterone on muscle size and strength in normal men. N Engl J Med 1996; 335(1):1–7.

14. Bhasin S, Woodhouse L, Casaburi R, et al. Testosterone dose-response relationships in healthy young men. Am J Physiol Endocrinol Metab 2001; 281(6): E1172-E1181.

15. Bhasin S, Woodhouse L, Casaburi R, et al. Old men are as responsive as young men to the anabolic effects of graded doses of testosterone on skeletal muscle. J Clin Endocrinol Metab 2004; 90(2):678–688.

16. Buena F, Swerdloff RS, Steiner BS, et al. Sexual function does not change when serum testosterone levels are pharmacologically varied within the normal male range. Fertil Steril 1993; 59(5):1118–1123.

17. Singh AB, Hsia S, Alaupovic P, et al. The effects of varying doses of T on insulin sensitivity, plasma lipids, apolipoproteins, and C-reactive protein in healthy young men. J Clin Endocrinol Metab 2002; 87(1): 136–143.

18. Bremner WJ, Vitiello MV, Prinz PN. Loss of circadian rhythmicity in blood testosterone levels with aging in normal men. J Clin Endocrinol Metab 1983; 56(6): 1278–1281.

19. Taieb J, Mathian B, Millot F, et al. Testosterone measured by 10 immunoassays and by isotope-dilution gas chromatography-mass spectrometry in sera from 116 men, women, and children. Clin Chem 2003; 49(8): 1381–1395.

20. Wang C, Catlin DH, Demers LM, et al. Measurement of total serum testosterone in adult men: comparison of current laboratory methods versus liquid chromatography-tandem mass spectrometry. J Clin Endocrinol Metab 2004; 89(2):534–543.

21. Vermeulen A, Verdonck L, Kaufman JM. A critical evaluation of simple methods for the estimation of free testosterone in serum. J Clin Endocrinol Metab 1999; 84(10):3666–3672.

22. Winters SJ, Kelley DE, Goodpaster B. The analog free testosterone assay: are the results in men clinically useful? Clin Chem 1998; 44(10):2178–2182.

23. Spratt DI, O'Dea LS, Schoenfeld D, et al. Neuroendocrine-gonadal axis in men: frequent sampling of LH, FSH, and testosterone. Am J Physiol 1988; 254(5 Pt 1):E658-E666.

24. Wang C, Swerdloff RS, Iranmanesh A, et al. Transdermal testosterone gel improves sexual function, mood, muscle strength, and body composition parameters in hypogonadal men. Testosterone Gel Study Group. J Clin Endocrinol Metab 2000; 85(8): 2839–2853.

25. Nankin HR. Hormone kinetics after intramuscular testosterone cypionate. Fertil Steril 1987; 47(6): 1004–1009.

26. Snyder PJ, Lawrence DA. Treatment of male hypogonadism with testosterone enanthate. J Clin Endocrinol Metab 1980; 51(6):1335–1339.

27. Gooren LJ. A ten-year safety study of the oral androgen testosterone undecanoate. J Androl 1994; 15(3): 212–215.

28. Wang C, Alexander G, Berman N, et al. Testosterone replacement therapy improves mood in hypogonadal men—a clinical research center study. J Clin Endocrinol Metab 1996; 81(10):3578–3583.

29. Wang C, Eyre DR, Clark R, et al. Sublingual testosterone replacement improves muscle mass and strength, decreases bone resorption, and increases bone formation markers in hypogonadal men—a clinical research center study. J Clin Endocrinol Metab 1996; 81(10): 3654–3662.

30. Dobs AS, Meikle AW, Arver S, et al. Pharmacokinetics, efficacy, and safety of a permeation-enhanced testosterone transdermal system in comparison with bi-weekly injections of testosterone enanthate for the treatment of hypogonadal men. J Clin Endocrinol Metab 1999; 84(10):3469–3478.

31. De Luca F, Argente J, Cavallo L, et al. Management of puberty in constitutional delay of growth and puberty. J Pediatr Endocrinol Metab 2001; 14(suppl 2): 953–957.

32. Houchin LD, Rogol AD. Androgen replacement in children with constitutional delay of puberty: the case for aggressive therapy. Baillieres Clin Endocrinol Metab 1998; 12(3):427–440.

33. Soliman AT, Khadir MM, Asfour M. Testosterone treatment in adolescent boys with constitutional delay of growth and development. Metabolism 1995; 44(8): 1013–1015.

34. Amory JK, Matsumoto AM. The therapeutic potential of testosterone patches. Expert Opin Invest Drugs 1998; 7(12):1977–1988.

35. Qoubaitary A, Swerdloff RS, Wang C. Advances in male hormone substitution therapy. Expert Opin Pharmacother 2004; 6(9):1493–1506.

36. Cunningham GR, Cordero E, Thornby JI. Testosterone replacement with transdermal therapeutic systems. Physiological serum testosterone and elevated dihy-

drotestosterone levels. JAMA 1989; 261(17): 2525–2530.

37. Findlay JC, Place V, Snyder PJ. Treatment of primary hypogonadism in men by the transdermal administration of testosterone. J Clin Endocrinol Metab 1989; 68(2):369–373.

38. Findlay JC, Place VA, Snyder PJ. Transdermal delivery of testosterone. J Clin Endocrinol Metab 1987; 64(2): 266–268.

39. Behre HM, von Eckardstein S, Kliesch S, et al. Long-term substitution therapy of hypogonadal men with transscrotal testosterone over 7–10 years. Clin Endocrinol (Oxf) 1999; 50(5):629–635.

40. Snyder PJ, Peachey H, Hannoush P, et al. Effect of testosterone treatment on bone mineral density in men over 65 years of age. J Clin Endocrinol Metab 1999; 84(6):1966–1972.

41. Snyder PJ, Peachey H, Hannoush P, et al. Effect of testosterone treatment on body composition and muscle strength in men over 65 years of age. J Clin Endocrinol Metab 1999; 84(8):2647–2653.

42. de Lignieres B. Transdermal dihydrotestosterone treatment of 'andropause'. Ann Med 1993; 25(3):235–241.

43. Kunelius P, Lukkarinen O, Hannuksela ML, et al. The effects of transdermal dihydrotestosterone in the aging male: a prospective, randomized, double blind study. J Clin Endocrinol Metab 2002; 87(4):1467–1472.

44. Ly LP, Jimenez M, Zhuang TN, et al. A double-blind, placebo-controlled, randomized clinical trial of transdermal dihydrotestosterone gel on muscular strength, mobility, and quality of life in older men with partial androgen deficiency. J Clin Endocrinol Metab 2001; 86(9): 4078–4088.

45. Meikle AW, Arver S, Dobs AS, et al. Pharmacokinetics and metabolism of a permeation-enhanced testosterone transdermal system in hypogonadal men: influence of application site—a clinical research center study. J Clin Endocrinol Metab 1996; 81(5): 1832–1840.

46. Meikle AW, Mazer NA, Moellmer JF, et al. Enhanced transdermal delivery of testosterone across nonscrotal skin produces physiological concentrations of testosterone and its metabolites in hypogonadal men. J Clin Endocrinol Metab 1992; 74(3):623–628.

47. Arver S, Dobs AS, Meikle AW, et al. Long-term efficacy and safety of a permeation-enhanced testosterone transdermal system in hypogonadal men. Clin Endocrinol (Oxf) 1997; 47(6):727–737.

48. Kenny AM, Bellantonio S, Gruman CA, et al. Effects of transdermal testosterone on cognitive function and health perception in older men with low bioavailable testosterone levels. J Gerontol A Biol Sci Med Sci 2002; 57(5):M321-M325.

49. Kenny AM, Prestwood KM, Gruman CA, et al. Effects of transdermal testosterone on bone and muscle in older men with low bioavailable testosterone levels. J Gerontol A Biol Sci Med Sci 2001; 56(5): M266-M272.

50. Brocks DR, Meikle AW, Boike SC, et al. Pharmacokinetics of testosterone in hypogonadal men after transdermal delivery: influence of dose. J Clin Pharmacol 1996; 36(8):732–739.

51. Bennett NJ. A burn-like lesion caused by a testosterone transdermal system. Burns 1998; 24(5):478–480.

52. Jordan WP Jr. Allergy and topical irritation associated with transdermal testosterone administration: a comparison of scrotal and nonscrotal transdermal systems. Am J Contact Dermat 1997; 8(2):108–113.

53. Parker S, Armitage M. Experience with transdermal testosterone replacement therapy for hypogonadal men. Clin Endocrinol (Oxf) 1999; 50(1):57–62.

54. Wilson DE, Kaidbey K, Boike SC, et al. Use of topical corticosteroid pretreatment to reduce the incidence and severity of skin reactions associated with testosterone transdermal therapy. Clin Ther 1998; 20(2): 299–306.

55. Singh AB, Norris K, Modi N, et al. Pharmacokinetics of a transdermal testosterone system in men with end stage renal disease receiving maintenance hemodialysis and healthy hypogonadal men. J Clin Endocrinol Metab 2001; 86(6):2437–2445.

56. Yu Z, Gupta SK, Hwang SS, et al. Transdermal testosterone administration in hypogonadal men: comparison of pharmacokinetics at different sites of application and at the first and fifth days of application. J Clin Pharmacol 1997; 37(12):1129–1138.

57. Yu Z, Gupta SK, Hwang SS, et al. Testosterone pharmacokinetics after application of an investigational transdermal system in hypogonadal men. J Clin Pharmacol 1997; 37(12):1139–1145.

58. Jordan WP Jr, Atkinson LE, Lai C. Comparison of the skin irritation potential of two testosterone transdermal systems: an investigational system and a marketed product. Clin Ther 1998; 20(1):80–87.

59. Swerdloff RS, Wang C, Cunningham G, et al. Long-term pharmacokinetics of transdermal testosterone gel in hypogonadal men. J Clin Endocrinol Metab 2000; 85(12):4500–4510.

60. Wang C, Swerdloff RS, Iranmanesh A, et al. Effects of transdermal testosterone gel on bone turnover markers and bone mineral density in hypogonadal men. Clin Endocrinol (Oxf) 2001; 54(6):739–750.

61. Wang C, Cunningham G, Dobs A, et al. Long-term testosterone gel (AndroGel) treatment maintains beneficial effects on sexual function and mood, lean and fat mass, and bone mineral density in hypogonadal men. J Clin Endocrinol Metab 2004; 89(5):2085–2098.

62. McNicholas TA, Dean JD, Mulder H, et al. A novel testosterone gel formulation normalizes androgen levels in hypogonadal men, with improvements in body composition and sexual function. BJU Int 2003; 91(1):69–74.

63. Steidle C, Schwartz S, Jacoby K, et al. AA2500 testosterone gel normalizes androgen levels in aging males with improvements in body composition and sexual function. J Clin Endocrinol Metab 2003; 88(6): 2673–2681.

64. Marbury T, Hamill E, Bachand R, et al. Evaluation of the pharmacokinetic profiles of the new testosterone topical gel formulation, Testim, compared to AndroGel. Biopharm Drug Dispos 2003; 24(3):115–120.

65. Handelsman DJ, Conway AJ, Boylan LM. Pharmacokinetics and pharmacodynamics of testosterone pellets in man. J Clin Endocrinol Metab 1990; 71(1):216–222.

66. Wang C, Swerdloff R, Kipnes M, et al. New testosterone buccal system (Striant) delivers physiological

testosterone levels: pharmacokinetics study in hypogonadal men. J Clin Endocrinol Metab 2004; 89(8): 3821–3829.

67. Handelsman DJ, Mackey MA, Howe C, et al. An analysis of testosterone implants for androgen replacement therapy. Clin Endocrinol (Oxf) 1997; 47(3): 311–316.

68. Jockenhovel F, Vogel E, Kreutzer M, et al. Pharmacokinetics and pharmacodynamics of subcutaneous testosterone implants in hypogonadal men. Clin Endocrinol (Oxf) 1996; 45(1):61–71.

69. Liu PY, Wishart SM, Handelsman DJ. A double-blind, placebo-controlled, randomized clinical trial of recombinant human chorionic gonadotropin on muscle strength and physical function and activity in older men with partial age-related androgen deficiency. J Clin Endocrinol Metab 2002; 87(7):3125–3135.

70. Skakkebaek NE, Bancroft J, Davidson DW, et al. Androgen replacement with oral testosterone undecanoate in hypogonadal men: a double blind controlled study. Clin Endocrinol (Oxf) 1981; 14(1): 49–61.

71. Bagchus WM, Hust R, Maris F, et al. Important effect of food on the bioavailability of oral testosterone undecanoate. Pharmacotherapy 2003; 23(3):319–325.

72. Houwing NS, Maris F, Schnabel PG, et al. Pharmacokinetic study in women of three different doses of a new formulation of oral testosterone undecanoate, Andriol Testocaps. Pharmacotherapy 2003; 23(10):1257–1265.

73. Salehian B, Wang C, Alexander G, et al. Pharmacokinetics, bioefficacy, and safety of sublingual testosterone cyclodextrin in hypogonadal men: comparison to testosterone enanthate—a clinical research center study. J Clin Endocrinol Metab 1995; 80(12):3567–3575.

74. Baisley KJ, Boyce MJ, Bukofzer S, et al. Pharmacokinetics, safety and tolerability of three dosage regimens of buccal adhesive testosterone tablets in healthy men suppressed with leuprorelin. J Endocrinol 2002; 175(3):813–819.

75. Rolf C, Gottschalk I, Behre HM, et al. Pharmacokinetics of new testosterone transdermal therapeutic systems in gonadotropin-releasing hormone antagonist-suppressed normal men. Exp Clin Endocrinol Diabetes 1999; 107(1):63–69.

76. Wang C, Iranmanesh A, Berman N, et al. Comparative pharmacokinetics of three doses of percutaneous dihydrotestosterone gel in healthy elderly men—a clinical research center study. J Clin Endocrinol Metab 1998; 83(8):2749–2757.

77. Swerdloff RS, Wang C. Dihydrotestosterone: a rationale for its use as a non-aromatizable androgen replacement therapeutic agent. Baillieres Clin Endocrinol Metab 1998; 12(3):501–506.

78. Nieschlag E, Buchter D, Von Eckardstein S, et al. Repeated intramuscular injections of testosterone undecanoate for substitution therapy in hypogonadal men. Clin Endocrinol (Oxf) 1999; 51(6):757–763.

79. Zhang GY, Gu YQ, Wang XH, et al. A pharmacokinetic study of injectable testosterone undecanoate in hypogonadal men. J Androl 1998; 19(6):761–768.

80. von Eckardstein S, Nieschlag E. Treatment of male hypogonadism with testosterone undecanoate injected at extended intervals of 12 weeks: a phase II study. J Androl 2002; 23(3):419–425.

81. Behre HM, Nieschlag E. Testosterone buciclate (20 Aet-1) in hypogonadal men: pharmacokinetics and pharmacodynamics of the new long-acting androgen ester. J Clin Endocrinol Metab 1992; 75(5):1204–1210.

82. Amory JK, Anawalt BD, Blaskovich PD, et al. Testosterone release from a subcutaneous, biodegradable microcapsule formulation (Viatrel) in hypogonadal men. J Androl 2002; 23(1):84–91.

83. Bhasin S, Swerdloff RS, Steiner B, et al. A biodegradable testosterone microcapsule formulation provides uniform eugonadal levels of testosterone for 10–11 weeks in hypogonadal men. J Clin Endocrinol Metab 1992; 74(1):75–83.

84. Roy AK, Tyagi RK, Song CS, et al. Androgen receptor: structural domains and functional dynamics after ligand-receptor interaction. Ann N Y Acad Sci 2001; 949:44–57.

85. Negro-Vilar A, Jordan WP Jr. Selective androgen receptor modulators (SARMs): a novel approach to androgen therapy for the new millennium. J Clin Endocrinol Metab 1999; 84(10):3459–3462.

86. Segal S, Narayanan R, Dalton JT. Therapeutic potential of the SARMs: revisiting the androgen receptor for drug delivery. Expert Opin Investig Drugs 2006; 15(4): 377–387.

87. Sundaram K, Kumar N. 7alpha-methyl-19-nortestosterone (MENT): the optimal androgen for male contraception and replacement therapy. Int J Androl 2000; 23(suppl 2):13–15.

88. Cummings DE, Kumar N, Bardin CW, et al. Prostate-sparing effects in primates of the potent androgen 7alpha-methyl-19-nortestosterone: a potential alternative to testosterone for androgen replacement and male contraception. J Clin Endocrinol Metab 1998; 83(12):4212–4219.

89. Anderson RA, Martin CW, Kung AW, et al. 7Alpha-methyl-19-nortestosterone maintains sexual behavior and mood in hypogonadal men. J Clin Endocrinol Metab 1999; 84(10):3556–3562.

90. Anderson RA, Wallace AM, Sattar N, et al. Evidence for tissue selectivity of the synthetic androgen 7 alpha-methyl-19-nortestosterone in hypogonadal men. J Clin Endocrinol Metab 2003; 88(6):2784–2793.

91. Bhasin S, Bremner WJ. Clinical review 85: emerging issues in androgen replacement therapy. J Clin Endocrinol Metab 1997; 82(1):3–8.

92. Behre HM, Bohmeyer J, Nieschlag E. Prostate volume in testosterone-treated and untreated hypogonadal men in comparison to age-matched normal controls. Clin Endocrinol (Oxf) 1994; 40(3):341–349.

93. Jin B, Conway AJ, Handelsman DJ. Effects of androgen deficiency and replacement on prostate zonal volumes. Clin Endocrinol (Oxf) 2001; 54(4):437–445.

94. Jackson JA, Waxman J, Spiekerman AM, et al. Prostatic complications of testosterone replacement therapy. Arch Intern Med 1989; 149(10):2365–2366.

95. Bhasin S, Singh AB, Mac RP, et al. Managing the risks of prostate disease during testosterone replacement therapy in older men: recommendations for a standardized monitoring plan. J Androl 2003; 24(3): 299–311.

96. Rhoden EL, Morgentaler A. Risks of testosterone-replacement therapy and recommendations for monitoring. N Engl J Med 2004; 350(5):482–492.

97. Amory JK, Watts NB, Easley KA, et al. Exogenous testosterone or testosterone with finasteride increases bone mineral density in older men with low serum testosterone. J Clin Endocrinol Metab 2004; 89(2): 503–510.

98. Gruenewald DA, Matsumoto AM. Testosterone supplementation therapy for older men: potential benefits and risks. Am J Geriatr Soc 2003; 51(1): 101–115.

99. Bhasin S, Buckwalter JG. Testosterone supplementation in older men: a rational idea whose time has not yet come. J Androl 2001; 22(5):718–731.

100. Calof OM, Singh AB, Lee ML, et al. Adverse effects associated with testosterone replacement in middle-aged and older men: a meta-analysis of randomized, placebo-controlled trials. J Gerontol Biol Sci Med Sci 2005; 60(11):1451–1457.

101. Swerdloff RS, Blackman MR, Cunningham GR, et al. Summary of the Consensus Session from the 1st Annual Andropause Consensus 2000 Meeting. Bethesda, MD: The Endocrine Society, 2000:1–6.

102. Shahidi NT. Androgens and erythropoiesis. N Engl J Med 1973; 289(2):72–80.

103. Matsumoto AM, Sandblom RE, Schoene RB, et al. Testosterone replacement in hypogonadal men: effects on obstructive sleep apnoea, respiratory drives, and sleep. Clin Endocrinol (Oxf) 1985; 22(6):713–721.

104. Schneider BK, Pickett CK, Zwillich CW, et al. Influence of testosterone on breathing during sleep. J Appl Physiol 1986; 61(2):618–623.

105. Liu PY, Yee B, Wishart SM, et al. The short-term effects of high-dose testosterone on sleep, breathing, and function in older men. J Clin Endocrinol Metab 2003; 88(8):3605–3613.

106. Bagatell CJ, Bremner WJ. Androgen and progestagen effects on plasma lipids. Prog Cardiovasc Dis 1995; 38(3):255–271.

107. Bagatell CJ, Knopp RH, Vale WW, et al. Physiologic testosterone levels in normal men suppress high-density lipoprotein cholesterol levels. Ann Intern Med 1992; 116(12 Pt 1):967–973.

108. Jockenhovel F, Bullmann C, Schubert M, et al. Influence of various modes of androgen substitution on serum lipids and lipoproteins in hypogonadal men. Metabolism 1999; 48(5):590–596.

109. Whitsel EA, Boyko EJ, Matsumoto AM, et al. Intra-muscular testosterone esters and plasma lipids in hypogonadal men: a meta-analysis. Am J Med 2001; 111(4):261–269.

110. Alexandersen P, Haarbo J, Christiansen C. The relationship of natural androgens to coronary heart disease in males: a review. Atherosclerosis 1996; 125(1):1–13.

111. Phillips GB, Pinkernell BH, Jing TY. The association of hypotestosteronemia with coronary artery disease in men. Arterioscler Thromb 1994; 14(5): 701–706.

112. English KM, Steeds RP, Jones TH, et al. Low-dose transdermal testosterone therapy improves angina threshold in men with chronic stable angina: a randomized, double-blind, placebo-controlled study. Circulation 2000; 102(16):1906–1911.

113. Jaffe MD. Effect of testosterone cypionate on postexercise ST segment depression. Br Heart J 1977; 39(11): 1217–1222.

114. Rosano GM, Leonardo F, Pagnotta P, et al. Acute anti-ischemic effect of testosterone in men with coronary artery disease. Circulation 1999; 99(13):1666–1670.

115. Sigler LH, Tulgan J. Treatment of angina pectoris by testosterone propionate. N Y State J Med 1943; 43: 1424–1428.

116. Webb CM, Adamson DL, de Zeigler D, et al. Effect of acute testosterone on myocardial ischemia in men with coronary artery disease. Am J Cardiol 1999; 83(3):437–439, A439.

117. Webb CM, McNeill JG, Hayward CS, et al. Effects of testosterone on coronary vasomotor regulation in men with coronary heart disease. Circulation 1999; 100(16):1690–1696.

118. Wu SZ, Weng XZ. Therapeutic effects of an androgenic preparation on myocardial ischemia and cardiac function in 62 elderly male coronary heart disease patients. Chin Med J (Engl) 1993; 106(6):415–418.

119. Anderson RA, Bancroft J, Wu FC. The effects of exogenous testosterone on sexuality and mood of normal men. J Clin Endocrinol Metab 1992; 75(6): 1503–1507.

120. Tricker R, Casaburi R, Storer TW, et al. The effects of supraphysiological doses of testosterone on angry behavior in healthy eugonadal men—a clinical research center study. J Clin Endocrinol Metab 1996; 81(10):3754–3758.

36

Treatment of Erectile Dysfunction in Men with Heart Disease

Graham Jackson
Cardiothoracic Centre, St. Thomas' Hospital, London, England, U.K.

□ INTRODUCTION

Erectile dysfunction (ED) is common, affecting 52% of men aged 40 to 70 years and 75% of men over 65 years of age (1), with the prevalence predicted to rise to 322 million by the year 2025, presumably reflecting an aging population (2). Regarding ED as an inevitable part of the natural aging process, however, overlooks the fact that vascular disease increases in frequency with age, and vascular disease shares the same risk factors as ED (3). Similarly, blaming ED on increasing prostatic problems with age also fails to take into account the increased likelihood of vascular disease in the population vulnerable to prostatic disease.

Both vascular disease and diabetes are now recognized to be causes of ED in as many as 70% of organic cases (4). These findings have shifted the emphasis away from a purely urological management of ED, giving clinicians the opportunity to consider ED as an integral part of their cardiovascular risk assessment (3). Thus, within the context of a multidisciplinary approach, cardiologists must play an important role in the management of ED—not only because ED is common in cardiac patients but also because ED in the otherwise cardiovascularly asymptomatic male may, in fact, be an early marker of occult vascular disorder, in particular, coronary disease (5).

□ ED AND CARDIOVASCULAR RISK FACTORS
Endothelial Dysfunction

Endothelial dysfunction is a common denominator in erectile dysfunction (Fig. 1) (6). For normal vasodilatation to occur in the blood vessels that supply the penis, the endothelium must be intact and functioning normally. Once believed to be an inert monolayer of cells simply lining blood vessels, the endothelium is now recognized as having a primary role in the local regulation of vessel function and vascular homeostasis. Endothelial dysfunction is defined as an abnormal endothelial response that leads to a reduction in the bioavailability of nitric oxide (NO) and subsequently impaired vasodilatation. It has been found to be associated with several disorders of the cardiovascular system, including diabetes, hypertension, hyperlipidemia, heart failure, and cigarette smoking. The vascular endothelium acts as a "plasma-tissue barrier" and has a crucial role in controlling vascular function, with the balance between endothelium-derived vasodilators and vasoconstrictors determining vascular tone and the pathophysiologic consequences (7). In addition, the reduction in NO bioavailability can adversely affect platelet aggregation and promote vascular wall inflammation and smooth-muscle cell proliferation.

The clinical consequences of endothelial dysfunction include the development of atherosclerosis, acute coronary syndromes, cardiac failure, and erectile dysfunction. It is now recognized that a defect in the NO-cyclic guanosine 3'5'-monophosphate system in smooth-muscle cells is an early marker of systemic vascular abnormalities before the development of overt cardiovascular disease in men with erectile dysfunction (6).

Measures of endothelial dysfunction have been shown to be improved by drugs that benefit cardiovascular morbidity and mortality (e.g., angiotensin-converting enzyme inhibitors in cardiac failure; statin and angiotensin-converting enzyme inhibitors in ischemic heart disease) and by drugs used in the treatment of erectile dysfunction, heart failure, and diabetes [e.g., phosphodiesterase type 5 (PDE5) inhibitors] (7). Over the past decade, as the direct relationship of erectile dysfunction and endothelial dysfunction has become elucidated, it has become similarly apparent that erectile dysfunction may be treated with PDE5 inhibitors, which improve endothelial dysfunction by acting within the smooth-muscle cell (8).

Due to the large number of clinical conditions that are clearly related to endothelial dysfunction, it has become increasingly important to develop and validate the means of its evaluation as well as to determine whether improving endothelial dysfunction may in turn improve the long-term clinical outcome of conditions such as diabetes and cardiac failure. For further information on vascular dysfunction, see Chapter 25.

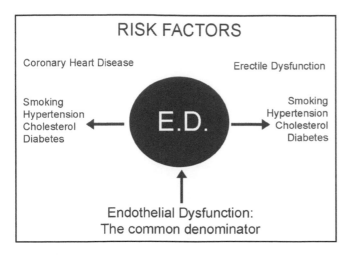

Figure 1   Endothelial dysfunction as the common denominator for erectile dysfunction and vascular disease. *Source*: From Ref. 6.

Cardiovascular Risk Factors

The shared risk factors between ED and vascular disease include smoking, hyperlipidemia, diabetes, hypertension, obesity, and a sedentary lifestyle. Endothelial dysfunction may affect all vascular beds, predisposing the patient to widespread atherosclerosis; thus, the close link between ED and vascular disease is readily explained.

In the Massachusetts Male Aging Study (MMAS) involving a large population-based random sample of 1290 healthy men aged 40 to 70 years, the age-adjusted probability of complete ED was 15% in treated hypertensives compared to 9.6% of the whole population (1). In another study, ED was reported in 17% of men with untreated hypertension in comparison with 25% of men who were receiving current antihypertensive treatment (9).

In the MMAS, smoking doubled the chance of ED developing over an eight-year follow-up period and increased the rate of occurrence from 15% to 20% in hypertensives. Smoking is well known as a risk factor for endothelial damage and vascular disease. Although cessation of smoking later in life may still be of some benefit to the 3- to 4-mm coronary arteries, it may be too late to reverse damage to the small (1–2 mm) penile arteries. Because the practice of smoking remains popular among young people who seem to ignore the heart and lung disease risks, perhaps focus should be placed on the reduction of midlife ED development.

Hyperlipidemia increases the risk of ED by 1.8 times, with a raised high-density lipoprotein (HDL) cholesterol level being protective (10). For every 1 mmol/L increase in cholesterol, there is an increase by a factor of 1.32 in the risk of developing ED. For every 1 mmol/L increase in HDL, there is a 0.38 risk factor decrease of ED. In contrast to what might be expected, lipid-lowering therapy does not benefit ED, and in some cases, can actually cause or exacerbate

ED—possibly due to a central action secondary to blood-brain barrier penetration (11).

Diabetics suffer from both endothelial and neurological ED, with ED prevalence recorded as high as 80% in those over 60 years of age (12). It is possible that early and vigorous glucose control might be preventative. In addition, the early use of statins and perhaps prophylactic PDE5 inhibitors as daily therapy theoretically could preserve endothelial function (13,14).

Given the shared risk factors, it is not surprising that ED is common in men with coronary artery disease (CAD) and increases in severity as the number of diseased coronary arteries increases. In the author's study of 132 men undergoing coronary angiography, the severity of the ED increased as the plaque burden increased, with 65% experiencing ED, 58% of whom developed ED before their cardiac symptoms (15). In a meta-analysis of four studies involving 1476 men with cardiovascular disease, the incidence of ED ranged from 39% to 64% (16).

In summary, one type of ED (endothelial dysfunction) develops as the result of damage from smoking, hypertension, diabetes, etc., which in turn causes the other type of ED (erectile dysfunction). The asymptomatic man should be evaluated for cardiac risk, and even the cardiac patient who does not complain of ED should be routinely asked about any sexual difficulties.

ED as a Marker of Occult CAD

In 2001, Kirby et al. posed the question: "Is erectile dysfunction a marker for cardiovascular disease?" (5). The short answer is, "Yes." The risk factors discussed above explain the common coexistence of cardiovascular disease and ED. In 1999, Pritzker presented a preliminary report entitled "The Penile Stress Test: A window to the hearts of man" (17). He reviewed the results of exercise stress testing, risk factor profiles, and, in selected cases, angiography in 50 men with ED, who had no cardiac symptoms or past history. Multiple cardiovascular risk factors were present in 80%, and of these men, exercise tests positive for ischemia were found in 28 of the 50 men. Coronary angiography was performed in 20 men and revealed left main stem or severe three-vessel disease in six men, moderate two-vessel disease in seven men, and significant single-vessel disease in seven men (Fig. 2). This study clearly showed the significant incidence of occult coronary disease in cardiologically asymptomatic men presenting with ED to a urological service. Others have reported similar findings and noted the occurrence of ED before cardiac symptoms developed (15). In a study comparing the velocity of cavernosal artery blood flow with the presence of ischemic heart disease in men with ED, a low peak systolic velocity (PSV) predicted the presence of CAD. A PSV below 35 cm/sec was associated with CAD in 41.9% of men and above 35 cm/sec in only 3.7% of men (18). This finding links to the theory presented by Montorsi

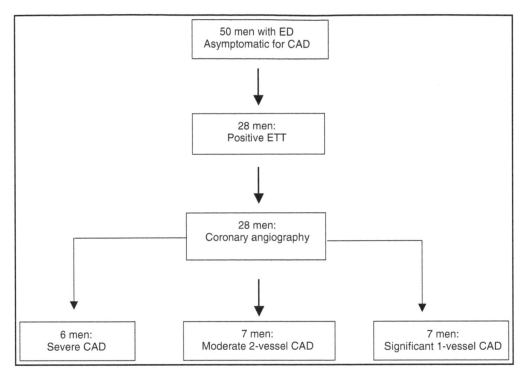

Figure 2 Silent coronary disease in men presenting with ED. *Abbreviations*: CAD, coronary artery disease; ED, erectile dysfunction; ETT, exercise tolerance test.

et al., relating symptomatic disease to artery diameter (Table 1) (19). The small size of the penile artery (1–2 mm), compared with the major coronary arteries (3–4 mm), carotid (5–8 mm) and femoral (6–8 mm) arteries, suggests that early disease in the penile vessels might have a greater impact on flow. The resulting ED may therefore represent an early manifestation of subclinical disease elsewhere.

In support of this concept, a series of 300 patients with acute chest pain and angiographically proven CAD were evaluated with a semistructured interview to assess their medical and sexual histories prior to presentation (20). The prevalence of ED among these patients was 49% ($n = 147$). In these 147 men with both ED and CAD, ED was experienced before CAD symptoms in 99 patients (67%). The mean time interval between the occurrence of ED and the occurrence of CAD was 38.8 months (range: 1–168 months).

Interestingly, all men with ED and type 1 diabetes developed sexual dysfunction before the onset of CAD symptoms. The authors do point out the absence of a control group with CAD and normal erections, but their findings clearly identify the need to assess cardiovascular risk in all males presenting with ED without obvious psychosexual etiology, especially in patients with diabetes.

Speel et al. evaluated 158 men aged 40 to 69 years with penile pharmacoduplex ultrasonography in order to determine whether there was cavernous arterial insufficiency and related these findings to the Framingham risk with the results extrapolated to the Dutch aging male population (21). Cavernous insufficiency identified a significantly increased risk of CAD in the group aged 50 to 59 years but not in the age groups of 40 to 49 years and 60 to 69 years. Overall, it was predicted that one in four men with ED aged 40 to 69 years and without known CAD would develop CAD over the next 12 years.

Roumeguére et al. compared 215 patients with ED and 100 patients without ED in order to evaluate undiagnosed hyperlipidemia and coronary risk (22). The prevalence of hypercholesterolemia was 70.6% versus 52% in the ED and non-ED groups ($p = 0.06$). Increased 10-year CAD risk was 56.6% versus 32.6% (ED vs. no ED; $p < 0.05$). Low HDL cholesterol and a high total cholesterol-to-HDL ratio, both established important risk markers for CAD, were identified as predictors of ED. This study suggested that ED might serve as a "sentinel event" for coronary heart disease.

Table 1 Artery Size and Atherothrombosis. A Significant Restriction to Flow in the Penile Arteries may be Subclinical in Larger Vessels

Artery	Diameter (mm)	Clinical Event
Penile	1–2	Erectile dysfunction
Coronary	3–4	Ischaemic heart disease
Carotid	5–7	TIA/Stroke
Femoral	6–8	Claudication

Abbreviation: TIA, transient ischemic attack.
Source: From Ref. 19.

Until clear-cut evidence is obtained from prospective trials that suggest the contrary, clinicians should be alert to the possibility of cardiovascular risk in men with no apparent cardiac symptoms other than ED (23). ED may provide an opportunity to evaluate other risk factors, including blood glucose, lipid profile, and blood pressure. Thus, ED is one of the many windows of opportunity that may serve to reduce the burden of cardiovascular disease (24).

☐ MANAGING ED IN THE CARDIAC PATIENT

Potential questions that patients may pose to a clinician include the following:

- Is sex safe?
- Can ED be safely treated?

Both these questions can be answered using statistical data available in the literature. It should be emphasized, however, that statistics can only provide a general guide, and clinical advice must always be tailored to the particular medical condition of the individual patient. Guidelines and clinical judgment should be complimentary tools and not mutually exclusive.

Is Sex Safe?

Using ambulatory heart rate and electrocardiogram (ECG) and blood pressure monitoring, cardiac responses during sex have been found to be no different from other daily physical activities such as driving to work, walking to the metro station, and climbing stairs (25). For couples in a long-standing relationship, the average peak heart rate during sex is between 110 and 130 beats/min, with peak systolic blood pressure between 150 and 180 mmHg. When expressed as the metabolic equivalent of energy expended in the resting state (METS), sexual intercourse is associated with a workload of 3 to 4 METS, peaking at orgasm. Younger couples who engage in more vigorous sexual activity may expend as many as 5 to 6 METS. The average duration of sex is 5 to 15 minutes, and the peak exercise period rarely extends beyond three minutes. Therefore, sex should not be considered a sustained or extreme cardiovascular stress, although there is the caveat that casual sex with a new partner may actually involve a greater cardiac workload because of greater excitement and lack of familiarity. An age discrepancy within the couple may lead to a mismatch of activity level and expectations. For further information on cardiac responses to sexual activity, see Chapter 7.

It should be emphasized that coital death is rare. In fact, frequent sexual activity is associated with longevity and regular physical exercise reduces sexually related cardiac events. Even though the sudden death rate during sex is a very small proportion of all sudden deaths (between 0.6% and 1.7%), in 75% of these cases, the deaths occurred during extramarital sex, and 95% of these occurred in men. The setting was invariably that of an older male and a younger female after having too much to eat and too much to drink (26,27).

In the clinic outpatient or family practice setting, simple practical guidelines can be constructed by equating the number of METS used during sex to other activities (Table 2). One of the most useful is the comparison with walking one mile (1.5 km) over flat terrain in 20 minutes or 15 minutes of walking plus two flights of stairs (28).

Patients, by the nature of their individuality, may not always be clear about their ability, and doubts exist about the advice needed. In these cases, exercise testing is useful. For middle-aged couples in a stable relationship, a sexual act is equivalent to three to four minutes of the Bruce treadmill protocol, which can provide important reassurance and help in advising not only on the safety of sex but also on the treatment of ED (28). If a man (or woman) can manage four minutes on the treadmill (5–6 METS allowing a safety margin) without significant ischemia, arrhythmia, or a fall in systolic blood pressure, sex will be safe; similarly, ED therapy for the male will be safe in these circumstances.

A useful study by Drory compared the cardiovascular response during sex using ambulatory ECGs versus a bicycle exercise test (26). One-third of men had ischemia during sex on the ambulatory ECG, and all had ST changes of ischemia on the exercise test. No patient had ischemia during sex if the exercise test was normal and all ischemic episodes during sex were associated with a rise in heart rate. This suggests the role of a proven heart rate–lowering anti-ischemic drug such as verapamil or diltiazem in reducing ischemia during sex as well as other physical activities.

Patients, who cannot exercise on a treadmill because of mobility problems such as arthritis, especially of the knees, can be evaluated using pharmacological stress testing and nuclear cardiology or echocardiography. A man who cannot fulfill the

Table 2 MET Equivalents—Comparing Sex to Other Activities

Daily activity	MET score rating
Sexual intercourse with established partner	
Lower range (normal)	2–3
Lower range orgasm	3–4
Upper range (vigorous activity)	5–6
Lifting and carrying objects (9–20 kg)	4–5
Walking one mile for 20 min on level ground	3–4
Golf	4–5
Gardening (digging)	3–5
DIY: wallpapering, etc.	4–5
Light housework, e.g., ironing, polishing	2–4
Heavy housework: e.g., making beds, scrubbing floors, cleaning windows	3–6

Abbreviations: DIY, do-it-yourself; MET, metabolic equivalent of energy.

criteria for safe cardiovascular sex should be evaluated further by angiography in order to consider percutaneous or surgical intervention. Significantly symptomatic patients should have all the options available to remove their limitations with a full discussion of risk and benefit.

Sexual activity does pose a small but definite risk of a cardiac event, usually a myocardial infarction, rather than a life-threatening arrhythmia. Less than 1% of myocardial infarctions occur during sex, but although there is a slightly increased (2.5 times) risk for the two hours after sex, the absolute risk is low. Two large studies from the United States and Sweden show similar degrees of risk, with the same relative risk for those with a previous cardiac history and no increased risk for the physically fit (0.7) compared to the sedentary (4.4) (29,30). The potential benefit of being able to engage in safer sex from a cardiac standpoint presents yet another good reason for maintaining a healthy, active lifestyle.

Based on the Framingham estimates of a 1% annual absolute risk of a myocardial infarction in a 50-year-old, nonsmoking man without diabetes, weekly sex increases the annual absolute risk to 1.01% in men without a previous cardiac history and to 1.1% in those with a previous cardiac history. Since previous plaque rupture is invariably the mechanism, this reemphasizes the fact that lifestyle changes to reduce cardiovascular risk will also reduce the risk during sex.

Can ED Be Safely Treated?

There is no evidence that treating ED increases cardiac risk providing that the patient is properly assessed and the couple appropriately counselled (28). Often, men will seek medical advice without their partners, but couples therapy should be strongly encouraged. It should be emphasized that the treatment of ED is only one component of maintaining a healthy sexual life, and that advice and support are just as essential to the patient's overall sexual management.

There are guidelines for the advisement and treatment of cardiovascular patients presenting with ED. In the author's Male Cardiovascular Sexual Health Clinic, 370 men with ED were assessed using the British Consensus (28), and 80% were found to fall into the low-risk category (Table 3). Men in the intermediate- and high-risk groups, however, should not be denied advice, but should also be offered a full cardiac evaluation in order to reduce their risk and allow sexual activity to resume safely.

Drug Therapy
PDE5 Inhibitors

Sildenafil has transformed the management of ED substantially since its introduction. It inhibits PDE5 degradation of cGMP, the most active vasodilating agent within the cavernous tissues of the penis, promoting blood flow into the penis and thus restoring erectile function. Vardenafil and tadalafil are newer PDE5 inhibitors with similar effects. Hemodynamically, PDE5 inhibitors have mild nitrate-like actions (sildenafil was originally intended to be a drug for mild angina). Because PDE5 is present in smooth-muscle cells throughout the vasculature and the NO/cGMP pathway is involved in the regulation of blood pressure, PDE5 inhibitors have a modest hypotensive action. In healthy subjects, a single dose of 100 mg sildenafil transiently

Table 3 Management Guide According to Graded Cardiac Risk

Grading or risk	Cardiovascular status upon presentation	ED management recommendations
Low risk	Controlled hypertension Asymptomatic ≤ 3 risk factors for CAD—excluding age and gender Mild valvular disease Minimal/mild stable angina Post successful revascularization CHF (I)	Manage within the primary care setting Review treatment options with patient and his partner (where possible)
Intermediate risk	Recent MI or CVA (i.e., within last 6 wks) LVD/CHF (II) Murmur of unknown cause Moderate stable angina Heart transplant Recurrent TIAs Asymptomatic but > 3 risk factors for CAD—excluding age and gender	Specialized evaluation recommended (e.g., exercise test for angina and echo for murmur) Patient to be placed in high- or low-risk category, depending upon outcome of testing ED treatment can be initiated with exercise testing recommended to stratify risk
High risk	Severe or unstable or refractory angina Uncontrolled hypertension (SBP > 180 mmHg) CHF (III, IV) High-risk arrhythmias Hypertrophic cardiomyopathy Moderate/severe valve disease	Refer for specialized cardiac evaluation and management Treatment for ED to be deferred until cardiac condition is established and/or specialist evaluation completed

Abbreviations: CAD, coronary artery disease; CHF, congestive heart failure defined with NYHC stages I–IV; CVA, cerebral vascular accident; ED, erectile dysfunction; LVD, left ventricular dysfunction; MI, myocardial infarction; SBP, systolic blood pressure; TIA, transient ischemic attack.

lowered blood pressure by an average of 8.5/5.5 mm Hg, with a return to baseline six hours post dose. There was no effect on heart rate (31).

NO is an important neurotransmitter throughout the vasculature in that it is involved in the regulation of vascular smooth-muscle relaxation. It should be noted that a clinically important synergistic interaction could occur with the administration of oral and sublingual nitrates, which can result in a profound fall in blood pressure. The mechanism involves the increase of cGMP formation by activating guanylate cyclase and PDE5 inhibition, thus decreasing cGMP breakdown by inhibiting PDE5 (32). Concomitant administration of PDE5 inhibitors and nitrates is contraindicated, and this recommendation also extends to other NO donors such as nicorandil. Clinical guidelines regarding the timing of nitrate use post PDE5-inhibitor administration and/or the initiation of a PDE5 inhibitor after cessation of oral or sublingual nitrates are not available, but recent studies are helpful. In a study involving healthy volunteers, administration of 100 mg dosage of sildenafil did not react with sublingual nitrates given six hours post use due to the drug's short half-life (see below). Even tadalafil, with its long half-life, did not react at 48 hours. No data are yet available for vardenafil, but because its half-life is similar to that of sildenafil, a similar result is to be expected. Oral nitrates are not prognostically important drugs; so, their use can be discontinued and, if needed, alternative agents substituted. After oral nitrate cessation, and provided there has been no clinical deterioration, PDE5 inhibitors can be used safely. It is recommended that the time interval prior to PDE5 inhibitor use is five half-lives, which is the equivalent of five days for the most popular once-daily oral nitrate agents.

When comparing the three PDE5 inhibitors, clinically relevant differences are detected in PDE half-life. Tadalafil has a half-life of 17.5 hours, with a period of responsiveness of 36 hours or longer, whereas sildenafil and vardenafil have durations of action of four to six hours. Onset of action following sexual stimulation is approximately 30 minutes, with maximal effect achieved at one hour with sildenafil and vardenafil, and one to two hours with tadalafil. Although tadalafil's absorption is not influenced by food, sildenafil and vardenafil are affected by a fatty meal due to delayed gastric emptying, and thus are more effective if taken at least two hours have elapsed after food intake.

Sildenafil was the first oral PDE5 inhibitor treatment for ED, and it has been the most extensively evaluated. Overall success rates in cardiac patients of 80% and above have been recorded, with no evidence of tolerance (decreasing effect over time). Diabetic patients with more complex and extensive pathophysiology have an average success rate of 60% with or without additional risk factors. To date, the use of sildenafil is not associated with any excess risk of myocardial infarction, stroke, or mortality in randomized trials or open label and outpatient monitoring studies.

In patients with stable angina, there is no evidence of an ischemic effect due to coronary steal. In one large exercise study, compared with double-blind placebo, 100 mg of sildenafil increased exercise time and diminished ischemia (33). A study of hemodynamic effects in men with severe CAD identified no adverse cardiovascular effects and a potentially beneficial effect on coronary blood flow reserve (31). Studies in diabetic and nondiabetic patients have demonstrated improved endothelial function both acutely and after chronic oral dosing, which may have implications beyond the treatment of ED (14). Hypertensive patients on monotherapy or multiple therapies have experienced no increase in adverse events, with the exception of patients on doxazosin, a nonselective α-blocker. Occasional postural effects have occurred when sildenafil was taken within four hours of doxazosin 4 mg; so, an advisory to avoid this time interval is now in place. Sildenafil has also been proven effective in heart failure patients who were deemed suitable for ED therapy. The incidence of ED in heart failure subjects is 80%; so, this finding is of major clinical importance. Sildenafil dose is on average 50 mg, with 25 mg advised initially in patients older than 80 years, owing to delayed excretion. The 100 mg dose may be required for the treatment of diabetic patients.

Sildenafil's short half-life makes it the drug of choice in the more severe cardiac patients, allowing early use of support therapy if an adverse clinical event occurs. Its quick onset of action and predictable duration suit many patients; nonetheless, some couples do complain of a lack of spontaneity—most often, the complainant tends to be the patient's partner.

Tadalafil has also been extensively evaluated in cardiac patients and has a similar safety and efficacy profile as sildenafil. Studies have shown no adverse effects on cardiac contraction, ventricular repolarization, or ischemic threshold (34). A similar hypotensive effect has been recorded with doxazosin, using 8 mg dosage; so, caution is needed. Because hypotension does not occur in the supine position and as tadalafil has a long half-life, it is suggested that tadalafil be taken in the morning and doxazosin in the evening. There is no interaction with the selective α-blocker tamsulosin, which can therefore be prescribed as an alternative to doxazosin for benign prostatic hypertrophy. Specific recommendations for tadalafil (at 10 and 20 mg doses) are similar to sildenafil, apart from food not affecting the onset of activity. Sexual activity, however, should be avoided within two hours of a heavy meal, since it would be occurring at the time of increased cardiac work required for food digestion.

Because of its long half-life, tadalafil may not be the first choice for the more complex cardiac cases. Because 80% of cardiac cases stratify into low risk, however, it is a viable alternative for the majority of patients. Tadalafil's long half-life may also alleviate issues related to nonspontaneous sexual interactions when compared to sildenafil.

Because vardenafil has a very similar molecular structure as sildenafil, it is not surprising that they have similar clinical profiles. One study has reported no impairment of exercise ability in stable CAD patients at 10 mg dosage (35). Similar clinical efficacy for all three agents has been observed in diabetic patients. For further information on this drug class, see Chapter 29.

Apomorphine

Apomorphine is a D_1D_2 dopamine-receptor agonist acting specifically in the paraventricular and supraoptic nuclei of the hypothalamus. The subsequent triggering of neural outflow stimulates the spinal cord and parasympathetic outflow increases, leading to smooth-muscle relaxation. It is administered sublingually in 2- or 3-mg dosages and acts rapidly, with its peak effect occurring in 15 to 20 minutes. This allows a rapid erectile response if sexual activity begins. Its overall efficacy, however, is less than the PDE5 inhibitors and is confined to the milder cases of ED. Compared with placebo in nondiabetic patients, the percentage of attempts resulting in an erection firm enough for sexual intercourse using 2 or 3 mg of apomorphine was 47% versus 34.8% ($p < 0.001$). Safety has been established in patients with hypertension, CAD, hyperlipidemia, and diabetes. No significant cardiovascular drug interactions have been recorded, and concomitant nitrate use is not a contraindication (36).

In clinical practice, the response to apomorphine has been disappointing in comparison with the PDE5 inhibitors, and this is almost certainly due to the deficit in erectile function being mainly peripheral (at the endothelial level) rather than central. It is no longer promoted for the treatment of ED because of poor patient responses, particularly in cardiac patients. For further information on this drug, see Chapter 29.

Injection Therapy

Direct intracavernosal injection of vasodilating agents began in the 1980s. Prostaglandin E1 is a natural substance that relaxes smooth-muscle cells and dilates the arterioles, increasing blood flow into the penis. Alprostadil is a commercially available form of prostaglandin E1 that is effective in 5 to 15 minutes, with an erection that usually lasts 30 minutes but occasionally may persist for several hours. The starting dose is 1.25 µg, and can be increased to 20 µg, depending on effect. It is important that patients be taught the correct technique for injection; men with poor dexterity (e.g., arthritic hands or tremor) will need their partner's help with the injection. In fact, partners may often perform the injection as part of the sexual activity. On removal of the needle, firm pressure is applied and the drug should be gently massaged into the penis for approximately 30 seconds. Men on anticoagulants, however, should compress the injection site for 5 to 10 minutes.

The resulting erection occurs without stimulation, although stimulation may enhance its effects. The erections are occasionally painful, but usually feel natural. It is recommended that this treatment not be used more frequently than every four days.

Alprostadil is effective in up to 80% of the cases and is associated with a return to spontaneous erections in 35%. It is safe and effective in diabetic patients who are used to self-injection of insulin. Although its efficacy rates are impressive, the discontinuation rate for alprostadil is high, with local pain and loss of spontaneity being the most commonly cited reasons. For further information on this type of therapy, see Chapter 30.

Transurethral Therapy

Intraurethral therapy of alprostadil presents an alternative to injections. Medicated Urethral System for Erection (MUSE) is a single-use, transurethral system that involves the insertion of a 1.4-mm pellet into the urethra using a hand-held applicator just after micturition and about 15 minutes prior to sexual activity. As with injection therapy, the patient must be taught the correct technique of insertion. Patients should receive an initial dose of 250 µg with dosage titration between 125 and 1000 µg under medical supervision until the patient achieves a satisfactory response. These numbers are much higher than with injection therapy due to the fact of drug loss in the general circulation. A maximum of two doses are allowed per 24-hour period. Once the correct dose has been identified, success rates of up to 60% have been recorded, although in a comparative study with injections, this fell to 43% (injections, 70%). For further information on transurethral therapy, see Chapter 30.

Nondrug Therapy
Psychosexual Therapy

If psychogenic ED is present, appropriate counseling should be arranged. Even organic cases of ED may have a psychological component secondary to the dysfunction itself. Cooperative teamwork between the physician and the therapist is valuable when the organic and psychological causes of ED overlap. For further information on psychological interventions in erectile dysfunction, see Chapters 27 and 28.

Vacuum Constriction Devices

The vacuum constriction device is a long-established means of treating ED. It is a noninvasive method that produces an erection by creating a pressure vacuum of up to 250 mmHg, causing blood flows into the penis. The erection is then maintained with the placement of a rubber constriction ring at the base of the penis. The constriction ring must not be left in place longer than 30 minutes, since ischemic damage could occur.

It should be recognized that a significant hematoma (minor in 10% of cases) may occur in men on anticoagulants; so, this is a relative contraindication. Specific training and advice before commencing the use of a vacuum device are needed. Vacuum devices are also not recommended for men with penile curvature. For further information on vacuum devices, see Chapter 32.

Surgical Treatment

When all else fails or when there is a history of trauma, penile surgery offers another therapeutic route. Cardiac patients should not be denied this option. Clearly, specialist referral and advice is needed and referral to the urologist is advised, with the cardiologist outlining the risk from a cardiac perspective.

☐ QUICK GUIDE TO SPECIFIC CARDIAC CONDITIONS AND SEX

Hypertension

- This is not a contraindication to sex when controlled.
- Controlled patient: antihypertensives (single or multiple) are not a contraindication, but use caution with doxazosin (and other nonselective α-blockers) and PDE5 inhibitors.
- All ED therapies can be utilized.
- Antihypertensives least likely to cause ED are the angiotensin II receptor antagonists and doxazosin.

Angina

- For stable patients, there is minimal risk for sex or ED therapy.
- Nitrates and Nicorandil are contraindications to PDE5 inhibitors. On most occasions, these can safely be discontinued.
- Heart rate-slowing drugs are the most effective antianginal agents: verapamil, diltiazem.
- Use an exercise ECG to stratify risk if unsure.

Post-Myocardial Infarction

- Use pre- or post-discharge exercise ECG to guide advice; no need to delay sex resumption if satisfactory.
- Advise gentle return to allow for loss of confidence by both patient and partner.
- Rehabilitation programs are a positive advantage.
- Avoid sex in the first two weeks (period of maximal risk).

Post Surgery or Percutaneous Intervention

- If successful, risk is low.
- Sternal scar may be painful; advise side-to-side position or patient in top position.
- Use exercise ECG, if unsure of ability.

Cardiac Failure

- The risk is low if ability is good.
- If symptomatic, adjust medication accordingly; patient may need to be the more passive partner.
- If severely symptomatic, sex may not be possible owing to physical limitation and can occasionally trigger decompensation.

- An exercise program can facilitate the return to sex; physically fit equals sexually fit.

Valve Disease

- For mild cases, there is no increased risk.
- Antibiotic prophylaxis is not needed.
- Significant aortic stenosis may lead to sudden death and can be worsened by the vasodilatory effects of PDE5 inhibitors.

Arrhythmias

- Controlled atrial fibrillation is not an increased risk depending on cause and exercise ability.
- Warfarin does not contraindicate the vacuum device but care is needed and caution is required with injections.
- Complex arrhythmias: arrange for 24- to 48-hour ambulatory ECG monitoring and exercise testing. Treat and retest.
- Pacemakers are not a contraindication.
- With implanted defibrillators, use exercise test for safety before advising. This is usually not a problem.

Other Conditions

- For pericarditis, await full recovery; there is no specific increased risk thereafter.
- With peripheral vascular disease, stroke, or transient ischemic attacks (TIAs), there is increased risk of myocardial infarction; therefore, screen.
- With hypertrophic obstructive cardiomyopathy, there is increased risk of syncope and sudden death on exercise. Exercise ECG is advised. PDE5 and alprostadil may increase the degree of obstruction owing to vasodilatory effects. Test dose under hospital supervision is recommended.

An assessment algorithm (Table 3) summarizes management guidelines.

☐ CONCLUSION

Cardiac patients may have anxieties about sexual activity because of their false belief of substantially increased risk. ED is common in cardiac patients because of the shared risk factors that adversely impact endothelial function. Signs of ED often present before overt cardiac symptoms develop; therefore, cardiac workups may be warranted for these patients even without relevant cardiovascular histories. There is now increasing awareness of therapy for ED, but many patients remain reluctant to come forward for advice. The question of sexual activity and ED therapy should be raised by health-care professionals as a routine part of the management of cardiac patients. Treatment is available. With reassurance, support, and careful explanation, sexual relationships can be enjoyed by cardiac patients who receive appropriate advice.

□ REFERENCES

1. Feldman HA, Goldstein I, Hatzichristou DG, et al. Impotence and the medical and psychosocial correlates: results of the Massachusetts Male Aging Study. J Urol 1994; 151(1):54–61.

2. Ayta IA, McKinlay JB, Krane R. The likely worldwide increase in erectile dysfunction between 1995 and 2025 and some possible policy consequences. BJU Int 1999; 84(1):50–56.

3. Solomon H, Man J, Wierzbicki AS, et al. Erectile dysfunction: cardiovascular risk and the role of the cardiologist. Int J Clin Pract 2003; 57(2):96–99.

4. Lue TF. Erectile dysfunction. N Engl J Med 2000; 342(24):1622–1626.

5. Kirby M, Jackson G, Betteride J, et al. Is erectile dysfunction a marker for cardiovascular disease? Int J Clin Pract 2001; 55(9):614–618.

6. Solomon H, Man JW, Jackson G. Erectile dysfunction and the cardiovascular patient: endothelial dysfunction is the common denominator. Heart 2003; 89(3):251–253.

7. Hurairah H, Ferro A. The role of the endothelium in the control of vascular function. Int J Clin Pract 2004; 58(2):173–183.

8. Kraiser DR, Billups K, Mason C, et al. Impaired brachial artery endothelium-dependent and independent vasodilatation in men with erectile dysfunction and no other clinical vascular disease. J Am Coll Cardiol 2004; 43:179–184.

9. Bulpitt CJ, Dollery CT, Carne S. Change in symptom of hypertensives patient after referral to hospital clinic. Br Heart J 1976; 38:121–128.

10. Wei M, Macera CA, Davis DR, et al. Total cholesterol and high density lipoprotein cholesterol as important predictors of erectile dysfunction. Am J Epidemiol 1994; 140(10):930–937.

11. Rizvi K, Hampson JP, Harvey JN. Do lipid-lowering drugs cause erectile dysfunction? A systematic review. Fam Pract 2002; 19(1):95–98.

12. Saenzed de Tejada IS, Goldstein I, Azadzoi K, et al. Impaired neurogenic and endothelium mediated relaxation of penile smooth muscle from diabetic men with impotence. N Engl J Med 1989; 320(16):1025–1030.

13. Reffelman T, Kloner RA. Therapeutic potential of phosphodiesterase 5 inhibition for cardiovascular disease. Circulation 2003; 108(2):239–244.

14. Jackson G. PDE5 inhibitors: looking beyond ED. Int J Clin Pract 2003; 57(3):159–160.

15. Solomon H, Man JW, Wierzbicki AS, et al. Relation of erectile dysfunction to angiographic coronary artery disease. Am J Cardiol 2003; 91(2):230–231.

16. Bortolotti A, Parazzini F, Colli E, et al. The epidemiology of erectile dysfunction and its risk factors. Int J Androl 1997; 20(6):323–334.

17. Pritzker M. The penile stress test: a window to the hearts of man? Circulation 1999; 100(suppl I):P3751.

18. Kawanishi Y, Lee KS, Kimura K, et al. Screening of ischaemic heart disease with cavernous artery blood flow in erectile dysfunction patients. Int J Impot Res 2001; 13(2):100–103.

19. Montorsi P, Montorsi F, Schulman CC. Is erectile dysfunction the 'tip of the iceberg' of a systemic vascular disorder? Eur Urol 2003; 44(3):352–354.

20. Montorsi F, Briganti A, Salonia A, et al. Erectile dysfunction prevalence, time of onset and association with risk factors in 300 consecutive patients with acute chest pain and angiographically documented coronary artery disease. Eur Urol 2003; 44(3): 360–364.

21. Speel TGW, van Langen H, Meuleman EJH. The risk of coronary heart disease in men with erectile dysfunction. Eur Urol 2003; 44(3):366–371.

22. Roumeguére Th, Wespes E, Carpentier Y, et al. Erectile dysfunction is associated with a high prevalence of hyperlipidaemia and coronary heart disease risk. Eur Urol 2003; 44(3):355–359.

23. O'Kane PD, Jackson G. Erectile dysfunction: is there silent obstructive coronary artery disease? Int J Clin Pract 2001; 55(3):614–618.

24. Jackson G. Erectile dysfunction: a window of opportunity for preventing vascular disease? Int J Clin Pract 2003; 57(9):747.

25. Jackson G. Sexual intercourse and angina pectoris. Int Rehabil Med 1981; 3(1):35–37.

26. Drory Y. Sexual activity and cardiovascular risk. Eur Heart J Suppl 2002; 4(suppl H):H13-H18.

27. Jackson G. Sex, the Heart and Erectile Dysfunction. London: Taylor and Francis, 2004.

28. Jackson G, Betteridge J, Dean J, et al. A systematic approach to erectile dysfunction in the cardiovascular patient: a consensus statement—update 2002. Int J Clin Pract 2002; 56(9):663–671.

29. Muller JE, Mittleman A, Maclure M, et al. Triggering myocardial infarction by sexual activity: low absolute risk and prevention by regular physical exertion. JAMA 1996; 275(18):1405–1409.

30. Möller J, Ahlbom A, Hulting J, et al. Sexual activity as a trigger of myocardial infarction: a case crossover analysis in the Stockholm Heart Epidemiology Programme (SHEEP). Heart 2001; 86(4):387–390.

31. Gillies HC, Roblin D, Jackson G. Coronary and systemic haemodynamic effects of sildenafil citrate: from basic science to clinical studies in patients with cardiovascular disease. Int J Cardiol 2002; 86:131–141.

32. Giuliono F. Phosphodiesterase type 5 inhibition in erectile dysfunction: an overview. Eur Heart J Suppl 2002; 4(suppl H):H7-H12.

33. Fox KM, Thadani U, Ma PTS, et al. Sildenafil citrate does not reduce exercise tolerance in men with erectile

dysfunction and chronic stable angina. Eur Heart J 2003; 24(24):2206–2212.

34. Kloner RA, Mitchell M, Emmick JT. Cardiovascular effects of tadalafil. Am J Cardiol 2003; 92(9A):37M–46M.

35. Thadani U, Smith W, Nash S, et al. The effect of vardenafil, a potent and highly selective phosphodiesterase 5 inhibitor for the treatment of erectile dysfunction, on the cardiovascular response to exercise in patients with coronary artery disease. J Am Coll Cardiol 2002; 40(11):2006–2012.

36. Heaton JPW. Key issues from the clinical trials of apomorphine SL. World J Urol 2001; 19(1):25–33.

37

Treatment of Sexual Dysfunction in Patients with Prostate Cancer

John J. Mulcahy

Department of Urology, Indiana University School of Medicine, Indianapolis, Indiana, U.S.A.

□ INTRODUCTION

Prostatic adenocarcinoma is now the number one cancer found in men. Approximately 230,000 new cases will be diagnosed in 2006. As one ages, the incidence of the disease increases: it is estimated that by age 60, one in three men will have a focus of prostate cancer present, while half of all men in their eighth decade will harbor this tumor. Prostate cancer is usually slow growing, and most men who have this tumor will die of another cause.

Erectile dysfunction is another very common problem in the male population, and it, too, increases in incidence with aging. It is estimated that at least one-half of American men between the ages of 50 and 70 are affected by erectile dysfunction (1). Diseases and conditions such as hypertension, abnormal serum lipids, diabetes mellitus, smoking, and obesity contribute to the problem, and in those with these diseases and conditions, erectile dysfunction occurs earlier in life and to a greater degree. For more detailed information on sexual dysfunction and these various conditions, see chapters in Part II: Pathophysiology of Male Sexual Dysfunction, Section III: Organic Factors.

Many of the treatments available for prostate cancer have a negative influence on a man's erections and, in addition, he may have comorbid conditions that contribute to vascular disease and further reduction in potency.

When evaluating effects of proposed treatments of prostate cancer on erectile function, one must also keep in mind that men tend to minimize their erectile inability—i.e., they are not prone to confess their personal failings, which they believe would make them appear inferior or less desirable compared with other men, especially in the eyes of the opposite sex. For these reasons, men do not consistently admit the fact of their impotence when answering questionnaires or when interviewed during post-treatment office visits. A more accurate assessment of erectile ability can usually be obtained from the wife or partner, especially one who regards sexual activity in a positive light.

□ TREATMENTS FOR PROSTATE CANCER

There are a number of treatments available for prostate cancer, and the applicability of each treatment depends on the stage and grade of tumor when the disease is detected. Prostate-specific antigen (PSA) was introduced as a screening test for prostate cancer over two decades ago, and with its recent application as a common screening test in men over age 50, the incidence of detecting early disease has increased markedly (2). As more men are presenting early for screening and tumors are discovered when they are still confined to the prostate, they are also more amenable to curative treatments.

Radical Prostatectomy

Definitive treatment of a cancerous prostate would be its total removal if the tumor is confined to the gland. Over 20 years ago, few of these extirpative procedures of the prostate were performed because most tumors were found in an advanced metastatic state. In addition to PSA as a marker for early detection, the development and widespread use of nerve-sparing radical prostatectomy has reduced the incidence of postoperative erectile dysfunction, which in the past had been almost universal. In 1983, Walsh and Donker defined the anatomy of the autonomic nervous system related to erectile function as it coursed over the rectal wall adjacent to the prostate (3). In addition to those undergoing radical prostatectomy, patients subjected to distal colectomy for carcinoma or ulcerative colitis or cystoprostatectomy for bladder cancer are also subject to injury of these nerves. When considering potency preservation, the success of any given procedure is not dependent only on sparing these nerves because the age of the patient and the presence or absence of comorbid diseases also play significant roles in determining surgical outcome. In patients in their fifth decade with tumor confined to one lobe of the prostate, the recovery rate of sexual potency at 12 months is 83% if both nerves are spared during prostate removal (4). In men in their sixth decade, however, the recovery rate drops to 60%. Less than 50% of men older than age 70 will have erections restored under these circumstances. In those with more extensive disease involving both lobes of the prostate, the post-operative potency rate in men in the sixth decade decreases substantially to 38%. Catalona and Basler reported on 295 men with a mean age of 64 years (5). Bilateral nerve-sparing prostatectomy was performed in 236 cases with 63% preservation of potency, and unilateral nerve-sparing surgery performed in 59 cases resulted in a potency rate of 41%. When potency outcomes are reported by those other than the surgeon, however, the results have been less positive. In a series of 69 such men who underwent the bilateral nerve-sparing procedure, just 31% reported postoperative potency (6). Of 203 patients undergoing unilateral nerve-sparing prostatectomy, only 13% reported erections useful for intercourse after the surgery. A multi-institutional study was conducted by Pfizer (7). Men with good erections by questionnaire and nocturnal penile tumescence monitoring using Rigiscan were recruited prior to bilateral nerve-sparing radical retropubic prostatectomy. Starting at two months postoperatively, one group was given a daily Viagra® (sildenafil citrate) and a control group was given a daily placebo. At eight months, erections were reevaluated using questionnaire and Rigiscan testing. The sildenafil group showed 27% of patients maintained usable erections, compared to 4% of patients in the control group.

The question also arises as to whether the blood supply to the erectile mechanism may be interrupted by total prostatectomy. Data regarding the presence of an accessory pudendal artery, which may or may not be sacrificed during the performance of the procedure, has not been conclusive (8). The blood supply to the cavernous arteries is not impaired during prostate removal.

Patients are offered radical prostatectomy if the tumor appears to be organ confined and there appears to be a reasonable life expectancy of at least 10 years. Most urologists do not recommend this option to men beyond their mid-70s. In addition to a less than 10-year life expectancy at this juncture, prostate tumors tend to grow more slowly, and patients will usually die of some other cause.

External Beam Radiotherapy

An alternative treatment to radical prostatectomy for locally confined prostate cancer has been external beam radiation. This modality is popular among patients who do not wish to undergo the risks of urinary incontinence or impotence, which are potential sequelae following prostate removal. Potency rates documented after external beam radiation vary between 20% and 80% (9). Explanations for this large discrepancy include a lack of prospective data, variability in radiation dosing and delivery, and scant long-term follow-up. External beam radiation is thought to initiate erectile dysfunction by accelerating microvascular angiopathy,

which causes cavernosal fibrosis and dysfunction. This process may take five or six years to develop, and most of the data on erectile abilities following this modality were obtained in the first two years. External beam radiation was sometimes advised in older patients beyond the mid-70s who were not considered candidates for radical prostatectomy due to their advanced age. Another group who frequently received this treatment modality included patients whose surgical specimens at radical prostatectomy showed margins positive for tumor.

Brachytherapy

Over a decade ago, brachytherapy was introduced as an alternative treatment for confined prostate cancer. Using this technique, Pd-103 or I-125 seeds are strategically placed using ultrasound guidance and a grid into the prostate (10). These radioactive seeds emit radiation in a localized area, and if properly placed according to the grid, this radiation will be distributed to the prostate completely, with surrounding structures being spared the radiation effect. This treatment was originally recommended for patients with small prostates, with relatively low tumor grade and stage. In the 15 years since its introduction, however, the survival data compared with radical prostatectomy are very similar. Brachytherapy has become a very popular modality for treating men with localized prostate cancer. Avoidance of radical surgery and a markedly reduced possibility of both urinary incontinence and erectile dysfunction are the prime reasons that this treatment has been consumer driven. Recent data revealed that preservation of potency using this modality was 79% at three years and 59% at six years (11). If patients elect radiation treatment, brachytherapy combined with external beam radiation has been advised when the PSA is greater than 10, the Gleason score is 7 or higher, and the tumor is extensive or found in both lobes of the prostate. Under these conditions, the incidence of erectile dysfunction following the two treatments can be expected to be higher than it is with each treatment administered alone.

For further information on the effects of radiation on sexual function, see Chapter 20.

Hormonal Ablation

When there is evidence that the prostate tumor has spread beyond the confines of the gland and the patient is not a candidate for a curative procedure, disease progression may be arrested by hormonal ablation. Over 80% of prostate tumors do respond to the removal of male hormone (testosterone) (12), as monitored by serum PSA. The most common method today of removing male hormone is the use of an luteinizing hormone-releasing hormone (LHRH) agonist. These agents act by keeping the levels of testosterone low and are administered as a subcutaneous injection of implant at one-month, three-month, or yearly intervals. Lowering the testosterone level will frequently result in a lethargic feeling, diminished sexual drive, and decreased erectile ability; however, sexual function may be possible despite the low male hormone.

Cryotherapy

Freezing the prostate in an attempt to kill the cancerous cells has had a recent resurgence (13), but the almost universal development of erectile dysfunction and disastrous complications such as urinary incontinence and rectourethral fistulae have limited its application in the past. Newer technology has resulted in fewer complications and the use of this therapy appears to be increasing.

Watchful Waiting

A patient in whom prostate cancer is discovered in his mid-70s or later may best be advised to follow a course of watchful waiting. At that age, tumor progression is slow and life expectancy is relatively short. Certainly, periodic monitoring of serum PSA would be advisable, and if rapid progression of tumor growth were detected, appropriate treatments to arrest this growth could be undertaken. Conversely, a patient in his 40s or 50s in whom prostate cancer is found, who is otherwise healthy with a normal life expectancy would be ill-advised to follow this approach because it would then be very likely that within 15 to 20 years, he would have to deal with the unpleasant metastatic complications of prostate cancer such as bone pain, lymphedema, and voiding difficulties.

☐ TREATMENTS FOR ERECTILE DYSFUNCTION IN PROSTATE CANCER PATIENTS
Ejaculation

As men age or undergo surgical procedures that result in the loss of erection, ejaculation is usually preserved. This function consists of two components: "emission," or the placement of semen in the prostatic urethra, and "ejaculation," or the forceful expulsion of semen to the urethra and out the urethral meatus in a rhythmic fashion. During emission, the bladder neck or internal sphincter closes, and the prostatic muscles contract with the resultant expressing of semen or prostatic fluid into the prostatic urethra. During the ejaculatory phase, the rhythmic contraction of the vas deferens propels sperm to the prostatic urethra to mix with the seminal fluid and the rhythmic contraction of the bulbocavernosus and ischiocavernosus muscles propels the semen in spurts along the urethra and out the meatus. For further information on ejaculation, see Chapter 3.

With radical prostatectomy, the emission phase is lost, since there is no prostate to expel semen into the urethra and the vas deferens has been ligated. The ejaculatory phase, however, may be preserved and patients following radical prostatectomy will frequently reach climax with adequate sexual stimulation. There is a feeling of pleasure and relief with the rhythmic contractions of the bulbous muscles but no elimination of fluid.

Other forms of treatment for prostate cancer, such as external beam therapy and brachytherapy do not significantly affect ejaculation per se. Premature ejaculation does not seem to be age dependent because it appears to be equally prevalent in younger and older men. Less direct, tactile stimulation prior to penetration, the use of distracting maneuvers such as the squeeze technique (see Chapter 28), and biofeedback exercises have all been used in the past with modest success. Recently, it has been found that the selective serotonin reuptake inhibitors (SSRIs) such as Paxil (paroxetine) 20 mg, given two to four hours prior to ejaculation, have been effective in 80% of the cases in prolonging ejaculatory latency (14). For further information on the physiology of male sexual dysfunction, see Chapter 10.

Counseling

As mentioned previously, prostate cancer is a disease of aging and is almost unheard of before the age of 40. As men reach this milestone, erections become less reliable. It should be noted, however, that each man's particular environmental circumstance plays a major role in whether erection can be satisfactorily achieved. For example, if the patient is rested, erections will be easier to produce than when he is tired. Similarly, if the patient is distracted by pain, career or financial worries, or other such concerns, he will be unable to focus on sexual activity. This is in contrast to a man's younger years—i.e., the teens and twenties—during which concentration is not very necessary to achieve an erection. In young men, only slight stimulation is necessary to achieve a complete erection rapidly. Also, as one ages, the importance of a partner's participation becomes greater, and with the partner's help, an erection will be more readily achieved. In addition to these environmental influences, comorbid features such as smoking, obesity, diabetes mellitus, hypertension, and hyperlipidemia that may further contribute to erectile dysfunction should be discussed and appropriate treatment and a change in lifestyle advised. Even though the treatments of prostate cancer may have a detrimental effect on erections, such counseling may be very beneficial in improving marginal erectile function. For further information on the counseling of sexual dysfunction, see Chapter 27.

Male Hormone Replacement

Male hormone, testosterone, is below the normal level in 7% of men below age 60 and 20% of men above age 60 (15). The gradual decline of testosterone levels with age, termed "andropause," occurs at about 1% per year (16). If this circumstance occurs, sex drive may be low, erections may be problematic, and energy level or enthusiasm for the activities of life may be reduced. Replacement of the male hormone may improve each of these three problems. As previously discussed, one treatment of advanced prostate cancer is the reduction/removal of testosterone. To date, such a study has never been done, but by inference, testosterone in the normal range—or even in the supraphysiologic range, which may occur with intramuscular replacement—may stimulate the growth of prostate cancer. Hence, it is recommended that patients with known prostate cancer not be given testosterone replacement as a treatment for sexual dysfunction unless the cancer is considered cured and it is believed that the individual patients in question would comply completely with follow-up evaluations. For further information on hormone replacement, see Chapters 29 and 35.

Vasoactive Medications

The penis is composed of two twin erectile chambers, the corpora cavernosa, which are surrounded by an elastic membrane called the tunica albuginea that stretches with an erection until the cavities become three times larger in size as this covering reaches its limit of stretch. The components of these two cavities are numerous cul-de-sacs, or endothelial-lined spaces surrounded by smooth muscle. For further information on the anatomy and physiology of the penis, see the chapters in Part I of this volume.

Agents that cause relaxation of this smooth muscle are very effective in allowing blood to flow into the penis, expanding the sinusoids and compressing subtunical venules to hold blood in the penis and to generate an erection. Conversely, agents that cause contraction of the smooth muscle are effective in reducing a prolonged erection (priapism). In recent years, a number of agents have emerged in various forms that affect the smooth muscle surrounding the sinusoids. As with many muscle cells elsewhere in the body, when the calcium content of the cell is lowered, the penile smooth muscle will relax. There are various transmitter substances, which, when released from nerve endings, will diffuse across the intercellular space to stimulate the enzyme systems within these smooth-muscle cells, eventually resulting in the loss of calcium from the cell and producing muscle relaxation. Nitric oxide has recently been discovered as one of the major transmitters that affects this action in penile smooth-muscle cells (17).

Oral Medications

The recent introduction of sildenafil citrate (Viagra®) and subsequently vardenafil (Levitra®) and tadalafil (Cialis®) has revolutionized the treatment of erectile dysfunction (18). These compounds are type V phosphodiesterase inhibitors, and under the influence of sexual stimulation, have been found to be beneficial in enhancing and prolonging erections. When nitric oxide is released from nerve terminals, it diffuses across the interspace to the penile smooth-muscle cell, where it influences the guanyl cyclase enzyme system. This converts GTP to cyclic GMP, which results in decreased intracellular calcium concentration and smooth-muscle relaxation. Type V phosphodiesterase is the enzyme that degrades cyclic GMP to its metabolite. When this enzyme is inhibited by these compounds, cyclic GMP levels stay high, calcium stays out of the cell, and the smooth muscle stays relaxed. For further information on the physiology of erection, see Chapter 3.

For the three available type V phosphodiesterase inhibitors to work effectively, sexual stimulation is necessary and the penile nerves need to be intact in order to release nitric oxide. Absorption of these agents in the gastrointestinal tract is relatively rapid, and effects are sometimes seen in as short a time as 20 minutes after ingestion. Peak absorption occurs at 0.8 hours, and the drug's half-life is between four and five hours for sildenafil and vardenafil. The window of opportunity for sexual activity with both of these agents is usually even beyond the five-hour half-life noted. By 24 hours, they are completely gone from the body. Tadalafil has a longer half-life of 17 hours and may be effective for up to 36 hours after ingestion. Overall, the success rate with the type V phosphodiesterase inhibitors has been 80% in psychogenic impotence and about 60% in organic erectile dysfunction. Generally, the two groups of patients who do not respond as well to phosphodiesterase inhibitors are those with diabetes mellitus (see Chapter 14) and those who have had radical prostatectomy. In clinical trials, the response in the latter group was 43% (19). If bilateral nerve-sparing prostatectomy has been performed, the response rate with sildenafil in patients who were previously potent is 72% (20). If only one nerve was spared during the prostate ablative procedure, the response rate with sildenafil falls to the range of 50%. If both nerves were removed during the prostatectomy, only a 15% positive response is seen. These drugs have also been effective to some degree in patients whose erections have been diminished following brachytherapy or external beam radiation. Side effects of these medications include headache, flushing, and dyspepsia. These side effects are uncommon and usually very well tolerated. They also tend to diminish with time as patients continue to take the medication. There have been a number of deaths reported in conjunction with the use of these drugs, but more recent studies have shown that they have no significant effect on the heart. A study of patients with cardiac disease measured cardiac dynamics before and after ingestion of sildenafil and found no difference—i.e., no effect of this medication on the heart muscle and function (21). For further information on sexual dysfunction in cardiac patients, see Chapters 7 and 36. It should be noted, however, that there has been some synergy of type V phosphodiesterase inhibitors with nitrates in lowering the blood pressure, and for this reason, the American College of Cardiology has recommended that nitrates and these medications not be used simultaneously (22). In addition, phosphodiesterase inhibitors should be used with extreme caution in patients with congestive heart failure, myocardial disease, or in those on a complex antihypertensive regimen. In one set of clinical trials, no priapism was seen in patients using sildenafil; this was, however, a controlled group, and the medications that patients were taking in addition to the trial drug were limited. Now that these compounds are readily available, patients are using cocktails or mixtures with other treatments that enhance erections. In addition, they may be using these medications combined with other medicines that predispose to priapism, such as thioridazine (Mellaril), trazodone, or the phenothiazine compounds. Under these circumstances, prolonged, painful, and unwanted erections have been seen.

The advent of sildenafil in 1998 has broadened the awareness of erectile dysfunction as a problem related to various disease processes. This awareness has brought many new patients into the clinic for treatment. Before the introduction of sildenafil, yohimbine (Yocon) was the most commonly prescribed treatment for erectile dysfunction. Most studies, however, have failed to demonstrate any significant benefit of yohimbine over placebo in the treatment of poor erections (23). A number of other oral preparations are now under study and in clinical trials for the treatment of erectile dysfunction. For further information on phosphodiesterase inhibitors, see Chapter 29.

Intracorporal Injections

At the American Urological Association meeting in Las Vegas in 1983, Dr. Giles Brindley, a British pharmacologist, dramatically and memorably illustrated the effectiveness of intracorporal injections of papaverine by demonstrating to the audience his own erection induced by this medication (24). Following this graphic display, the use of this agent and other intracorporal injections rapidly gained popularity. Now, papaverine, phentolamine, and prostaglandin E_1 (PGE_1) (Caverject) (EDEX) alone or in combination are used effectively in generating an erection with up to 80% success (25). Both papaverine and PGE_1 act directly on penile smooth-muscle cells via the cyclic AMP pathway to cause smooth-muscle relaxation by decreasing intracellular calcium. When injected into one portion of the penis, this effect is rapidly spread throughout the entire length of both corporal bodies by gap junction or cell-to-cell transmission. Phentolamine is a selective α-adrenergic adrenoceptor blocker that inhibits sympathomimetic amines such as norepinephrine and blocks contraction of penile smooth-muscle cells. It acts synergistically with papaverine and PGE_1, but has not been practically effective by itself in generating an erection by intracorporal injection. Almost 90% of patients following nerve-sparing radical prostatectomy will respond to intracavernosal PGE_1, in contrast to only 66% of patients who have had non–nerve-sparing

procedures (26). In addition, nearly 25% of the nerve-sparing prostatectomy patients who have responded did so at a low dose of PGE_1, in contrast to those with non–nerve-sparing procedures, who required high doses of the same medication. PGE_1 may result in pain in some patients, and this is particularly distressing in cases of neurapraxia, which may be seen following prostatectomy. Montorsi et al. (27) have shown that instituting intracavernous injections of PGE_1 very shortly (two months) after performing radical prostatectomy will result in a return of spontaneous erections without medication at one year in 67% of patients. In a controlled group that was not treated with intracavernous injections of PGE_1, only 20% of patients noted the spontaneous return of erections by that time interval. The exact mechanism for this is unknown, but it may be related to the prevention of a buildup of transforming growth factor-β (TGF-β) in the low oxygen states associated with reduced penile blood flow. This leads to the occurrence of fibrosis in penile muscles (28).

In the aging patient, it is well known that the more erections are used, the better they tend to work. Abstinence from sexual activity for a period of time as is necessitated by a surgical procedure and the subsequent recovery period is certainly contributory to sexual dysfunction in this regard. When approaching patients who are impotent before nerve-sparing prostatectomy, the surgeon should be aware that pharmacotherapy afterward will be more effective if the nerves have been spared. Priapism or prolonged painful erection has been seen about 7% of the time with papaverine and phentolamine and about 1% of the time using PGE_1. Such erections are usually easily reversed using dilute sympathomimetic amine solutions such as epinephrine or phenylephrine injected intracorporally. The incidence of development of corporal fibrosis (i.e., penile plaques) varies from 1.9% to 16% in patients using a pharmacologic erection program. This can be minimized by less frequent use (less than twice a week), varying the site of injection, and compressing the site of injection for a period of about 30 seconds to prevent internal bleeding. Long-term follow-up studies with patients on intracorporal injections show a relatively high dropout rate in the range of 70% over three years. Reasons for discontinuation of therapy include a desire for a permanent treatment alternative, fear of injections with needles, poor response, lack of a suitable partner, comorbid health conditions precluding comfortable positions for intercourse, and loss of sexual spontaneity. For further information on intracorporal injections, see Chapter 30.

Intraurethral Therapy

The effectiveness of injectable intracorporal forms of therapy over the last 15 years has encouraged the development of more acceptable and appealing delivery systems for these medications. Some men are opposed to the use of a needle placed in the penis to deliver medication, and this has contributed to the high dropout rate for patients who are prescribed intracorporal injections. Medicated urethral system for erections (MUSE) was introduced in early 1997 as an alternative method of delivering PGE_1 to the erectile bodies (29). After urination, an applicator is placed about 1.5 in. into the urethra. After pushing a button, a pellet of PGE_1 approximately the size of a grain of rice is deposited in the urinary tract. Absorption occurs in the corpus spongiosum; through venous communications between the corpus spongiosum and the corpora cavernosa, some of this medication gains entry into the erectile bodies. PGE_1 then acts on the adenosine triphosphate system to decrease intracellular calcium and relax the penile smooth-muscle cells. Because of this direct action, intact innervation of the erectile mechanism is not necessary. To enhance delivery of this compound into the erectile body, a constricting band (ACTIS) at the base of the penis should be used. Penile, urethral, testicular, and perineal pain may be seen in up to 50% of the patients. Although hypotension and syncope rarely occur, this medication should be nonetheless applied while sitting to avoid falling. The effectiveness of MUSE at providing an erection that can be used for intercourse is in the range of 30% to 40%. A MUSE-induced erection is rarely rigid but may be described as a swollen penis that does not buckle when it is used for vaginal penetration with some assistance. MUSE may be useful in some patients following radical prostatectomy, who have not responded to type V phosphodiesterase inhibitors. This medication has also been used in conjunction with oral medication to provide additional support when adequate rigidity is not provided by one treatment alone. In addition, the use of MUSE with a previously placed penile implant has provided some increase in girth and length as engorgement of the glans penis and corpus spongiosum readily occurs with its use. Such increases in size, however, have only been in the range of 1 cm and each application costs approximately $20. For further information on intraurethral therapy, see Chapter 30.

Vacuum Erection Devices

Vacuum erection therapy as a treatment for impotence had been used sporadically with homemade devices until the pioneering work of Geddings Osbon, who obtained Food and Drug Administration (FDA) approval for such a device in 1982. Over the next decade, primarily through the efforts of the Osbon Corporation, these constriction devices became a definite player in the treatment of erectile failure. Initial reports of Witherington (30) and Nadig et al. (31) have claimed success and satisfaction in over 90% of the patients using these devices. In a series of 45 patients of Gilbert and Gingell, 84% reported adequate rigidity, but only 27% were satisfied with the device (32). This experience was reinforced by Earle et al., who reported a satisfaction rate as low as 9% (33). The key to patient satisfaction with this treatment is the careful

instruction of patients and adequate practice in removing the ring from the cylinder before the seal at the penoscrotal junction is broken to allow maintenance of penile rigidity. Common reported side effects include pain on ejaculation, inability to ejaculate, petechiae or bruising of the penis, and numbness during erection. Partners will frequently relate that the resulting erection is unpleasantly cold. The recommended maximum time period that the constriction ring may remain in place is 30 minutes. Even if this device is left on for longer periods—i.e., if the patient falls asleep with the ring in place—blood flow will continue at a very slow rate, but this volume is usually adequate to prevent necrosis of the penis.

The major advantage of the vacuum device is its relative margin of safety when compared to pharmacologic or surgical treatments of erectile dysfunction. Serious problems such as skin necrosis have only occurred with misuse. The relative safety of vacuum devices has encouraged the FDA to remove them from the list of prescribed devices, and they are now sold over the counter. Older patients in a stable marital relationship, who have failed in restoring erections with the use of medications, tend to choose the vacuum device when they are not inclined toward the surgical placement of a penile prosthesis. For further information on vacuum erection devices, see Chapter 32.

Penile Prostheses

Effective penile prostheses were first introduced to the impotence marketplace in the early 1970s. Prior to this, there was no effective treatment for the unfortunate patient who had significant erectile dysfunction. Since less aggressive forms of treatment such as vacuum devices and medications were introduced, the market share of penile prostheses has become smaller; however, they do provide a predictable and reliable means of restoring erectile function, and the satisfaction rate among patients and partners who use penile prostheses has been the highest of all treatment modalities for erectile dysfunction, in the level of 85% (34,35). The small percentage of patients who report disappointment with this modality typically have unrealistic expectations regarding penile size, sensitivity, and arousal. Malfunctions may occur due to either wearing of parts or breakdown of the coverings of the erectile body or the skin of the scrotum, with the resulting extrusion of prosthetic parts. A recent multicenter study of 372 patients with the AMS-700 CX (American Medical Systems) prosthesis shows a mechanical reliability of 92% at 3 years, 85% at 5 years, and 71% at 10 years (36). Patient selection, proper sizing, placement by an experienced surgeon, and prompt attention to problems that may develop are of paramount importance in assuring success and satisfaction. Silicone and polyurethane used in the construction of these devices have not had detrimental effects on the body as shown in studies of patients with breast implants (37). Despite this, the FDA mandated that

AMS and the Mentor Corporation conduct prospective clinical trials (36) to document the safety, efficacy, and patient satisfaction of these devices. These studies have provided no evidence related to the presence of these foreign bodies, which would be considered detrimental to the patient's health. In the past, while infection of a penile prosthesis has been uncommon—in the range of 1% to 3% (38)—when it occurs, however, it is a catastrophic occurrence that necessitates immediate removal of the device. Recent experience with salvage procedures in which the infected prosthesis is removed completely, the wound thoroughly cleansed, and a new device placed at the same procedure, has shown successful outcomes in about 82% of the patients with up to eight years of followup (39).

An additional advantage of these devices is that they can be satisfactorily placed in patients following external beam therapy or brachytherapy for prostate cancer. They are also sometimes placed in patients following radical prostatectomy in conjunction with an artificial urinary sphincter, which is used to control incontinence if it develops following this procedure. For further information on penile prostheses, see Chapters 33 and 41.

□ SUMMARY

Erectile dysfunction in patients with prostate cancer is a common problem that is seen more frequently in older patients in whom erectile dysfunction may already be present. Further, many of the treatments used for prostate cancer can result in erectile dysfunction. A multitude of treatment modalities, however, are now available for the treatment of sexual dysfunction in prostate cancer patients, including medications, nonsurgical vacuum devices, and surgical penile implants. Almost any patient can be restored to erectile abilities if he is sufficiently motivated to pursue adequate treatment.

□ REFERENCES

1. Feldman HA, Goldstein I, Hatzichristou DG, et al. Impotence and its medical and psychological correlates: results of the Massachusetts Male Aging Study. J Urol 1994; 151(1):54–61.

2. Wang MC, Valenzuela LA, Murphy GP, et al. A simplified purification procedure for human prostate antigen. Oncology 1982; 39(1):1–5.

3. Walsh, PC, Donker PJ. Impotence following radical prostatectomy: insight in etiology and prevention. J Urol 2002; 167(2 Pt 2):1005–1010.

4. Quilan, PM, Epstein JI, Carter BS, et al. Sexual function following radical prostatectomy: influence of preservation of neurovascular bundles. J Urol 1991; 145(5): 998–1002.

5. Catalona WJ, Basler JW. Return of erections and urinary continence following nerve sparing radical retropubic prostatectomy. J Urol 1993; 150(3):905–907.

6. Geary ES, Dendenagh TE, Frehia FS, et al. Nerve sparing radical prostatectomy: a different view. J Urol 1995; 154(1):145–149.

7. Padma-Nathan H, McCullogh A, Giuliano F, et al. Postoperative nightly administration of sildenafil citrate significantly improved return of normal spontaneous erectile function after bilateral nerve-sparing radical prostatectomy. J Urol 2003; 4(suppl 1):375.

8. Polascik TJ, Walsh PC. Radical retropubic prostatectomy: the influence of accessory pudendal arteries on the recovery of sexual function. J Urol 1995; 154(1):150–152.

9. Siegel T, Moul JD, Spevak M, et al. The development of erectile dysfunction in men treated for prostate cancer. J Urol 2001; 165(2):430–435.

10. Blasko JC, Ragde H, Luse RW, et al. Should brachytherapy be considered a therapeutic option in localized prostate cancer? Urol Clin North Am 1996; 23(4):633–650.

11. Stock RG, Kao J, Stone NN. Penile erectile function after permanent radioactive seed implantation for treatment of prostate cancer. J Urol 2001; 165(2):436–439.

12. Huggins C, Hodges CV. Studies on prostatic cancer. 1. The effect of castration, estrogen and of androgen injection on serum phosphates in metastatic carcinoma of the prostate. Cancer Res 1941; 1:293–297.

13. Connolly JA, Shinohara K, Presti JC, et al. Should cryosurgery be considered a therapeutic option in localized prostate cancer? Urol Clin North Am 1996; 23(4):623–631.

14. Waldinger M, Hergeveld M, Zwinderman A. Paroxetine treatment of premature ejaculation: a double-blind randomized placebo-controlled study. Am J Psychiatry 1994; 151(9):1377–1379.

15. Ferrini RL, Barrett-Connor E. Sex hormones and age: a cross-sectional study of testosterone and estradiol and their bioavailable fractions in community-dwelling men. Am J Epidemiol 1998; 147(8):750–754.

16. Vermeulen A. The male climaterium. Ann Med 1993; 25:531–534.

17. Rajfer J, Aronson EJ, Bush PA, et al. Nitric oxide as a mediator of the corpus cavernosum in response to non-cholinergic, non-adrenergic neurotransmission. N Engl J Med 1992; 326(2):90–94.

18. Goldstein I, Lue TF, Padma-Nathan H, et al. Oral sildenafil in the treatment of erectile dysfunction. N Engl J Med 1998; 338(20):1397–1404.

19. Data on File, Pfizer Inc. Sandwich, Kent, U.K.

20. Zippe CD, Pasqualotto FF, Agarwals, et al. Impact of bilateral neurovascular bundles on response to Viagra following radical prostatectomy [abstr]. J Urol 2000; 163:893A.

21. Herrmann HC, Chang G, Klugherz BD, et al. Hemodynamic effects of sildenafil in men with severe coronary artery disease. N Engl J Med 2000; 342(22): 1622–1626.

22. Kloner RA, Jarow JP. Erectile dysfunction and sildenafil citrate and cardiologists. Am J Cardiol 1999; 83(4):576–582.

23. Susset JG, Tesier CD, Winze J. Effect of yohimbine hydrochloride on erectile impotence: a double blind study. J Urol 1989; 141(6):1360–1363.

24. Brindley GS. Pilot experiments on the action of drugs injected in the human corpus cavernosum penis. Br J Pharmacol 1986; 87:495–500.

25. Porst H. The rationale for prostaglandin e1 in erectile failure: a survey of worldwide experience. J Urol 1996; 155(3):802–815.

26. Chung WS, Lieskovsky G, Skinner DG, et al. The value of a nerve sparing approach in post-operative response to intracavernosal phamacotherapy following radical prostatectomy [abstr]. J Urol 1993; 149:231A.

27. Montorsi F, Guazzoni G, Barbieri L, et al. Recover of spontaneous erectile function after nerve sparing radical prostatectomy with and without early intracavernous injections of prostaglandin E-1: results of a prospective randomized trial [abstr]. J Urol 1996; 155:628A.

28. Nehra A, Nugent M, Pabby A, et al. An in vivo model for transforming growth factor–β1 induced corporal fibrosis: implications for penile ischemia associated fibrosis [abstr]. J Urol 1996; 155:1243A.

29. Padma-Nathan H, Hellstrom WJG, Kaiser FE, et al. Treatment of men with erectile dysfunction with transurethral alprostadil. N Engl J Med 1997; 336:1–7.

30. Witherington R. Suction device therapy in the management of erectile impotence. Urol Clin North Am 1988; 15(1):123–128.

31. Nadig PW, Ware JC, Blumoff R. Non-Invasive device to produce and maintain an erection-like state. Urology 1986; 27(2):126–131.

32. Gilbert HW, Gingell JC. Vacuum constriction devices: second-line conservative treatment for impotence. Br J Urol 1992; 70(1):81–83.

33. Earle CM, Seah M, Coulden SE, et al. The use of the vacuum erection device in the management of erectile impotence. Int J Impot Res 1996; 8(4):237–240.

34. Kabalin JN, Kou JC. Long-term followup and patient satisfaction with the Dynaflex self-contained inflatable penile prosthesis. J Urol 1997; 158(2):456–459.

35. Fallon B, Ghanem H. Sexual performance and satisfaction with penile prostheses in impotence of various etiologies. Int J Imp Res 1990; 2:35–42.

36. Carson CC, Mulcahy JJ, Govier FE. Efficacy, safety, and patient satisfaction outcomes of the AMS 700CX inflatable penile prosthesis: results of a long-term multicenter study. J Urol 2000; 164(2):376–380.

37. Sherine GE, O'Fallon WM, Kurland LT, et al. Risk of connective tissue diseases and other disorders after breast implantation. N Engl J Med 1994; 330: 1697–1702.

38. Carson CC. Infections in genitourinary prostheses. Urol Clin North Am 1989; 16(1):139.

39. Mulcahy JJ. Long-term experience with salvage of infected penile implants. J Urol 2000; 163(2):481–482.

Treatment of Sexual Dysfunction in Men with Spinal-Cord Injury and Other Neurologic Disabling Diseases

Manoj Monga
Department of Urologic Surgery, University of Minnesota, Minneapolis, Minnesota, U.S.A.

□ INTRODUCTION

Neurogenic dysfunction is estimated to be a major contributing factor in 20% of patients with erectile dysfunction (ED) (1). The sequelae of neurologic disorders may affect sexual functioning in an indirect manner. For example, patients with neurologic disorders may have language, auditory, visual, or sensory deficits, which could make it difficult to comprehend sexual cues, to experience cognitive and sensory stimulation, and to express their sexual desires, feelings, and interests. Fatigue, weakness, ataxia, and spasticity may also interfere with sexual functioning (2). Men with multiple sclerosis (MS) reported fatigue (47%), muscle weakness (32%), muscle spasms (10%), loss of sensation (13%), and pain (16%) as generalized conditions contributing to their sexual dysfunction (3). Patients may also fear poor performance that results in rejection from their partners, and further, that any deterioration in sexual relations may lead to progression of their neurologic disease, such as precipitating a second cerebrovascular accident (CVA) (4). Additionally, changes in the partner's perception of the patient with regard to his neurologic disorder may alter the partner's attitude toward the place for sexuality in their relationship. Neurological diseases can thus have a profound impact on the patient's relationship with his partner as well as his personal self-image.

Many of the factors predisposing to neurologic disorders overlap with the risk factors for ED. For example, smoking, hypertension, and diabetes mellitus may result in vascular and neurological changes that can lead to both CVA and ED. As part of normal aging, the penile sensory thresholds become elevated, serum testosterone levels decrease, penile nitric oxide synthase (NOS) activity decreases, and alterations in corporal collagen leads to veno-occlusive dysfunction and decreased neuronal transmission. Therefore, the pathophysiology of ED in neurologic disabling diseases is multifactorial, reflecting the combination of vascular, neurological, hormonal, psychological, and age-related changes in the penis that characterize ED in the general population.

This chapter will first briefly outline the neuroanatomy and physiology of erectile function with the goal of focusing on the evaluation and treatment of male sexual functioning in patients who have sustained neurological injury. The words of Alex Comfort should be heeded: "Nobody is too disabled to derive some satisfaction and personal reinforcement from sex. Human sex is widely versatile and hardly limited to the genitalia" (5).

□ BACKGROUND: NEUROANATOMY AND PHYSIOLOGY OF ERECTILE FUNCTION

Sexual excitation is the result of integrated tactile, visual, auditory, and olfactory stimulation, as modulated cognitively by societal, cultural, and behavioral norms. The physical response to sexual excitation, however, requires intact autonomic and somatic nervous systems. Somatosensory receptors in the penis converge to form the dorsal nerve of the penis, which joins the pudendal nerve. Stimulation of the dorsal nerve of the penis is transmitted through low-threshold pudendal sensory fibers and results in long latency discharges in the cavernous nerves, suggesting a polysynaptic reflex response (6). Afferents for the spinal interneuronal reflex pathway terminate in the medial portions of the lumbosacral spinal gray matter (7). Somatic motor neurons of the pudendal nerve originate in the second-through-fourth sacral spinal-cord segments (Onuf's nucleus).

Ascending sensory stimulation from the penis (touch, pain, pressure, temperature, and proprioception) is transmitted via the pudendal nerve to the spinothalamic and spinoreticular tracts of the spinal cord and then to the posterolateral and medial thalamus and brainstem reticular formation, respectively. Cortically evoked potentials are highest in the midline (Cz-2) sensory cortex following electrical stimulation of the dorsal nerve of the penis (8). Descending inhibition of spinal sexual reflexes is mediated by serotonin-dependent tonic inhibitory control from the nucleus paragigantocellularis in the brainstem (9,10).

The medial preoptic area of the hypothalamus (MPOA) is an important integration site that provides supraspinal control of the erectile response. MPOA lesions will prevent male copulatory behavior but have no effect on nocturnal penile erections or masturbation (11,12). The MPOA receives sensory input from the locus coeruleus, α-2 adrenergic inhibition from the medial amygdala in the forebrain, and stimulation through dopaminergic stimulatory paths (central D2-dopamine receptors). Visually evoked sexual stimulation results in increased activity in the right insula and right inferior frontal and left anterior cingulate paralimbic cortical areas (13). The MPOA receives input from the periaqueductal gray in the midbrain during copulation. This area of the midbrain has a high density of androgen receptors, and electrolytic lesions in this area result in faster copulation (14,15). The MPOA also connects with the paraventricular nucleus, which stimulates oxytocin secretion during sexual arousal (16). Both electrical stimulation of the paraventricular nucleus (PVN) and central nervous system infusion of oxytocin result in a penile erection (17,18). Stimulation of the MPOA results in a parasympathetically mediated erection (19).

The nonadrenergic, noncholinergic neural pathways stimulate an erection by the production of nitric oxide by NOS. Immunohistochemical studies have also demonstrated the presence of NOS within the lumbosacral spinal cord. Nitric oxide results in relaxation of the cavernosal smooth muscle and cavernosal arteries through a cGMP-mediated pathway (20).

Detumescence of the penis results following sympathetic-mediated contraction of the smooth muscle and cavernosal arteries in the corpora cavernosa of the penis.

For further details on the neuroanatomy, neurophysiology, and neuroendocrine control of erectile function, see chapters in Part I of this volume.

☐ CLINICAL EVALUATION OF ED PATIENTS WITH SPINAL-CORD INJURY OR OTHER NEUROLOGIC DISABLING DISEASES
History and Physical Examination

The assessment of the patient presenting with sexual dysfunction should be no different from any other standard evaluation in that the patient history and physical examination are of utmost importance, particularly since sexual complaints are often largely subjective observations. A significant portion of the history should consider the degree, if any, of psychogenic overlay to the underlying organic dysfunction. Depression may be a significant correlate with ED in neurologically impaired patients (21). The physical exam should include the inspection of hormone-dependent secondary sexual characteristics such as vocal tone, muscle development, and hair distribution. Peripheral visual fields are evaluated to detect any potential mass-occupying lesion in the sella tursica.

The breasts are inspected and palpated for gynecomastia. Palpation of femoral and lower extremity pulses provides insight into the vascular status of the man. The prostate is palpated for asymmetry or nodularity that would indicate the possibility of occult prostate cancer. For further guidelines on performing a history and physical exam in patients with ED, see Chapter 22.

Neurologic Examination

The focused neurologic examination of patients presenting with sexual dysfunction includes an evaluation of perianal sensation and rectal sphincter tone. The bulbocavernosus reflex (BCR) establishes the integrity of the pudendal nerve and sacral arc and is performed by inspection or palpation of the rectal sphincter while compressing the glans penis (22). Loss of the BCR correlates with ED in spinal-cord injury (SCI) and MS (23). Other studies suggest that loss of the BCR does not correlate with ED in MS (24). Pyramidal dysfunction in the lower extremity may correlate with ED in the neurologically impaired (23,25); however, the severity of pyramidal dysfunction does not correlate with the degree of ED. For further details on the neurologic examination, see Chapter 26.

Laboratory Values

Total or free testosterone levels should be evaluated in all individuals over the age of 50 as well as those with signs or symptoms that suggest an underlying hormonal imbalance, such as decreased libido or testicular atrophy. A serum prolactin level would be ordered if the patient complains of headaches, if visual field disturbances are noted on physical examination, or if the serum testosterone level is noted to be low. A serum prostate-specific antigen (PSA) should be tested in men over the age of 50 or prior to initiation of androgen supplementation to exclude the presence of an occult prostate cancer. No specific link between CVA and hypogonadism has been identified (26). For further information on laboratory testing, see Chapter 22.

Additional Evaluations

Objective testing does not often have a role in the routine evaluation and therapy of ED presenting with concomitant neurologic disorders; however, these special investigations may be helpful in select cases or for investigational purposes. Nocturnal penile tumescence (NPT) monitoring, for example, is helpful in evaluating the integrity of the pelvic nerves' efferent component of erectile function in order to differentiate neurogenic and psychogenic impotence in SCI and other neurologic disorders (27). NPT has been reported to be normal in the majority of patients with MS (24); however, more restrictive criteria for normality (rigidity ≥ 80%, duration > 30 minutes) may be needed to differentiate between psychogenic and neurogenic etiologies in patients with MS (28). For further information on NPT monitoring, see Chapter 23.

The pudendal nerve afferent circuit can be measured by evaluating the vibration perception threshold of the penile skin with penile biothesiometry (1). Vascular inflow can be measured noninvasively with Doppler ultrasound and the veno-occlusive mechanism can be assessed with dynamic infusion cavernosometry (29). Single potential analysis of cavernous electrical activity (SPACE) using needle electrodes in the corpora cavernosa can measure abnormal autonomic activity in the corpora (30). Sympathetic skin response recordings of the perineal skin can assess the thoracolumbar sympathetic outflow, which has been shown to correlate with preservation of psychogenic erections in SCI (31). The pudendal nerve afferent pathway may be evaluated with dorsal nerve somatosensory-evoked potential testing (1). Abnormalities in posterior tibial cortical-evoked potentials have been demonstrated to correlate with ED in men with MS and may serve as a surrogate measure of pudendal cortical-evoked potentials (23). Neurophysiological results, however, did not correlate with the severity of ED. Other studies have reported no correlation between pudendal-evoked potentials or motor-evoked potentials of the bulbocavernosus muscle and the presence or severity of ED in MS (24). For further information on these specialized evaluations, see Chapter 26.

☐ MANAGEMENT AND CLINICAL RESULTS OF ED IN PATIENTS WITH SCI AND OTHER NEUROLOGIC DISABLING DISEASES
Psychological Counseling and Behavior Modification

Sexual preferences may change following the development of neurologic disease. Men with SCI are less likely to engage in intercourse (54%) than in oral sexual activities (78%) (32). An inability to discuss sexuality with the spouse correlates significantly with a decrease in coital frequency and increase in sexual dissatisfaction in men with CVA (33); further, the partner's desire for sex has been shown to correlate with the frequency of sexual activity after SCI (32).

The management of ED in neurologically disabled patients requires empathy, sensitivity, and respect. Proactive counseling by health-care providers for men with physical disabilities should be encouraged, and subjects such as love, intimacy, and sexual expression should be addressed. A coordinated, compassionate approach is needed to help preserve the relationship between the patient and his partner. Social discord in the relationship may indicate the need for joint counseling with a physiatrist, urologist, gynecologist, social worker, marital counselor, clergyman, or psychiatrist. A survey of men with MS reported that only 21% had received counseling about sexual issues, and only 11% had discussed these issues with their physicians (3).

The couple should be reassured regarding the safety of sexual activities in relation to their neurologic

disorder. Certain sexual positions may be recommended based on the specific neurologic deficit. For example, hemiplegics may find that lying on the affected side allows the unaffected arm to caress his partner, and with a pillow to support his back, rear entry may be possible (34). Alternatively, a partner-superior position may facilitate sexual relations in most circumstances. Patients who suffer from fatigue should be encouraged to rest frequently during the day and experiment with sexual relations at varying times of the day (2). Warm baths prior to sexual activity may help decrease spasticity (2). The couple should also be encouraged to experiment with sensate focusing and increased foreplay. Nipple stimulation will result in sexual arousal in 75% of paraplegics and 50% of quadriplegics (35). The health-care provider may stimulate a broader dialogue between the couple in order to evaluate their wants and needs.

An important component of counseling is reassurance that a wide range of treatment options is available. The "ED Pyramid" was designed to portray to the couple the step-incremental approach to the therapy of ED (Fig. 1).

General Rehabilitative Efforts

The patient should be encouraged to participate in a rehabilitative graduated exercise program because improvements in overall health will also be beneficial for sexual functioning. Gains in functional status and coping skills will translate into a higher self-esteem and improved relationship dynamics. Retraining of cognitive, sensory, and perceptual deficits may overcome difficulties with comprehension and expression of sexual cues and integration of cognitive and sensory stimulation.

Specific ED Treatment Strategies for Patients with Common Neurologic Conditions
Spinal-Cord Injury

It is estimated that traumatic SCI in socioeconomically advanced countries has an annual incidence rate of three individuals per 100,000 (36). Of the victims, 82% are males, and the majority is in their prime reproductive years (mean age 26 years) (37).

In general, sexual desire decreases after SCI; however, 78% to 80% of men report that their sexual desire remains appropriate or high (32,35). Preservation of libido is independent of preserved genital sensation (32). Sexual arousal remains normal or high in 81% of men with SCI, and arousability does not correlate with level or completeness of injury (32).

Sexual functioning following SCI depends on both location and extent of the injury. Reflexogenic erections are preserved in 93% to 95% of SCI patients with complete upper-motor neuron (UMN) lesions and 93% to 99% with incomplete UMN lesions. Psychogenic erections are achieved in only 9% of complete UMN lesions and 48% of incomplete UMN lesions. Reflexogenic erections are preserved in 0% to

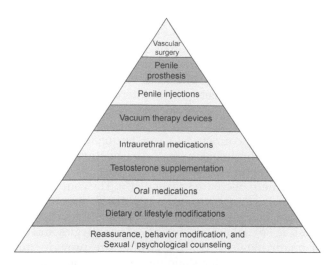

Figure 1 The ED Pyramid. An important component of counseling is reassurance that a wide range of treatment options is available for ED. The "ED Pyramid" was designed to portray to the couple the step-incremental approach to the therapy of ED. *Abbreviation*: ED, erectile dysfunction.

12% of patients with complete lower-motor neuron (LMN) lesions; however, 24% to 26% maintained the ability to have psychogenic erections. Of patients with incomplete LMN lesions, 90% could achieve an erection (38,39). All patients with lesions caudal to the 12th thoracic cord segment achieve a psychogenic erection irrespective of severity of the lesion (27).

As erectile function relies on an intact sensory and autonomic nervous system, SCI may have a direct impact on sexuality. Complete spinal-cord transection does not prevent sexual arousal and climax because the erectile response is coordinated at the spinal level (40). Reflexogenic erections are mediated via pathways in the sacral spinal cord and involve the parasympathetic nervous system. Psychogenic erections involve communication between cortical stimuli and both sympathetic and parasympathetic centers in the spinal cord.

In an animal model, after T-10 spinal-cord transection, alterations in the nitric oxide system have been demonstrated. A threefold increase in NOS mRNA was demonstrated in the penis and pelvic ganglia after spinal-cord transection. Disruption of serotonin-mediated tonic inhibitory control from the nucleus paragigantocellularis in the brainstem after spinal transection may reduce the sensory threshold and facilitate the onset and number of erectile responses (9,10). From a clinical standpoint, these changes would suggest that SCI would render the patient supersensitive to the effects of agents such as sildenafil that promote the nitric oxide–mediated erection (41).

ED in the SCI patient is primarily neurogenic because the prevalence of other risk factors such as hypertension and diabetes is low in this young population; however, psychogenic ED may be identified as the primary etiology in up to 10% of men with SCI (27).

Sildenafil (Viagra®) was released in March 1998. Within the first year, over 10 million prescriptions were filled. As a competitive and selective inhibitor of cGMP-specific phosphodiesterase 5, the primary phosphodiesterase in cavernosal tissue, sildenafil increases cGMP levels, resulting in an increase in cavernosal tumescence and rigidity (6). Efficacy in unselected populations has ranged from 68% to 71% (42). Reported side effects include headache (7–25%), flushing (7–34%), dyspepsia (1–11%), rhinitis (4–19%), and visual disturbances (1–6%) (42). Sildenafil is used "on demand" about 20 to 60 minutes prior to intercourse.

Stable cardiovascular disease is not a contraindication to the use of sildenafil. The concomitant use of nitrates and sildenafil, however, is an absolute contraindication. Patients with a significant cardiac history and sedentary lifestyle should institute a behavioral modification program prior to receiving sildenafil. This should incorporate a graduated exercise program, dietary modification, tobacco cessation, and weight loss. For further details on the treatment of sexual dysfunction specifically in the cardiovascular patient, see Chapter 36.

A placebo-controlled study of men with an intact reflexogenic erectile response following traumatic SCI of the lower thoracic and lumbar spinal cord provided objective and subjective evidence of the efficacy of sildenafil in men with SCI (37,43). Penile-base rigidity and penile-tip rigidity of greater than 60% was significantly more common with sildenafil (65% and 46%, respectively) compared to placebo (8% and 4%) (43). Subjective improvement in erections was reported in 75% of men on sildenafil as compared to 7% on placebo (37). Subsequent placebo-controlled studies demonstrated 64% of patients with no residual erectile function (reflexogenic or psychogenic) and 78% of patients with residual erectile function noted improvement in erection, frequency of vaginal penetration, and frequency of maintained erection (44–46). Other studies have suggested an efficacy of 93% in men with SCI, with ongoing long-term use of the medication by 88% of the men (31). Only 2 of 41 patients in this study, however, had a prior loss of both reflexive and psychogenic erections, and patients enrolled in the study were preselected by a positive response to intracavernosal prostaglandin E_1 (PGE$_1$). The most common dose required to optimize response in this study was 50 mg (58%); however, patients with complete lesions were more likely to require higher doses (55%) than patients with incomplete lesions (29%). A trend was noted toward higher dose requirements for men with LMN lesions as compared to those with UMN lesions.

Sildenafil treatment resulted in a median of 55% of successful attempts at sexual intercourse (46). Improvements in quality-of-life parameters relating to mental health, general well-being, depression, and anxiety in men with SCI also occurred with sildenafil (47). Treatment-related side effects in men with SCI included headaches (7–17%), flushing (5–7%), dizziness (5%), dyspepsia (2–3%), rhinitis (2%), and transient changes in visual hues or blurred vision (2%) (31,46). For more general information on sildenafil, see Chapter 29.

Though topical formulations of vasoactive agents are an active area of investigation, to date no formulation has demonstrated sufficient, reliable clinical responses to justify further development. Topical agents have included nitroprusside, nitroglycerin, minoxidil, PGE_1, and vasoactive intestinal peptide (VIP). Although a topical PGE_1 gel produced increases in mean cavernous artery flow velocity and diameter, an erection sufficient for penetration was observed in only two of eight spinal cord–injured patients tested (48). Minoxidil 2% solution produced minimal or no success both objectively and subjectively in men with SCI (49). Topical nitroglycerin resulted in an erection adequate for vaginal penetration in only 29% of SCI men who had responded to intracavernosal papaverine. Side effects included hypotension and headache (50). For further information on these topical agents, see Chapter 30.

Medicated Urethral System for Erection (MUSE®) is a novel intraurethral delivery system that involves the administration of an intraurethral PGE_1 suppository. Initial studies that reported a 65% success rate with MUSE excluded patients with SCI (51). The effects of MUSE are dampened by systemic absorption of the medication through the well-vascularized corpus spongiosum before the PGE_1 reaches the corpora cavernosa. Systemic absorption of prostaglandin after the insertion of MUSE can result in orthostatic hypotension and syncope. The use of a venous constrictive band at the base of the penis prior to insertion of MUSE is recommended to prevent systemic absorption. Transient hypotensive episodes (systolic decrease of 20 mmHg and/or diastolic decrease of 10 mmHg) were effectively prevented in all SCI patients who used a constricting band (52). For additional information on intraurethral agents, see Chapter 30.

A variety of other vasoactive agents including papaverine, phentolamine, and PGE_1 have been used for intracavernosal therapy for ED. A 27-gauge needle is inserted into the corpora cavernosum. Intracavernosal injection therapy requires a degree of visual acuity and manual dexterity that may be decreased in a patient with a neurologic disorder. In these situations, the partner may be trained in injection technique.

The use of intracavernosal injections of papaverine, phentolamine, and PGE_1 in SCI results in a success rate over 95%, which is defined as an erection adequate for penetration (53–55). Men with SCI may be supersensitive to intracavernosal vasoactive agents due to receptor upregulation and the lack of vascular disease in this relatively young population. The release of erection-inducing neurotransmitters from the parasympathetic nerves may be enhanced in neurologic disorders. Neurologic disorders may interfere with tonic discharge from the sympathetic nervous system that maintains and restores detumescence. Therefore, patients with SCI should be started on lower dosages of medication (papaverine 7.5 mg or PGE_1 2 μg) to decrease the risk of priapism (56,57). Lower dose

requirements have been demonstrated in patients with LMN lesions compared with UMN patients (58).

Because SCI patients require lower dosages of intracavernosal agents for adequate erection and engage in fewer sexual acts per week than a cohort of vascular or psychogenic patients, their risk of penile fibrosis may be reduced (59,60). Papaverine is associated with a higher rate of fibrosis when compared to PGE-1. Although the development of penile fibrosis is dose dependent, the duration of therapy does not correlate with the risk of fibrosis. When fibrosis develops, discontinuation of the medication for three to four months is recommended. For additional information on intracavernosal agents, see Chapter 30.

The use of vacuum erection devices requires adequate manual dexterity or a partner who is willing to incorporate the use of the device into foreplay. Small battery-operated models may be most appropriate in men with neurologic deficits. Erections adequate for vaginal penetration with the use of the vacuum erection device were reported by 93% and 76% men with SCI at three and six months, respectively. Premature detumescence was the most common complaint. Other side effects included ecchymosis (46%), petechiae (77%), skin edema (38%), abrasions (31%), discomfort (13%), and leg spasms (7%) (61,62). For further information on vacuum erection devices, see Chapter 32.

Special considerations regarding the use of penile prosthesis in men with neurologic disorders include the potential for increased risk of infection associated with neurogenic bladder dysfunction and the increased risk of erosion and extrusion of the prosthesis due to impaired sensation (63,64).

The insertion of penile prostheses in men with SCI may be associated with significant complications. Dietzen et al. followed 30 SCI patients who underwent implantation of penile prostheses and reported high rates of mechanical failure (43%), infection (37%), prosthesis extrusion (10%), and hematoma formation (7%) (65). Other investigators have reported a 25% prosthesis-extrusion rate (66). Similarly, Kabalin and Kessler reported a 25% explantation rate for infection or erosion of the prosthesis (67). Iwatsubo et al. reported a 5% complication rate; however, the majority of patients reported either no benefit (48%) or no dissatisfaction (11%) with the penile prosthesis (68).

Field electrical implant stimulation of the anterior root of S2 results in a full erection in 60% of men with SCI (69); however, since the Food and Drug Administration–approved implants for bladder dysfunction utilize two channel electrodes targeted at S3 and S4, the expected effects on sexual function will be significantly less. For further information about penile prosthetics, see Chapters 33 and 41.

Stroke (CVA)

The impact of CVA on sexual functioning is well documented. Long-term follow-up of married men four to six years following CVA demonstrated that 68% were dissatisfied with their sex life (70). Normal libido was reported by only 21% of men after CVA compared to 75% of men prior to CVA (4). A decrease in libido was reported by 57% of CVA patients and 65% of their spouses (33). An interview study of subjects who have been CVA patients for less than six years demonstrated that CVA diminishes libido as well as coital frequency. The decline in sexual functioning was more common in patients with right-sided weakness as compared to those with left-sided weakness (71). Other studies confirmed that a decrease in libido was more prevalent in subjects with dominant hemispheric lesions (72); however, some studies have not supported this observation (4,26).

Cessation of coital activity has been reported by 41% to 64% of men post-CVA (4,26). Only 45% of men remained sexually active post-CVA compared to 79% of men before CVA (33). Cessation of foreplay was reported by 31% of men after CVA (26). Difficulty in achieving an erection or premature ejaculation after CVA has been reported by 62% to 64% and 35% of the men, respectively (4,73).

Sexual dysfunction and changes in coital frequency after CVA have been shown to correlate with the degree of cutaneous sensibility impairment, level of dependency in activities of daily living, and degree of motor impairment (34,74). Although loss of expressive communicative abilities contributes to problems with sexual adjustment in aphasic patients, the preservation of good auditory comprehension and nonverbal communication ability provides an avenue for sexual readjustment (74).

Some studies have suggested that dominant hemispheric lesions result in a more severe decrease in libido (71) whereas others have reported no significant correlation between sexual function in men after CVA and side of lesion (4,26). Patients with temporal lobe lesions may exhibit hypersexuality and deviant sexual behavior as characterized in the Kluver-Bucy syndrome (75).

Multiple Sclerosis

Multiple sclerosis (MS) is a chronic, progressively degenerative neurological disease of young adults (76), most commonly occurring during the reproductive years between the ages of 20 and 40 (2,76). Considering this age group, it is not surprising, then, that 87% of men with MS report that sexual issues are of great importance to them (3).

MS is an inflammatory process marked by focal demyelination and plaque formation in the central nervous system (76); thus, ED is an unusual presenting symptom in MS, more commonly occurring considerably after the onset of urinary symptoms (23).

Sexual dysfunction is reported by 75% to 91% of men with MS. A decrease in coital frequency subsequent to the diagnosis of MS has been reported by 58% to 76% of men (3,21,25,77,78). ED in MS is believed to be the result of lesions in the lateral horns of the dorsolumbar cord, the most common site affected by MS.

This hypothesis is supported by the observations that pudendal and tibial cortical-evoked potentials and BCRs are abnormal in the majority of men with ED and MS (23,79). Decreased sensation has been shown to correlate with a decrease in libido (77).

MS lesions in the brain may also affect libido (2). The observation that duration or severity of disease does not correlate with ED suggests that location of plaque is a more important variable than extent of involvement (2,21,23,77,79).

Severity of sexual dysfunction fluctuates with exacerbations of MS. Of the patients, 38% reported fluctuation in the degree of sexual dysfunction and 47% reported fluctuation in libido that mirrored changes in their MS activity. Sexual dysfunction was felt to be causing marital problems in 33% of the men with MS (21). No association with duration of disease or degree of disability was identified (21,23,77,79).

A recent study compared the frequency of sexual dysfunction in men with MS to age-matched healthy controls and patients with chronic musculoskeletal disease (3). Absence of sexual intercourse over the preceding year was reported by 25% of MS patients compared to 9% in the chronic disease group and 5% in the healthy group. ED was reported by 63% of the men with MS when compared to 13% of the group with chronic disease and 15% of the healthy group. Ejaculatory dysfunction was reported by 50% of the men with MS compared to 3% of the group with chronic disease and 15% of the healthy group. Finally, a decrease in libido was noted by 40% of men with MS, compared to 9% with chronic illness and 10% of healthy controls. Men with MS were more likely to report worsening of ED with progression of their disease (55%) compared to men with musculoskeletal chronic illnesses.

Other studies report that decreased libido (43–48%), ED (63–81%), orgasmic dysfunction (44–64%), decreased penile sensation (55–72%), and premature ejaculation (25%) were common complaints (21,77,78). Sexual dysfunction correlated significantly with pyramidal signs and spasticity in the lower extremities as well as urinary dysfunction. Some studies have suggested a link between ED and depression in patients with MS (21) whereas others have not (77); however, sexual dysfunction was noted in approximately 50% of patients without spasticity or urinary dysfunction (77).

A randomized double-blind, placebo-controlled, flexible-dose study of 217 men with MS demonstrated improved erections in 89% of men with sildenafil compared to 24% on placebo (80). Significant improvements in quality of life and measures of satisfaction with sexual life, partnership relations, family life, and social life were noted (81). Side effects in men with MS included headache (23%), flushing (13%), and rhinitis (5%) (80). For more general information on sildenafil, see Chapter 29.

Surprisingly, corticosteroid treatments that were started for problems other than sexual dysfunction resulted in improved sexual functioning in many patients. A retrospective patient survey suggested an observed improvement in sexual performance in response to corticosteroids in up to 40% of the patients (21). Corticosteroids were proposed to affect spinal-cord plaque inflammation and the production of edema as well as more general effects such as fatigue and depression (21).

Betts et al. reported a 98% success rate with intracorporeal injections of papaverine in men with MS, with 62% of men continuing on medication (23). Kirkeby et al. reported a 93% success rate with intracorporeal papaverine, with 79% of men using ongoing therapy (82). Dosage needed for a satisfactory response ranged from 7 to 80 mg (mean = 30 mg, median = 20 mg), with no apparent relationship between the dose required and the degree of neurologic disability (23). Other studies have suggested an inverse relationship between the degree of disability and the dosage of papaverine needed to produce an erection, due to "autonomic hypersensitivity" (79,82). Complications at two-year followup included priapism (managed with corporal aspiration) (24%) and development of a fibrotic plaque (2%) (23). Spontaneous recovery of erections during therapy was an uncommon observation (2%).

It has been proposed that vibratory stimulation may improve decreased genital sensation associated with MS; however, clinical data to support this approach is currently lacking (76).

Parkinson's Disease

Only 73% of patients with Parkinson's disease (PD) reported satisfaction with their current sex lives compared to 88% of age- and sex-matched community-derived controls (83). A decrease in coital frequency with the onset of PD has been reported by 80% of the men (43). Other studies have reported no difference in the frequency of intercourse in men with PD when compared to age-matched controls (83).

ED has been reported in 54% to 60% of men with PD, with no significant increases noted in ejaculatory dysfunction (43,84). It has been proposed that ED in PD is a symptom of a generalized autonomic dysfunction (84). In general, PD-related sexual dysfunction is thought to involve a decrease in limbic and hypothalamic dopaminergic activity, reduction in dopamine D_2 receptor function, and reduction in hypothalamic oxytocin production (85,86). Reduced dopaminergic stimulation from the brainstem may decrease the number of oxytocin-secreting neurons in the hypothalamic paraventricular nucleus (87).

Some studies report no decrease in libido (84) whereas others report a decrease in libido in 44% of the men (43). An increase in libido may occur in 1% to 50% of patients treated with levodopa (88). Hypersexuality is a rare occurrence in men being treated for PD and appears to correlate with an early onset of PD (88). Hypersexuality has been reported in patients being treated for PD with levodopa, dopamine agonists, and deprenyl. It has been postulated that the hypersexuality is the consequence of dopaminergic stimulation of libido and inhibition of prolactin secretion (88). Some patients demonstrated a dose-dependent onset of hypersexuality, and in all cases, hypersexuality resolved upon discontinuation of the anti-Parkinsonian medication (88).

An open-label pilot study ($n = 10$) and a placebo-controlled pilot study ($n = 10$) have reported improved sexual functioning and sexual satisfaction with sildenafil in men with PD (89,90). Sildenafil should be used with caution in men with PD and autonomic dysfunction (multiple system atrophy) because precipitous drops in blood pressure may occur (90).

Two cases of sexual arousal and spontaneous nocturnal erections occurring 12 to 24 hours following administration of transcranial picotesla flux density electromagnetic field stimulation of dopamine D_2 receptor sites have been reported in the literature (85).

Apomorphine is another sublingual medication under development. This drug was reportedly utilized as an emetic since the late nineteenth century and subsequently as a sedative in the early 1900s (91). As a central-acting dopaminergic agonist, it was utilized in trials for PD. Apomorphine, therefore, may be ideally suited for patients with neurologic disorders such as PD. Sublingual apomorphine stimulates a spontaneous erection within 15 to 30 minutes of ingestion. Clinical trials suggest a 60% to 70% efficacy rate, with the main side effect being nausea (30%) (92). A series of five PD patients with satisfactory erectile responses to subcutaneous apomorphine has been reported; significantly, one patient was able to resume sexual relations after 14 years of inactivity (86).

☐ FUTURE THERAPEUTIC DIRECTIONS

Most pharmaceutical companies maintain in the product pipeline some type of oral agent for ED in varying stages of development. The major thrust of current research is to develop a more specific PDE-5 inhibitor that might act faster with fewer side effects. For detailed specificities and comparison tables for each of the currently available PDE-5 inhibitors, see Chapter 29.

Identification of a penile-specific neuronal NOS gene on Intron 16 of chromosome 17 may open the avenue to more specific pharmacological and possibly gene therapy-directed intervention. Iontophoresis and electroporation may improve delivery of topical formulations to the corpora cavernosa.

Goal-directed therapy will remain the mainstay of treatment of ED in men with or without neurologic disorders. The choice of therapy is often defined more by the patient's current sexual relationship and the needs and desires of both the patient and the partner as it is by the underlying neurological disease. Therapy for ED, therefore, should be tailored to the preferences and goals of the couple. The impact of sexual dysfunction on quality of life, self-esteem, and social relations should not be underestimated.

□ REFERENCES

1. Padma-Nathan H. Neurologic evaluation of erectile dysfunction. Urol Clin N Am 1988; 15(1):77–80.

2. Grana EA. Sexuality issues in multiple sclerosis. Physical Med Rehab: State of the Art Reviews 1995; 9(4):377–385.

3. Zorzon M, Zivadinov R, Bosco A, et al. Sexual dysfunction in multiple sclerosis: a case-control study. I. Frequency and comparison of groups. Mult Scler 1999; 5(6):418–427.

4. Monga TN, Lawson JS, Inglis J. Sexual dysfunction in stroke patients. Arch Phys Med Rehabil 1986; 67(1): 19–22.

5. Comfort A. Foreword. In: Mooney TO, Cole TM, Chilgren RA, eds. Sexual Options for Paraplegics and Quadriplegics. Boston: Little Brown, 1975.

6. Goldstein I, Lue TF, Padma-Nathan H, et al. Oral sildenafil in the treatment of ED. N Engl J Med 1998; 338: 1397–1404.

7. Fedirchuk B, Song L, Downie JW, et al. Spinal distribution of extracellular field potentials generated by electrical stimulation of pudendal and perineal afferents in the cat. Exp Brain Res 1992; 89(3):517–520.

8. Geurit JM, Opsomer RJ. Bit-mapped imaging of somatosensory evoked potentials after stimulation of the posterior tibial nerves and dorsal nerve of the penis/clitoris. Electroencephalogr Clin Neurophysiol 1991; 80(3):228–237.

9. Marson L, McKenna KE. The identification of a brainstem site controlling spinal sexual reflexes in male rats. Brain Res 1990; 515(1–2):303–308.

10. Marson L, McKenna KE. A role for 5-hydorxyptryptamine in descending inhibition of spinal sexual reflexes. Exp Brain Res 1992; 88(2):313–320.

11. Schmidt MH, Valatx JL, Sakai K, et al. Role of the lateral preoptic area in sleep-related erectile mechanisms and sleep generation in the rat. J Neurosci 2000; 20(17): 6640–6647.

12. Slimp JC, Hart BL, Goy RW. Heterosexual, autosexual and social behavior of adult male rhesus monkeys with medial preoptic-anterior hypothalamic lesions. Brain Res 1975; 142(1):105–122.

13. Stoleru S, Gregoire MC, Gerard D, et al. Neuroanatomical correlates of visually evoked sexual arousal in human males. Arch Sex Behav 1999; 28(1):1–21.

14. Greco B, Edwards DA, Zumpe D, et al. Androgen receptor and mating-induced fos immunoreactivity are co-localized in limbic and midbrain neurons that project to the male rat medial preoptic area. Brain Res 1998; 781(1–2):15–24.

15. Barfield RJ, Wilson C, McDonald PG. Sexual behavior: extreme reduction of post-ejaculatory refractory period by midbrain lesions in male rats. Science 1975; 189(4197):147–149.

16. Carmichael MS, Warburton VL, Dixen J, et al. Relationships among cardiovascular, muscular and oxytocin responses during human sexual activity. Arch Sex Behav 1994; 23(1):59–79.

17. Chen KK, Chan JYH, Chang LS, et al. Elicitation of penile erection following activation of the hippocampal formation in the rat. Neurosci Lett 1992; 141(2): 218–222.

18. Argiolas A, Melis MR, Gessa GL. Oxytocin: an extremely potent inducer of penile erection and yawning in male rats. Eur J Pharmacol 1986; 130(3):265–272.

19. Giuliano F, Bernabe J, Brown K, et al. Erectile response to hypothalamic stimulation in rats: role of peripheral nerves. Am J Physiol 1997; 273(6):R1990–R1997.

20. Burnett AL. Nitric oxide control of lower genitourinary tract functions: a review. Urology 1995; 45(6):1071–1083.

21. Mattson D, Petrie M, Srivastava DK, et al. Multiple sclerosis: sexual dysfunction and its response to medications. Arch Neurol 1995; 52(9):862–868.

22. Bors E, Blinn KA. Bulbocavernous reflex. J Urol 1959; 82:128–130.

23. Betts CD, Jones SJ, Fowler CG, et al. Erectile dysfunction in multiple sclerosis: associated neurological and neurophysiological deficits, and treatment of the condition. Brain 1994; 117(6):1303–1310.

24. Ghezzi A, Malvestiti GM, Baldini S, et al. Erectile impotence in multiple sclerosis: a neuorphysiological study. J Neurol 1995; 242(3):123–126.

25. Lilius HG, Valtonen E, Wikstrom J. Sexual problems in patients suffering from multiple sclerosis. Scand J Soc Med 1976; 4(1):41–44.

26. Sjogren K, Damber JE, Liliequist B. Sexuality after stroke with hemiplegia: I. aspects of sexual function. Scand J Rehabil Med 1983; 15(2):55–61.

27. Tay HP, Juma S, Joseph AC. Psychogenic impotence in spinal cord injury patients. Arch Phys Med Rehabil 1996; 77(4):391–393.

28. Staerman F, Guiraud P, Coeurdacier P, et al. Value of nocturnal penile tumescence and rigidity (NPTR) recording in impotent patients with multiple sclerosis. Int J Impot Res 1996; 8(4):241–245.

29. Padma-Nathan H, Kanellos A. The management of ED following spinal cord injury. Sem Urol 1992; 10: 133–137.

30. Stief CG, Hoppner C, Sauerwein D, et al. Single potential analysis of cavernous electrical activity in spinal cord injury patients. J Urol 1994; 151(2):367–372.

31. Schmid DM, Schurch B, Hauri D. Sildenafil in the treatment of sexual dysfunction in spinal cord-injured male patients. Eur Urol 2000; 38(2):184–193.

32. Alexander CJ, Sipski ML, Findley TW. Sexual activities, desire and satisfaction in males pre- and post-spinal cord injury. Arch Sex Behav 1993; 22(3):217–228.

33. Korpelainen JT, Nieminen P, Myllyla VV. Sexual functioning among stroke patients and their spouses. Stroke 1999; 30(4):715–719.

34. Fugl-Meyer AR, Jaasko L. Post-stroke hemiplegia and sexual intercourse. Scand J Rehabil Med 1980; 7:158–166.

35. Phelps G, Brown M, Chen J, et al. Sexual experience and plasma testosterone levels in male veterans after spinal cord injury. Arch Phys Med Rehab 1983; 64(2):47–52.

36. Kurtzke JF. Epidemiology of SCI. Neurologia-Neurocirugia-Psiquiatria 1977; 18(suppl 2–3):157–191.

37. Derry F, Dinsmore WW, Fraser M, et al. Efficacy and safety of oral sildenafil (Viagra) in men with ED caused by spinal cord injury. Neurology 1998; 51:1629–1633.

38. Bors E, Comarr AE. Neurological disturbances of sexual function with special reference to 529 patients with spinal cord injury. Urol Surv 1960; 110:191–221.

39. Comarr AE. Sexual function among patients with spinal cord injury. Urol Int 1970; 25(2):134–168.

40. McKenna KE, Chung SK, McVary KT. A model for the study of sexual function in anesthetized male and female rats. Am J Physiol 261(5 Pt 2):1276–1285.

41. Brock GB, Abdel-Baky TM, Begin L. Spinal cord injury is associated with a disturbance in the statement of penile nitric oxide synthase: a paraplegic animal model. J Urol 1998; 159(suppl):94.

42. Sadovsky R, Miller T, Moskowitz M, et al. Three-year update of sildenafil citrate (Viagra) efficacy and safety. Int J Clin Pract 2001; 55(2):115–128.

43. Maytom MA, Derry FA, Dinsmore WW, et al. A two-part pilot study of sildenafil (Viagra) in men with erectile dysfunction caused by spinal cord injury. Spinal Cord 1999; 37(2):110–116.

44. Derry F, Glass C, Dinsmore W. Sildenafil (Viagra): an oral treatment for men with ED caused by traumatic spinal cord injury—a 28 day, double blind, placebo controlled, parallel-group, dose-response study. Neurology 1997; 48:A215.

45. Holmgren E, Giuliano F, Hulting C. Sildenafil (Viagra) in the treatment of ED caused by spinal cord injury: a double blind, placebo-controlled, flexible dose, two-way crossover study. Neurology 1998; 50:A127.

46. Giuliano F, Hultling C, El Masry WS, et al. Randomized trial of sildenafil for the treatment of erectile dysfunction in spinal cord injury. Ann Neurol 1999; 46(1):15–21.

47. Hulting C, Guiliano F, Quirk F, et al. Quality of life in patients with spinal cord injury receiving Viagra (sildenafil citrate) for the treatment of erectile dysfunction. Spinal Cord 2000; 38(6):363–370.

48. Kim ED, McVary KT. Topical prostaglandin-E1 for the treatment of ED. J Urol 1995; 153(6):1828–1830.

49. Chancellor MB, Rivas DA, Panzer DE, et al. Prospective comparison of topical minoxidil to vacuum constriction device and intracorporeal papaverine injection in treatment of ED due to spinal cord injury. Urology 1994; 43(3):365–369.

50. Sonksen J, Biering-Sorensen F. Transcutaneous nitroglycerin in the treatment of erectile dysfunction in spinal cord injured. Paraplegia 1992; 30(8):554–557.

51. Padma-Nathan H, Hellstrom WJG, Kaiser FE, et al. Treatment of men with ED with transurethral alprostadil.

52. Bodner DR, Haas CA. Intraurethral alprostadil for treatment of ED in patients with spinal cord injury. Urology 1999; 53(1):199–202.

53. Bodner DR, Lindan R. The application of intracavernous injection of vasoactive medications for erection in men with spinal cord injury. J Urol 1987; 138:310–311.

54. Wyndaele JJ, deMeyer JM, de Sy WA, et al. Intracavernous injection of vasoactive drugs, an alternative for treating impotence in spinal cord injury patients. Paraplegia 1986; 24:271–275.

55. Chao R, Clowers DE. Experience with intracavernosal tri-mixture for the management of neurogenic ED. Arch Phys Med Rehabil 1994; 75:276–278.

56. Kapoor VK, Chahal AS, Jyoti SP, et al. Intracavernous papaverine for impotence in spinal cord injured patients. Paraplegia 1993; 31(10):675.

57. Earle CM, Keogh EJ, Ker JK, et al. Intracavernosal injection therapy for impotence due to spinal cord injury. Int J Impotence Res 1990; 2:297.

58. Sidi AA, Cameron JS, Dykstra DD, et al. Vasoactive intracavernous pharmacotherapy for the treatment of erectile impotence in men with spinal cord injury. J Urol 1987; 138(3):539–542.

59. Earle CM, Keogh EJ, Ker JK, et al. The role of intracavernosal vasoactive agents to overcome impotence due to spinal cord injury. Paraplegia 1992; 30(4):273–276.

60. Lloyd LK, Richards JS. Intracavernous pharmacotherapy for management of ED in spinal cord injury. Paraplegia 1989; 27:457–464.

61. Denil J, Ohl DA, Smythe C. Vacuum erection device in spinal cord injured men: patient and partner satisfaction. Arch Phys Med Rehabil 1996; 77(8):750–753.

62. Zasler ND, Katz PG. Synergist erection system in the management of impotence secondary to spinal cord injury. Arch Phys Med Rehabil 1989; 70(9):712–716.

63. Kaufman JJ, Lindner A, Raz S. Complications of penile prosthesis surgery for impotence. J Urol 1982; 128(6):1192–1193.

64. Rossier AB, Fam BA. Indication and results of semirigid penile prostheses in spinal cord injury patients: long-term follow-up. J Urol 1984; 131(1):59–62.

65. Dietzen CJ, Lloyd LK. Complications of intracavernous injections and penile prostheses in spinal cord injured men. Arch Phys Med Rehabil 1992; 73(7):652–655.

66. Van Arsdalen KN, Klein FA, Hackler RH, et al. Penile implants in spinal cord injury patients for maintaining external appliances. J Urol 1981; 126(3):331–332.

67. Kabalin JN, Kessler R. Infectious complications of penile prosthesis surgery. J Urol 1988; 139(5):953–955.

68. Iwatsubo E, Tanaka M, Takahashi K, et al. Non-inflatable penile prosthesis for the management of urinary incontinence and sexual disability of patients with spinal cord injury. Paraplegia 1986; 24:307–310.

Medicated Urethral System for Erection (MUSE) Study Group. N Engl J Med 1997; 336(1):1–7.

69. Brindley GS. The actions of parasympathetic and sympathetic nerves in human micturition, erection and seminal emission, and their restoration in paraplegic patients by implanted electrical stimulators. Proc R Soc Lond 1988; B235:111–120.

70. Viitanen M, Fugl-Meyer KS, Bernspan B, et al. Life satisfaction in long term survivors after stroke. Scand J Rehabil Med 1988; 20(1):17–24.

71. Kalliomaki JL, Markkanen TK, Mustonen VA. Sexual behavior after cerebral vascular accident: study of patients below age 60 years. Fertil Steril 1961; 12:156–158.

72. Goddess ED, Wagner NN, Silverman DR. Post-stroke sexual activity of CVA patients. Med Aspects Hum Sex 1979; 13:16–29.

73. Sjogren K, Fugl-Meyer AR. Adjustment to life after stroke with special reference to sexual intercourse and leisure. J Psychosom Res 1982; 26(4):409–417.

74. Sjogren K, Fugl-Meyer AR. Sexual problems in hemiplegia. Int Rehabil Med 1981; 3(1):28–31.

75. Monga TN, Monga M, Raina MS, Hardjasudarma M. Hypersexuality in stroke. Arch Phys Med Rehabil 1986; 67(6):415–417.

76. Stone B, Melman A. Management of sexual and bladder dysfunction in multiple sclerosis. J Neurol Rehabil 1989; 3:167–175.

77. Valleroy ML, Kraft GH. Sexual dysfunction in multiple sclerosis. Arch Phys Med Rehab 1984; 65:125–128.

78. Hennessey A, Robertson NP, Swingler R, et al. Urinary, faecal and sexual dysfunction in patients with multiple sclerosis. J Neurol 1999; 246(11): 1027–1032.

79. Kirkeby HJ, Poulsen EU, Petersen T, et al. Erectile dysfunction in multiple sclerosis. Neurology 1988; 38(9):1366.

80. Miller J, Fowler C, Sharief M. Viagra (sildenafil citrate) for the treatment of erectile dysfunction in men with multiple sclerosis [abstr 200]. Ann Neurol 1999; 46:497.

81. Fowler C, Miller J, Sharief M. Effect of sildenafil citrate (Viagra) on quality of life in men with erectile dysfunction and multiple sclerosis [abstr 198]. Ann Neurol 1999; 46:496.

82. Kirkeby HJ, Petersen T, Poulsen EU. Pharmacologically induced erection in patients with multiple sclerosis. Scand J Urol Nephrol 1988; 22(4):241–244.

83. Jacobs H, Vieregge A, Vieregge P. Sexuality in young patients with Parkinson's disease: a population based comparison with healthy controls. J Neurol Neurosurg Psychiat 2000; 69(4):550–552.

84. Singer C, Weiner WJ, Sanchez-Ramos JR. Autonomic dysfunction in men with Parkinson's disease. Eur Neurol 1992; 32:134–140.

85. Sandyk R. AC pulsed electromagnetic fields-induced sexual arousal and penile erections in Parkinson's disease. Int J Neurosci 1999; 99:139–149.

86. O'Sullivan JD, Hughes AJ. Apomorphine-induced penile erections in Parkinson's disease. Mov Disord 1998; 13(3):536–539.

87. Purba JS, Hofman MA, Swaab DF. Decreased number of oxytocin-immunoreactive neurons in the paraventricular nucleus of the hypothalamus in Parkinson's disease. Neurology 1994; 44(1):84–89.

88. Uitti RJ, Tanner CM, Rajput AH, et al. Hypersexuality with antiparkinsonian therapy. Clinical Neuropharmacol 1989; 12(5):375–383.

89. Zesiewicz TA, Hauser RA, Helal M. Sildenafil citrate (Viagra) for the treatment of erectile dysfunction in men with Parkinson's disease. Mov Disord 2000; 15(2): 305–308.

90. Hussain IF, Brady CM, Fowler CJ. Sildenafil for the treatment of erectile dysfunction in parkinsonism. BJU Int 2000; 85(suppl 5):14(abstr P33).

91. Apomorphine for the management of motor fluctuations in Parkinson's Disease: a CME monograph based on a kickoff seminar held at The Movement Disorder Society's 9th International Congress on Parkinson's Disease and Movement Disorders. New Orleans, LA: March 5, 2005.

92. Eardley I. New oral therapies for the treatment of ED. Br J Urol 1998; 81:122–127.

39

Treatment of Sexual Dysfunction in Male Cancer Survivors

Judith Shell
Osceola Cancer Center, Kissimmee, Florida, U.S.A.

□ INTRODUCTION

According to the American Cancer Society (1), approximately 63% of people diagnosed with cancer today will be alive for five or more years past the time of their initial diagnosis, depending on the type and stage of cancer. Of those who survive, between 10% and 90% report sexual problems, depending on the patient's gender, the diagnosis, and the choice of treatment pursued (2–4). Interestingly, Alfonso et al. (5) reported that sexual dysfunction was more common in males (82%) than in females (61%) in both experimental and control groups of cancer patients tested. Traditionally, men are more subject to the pressures of unrealistic societal expectations regarding their sexuality, from the maintenance of an outwardly "tough" and emotionally invulnerable exterior to the concerns about maximizing penis size and the ability to achieve and maintain erections. Nowhere greater than in the face of illness, however, is a man's sexuality tested as truly, and when the limits of physical capability fall short of perceived expectations, a man's self-worth may be severely affected. Thus, the maintenance of sexual function is of great importance to many male cancer patients. One study revealed that in order to preserve erectile function after prostate cancer, 68% of men claimed they would be willing to trade away a 10% greater chance of survival for a treatment that would offer better future sexual function (6).

Because intact sexual function is such a vital part of what comprises quality of life, it is the responsibility of health-care providers to integrate sex education and appropriate interventions into the routine care of cancer survivors by fostering communication between the patient, the patient's partner, and the health-care team, regardless of age, marital status, or sexual orientation. This chapter will provide clinical guidelines (summarized in Tables 1–5) for the sensitive and appropriate treatment of sexual dysfunction in male cancer patients, giving special attention to the obstacles most commonly encountered in treatment based on age and type of cancer diagnosis.

□ TIMING AND FOCUS OF TREATMENT

Due to the heightened awareness of the existence of sexual dysfunction in cancer survivors that has been made possible by a more receptive societal attitude and an increased demand for the open discussion of sexuality, more attention in the literature has been given to the implementation of sexual rehabilitation before, during, and after cancer treatment. If sexual function is addressed during all phases of clinical treatment, the patient and partner will realize that it is both normal and appropriate to have concerns about maintaining a sexual relationship despite ongoing cancer treatment. For many patients who have partners, intimacy may not only be a comfort but also an affirmation of life. Some patients, however, may decide that being sexually active is no longer important to them, and this is also a normal, healthy choice. The clinical practitioner should be aware that this latter group of patients may still enjoy being "sexual" without actually engaging in intercourse and thus may still have sexuality concerns to be addressed.

Not all patients have partners, nor does every patient wish to have a partner. Further, health-care providers should be careful not to make inaccurate assumptions regarding the sexual orientation of a patient. Frequently, gay men choose not to disclose their sexual orientation in the health-care setting because they fear the repercussions of negative attitudes, particularly if the provider is clearly "heterosexist" in all of his or her remarks (15,16). Consequently, the couple may not feel comfortable demonstrating love and affection toward each other during office or hospital visits, which may lead to the partner being excluded from decision making. It is the clinician's responsibility to be knowledgeable about each individual patient and to provide care in a nonjudgmental manner.

The experience of having cancer, even when the disease itself is in remission, can induce an undercurrent of foreboding that may encroach upon all aspects of couples' lives. Couples often react either by pulling away from one another or by clinging even more closely together (17). Couples adapt best when they

Table 1 Factors that Obstruct Communication Between Physicians and Cancer Patients

A shortage of information or specialized training
Discomfort talking about sex
Inflexible opinions about sexuality
Fear that a focus on sexuality will insult or trouble the patient
Presumption that patient's sexual capabilities are ended due to the illness
Supposition that someone else has counseled the patient regarding sexual matters
Assumption that the patient has no concerns because they have asked no questions

Source: From Ref. 7.

Table 3 Brief Assessment Questions of Sexual Function in Male Patients with Cancer

Has having cancer (or its treatment) interfered with your being a father (partner, husband)?
Has your cancer (or its treatment) changed the way you see yourself as a man?
Has your cancer (or its treatment) caused any change in your sexual functioning (sex life)?
Do you expect your sexual functioning (sex life) to be changed in any way after you leave the hospital (after treatment is finished)?

Source: From Ref. 9.

face the cancer experience in an empowering manner, trying to live more fully rather than constraining their relationship. This sometimes means revising the nature of their intimacy to include, rather than avoid, issues of disability and threatened loss.

☐ LIFE-STAGE PSYCHOSOCIAL DEVELOPMENT
Overview

A man's sexuality and feelings of masculinity are integral to his self-esteem and remain so throughout the life cycle. Young, middle-aged, and older adults alike often wish to maintain sexual interest and activity. Cancer can affect men throughout the life cycle from adolescence into older adulthood. Therefore, it is essential for practitioners to tailor their treatment approaches according to the projected impact that cancer may have on the specific life stage in which it occurs, thus promoting the expedient assessment of the nature and extent of sexual rehabilitation required in men with cancer.

Adolescence

From a psychosexual perspective, it is during adolescence that one attempts to acquire a sense of identity independent from his family. The development of secondary sexual characteristics and functions, such as the control of ejaculation, provides new frontiers to explore and conquer. Mastery is gained of the emerging struggle between logical restraint and heightened sexual

impulse (18). The opinions of peers exert a vital influence on adolescent self-esteem, and the maintenance of appearances for friends, neighbors, and schoolmates takes on an overwhelming significance.

The loss of a testicle to cancer in adolescence can be devastating to a boy's self-image and to his peer interdependence. Sports, a common bonding activity for many teens, may no longer be considered a viable pastime for postorchiectomy patients because locker rooms are often used to compare each other's physical development. Similarly, the side effects of conventional chemotherapy for disorders such as Hodgkin's disease or leukemia may be even more severe: short-term effects such as nausea and vomiting, hair loss, pain, and fatigue will commonly preclude the normal activities (movies, dances, clubs, and part-time jobs) in which teens usually participate with enthusiasm. Long-term side effects such as lifelong

Table 2 "A.L.A.R.M." Assessment Method of Sexuality in Male Patients with Cancer

A = Activity	Frequency of sexual activity
L = Libido/desire	Changes in desire or interest in sexual activity
A = Arousal/orgasm	Changes in ability to get an erection and ability to ejaculate with sexual excitement
R = Resolution	Changes in the sense of release of tension or sexual contentment after intercourse
M = Medical history	Description of history relative to disruption of sexual activity

Source: From Ref. 8.

Table 4 Suggested Scheme for Assessment of Sexual Function in Male Patients with Cancer

Component	Process
Privacy	Do not discuss when making rounds or if the roommate is present; move to another room or a private area if possible
Confidentiality	Usual practice is to meet with the patient first and then include the partner with permission. This decreases anxiety
Obtain sexual history early	Ascertain sexual function before disease occurred; the psychological status of the patient; and the relationship with and attitude of his sexual partner
Avoid overreaction	Listen attentively with genuine interest; this conveys acceptance
Move from less sensitive (general) questions to more sensitive (specific) issues	Introduce concept during other informational/educational conversations
Determine patient goals	Clear and detailed information assist in patient/partner decisions and helps to anticipate problems
Realize when a problem is too complex	Refer the patient to a sex therapist, preferably one who is certified as Assoc. of Sex, Education, Counseling, and Therapy (ASSECT)

Source: From Refs. 10–12.

Table 5 Precautions and Behavioral and Sexual Adaptations for Males with Cancer

Head and neck

Before sexual activity, clean tracheostomies and shield with cover (Byram Health Care Center, Inc. Greenwich, Connecticut, U.S.A., 800-354-4054). Men may also wish to wear a dickey

Artificial saliva (Moi-Stir, Xerolube) and sugarless mints help to freshen breath and lubricate a dry mouth

Fragrance may not be appreciated since the patient may have a decreased sense of smell; however, candles, scented or not, will enhance ambience

Partners may be fearful of obstructing the patient's air supply; so, various positions may need to be tried (13)

Hematologic malignancies

Caution patients with neutropenia or thrombocytopenia against oral, penile, and anal manipulation. Suggest nonperformance activities such as a warm bubble bath together with candlelight, romantic music, and some wine (in plastic glasses)

Suggest the planning for a sexual interlude after antiemetics have taken effect, and advice avoiding heavy meals and alcohol

Advise a supine or side-lying position for intercourse to decrease fatigue, because this uses less energy. A nap may also be helpful

Emphasize the importance of contraception during chemotherapy; encourage sperm banking before chemotherapy begins or within the first 10–14 days (14). If quality or quantity of preserved sperm is too low for intrauterine insemination, in vitro fertilization or intracytoplasmic sperm injection (ICSI) may be used (14)

Prostate cancer

Arousal may be stimulated through use of non-androgen-dependent mechanisms such as erotic books, pictures, or videos

Stimulation may also occur with long periods of foreplay that include a change in environment (an inexpensive motel or house sitting for a friend), a romantic dinner, and showering together

Mutual masturbation may help the patient reach orgasm and ejaculation if erection is not possible. By inserting a partially erect penis into the vagina and flexing the perineal muscles, a female partner may help with an erection

The bladder should be emptied before intercourse if incontinence is a problem. If an accident should occur, remind the partner that urine is sterile and can be washed off easily, perhaps in the shower together

Medication and mechanical devices are available (see other chapters in Part IV)

Testicular cancer

If physiologically possible, intercourse may be resumed about 6 wks after pelvic surgery

Sperm banking should be encouraged if the patient is interested

Normal sexual desire and pleasurable sensations will most likely continue. If testosterone levels are decreased, hormone replacement therapy may be necessary after treatment is finished

A man may be embarrassed after the loss of a testicle; saline implants are now available

Partners may need to be reminded that cancer cannot be transmitted through sexual activity and if radiation therapy is being used, they will not be contaminated

Penis cancer

Men should be reminded that it is possible to experience erection and normal or near-normal intensity of orgasms if partial penectomy has occurred

If the penis is removed entirely, the mons pubis, perineum, and scrotum can still be stimulated and orgasms attained with pleasurable contractions

Colorectal cancer (ostomy present)

Empty the pouch and ensure the seal. If the ostomy is dry or controllable with irrigation, a cap or mini pouch may be attached

Avoid foods that cause gas and strong odors or foods that cause loose stool for 6–12 hr before intercourse. Deodorize the pouch with 1 or 2 drops of Banish. In case the stoma should produce unflattering noises, have a humorous response ready to prevent embarrassment

An attractive pouch can be worn to camouflage fecal material

It is wise to have the bed protected with a rubber sheet and towel on top in case pouch leakage occurs

Different positions should be explored other than the missionary position, which may irritate or rub the stoma

Lung cancer

Experience sexual closeness that does not necessarily lead to intercourse, which may exacerbate fatigue and dyspnea

To prevent bronchospasm, decrease or eliminate environmental irritants such as perfumes, colognes, and hairsprays

Avoid long, slow kisses on the mouth because patients can become fearful of not getting enough oxygen

To reduce exertion during sexual activity, encourage the use of a waterbed; movement is created without effort

Emotional intimacy

Focus on the development of increased intimacy in the relationship rather than simply thinking about sex

Encourage communication between partners about their respective daily activities (jobs, relationships, feelings, etc.)

Encourage patients to hold realistic expectations of themselves and their mate about sexual performance

Time for fun and companionship with a partner should be planned

Source: From Ref. 11.

immunosuppression, cardiomyopathy, pulmonary fibrosis, and renal failure may all exert a substantial impact on current and future sexuality, causing infertility, a reduction in growth, and oppressive changes in physical characteristics (19). Olivo and Woolverton (18) reported that childhood cancer survivors are 20 times more likely to incur another new cancer during their lifetime. Each subsequent visit to the hospital or outpatient center further intrudes on a teenager's sense of privacy, and as both the disease and its treatment may serve to sequester the patient from full participation in peer-related social activities, a diagnosis of cancer at this stage can have overwhelming long-term psychological and psychosexual consequences. A young man with a history of adolescent cancer may become fearful of his own ability to establish an intimate relationship, father children, raise a family, build a career, and maintain a sense of self-esteem. Often, a complete avoidance of sexual relationships is exhibited due to a maintained fear of deceiving a new partner.

Young Adults

During young adulthood, a man begins to experience the dichotomy between intimacy and isolation (20). At this stage, men exhibit greater levels of self-confidence and often experience increased vocational effectiveness, interpersonal security, and sexual satisfaction. The most formidable psychosexual task during this period is that of sexual adequacy and performance, although fertility and parenting concerns may also be present (21) as well as more general stressors regarding business and financial status. In general, however, this group is typically secure in the understanding of their individual identities.

The occurrence of cancer during this period, however, threatens body image, social status, role effectiveness, and self-esteem, and it may substantially influence whether or not the patient chooses to develop a lasting relationship that will eventually lead to marriage and family. In this age group, Hodgkin's disease is common, and colon and lung cancer may begin to occur, along with kidney and bladder cancer; testicular cancer will still pose a threat.

Middle Adulthood

In middle adulthood, men begin the process of developing and maintaining a sense of self-esteem in the face of despair because they must adjust to diminished levels of energy, competence, and possibly "empty nest syndrome" (20). Similarly, age-related bodily deteriorations may result in a diminished capacity to engage in physical activities for as long as or as aggressively as before, causing distress. There may be additional stress of being in the "sandwich generation," in which a man may be responsible for the financial and physical care of both his elderly parents and his college-aged children. Another potentially threatening new psychosexual problem of this period may be the onset of erectile dysfunction (ED) (including longer time to erection, less firm erection, and difficulty in maintaining an erection).

At this stage, a diagnosis of cancer will add another level of stress that can further drain energy, raising new questions about adequacy and self-worth. Prostate cancer is a major threat to this age group—not only to longevity but also to sexuality, since many standard prostate cancer treatments will also cause impotence problems as a side effect (22). Other common cancer risks in this group are those of the colon and the lung as well as lymphoma.

The Older Adult

The loss of friends and family can cause older adults to reconsider the fact of their own mortality. Men must adjust to the social stigma of being "old" along with the physical aggravations of painful arthritis, decreased visual acuity, and reduced hearing. As the "baby boomer" generation has aged, however, many of these preconceived notions about the older adult have been radically altered, as is evidenced by greater numbers of baby boomers participating in marathons, opting for liposuction and other cosmetic surgery, and staying sexually active (23).

Other major psychosexual tasks for this age group include adjustments to retirement and reduced income (24). While attempting to manage these tasks, there will be less energy for and a decreased interest in sex and intimate relationships.

In this age group, men may be faced with the long-term problems associated with prostate cancer. While managing recurrence, the constant application of androgen suppression may cause not only impotence but also emotional volatility. Radiation and chemotherapy will compound these emotional problems. Colon and lung cancers may also be concurrent problems.

□ FACTORS AFFECTING SEXUAL FUNCTION IN MEN WITH CANCER
Treatment-Related Factors Secondary to Surgery
Colorectal Cancer

Surgery, with or without chemotherapy, continues to be the mainstay of treatment for cancer of the colon—the second most common malignancy in the United States (2,10). Resection of colorectal tumors using an abdominoperineal (AP) or a high or low anterior approach with pelvic lymphadenectomy can cause major problems with male sexual function. Damage to the parasympathetic nervous system during intestinal surgery can interfere with the ability to achieve an erection. Injury to the sympathetic nervous system can impair the ejaculatory response and precipitate retrograde or diminished ejaculation (2). Since erection and ejaculation are controlled by different neural pathways, a man may be able to achieve erection but may be unable to ejaculate or vice versa. Even if a man cannot ejaculate, orgasm may still be possible, as has been observed in men who are paraplegic (25). The prevalence of sexual dysfunction increases with more extensive surgery. Koukouras et al. (26) studied 60 sexually active men who underwent high anterior resection, low anterior resection, or AP resection, in order of invasiveness. Patients with AP resection had the highest reported sexual problems, with 65% becoming sexually inactive, 50% reporting an inability to ejaculate, and 45% losing erectile ability. Although nerve-sparing procedures may offer some protection, one study has acknowledged that partial-to-complete ED was still noted in 44% of patients who underwent this type of operation; however, it should be noted that of these, 33% of the study participants had already experienced some type of sexual dysfunction preoperatively (27).

For men who must endure colostomy placement, many valid concerns may develop regarding hygiene and body image, including the loss of bowel control, the need to wear an external collection device, and the potential public embarrassment related to undesired noise, odors, and colostomy leakage. The resulting fear of rejection can be overwhelming and may significantly impact an individual's sense of masculinity and sexuality. To prevent a pattern of sexual avoidance, it is imperative that the health-care provider proactively manages any occurrences of depression, anxiety, or other social dysfunction in these patients.

Bladder Cancer

The incidence of bladder cancer is greatest in older men. Cystectomy is not necessary for superficial non-invasive tumors, because they are usually treated topically with bacilli Calmette-Guérin (BCG) (10). Repeated cystoscopies must be performed to instill the BCG, however, and this can cause urethral irritation and pain with erection and ejaculation (28). Sexual partners may express concern about becoming "contaminated" with the medication and thus avoid intercourse, causing distress in the patient.

If the bladder tumor is invasive, cystectomy with prostate resection remains the treatment of choice, with or without radiation therapy (29). Either a stoma (urostomy) and ostomy appliance or a continent urinary reservoir will be placed that requires frequent catheterization. As in the case of ostomies placed as the result of a colostomy, body image is affected; specific sexual dysfunctions that may occur are similar to those seen with radical prostatectomy (see below), including difficulty achieving and/or maintaining erections. Because the prostate is also removed, there can be no ejaculate with orgasm, and the sensation of orgasm itself may be diminished. Nordstrom and Nyman (30) studied 40 men who underwent ileal conduit urinary diversion surgery and found that 90% of the men sexually active before surgery could not attain erection after bladder resection. Yet, 41% were able to masturbate to orgasm, albeit without erection.

Prostate Cancer

Treatment for prostate cancer continues to improve, resulting in fewer unwanted side effects such as impotence. It must be emphasized, however, that all forms of cancer treatment are frequently accompanied by some degree of psychosexual detriment to self-image and sexual function. Further, since 80% of prostate cancer cases are diagnosed in men aged 65 years and older, several additional factors not directly related to prostate cancer treatment may also contribute to the presence of sexual dysfunction, including the fact of advanced age itself, retirement, loss of a spouse, previous medical history, and concomitant medical/pharmacological therapy for other chronic systemic illnesses such as hypertension or diabetes (10). Therefore, the clinician should realize that post-treatment ED is not always therapy induced, and other potential causes may need to be addressed. (For further information on the effects of pharmacotherapy on sexual function, see Chapter 19.)

Early-stage prostate cancer is commonly treated with surgery or radiation therapy; radical surgery bears nearly an 85% risk of ED, while radiation therapy alone has about a 50% risk (31). The high association of sexual dysfunction with radical prostatectomy is due to the potential risk of injury to the branches of the pelvic plexus. Similarly, removal of the seminal vesicles and transection of the vas deferens results in the total lack of semen, emission, or ejaculation (32). For these reasons, the use of nerve-sparing surgical techniques has gained increasing popularity, but one study has found that the incidence of ED with these types of procedures remains up to 79% (33). This figure is substantially higher than those of other studies, in which the incidence was reported between 32% and 58% (34,35). Because the true extent of the tumor may be unknown until the time of surgery, it is not always possible to utilize nerve-sparing techniques. Even if nerve-sparing surgery is performed, erectile function may not be restored for up to six months in some men. On the other hand, after radiation therapy, ED often does not become evident until six months have elapsed after treatment. A meta-analysis of 40 articles compared surgery [including radical prostatectomy, a nerve-sparing procedure (unilateral or bilateral)], and radiotherapy. Taking pretreatment erectile function into consideration, findings determined that there is a reduced rate of treatment-induced ED with radiotherapy compared to surgery (36).

Advanced stages of prostate cancer require hormone manipulation and often bilateral orchiectomy. Clearly, the surgical removal of both testicles will have more devastating repercussions to the body image than the side effects resulting from oral or injected agents that suppress androgen production and/or action. Patients may be offered saline implants and should be strongly encouraged to consult a sex therapist if a desire for sexual activity remains.

Testicular Cancer

Testicular cancer most often affects younger men from the ages of 17 to 34. Because the presence of testicular cancer often results in significantly lower sperm counts and quality even before the initiation of treatment begins (37), a diagnosis of testicular cancer can be particularly devastating since many men attempt to start families during this period.

Men between the ages of 40 and 50 years may be at risk for the seminomatous type of testicular cancer. Treatment consists of the removal of the affected testicle followed by bilateral retroperitoneal lymphadenectomy (RLND) and radiotherapy. If metastasis is present, chemotherapy is then initiated (2,10). Unilateral orchiectomy alone with subsequent monitoring for metastases may be sufficient treatment for nonseminomatous tumors. Nerve-sparing surgery may be attempted to preserve fertility.

Side effects of unilateral orchiectomy include interference with ejaculation, arousal, and ability to reach orgasm and even a decrease in libido (38,39). RLND typically damages the sympathetic ganglia, resulting in "dry orgasms" due to retrograde ejaculation. If retrograde ejaculation cannot be reversed, it may be possible to harvest viable sperm from a sterile sample of postorgasmic urine for use in artificial insemination (11). Ofman (10) reports that this patient population often experiences great levels of overall sexual distress; some demonstrate a drastic decline in sexual activity, while others cease sexual activity completely.

Penile Cancer

Even an early penile lesion can cause discomfort and embarrassment, and the partner may express a fear of contracting the disease through sexual intercourse. If detected early, topical chemotherapy, interstitial implant, or laser fulguration may be adequate treatment, and any resulting sexual dysfunction will be minimal. Because men tend not to seek early treatment of this disease, however, partial or total penectomy will often be required to control cancer of the penis. Clearly, such surgical treatment threatens the ability to function sexually; however, with proper education and counseling, both the patient and his partner can learn to adjust to the impairment and achieve satisfaction in various ways. With partial penectomy, the penile stump can usually become erect with stimulation, and is typically long enough for penetration and antegrade ejaculation (11,40). If the entire glans penis requires removal, stimulation to orgasm can still usually occur (40,41), and a perineal urethrostomy can be created behind the scrotum. Ejaculation then occurs through the perineal urethrostomy at orgasm.

Treatment-Related Factors Secondary to Systemic Chemotherapy
Hematological Cancers

Although many studies related to male sexuality have been performed regarding prostate and testicular cancers, little has been accomplished in this field regarding most other malignancies. Leukemia and lymphomas can strike any age group, but myeloma usually occurs in older men. Although chemotherapy is the treatment mainstay of these types of disorders, a biopsy is always required to confirm the finding. Chemotherapy is often administered in high doses, with subsequent blood or marrow transplantation (BMT). Even when given in standard doses, however, chemotherapy (particularly the alkylating agents) can cause adverse affects on sperm-forming germ cells, resulting in azoospermia or decreased sperm counts (Table 6). Decreased testosterone production and difficulty with erections may also result (14). These effects are sometimes temporary during standard chemotherapy and may return to baseline after treatment has subsided.

Immediately after chemotherapy, men may experience a decreased desire for sexual intimacy due to increased weakness and fatigue, intermittent nausea

Table 6 Chemotherapy Agents that Cause Adverse Sexual Side Effects

Drug class	Chemotherapy drug
Alkylating agent	Busulfan melphelan
	Chlorambucil nitrogen mustard
	Cisplatin temozolomide
	Cyclophosphamide thiotepa
Nitrosureas	Carmustine
	Lomustine
Vinca alkaloid	Vinblastine
Miscellaneous agent	Procarbazine

Source: From Ref. 14.

and vomiting, and possible diarrhea or constipation (11). After approximately three weeks, alopecia may occur, and this type of defacement can destroy self-image and the sense of masculinity. The prolonged hospitalization often required for the treatment of acute leukemias can also create a lack of privacy.

In the case of BMT and its accompanying supralethal doses of chemotherapy, sexual difficulties may ensue that are not reversible, particularly in regard to fertility. For up to 18 years after completion of BMT, researchers have reported rates of sexual dysfunction between 20% and 44% in quality-of-life outcome studies across genders (4,42,43). These difficulties include ED caused by peripheral neuropathies, decreased libido associated with hyperprolactinemia (likely caused by damage to the hypothalamus), and changes in hormone levels that may cause disruption in the sexual response cycle at the phases of desire, arousal, or orgasm (44). Mumma et al. (45) correlated increased psychological distress with decreased sexual satisfaction, poor body image, and an increased disruption in sexual relationships in a study of BMT recipients. Individually variable social factors influencing intimate partner relationships may include partner uncertainty and anxiety, difficulty communicating, and role shifting within the couple during treatment and recovery (46). During BMT, the sexual partner often assumes the role of caregiver, and this can also have an adverse affect on the relationship due to the new intensified dependence placed upon the sexual partner by the patient. Reestablishing intimacy can be difficult, at best, since there has been little chance for privacy due to prolonged treatment and hospitalization.

Lung Cancer

Lung cancer is one of the most commonly diagnosed malignancies per annum. Treatment for lung cancer includes possible surgery, chemotherapy, and/or radiation therapy, with chemotherapy being used most often as a palliative measure for advanced disease.

The possibility of malignancy, an uncertain prognosis, and the resultant psychosocial and emotional distress are all issues that require lifestyle adjustments (11). Treatment with chemotherapy can be devastating, particularly if the patient begins in a debilitated state. Changes in role function, inability to continue working, and/or deflated body image as the result of an altered appearance and/or fatigue can threaten the individual with the loss of masculinity, along with the loss in physical sexual functioning. Here, also, nausea and vomiting, hair loss, and increased shortness of breath due either to the tumor or to the low hemoglobin can also increase fatigue. These cumulative symptoms are not only troublesome but can also create a lack of sexual desire and even cause the patient to withdraw from intimacy, affection, and physical gratification.

There is a paucity of research in the area of sexuality and lung cancer. A Canadian study examined psychiatric illness and psychosocial concerns in 52 newly diagnosed lung cancer patients, 75% male and 25% female. Only 1 out of 20 outcome measures (loss of libido) was related to the patients' sexuality (47). Results indicated that this patient population often experienced symptoms of potential psychiatric significance and psychosocial concerns. Twenty-five patients (48%) acknowledged loss of libido, and 27% of these considered the problem to be "severe" (47).

Another quality of life study assessed adult survivors of lung, colon, and prostate cancer. Significant physical, psychosocial, sexual, and marital problems were reported in all three groups (48). Notably, lung cancer survivors experienced more problems than the other survivors. The author [Shell JA. The longitudinal effects of cancer treatment on sexuality in individuals with lung cancer. Michigan State University, East Lansing, Michigan, U.S.A. 2002 (unpublished doctoral dissertation)] reported on 59 patients (32 males) at three points in time over a period of four months. Sexual function was measured by the Derogatis Interview for Sexual Function Self-Report (DISF-SR) (49). Sexual function (sexual cognition/fantasy, sexual arousal, sexual behavior/experiences, orgasm, and drive and relationship) worsened with treatment, particularly between times one and two. Other variables that affected sexual function were age, gender, and mood status.

Head and Neck Cancer

Alcohol is often a contributing factor that predates the development of head and neck cancer, and may also contribute to problems with sexual function. ED is prominent in those who consume large amounts of alcohol, and impotence may continue indefinitely in chronic abusers.

Little research has been carried out relative to the specific impact of head and neck cancer on sexuality. Even though this type of cancer does not affect the sexual organs directly, Siston et al. (50) have recognized the significant need to address sexual function in this population because the qualities of desire, arousal, erection, and orgasm can be affected indirectly by the combination chemotherapy (and radiotherapy) required for treatment (2). Further, as many of these

cancers can affect and subsequently disfigure the face, this population may feel grossly unattractive and often will develop difficulties with simple tasks such as talking, eating, and even breathing (11). Consequently, when faced with the arduous task of rehabilitation due to significant cosmetic and nonsexual functional impairments, patients may give little attention to rejuvenating intimacy with a partner. In fact, a partner may be repulsed by the sight and smell of the patient in the late stages of the disease. Nevertheless, sexual problems may still occur in the absence of severe disfigurement; patients without extensive disfigurement in one study experienced no sex drive (33%), no intercourse (40%), erectile problems (60%), and no orgasm (50%). Although one half were content with their partner, the majority masturbated, and only 20% enjoyed their present sexual functioning (51).

Treatment-Related Factors Secondary to Radiation Therapy
Effects of Radiotherapy to the Upper Body

The effects of radiotherapy are localized and depend on many factors such as area of treatment, volume of tissue irradiated, total dose, type of radiation given, and individual patient differences. Because radiation therapy mainly affects rapidly dividing cells, the epithelial tissues (e.g., mucous membranes and skin) are the most susceptible (52). Early side effects may occur within two weeks and may not subside until two to three weeks after therapy completion; late reactions can occur even years later (52).

Radiation to the head and neck area can cause severe problems with xerostomia, chewing, swallowing, and talking; pain may be severe and the treatment provider must be prepared to provide measures of analgesia (52). Oral sex may be difficult due to decreased amounts of saliva production, and the use of artificial saliva is not acceptable to many patients. Further, decreased taste and swallowing function may cause the patient to eat less, resulting in weight loss and poor body image. Skin changes will accompany radiotherapy, and this may be particularly embarrassing if the reddened and peeling treatment areas are readily visible on the head and neck. Treated areas of the chest and back can also become sore and painful—additional detriments to the maintenance of intimate relationships.

Monga et al. (3) conducted a study with 55 head-and-neck cancer patients following radiation therapy, of whom 54 were men. While the majority (58%) reported arousal problems (including orgasmic problems and/or not participating in sexual intercourse), 85% reported maintaining an interest in sex, and most patients were able to fantasize. Over half of the patients were content with their present sexual partners, and 49% were satisfied with their current sexual functioning.

Treatment for lung and esophageal cancers and lymphomas may also include radiation therapy to the chest area. Subsequently, esophagitis and radiation pneumonitis can occur, with the accompanying development of a cough. Coughing can be one of the most problematic and aggravating side effects for patients because a poorly controlled cough can ultimately lead to shortness of breath and fatigue, requiring the cessation of sexual activity. The focus of the relationship may need to change to a sexual closeness that does not necessarily lead to intercourse.

Effects of Radiotherapy to the Lower Body

Radiotherapy to the lower body is primarily administered to men with colorectal, prostate, and testicular cancers. In the instance of colorectal and prostate tumors, it is thought that radiation causes ED via the constriction of vessels and the development of atherosclerosis, resulting in decreased arterial blood supply to the penis (2,53). Several other researchers have found that there is a correlation between the external beam radiotherapy and brachytherapy-induced ED and the amount of the radiation dose to the bulb of the penis (54,55). A possible mechanism for this correlation was proposed by Stipetich et al. (56): that increasing doses of radiation therapy to the bulb of the penis could potentially decrease the number of nitric oxide–producing cells.

Of those who received external beam radiation to the pelvis for prostate cancer, approximately 40% to 60% reported a gradual loss of the ability to achieve or maintain an erection over a period of 6 to 12 months after treatment (57). It is well known, however, that men who are more sexually active before the initiation of radiation therapy have fewer problems when treatment terminates (2,53). Beard et al. (58) described the complications after external-beam irradiation in prostate patients who underwent small-field therapy (i.e., radiation only of the prostate, seminal vesicles, and a small margin of surrounding tissues) or conformal irradiation: they had fewer problems with impotence and bowel tenderness than those who had whole-pelvis treatment (20% vs. 44%).

The testis is rarely irradiated directly. Even a single radiation dose of 6 to 9.5 Gy will result in permanent sterility (2). Dose-dependent consequences on germ cells during radiotherapy are related to their stage of maturation. Some studies have shown residual oligospermia and a decrease in seminal volume after fertility returns. The recovery of sexual function, including spermatogenesis, is highly variable and thought to occur within 1 to 45 years after treatment ceases (59).

Treatment-Related Factors Secondary to Hormone Manipulation

Men with advanced-stage prostate cancer are usually treated with androgen deprivation. This treatment is also being used in clinical trials with early-stage disease (60). Treatment usually consists of antiandrogen agents such as flutamide, with or without a luteinizing hormone–releasing hormone (LH-RH) analogue that suppresses pituitary secretion of LH, consequently reducing testicular production of testosterone. Estrogen is used less frequently. It should be noted that all of these androgen inhibition treatments produce unwanted sexual side effects. The antiandrogens reduce testosterone levels or actions, resulting in the loss of libido, problems achieving erection, decreased semen production, diminished spermatogenesis, difficulty in attaining orgasm, hot flashes, and mood swings (2,61). The use of estrogen creates the additional problems of gynecomastia, feminization, penile and testicular atrophy, and ED (14). One study examined sexual function in men who were being treated with either radiotherapy alone or radiotherapy and androgen deprivation ($n = 67$). Mean followup was 2.6 years compared to age-matched controls ($n = 48$). Results revealed that the radiotherapy-only and control groups were significantly superior to the radiotherapy/androgen deprivation therapy group in all areas of sexual function (60).

□ CONCLUSION

Being identified as a cancer patient often strips patients of their individual identities, and thus, they may "become" their illnesses. In general, however, men are not only interested in overall quality of life but also wish to preserve the quality of their sexual life. Depending on the type of cancer and treatment employed, specific physiological and psychological changes will interfere with an individual's sense of masculinity and normal sexual function. Although much of the current literature focuses on the incidence of sexual dysfunction in cancer patients, more randomized, controlled studies are needed in order to determine how best to prevent or ameliorate sexual side effects and infertility as the result of cancer treatment. If information is provided compassionately before treatment begins, as well as during and after treatment, the impact of psychosexual side effects may be diminished or eliminated altogether.

□ REFERENCES

1. American Cancer Society. Cancer facts and figures 2004. Basic Cancer Facts. Atlanta, GA: American Cancer Society, 2004.
2. Monga U. Sexuality in cancer patients. Arch Phys Med Rehab 1995; 9:417–442.
3. Monga U, Tan G, Ostermann HJ, et al. Sexuality in head and neck cancer patients. Arch Phys Med Rehab 1997; 78(3):298–303.
4. Syrjala KL, Roth-Roemer SL, Abrams JR, et al. Prevalence and predictors of sexual dysfunction in long-term survivors of marrow transplantation. J Clin Oncol 1998; 16(9):3148–3157.
5. Alfonso C, Cohen MA, Levin M, et al. Sexual dysfunction in cancer patients: a collaborative psychooncology project. Int J Mental Health 1997; 26:90–98.
6. Singer PA, Tasch ES, Stocking C, et al. Sex or survival: trade-offs between quality and quantity of life. J Clin Oncol 1991; 9(2):328–334.
7. Shell JA. Do you like the things that life is showing you? The sensitive self-image of the person with cancer. Oncol Nurs Forum 1995; 22(6):907–911.
8. Anderson BL. How cancer affects sexual functioning. Oncology 1990; 4(6):81–94.
9. McPhetridge L. Nursing history: one means to personalize care. Am J Nurs 1968; 68(1):73–76.
10. Ofman US. Disorders of sexuality and reproduction. In: Berger A, Portenoy RK, Weissman DE, eds. Principles and Practice of Supportive Oncology. Philadelphia: Lippincott Williams & Wilkins, 1998.
11. Shell JA. Impact of cancer on sexuality. In: Otto S, ed. Oncology Nursing. 4th ed. St. Louis: Mosby, Inc. 2001: 973–999.
12. Nashimoto PW. Sex and sexuality in the cancer patient. Nurse Pract Forum 1995; 6(4):221–227.
13. Schover LR. Sexuality and Cancer: For the Man Who Has Cancer and His Partner. Atlanta, GA: American Cancer Society, 2001.
14. Leonard M, Hammelef K, Smith GD. Fertility considerations, counseling, and semen cryopreservation for males prior to the initiation of cancer therapy. Clin J Oncol Nurs 2004; 8(2):127–145.
15. American Association of Physicians for Human Rights. Anti-gay discrimination in medicine: results of a national survey of lesbian, gay, and bisexual physicians. San Francisco, 1994.
16. American Medical Association, Council on Scientific affairs. Health care needs of gay men and lesbians in the United States. J Am Med Assoc 1996; 275(17): 1354–1359.
17. Rolland J. In sickness and in health: the impact of illness on couples' relationships. J Marital Family Ther 1994; 20:327–347.
18. Olivo EL, Woolverton K. Surviving childhood cancer: disruptions in the developmental building blocks of sexuality. J Sex Education Ther 2001; 26(3): 172–181.
19. DeLaat CA, Lampkin BC. Long-term survivors of childhood cancer: evaluation and identification of sequelae of treatment. Cancer J Clin 1992; 42(5):263–282.
20. Schain WS. Sexual problems of patients with cancer. In: Devita VT, Hellman S, Rosenberg S, eds. Cancer: Principles and Practice of Oncology. 2nd ed. Philadelphia: Lippincott, 1985.
21. Shell JA, Bell K, Dougherty M. Gonadal toxicities. In: Liebman M, Camp-Sorrel D, eds. Multimodal Therapy in Oncology Nursing. St. Louis: Mosby Inc., 1996.
22. Monga U, Kerrigan AJ, Garber S, Monga TN. Pre- and post-radiotherapy sexual functioning in prostate cancer patients. Sexual Disab 2001; 19(4):239–252.
23. National Council on Aging. Healthy sexuality and vital aging. Washington, DC, 1998.
24. Shell J. Sexuality issues for the older adult with cancer. In: Cope D, Reb A, eds. An Evidence-Based Approach to the Treatment and Care of the Older Adult with Cancer. Pittsburgh, PA: Oncology Nursing Press, 2006; 439–464.
25. Masters W, Johnson V, Kolodny R. Heterosexuality. New York: Harper Perennial, 1994.
26. Koukouras D, Spiliotis J, Scopa CD, et al. Radical consequence in the sexuality of male patients operated for colorectal carcinoma. Eur J Surg Oncol 1991; 17(3): 285–288.
27. Mancini R, Cosimelli M, Filippini A, et al. Nerve-sparing surgery in rectal cancer: feasibility and functional results. J Exp Clin Cancer Res 2000; 19(1):35–40.
28. Ofman US. Preservation of Function in Genitourinary Cancers: Psychosexual and Psychosocial Issues. New York: Marcel Dekker, Inc., 1995.
29. Little FA, Howard GC. Sexual function following radical radiotherapy for bladder cancer. Radiother Oncol 1998; 49(2):157–161.
30. Nordstrom GM, Nyman CR. Male and female sexual function and activity following ileal conduit urinary diversion. Br J Urol 1992; 70(1):33–39.
31. Schover LR. Sexual rehabilitation after treatment for prostate cancer. Cancer 1993; 2(suppl 3):1024–1030.
32. Lind J, Nakao SL. Urologic and male genital cancers. In: Groenwald SL, Frogge MH, Goodman M, et al. eds. Cancer Nursing: Principles and Practice. 2nd ed. Boston: Jones & Bartlett, 1990:1026–1076.
33. Talcott JA, Rieker P, Clark JA, et al. Patient-reported impotence and incontinence after nerve-sparing radical prostatectomy. J Natl Cancer Instit 1997; 89(15): 1117–1123.
34. Quinlan DM, Epstein JL, Carter BS, et al. Sexual function following radical prostatectomy: influence of preservation of neurovascular bundles. J Urol 1991; 145(5):998.
35. Walsh PC. Radical prostatectomy, preservation of sexual function, cancer control: the controversy. Urol Clin North Am 1987; 14(4):663–673.

36. Robinson JW, Dufour MS, Fung TS. Erectile functioning of men treated for prostate carcinoma. Cancer 1997; 79(3):538–544.

37. Lass A, Akagvbosu F, Abusheikha N, et al. A programme of semen cryopreservation for patients with malignant disease in a tertiary infertility centre: lessons from 8 years' experience. Hum Reprod 1998; 13(11): 3256–3261.

38. Arai Y, Kawakita M, Okada Y, et al. Sexuality and fertility in long-term survivors of testicular cancer. J Clin Oncol 1997; 15(4):1444–1448.

39. Jonker-Pool G, van Basten JP, Hoekstra HJ, et al. Sexual functioning after treatment for testicular cancer: comparison of treatment modalities. Cancer 1997; 80(3): 454–464.

40. Smith D, Babaian R. The effects of treatment for cancer on male fertility and sexuality. Cancer Nurs 1992; 15(4): 271–275.

41. Witkin MH, Kaplan HS. Sex therapy and penectomy. J Sex Marital Ther 1983; 8(3):209–221.

42. Bush NE, Haverman M, Cobleigh MA. Quality of life of 125 adults surviving 6–18 years after bone marrow transplantation. Social Sci Med 1995; 40(4):479–490.

43. Marks DI, Friedman SH, Carpini LD, et al. A prospective study of the effects of high-dose chemotherapy and bone marrow transplantation on sexual function in the first year after transplant. Bone Marrow Transpl 1997; 19(8):819–822.

44. Molassiotis A, van den Akker OB, Milligan DW, et al. Gonadal function and psychosexual adjustment in male long-term survivors of bone marrow transplantation. Bone Marrow Transpl 1995; 16(2):253–259.

45. Mumma GH, Mashberh D, Lesko LM. Long-term psychosexual adjustment of acute leukemia survivors: impact of marrow transplantation versus conventional chemotherapy. Gen Hosp Psychiatry 1992; 14(1):43–55.

46. Tierney DK. Sexuality following hematopoietic cell transplantation. Clin J Oncol Nurs 2004; 8(1):43–47.

47. Ginsberg M, Quirt C, Ginsberg A, et al. Psychiatric illness and psychosocial concerns of patients with newly diagnosed lung cancer. Canadian Med Assoc 1995; 152(5):701–708.

48. Schag C, Ganz P, Wing D, et al. Quality of life in adult survivors of lung, colon, and prostate cancer. Quality Life Res 1994; 3(2):127–141.

49. Derogatis LR. The DISF/DISF-SR Manual. Baltimore: Clinical Psychometric Research, 1987.

50. Siston AK, Schlesser R, Vokes E, et al. Sexual functioning and head and neck cancer. J Psychosoc Oncol 1997; 15:107–111.

51. List MA, Ritter-Sterr C, Landsky SB. A performance status scale for head and neck cancer patients. Cancer 1990; 66:564–569.

52. Iwamoto R. Radiation therapy. In: Otto S, ed. Oncology Nursing. 4th ed. St. Louis: Mosby, Inc., 2001:606–637.

53. Banker FL. The preservation of potency after external beam irradiation for prostate cancer. Int J Rad Oncol Biol Phys 1998; 15(1):219–220.

54. Fisch BM, Pickett B, Weinberg V, et al. Dose of radiation received by the bulb of the penis correlates with risk of impotence after three-dimensional conformal radiotherapy for prostate cancer. Urology 2001; 57(5): 955–959.

55. Merrick GS, Wallner K, Butler WM, et al. A comparison of radiation dose to the bulb of the penis in men with and without prostate brachytherapy-induced erectile dysfunction. Int J Rad Oncol Biol Phys 2001; 50(3): 597–604.

56. Stipetich RL, Abel LJ, Blatt HJ, et al. Nursing assessment of sexual function following permanent prostate brachytherapy for patients with early-stage prostate cancer. Clin J Oncol Nurs 2002; 6(5):271–274.

57. Hanks GE, Myers CE, Scardino PT. Cancer of the prostate. In: DeVita V, Hellman S, Rosenberg S, eds. Cancer: Principles and Practice of Oncology. 4th ed. Philadelphia: J.B. Lippincott, 1993.

58. Beard CJ, Propert KJ, Rieker PP. Complications after treatment with external-beam irradiation in early-stage prostate cancer patients: a prospective multiinstitutional outcomes study. J Clin Oncol 1997; 15(1): 223–229.

59. Kuczyk M, Machtens S, Bokemeyer C, et al. Sexual function and fertility after treatment of testicular cancer. Curr Opin Urol 2000; 10(5):473–477.

60. Brunner DW, Hanlon A, Nicolaou N, et al. Sexual function after radiotherapy + androgen deprivation for clinically localized prostate cancer in younger men (age 50–65) [abstr]. Oncol Nurs Forum 1997; 24:327.

61. Waxman ES. Sexual dysfunction following treatment for prostate cancer: nursing assessment and interventions. Oncol Nurs Forum 1993; 20(10):1567–1571.

Penile Arterial Reconstruction

Gemma Viola Fantini
Department of Urology, University Vita-Salute San Raffaele, Milan, Italy

Abdullah Armagan
Department of Urology, Faculty of Medicine, Suleyman Demirel University, Isparta, Turkey

Ricardo Munarriz
Department of Urology, Boston University School of Medicine, Boston, Massachusetts, U.S.A.

Irwin Goldstein
Department of Sexual Medicine, Alvarado Hospital, San Diego, California, U.S.A.

□ INTRODUCTION

Erectile dysfunction (ED) is defined as the consistent inability to obtain or maintain a penile erection satisfactory for sexual intercourse (1). Community epidemiologic studies have revealed that 52% of men aged 40 to 70 years have one of the following forms of impotence: self-reported (17%), moderate (25%), and clinically complete (10%) (2). Although there are a large variety of surgical and nonsurgical options available for the treatment of these patients, penile revascularization is the only modality that has the capability of restoring fully natural penile erections without necessity of external mechanical devices, chronic use of vasoactive medication, or surgical placement of internal penile prosthetic devices.

Historically, the first cases of penile arterial bypass surgery for ED were reported by Michal in the early 1970s. He anastomosed the inferior epigastric artery directly to the corpora cavernosal artery (3). Subsequent modifications by Virag et al. resulted in a multitude of procedures that included the use of the deep dorsal vein as the recipient vessel (4–6). Crespo et al. presented procedures for revascularization of the cavernous artery directly using the inferior epigastric artery as a donor source (7,8). Lack of standardized techniques and selection criteria may have contributed to the current low popularity of arterial revascularization such that no single procedure has been universally accepted.

An example of a typical candidate for penile vascular reconstruction would be the case of a young male without classic vascular risk factors (diabetes, hypertension, and hypercholesterolemia), who has cavernosal arterial insufficiency secondary to blunt perineal trauma (bicycle riding) or pelvic fracture. Penile vascular reconstruction is often very successful in such a case.

The overall goal of penile revascularization is to increase the cavernosal arterial perfusion pressure by bypassing the obstructive arterial lesion in the hypogastric-cavernous arterial bed. Part of the failure of revascularization surgery may be that many of those patients in whom revascularization is used have significant end-organ disease already, such that revascularization is doomed to failure even though vascular lesions may be part of the pathologic process. In addition, in some arterialization surgery, there is a problem because of poor runoff after rearterialization for damaged arterial systems. The corpora cavernosa are areas of very high resistance, and, unless adequate runoff into the corpora tissue is present, vascular surgery may again be doomed to failure.

□ DIAGNOSIS

The diagnostic algorithm is aimed at ensuring that this operation is performed on the ideal candidate. All young patients with a history suggestive of trauma-associated ED undergo a comprehensive history and physical examination. The patient's history is characterized by (*i*) strong libido, (*ii*) consistent reduction in erectile rigidity during sexual activity, (*iii*) increased erection rigidity during morning erections, (*iv*) variable sustaining capability with the best maintenance of rigidity during early morning erections, and (*v*) poor spontaneity of erections, taking much effort and excessive time to achieve a poorly rigid erectile response.

Standard endocrinologic and psychologic evaluations are mandatory to rule out complex endocrinopathies or psychogenic ED. In addition, a nocturnal penile tumescence test may be conducted in an attempt to rule out neurogenic and psychogenic ED.

Penile duplex Doppler ultrasonography (DDU) provides diagnostic hemodynamic data such as decreased cavernosal peak systolic velocities with normal resistive index and preoperative information such as (*i*) presence of communicating branches from the dorsal to the cavernosal artery (Fig. 1A) and (*ii*) direction of flow through septal communicators (Fig. 1B), and dorsal artery diameters and peak systolic velocities, which are critical in the selection of the best recipient dorsal artery.

Finally, vascular assessment by dynamic infusion cavernosometry/cavernosography (DICC) is required to demonstrate arterial pressure gradients between the brachial artery and the cavernosal arteries and the normal veno-occlusive parameters (flow-to-maintain values, pressure decay values).

Selective internal pudendal arteriography is then performed to document the presence of (*i*) an occlusive lesion in one or both hypogastric-cavernous arterial beds (Fig. 1C), (*ii*) an inferior epigastric artery of sufficient length to allow anastomosis to the dorsal artery (Fig. 1D), and (*iii*) a communication branch(es) between the dorsal artery and the cavernosal artery distal to the occlusion that will allow the inflow of new blood and the development of increased intracorporal pressure.

For more detailed information on the evaluation of the male patient with sexual dysfunction, see the chapters in Part III: Investigation of Male Sexual Function.

□ OPERATIVE TECHNIQUE

Penile vascular surgery is performed with the patient under general anesthesia, intubated with complete muscle relaxant or spinal anesthesia, which facilitates harvesting the donor vessel.

Because this operation may last in excess of five hours, great care must be taken in positioning and padding the limbs, particularly the neurovascular points on the upper limbs. In addition, alternating the position of the blood pressure cuff periodically throughout the procedure may decrease the possibility of transient nerve palsies. The authors of this chapter have placed patients in the supine position with their arms secured next to their body. The patient's abdomen and genitalia are carefully shaved, prepped, and draped, then followed with placement of a 16-Fr Foley catheter using sterile technique. The patient is given one dose of

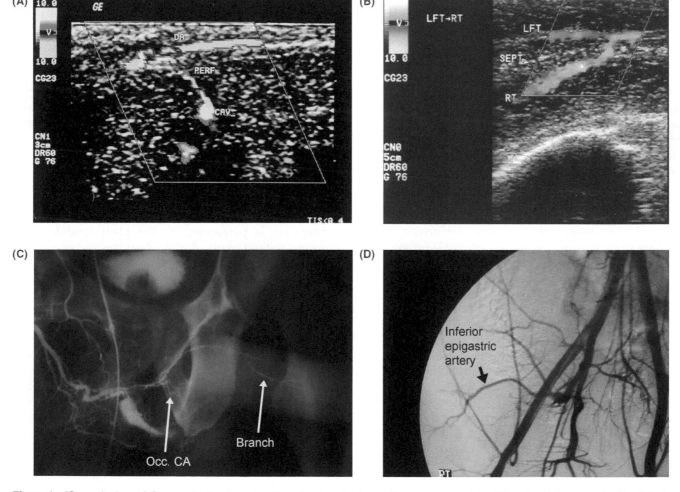

Figure 1 (*See color insert.*) Communicating branches from the dorsal artery to the cavernosal artery (**A**) and septal communication (**B**), documented by penile DDU. Selective internal pudendal arteriogram documenting obstruction of cavernosal artery and a dorsal perforating branch (**C**) and inferior epigastric artery with good length and no branches (**D**).

preoperative antibiotics (cefazolin or vancomycin, if allergic to penicillin).

From a technical standpoint, the operation can be divided into three stages: dorsal artery dissection, inferior epigastric artery harvesting, and microsurgical anastomosis.

To maximize operative exposure, a meticulous technique, a headlight, surgical loupes (during the dorsal artery dissection and harvesting of the inferior epigastric artery), and a ring retractor with its elastic hooks are used. In addition, a hand-held Doppler probe is an excellent accessory tool for monitoring of the dorsal artery and checking for runoff into revascularized arteries.

Dorsal Artery Dissection

A semilunar scrotal incision, two fingerbreadths from the base of the penis, is made on the side opposite to the planned abdominal incision for inferior epigastric artery harvesting. This incision is carried down through the dartos layer using cautery. This incision offers (i) an excellent proximal and distal exposure of the penile neurovascular bundle, (ii) the ability to preserve the fundiform and suspensory ligaments preventing penile shortening, and (iii) the absence of unsightly postoperative scars on the penile shaft or at the base of the penis.

The ipsilateral tunica albuginea is subsequently identified at the midpenile shaft. With the penis stretched, blunt finger dissection along the tunica albuginea is performed in a distal direction deep and inferior to the spermatic cord structures along the lateral aspect of the penile shaft avoiding injury to the fundiform ligament. The penis is then inverted through the skin incision, with care taken to push the glans in fully. The penis must not be tumesced during this maneuver. If a partial erection is present, intracavernosal α-adrenergic agonist (100 μg phenylephrine) should be administered. Blunt finger dissection around the distal penile shaft enables a plane to be established between Buck's fascia and Colles' fascia, and a Penrose drain is secured in this plane.

Exposure of the neurovascular bundle and, in particular, the right and left dorsal penile arteries, is now performed. The arteries are usually obvious, located on either side of the deep dorsal vein and surrounded by the dorsal nerves. Isolation of the dorsal penile arteries for such arterial bypass surgery requires limited dissection at this time in the procedure; thus ischemic, mechanical, and thermal trauma to the dorsal penile arteries may be minimized. To avoid injurious vasospasm, topical papaverine hydrochloride irrigation is applied frequently. In this way, preservation of endothelial and smooth-muscle cell morphology during dorsal artery preparation is ensured. This is very critical because the room temperature of the operating room, the use of room temperature irrigating solution, and even the skin incision can induce vasoconstriction, spasm, and possible endothelial cell

damage. For intraluminal irrigation, a dilute papaverine, heparin, and electrolytic solution, believed to be capable of inhibiting the early development of myointimal proliferative lesions during surgical preparation, is used.

The right and left dorsal penile arteries are first identified in the midpenile shaft. Their courses are followed proximally underneath the fundiform ligament, with care being taken to leave the fundiform ligament intact. A fenestration is fashioned in the fundiform ligament proximally, usually near the junction of the fundiform and suspensory ligaments at a location where the pendulous penile shaft becomes fixed proximally. Blunt dissection is performed under the proximal aspect of the fundiform ligament above the pubic bone toward the external ring. This dissection enables the inferior epigastric artery to pass from its abdominal location to the appropriate location in the penis while simultaneously preserving the fundiform ligament. The penis is placed back on its normal anatomical position and the inguinoscrotal incision is temperately closed with staples.

Harvesting of the Inferior Epigastric Artery

A transverse semilunar abdominal incision following Langer's lines is the preferred incision, though a paramedian incision can be used especially if the desired inferior epigastric artery is short and has several branches or if the patient habitus precludes a standard transverse incision. The transverse incision provides excellent operative exposure of the inferior epigastric artery and heals with a more cosmetic scar compared to that observed with paramedian skin incisions. The starting point of the transverse incision is approximately 11/16 of the total distance from the pubic bone to the umbilicus in the midline. It extends laterally along the skin lines for approximately 5 cm. The rectus fascia is incised vertically. The junction between the rectus muscle and underlying preperitoneal fat is identified and the preperitoneal space is entered. The rectus muscle is reflected medially.

The inferior epigastric artery and its two accompanying veins are located beneath the rectus muscle in the preperitoneal plane. The ring retractor is again utilized to optimize operative exposure. It is critical to harvest an inferior epigastric artery of sufficient length to prevent tension on the microvascular anastomosis. Application of topical papaverine is utilized on the inferior epigastric artery throughout the dissection. Thermal injury is avoided using low current microbipolar cautery set at the minimum level necessary for adequate coagulation, and the vasa vasora are preserved by dissecting the artery en bloc with its surrounding veins and fat. Dissection of the inferior epigastric is required from its origin at the level of the external iliac artery to a point at the level of the umbilicus. It is at this point that the artery bifurcates. In the past, every effort was made to use the bifurcation where possible to allow anastomoses to both dorsal arteries, but we have not seen a significant improvement in erectile function in patients who underwent anastomosis of the inferior epigastric artery to both dorsal arteries when compared to patients who had a single anastomosis. The authors, more recently, performed a single anastomosis minimizing surgical time and preserving a dorsal artery in case a second penile revascularization is desired.

The transfer route of the neoarterial inflow source is prepared from the abdominal perspective prior to transecting the vessel distally (the penile transfer route has previously been dissected). The temporary scrotal staples are removed and the penis is reinverted. The internal ring on the side of the harvested artery is identified lateral to the origin of the inferior epigastric artery. Using blunt finger dissection through the inguinal canal, a long fine vascular clamp is passed through the fenestration in the fundiform ligament, the external and internal inguinal rings, and a Penrose drain is placed to protect this transfer route.

The donor vascular bundle is transected at the level of the umbilicus between two Ligaclips and is carefully inspected for any proximal bleeding points. The long fine vascular clamp is brought through the internal inguinal ring again, this time to grasp the end of the transected inferior epigastric artery. The inferior epigastric vascular bundle is transferred to the base of the penis. It should be briskly pulsating and of adequate length. The origin of the inferior epigastric artery should be inspected for kinking or twisting. Following the achievement of complete hemostasis, closure of the abdominal wound is performed in two layers. The rectus fascia is closed utilizing a running 0 polyglycolic acid suture, with one suture started at either end of the incision. The skin edges are apposed using skin staples.

Microvascular Anastomosis

A ring retractor and the associated elastic hooks are utilized once again on the inguinoscrotal incision and the fenestration of the fundiform ligament to gain exposure of the proximal dorsal neurovascular bundle. The pulsating inferior epigastric artery is placed against the recipient dorsal penile arteries, and a convenient location is selected for the vascular anastomosis. The anastomosis (or anastomoses) is (are) created based on the arteriographic and duplex Doppler ultrasound findings. An end-to-end anastomosis is best under conditions whereby dorsal penile artery communications exist with the cavernous artery. In addition, an end-to-end anastomosis transfers perfusion pressure more effectively than end-to-side anastomosis with less turbulence. It has been the authors' experience that ligation of both dorsal penile arteries to perform bilateral proximal end-to-end anastomoses has not ever caused ischemic injury to the glans penis.

The appropriate dorsal penile artery segment is freed from its attachments to the tunica albuginea, with care being taken to avoid injury to any communicating branches of the cavernosal artery. Vascular hemostasis of this segment of the dorsal penile artery may be achieved with either gold-plated (low-pressure) aneurysm vascular clamps or vessel loops under minimal tension for the minimal operating time. The only location where the adventitia must be carefully removed is at the site of the vascular anastomosis, i.e., the distal end of the inferior epigastric artery and the free end of dorsal artery, in order to avoid causing subsequent thrombosis. If segments of adventitia enter the anastomosis, patency of the anastomosis is in jeopardy because adventitia activates clotting factors from the extrinsic clotting system. The remaining adventitia should be preserved in the vessels because the vasa vasorum provide a nutritional role to the vessel wall. The preservation of the adventitia is additionally important in terms of vessel innervation.

A plastic, colored background material is used to aid in vessel visualization under the microscope. An end-to-end anastomosis is performed between the inferior epigastric artery and the dorsal artery using interrupted 10-0 nylon sutures (single-armed, 100-µm, 149° curved needle) under 10× magnification. Following release of the temporary occluding vascular clamps (or vessel loops) on the dorsal penile artery, the anastomosed segment should reveal arterial pulsations along its length and retrograde into the inferior epigastric artery. Such an observation implies a patent anastomosis. At this time, the inferior epigastric artery gold-plated aneurysm clamp may be removed. The intensity of the arterial pulsations in the anastomosis usually increases. Occasionally, the application of a small amount of hemostatic material may be needed to aid in promoting hemostasis from suture needle holes in the vessel walls. After complete hemostasis has been achieved and correct instrument and sponge counts are assured, closure of the inguinoscrotal incision may begin. The dartos layer is reapproximated using a 3-0 polyglycolic acid suture in a running fashion. The skin edges are closed with skin staples. The Foley catheter is left for closed-system gravity drainage overnight.

Modifications of the above-described procedure may be utilized. The most common alternative, arterial anastomosis, is an end-to-side anastomosis between the inferior epigastric artery and the dorsal penile artery. A 10-0 is placed along the longitudinal axis of the dorsal penile artery in a 1-mm segment in the region of the intended anastomosis. After placing tension on the suture, an oval section of the artery wall is excised with curved microscissors, resulting in a 1.2 to 1.5 mm horizontal arteriotomy. A temporary 2-Fr silastic stent is placed within the arteriotomy for clearer definition of the vessel lumen. The sutures are placed initially at each apex of the anastomosis and then subsequently three to five interrupted sutures are placed on each side wall. All sutures used to complete the anastomosis are made equidistant from each other to avoid an uneven anastomosis. One side of the anastomosis is completed prior to commencing the other side. If a temporary vascular stent is used, it is removed following placement of all sutures. The use of a temporary vascular stent enables careful inspection of the vessel back wall.

☐ COMPLICATIONS

Superficial ecchymosis and penile edema are not unusual or debilitating. Wound infections are rare and generally can be managed with oral antibiotics. Arterial bleeding is extremely rare and is generally due to bleeding from a small branch of the inferior epigastric artery or from the anastomosis. Mechanical disruption of the microvascular anastomosis has been reported by Hatzichristou and Goldstein (9). This disruption of the microvascular anastomosis and subsequent uncontrolled arterial hemorrhage may occur from blunt trauma in the first few postoperative weeks following coitus, masturbation, or from accidents. Consequently, resumption of sexual activity should not begin until six weeks after this surgery.

Penile numbness or pain due to injury to the nearby dorsal nerve may occur (10). Penile sensation

fully returns 12 to 18 months after surgery if no major penile sensory nerve has been significantly severed.

Penile shortening due to scar entrapment may be experienced in as many as 20% of the patients, but preservation of the suspensory and fundiform ligaments has markedly diminished penile shortening in our series. Occasionally, penile shortening due to severe scar entrapment may require subsequent scar release surgery and the use of relaxing Z-plasty incisions or scrotal flap coverage.

Another complication of deep dorsal penile vein arterialization (rare, in our experience), is glans hyperemia, which occurs when a communicating vein from the revascularized deep dorsal vein to the glans in the distal dissection is missed (9). Surgical exploration and ligation of the arterialized communicator resolves the problem.

☐ RESULTS

Of the 31 publications on penile revascularization surgery reviewed by the American Urologic Association (AUA) committee, only 4 reports of a total of 64 patients

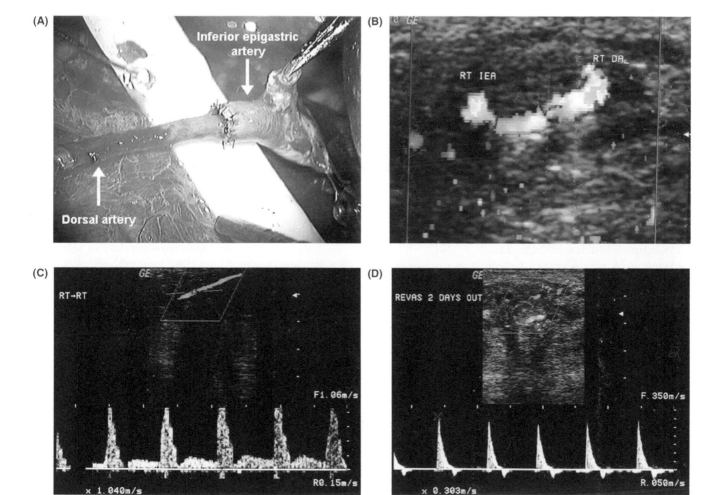

Figure 2 (*See color insert.*) (**A**) Microsurgical anastomosis between the inferior epigastric artery and the dorsal artery using an end-to-end technique. Penile duplex Doppler color ultrasound documenting anastomotic patency (**B**) and high peak systolic velocities at anastomosis (**C**, **D**).

met the peer review criteria: (*i*) age below 55 years, (*ii*) absence of major vascular risk factors (diabetes, tobacco, etc.), (*iii*) a minimum follow-up of one year, (*iv*) classic findings by penile duplex Doppler ultrasound, DICC, cavernosography, and selective internal pudendal arteriography, and (*v*) objective follow-up data (Fig. 2). These reports document a success rate of 36% to 91%, which has led some to question the possible benefits from this type of surgery (11–14).

In the authors' experience, young men free of classic vascular risk factors and with pure cavernosal arterial insufficiency secondary to blunt perineal trauma, who undergo microvascular arterial bypass surgery (inferior epigastric artery to dorsal artery) experience a significant improvement in erectile function, sexual distress, mood, and overall satisfaction.

More specifically, the authors have reported mean preoperative penile rigidity, International Index of Erectile Function (IIEF), Erectile Function (EF) domain, Q3, Q4, Sexual Distress Scale (SDS), CES-D of 40%, 35.9 ± 14.1, 12.8 ± 6.5, 2.2 ± 1.4, 2.1 ± 1.4, 37.1 ± 11.4, and 39.9 ± 15.3, respectively. The postoperative penile rigidity, IIEF, EF domain, Q3, Q4, SDS, CES-D, and Erectile dysfunction inventory of treatment rdirfaction (EDITS) were 74.4%, 58.1 ± 14.7, 24 ± 7.2, 4 ± 1.6, 3.9 ± 1.5, 18.4 ± 13.4, and 18.4 ± 6.8, respectively. All pre- and postoperative differences were significant. In addition, 91% of the subjects would recommend Microarterial bypass surgery (MABS) to other patients. Postoperative complications included inguinal hernia (1/50), penile shortening (12/60; 0.29 in.), and penile pain (4/50).

□ REFERENCES

1. National Institutes of Health Consensus Statement. Development Panel on Impotence. JAMA 1993; 270: 83–90.

2. Feldman H, Goldstein I. Impotence and its medical and psychosocial correlates: results of the Massachusetts Male Aging Study. J Urol 1994; 151(1):457–467.

3. Michal V, Kramer R, Popischal J, et al. Direct arterial anastomosis on corporal cavernosa penis in therapy of erectile dysfunction. Rozhl Chir 1973; 52:587–590.

4. Virag R, Zwang G, Dermange H, et al. Vasculogenic impotence: a review of 92 cases with 54 surgical operations. Vasc Surg 1981; 15:9–17.

5. Virag R. Revascularization of the penis. In: Bennett AH, ed. Management of Male Impotence. Baltimore: Williams & Wilkins, 1982:219–233.

6. Hauri D. A new operative technique in vasculogenic erectile impotence. Wold J Urol 1986; 4(4):237–249.

7. Crespo E, Soltanik E, Bove D. Treatment of vasculogenic sexual impotence by revascularizing the cavernous

and/or dorsal arteries using microvascular techniques. Urol 1982; 20(3):271–275.

8. Konnak JW, Ohl DA. Microsurgical penile revascularization using the central corporeal penile artery. J Urol 1989; 142(2 Pt 1):305–308.

9. Hatzichristou DG, Goldstein I. Arterial bypass surgery for impotence. Curr Opin Urol 1991; 1:144–148.

10. Zorgniotti AW, Lizza EF. Complications of penile revascularization. In: Zorgniotti AW, Lizza EF, eds. Diagnosis and Management Of Impotence. Philadelphia: B.C. Decker, 1991.

11. Ang LP, Lim PH. Penile revascularization for vascular impotence. Singapore Med J 1997; 38(7):285–288.

12. Grasso M, Lania C, Castelli M, et al. Deep dorsal vein arterialization in vasculogenic impotence: our experience. Arch Ital Urol Nefrol Androl 1992; 64(4):309–312.

13. Jarow JP, DeFranzo AJ. Long-term results of arterial bypass surgery for impotence secondary to segmental vascular disease. J Urol 1996; 156(3):982–985.

14. Kayigil O, Ahmed SI, Metin A. Deep dorsal vein arterialization in pure caverno-occlusive dysfunction. Eur Urol 2000; 37(3):345–349.

41

Advances in Phallic Reconstruction

Culley C. Carson and Ash Kshirsagar

Division of Urology, Department of Surgery, University of North Carolina School of Medicine, Chapel Hill, North Carolina, U.S.A.

□ PENILE ENLARGEMENT SURGERY
Introduction

The penis is a unique, complex, and dynamic organ. It must perform the important tasks of urine passage, erection, vaginal penetration, and ejaculate delivery. Equally important, the penis must be able to appreciate both tactile and erogenous sensation. All these functions can be achieved by this one organ because it has an intricate interposition of vascular, neural, erectile, and urothelial tissues.

In the past, surgery to increase penile size has been performed to correct congenital and acquired deformities of the penis. These techniques were developed to treat patients with conditions such as bladder extrophy, epispadius, buried penis, or hidden penis or to facilitate continence mechanisms in patients with spinal cord injuries (1–6). Now, there is increasing interest in performing penile enlargement surgery for normal men who desire a larger penis (6–9). The practice of penile enhancement surgery is limited by the cosmetic motivation of patients as well by the number of surgeons who perform these procedures. Long-term results and outcomes continue to be established (6,7,10–13).

History and Development

Penile enlargement surgery has evolved out of treatments for congenital disorders that are associated with a small penile length (1–4,14). These conditions are usually diagnosed and corrected in childhood. "Buried penis" is one such congenital disorder where a normal size penis appears small. The penis does not attain a normal external length because of retraction of the shaft proximally into the body by the shaft skin. Upon palpation, the corporal bodies and shaft can be appreciated to be of normal size. There is, however, an inadequate amount of penile skin available to cover the shaft. Tension from the skin pulls the shaft proximally toward the pubis, decreasing the visible external portion of the penis. Additionally, abnormal fibrous bands of Dartos fascia at the penile base tether the shaft to the pubic region and further prevent the shaft from attaining its full external length. Surgical intervention involves release of the Dartos bands, which allows for distal extension of the shaft. Next, skin grafting or skin advancement is performed to increase the amount of shaft skin. The skin can be harvested from the prepuce or suprapubic region or from skin grafts. Providing this additional shaft skin allows the penis to attain its full external length (3).

"Hidden penis" is a similar congenital condition in which a penis of normal length appears smaller than its true size. As with buried penis, the shaft is tethered by abnormal fibrous bands of Dartos fascia at the base of the penis. This condition is distinct from buried penis in that there is an adequate amount of penile skin to cover the shaft. Patients with hidden penis, however, also have excessive adipose tissue in the suprapubic region that surrounds the base of the shaft. This excess adipose tissue decreases the visible length of the pendulous penis. Surgical management involves release of the restrictive Dartos bands as well as resection of the excess suprapubic fat. Surgery increases the external length and visibility of the normal penis. In obese patients who do not have the restricting bands of Dartos fascia, simple weight loss may increase both the visible and functional length of the penis (4,10).

More invasive penile enlargement surgery is required in patients who suffer from bladder extrophy—a congenital condition in which the anterior abdominal wall fails to close prior to birth. The bladder is left exposed and opens onto the abdomen. These patients also suffer from epispadius and a decreased visible penile length. In normal males, the proximal ends of both corporal bodies are attached to the pubis and lie relatively parallel to one another. In extrophy patients, the pubic rami are separated from one another. The corporal bodies must first bridge the gap between the pubic rami prior to joining together in the shaft. Less corporal tissue is therefore available to contribute to the external shaft. Penile lengthening is performed by dissection of the corpora off of their attachments to the pubic rami. The proximal ends of the corpora are brought together and advanced in an anterior and medial fashion. The coprora are then secured and anchored to the fibrous band of tissue connecting the pubic rami. The surgery increases the amount of corporal tissue in the external penile shaft (1,2). While surgical descriptions are clear, there remains a need for long-term functional results.

Indications for Penile Enlargement Surgery

In the past few years, there has been a growing interest in surgery to increase penile size in normal men for cosmetic purposes. Over 10,000 men in the United States have undergone some type of surgery to increase penile size (6,7). Unlike congenital or acquired medical conditions, indications for cosmetic surgery are not concrete. A patient's desire to undergo penile enlargement surgery is often personal and may be confounded by psychological issues (6–8).

Normal penile length is a variable and subjective measure that can differ among cultures and races. Some studies have attempted to establish standards for penile size (8,10). One study specifically investigated penile length as an indication for penile enlargement surgery (10). It suggests that surgery may be an option for those individuals who fall below two standard deviations of normal penile size, but only if the patient has a strong desire. Using these cutoff points in the study population, the lower limits of normal for penile length is less than 4 cm in a flaccid penis and less than 7.5 cm of length in an erect penis. These guidelines, however, are not intended to be concrete or applied universally: other series have used different lengths to define normal (15). It is essential to remember that flaccid penile length does not always correlate with the erect or functional length. Furthermore, adequate penile size, either flaccid or erect, is often a personal and subjective judgment (10).

In some men, perceptions of small phallic size may stem from low self-esteem or depression. Often, these feelings manifest from experiences in childhood or adolescence, but seem to be antecedent to adulthood (16). All patients who seek penile enlargement surgery should undergo, at the very least, a cursory psychological evaluation to identify any significant pathology. Some men who feel their penile size is small relative to others often have unrealistic assessments of normal. Educating patients as to what is normal as well as unbiased assessment of their penile size has been proven to ameliorate misperceptions and, in some men, obviate the need to undergo surgery (15,16). Surgery may be of no benefit to psychiatrically troubled men or men with unrealistic expectations of normal. Still, there are men who are mentally stable, who feel that increasing penile size may help with their confidence and may even enhance the quality of intercourse. Since there are no definitive or concrete indications, the decision to undergo penile enlargement surgery remains a personal one. This desire may be considered analogous to the desire in women who seek breast augmentation for cosmetic purposes. Surgery cannot remedy deep psychological deficits; however, it may enhance the self-image and interpersonal interactions in certain individuals with realistic expectations regarding increase in actual size (8,9). Individuals who seek out these procedures, however, must be willing to accept the risks of complications.

Methods

Penile Lengthening Surgery

Penile lengthening surgery involves increasing the length of the pendulous or external portion of the penis. The goal is to increase both the length of the visible shaft and the functional length available for sexual intercourse. Both goals are thought to be achieved by surgical release of the suspensory ligament. The suspensory ligament is a fibrous band of connective tissue that originates from the lower abdominal wall and suprapubic region. It envelops the Dartos fascia of the shaft base (Fig. 1), providing support to the penis by anchoring the proximal shaft to the pubic bone and suprapubic region. Dissection of the suspensory ligament off of the periostium of the pubic bone facilitates anterior inferior displacement of the corporal bodies (1,2,7–9). This allows for a greater percentage of the corporal body length to be available externally. Penile lengthening surgery is performed through a suprapubic approach that provides for excellent visualization and exposure of the suspensory ligament at the dorsal penopubic junction. This approach also avoids unnecessary damage to the dorsal venous complex or neurovascular bundle.

Some surgeons advocate that dissection of the suspensory ligament alone does not adequately increase penile length. The use of penile weights, along with surgery, is thought to result in a significant increase in penis size. Weights are attached to the distal end of the penis in order to stretch it and facilitate penile growth. The amount of weight can be increased gradually over the course of months (8,9).

Forward displacement of the penis after suspensory ligament release creates a space in the suprapubic subcutaneous tissue as well as skin between the shaft and the pubic bone. This space must be filled in order to prevent reattachment of the corporal bodies after their release: otherwise any gain from surgery may be subsequently lost. Often, the corporal bodies and pubis are kept separated by a fat pad interposition or by placing a piece of Gore-Tex at this site (8,9). The surface created by this space must also be covered by skin. Simple realignment of the incision line is not possible. It will cause the shaft skin to be under tension. As in patients with buried penis, this will restrict the penis from attaining it full external potential length. This tension may also bring the corpora closer to the pubis, predisposing to reattachment. Skin advancement flaps are necessary to cover this newly freed area (8). Two flap techniques, the inverted V-Y plasty and the double Z plasty, have been routinely used for skin advancement in penile enlargement surgeries (Figs. 1 and 2). Both techniques facilitate suprapubic access to the suspensory ligament with suprapubic flap advancement at the time of closure.

Initially, the inverted V-Y plasty was performed for skin advancement in penile lengthening surgery. This method involves advancement of a flap of suprapubic skin onto the newly extended dorsal shaft. An

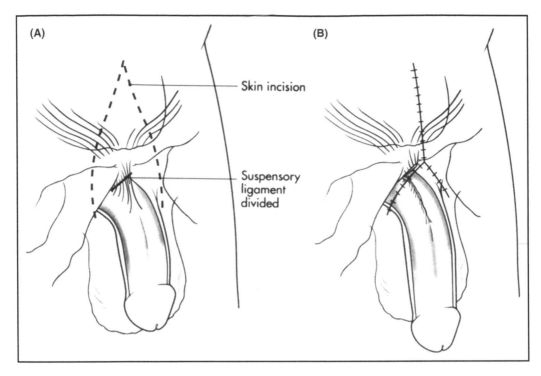

Figure 1 (**A**) Location of the suspensory ligament. The dashed line indicates the location for the incision of the "V" portion of the inverted V-Y plasty. (**B**) Illustration of the penis after suspensory ligament release and skin advancement with closure of the incision as an inverted "Y." *Source*: From Ref. 6.

incision in the shape of an inverted V is made in the suprapubic region superior and lateral to the shaft base (Fig. 1A). The suprapubic skin between the arms of the V is advanced onto the newly expanded dorsum of the penis. The apex of the V is then sewn together to form the base of the Y. Sewing together the base of the V reapproximates the lateral margins of the incision and covers the deficit left by the donor flap. The long arms of the V are shortened and form the arms of the Y (Fig. 1B). Due to mixed cosmetic results from the inverted

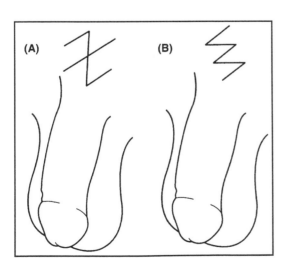

Figure 2 (**A**) The double Z plasty technique of skin advancement prior to skin advancement. (**B**) Closure of the incision after skin advancement. *Source*: From Ref. 7.

V-Y plasty, a double Z plasty has been employed as an alternative for skin advancement (Fig. 2) (7,9). This technique also employs transposition of a suprapubic flap on to the dorsum of the penis. An incision, comprising a Z with a line through it, is made in the suprapubic region. After dissection of the suspensory ligament and flap advancement, the incision is reapproximated and closed in a zigzag line. Regrowth of pubic hair over the suprapubic region should cover both types of incisions.

There is another technique for penile enhancement that does not focus on suspensory ligament release in order to gain length. This technique involves placing a rib cartilage graft between the distal corporal bodies and the glans. Through a subcoronal incision, the glans is dissected off from the distal coropora. The glans is left attached to the urethra ventrally and the neurovascular bundle dorsally. Autologous rib cartilage is secured in the space between the glans cap and distal corpora. Subcutaneous penile tissue is placed over the rib cartilage to provide a vascular supply (12).

Some surgeons who perform enlargement surgeries inform their patients that the outcomes are variable and that certain individuals may not obtain any true increase in length (8). Reports of techniques that rely on suprapubic release have suggested an increase in length from 2.2 up to 3.8 cm (8), but other series report varied results (11,13). Results for rib cartilage graft interposition technique report durable increase in length from 2 to 4 cm at around three years (12).

Girth Enhancement

As with penile lengthening procedures, surgery has been attempted to increase penile girth. Girth enhancement surgery focuses on the use a patient's own fat to increase the diameter of the penis. The autologous fat is harvested through liposuction and is reinjected underneath the Dartos fascia. Multiple incisions made at the corona and penile base are necessary to inject fat along the shaft (7). The challenge in girth enhancement surgery involves obtaining an even, smooth circumferential distribution of the transplanted fat. This is technically difficult because there is a tendency for the fat to be absorbed, undergo necrosis, or migrate laterally between tissue planes (7–9).

New advances in penile girth enhancement surgery have been described using dermal fat pad grafts. In this technique, de-epithelialized fat pads with a layer of dermis can be harvested from either the lateral groin or the gluteal creases. The penis is circumferentially degloved by separating the skin and Dartos layers from Buck's fascia. The dermal fat pads are then placed in longitudinal strips along the penis from the base to the corona. The dermal side is placed on the outside and will oppose the Dartos fascia; the fat side will border Buck's fascia. This arrangement gives the penis a more even and natural texture as the dermal aspect of the graft is smoother than the surface apposing Buck's fascia. The spongiosum is left uncovered from the grafts to prevent any urethral injury or constriction. The dermal fat pads are sewn together and to Buck's fascia longitudinally along the dorsum of the penis. Along the ventral aspect of the penis, the lateral wings of the grafts are sewn to Buck's fascia at the corpospongiosal border. The grafts are placed tension free in order not to restrict the penis during an erection. The maximal thickness of the harvested tissue can be no greater than 1 cm. Anything thicker will not allow graft uptake and is more susceptible to ischemia. A pad thicker than 1 cm will also prevent the Dartos as well as the shaft skin from being advanced over the graft and reattached in a tension-free manner. Dermal fat pads offer a new alternative for girth enhancement surgery. These grafts have a better chance for growth because they receive blood from Dartos and Buck's fascia until neovascularization occurs.

The results of girth enhancement surgery, including durability and complications as well as increases in diameter, are varied and continue to be established (7–9,13,14). Results from adipose tissue injection are often asymmetrical because of fat cell migration, reabsorption, and necrosis. The use of dermal fat pad grafts, however, has been reported to uniformly increase the penile diameter from 2.2 up to 4.4 cm (8).

Results of Enlargement Surgeries
Risks and Complications of Penile Lengthening

A comprehensive knowledge of complications resulting from these specialized procedures is limited because an unquantified number of complications are not reported in the literature. Reports have surfaced, however, detailing some common complications resulting from these types of surgery (6,7,14).

All surgical procedures that involve closure of an incision carry risk. Complications from skin closure include infection, separation, and tissue breakdown. Penile enlargement surgery is no different. There have been reports of wound infections leading to patient hospitalization and skin breakdown necessitating additional surgical scar revision. One report of the formation of an abscess that led to the development of suprapubic and perianal fistulas highlights the potential severity of these complications (6). Additionally, patients who have undergone lengthening procedures have reported sexual dysfunction, painful erections, painful intercourse, and, paradoxically, even penile shortening (6,7,14). Some patients have been found to have a documented paresthesia with decreased light touch and vibratory discrimination along the shaft (6). It has been speculated that the dorsal nerve of the penis could be injured during suprapubic dissection of the suspensory ligament. Decreased sensation or pain in the shaft may limit enjoyment of sexual intercourse. These complications can cause or compound preexisting psychological problems such as poor self body image or decreased self-esteem and have been reported to lead to erectile dysfunction (6,7,14).

Patients have also relayed dissatisfaction with hypertrophic scar formation along the incision (6,7). For some, pubic hair will not cover these scars (14), and these patients are left with a relatively hairless and large scar in the middle of normal hair-covered skin. Flaps carry an increased risk for these complications as their native blood supply may be compromised. The blood and lymphatic flow of the flap is disrupted along its undersurface and three of the flap's four borders. In the inverted V-Y flap, for example, lymphatic and blood flow is dependent upon the penopubic border. The potential for lymph edema and ischemia can impair wound-healing, leading to wound separation or to the formation of these large, adherent scars (8).

Certain complications have been attributed specifically to the design of inverted V-Y skin advancement flap. The procedure involves moving a piece of suprapubic skin onto the dorsal base of the penis to cover the newly released shaft. Along with the suprapubic skin, lateral scrotal skin is also raised up on to the penis. As the suprapubic and scrotal skin is hair covered and normal shaft skin is not, the V-Y advancement may cause a protuberance of pubic hair on the shaft. The hair is not uniform and may leave a poor cosmetic appearance. The shaft can also appear deformed as the thick suprapubic skin and the wrinkled scrotal skin replace the smooth, thin skin of the proximal shaft. The texture of the proximal shaft becomes similar to that of the scrotum. This has been called "scrotalization," and is a significant complaint among some patients (Fig. 3) (6,9,14). Suprapubic skin also has a greater amount of underlying fat than does penile skin (8). For this reason, the flap sometimes gives the appearance of a hump on the dorsal penis. Patients complain that both the scrotalization and the dorsal hump reduce the amount of smooth shaft. In some, this makes the penis appear smaller despite any length gained from the release of the suspensory ligament (14).

The skin closures that form the arms of the Y also have the potential to lead to a cosmetically poor result. In certain patients, these lines are thicker and more pronounced than the surrounding tissue. Reapproximation of the incision leads to a raised ridge of skin superior and lateral to the penis. The appearance of bilateral ridges on either side of the penis has led to the evolution of the term, "scrotal dog ears" (7–9,14). The cosmetic result is so poor in some patients that they have had to undergo additional surgery to resect these ridges (14). One technique to prevent these dog ears is to perform Z plasties on the anterior scrotum just underneath the penoscrotal junction (13). A handful of men who have undergone rib cartilage interposition have reported moderate penile curvature that was treated with penile stretch and vacuum erection devices (12).

Corrective Surgery for Penile Enlargement Complications

Some patients have reported an overall dissatisfaction from surgery. They are either unhappy with the cosmetic result of the skin advancement procedure or dissatisfied by an inadequate increase in penile length. These feelings may stem from unreal expectations that patients have prior to the surgery. This has led certain individuals to seek out corrective surgery to improve the cosmetic result. Revision of the cosmetic defects have included resection of the "dog ears." Others have attempted to use topical steroids to treat the hypertrophic scar or have undergone surgical scar resection. Obtaining an adequate cosmetic result through surgical reversal is difficult and may require more than one surgery. It is important to note that any further surgery also carries with it additional risk and may not completely reverse the results of the initial surgery.

A few patients have been so displeased with the cosmetic results that they have undergone complete reversal of the skin advancement. Reversal involves resection of the scar or base of the inverted Y. The arms of the Y are incised to separate the penis from the skin of the penile base and suprapubic region. The skin advancement flap that is on the penile dorsum is then repositioned into its original position on the suprapubic region. The skin is reapproximated and closed in the shape of a V. Surgical reversal may be impossible for patients who do not have adequate dorsal shaft skin to pull up onto the suprapubic region (6,7,14). During the penile lengthening procedure, some surgeons will remove any new distal foreskin created by the skin advancement procedure. After lengthening surgery, there is an insufficient amount of skin available to cover the shaft and for flap reversal. Reversal may

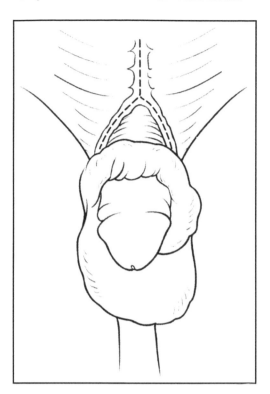

Figure 3   Scrotalization after a skin advancement using the inverted V-Y plasty. *Source*: From Ref. 6.

cause the penis to retract proximally toward the pubis, giving it a smaller visible and functional length (14).

Results of Girth Enhancement Surgery
Risks and Complications of Girth Enhancement Surgery

Penile girth enhancement surgery also has unique complications. Patients who have undergone fat injection have reported an uneven, bumpy, and irregular appearance to the shaft. This can be caused by asymmetric injection, migration, or reabsorption of the transposed fat. The penis does not have any tissue in between the Dartos and Buck's fascial layers to prevent lateral migration of the fat. The injected fat may easily move between tissue planes and has been noted to coalesce into large globules. This has led to difficulty with intromission in certain individuals (6). Further asymmetry can be caused by necrosis of the injected fat. Fat necrosis leads to fibrosis and calcification deposits that further disfigure the smooth shaft skin. In some, it has even caused pain. Others have noted a decreased amount of sensation under the fat deposits. Overall, fat injections tend to have a poor durable result because of reabsorption, necrosis, and migration (6–9,14). The use of dermal fat pads to increase penile girth is a relatively new procedure. Potential complications may include poor graft take and subsequent graft necrosis. There is also the risk of fibrosis and scarring of the grafts that can theoretically interfere with erection, sensation, and micturition.

Corrective Surgery for Girth Enhancement Procedures

Corrective surgery involves resection of the previously transplanted fat through a circumcision incision, through an incision along the median raphe, or through an inverted V-Y flap incision if a penile lengthening procedure is also being reversed. It may not be possible, however, to resect the fibrotic plaques or the calcified deposits. Resecting previously injected fat can also leave dimples along the shaft. Corrective surgery also carries additional risk: a median raphe incision may insult any previously undisturbed Dartos. This tissue layer provides the blood flow to the shaft in those patients who have undergone an inverted V-Y plasty. Compromising blood flow to this region could lead to ischemic necrosis of the flap (7,14).

□ PENILE RECONSTRUCTION
Introduction

Congenital absence or loss of the penis due to trauma, infection, or the treatment of penile malignancies can impair normal penile physiologic function. The resulting psychosocial morbidity may be equally devastating. Phalloplasty, the surgical reconstruction of the penis, can replace an absent penis or augment a damaged penis.

The principles behind phalloplasty involve using a patient's own tissue to create a neophallus that can perform functions similar to that of the normal penis. In the past, surgeons have used a combination of flap transfer techniques, recruiting tissue from the scrotum, groin, or abdomen to create a neophallus. These methods were met with limited success. Advances in microvascular surgery have allowed for better aesthetic and functional results in phalloplasty. Despite many different surgical methods that can be employed and a variety of donor tissues available, the goals of phalloplasty are common:

1. The surgical creation of a neophallus should be a one-stage procedure.
2. The neophallus should be able to provide both tactile and erogenous sensation.
3. The neophallus should have a neourethra extending to the distal shaft that will allow urination from a standing position.
4. The neophallus should be aesthetically acceptable.
5. The neophallus should be of enough length, girth, and rigidity to allow for intercourse.

Although all surgical techniques cannot meet these goals, the creation of a functional penis that is aesthetically pleasing is possible. Advances in surgery continue to be made and will ultimately improve on all aspects of phalloplasty (17–21).

History of Phalloplasty

Historically, there have been a variety of surgical techniques employed to create a new penis. Surgeons have used a variety of donor tissues from the scrotum, groin, or abdomen in an attempt to create a phallus that looks and performs like the native penis. The aesthetic and functional results, however, have been limited (22–32).

Early attempts at penile reconstruction employed scrotal tissue to create a neophallus for patients who had suffered penile transection from trauma or for the treatment of a penile disease (22–24). One technique uses the scrotal skin to create the neourethra, and, in a later stage, employs the underlying scrotal tissue to create a neophallus. Initially, parallel incisions are made on either side of the scrotal median raphe. The medial margins of each incision are brought over a Foley catheter and sewn together to create the lumenal surface of the neourethra. The lateral skin margins are then brought together and sewn in place over the catheter and the first suture line. Both the lumenal and external surfaces of the new tube consist of scrotal skin. Next, the distal aspect of the native urethra and the proximal portion of the neourethra are sewn together. A perineal urethrostomy is performed to divert urine and allow the urethral anastomosis to heal. Initially, the neourethra is left attached to the scrotum as the highly vascularized scrotal tissue provides the necessary blood supply to the anastomosis and neourethra (22).

The neourethra is given time to heal and, after a few weeks, a second and final surgery is performed. The neophallus is created from the thick connective tissue of the scrotal septum located just under the neourethra. Two parallel or zigzag incisions are made into the scrotal skin on either side of the neourethra. The incisions are carried down through the subcutaneous tissue into the scrotal septum. The incisions are then brought together along the underside of the neourethra, creating a cylinder of tissue. At this time, a rib cartilage graft or long piece of acrylic is inserted along the undersurface of the shaft in order to provide rigidity. The medial skin borders of the incision are then sewn together over the rib cartilage graft or acrylic, thereby closing the ventral surface of the neophallus. The lateral borders of the scrotal incision are also reapproximated and sewn together to close the now separate scrotum (22).

This procedure created a new phallus that allowed the patient to urinate from a standing position. There were, however, many limitations to this technique. First, the surgery required more than one stage. Durable rigidity necessary for intercourse was not obtained as the rib graft warped or was absorbed over time. In some, the acrylic implants caused overlying skin breakdown from pressure, with implant extrusion (22). The size and aesthetic result of the neophallus were also not reported.

A similar technique using scrotal skin successfully employed rib grafts to provide rigidity. In this technique, the proximal end of the rib was sewn to the distal remnant of the cavernosal tissue and covered with skin. This anchored the graft and provided blood flow necessary to sustain the rib over time. The patient was able to have intercourse with this method of phalloplasty. This technique, however, fell short of meeting other important goals for penile reconstruction (17–21,33). It was a multistep procedure with limited aesthetic results: the skin of the neophallus was wrinkled and not smooth like a normal penis. Long-term assessment of durability was limited. The patient also relied on a perineal urethrostomy for micturition since a neourethra was not created with this technique of phalloplasty (23).

Subsequent attempts at phalloplasty have incorporated gracilis muscle flaps (25–28). The gracilis muscle is a long, narrow, superficial muscle that courses along the medial aspect of the thigh. The muscle aids with adduction, flexion, and medial rotation of the leg. The gracilis is useful but not critical to the leg because other muscles also perform these movements. The proximity, innervation, vasculature, and complimentary function of the gracilis make it an excellent choice for the use as a flap. One phalloplasty technique incorporates both right and left gracilis muscles to create a new penis. The muscles are dissected free of adjacent fascia and transected distally. The distal ends of each muscle are pulled underneath the groin skin and brought together into the pubic area. The proximal ends of each gracilis flap are sewn to the remaining native cavernosal tissue and secured to the pubic region. The right and left gracilis muscles are then sewn together along the dorsum in a longitudinal manner to create a neophallus. The neourethra is created from an abdominal full thickness skin graft that is tubularized around a Foley catheter. The neourethra is positioned ventrally between the right and left gracilis muscles. Scrotal skin flaps are then mobilized to cover the proximal portion of the neophallus, and split thickness skin grafts are used to cover the remainder of the shaft (28). Although the phallic reconstruction with a neourethra can be performed in one stage, sensation to the neophallus is limited. Furthermore, aesthetic results and long-term evaluation of rigidity for this method of phalloplasty were not reported. Variations of this technique have used myocutaneous grafts or grafts containing the gracilis muscle with its overlying skin to create a neophallus. Using a myocutaneous graft increases the girth and bulk of the neophallus as subcutaneous fat and tissue is brought along with the gracilis muscle (27). Rigidity necessary for intercourse can be obtained by using a penile prosthesis that can be inserted after the neophallus has had time to heal (29).

Tissue flaps from the abdomen have also been utilized in phalloplasty. These techniques are multistep procedures that incorporate a tube with in a tube motif (28,30). The first step involves creation of a neourethra out of abdominal skin. A Foley catheter is laid obliquely onto a lateral portion of anterior abdominal skin. Parallel incisions are made alongside either edge of the catheter. The medial skin borders of each incision are brought over the catheter and sewn together to create a tube of skin that will become the neourethra. The two lateral skin edges are then pulled together over the neourethra and are sewn to one another. The catheter is secured into place on the abdomen and the new urethra is given time to heal. In a second procedure, rectangular skin flaps along either side of the neourethra are created. The skin flaps are freed from the underlying abdominal musculature and fascia. The lateral ends of both flaps are brought together underneath the neourethra and sewn together to create the neophallus. The tube in a tube structure is left attached to the abdomen by both the superior and the inferior pedicles in order to allow the neophallus to heal. Skin grafts are used to cover the areas left by the flaps (31).

In a third procedure, the superior pedicle of the neophallus is released from the abdomen and is sewn to the pubic region to become the proximal shaft. It is during this stage that the neourethra is attached to the distal native urethra. The inferior pedicle is left attached to the abdomen. Urine is diverted until a fourth surgery, at which time the inferior abdominal pedicle of the neophallus is released from the abdominal wall to become the distal shaft. The use of tubed abdominal flaps in phalloplasty has proven to be suboptimal: it requires many involved surgical procedures and falls short of creating a phallus with sensate or erectile capability. The aesthetic appearance of the neophallus is also not similar to that of a native penis (26).

Current Concepts in Phalloplasty

Over the last several years, advances in microvascular surgery have led to the use of free tissue flaps for phalloplasty. Free tissue flaps can be shaped into an aesthetically superior phallus with the capacity for sensation and urine passage (17–20,33,34). The addition of a penile prosthesis during phalloplasty or in a second stage can further provide necessary erectile capacity (17,18,35–37). The superior results from the use of microvascular free flaps have led to the adoption of this technique as the standard for phalloplasty (17–20,33).

Free flaps can be harvested from many parts of the body. In penile reconstruction, the nondominant arm has become the donor area of choice (Fig. 4A). The arm has redundant blood flow, which will enable vessels to be harvested without ischemic compromise or venous congestion of the donor site. The skin and subcutaneous tissue is relatively smooth, can be easily manipulated, and contains a minimal amount of hair. Superficial cutaneous nerves can be readily identified and attached to nerves at the recipient area to create a sensate neophallus (18–20,23). Additionally, the donor area is receptive to skin grafts and heals well (Fig. 4B).

Prior to grafting, the arm must be carefully evaluated. The donor area must have an adequate amount of surface area and subcutaneous tissue. Doppler ultrasonography is used to assess vessel patency and to mark the vessels that will be transposed. Occasionally, ultrasonography is insufficient and angiography may be necessary to fully evaluate the anatomy and patency of the vessels (18,19). The Allen test must also be performed on each patient to assure sufficient

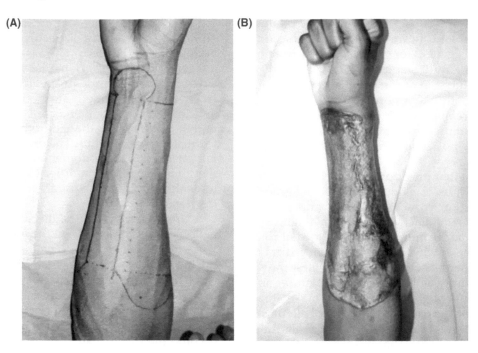

Figure 4 (**A**) Marking the nondominant forearm prior to phalloplasty. The less hirsute ulnar surface will be used to create the neourethra. (**B**) Picture of the same patient's forearm after the split thickness skin grafts to the donor site have healed.

collateral blood flow to the forearm and hand. An area of limited hair is best used because a hairy surface predisposes the neourethra to infections and to the formation of calculi, strictures, or fistulas (17–19).

Phalloplasty Utilizing Forearm Grafts

The original design for phalloplasty using microvascular free flaps is based upon a graft containing the radial artery (Fig. 5A) (34). The radial surface of the forearm is shaped into a neophallus using a tube within a tube motif. The flap is centered around the radial artery and covers an area that is approximately 15 to 18 cm long and 14 to 16 cm wide and contains the skin and subcutaneous tissue of the forearm (17). The flap is elevated and neophallus is created on the arm to allow for continuous perfusion by the radial artery. After harvesting and transposition to the pubic region, the radial artery will provide all necessary blood flow to the newly created penis. The cephalic vein and the venae comitantes of the radial artery, which are harvested as part of the flap, provide the venous drainage (19,20,34).

At the start of surgery, the skin and subcutaneous tissue are outlined and elevated off of the arm (Fig. 4A). Next, the radial artery and the venous vasculature are carefully dissected free from their inferior attachments. During the dissection, careful attention is paid to identifying and preserving the lateral antebrachial nerve and the medial antebrachial nerve. These nerves will be coapted to the nerves of the pubic region to provide sensation to the neophallus. Once the flap is completely elevated, a 3-cm to 4-cm longitudinal strip on the ulnar surface of the flap is

marked off. This portion of the flap is to become the neourethra. The ulnar surface is chosen because it is less hirsute than the radial surface of the flap. The ulnar surface is separated from the radial surface by a 0.5-cm to 1.0-cm longitudinal strip of skin that is de-epithelialized. The ulnar surface is wrapped around a Foley catheter and sewn to itself to create a tube (Fig. 5B). A two-layered closure is used: the first layer is skin to skin and the second overlying closure secures the subcutaneous tissue to itself. Once the neourethra has been created, the radial aspect of the flap is brought around the neourethra and sewn to itself, thereby completing the tube within a tube motif (Fig. 5C). This method of phalloplasty is commonly referred to as the Chinese design or method (17,18,34).

Since its introduction and widespread implementation, the radial artery forearm flap has undergone several modifications. One variant centers the skin of the neourethra over the radial artery itself (Fig. 6A). The Foley catheter is placed along the longitudinal axis of the radial artery. The skin is brought up on either side of the catheter and sewn together to form the neourethra (Fig. 6B). Two narrow lateral flaps on either side of the neourethra remain. These flaps are brought around each side of the neourethra and are sewn together to create the neophallus (Fig. 6C). This phalloplasty technique was designed to provide the greatest possible blood flow to the neourethra in order to reduce the risk of stricture and fistula formation (17,18,20). One disadvantage of this flap design, however, is that there are two visible suture lines along the shaft of the neophallus (Fig. 6D). To increase rigidity, the flap design may also include partial resection of the radius bone. If radius is to be harvested, approximately 10 to 13 cm of bone that is one-third the diameter of the radius is resected. This bone is left attached to the flap's vasculature and is incorporated within the neophallus (20). The use of bone grafts for rigidity, however, is controversial as bone grafts are prone to warping and absorption (22,36,38).

Another variant of the radial free flap is the "Cricket-Bat" design (Fig. 7) (17,18,39). In this variant, the neourethra and the neophallus are centered in tandem along the axis of the radial artery. The handle, or distal portion of the flap, is sewn into a tube over a catheter to create the neourethra. Then, the neourethra is folded under the body of the bat, which is the broader, proximal aspect of the flap. The neourethra is attached to the native urethra prior to the creation of the neophallus. The lateral flap edges of the wider, more proximal portion of the arm are then wrapped around either side of the neourethra and sewn together along the ventral surface of the neophallus. The "Cricket-Bat" technique is advantageous in that both the neourethra and the neophallus receive maximum blood flow from the radial artery. Additionally, the urethral anastomosis is technically easier because of

excellent exposure and visualization of the urethra (18,39). This free flap motif has been criticized, however, because the creation of both the neophallus and the neourethra from one tandem segment leads to a shorter penis. Furthermore, creation of the neourethra from the more hairy radial surface will predispose it to infections as well as calculi, strictures, and fistula formation (17,18).

In an attempt to create a less hair-filled neourethra, one technique describes a free-flap method centered around the ulnar artery (Fig. 8). A similarly sized flap is raised over the surface of the ulnar artery. A neourethra is then tubularized along the longitudinal axis of the ulnar artery. As in the modified radial technique, the lateral wings of the flap are brought around either side of the neourethra to complete the neophallus. The ulnar artery is then transected and transposed to the pubic region. The nerves are the same as those employed in the radial forearm graft. Some surgeons prefer this technique because the ulnar skin surface is smoother and less hirsute. Additionally, the larger diameter of the ulnar artery is thought to provide superior blood flow (17–19,21).

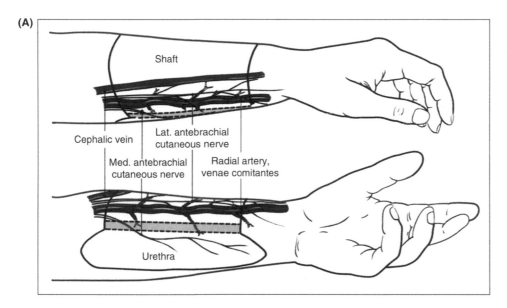

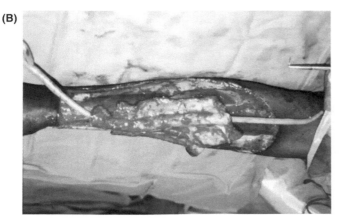
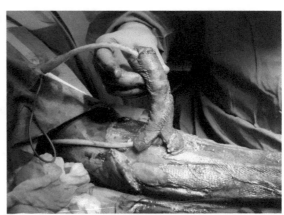

Figure 5 (A) The "Chinese flap" design that uses the radial artery and forearm surface. *Source*: From Ref. 18. (B) The neourethra is created over a Foley catheter while still being perfused by the forearm. (C) The neophallus is created while still being perfused by the forearm.

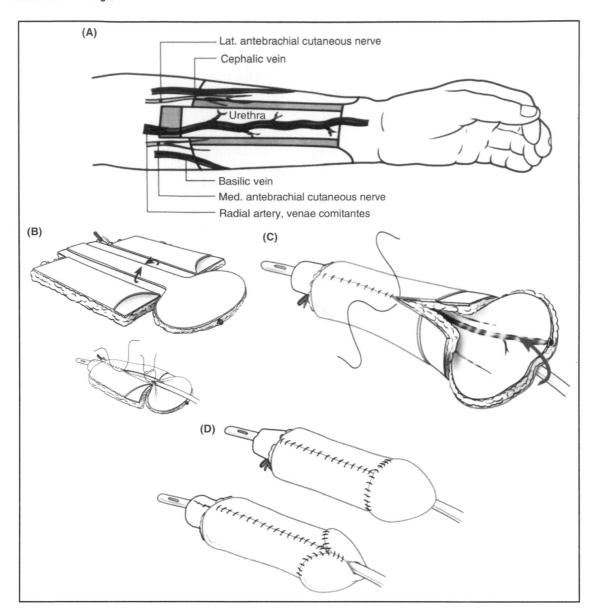

Figure 6 (**A**) The modified radial artery forearm flap. (**B**) The neourethra is centered over the artery. (**C**) Two lateral skin flaps on either side of the neourethra are used to create the neophallus. (**D**) The completed neophallus. Two longitudinal suture lines remain as two flaps are brought around either side of the neourethra. *Source*: From Ref. 18.

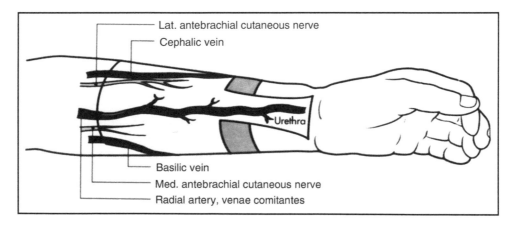

Figure 7 The "cricket bat" motif. The neourethra and neophallus are created from a tandem segment of tissue that lies above the radial artery. *Source*: From Ref. 18.

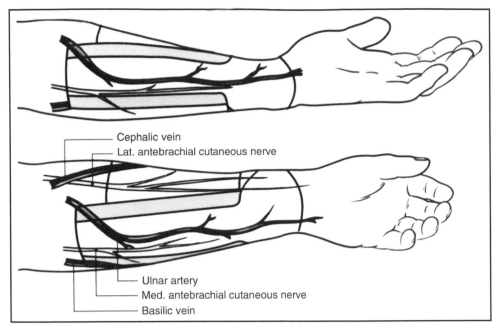

Figure 8 The ulnar artery forearm flap is designed around the ulnar artery and its venae comitantes. *Source*: From Ref. 18.

Phalloplasty Utilizing the Lateral Arm Free Flap

Forearm flaps have been widely used for phalloplasty, with good results. The flaps, however, are not without limitations and complications. The forearm skin is often thin. It may not be thick enough to provide for an adequate aesthetic and functional girth. This can hinder the placement of a penile prosthesis and may predispose to prosthesis extrusion. Prosthesis placement must also be performed later as a separate surgical procedure. The forearm skin often contains thick hair. Hair within the neourethra has been attributed to

infections as well as the formation of calculi, strictures, and fistulas. Once the flap has been harvested, the forearm may have cold intolerance and decreased sensation. Furthermore, the donor site is quite visible and difficult to hide (17,18,21,33).

Use of the lateral arm free flap is another alternative in microvascular phalloplasty (17,21,33). This free flap uses the skin and subcutaneous tissue along the lateral surface of the upper arm to create a neophallus. The flap is centered around the posterior radial collateral artery, its venae comitantes, and the posterior cutaneous nerve (Fig. 9). Some surgeons advocate

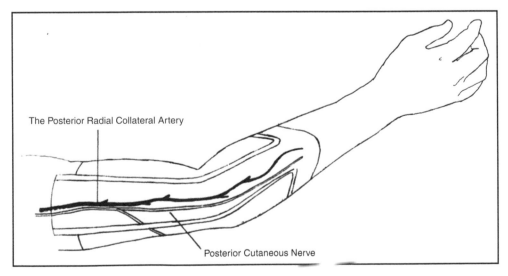

Figure 9 The lateral arm free flap. The flap is centered around the posterior radial collateral artery and its venae comitantes and employs the posterior cutaneous nerve of the arm for nerve coaptation.

that the use of this donor area leads to a superior result (17,21,33). The thicker subcutaneous tissue provides increased girth and protection to the new phallus. The flap can be extended below the elbow to obtain additional length. The paucity of hair on the skin surface is also thought to decrease complications in the neourethra. Furthermore, prosthesis placement may be possible at the time of phalloplasty (17,21,33).

The larger size of the neophallus stems from a fundamental difference in graft design: the use of a prefabricated urethra. Unlike the radial and ulnar forearm grafts, the lateral arm graft temporally separates the construction of the neourethra and the neophallus into a two-stage process. The first stage involves the creation of a neourethra. A full-thickness skin graft obtained from the abdomen, groin, or flank is used to make the neourethra. The graft is sewn together around a Foley catheter, creating a tube with the interior lining consisting of skin surface. Next, an incision is made along the upper arm down to the lateral intermuscular septum. Care is taken not to extend the incision beyond the posterior radial collateral artery. The neourethra and Foley catheter are then inserted into this space. The incision along the lateral arm surface is then closed over the neourethra and catheter. The proximity of the posterior radial collateral artery allows for excellent healing of the neourethra. This positioning will further serve the neourethra after flap transfer as the proximity of the vasculature is thought to decrease the incidence of stricture formation. The neourethra is allowed to heal for three to six months, during which time the patient periodically removes the catheter to irrigate the lumen. Endoscopic evaluation of the neourethra is also performed to assess graft take and to identify strictures. This will allow for any modification prior to flap transfer. The presence of a fully vascularized and patent neourethra is established prior to the second surgical procedure (17,21,33).

In the second surgery, a lateral arm flap containing the neourethra is elevated along the axis of the posterior radial collateral artery. An area of 12 × 35 cm of tissue is used to create the neophallus. After elevation, the lateral wings of the flap are brought around either side of the neourethra to create the neophallus. Care is taken to identify and preserve the posterior cutaneous nerve. A penile prosthesis can be placed at the time of transfer to the pubic region. The larger girth of the neophallus can readily accommodate the prosthesis. Since the urethra is preformed, there is also a decreased risk of the prosthetic rods interfering with its healing (17,21,33).

If the width of the graft that can be taken from the upper arm is greater than 18 cm, some surgeons advocate a one-stage reconstruction without the use of a prefabricated neourethra (17,21,33). This design is similar to the forearm flaps in that the neourethra is centered along the artery and is made from the flap tissue itself and not from transposed skin. After construction of the neourethra, the two lateral edges are brought on either side of the neourethra to finish the tube within a tube motif. Although this method has the advantage of being a one-stage repair resulting in a larger neophallus, the advantages of having a prefabricated neourethra are lost. Furthermore, insertion of a prosthesis may interfere with normal healing of the neophallus (17,33).

Transfer of the Neophallus

While the neophallus is being constructed on the arm, the pubic region should be concurrently prepared to accept the graft. Initially, the vasculature of the recipient site is identified and made ready to be attached to the graft vessels. The inferior epigastric artery and vein are the vessels of choice (Fig. 10) (17,18,22,30,33). Once identified, they are dissected upward toward their origin underneath the abdominal musculature in order to gain as much length as possible. Upon transfer of the neophallus, the graft vessels are anastomosed to the artery and vein. Occasionally, additional venous drainage is necessary to service the graft. The patient's nondominant saphenous vein can be transposed to the pubic region to accept any additional venous return. The inferior epigastric vessels may not always be available to accept the graft due to obliteration or thrombus. If necessary, arterial supply can be provided by the femoral artery through a saphenous vein graft interposition. Venous drainage can also be diverted to the saphenous vein (Fig. 11) (17–19). If the inferior epigastric vessels are known to be unavailable prior to surgery, an arteriovenous (A-V) fistula is created between the femoral artery and saphenous vein prior to the phalloplasty. The A-V fistula is then allowed to mature. During flap transfer, the A-V fistula is transected and attached to the respective arterial and venous connections of the graft (17,33).

Urethral reanastomosis is a critical step in the transfer process. In men undergoing penile reconstruction, the neourethra is attached directly to the residual native urethra. The anastomosis is fashioned using a two-layer closure over a Foley catheter draining the bladder. In transgender surgery, the native urethra is intact but not long enough for direct anastomosis because of its posterior and oblique position. Bilateral flaps elevated from the labia minora are sewn together over a catheter to extend the length of the urethra (17,18,21,33). The neourethra of the graft is then sewn to this urethral extension. In both penile reconstruction and transgender surgery, a gracilis flap can be elevated and wrapped around the urethral anastomosis to decrease the risk of fistula formation (Fig. 12) (17–19).

In genetic males, the remainder of the graft is secured to the penile stump. The fascial layers in the neophallus are sewn to the corporal bodies and the penile fascia. The skin is easily approximated and closed. In transgender surgery, the task of securing the penis to the patient is more complex. A horizontal incision is made just above the vagina and is carried down to the pubic bone (Fig. 13). A second vertical incision is made, starting in the middle of the first incision, and

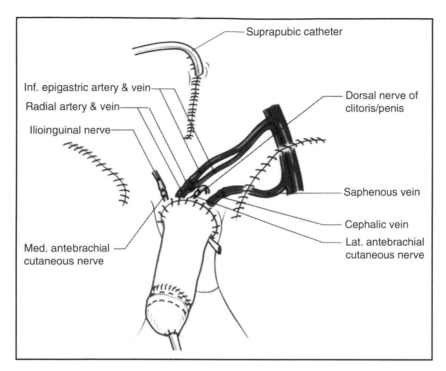

Figure 10 The vascular anastomosis of the neophallus to the inferior epigastric artery and vein. The cephalic vein is attached to the saphenous vein in order to accommodate the additional venous flow. The purpose of the incision (two shown, one is theoretical, to indicate this procedure may be performed on either side) is to allow access to the recipient vessels for the anastomosis. The suprapubic catheter is used to divert urine. *Source*: From Ref. 18.

carried down to the superior aspect of the vagina (17). After urethral anastomosis, the tissue is positioned into a bipedicle flap that is attached to the fascia and skin of the neophallus (17,33). The fascia of the neophallus can also be sutured to the pubic bone periostium in order to provide additional support.

Nerve coaptation in the neophallus is an extremely essential part of phalloplasty. Providing sensation allows for both protection of the neophallus and participation in sexual intercourse. In genetic males undergoing reconstruction, the right and left dorsal penile nerves are preferentially selected (Fig. 14). These

nerves are branches of the internal pudendal nerve and provide tactile and erogenous sensation. During graft transfer, these nerves are attached to the medial and lateral cutaneous nerves of the forearm or the posterior cutaneous nerves, if a lateral arm flap has been employed. In transgender patients, the clitoris is degloved and the branches of the internal pudendal nerves are isolated. The right and left branches of these nerves are coapted to the nerves of the neophallus. If the nerve length is insufficient, neural interposition grafts can be placed to connect the nerves of the neophallus to the pudendal nerves. Nerve anastomosis to

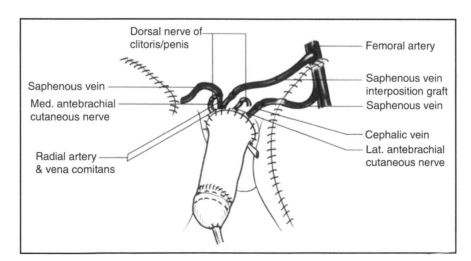

Figure 11 When the inferior epigastric artery and vein are unavailable, the blood flow to the neophallus can be provided by the femoral artery through a saphenous vein interposition graft. Two incisions (one theoretical) are shown to indicate that this procedure may be performed on either side. *Source*: From Ref. 18.

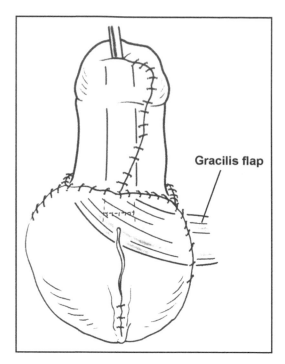

Figure 12 A Gracilis muscle flap from the patient's nondominant leg can be raised and wrapped around the urethral anastomosis to provide additional support and to decrease the incidence of fistula formation. *Source*: From Ref. 18.

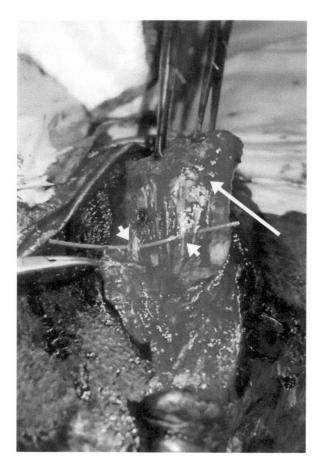

Figure 14 The dorsal penile nerves (*arrowheads*) are isolated at the recipient site and can provide erogenous sensation to the neophallus after nerve coaptation. Arrow shows penile stump: native corporal stump covered with Buck's and Dartos fascia.

the dorsal penile nerves in men, or to the internal pudendal branches on the clitoris in women, allows for both erogenous and tactile sensation in the neophallus. If nerve anastomosis to branches of the internal pudendal nerve is not possible, the nerves on the

neophallus may alternatively be coapted to branches of the ilioinguinal or iliofemoral nerves to provide tactile sensation. Erogenous sensation, however, may not be attained (17–19,21,33,34).

Implantation of a Penile Prosthesis

Attaining rigidity sufficient for sexual intercourse remains a long-standing challenge in phalloplasty (17,18,23–25). Previous mechanisms for obtaining rigidity include the placement of cartilage, bone, or acrylic rods into the neophallus at the time of surgery (19,22–24,35,36,38). These attempts, however, have met with limited success. Cartilage and bone tend to bend, fracture, or be absorbed over time. Acrylic rods have caused tissue breakdown and pressure necrosis along the shaft. These mechanisms are also socially unacceptable as the neophallus remains in a constantly erect state. Some surgeons do not advocate the use of internal stiffening devices in patients who have undergone phalloplasty, because the risks of infection, prosthesis extrusion, and damage to the neourethra are thought to be too great. These surgeons feel that rigidity can be safely attained by external stiffening devices such as splints, re-enforced condoms, or

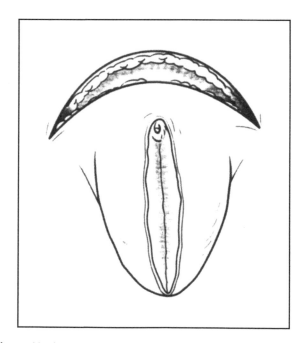

Figure 13 In transgender patients, a horizontal incision is made in the suprapubic region in preparation for flap transfer. *Source*: From Ref. 18.

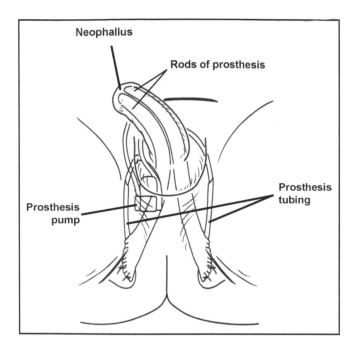

Figure 15 Installation of a penile prosthesis. *Source*: From Ref. 18.

vacuum assist devices (24). Patients, however, may not attain the degree of rigidity necessary for sexual intercourse and current practice advocates the use of a penile prosthesis to obtain rigidity in phalloplasty (Fig. 15) (17,18,23,33,38).

In most patients, superior erectile function can be obtained with careful surgical placement of a penile prosthesis. If the neophallus is large enough, prosthesis placement can be done during phalloplasty (21,33). More often, however, it is performed as a second surgical procedure in order to allow the initial phalloplasty to heal. There are advantages to waiting: a healed neourethra will decrease the incidence of infection. Waiting will also allow the contractile forces within the tissue to subside. Perhaps most important, it also allows adequate time for the development of sensation along the shaft. Sensation is a prerequisite to prosthesis placement, as it will allow for protection of the neophallus (18,34,36).

The types of penile prosthetics used in phalloplasty have been modified for this specialized indication. In patients who have undergone phalloplasty, a major concern of prosthesis placement is the risk of extrusion. In normal males who are being treated purely for erectile dysfunction, the prosthesis cylinders are placed within the corpora. The corporal body is a thick fibrous structure that contains and prevents migration or extrusion of the cylinders. In the neophallus, while proximal corpora may be present, there is not any native corpora or other tissue to contain the

cylinders distally. The risk of extrusion is therefore greater. In patients who have undergone phalloplasty, an artificial tunica is created to prevent migration and extrusion of the rods. The neotunica is made of Gore-Tex that encompasses each cylinder. The sleeve of Gore-Tex is closed both proximally and distally to form a protective pocket at each end of the prosthesis. Along the body of the cylinders, longitudinal strips of Gore-Tex are cut out. These holes prevent the buildup of fluid within the neotunica and decrease the risk of infection (17,35,36).

Placement of a prosthesis into a neophallus is similar to the placement in a normal male. Semirigid rods can be used but more often an inflatable penile prosthesis is placed because it better simulates normal erectile function and is less likely to extrude. A transverse infrapubic or penoscrotal incision is made to gain access into the base of the shaft. Care must be taken to avoid injury to the neourethra, vessels, and nerves of the neophallus. A Foley urethral catheter is not placed as it may increase the risk of urethral injury. Once the base of the penis is reached, blunt dissection with either Metzenbaum scissors or urethral dilators is performed to create a longitudinal space along the inside of shaft. This space is then widened using Brooks dilators or by using a urethratome. Once there has been adequate dilation, the cylinder and its surrounding neotunica are placed inside the newly created space. If the neophallus is large enough, a parallel space is made and a second cylinder is implanted. Although the placement of two cylinders is ideal, most neophalluses can only accommodate one cylinder (18,33,35,36).

In men who have suffered penile loss, a proximal pocket of neotunica is not necessary. The proximal ends of the cylinders are inserted in to the remnants of the corporal bodies. A circular cuff of the Gore-Tex neotunica is circumferentially sutured to the corporal tissue. The corporal bodies provide a strong secure base for the cylinders. The proximal ends of the neotunica are also anchored to the ishium using Gore-Tex sutures (18,35,36). Additional stability can be obtained by suturing the neotunica to the pubic symphysis. In transgender patients, the cylinders and neotunica are placed within the shaft in the same manner. Securing the prosthesis, however, is more challenging as there is not any native corporal tissue available to which the rods may be secured. In these patients, the proximal pocket of the Gore-Tex neotunica is essential. If one is using an inflatable penile prosthesis, the tubing at the proximal cylinder exits the neotunica through a prefabricated hole (Fig. 15). The location of the reservoir remains the same and it is placed in the Space of Retzius (17,18,35,36). The pump is placed in the scrotum in men and in the neoscrotum in transgender patients (18).

□ REFERENCES

1. Kelly JH, Eraklis AJ. A procedure for lengthening the phallus in boys with extrophy of the bladder. J Pediatric Surg 1971; 6(5):645–650.

2. Johnston JH. Lengthening of the congenital or acquired short penis. Br J Urol 1974; 46(6):685–688.

3. Wollin M, Duffey PG, Malone PS, et al. Buried penis: a novel approach. Br J Urol 1990; 65(1):97–100.

4. Horton CE, Vorstman B, Teasley D, et al. Hidden penis release: adjunctive suprapubic lipectomy. Ann Plast Surg 1987; 19(2):131–135.

5. Kabalin JN, Rosen J, Perkash I. Penile advancement and lengthening in spinal cord injury patients with retracted phallus who have failed penile prosthesis placement alone. J Urol 1990; 144(2 Pt 1):316–318.

6. Wessells H, Lue TF, McAninch JW. Complications of penile lengthening and augmentation seen at 1 referral center. J Urol 1996; 155(5):1617–1620.

7. Carson CC, Kirby RS, Goldstein I. Textbook of Erectile Dysfunction. Oxford: Isis Medical Media Ltd., 1999: 507–514.

8. Alter GJ. Augmentation phalloplasty. Urol Clin North Am 1995; 22(4):887–902.

9. Alter GJ. Penile enlargement surgery. Techniques Urol 1998; 4(2):70–76.

10. Wessells H, Lue TF, McAninch JW. Penile length in the flaccid and erect states: guidelines for penile augmentation. J Urol 1996; 156(3):995–997.

11. Spyropoulos E, Christoforidis C, Borousas D, et al. Augmentation phalloplasty surgery for penile dymorphophobia in young adults: considerations regarding patient selection, outcome evaluation and techniques applied. Eur Urol 2005; 48(1):121–128.

12. Perovic SV, Djordjevic MLJ. Penile lengthening. Br J Urol 2000; 86(9):1028–1033.

13. Panfilov DE. Augmentative phalloplasty. Aesth Plast Surg 2006; 30:193–197.

14. Alter GJ. Reconstruction of deformities resulting from penile enlargement surgery. J Urol 1997; 158(6): 2153–2157.

15. Shamloul R. Treatment of men complaining of short penis. Urology 2005; 65(6):1183–1185.

16. Mondaini N, Ponchietti R, Gontero P, et al. Penile length is normal in most men seeking penile lengthening procedures. Int J Impot Res 2002; 14(4):283–286.

17. Aston SJ, Beasley RW, Thorne CHM. Grabb and Smith's Plastic Surgery. Philadelphia: Lipincott-Raven Publishers, 1997:1111–1119.

18. Carson CC, Kirby RS, Goldstein I. Textbook of Erectile Dysfunction. Oxford: Isis Medical Media Ltd., 1999: 589–598.

19. Gilbert DA, Schlossberg SM, Jordan CH. Ulnar forearm phallic construction and penile reconstruction. Microsurgery 1995; 16(5):314–321.

20. Biemer E. Penile construction by the radial arm flap. Clin Plast Surg 1988; 15(3):425–430.

21. Khouri RK, Young VL, Casoli VM. Long-term results of total penile reconstruction with a prefabricated lateral arm free flap. J Urol 1998; 160(2):383–388.

22. Goodwin WE, Scott WW. Phalloplasty. J Urol 1952; 68(6):903–908.

23. Morales PA, O'Conner JJ, Hotchkiss RS. Plastic reconstructive surgery after total loss of the penis. Am J Surg 1956; 92(3):403–408.

24. Chappell BS. Utilization of scrotum in reconstruction of penis. J Urol 1953; 69(5):703–707.

25. Horton CE, McCraw JB, Devine CJ, et al. Secondary reconstruction of the genital area. Urol Clin North Am 1977; 4(1):133–141.

26. Hester TR, Hill HL, Jurkiewicz MJ. One-stage reconstruction of the penis. Br J Plast Surg 1978; 31(4): 279–285.

27. Persky L, Resnick M, Desprez J. Penile reconstruction with gracilis pedicle grafts. J Urol 1983; 129(3): 603–605.

28. Orticochea M. A new method of total reconstruction of the penis. Br J Plast Surg 1972; 25(4):347–366.

29. Hoopes JE. Surgical construction of the male external genitalia. Clin Plast Surg 1974; 1(2):325–334.

30. Gillies H, Harrison RJ. Congenital absence of the penis. Br J Plast Surg 1948; 1(8):8–28.

31. Puckett CL, Montie JE. Construction of male genitalia in the transsexual using a tubed groin flap for the penis and a hydraulic inflation device. Plast Reconst Surg 1978; 61(4):523–530.

32. Julian R, Klein MH, Hubbard H. Management of a thermal burn with amputation and reconstruction of the penis. J Urol 1969; 101(4):580–586.

33. Young VL, Khouri RK, Lee GW, et al. Advances in total phalloplasty and urethroplasty with microvascular free flaps. Clin Plast Surg 1992; 19(4): 927–938.

34. Chang TS, Hwang WY. Forearm flap in one-stage reconstruction of the penis. Plast Reconst Surg 1984; 74(2):251–258.

35. Jordan GH, Alter GA, Gilbert DA, et al. Penile prosthesis implantation in total phalloplasty. J Urol 1994; 152 (2 Pt 1):410–414.

36. Alter GJ, Gilbert DA, Schlossberg SM, et al. Prosthetic implantation after phallic reconstruction. Microsurgery 1995; 16(5):322–324.

37. Levine LA, Zachary LS, Gottleib LJ. Prosthesis placement after total phallic reconstruction. J Urol 1993; 149(3):593–598.

38. Hage JJ, Bloem JJAM, Bouman FG. Obtaining rigidity in the Neophallus of female-to-male transsexuals: a review of the literature. Ann Plast Surg 1993; 30(4): 327–333.

39. Semple JL, Boyd JB, Farrow GA, et al. The "Cricket Bat" flap: a one stage free forearm phalloplasty. Plast Reconst Surg 1991; 88(3):514–519.

42

Tissue and Molecular Engineering in the Treatment of Male Sexual Dysfunction

Joerg Wefer, Michael C. Truss, Armin J. Becker, and Christian G. Stief
Department of Urology, Hannover Medical School, Hannover, Germany

□ INTRODUCTION

In recent years, new developments in cell culture techniques, an increasing knowledge about genes and their effects in the mammalian organism, and the discovery of growth factors as important stimulators of tissue proliferation and differentiation have led to new experimental approaches in the treatment of erectile dysfunction (ED). This chapter introduces the recent advances in the treatment of ED via tissue engineering, growth factor treatment, and gene therapy, highlights the results of pioneering experiments, and offers a glimpse into the future of these techniques.

□ TISSUE ENGINEERING

The restoration of sufficient erectile function in patients who are refractory to conservative treatment options remains a medical challenge. The efficacy and safety of medical therapies continue to be suboptimal in some patients, and the results of penile vascular surgery, both arterial and venous, remain unsatisfactory. Despite good results with implantable semirigid or inflatable penile prostheses, the issues of patient acceptance, biocompatibility, and biomechanical complications (e.g., implant infection, penile perforation, or mechanical dysfunctions) present significant barriers to their widespread implementation.

Tissue engineering is proving to be an alternative to the abovementioned operative treatments. Since the last decade, models have been established in which tissue engineering applications for the treatment of ED are being developed. Tissue engineering for the treatment of ED involves the creation of structural and implantable corporal tissue, engineered penile prostheses, and the development of other engineered penile components (e.g., urethra or tunica albuginea) for complete phallic reconstruction.

Engineering of Corporal Tissue

Initial experiments involved the in vivo growth of either corporal smooth muscle or sinusoidal endothelial cells in organ cultures. These were performed on different scaffolds such as biodegradable polymers and collagen gel. It has been shown that engineered corporal smooth muscle subcutaneously implanted in athymic mice not only survived but also grew and induced vascularization by the host (1,2).

Next to be investigated was the seeding and growth of both corporal smooth muscle and endothelium on biodegradable copolymers. The engineered smooth muscle/endothelium constructs were again implanted subcutaneously in athymic mice. Graft survival after transplantation was demonstrated, as well as rapid graft vascularization due to capillary formation in the graft, facilitated by the endothelium (3).

The availability of an acellular three-dimensional scaffold for structural corpus cavernosum growth is crucial. This can be achieved easily by processing donor corpus cavernosa using cell lysis techniques. Three-dimensional acellular matrices are seeded with smooth muscle cells and endothelial cells. The seeded matrices can then be implanted subcutaneously in athymic mice. The growth of a structural vascularized corpus cavernosum with appropriate cell architecture can be achieved within four weeks postimplantation (3); however, the engineered corpora cavernosa still lack nerve fibers and connective tissues to provide a fully functional organ.

Engineering of Penile Prostheses

In an initial experiment, bovine cartilage was harvested, seeded, and grown on cylindrical acid polymer rods. Extensive biomechanical testing of the cartilage cylinder revealed high pressure and tensile stability. The cartilage rods showed complete mechanical stress relaxation after application of mechanical forces without significant structural damages (4).

In a further experiment, autologous cartilage was retrieved from rabbit ear and the harvested chondrocytes were seeded on polymer rods. These rods were implanted into the corporal spaces of the same rabbits. Within two months, the polymers were fully degraded and rod-shaped solid cartilaginous structures had formed in vivo. This experiment demonstrated the feasibility of the in vitro engineering plus in vivo development of autologous biological penile prostheses (5).

Repair of the Tunica Albuginea and Urethra

It has been demonstrated that using an organ-specific homologous acellular matrix graft in the urogenital tract leads to good results, by serving as a scaffold for target-organ–promoted cellular regeneration (6–14). Acellular organ grafts (e.g., acellular bladder, urethra, and tunica albuginea) are easy to produce using cell lysis techniques. In a rabbit model, segmental defects of the complete urethra were created and the defect was repaired with the tubular-structured acellular urethra matrix graft. Within weeks after surgery, the graft was lined completely with urothelium; within three months, the regeneration of smooth muscle structures in the graft was observed. There was no occurrence of urethral stricture in any of the grafted animals (6).

In another experiment in rabbits, a defect in the tunica albuginea of the penis was created and an acellularized tunica albuginea matrix patch was used to cover the defect. Within three months after surgery, there was no significant difference between patch regenerate and neighboring tunica albuginea regarding cell number, collagen, and elastin content. Although some animals had reduced penile rigidity or curved erections after surgery, the overall functional outcome was deemed satisfactory (15).

The Future of Tissue Engineering for ED

The development of tissue engineering in urology will provide additional therapeutic strategies for ED. Severe forms of ED may be treatable with tissue engineering techniques. After a biopsy of the target tissue, healthy autologous cells could be isolated and grown in a cell culture system. These cultured cells could then be seeded on structural scaffolds made of acellular tissue or degradable polymeric matrices, and the cell/matrix construct implanted back into the host. Although only certain genital structures such as cavernous tissue, urethra, and tunica albuginea can be reconstructed in experiments at present, complete functional phallic reconstruction using bioengineering techniques might be possible in the future.

☐ GROWTH FACTORS

Growth factors are an interesting new area in the treatment of ED (16). Most growth factors are proteins that regulate various cell functions in the organism and may be expressed basally or in response to a challenge (e.g., trauma). Growth factors act in an endocrine, paracrine, or autocrine way to inhibit cellular activity or stimulate cell proliferation, differentiation, or certain cellular functions (17,18). Growth factors of interest include the groups/families of insulin-like growth factor (IGF), human growth hormone (hGH), vascular endothelial growth factor (VEGF), fibrocyte growth factor, nerve growth factor (NGF), transforming growth factor (TGF), brain-derived neurotrophic factor (BDNF), and platelet-derived growth factor (18–24). Work with IGF, hGH, NGF, and VEGF is reviewed below.

Insulin-like Growth Factor

IGF acts on many tissues and has been implicated in maintenance and regeneration of the nervous system (25). In one rat experiment, regeneration of nitric oxide synthase (NOS)-containing nerves was studied (26). Researchers disrupted the continuity of the cavernous nerve by neurotomy. Six months after nerve damage, there was a significantly greater maximal intracavernous pressure response to electrostimulation versus one month postoperatively. This correlates with significantly increased expression of IGF-1 and TGF-β2 during nerve regeneration as measured by reverse transcription–polymerase chain reaction. While IGF-1 is likely to enhance the regeneration of the damaged nerve, as reflected by the improvement in function and number of NOS-positive nerve fibers, the role of TGF-β2 and its growth regulating effect remains unclear.

Treatment of diabetic rats with insulin and IGF-1 can improve the intracavernous pressure response to electrostimulation of the major pelvic ganglion (27). Insulin and IGF-1 appear to function as vasodilators. Although the level of gene expression for IGF-binding proteins is increased during diabetes, treatment with IGF-1 reduces the IGF-binding protein expression to normal (nondiabetic) levels. Overexpression of IGF-binding protein 3 and 4 seems to have a vasoconstricting effect on the corpus cavernosum. The key results of these experiments are that insulin deficiency may result in upregulation of vasoconstrictive proteins (i.e., IGF-binding proteins) and downregulation of vasodilating proteins such as IGF.

Human Growth Hormone

Treating hGH-deficient adult patients with recombinant hGH is known to stimulate hepatic IGF synthesis and to increase nitric oxide (NO) and cyclic guanosine monophosphate (cGMP) synthesis. Tissue bath experiments with human corpus cavernosum revealed a relaxing effect of hGH on corpus cavernosum strips as well as an ability to elevate intracellular levels of cGMP. In healthy potent volunteers, it was found that blood levels of hGH increase significantly during the development of an erection. These results suggest that penile erection may be induced by the growth hormone through its cGMP-stimulating activity on human cavernosum smooth muscle (28).

Nerve Growth Factor

NGF is a neurotrophic protein that is known to maintain the survival and differentiation of sympathetic and sensory neurons and to enhance regeneration of damaged nerves (29). NGF is usually released by tissues that are innervated by the neurites (terminal axons/dendrites) of sympathetic and sensory nerve cells. NGF uptake by the neurites is followed by its transport to the cell body where it exercises its effect.

Following cavernosal nerve freezing in rats, it was found that NGF expression in penile tissue was persistently increased; however, the NGF expression in the major pelvic ganglion was decreased, most likely due to blocked retrograde transport in the damaged nerve (30). In a different experiment, it was shown that less NGF is expressed in the penile tissue of old rats compared to young rats. This implies that endogenous penile/cavernosal nerve repair may be reduced in older organisms and may contribute, at least in part, to the development of ED frequently seen in older age (31).

The use of exogenous NGF was tested in a rat model, where a segmental defect of the cavernous nerve was created (32). The nerve defect was treated locally with NGF-loaded copolymers, either alone, with autologous nerve grafts, or with amniotic membrane grafts. Rats with no treatment of the nerve defect were not able to mate with female rats or to develop erections. A stepwise improvement in electrically induced erections was observed in rats treated with NGF alone, nerve graft alone, or the combination of NGF and nerve graft. Restoration of sexual behavior was found to follow the same pattern of erections observed with electrical stimulation. Thus, local adjuvant NGF administration during nerve transplantation for neurogenic impotence was found to markedly improve the therapeutic result of nerve grafting, most likely due to its ability to direct axonal regeneration of the graft within the host nerve. Phase I clinical studies for nerve grafting after cavernosal nerve damage are underway (33), and administration of NGF copolymers during such surgical interventions may prove useful.

Vascular Endothelial Growth Factor

VEGF is one of several polypeptides that have significant angiogenetic effect in vitro and in vivo (34). VEGF may well be one of the most potent growth factors and it is thought to play an important role in embryonal vasculogenesis and the maintenance of vascular structures in the adult organism, as well as in the formation of new vascular structures in cases of pathologic vascular alteration in ischemic tissues. Administration of VEGF in animal experiments and in clinical pilot studies resulted in a marked increase in tissue vascularization.

Extensive analyses of VEGF transcripts of human or rat cavernosal tissue using reverse transcription–polymerase chain reaction revealed that a number of VEGF isoforms are expressed in the cavernosal tissue. The splice variant VEGF164 appeared to be the most abundant isoform in the penis, while other tissues contained a higher abundance of other isoforms (35).

In a rabbit model of hyperlipidemic-induced ED, the animals received a single injection of VEGF intravenously. This single dose of VEGF was shown to produce recovery of erectile function for at least six weeks, as measured by tissue bath studies of corporal tissue (36). It was further shown that the intracavernosal injection of VEGF in hyperlipidemic rabbits not only protected them from developing ED when given a hypercholesteremic diet, but also restored endothelial-dependent and endothelial-independent corporal smooth muscle relaxation (37,38). In a different experiment, bilateral ligation of the internal iliac arteries produced traumatic arteriogenic ED. A single dose of VEGF injected intracorporally minutes after induction of the injury had a marked protective effect on erectile function by facilitating erectile recovery within six weeks as illustrated by the recovery of NOS-positive nerve fibers and significantly higher intracavernous pressure observed after electrostimulation (39).

☐ THE FUTURE OF GROWTH FACTOR THERAPY FOR ED

Although there are many unanswered questions about the influence of growth factors on the growth, regeneration, and physiology of penile tissue, it is known that these growth factors play roles as "additives," from cell culture studies of penile tissue. Gaining facility with the interactive aspects of growth factors and tissues will enable a better understanding of the pathophysiology of ED and help establish growth factors as a valuable diagnostic tool. Changes in the expression of certain growth factors, as well as their receptors and binding proteins, may lead to an improved differential diagnosis of neurogenic or angiogenic ED. Furthermore, growth factors might become a new therapeutic option; for example, IGF could be administered in diabetes-induced ED, VEGF could be used in angiogenic ED, and NGF in neurogenic ED. Determining the optimal dose and administration route of growth factors will be another challenge in ED research. Also, side effects of growth factors must be elucidated before growth factors can be used for ED treatment.

☐ GENE THERAPY

Gene therapy is based on the concept of transferring selected genes (with an identified function and/or gene product) into a host with the aim of normalizing the function of various diseased cells or tissues (40–43), including penile tissue (44).

To perform gene therapy, an optimal vector to transfer a gene to a target (i.e., penile tissue) remains to be identified. Although adeno- and retrovirus vectors are most effective in gene transfer, they can produce an immune response in the targeted organism and injure transfected cells. Naked DNA in liposomes or as plasmids does not provoke an immune response, but they are less effective regarding the success of gene transfer (40). This disadvantage might be compensated for by the presence of gap junctions in the penis, allowing the cellular syncytium to react to the gene introduction in only a small percentage of the targeted cells (45,46).

So far, gene therapy experiments for the treatment of ED have included growth factor, NOS, and potassium channels. Results of these experiments are discussed below.

Growth Factor Gene Therapy

In a rat model, nerve damage was created by bilateral cavernous nerve freezing. Following nerve injury, an intracavernous injection of an adeno-associated virus carrying the BDNF gene was given; as a control, some animals were injected with an adeno-associated virus carrying a marker gene *LacZ*. In the BDNF group, maximal intracavernous pressure during electrical stimulation of the major pelvic ganglia was significantly greater than in the *LacZ* group after four and eight weeks. Additionally, there were noticeably more nerve fibers positive for NADPH and nNOS in the dorsal nerves, and in the cavernous tissue of BDNF-treated animals compared to *LacZ*-treated animals. The nNOS content in the major pelvic ganglia was also significantly higher in BDNF-treated animals. It was concluded that BDNF gene therapy could prevent the degeneration of nNOS-containing neurons in the major pelvic ganglia and facilitate the regeneration of nNOS-containing nerve fibers in penile tissue, thus enhancing the recovery of erectile function after nerve damage (47).

In another experiment, penile venous leakage was created by castrating rats. The animals were treated with either testosterone, VEGF protein (via intracavernous injection), or intracorporal injection of adeno-associated virus carrying the VEGF gene. Nine weeks after treatment, markedly higher intracavernosal pressures were observed by functional cavernosometric evaluation during papaverine-induced erection in all three treatment groups compared to untreated controls. These results indicated the efficacy of VEGF in preventing veno-occlusive dysfunction of the corporal tissue after castration. Thus indirect VEGF delivery via gene transfer showed a therapeutic effect similar to that seen by direct delivery of VEGF protein via injections (48).

NOS Gene Therapy

It is thought that vasodilator NO may enhance erectile function. Thus, it might be possible to use gene therapy to increase endothelial NOS (eNOS) expression. To test this, an adenovirus containing the *eNOS* gene was injected into the corpus cavernosum of aged rats (49). One day after injection, protein blots showed that eNOS protein had increased in the corporal tissue; assays showed cGMP levels increased also. Treated rats showed increased intracavernosal pressures after cavernosal nerve stimulation and greater erectile responses to acetylcholine and zaprinast. Thus, gene therapy with eNOS appears to enhance erectile response from both electrical and pharmacological stimulation.

Potassium Channel Gene Therapy

Potassium channels (K-channels) are thought to participate in the modulation of both contraction and relaxation responses in corporal smooth muscle. In a rat model, aged rats received a potassium channel gene transfer (human smooth muscle maxi-K channel hSlo) (50). Gene transfer was achieved by a "single shot" injection of naked cDNA into the cavernous tissue. Nerve-stimulated intracavernous pressure evaluation of the treated animals revealed a greater pressure response compared to age-matched controls. These effects were apparent for a minimum of one to three months postinjection. The effect of this gene transfer was presumably due to the improved hyperpolarizing ability of the corporal smooth muscle cells that had incorporated and expressed the foreign human K-channel gene. Gene therapy–mediated K-channel alteration may be a useful treatment modality in the future, especially since the effect of gene therapy in this study was maintained over a long period (one to three months) after a single injection.

The Future of Gene Therapy for ED

The described studies indicate the feasibility and efficacy of different gene therapy strategies in treating ED. The corporal tissue is particularly well suited for gene therapy since the penis is positioned externally and is thereby easily accessible. It can be partially and temporarily separated from the general circulation by placing a tourniquet around it to prevent the spread of gene therapeutics to the whole body, although this may limit the gene transfer to the target organ. Because the penile smooth muscle cells have a low turnover rate, the effect of gene therapy may last for an extended period of time.

Based on the individual pathophysiologic mechanism of ED (e.g., diabetic, neuropathic, vasculogenic), gene therapy may be individually tailored for each patient, accessing not only one gene at a time, but also sometimes two, three, or more genes simultaneously.

Although the best method of gene transfer (virus-mediated, naked DNA, liposomes, etc.) remains to be elucidated, and side effects of gene therapy need to be evaluated extensively, the future of gene therapy seems bright. Now that the human genome has been described, many "new" genes will be identified as playing a role in erectile function and dysfunction, opening the door for new targets for gene therapy.

□ CONCLUSION

Several new treatment modalities for ED are currently under experimental evaluation. Tissue engineering may provide new solutions for the restoration of the targeted organ in cases of genital injury, malformation, or severe organic impotence. Promising studies have been published that demonstrate the ability of engineered penile organ components to restore corporal tissue, the urethra, and the tunica albuginea. Additionally, the feasibility of constructing and implanting biologic penile prostheses (i.e., cartilage rods) has been explored and may serve as another future treatment option.

Growth factors also have been successfully used in experiments to improve erectile function under pathological conditions. IGF seems to have a positive effect on neuronal regeneration of the cavernous nerve besides having a vasodilating effect on the cavernous tissue. hGH also has a vasodilating effect on cavernous tissue by influencing intracellular cGMP level. NGF has been shown to positively influence the maintenance and repair of the cavernous nerve. VEGF has been shown to be one of the most potent members of the group of growth factor proteins, not only for its role in preventing vascular ED in pathological models, but also for its ability to restore erectile function in vasculogenic impotence. Although many questions about the dose and optimal administration of growth factors remain currently unanswered, these peptides will certainly become useful tools in the diagnosis and treatment of vasculogenic and neurogenic ED.

Finally, gene therapy for treating ED has shown early promise. Transfer of the BDNF gene into penile tissue has positively influenced the restoration of erectile function after cavernosal nerve damage. VEGF gene transfer has also been shown to have a positive impact on the restoration of sexual function in a vasculogenic impotence model. Gene therapy with the NOS gene can increase local concentrations of the vasodilator NO. Likewise, gene therapy using K-channels appears to improve erections. However, a number of questions about gene therapy for ED remain open. The optimal (i.e., most efficient and safe) method of gene transfer remains to be found; also, promising genes have to be identified before this revolutionary treatment modality can be clinically applied.

□ REFERENCES

1. Kershen RT, Yoo JJ, Moreland RB, et al. Novel system for the formation of human corpus cavernosum smooth muscle tissue in vivo. J Urol 1998; 159(1):156.

2. Yoo JJ, Park HJ, Atala A. Tissue-engineering applications for phallic reconstruction. World J Urol 2000; 18(1):62–66.

3. Park HJ, Yoo JJ, Kershen RT, et al. Reconstitution of human corporal smooth muscle and endothelial cells in vivo. J Urol 1999; 162(3 Pt 2):1106–1109.

4. Yoo JJ, Lee I, Atala A. Cartilage rods as a potential material for penile reconstruction. J Urol 1998; 160(3 Pt 2):1164–1168.

5. Yoo JJ, Park HJ, Lee I, et al. Autologous engineered cartilage rods for penile reconstruction. J Urol 1999; 162(3 Pt 2):1119–1121.

6. Sievert KD, Bakircioglu ME, Nunes L, et al. Homologous acellular matrix graft for urethral reconstruction in the rabbit: histological and functional evaluation. J Urol 2000; 163(6):1958–1965.

7. Sievert KD, Tanagho EA. Organ-specific acellular matrix for reconstruction of the urinary tract. World J Urol 2000. 18(1):19–25.

8. Probst M, Piechota HJ, Dahiya R, et al. Homologous bladder augmentation in dog with the bladder acellular matrix graft. BJU Int 2000; 85(3):362–371.

9. Probst M, Dahiya R, Carrier S, et al. Reproduction of functional smooth muscle tissue and partial bladder replacement. Br J Urol 1997; 79(4):505–515.

10. Piechota HJ, Dahms SE, Nunes L, et al. In vitro functional properties of the rat bladder regenerated by the bladder acellular matrix graft. J Urol 1998; 159(5): 1717–1724.

11. Dahms SE, Piechota HJ, Nunes L, et al. Free ureteral replacement in rats: regeneration of ureteral wall components in the acellular matrix graft. Urology 1997; 50(5):818–825.

12. Chen F, Yoo JJ, Atala A. Experimental and clinical experience using tissue regeneration for urethral reconstruction. World J Urol 2000; 18(1):67–70.

13. Chen F, Yoo JJ, Atala A. Acellular collagen matrix as a possible "off the shelf" biomaterial for urethral repair. Urology 1999; 54(3):407–410.

14. Atala A, Guzman L, Retik AB. A novel inert collagen matrix for hypospadias repair. J Urol 1999; 162(3 Pt 2):1148–1151.

15. Wefer J, Schlote N, Sekido N, et al. Tunica albuginea matrix graft for penile reconstruction in the rabbit: a model for treating Peyronie's Disease. BJU Int 2002; 90(3):326–331.

16. Lue TF. Future treatment for ED: growth factors and gene therapy. Int J Impot Res. 1999; 11(suppl 1): S56–S57.

17. Alison MR, Wright NA. Growth factors and growth factor receptors. Br J Hosp Med 1993; 49(11):774–775.

18. Herndon DN, Nguyen TT, Gilpin DA. Growth factors. Local and systemic. Arch Surg 1993; 128(11): 1227–1233.

19. Hafez B. Recent advances in clinical/molecular andrology. Arch Androl 1998; 40(3):187–210.

20. Yakar S, Liu JL, Le Roith D. The growth hormone/insulin-like growth factor-I system: implications for organ growth and development. Pediatr Nephrol 2000; 14(7):544–549.

21. See WA. Commentary on growth factors: the bread-and-butter cytokines of urology. J Urol 1994; 152(6 pt 1): 1942.

22. Pressler LB, Burbige KA, Connor JP. Molecular advances in pediatric urology. Urology 1995; 46(6): 888–898.

23. Kaplan DR, Miller FD. Neurotrophin signal transduction in the nervous system. Curr Opin Neurobiol 2000; 10(3):381–391.

24. Finkbeiner S. Calcium regulation of the brain-derived neurotrophic factor gene. Cell Mol Life Sci 2000; 57(3): 394–401.

25. Dore S, Kar S, Quirion S. Rediscovering an old friend, IGF-1: potential use in the treatment of neurodegenerative diseases. Trends Neurosci. 1997; 20(8):326–31.

26. Jung GW, Kwak JY, Kim IH, et al. The role of growth factor on regeneration of nitric oxide synthetase (NOS)-containing nerves after cavernous neurotomy in the rats. Int J Impot Res 1999; 11(4) 227–235.

27. Abdelbaky TM, Brock GB, Huynh H. Improvement of erectile function in diabetic rats by insulin: possible role of the insulin-like growth factor system. Endocrinology 1998; 139(7):3143–3147.

28. Becker AJ, Uckert S, Stief CG et al. Possible role of human growth hormone in penile erection. J Urol 2000; 164(6):2138–2142.

29. Terenghi G. Peripheral nerve regeneration and neurotrophic factors. J Anat 1999; 194(Pt 1):1–14.

30. El-Sakka A, Hassan MU, Bakircioglu ME, et al. Possible molecular mechanisms of cryoablation-induced impotence in a rat model. Urology 1998; 52(6):1144–1150.

31. Dahiya R, Chui R, Perinchery G, et al. Differential gene expression of growth factors in young and old rat penile tissues is associated with erectile dysfunction. Int J Impot Res 1999; 11(4):201–206.

32. Burgers JK, Nelson RJ, Quinlan DM, et al. Nerve growth factor, nerve grafts and amniotic membrane grafts restore erectile function in rats. J Urol 1991; 146(2): 463–468.

33. Chang DW, Wood CG, Kroll SS, et al. Cavernous nerve reconstruction to preserve erectile function following non-nerve-sparing radical retropubic prostatectomy: a prospective study. Plast Reconstr Surg 2003; 111(3):1174–1181.

34. Li WW, Talcott KE, Zhai AW. The role of therapeutic angiogenesis in tissue repair and regeneration. Adv Skin Wound Care 2005; 18(9):491–500.

35. Burchardt M, Burchardt T, Chen MW, et al. Expression of messenger ribonucleic acid splice variants for vascular endothelial growth factor in the penis of adult rats and humans. Biol Reprod 1999; 60(2): 398–404.

36. Rao D, Byrne R, Henry G, et al. Duration of VEGF effect in the restoration of corporal vasoactive function. Int J Impot Res 2000; 12(suppl 3):S63.

37. Henry GD, Byrne RR, Huynh TT, et al. Intracavernosal vascular endothelial growth factor protects endothelial dependent corporal smooth muscle relaxation: a preliminary study. Int J Impot Res 1999; 11(suppl 1):S68.

38. Byrne RR, Henry GD, Huynh TT, et al. Intracavernosal vascular endothelial growth factor restores corporal smooth muscle response to nitric oxide. Int J Impot Res 1999; 11(suppl 1):S68.

39. Lee MC, El-sakka A, Bakircioglu ME, et al. The effect of vascular endothelial growth factor on a rat model of arterial impotence. J Urol 2000; 163(suppl 4):198.

40. Rochlitz CF. Gene therapy of cancer. Swiss Med Wkly 2001; 131(1–2):4–9.

41. High KA. Gene therapy: a 2001 perspective. Haemophilia 2001; 7(suppl 1):23–27.

42. Hauser H, Spitzer D, Verhoeyen E, et al. New approaches towards ex vivo and in vivo gene therapy. Cell Tiss Organs 2000; 167(2–3):75–80.

43. Gottschalk U, Chan S. Somatic gene therapy. Present situation and future perspective. Arzneimittelforschung 1998; 48(11):1111–1120.

44. Andersson KE. Penile erectile function: recommendations for future research. Int J Impot Res 2000; 12(suppl 4):S163–S167.

45. Christ GJ, Melman A. The application of gene therapy to the treatment of erectile dysfunction. Int J Impot Res 1998; 10(2):111–112.

46. Christ GJ. Gap junctions and ion channels: relevance to erectile dysfunction. Int J Impot Res 2000; 12(suppl 4): S15–S25.

47. Bakircioglu ME, Lin CS, Fan P, et al. The effect of adeno-associated virus mediated brain derived neurotrophic factor in an animal model for neurogenic impotence. J Urol 2001; 165(6 Pt 1):2103–2109.

48. Rogers R, Meyer T, Lin CS, et al. Intracavernosal VEGF and AAV-VEGF gene prevents ED in a rat model of venous leakage impotence. Int J Impot Res 2000; 12(suppl 3):S63.

49. Champion HC, Bivalacqua TJ, Hyman AL, et al. Gene transfer of endothelial nitric oxide synthase to the penis augments erectile responses in the aged rat. Proc Natl Acad Sci USA 1999; 96(20):11648–11652.

50. Christ GJ, Rehman J, Day N, et al. Intracorporal injection of hSlo cDNA in rats produces physiologically relevant alterations in penile function. Am J Physiol 1998; 275(2 Pt 2):H600–H608.

Effect of Sexual Dysfunction and Its Treatment on Quality of Life of Affected Men

Marita P. McCabe

School of Psychology, Deakin University, Burwood, Victoria, Australia

□ INTRODUCTION

Male sexual dysfunction is a condition that affects a large number of men, and, due to the sensitive nature of the problem, is likely to have an impact on both their individual well-being and broader aspects of their social and relationship functioning. The types of sexual dysfunctions experienced by men can be categorized according to the male sexual response cycle and include disorders of desire, erection, ejaculation, and orgasm (1). These conditions may be primary or secondary, situational or global. They may occur in response to particular life stressors or may be due to a range of physical factors. There is also a relationship between age and sexual dysfunction, particularly erectile dysfunction. Whatever the cause of sexual dysfunction, each may cause significant distress in the lives of males with these problems, as well as their partners.

This chapter will evaluate the impact of sexual dysfunction and its treatment on the quality of life of men. Given the dearth of research on the general well-being of men with sexual dysfunction, a consideration of future research directions in this area will also be provided.

□ IMPACT OF SEXUAL DYSFUNCTION ON THE QUALITY OF LIFE OF MEN

There has been limited research that has examined the impact of male sexual dysfunction on quality of life. Primarily, research has focused on a description of sexual dysfunctions, etiology of these dysfunctions, and an evaluation of the effectiveness of treatments for sexual dysfunction. The literature that is available will be discussed under three headings: the impact of sexual dysfunction on individual quality of life, the relationship between sexual dysfunction and depression, and the impact of sexual dysfunction on relationships.

Impact of Sexual Dysfunction on Individual Quality of Life

Laumann et al. (2) demonstrated that the presence of sexual dysfunction had an effect on quality of life, but that this impact was greater for dysfunctional women than for dysfunctional men. The low levels of well-being (low feelings of physical and emotional satisfaction and low feelings of happiness) were significant for men with erectile dysfunction but not for men experiencing premature ejaculation.

A number of earlier studies examined variables associated with sexual dysfunction and overall well-being. Bell and Bell (3) and Masters and Johnson (4) found that sexual satisfaction was associated with both life satisfaction and well-being. A more recent study conducted by Donnelly (5) found no relationship between reduced sexual activity (which is frequently associated with sexual dysfunction) and either of these measures of quality of life. Donnelly's results, however, were drawn from responses to a single item regarding well-being, and so they may not adequately represent findings in relation to the impact of sexual dysfunction on quality of life.

McCabe (6) investigated the relationship between sexual dysfunction and quality of life among men and women. A multidimensional measure of quality of life was used in this evaluation. The following objective and subjective assessments of seven domains were obtained: material well-being, health, productivity, intimacy, safety, place in the community, and emotional well-being. Sexually functional men ($n = 43$) were compared on these quality-of-life measures to men with premature ejaculation ($n = 43$), erectile dysfunction ($n = 47$), and lack of sexual desire ($n = 24$). All respondents were currently involved in heterosexual relationships, and there were no differences between the functional and dysfunctional groups in the number of respondents who were in married and de facto relationships.

Consistent with earlier findings, quality of life was more strongly associated with sexual dysfunction for women than it was for men. Men with both premature ejaculation and erectile dysfunction experienced deficits when compared to sexually functional respondents in the areas of health, intimacy, and safety. Men with erectile dysfunction also experienced problems in the areas of emotional well-being and their perceived places in the community. Surprisingly, men with a lack of sexual desire did not experience as many deficits in objective levels of well-being, with the only difficulties being encountered in the areas of health and intimacy.

Further interesting findings were obtained in the subjective dimensions of quality of life. Men with both premature ejaculation and erectile dysfunction experienced a lack of satisfaction with each of the seven domains of quality of life, except for their productivity. On the other hand, men with a lack of sexual desire only experienced lower levels of satisfaction with the levels of intimacy in their relationships and their levels of safety.

These findings indicate that sexually dysfunctional men experienced deficits in their objective levels of well-being, as well as satisfaction with their lives in the areas of intimacy and emotional well-being, and, to a lesser extent, in their levels of health and safety. Sexual dysfunction, however, was not associated with a reduction in life quality in other areas such as productivity and place in the community. This was particularly the case for men with low levels of sexual desire.

The results of this study may indicate that men with sexual dysfunction can continue to achieve in their work and community involvements; in fact, they may channel their energies into these activities to escape confronting their sexual dysfunction. Alternatively, the sexual dysfunction may have originally developed because they pursued these activities and so did not put sufficient time into their relationships.

Interestingly, men with low levels of sexual desire, when compared to nondysfunctional respondents, were the least likely to experience problems in both the objective and the subjective dimensions of the quality of their lives, except for interpersonal relationships. This is despite the fact that these men experience what is purported to be the most severe form of sexual dysfunction (7). These findings suggest that these men are experiencing levels of achievement and satisfaction in their lives that are quite independent of their sexual functioning; i.e., their sexual dysfunction has little impact on their lives in areas other than their interpersonal relationships. These men may have separated their external lives from their personal lives, thereby preventing difficulties in one area from flowing over to difficulties in the other area.

If these proposals are correct, men with low sexual desire may be less motivated to go through the difficult therapeutic steps to address their sexual problems and, therefore, may be more resistant to therapy than men experiencing other types of sexual dysfunction. These lower levels of motivation may partly explain why treatment strategies that focus on the desire phase are less effective for sexual dysfunction than those that focus on the orgasm or arousal phase.

A recent British study (8) demonstrated that sexual dysfunction had a greater impact on the social and psychological functioning of women, whereas physical or medical problems were more greatly impacted in men with sexual dysfunction. This finding may indicate reluctance on the part of men to acknowledge their psychological reaction to having a sexual dysfunction and their greater focus on the physical factors associated with sexual dysfunction (e.g., prostate problems, hypertension, and diabetes).

Other studies have indicated some deficits in the quality of life of men with sexual dysfunction, but the problems are not as broad ranging as one may expect. For example, a Danish study (9) demonstrated that men with sexual difficulties experienced deficits of between 1.2% and 19.1% in their quality-of-life measures compared to men from the general population. For example, the authors found that general well-being, satisfaction with life, and overall happiness were lower among both men and women who experienced lower levels of sexual activity. Men who experienced all types of sexual dysfunction reported lower levels of overall quality of life than men without sexual dysfunction (ranging from 1.8% below the mean for men with premature ejaculation, to 3% for men with erectile problems, to 6.9% below the mean for men with reduced sexual desire).

The results of these studies would suggest that sexual dysfunction is associated with a reduced quality of life, at least for some men. There is some confusion in the literature on the extent of problems in this area. The conclusions that are drawn are largely dependent on the nature of the sample participating in the study (clinical and general population survey), the types of questions that are asked, the method of data collection (interviews and questionnaires), and the nature of the sexual dysfunction. These issues will be discussed in greater detail at the end of this chapter.

Whatever the extent of the impact of male sexual dysfunction on quality of life, both Ventegodt (9) and Rosen (10) indicate that this is an important dimension to be considered in clinical studies. Treatment programs need to consider the association between quality of life and sexual dysfunction in both the development of the treatment program and the measures of the effectiveness of treatment.

Depression and Quality of Life

A number of studies have examined the association between sexual dysfunction and depression. In particular, depression has been shown to be strongly associated with low levels of sexual desire. Although depression is not a direct aspect of quality of life, it is included in this discussion because depressed people are more likely to evaluate their lives negatively, and so may perceive that their lives are not functioning as well as others, at least in some domains. This effect is likely to be stronger for women than for men but is still likely to have some impact on both genders.

In a discussion of the association between depression and sexual desire, Phillips and Slaughter (11) reported that people with depression have a higher prevalence of sexual dysfunction, including lowered libido, than people from the general population. They further noted that for some people, although their depression improves after treatment with medication, their sexual dysfunction remains. In fact, the authors reported that about half of the patients taking medication for depression reported a decline in libido after commencing medication.

Harrison et al. (12) also reported from their results using a double-blind clinical trial that 30% to 40% of patients taking antidepressants reported a decline in sexual desire, whereas only 6% of patients taking placebo experienced the same results. Reductions in desire could result directly from the underlying depression, or it may be a complication of the medication itself. Hirschfeld (13) noted that it is difficult to determine the level of sexual dysfunction among people with depression, but in men, it is most likely to have a negative impact on sexual interest, erectile functioning, and ejaculation (leading to retarded or delayed ejaculation).

From the data it is difficult to determine the nature of the cause–effect relationship between sexual dysfunction and depression in males. Whatever the initial problem (depression or sexual dysfunction), however, they are likely to affect each other, resulting in exacerbation of the original problem.

Hirschfeld (13) presented data that indicated that selective serotonin reuptake inhibitors (SSRIs) are most likely to impact the arousal or orgasm phases but do not affect the desire phase of the response cycle nearly as much. Other psychotropic medications (monoamine-oxidase inhibitors, tricyclic antidepressants, etc.) have also been shown to have a strong impact on all phases of the sexual response cycle, particularly the desire phase. In fact, both Hirschfeld (13) and Ellison (14) proposed that the medications of choice for depression, if one is to avoid associated high levels of sexual dysfunction, should be bupropion, nefazodone, and mirtazapine. (For further information on the effects of SSRIs and other psychotropic medications, see Chapter 19.)

The above literature is difficult to evaluate due to a number of methodological problems. Many of the studies that have examined the association between sexual dysfunction and depression do not attempt to determine the direction of the relationship. Further, there is often no baseline measure taken of sexual dysfunction before antidepressants are prescribed, and so the impact of these medications is frequently based on retrospective recall. Most studies are also based on clinical data, and so the physician is not blind to the study design and may shape the responses of participants. Finally, respondents may not feel comfortable discussing their levels of sexual dysfunction, particularly if the physician does not question them about their problems in this area. Therefore, there may be an underreporting of the number of patients with depression experiencing sexual dysfunction and also the association between medication and the development of sexual problems. Clearly, better designed studies need to be conducted in order to obtain a more accurate understanding of the association between depression and sexual dysfunction in males and the impact of the various types of antidepressant medication on

sexual functioning in terms of both short-term and long-term use.

Impact of Sexual Dysfunction on Relationships

Research studies have demonstrated that a central aspect of quality of life is the nature of both the objective and the subjective dimensions of intimate relationships. In fact, the literature reviewed earlier in this chapter demonstrated a negative association between intimate relationships and quality of life for men with sexual dysfunctions that centers on all phases of the sexual response cycle. In this section, we will review studies that have examined the association between relationship quality and sexual dysfunction more closely.

Although they did not specifically focus on the association between sexual dysfunction and relationship satisfaction, DiBartolo and Barlow (15) found no relationship between marital satisfaction and the clinician's ratings of psychogenic impairment among men with erectile disorder. Spouses' marital satisfaction was also not related to these ratings. These findings are surprising, as other research would suggest that men with a strong psychogenic component to their sexual dysfunction would also experience high levels of marital distress (6–8); however, the results from the DiBartolo and Barlow (15) study should be treated with caution, because the measure of marital distress was completed by the participants, and the rating of psychogenic contribution to the sexual dysfunction was completed by the clinician (on a 5-point rating scale). Further, the study sample was small, including only 32 men with erectile dysfunction and 18 spouses.

Korenman (16) conducted a review of the literature that related to the association between erectile dysfunction and relationship quality and found that the evidence indicates that there is a relationship between this disorder and the quality of life of both the patient and his partner. As a result of the anger or anxiety associated with the disorder from either or both partners, the relationship frequently becomes impaired. Korenman emphasized the ripple effect of erectile dysfunction into other aspects of people's lives and encouraged physicians to discuss feelings and reactions to sexual dysfunction with both patients and their partners to prevent this from occurring.

Korenman's conclusions are drawn on a very limited numbers of studies that have explored the association between sexual dysfunction and relationship quality among men. Some of the treatment studies that are reviewed later in this chapter examine the impact of treatment on both sexual dysfunction and relationship functioning. Further studies, however, need to be conducted to obtain a better understanding of how this dimension of well being relates to sexual dysfunction in men. It is also important to better understand how sexual dysfunction impacts the life quality of partners of men with sexual dysfunction.

An understanding of these issues will provide information on the motivation of patients and their partners in seeking treatment for sexual problems and will thus better direct treatment programs on what dimensions should be addressed in therapy.

□ COMMON TREATMENTS FOR MALE SEXUAL DYSFUNCTION

The various treatment approaches for male sexual dysfunction are discussed in detail in Part IV of this volume. A brief summary of both the medical and the psychological approaches to treating male sexual dysfunction and the impact of different approaches on the quality of life of patients and their partners are provided.

Medication for the Treatment of Sexual Dysfunction

Various pharmacologic approaches are currently in use for the treatment of male sexual dysfunction. The main medications have focused on problems in the arousal and orgasm phases of the sexual response cycle. Treatments for erectile disorder include penile implants, injection therapy, and oral medications. There are advantages and disadvantages of each of these interventions, with oral treatment being the least invasive approach.

There are a number of drugs that have been used in the treatment of premature ejaculation, including dopamine antagonists, antidepressants, benzodiazepine anxiolytics, and a number of other agents (17). Balon (18) also noted the usefulness of antidepressant medication in cases for which psychological treatment was not effective, when the patient refused psychological intervention, or when partners were not willing to take part in treatment.

Disorders of sexual desire have been found to be the most resistant sexual dysfunction to treatment among both men and women. Outside of androgen treatment, few medical treatments have been developed to treat disorders in the desire phase.

It would appear that medical treatments for sexual dysfunction in men have become more popular in recent years. This is partly due to the less intrusive nature of the newer oral medications and to the publicity associated with the medical treatment of sexual dysfunction in males, most particularly, the treatment of erectile dysfunction.

Psychological Treatments for Sexual Dysfunction

The most common psychological interventions for male sexual dysfunction are various types of cognitive behavioral therapies. (For further information on this topic, see Chapter 27.) For erectile disorders, these therapies focus on general arousal techniques and take the pressure off the need to achieve an erection. For premature ejaculation, they focus on slowing down the sexual interaction, so that the man is trained to tune into his arousal levels and control his ejaculatory response.

Hawton et al. (19) found that cognitive behavioral treatment provided a relatively good long-term outcome for the treatment of erectile dysfunction but a poorer outcome for the treatment of premature ejaculation. McCabe (20) found that cognitive behavioral therapy was effective for half of the respondents who experienced erectile dysfunction and for 75% of the respondents who experienced premature ejaculation. This type of therapy was not as effective for men with retarded ejaculation (only effective with 20% of participants), and no men with lack of sexual interest completed therapy.

The effectiveness of therapy appears to depend on a range of factors, other than the actual disorder. It would appear that the length of time the problem has been in place, the extent to which the man experiences multiple sexual problems, his attitudes toward therapy, whether or not his partner also has a sexual dysfunction, and the quality of his relationship with his partner all influence the success or otherwise of therapy.

□ IMPACT OF TREATMENT ON QUALITY OF LIFE OF MEN

The effectiveness of most forms of interventions for male sexual dysfunction has not been subject to adequate evaluation. The evaluations that have been conducted frequently concentrate only on the remediation of the sexual problem and fail to examine the overall quality of life of participants. Due to the large range of factors responsible for the onset of sexual dysfunction and the fact that sexual dysfunction impacts a number of life areas, one would expect that treatment would also impact areas outside of sexual functioning.

The following discussion reviews the literature available regarding the impact of treatment on both the individual quality of life of men with sexual dysfunction and the impact of treatment on their relationships.

Individual Quality of Life

Treatment is most likely to be effective with men who experience sexual problems in the arousal or orgasm phases of the sexual response cycle. McCabe (20) found that a large percentage of men who completed a cognitive behavioral program for sexual dysfunction still experienced problems at the end of therapy. In fact, 35.5% of males still experienced sexual dysfunction 75% to 100% of the time at the end of therapy. This was a substantial shift, however, from the levels of sexual dysfunction pretherapy, in which 100% of the men experienced sexual dysfunction 75% to 100% of the time. The results of this study suggested that men seek help for their sexual problems only when they are well entrenched, more likely to impact other aspects of their lives (6), and more resistant to change.

McCabe (21) examined the outcomes of therapy for men with low sexual desire. Successful therapy was found to be associated with a broadening of the men's sexual repertoire, a development of more positive attitudes to sex, the men perceiving themselves positively as a sexual person, a development of an emotional self, and experiencing sex within an emotional relationship. Given the substantial nature of these changes, it is clear why many attempts to treat inhibited sexual desire are unsuccessful. Although the outcomes of therapy lead to significant changes in the man's attitudes toward himself, his sexuality, and his capacity to experience emotions, these changes are so fundamental to the man's core personality, they are not readily amenable to change.

Although changes after therapy lead to significant improvements in the quality of life of men that go well beyond the sexual arena, it requires highly motivated patients to achieve these gains. Successful therapy is associated with a change in attitude to sex, a greater enjoyment in sexual activities, and more positive feelings about one's own sexuality. The extent to which more broad-ranging changes occur in the individual quality of life of men after therapy requires further investigation.

Relationship Quality

A couple's relationship is often tied in with the development and maintenance of a sexual dysfunction. The partner may also be experiencing a sexual dysfunction and may thus be reluctant for the man's problem to be resolved. For example, if the partner of a man with premature ejaculation is experiencing inhibited sexual desire, she may be reluctant for him to be treated for this condition, since she would not want the sexual interaction to be extended. Sexual dysfunction may also create an emotional distance in the relationship, so that neither partner needs to confront their feelings of anger or confront the fact that they are not in love with their partner. Sexual dysfunctions can also be used to control a relationship or to exert power over the partner. For example, a woman may exhibit inhibited sexual desire and withhold an interest in sex so that she has power in at least some aspect of her relationship with her partner. Given the number of ways that sexual dysfunction can impact a relationship, it is easy to see why a partner may be reluctant to participate in treatment, or may actively sabotage the treatment process. In order for treatment to be successful, there needs to be willingness between both partners to develop a renewed sense of emotional involvement, with the associated risks that this entails.

The quality of the relationship, as well as the needs of his sexual partner, should be addressed in the treatment of sexually dysfunctional men. It has been shown that sexual and relationship problems are linked, and that effective therapy for men leads to an improvement in their relationship.

There have been few studies that have examined the effect of treatment on relationship issues. Since relationship problems have been shown to be related to the onset and maintenance of sexual problems in men (6), it would be expected that remediation of the sexual problem would also lead to an improvement in relationship functioning.

Medical treatments of male sexual problems, which are targeted specifically on the sexual disorder, are not designed to address relationship issues. There may be an improvement in relationship functioning as the sexual problem is resolved, or the difficulties encountered in the relationship may persist. Long-term evaluation of these interventions, with a consideration of broader individual and social functioning, will identify the extent to which these interventions lead to an improvement in individual quality of life and relationship functioning.

Many psychological treatments are designed to intervene at the relationship level, as well as target individual factors related to the development and maintenance of the sexual problem. There has been inadequate evaluation, however, of the effectiveness of these treatments and the impact of improvement in sexual functioning on the overall functioning of the individual. Since these programs frequently focus on sexual and verbal communication between the partners, as well as resolution of individual and relationship issues, it would be expected that, for successful interventions, there would be an improvement in the relationship quality, and in both partners' satisfaction with their relationship.

□ CONCLUSION

Sexual dysfunction impacts the quality of life of men. The impact appears to be greater for men with premature ejaculation and erectile disorder than for men with disorders of sexual desire. The more visible signs of problems experienced by men with either arousal or orgasm phase disorders may cause distress to these men and have a ripple effect into other aspects of their quality of life. In contrast, men with desire phase disorder seem to separate their sexual functioning from other aspects of their lives. They appear to maintain high levels of life quality despite their sexual problems.

The quality of relationships among men with desire disorders, however, is influenced by their sexual dysfunction. Their levels of intimacy are lower than other groups, and they appear to have "shut down" emotionally as well as sexually. Men with other types of sexual dysfunction also experience lower-quality relationships, particularly in terms of their levels of intimacy.

Studies that relate the impact of treatment on quality of life are extremely limited. It does appear, however, that successful treatment of sexual dysfunction in men has a positive effect on other aspects of their lives and relationships. Men with disorders of sexual desire appear to be reluctant to seek treatment for their problems and appear to be less motivated to complete treatment. This may be due to the major changes that need to be made in their lives at both the individual and the relationship levels in order for treatment to be successful. Alternatively, it may be due to the fact that these disorders do not have the same impact on other aspects of their lives as disorders in the arousal or orgasm phases.

☐ FUTURE DIRECTIONS

As outlined throughout this chapter, there is limited research on the impact of sexual dysfunction and its treatment on the quality of life of males experiencing these disorders. The studies that have been conducted present inconsistent results. This is primarily due to the limited range of quality-of-life dimensions examined in research and treatment studies, the limited sample sizes participating in these studies, and the selected groups from which participants are recruited. These methodological difficulties limit our understanding of the relationship between quality of life and sexual dysfunction and prevent accurate generalizations from being made. An understanding of the quality of life of men who experience sexual dysfunction is important in terms of providing information about the motivation of these men for treatment and areas to be targeted in treatment programs.

Sexual dysfunction is not just confined to difficulties in the sexual functioning of males. It has an impact on how males feel about themselves and their relationships. It also has an impact on how their partners feel about themselves and their relationship. In order to obtain a better understanding of sexual dysfunction, it is important to obtain a better evaluation of what the dimensions of well-being are, so that they can be assessed more systematically among men with sexual dysfunction, as well as their partners. These data will then identify dimensions that need to be addressed in the treatment of sexual problems.

Direct treatment of sexual dysfunctions may have a ripple effect, such that other dimensions of well-being are improved with the treatment of the sexual problem. Treatment, however, is much more likely to be effective if it also targets other difficulties associated with the sexual dysfunction in the lives of both the man and his partner. This multifaceted approach to treatment is not only more likely to lead to resolution of the sexual problem but will also be more likely to enhance the quality of life of men with sexual dysfunction, as well as improve their relationship satisfaction.

A consideration of the above issues is important for all conceptualizations and treatment programs for sexual dysfunction in men, whether they are primarily focused on physical/medical approaches or psychological approaches. Sexual dysfunction cannot be conceptualized as an isolated problem, but it needs to be considered within the broader context of a man's life. Further research in this area will lead to strategies to improve both the quality of life of men with sexual dysfunction and the quality of life of his partner.

☐ REFERENCES

1. American Psychiatric Association. Diagnostic and Statistical Manual of Mental Disorders Text Revision. 4th ed. Washington, DC: American Psychiatric Publishing, Inc., 2000:535–566.

2. Laumann EO, Paik A, Rosen RC. Sexual dysfunction in the United States: prevalence and predictors. JAMA 1999; 281(6):537–544.

3. Bell RR, Bell PL. Sexual satisfaction among married women. Med Aspects Hum Sex 1972; 6:136–144.

4. Masters WH, Johnson VE. Human Sexual Inadequacy. New York: Little Brown & Co., 1970.

5. Donnelly DA. Sexually inactive marriages. J Sex Res 1993; 30(2):171–179.

6. McCabe MP. Intimacy and quality of life among sexually dysfunctional men and women. J Sex Mar Ther 1997; 23(4):276–290.

7. McCarthy BW. Bridges to sexual desire. J Sex Educ Ther 1995; 21:132–141.

8. Dunn KM, Croft PR, Hackett GI. Association of sexual problems with social, psychological, and physical problems in men and women: a cross sectional population survey. J Epidemiol Community Health 1999; 53(3): 144–148.

9. Ventegodt S. Sex and quality of life in Denmark. Arch Sex Behav 1998; 27(3):295–307.

10. Rosen RC. Quality of life assessment in sexual dysfunction trials. Int J Impot Res 1998; 10(suppl 2): S21–S23.

11. Phillips RL Jr, Slaughter JR. Depression and sexual desire. Am Fam Physician 2000; 62(4):782–786.

12. Harrison WM, Rabkin JG, Ehrhardt AA, et al. Effects of antidepressant medication on sexual function: a controlled study. J Clin Psychopharmacol 1986; 6(3): 144–149.

13. Hirschfeld RM. Care of the sexually active depressed patient. J Clin Psychiatry 1999; 60(suppl 17):32–35.

14. Ellison JM. Antidepressant-induced sexual dysfunction: review, classification, and suggestions for treatment. Harv Rev Psychiatry 1998; 6(4):177–189.

15. DiBartolo PM, Barlow DH. Perfectionism, marital satisfaction, and contributing factors to sexual dysfunction in men with erectile disorder and their spouses. Arch Sex Behav 1996; 25(6):581–588.

16. Korenman SG. New insights into erectile dysfunction: a practical approach. Am J Med 1998; 105(2): 135–144.

17. Metz ME, Pryor JL, Nesvaci LJ, et al. Premature ejaculation: a psychophysiological review. J Sex Mar Ther 1997; 23(1):3–23.

18. Balon R. Antidepressants in the treatment of premature ejaculation. J Sex Mar Ther 1996; 22(2):85–96.

19. Hawton K, Catalan J, Martin P, et al. Long-term outcome in sex therapy. Behav Res Ther 1986; 24(6):665–675.

20. McCabe MP. Evaluation of a cognitive behavior therapy program for people with sexual dysfunction. J Sex Mar Ther 2001; 27(3):259–271.

21. McCabe MP. A program for the treatment of inhibited sexual desire in males. Psychotherapy 1992; 29:288–296.

INDEX

T - #0549 - 071024 - C8 - 279/216/26 - PB - 9780367389093 - Gloss Lamination